Thoracic
Anesthesia

Third Edition
Thoracic Anesthesia

Edited by

Joel A. Kaplan, MD
Vice President for Health Affairs;
Dean, School of Medicine;
and, Professor of Anesthesiology
University of Louisville
Louisville, Kentucky

Peter D. Slinger, MD, FRCPC
Professor of Anesthesia
University of Toronto
Toronto, Ontario
Canada

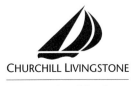

CHURCHILL LIVINGSTONE

An Imprint of Elsevier

CHURCHILL
LIVINGSTONE
An Imprint of Elsevier

The Curtis Center
Independence Square West
Philadelphia, Pennsylvania 19106-3399

NOTICE

Anesthesiology is an ever-changing field. Standard safety precautions must be followed, but as new research and clinical experience broaden our knowledge, changes in treatment and drug therapy may become necessary or appropriate. Readers are advised to check the most current product information provided by the manufacturer of each drug to be administered to verify the recommended dose, the method and duration of administration, and contraindications. It is the responsibility of the licensed prescriber, relying on experience and knowledge of the patient, to determine dosages and the best treatment for each individual patient. Neither the publisher nor the author assumes any liability for any injury and/or damage to persons or property arising from this publication.

ISBN-13: 978-0-443-06619-1
ISBN-10: 0-443-06619-1

Acquisitions Editor: Allan Ross
Developmental Editor: Josh Hawkins
Project Manager: Peggy Fagen
Designer: Amy Buxton

Printed in the United States of America

Last digit is the print number: 9 8 7 6 5 4 3

To our families and loved ones for their support and understanding,

and

To the pioneers of thoracic anesthesia and surgery;
they led the way for our students, who will continue the journey.

Joel A. Kaplan, MD
Peter D. Slinger, MD

CONTRIBUTORS

Kenneth J. Abrams, MD, MBA
Associate Professor, Anesthesiology, Mount Sinai School of Medicine, New York, New York

Bernard B. Baez, MD
Chief Resident, Anesthesiology, Mount Sinai School of Medicine, New York, New York

Jonathan L. Benumof, MD
Professor, Department of Anesthesia, University of California, San Diego, California

Simon C. Body, MD, ChB
Assistant Professor, Anesthesia, Harvard Medical School, Boston, Massachusetts

Sorin J. Brull, MD
Professor, Anesthesiology, University of Arkansas for Medical Science, Little Rock, Arkansas

Jean S. Bussières, MD, FRCPC
Anesthesiologist, Clinical Professor, Anesthesiology, University Heart and Lung Institute, Laval University, Québec City, Canada

Javier H. Campos, MD
Professor, Anesthesiology, Director of Cardiothoracic Anesthesia, University of Iowa Health Care, Iowa City, Iowa

I. D. Conacher, MB, ChB, MRCP, FFARCS
Consultant, Thoracic Anesthetist, Freeman Hospital, Newcastle-upon-Tyne, United Kingdom

Jan Ehrenwerth, MD
Professor, Anesthesiology, Yale University School of Medicine, New Haven, Connecticut

James B. Eisenkraft, MD
Professor, Anesthesiology, Mount Sinai School of Medicine, New York, New York

Brendan T. Finucane, MD
Professor, Anesthesiology and Pain Medicine, University of Alberta, Alberta, Canada

Thomas J. Gal, MD
Professor, Anesthesiology, University of Virginia, Charlottesville, Virginia

Richard L. Goldwin, MD, FACR
Assistant Professor, Radiology, University of Louisville School of Medicine, Louisville, Kentucky

Katherine P. Grichnik, MD
Associate Professor, Anesthesiology, Duke University, Durham, North Carolina

Philip M. Hartigan, MD
Assistant Professor, Anesthesia, Director of Thoracic Anesthesia, Brigham & Women's Hospital, Harvard Medical School, Boston, Massachusetts

Paul M. Heerdt, MD, PhD, FAHA
Associate Professor, Anesthesiology and Pharmacology, New York Presbyterian Hospital, Cornell University, New York, New York

Thomas L. Higgins, MD, FACP, FCCM
Associate Professor, Medicine and Anesthesiology, Baystate Medical Center, Tufts University, Springfield, Massachusetts

Rajiv M. Jhaveri, MD
Assistant Professor of Anesthesia and Director of Thoracic Transplantation Anesthesia, Johns Hopkins University, Baltimore, Maryland

Roger A. Johns, MD
Professor, Anesthesiology, Johns Hopkins University, Baltimore, Maryland

Michael R. Johnston, MD, FRCSC
Associate Professor, Surgery, University of Toronto, Toronto, Canada

Burkhard Lachmann, MD, PhD
Professor, Anesthesiology, Erasmus University, Rotterdam, The Netherlands

Carol L. Lake, MD, MBA, MPH
Professor and Chair, Anesthesiology, Associate Dean for Health Sciences Continuing Education, University of Louisville, Louisville, Kentucky

Harish S. Lecamwasam, MD
Chief Resident, Fellow in Critical Care, Anesthesia and Critical Care, Massachusetts General Hospital, Harvard University, Boston, Massachusetts

Guy M. Lerner, MD
Associate Professor, Anesthesiology, University of Louisville,
Louisville, Kentucky

William McIvor, MD
Assistant Professor, Anesthesiology, University of Pittsburgh,
Pittsburgh, Pennsylvania

Marshall Murphy, MD
Associate in Cardiothoracic Anesthesiology, Emory
University School of Medicine, Atlanta, Georgia

Paul S. Myles, MB, BS, MD, MPH, FCARCSI, FANZCA
Associate Professor and Head of Research, Anesthesia and
Pain Management, Alfred Hospital, Monash University,
Prahran, Australia

Steven M. Neustein, MD
Associate Professor, Anesthesiology, Mount Sinai School of
Medicine, New York, New York

Peter J. Papadakos, MD, FCCM, FCCP
Associate Professor, Anesthesiology and Surgery, Director of
Critical Care Medicine, University of Rochester, Rochester,
New York

James G. Ramsay, MD
Professor, Anesthesiology, Emory University School of
Medicine, Atlanta, Georgia

James C. Reed, MD, FACR
Professor, Radiology, University of Louisville, School of
Medicine, Louisville, Kentucky

Peter D. Slinger, MD, FRCPC
Professor of Anesthesia, University of Toronto, Toronto,
Canada

Jeffrey T. Smok, MD
Instructor, Department of Anesthesiology, University of
Pittsburgh, Pittsburgh, Pennsylvania

David John Sugarbaker, MD, FCCP
Chairman, Thoracic Surgery, Brigham and Women's Hospital,
Chief of Surgical Oncology, Dana Farber Cancer Center,
Boston, Massachusetts

Erin A. Sullivan, MD
Associate Professor, Anesthesiology and Critical Care
Medicine, Pittsburgh, Pennsylvania

Anastasios N. Triantafillou, MD
Staff Anesthesiologist, Tufts-New England Medical Center,
Boston, Massachusetts

Edda M. Tschernko, MD
Associate Professor, Anesthesia and Critical Care Medicine,
University of Vienna, Vienna, Austria

Roger S. Wilson, MD
Professor and Chairman, Anesthesiology and Critical Care
Medicine, Memorial Sloan-Kettering Cancer Center,
New York, New York

PREFACE TO THE THIRD EDITION

THE third edition of *Thoracic Anesthesia* was written for the purpose of continuing to improve the perioperative management of patients undergoing noncardiac thoracic surgery. Since the publication of the first edition in 1983 and the second edition in 1991, the subspecialty has continued to grow at a rapid pace and evolved from its historical emphasis on infectious diseases, to dealing with cancer, and now to the beginnings of surgery in end-stage lung disease. In order to maintain its place as the standard reference textbook in the field, this edition has been completely revised, expanded, and updated.

The material in this book was written by the acknowledged international authorities in each specific area related to thoracic anesthesia. The authors come from leading academic departments in the United States, Europe, Australia, and Canada. Peter Slinger, M.D., the well-known and highly respected Canadian expert in thoracic anesthesia, has joined me as Associate Editor of the third edition. Dr. Slinger also serves as Associate Editor of *Thoracic Anesthesia* for the *Journal of Cardiothoracic and Vascular Anesthesia*. His knowledge of the latest practices from around the world has contributed markedly to the development of the international perspective reflected in this book. This multi-authored, international text provides authoritative information on a broad and comprehensive scale that is not possible in single-authored books.

The third edition of *Thoracic Anesthesia* is the most comprehensive and up-to-date collection of material in the field. Each chapter aims to provide the scientific foundation in the area, as well as the clinical basis for practice. All of the chapters have been coordinated in an effort to minimize unnecessary duplication and conflicting opinions. Whenever possible, material has been integrated from the fields of anesthesiology, pulmonary medicine, thoracic surgery, critical care medicine, and physiology and pharmacology to present a complete clinical picture. Thus the book should continue to serve as the definitive text in the field for anesthesia residents, thoracic anesthesia fellows and attendings, thoracic surgeons, intensivists, and others interested in the management of patients for noncardiac thoracic surgery.

The content of the book ranges from the preoperative assessment of the thoracic surgery patient, through the anesthetic and intraoperative management, plus the postoperative care in the intensive care unit. The book is organized into four parts, consisting of 20 chapters with hundreds of illustrations. The four major areas covered are (1) preoperative respiratory assessment for thoracic surgery, (2) respiratory physiology and pharmacology, (3) specific anesthetic considerations for different types of thoracic surgery, and (4) postoperative management. Throughout, the emphasis is on the understanding of respiratory physiology and how disease states in an anesthetized open-chest patient with one-lung ventilation may alter this physiology. The latest techniques and equipment utilized in newer forms of surgery, such as lung volume reductions, single- and double-lung transplantations, and video-assisted thoracic surgery (VATS), are discussed. All aspects of patient care are presented in the belief that preoperative and postoperative care are as important as intraoperative management.

The first edition of *Thoracic Anesthesia* began with forewords written by Professor Mushin from England and Dr. Lichtmann and colleagues from the George Washington University School of Medicine. Dr. Mushin pointed out that "thoracic anesthesia is still a rapidly developing science" and that "it is almost impossible for anyone not a specialist in this field to keep abreast of new developments." Thus "there is a continued need to set down the accumulated experience of those who work in this field so that their great skill and knowledge can be disseminated both to their colleagues and to the rising generation of anesthesiologists." This edition of *Thoracic Anesthesia* is a continuation of the effort to keep anesthesiologists informed of the latest developments in the field.

Dr. Lichtmann and colleagues discussed the events immediately following the assassination attempt of President Reagan in 1981, which led to his emergency thoracic surgical procedure. They discussed the development of thoracic anesthesia techniques and their application in this highly successful operative procedure. It is well recognized that they made a significant contribution to saving the President's life. In fact, the development of the subspecialty of thoracic anesthesia has been responsible for reducing mortality and improving care for all patients undergoing noncardiac thoracic surgery, and it has been one of the major forces behind the surgeon's ability to handle bigger challenges with better results during both war and peace.

I gratefully acknowledge the contributions made by the authors of the individual chapters. They are the experts who have made the field of thoracic anesthesia come alive at the academic medical centers and are the teachers of our young colleagues practicing anesthesiology around the world. This book would not have been possible without their hard work and expertise.

My sincere appreciation also goes to my administrative assistants, Daniel Alkofer and Connie Schenck, whose long hours helped make this text a reality. In addition, thanks are in order to the secretaries of the contributing authors who sent us the original manuscripts from their institutions. I would also like to thank Allan Ross, Executive Editor, for making the transition to Elsevier so easy for all of us.

Finally, thanks go to Norma for again acting as Editor-in-Chief between rounds of beating us on the links!

Joel A. Kaplan, MD
Peter Slinger, MD

PREFACE TO THE SECOND EDITION

THE second edition of *Thoracic Anesthesia* was written for the purpose of further improving anesthetic management of patients undergoing noncardiac thoracic surgery. Since the publication of the first edition of *Thoracic Anesthesia* in 1983, the field has continued to grow at a rapid pace. In order to maintain its place as the standard reference textbook in the subspecialty, this edition has been completely revised, expanded, and updated. The material in this book was written by the acknowledged experts in each specific area of thoracic anesthesia. It is the most authoritative and up-to-date collection of material in the field. Each chapter aims to provide the scientific foundation in the area, as well as the clinical basis for practice. All of the chapters have been coordinated in an effort to avoid unnecessary duplication and conflicting opinions. Whenever possible, material has been integrated from the fields of anesthesiology, pulmonary medicine, thoracic surgery, critical care medicine, and pharmacology to present a complete clinical picture. Thus the book should continue to serve as the definitive text in the field for anesthesia residents, thoracic anesthesia fellows and attendings, thoracic surgeons, intensivists, and others interested in the management of patients for noncardiac thoracic surgery.

The content of the book ranges from the preoperative assessment of the thoracic surgery patient to the anesthetic, monitoring, and intraoperative support needed, plus the postoperative care of the patient in the intensive care unit. The book is organized into four parts, consisting of 26 chapters and hundreds of illustrations. The four major areas covered are (1) preoperative assessment and management, (2) respiratory physiology and pharmacology, (3) specific anesthetic considerations, and (4) postoperative management. Throughout, the emphasis is on the understanding of respiratory physiology and how disease states in an anesthetized open-chest patient with one-lung ventilation may alter this physiology. The latest techniques and equipment are discussed in the areas of intraoperative monitoring, endobronchial intubation, tracheostomy, and mechanical ventilation. All aspects of patient care are presented in the belief that preoperative and postoperative management of the patient are as important as intraoperative management.

The first edition of *Thoracic Anesthesia* began with forewords written by Professor Mushin from England and Dr. Lichtmann and colleagues from the George Washington University School of Medicine. Dr. Mushin pointed out that "thoracic anesthesia is still a rapidly developing science" and that "it is almost impossible for anyone not a specialist in this field to keep abreast of new developments." Thus "there is a continued need to set down the accumulated experience of those who work in this field so that their great skill and knowledge can be disseminated both to their colleagues and to the rising generation of anesthesiologists." This edition of *Thoracic Anesthesia* is a continuation of the effort to keep anesthesiologists informed of the latest developments in the field.

Dr. Lichtmann and colleagues discussed the events immediately following the assassination attempt of President Reagan in 1981, leading to his emergency thoracic surgical procedure. They discussed the development of thoracic anesthesia techniques and their application in this highly successful operative procedure. It is well recognized that they made a significant contribution to saving the President's life. In fact, the development of the subspecialty of thoracic anesthesia has been responsible for reducing mortality and improving care for all patients undergoing noncardiac thoracic surgery and has been one of the major forces behind the surgeon's ability to handle bigger challenges with better results during both war and peace.

I gratefully acknowledge the contributions made by the authors of the individual chapters. They are the experts who have made the field of thoracic anesthesia come alive at the major medical centers and are the teachers of our young colleagues practicing anesthesiology around the world. This book would not have been possible without their hard work and expertise.

My sincere appreciation also goes to my secretaries, Joanie Esbri-Cullen and Margorie Fraticelli, whose long hours helped make this text a reality. In addition, thanks are in order for the secretaries of the contributing authors who sent us the original manuscripts from their institutions. I would also like to thank Tony Tracy, President of Churchill Livingstone Inc., for her support with this project, and David Terry, for his hard work in putting together all the piece of the book.

Finally, my thanks go to Norma for again acting as Editor-in-Chief!

Joel A. Kaplan, MD

PREFACE TO THE FIRST EDITION

THIS book was written to improve anesthesia care for all patients undergoing thoracic surgery. The text reflects the experience of the Division of Cardiothoracic Anesthesia at the Emory University School of Medicine, as well as that of experts from the University of California-San Diego, Harvard University, Loyola University, Mount Sinai School of Medicine, and the University of Florida. The book presents methods, materials, philosophies, attitudes, and fundamentals whose use will provide safe, individualized anesthetic care.

The scope of the book ranges from the historical background to the modern practice of thoracic anesthesia and surgery, including new modes of postoperative ventilation and oxygenation. The book focuses on the patient undergoing a thoracotomy, beginning with the preoperative evaluation and preparation for surgery and continuing through to the intraoperative management and postoperative respiratory care. It is organized into five parts, consisting of 21 chapters and hundreds of illustrations and x-rays. The five major areas covered are (1) thoracic anesthesia and surgery, (2) assessment of the patient, (3) cardiopulmonary physiology, (4) specific anesthetic considerations, and (5) postoperative intensive care. Throughout, the emphasis is on understanding respiratory physiology and how disease state and an open chest with one-lung ventilation may later this physiology. The latest techniques and equipment are discussed in the areas of intraoperative monitoring, endobronchial intubation, pulmonary lavage, tracheostomy, pacemakers, and mechanical ventilators. All aspects of patient care are presented in the belief that preoperative and postoperative management of the patient are as important as intraoperative management.

The material in this book is an overview of the highly specialized field of thoracic anesthesia. Many medical disciplines including surgery, radiology, pediatrics, and internal medicine have contributed to the development of this text and the new subspecialty in thoracic anesthesia. Therefore this work may serve as a source book for use by anesthesia residents and fellows, anesthesiologists interested in the field of thoracic anesthesia, intensivists, thoracic surgeons, pulmonary medicine specialists, and other physicians dealing with thoracic surgical patients.

I gratefully acknowledge the help of my fellow anesthesiologists at Emory for the expertly written chapters they have contributed to this book. In addition, I would like to thank my colleagues in surgery and medicine for their outstanding contributions, and most of all, I wish to express my deep appreciation to the expert anesthesiologists from other institutions whose contributions give this text balance.

My sincere appreciation goes, in addition, to my executive secretary Patricia Bailey, to Judy Hawkins and Cindy Lewis, and to the rest of our secretarial staff who spent many long hours preparing this manuscript for publication.

And, finally, my thanks to my wife, Norma, who again managed to edit a manuscript between tennis sets!

Joel A. Kaplan, MD

CONTENTS

Preoperative Evaluation of the Thoracic Surgery Patient

Peter D. Slinger, MD, FRCPC
Michael R. Johnston, MD, FRCSC

PREOPERATIVE anesthetic assessment before chest surgery is a continually evolving science and art. Recent advances in anesthetic management, surgical techniques, and perioperative care have expanded the group of patients now considered to be operable (Figure 1-1).[1] This chapter primarily focuses on preanesthetic assessment for pulmonary resection surgery in cancer patients. The principles described also apply to all other types of nonmalignant pulmonary resections and to other types of chest surgery. The distinguishing factor is that in patients with malignancy, the risk/benefit ratio of canceling or delaying surgery pending other investigation or therapy is always complicated by the risk of further spread of cancer during any extended interval before resection. Surgery in these cases is never truly "elective."

Although 87% of patients with lung cancer will die of their disease, the 13% cure rate represents approximately 26,000 survivors per year in North America. Surgical resection is responsible for essentially all of these cures. A patient with a *resectable* lung cancer has a disease that is still local or local–regional in scope and can be encompassed in a plausible surgical procedure. An *operable* patient is someone who can tolerate the proposed resection with acceptable risk.[2] The following general points should be appreciated in the assessment of pulmonary resection patients:

1. *Disjointed assessment*—Until recently, preanesthetic management was part of a continuum in which a patient was admitted preoperatively for testing and the management plan evolved as test results were returned. Currently, however, the reality of practice patterns in anesthesia is that a patient is commonly assessed initially in an outpatient clinic, often by someone other than the member of the anesthesia staff who will actually administer the anesthesia. The actual contact with the responsible anesthesiologist may take place only 10 to 15 minutes before induction. It is necessary to organize and standardize the approach to preoperative evaluation for these patients into two temporally disjointed phases: the initial assessment in the outpatient clinic and the final assessment on the day of admission. This chapter describes the unique elements vital to each assessment.

2. *Short-term vs. long-term survival*—Although a great deal of research has been done on long-term survival (6 months to 5 years) after pulmonary resection surgery, there has been a comparatively small volume of research on the short-term outcome (less than 6 weeks) of these patients. This research area is currently very active, however, and several available studies can be used to guide anesthetic management in the immediate perioperative period in which management has an influence on outcome.

3. *"Lung-sparing" surgery*—An increasing number of thoracic surgeons are now being trained to perform lung-sparing resections such as sleeve lobectomies or segmentectomies. The postoperative preservation of respiratory function has been shown to be proportional to the amount of functioning lung parenchyma preserved.[3] To assess patients with limited pulmonary function, the anesthesiologist must understand these newer surgical options in addition to the conventional lobectomy or pneumonectomy.

4. *Anesthesiologist's responsibilities*—Anesthesiologists are not gatekeepers. It is rarely the anesthesiologist's function to assess these patients to decide who is or is not a viable candidate for operation. In the majority of situations, the anesthesiologist will be seeing the patient at the end of a referral chain that extends from a chest or family physician to a surgeon. At each stage, there should have been a discussion of the risks and benefits of surgery. It is the anesthesiologist's responsibility to use the preoperative assessment to identify those patients at elevated risk and then to focus perioperative management resources on the patients at highest risk to improve their outcome. This is the primary function of the preanesthetic assessment.

Prethoracotomy assessment naturally involves all of the factors of a complete anesthetic assessment—past history, allergies, medications, upper airway evaluation, and so on. To assess patients for thoracic anesthesia, it is necessary to have an understanding of the risks specific to this type of surgery. The major cause of perioperative morbidity and mortality in the thoracic surgical population is respiratory complications. Major respiratory complications include atelectasis, pneumonia, and respiratory failure, which occur in 15% to 20% of patients and account for the majority of the expected 3% to 4% mortalities.[4] The thoracic surgical population differs from other adult surgical populations in this respect. For other types of surgery, cardiac and vascular complications are the leading cause of early perioperative morbidity and mortality. Cardiac complications include, for example, arrhythmia and ischemia, which occur in 10% to 15% of the thoracic surgical population.[5] This chapter focuses on the additional information (beyond what is included in a standard anesthetic assessment) that the anesthesiologist needs to manage a pulmonary resection patient.

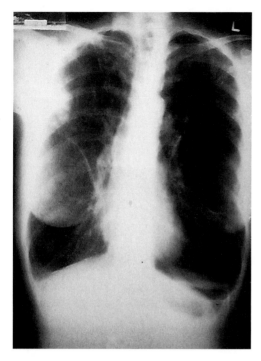

FIGURE 1-1 Preoperative chest x-ray of a 55-year-old female with severe bullous emphysema and a carcinoma of the upper lobe of the right lung. Preoperative FEV$_1$ = 25% predicted. Although this woman's pulmonary function does not meet traditional minimal criteria for a lung operation, she is now considered a potential candidate for bilateral combined cancer resection and emphysema surgery. (From Slinger PD, Johnston MR: *J Cardiothorac Vasc Anesth* 14:202, 2000.)

Assessment of Respiratory Function

The best assessment of respiratory function derives from a detailed history of the patient's quality of life. All thoracic surgery patients should have a preoperative baseline spirometric screening. (Figure 1-2).[6] An exception can be made for asymptomatic nonsmokers who are not scheduled for pulmonary

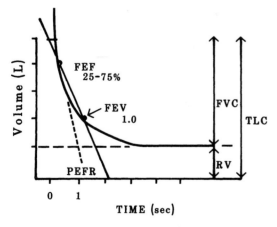

FIGURE 1-2 The expiratory spirogram plotting volume vs. time and the derived data (including the forced expiratory flow [FEF] from 25% to 75%) of the forced vital capacity (FVC), the forced expiratory volume at 1 second (FEV$_1$), and the peak expiratory flow rate (PEFR).

resection; unfortunately, because of the biology of lung cancer, these constitute a small minority of the patient population.

Because the anesthesiologist who will manage the case often must assimilate a great deal of information about the patient in a short period of time, it is very useful to have objective, standardized measures of pulmonary function that can be used to guide anesthetic management. It is also important to have this information available in a format that can be easily transmitted among members of the health-care team. Much effort has been spent in the attempt to find a single test of respiratory function that has sufficient sensitivity and specificity to predict outcome for all pulmonary resection patients. It is now clear that no single test will ever accomplish this because there are many factors that determine overall respiratory performance.[7] It is useful, however, to categorize the respiratory function into three related but somewhat independent areas: respiratory mechanics, gas exchange, and cardiorespiratory interaction. These can also be remembered as the basic functions of extracellular respiration, which are to transport the oxygen (1) to the alveoli, (2) into the blood, and (3) to the tissues (the process is reversed for carbon dioxide removal).

Respiratory Mechanics

Many tests of respiratory mechanics and volumes show a correlation with postthoracotomy outcome, for example, forced expiratory volume in 1 second (FEV$_1$), forced vital capacity (FVC), maximal voluntary ventilation (MVV), and residual volume/total lung capacity ratio (RV/TLC). It is useful to express these as a percentage of predicted volumes corrected for age, sex, and height (e.g., FEV$_1$ %). Of these, the most valid single test for postthoracotomy respiratory complications is the predicted postoperative FEV$_1$ (ppoFEV$_1$%), which is calculated as the following:

$$ppoFEV_1\% = preoperative\ FEV\ 1\% \times$$
$$(1 - \%\ functional\ lung\ tissue\ removed/100)$$

One method of estimating the percentage of functional postoperative lung tissue is based on a calculation of the number of functioning subsegments of the lung removed (Figure 1-3). Nakahara et al found that patients with a ppoFEV$_1$ more than 40% had either no or only minor respiratory complications after a lung resection.[4] Major respiratory complications were seen only in the subgroup with ppoFEV$_1$ less than 40% (although not all patients in this subgroup developed respiratory complications), and 10 out of 10 patients with ppoFEV$_1$ less than 30% required postoperative mechanical ventilatory support. These key threshold ppoFEV$_1$ values, 30% and 40%, are extremely useful to remember when managing lung resection patients. If the schema of Figure 1-3 seems overly complicated, it can be useful to consider the right upper and middle lobes combined as approximately equivalent to each of the other three lobes, with the right lung 10% larger than the left. These data of Nakahara are from work done in the 1980s, and recent advances—particularly the use of epidural analgesia—have decreased the incidence of complications in the high-risk group of patients.[4,8] However, ppoFEV$_1$ values of 40% and 30% remain useful as reference points for the anesthesiologist. The ppoFEV$_1$ is the most significant independent predictor of complications among a variety of historical, physical, and laboratory tests for these patients.[5]

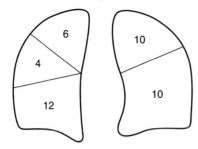

Lung segments

Total subsegments = 42

Example: Right lower lobectomy
Postoperative FEV$_1$ decrease = 12/42 (29%)

FIGURE 1-3 The number of subsegments of each lobe is used to calculate the predicted postoperative (ppo) pulmonary function. For example, after a right lower lobectomy, a patient with a preoperative FEV$_1$ (or D$_{LCO}$) at 70% of normal would be expected to have a ppoFEV$_1$ = 70% × (1-29/100) = 50%. (From Slinger PD, Johnston MR: *J Cardiothorac Vasc Anesth* 14:202, 2000.)

Complete pulmonary function testing in a pulmonary function laboratory will include assessments of lung volumes and airway resistance (Figures 1-4 to 1-6). These are more sensitive than an examination of the FEV$_1$-to-FVC ratio to distinguish between obstructive and restrictive lung pathologies and will confirm the clinical diagnosis of the underlying lung disease. These assessments also permit the anesthesiologist to optimize intraoperative management during both two-lung and one-lung ventilation by individualizing settings for mechanical ventilation according to the lung pathology.[9] There are two basic methods for measuring lung volumes: insoluble gas washout and plethysmography.

Lung Parenchymal Function

As important to the process of respiration as the mechanical delivery of air to the distal airways is the subsequent ability of the lung to exchange oxygen and carbon dioxide between the pulmonary vascular bed and the alveoli. Traditionally, arterial blood gas data such as Pao$_2$ less than 60 mmHg or Paco$_2$ more than 45 mmHg have been used as cutoff values for pulmonary resection. Cancer resections have now been successfully done or even combined with volume reduction in patients who do not meet these criteria, although they remain useful as warning indicators of increased risk.[10] The most useful test of the gas-exchange capacity of the lung is the diffusing capacity for carbon monoxide (D$_{LCO}$). Although the D$_{LCO}$ was initially thought only to reflect diffusion, it actually correlates with the total functioning surface area of the alveolar-capillary interface. This simple, noninvasive test, which is included with spirometry and plethysmography by most pulmonary function laboratories, is a useful predictor of perioperative mortality but not of long-term survival.[11] The corrected D$_{LCO}$ can be used to calculate a postresection (ppo) value using the same calculation as for the FEV$_1$ (Figure 1-3). A predicted ppoD$_{LCO}$ less than 40% correlates with an increased risk of both respiratory and cardiac complications and is to a large degree independent of the FEV$_1$ (Figure 1-7).[12]

Cardiopulmonary Interaction

The final, and perhaps most important, assessment of respiratory function is an assessment of the cardiopulmonary interaction. All patients should have some assessment of their

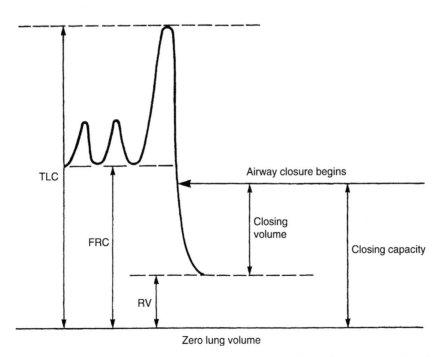

FIGURE 1-4 Complete pulmonary testing should include measurement of lung volumes to differentiate obstructive from restrictive lung disease. Measurement of volumes cannot be done by spirometry but will require either washout/dilution techniques of insoluble gases or plethysmography. (From Nunn JF: *Applied respiratory physiology,* Oxford, 1993, Butterworth Heinemann.)

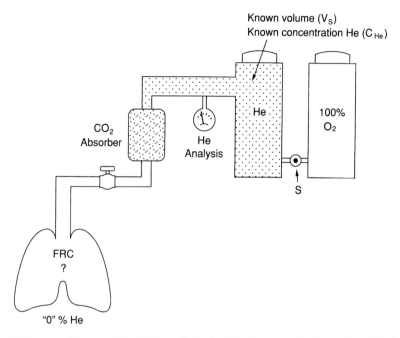

FIGURE 1-5 Diagram of the closed-circuit helium dilution technique for measuring lung volumes. The helium in the spirometer at the beginning of the test (a known volume and concentration) is "diluted" in proportion to the unknown volume in the lung (FRC). Washout techniques using other insoluble gases (xenon, nitrogen) can be used to measure other lung volumes such as closing volume. (From Tisi GM: *Pulmonary physiology in clinical medicine,* ed 2, Baltimore, 1983, Williams & Wilkins.)

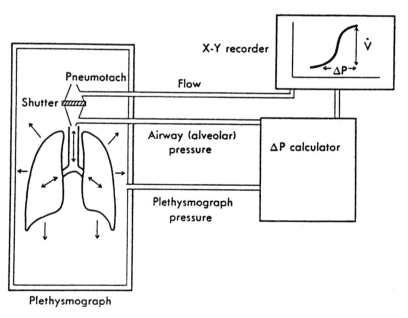

FIGURE 1-6 Diagrammatic representation of the measurement of airway resistance by whole-body plethysmography. Airway resistance = (atmospheric pressure − alveolar pressure)/flow. Flow (V̇) is measured directly by the Pneumotach. The pressure differential between the chamber and the alveoli is measured as follows: plethysmograph pressure is monitored by means of a sensitive manometer in the chamber; alveolar pressure is measured as airway pressure during intervals when no gas is flowing. A shutter occludes the airway momentarily, usually at the close of expiration, and a manometer monitors the falling pressure. The pressure differential is calculated and delivered to an appropriate display device (X-Y recorder or oscilloscope). (From Ruppel G: *Manual of pulmonary function testing,* St. Louis, 1975, Mosby.)

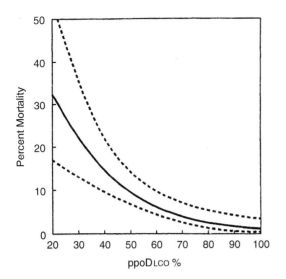

FIGURE 1-7 Estimated surgical mortality after major pulmonary resection as a function of the predicted postoperative diffusing capacity expressed as a percentage of predicted capacity (ppoD$_{LCO}$%). Dashed lines show 95% confidence intervals. (From Wang J et al: *J Thorac Cardiovasc Surg* 117: 581, 1999.)

cardiopulmonary reserves. The traditional (and still extremely useful) test in ambulatory patients is stair climbing.[13] Stair climbing is done at the patient's own pace but without stopping, and it is usually documented as a certain number of flights. There is no exact definition for a "flight," but 20 steps at 6 inches per step is a frequently referenced value. The ability to climb three flights or more is closely associated with decreased mortality and is somewhat associated with decreased morbidity. The ability to climb two flights corresponds to a maximal oxygen consumption (Vo$_2$ max) of 12 mL/kg/min. A patient unable to climb at least two flights is at extremely high risk.[14]

Formal laboratory exercise testing has become more standardized and thus more valid, and it is currently the "gold standard" for assessment of cardiopulmonary function.[15] Among the many cardiac and respiratory factors that are tested, the Vo$_2$ max is the most useful predictor of postthoracotomy outcome. Walsh et al have shown that in a high-risk group of patients (with a mean preoperative FEV$_1$ = 41%), there was no perioperative mortality if the preoperative Vo$_2$ max was greater than 15 mL/kg/min.[16] This is a useful reference number for the anesthesiologist. Only 1 in 10 patients with a Vo$_2$ max more than 20 mL/kg/min had a respiratory complication. Exercise testing can be modified in patients who are not capable of stair climbing, by using bicycle or arm exercises instead. Complete laboratory exercise testing is labor intensive and expensive. Recently, several alternatives to exercise testing have been demonstrated to have potential as replacement tests for prethoracotomy assessment.

The 6-minute walk test (6MWT) shows an excellent correlation with Vo$_2$ max and requires little or no laboratory equipment.[17] A 6MWT distance of less than 2000 ft correlates to a Vo$_2$ max less than 15 mL/kg/min and also correlates with a fall in oximetry (Spo$_2$) during exercise. Patients with a decrease of Spo$_2$ more than 4% during exercise (stair climbing two or three flights or the equivalent) are at increased risk of morbidity and mortality.[18]

The 6MWT and exercise oximetry may replace Vo$_2$ max for assessment of cardiorespiratory function in the future. Both of these tests are still evolving, and for the present, exercise testing remains the gold standard. Postresection exercise tolerance can be estimated based on the amount of functioning lung tissue removed. An estimated ppoVo$_2$ max less than 10 mL/kg/min may be one of the few remaining absolute contraindications to pulmonary resection. In a small series reported by Bollinger, mortality was 100% (three out of three) in patients with a ppoVo$_2$ max less than 10 mL/kg/min.[19]

After pulmonary resection, there is a degree of right ventricular dysfunction that appears to be proportional to the amount of functioning pulmonary vascular bed removed.[20] The exact etiology and duration of this dysfunction remain unknown. Clinical evidence of this hemodynamic problem is minimal when the patient is at rest but is dramatic when the patient exercises, leading to elevation of pulmonary vascular pressures, limitation of cardiac output, and absence of the normal decrease in pulmonary vascular resistance usually seen with exertion.[21]

Additional Useful Tests
VENTILATION/PERFUSION SCINTIGRAPHY

Prediction of pulmonary function after lung resection can be further refined by assessment of the preoperative contribution of the lung or lobe to be resected using ventilation/perfusion (V̇/Q̇) lung scanning.[22] If the lung region to be resected is nonfunctioning or minimally functioning, the prediction of postoperative function can be modified accordingly. This is particularly useful in pneumonectomy patients, and V̇/Q̇ scanning should be considered for any patient who has a ppoFEV$_1$ less than 40%. Because the V̇/Q̇ scanning is performed at rest, whereas the FEV$_1$ is a forced maneuver, there is always some degree of error in estimating the true eventual lung mechanics after a pulmonary resection. This extrapolation error, plus changes in lung and chest wall function secondary to lung remodeling and expansion after a pulmonary resection, lead to an underestimation of the eventual spirometric lung function. The long-term outcome spirometry values, however, are not as relevant for the anesthesiologist managing the patient in the perioperative period as are the simple ppoFEV$_1$% calculated from the preoperative FEV$_1$ and the amount of functioning lung tissue removed as assessed by the V̇/Q̇ scan.[22]

SPLIT-LUNG FUNCTION STUDIES

A variety of methods have been described for simulating the postoperative respiratory situation by unilateral exclusion of a lung or lobe using an endobronchial tube or blocker or by pulmonary artery balloon occlusion of a lung or lobe artery.[23] These and other varieties of split-lung function testing have also been combined with exercise in an attempt to assess the tolerance of the cardiorespiratory system to a proposed resection. Although these tests are used currently to guide therapy in certain individual centers, they have not shown sufficient predictive validity for widespread universal adoption in potential lung resection patients. One possible explanation for some predictive failures in these patients may be that the lack of a pulmonary hypertensive response to unilateral occlusion might represent a failing right ventricle misinterpreted as a good sign of pulmonary vascular reserve. Lewis et al have shown that in a group of patients with COPD (ppo FEV_1 less than 40%) undergoing pneumonectomy, there were no significant changes in the pulmonary vascular pressures intraoperatively when the pulmonary artery was clamped, but the right ventricular ejection fraction and cardiac output decreased.[24] Echocardiographic studies may offer more useful information than vascular pressure monitoring in these patients.[25] In the future, the combination of unilateral occlusion studies with echocardiography might become a useful addition to this type of preresection investigation. For the present, split-lung function studies have been replaced in most centers by a combination assessment involving $\dot{V}/\dot{Q}$ scanning, spirometry, DLCO, and exercise tolerance.

FLOW-VOLUME LOOPS

Routine spirometric measurements can be calculated from the flow-volume loop (Figure 1-8). Flow-volume loops can help identify the presence of a variable intrathoracic airway obstruction by evidence of a positional change in an abnormal plateau of the expiratory limb of the loop (Figure 1-9).[26] This can occur because of compression of a main conducting airway by a tumor mass. Such a problem might warrant induction airway management with awake intubation or maintenance of spontaneous ventilation.[27] In an adult patient capable of giving a complete history who does not describe supine exacerbation of cough or dyspnea, flow-volume loops are not required as a routine preoperative test. If airway compression is suspected, a CT scan of the chest and trachea is a more specific guide to therapy and provides more useful information to the anesthesiologist than do flow-volume loops.[28]

COMBINATION OF TESTS

No single test of respiratory function has shown adequate validity as a sole preoperative assessment.[29] Before surgery,

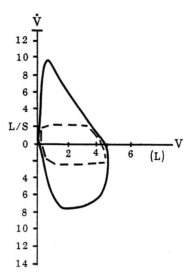

FIGURE 1-9 Changes in the flow-volume loop with airway obstruction. The dashed line during exhalation *(above baseline)* shows intrathoracic airway obstruction, while the dashed line during inspiration *(below baseline)* shows extrathoracic airway obstruction. When obstruction is seen in either expiration or inspiration but not in both, it is called a *variable airway obstruction*. Fixed obstruction throughout the respiratory cycle results in a "square" loop.

an estimate of respiratory function in the three areas of lung mechanics, parenchymal function, and cardiopulmonary interaction should be made for each patient. These three aspects of pulmonary function form the "three-legged stool" that is the foundation of prethoracotomy respiratory assessment (Figure 1-10). These data can then be used to plan intra- and postoperative management (Figure 1-11) and also to alter management plans when intraoperative surgical factors necessitate that a resection becomes more extensive than foreseen. If a patient has a ppoFEV$_1$ more than 40%, it should be possible for that patient to be extubated in the operating room at the conclusion of surgery assuming that the patient is alert, warm, and comfortable (AWaC). Patients with a ppoFEV$_1$ <40% usually comprise about 25% of an average thoracic

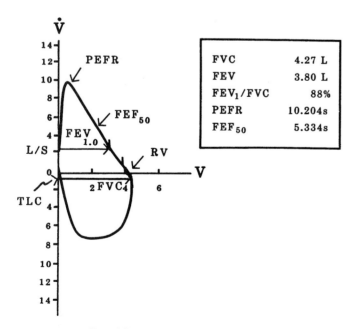

FIGURE 1-8 Normal flow volume loop showing peak expiratory flow rate (PEFR), forced expiratory volume at 1 second (FEV_1), and forced vital capacity (FVC). *FEF,* Forced expiratory flow. The values shown are within the normal range for a 20-year-old male, 170-cm height.

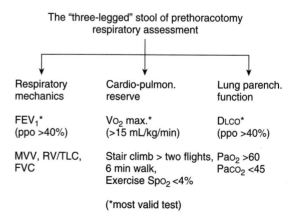

FIGURE 1-10 The "three-legged stool" of prethoracotomy respiratory assessment (* symbol indicates the most valid test; see text). (From Slinger PD, Johnston MR: *J Cardiothorac Vasc Anesth* 14:202, 2000.)

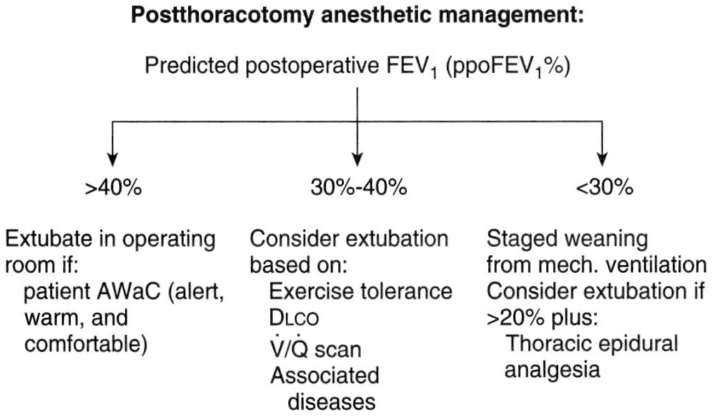

Postthoracotomy anesthetic management:

Predicted postoperative FEV_1 (ppoFEV_1%)

>40%	30%-40%	<30%

Extubate in operating room if:
    patient AWaC (alert, warm, and comfortable)
	Consider extubation based on:
	    Exercise tolerance
	    D_{LCO}
	    $\dot{V}$/Q scan
	    Associated diseases
		Staged weaning from mech. ventilation Consider extubation if >20% plus:
		    Thoracic epidural analgesia

FIGURE 1-11 Anesthetic management guided by preoperative assessment and the amount of functioning lung tissue removed during surgery. (From Slinger PD, Johnston MR: *J Cardiothorac Vasc Anesth* 14:202, 2000.)

surgical population. If the ppoFEV_1 is more than 30% and exercise tolerance and lung parenchymal function exceed the increased risk thresholds, then extubation in the operating room should be possible depending on the status of associated diseases (see Intercurrent Medical Conditions section). Those patients in this subgroup who do not meet the minimal criteria for cardiopulmonary and parenchymal function should be considered for staged weaning from mechanical ventilation postoperatively so that the effect of the increased oxygen consumption of spontaneous ventilation can be assessed. Patients with a ppoFEV_1 of 20% to 30% and favorable predicted cardiorespiratory and parenchymal function can be considered for early extubation if thoracic epidural analgesia is used (see Postoperative Analgesia section). Otherwise, these patients should have a postoperative staged weaning from mechanical ventilation. In the borderline group (ppoFEV_1 values from 30% to 40%) the presence of several associated factors and diseases that should be documented during the preoperative assessment will enter into the considerations for postoperative management.

Intercurrent Medical Conditions

Age

There appears to be no maximum age that is a cutoff for viable pulmonary resection. If a patient is 80 years of age and has stage I lung cancer, the chances of survival to age 85 are better with the tumor resected than without. In a series reported by Osaki et al,[30] the operative mortality in a group of patients ranging from 80 to 92 years of age was 3%, a very respectable figure. The rate of respiratory complications (40%), however, was double that expected in a younger population, and the rate of cardiac complications (40%), particularly arrhythmias, was nearly triple that which should be seen in younger patients. Although the mortality from lobectomy in the elderly is acceptable, the mortality from pneumonectomy (22% in patients more than 70 years), particularly pneumonectomy on the right lung, is excessive.[31] Presumably, the reason for this is the increased strain on the right ventricle of the heart caused by resection of the proportionally larger vascular bed of the right lung.

Cardiac Disease

Cardiac complications are the second most common cause of perioperative morbidity and mortality in the thoracic surgical population.

ISCHEMIA

Because the majority of pulmonary resection patients have a history of smoking, they already have at least one risk factor for coronary artery disease.[32] Elective pulmonary resection surgery, however, is regarded as an intermediate-risk procedure in terms of perioperative cardiac ischemia, which means that the outcomes are more favorable than those for accepted high-risk procedures such as major emergency or vascular surgery.[33] The overall documented incidence of postthoracotomy ischemia is 5% and peaks on day 2 or 3 after surgery.[34] This is approximately the level of risk that would be expected from a similar patient population having major abdominal, orthopedic, or other procedures. Beyond the standard history, physical, and electrocardiogram, routine screening testing for cardiac disease does not appear to be cost effective for all prethoracotomy patients.[35] Noninvasive testing is indicated for patients who have major clinical predictors of myocardial risk (unstable ischemia, recent infarction, severe valvular disease, significant arrhythmia) or intermediate predictors (stable angina, remote infarction, previous congestive heart failure, or diabetes) and also in the elderly (Table 1-1 and Figure 1-12).[36] Therapeutic options to be considered in patients with significant coronary artery disease are optimization of medical therapy, coronary angioplasty, or coronary artery bypass, either before or at the time of lung resection.[37] Timing of lung resection surgery after a myocardial infarction is always a difficult decision. Based on

---

TABLE 1-1

Clinical Predictors of Increased Cardiac Risk

MAJOR RISK
Unstable coronary syndromes
Recent myocardial infarction (7–28 days) with evidence of important ischemic risk by symptoms or noninvasive testing
    Unstable or severe angina (Canadian class III or IV)
Decompensated congestive heart failure
Significant arrhythmia:
    High-grade atrioventricular block
Symptomatic ventricular arrhythmias in the presence of underlying heart disease
    Supraventricular arrhythmias with uncontrolled ventricular rate
    Severe valvular disease

INTERMEDIATE RISK
Mild angina (Canadian class I or II)
Prior myocardial infarction by history or ECG
Compensated or previous congestive heart failure
Diabetes

MINOR RISK
Advanced age
Abnormal ECG (left ventricular hypertrophy, left bundle-branch block, ST-T abnormalities)
Rhythm other than sinus (e.g., atrial fibrillation)
Low functional capacity (e.g., inability to climb two flight of stairs)
History of stroke
Uncontrolled hypertension

From ACC/AHA task force on practice guidelines, *Anesth Analg* 82:854, 1996.

Cardiac risk assessment for thoracic surgery

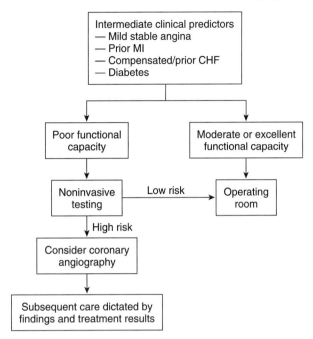

FIGURE 1-12 Prethoracotomy evaluation protocol for patients with intermediate predictors for perioperative myocardial ischemia. (From ACC/AHA Task Force on Practice Guidelines: *Anesth Analg* 82:854, 1996.)

the data of Rao et al and generally confirmed by recent clinical practice, limiting the delay to 4 to 6 weeks in a medically stable and fully investigated and optimized patient seems acceptable after myocardial infarction.[38] A delay of 2 to 4 weeks is recommended after coronary artery stenting.[39] The use of prophylactic β-blockers to reduce the risk of perioperative ischemia in thoracic surgical patients with known or suspected coronary artery disease in the absence of contraindications seems justified based on the recent literature.[40]

ARRHYTHMIA

Arrhythmias are a recognized complication of all pulmonary resection surgery. The incidence of arrhythmias approaches 50% of patients in the first week after surgery, when sophisticated detection techniques, such as continuous Holter monitoring, are used.[41] When documentation is limited to investigation of symptomatic patients, the diagnosed frequency falls to 15% to 20% of cases.[42,43] Of the supraventricular arrhythmias, 60% to 70% are atrial fibrillation; the remainder are atrial flutter and supraventricular tachycardia in approximately equal proportions. Several factors are known to correlate with an increased incidence of such arrhythmias; for example, extent of lung resection (60% of pneumonectomy patients, compared with 40% of lobectomy patients and 30% of patients undergoing nonresection thoracotomy) intrapericardial dissections, intraoperative blood loss, and age of the patient.[44-46] Patients undergoing extrapleural pneumonectomy are a high-risk group.[47]

Two factors in the early postthoracotomy period interact to produce atrial arrhythmias:

1. Increased flow resistance through the pulmonary vascular bed due to permanent causes (for example, lung resection)

or transient causes (such as atelectasis or hypoxemia), with attendant strain on the right side of the heart.

2. Increased sympathetic stimuli and oxygen requirements, which reach their peak on the second postoperative day as patients begin to mobilize.[48]

In pneumonectomy patients followed for 24 hours with right ventricular ejection reaction (RVEF) catheters, there was a significant fall of RVEF on the first postoperative day as compared with lobectomy patients.[49] This reduction in RVEF was accompanied by an increase in right ventricular size and pulmonary artery pressures. Pneumonectomy patients did not demonstrate the early postoperative increases in oxygen delivery, oxygen consumption, or cardiac index seen in lobectomy patients. This suggests that in some pneumonectomy patients, the right ventricle of the heart might be unable to adequately increase its output to meet the usual postoperative stress in the face of an increased afterload.

Pulmonary artery (PA) pressures and/or measures of pulmonary vascular resistance (PVR) alone do not yield a complete picture of the evolving hemodynamics in pneumonectomy patients. In pulmonary hypertension, significant falls in RVEF and cardiac output can occur after pulmonary artery clamping, without major accompanying changes in pulmonary pressures.[50] Also, patients who show no immediate postoperative changes in PA pressures evidence exaggerated postoperative increases in PA pressures and PVR during exercise.[51]

Transthoracic echocardiographic studies have shown that pneumonectomy patients develop an increase in right ventricular systolic pressure as measured by the tricuspid regurgitation jet (TRJ) on postoperative day two but not on postoperative day one.[52] Lobectomy patients did not show this increase, and neither group demonstrated increased right atrial or ventricular volumes. An increase in TRJ velocity has been associated with postthoracotomy supraventricular tachyarrhythmias.[53]

It is of interest to note that many patients will demonstrate their lowest oxygen saturation of the perioperative period on the second night after a thoracotomy.[54] The attendant increase in pulmonary vasoconstriction from this nocturnal hypoxemia may contribute to the postoperative dysfunction of the right side of the heart and explain the peak incidence of atrial arrhythmias on the second and third days after surgery.

Properly performed and interpreted pulmonary function tests can reliably predict adverse respiratory complications in the thoracic surgical population.[55] However, spirometry seems to have less value for determining which patients are at risk for arrhythmias. Preoperative exercise testing, which assesses the cardiopulmonary interaction, can predict postthoracotomy arrythmias.[19] Patients with COPD are more resistant to pharmacologic rate control when they develop postthoracotomy atrial fibrillation, and they often require multiple drugs.[56]

A wide variety of antiarrhythmics have been tried to decrease the incidence of atrial arrhythmias after lung surgery. The best known of these are digoxin preparations. It has now been clearly demonstrated in several randomized clinical trials that digoxin does not prevent arrhythmias after pneumonectomy or other intrathoracic procedures. A study by Ritchie et al found a 50% incidence of arrhythmias in the digoxin group (as opposed to a 30% incidence in the control group) and an 8% incidence of digoxin toxicity in the treatment group.[57]

Other agents that have been tried to prevent postthoracotomy arrhythmias include β-blockers, verapamil, and amiodarone.[58-60] All of these agents decrease arrhythmias in thoracic patients. On the other hand, they are all associated with side effects that preclude their widespread application in this surgical population. At present diltiazem is the most useful drug for postthoracotomy arrhythmia prophylaxis.[47] It seems that atrial arrhythmias are only a symptom of the dysfunctional right side of the heart, and preventing the symptom does not solve the underlying problem.

In a study of verapamil prophylaxis after thoracotomy, Lindgren et al found that in the control (placebo) group, patients who subsequently developed atrial tachyarrhythmias could be identified early in the postoperative period by their right ventricular response to the withdrawal of supplemental oxygen.[61] On the first day after surgery, a decrease of F_{IO_2} from 0.35 to 0.21 caused a significant rise of right ventricular end-diastolic pressure (RVEDP) in the arrhythmia subgroup from a mean of 4 to 8 mmHg, higher than the increase in the non-arrhythmia subgroup (0 to 2 mmHg). Of particular interest is that this rise occurred 1 day before the onset of arrhythmias. The clinical implication is that patients at high risk for atrial arrhythmias require both careful monitoring of oxygenation and optimization of postthoracotomy analgesia to improve pulmonary function in the postoperative period.[62]

Animal models of myocardial ischemia suggest that thoracic epidural analgesia (TEA) with local anesthetics can decrease the incidence and severity of arrhythmias.[63] This effect is thought to be due to increasing the myocardial refractory period, decreasing ventricular diastolic pressures, and improving endocardial/epicardial blood flow ratios. Unlike lumbar epidural analgesia, TEA has not been shown to exacerbate myocardial ischemia in patients with coronary artery disease.[64] There is some evidence from clinical studies to support the theory that TEA with local anesthetics decreases postthoracotomy arrhythmias.[65,66]

Renal Dysfunction

Renal dysfunction after pulmonary resection surgery is associated with a very high incidence of mortality. Gollege and Goldstraw reported a perioperative mortality of 19% (6/31) in patients who developed any significant elevation of serum creatinine in the postthoracotomy period, compared with a mortality rate of 0% (0/99) in those who did not show any renal dysfunction.[67] The factors that were highly associated ($p < 0.001$) with an elevated risk of renal impairment are listed in Table 1-2. Other factors that were statistically significant but less strongly associated with renal impairment included preoperative hypertension, chemotherapy, ischemic heart disease, and postoperative oliguria (less than 33 mL/hr). Nonsteroidal antiinflammatory agents (NSAIDs) were not associated with renal impairment in this series but are clearly

---

TABLE 1-2

Factors Associated with an Increased Risk of Postthoracotomy Renal Impairment

1. Previous history of renal impairment
2. Diuretic therapy
3. Pneumonectomy
4. Postoperative infection
5. Blood loss requiring transfusion

---

a concern in any thoracotomy patient with an increased risk of renal dysfunction. The high mortality in pneumonectomy patients from either renal failure or postoperative pulmonary edema emphasizes the importance of fluid management in these patients and the need for close and intensive perioperative monitoring, particularly in those patients who are on diuretics or have a history of renal dysfunction.[68]

Chronic Obstructive Pulmonary Disease

The most common concurrent illness in the thoracic surgical population is chronic obstructive pulmonary disease (COPD), which incorporates three disorders: emphysema, peripheral airways disease, and chronic bronchitis. Any individual patient may have one or all of these conditions, but the dominant clinical feature is impairment of expiratory airflow.[69] Assessment of the severity of COPD has traditionally been on the basis of the FEV_1% of predicted values. The American Thoracic Society currently categorizes stage I more than 50% predicted FEV_1 (this category previously included both mild and moderate COPD), stage II between 35% and 50%; and stage III less than 35%. Life expectancy may be less than 3 years in stage III patients over 60 years of age (Figure 1-13). stage I patients should not have significant dyspnea, hypoxemia, or hypercarbia, and other causes should be considered if any of these are present. Recent advances in the understanding of COPD that are relevant to anesthetic management include the following topics.

RESPIRATORY DRIVE

Major changes have occurred in the understanding of the control of breathing in COPD patients. Many stage II or III COPD patients have an elevated $PaCO_2$ at rest. It is not possible to differentiate these *CO₂-retainers* from nonretainers on the basis of history, physical examination, or spirometric pulmonary function testing (Figure 1-14).[70] CO_2 retention seems to be related to an inability to maintain the increased work of respiration (W_{resp}) required to keep the $PaCO_2$ at normal levels in patients with mechanically inefficient pulmonary function—it is not due primarily to an alteration of respiratory control mechanisms. It was previously thought that chronically hypoxemic/hypercapnic patients relied on a hypoxic stimulus for ventilatory drive and became insensitive to $PaCO_2$. This explained the clinical observation that COPD patients in incipient respiratory failure could be put into a hypercapnic coma by the administration of a high concentration of oxygen (F_{IO_2}). Actually, only a minor fraction of the increase in $PaCO_2$ in such patients is due to a diminished respiratory drive, because minute ventilation is basically unchanged.[71] The $PaCO_2$ rises because a high F_{IO_2} causes a relative decrease in alveolar ventilation and an increase in alveolar deadspace by the redistribution of perfusion away from lung areas of relatively normal $\dot{V}/\dot{Q}$ matching to areas of very low $\dot{V}/\dot{Q}$ ratio. This occurs because regional hypoxic pulmonary vasoconstriction (HPV) is decreased and also because of the Haldane effect.[72] Supplemental oxygen must, however, be administered to these patients postoperatively to prevent the hypoxemia associated with the unavoidable fall in functional residual capacity (FRC). The attendant rise in CO_2 should be anticipated and monitored. To identify these patients preoperatively, all stage II or III COPD patients need an arterial blood gas measurement.

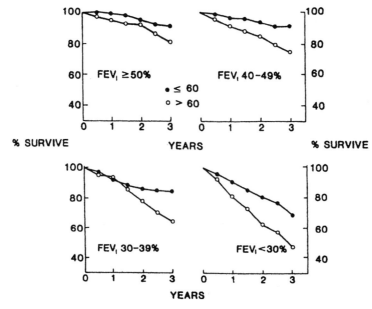

FIGURE 1-13 Three-year survival among COPD patients segregated by initial FEV_1% and age less than *(closed circles)* or greater than *(open circles)* 60 years. (From Anthonisen R: *Am Rev Resp Dis* 140:595, 1989).

NOCTURNAL HYPOXEMIA

COPD patients desaturate more frequently and severely during sleep than do normal patients.[73] This is due to the rapid, shallow breathing pattern that occurs in all patients during REM sleep. In COPD patients breathing air, shallow breathing causes a significant increase in the respiratory deadspace/tidal volume (V_D/V_T) ratio and results in reductions in alveolar oxygen tension (PA_{O_2}) and Pa_{O_2}. This is not the sleep apnea–hypoventilation syndrome (SAHS); there is no increased incidence of SAHS in COPD. In 8 of 10 COPD patients studied, the oxygen saturation fell to less than 50% at some time during normal sleep, and this fall was associated with an increase in pulmonary artery pressure.[74] This tendency to desaturate, combined with the postoperative fall in FRC and opioid analgesia, places these patients at high risk for severe hypoxemia postoperatively during sleep.

RIGHT VENTRICULAR DYSFUNCTION

Right ventricular (RV) dysfunction occurs in up to 50% of COPD patients.[75] The dysfunctional RV, even when

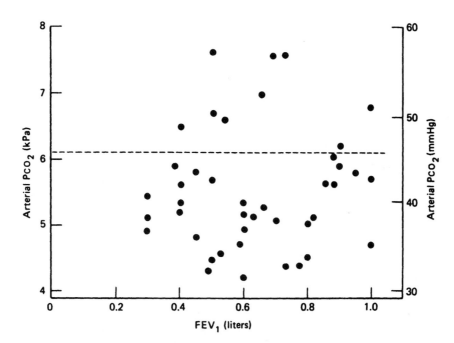

FIGURE 1-14 Relationship between arterial P_{CO_2} and FEV_1 in a group of stable hypercapnic *(top circles)* and nonhypercapnic *(bottom circles)* COPD patients. Note that there is a poor relationship between CO_2-retention and spirometry in COPD. (From Nunn J: *Applied respiratory physiology,* ed 4, Oxford, 1993, Butterworth Heinemann.)

hypertrophied, is poorly tolerant of sudden increases in afterload, such as the change from spontaneous to controlled ventilation.[76,77] RV function becomes critical in maintaining cardiac output as the pulmonary artery pressure rises. The RV ejection fraction does not increase with exercise in COPD patients as it does in normal patients. Chronic recurrent hypoxemia is the cause of the RV dysfunction and the subsequent progression to cor pulmonale. Patients who have episodic hypoxemia in spite of normal lungs (e.g., central alveolar hypoventilation, SAHS, etc.) develop the same secondary cardiac problems as COPD patients.[78] Cor pulmonale occurs in 40% of adult COPD patients with an FEV_1 less than 1 L and in 70% with FEV_1 less than 0.6 L.[75] It is now clear that mortality in COPD patients is primarily related to chronic hypoxemia.[79] The only therapy that has been shown to improve long-term survival and decrease right ventricular strain in COPD is oxygen. COPD patients who have resting Pao_2 less than 55 mmHg should receive supplemental home oxygen, as should those who desaturate to less than 44 mmHg with usual exercise.[69] The goal of supplemental oxygen is to maintain a Pao_2 of 60 to 65 mmHg. Compared to patients with chronic bronchitis, emphysematous COPD patients tend to have a decreased cardiac output and mixed venous oxygen tension while maintaining lower pulmonary artery pressures.[75] Pneumonectomy candidates with a $ppoFEV_1$ less than 40% should have transthoracic echocardiography to assess right ventricular heart function. Elevation of right ventricular pressures places these patients in a very high-risk group.[62]

BULLAE

Many patients with moderate or severe COPD develop cystic air spaces in the lung parenchyma known as *bullae*. These bullae will often be asymptomatic unless they occupy more than 50% of the hemithorax, in which case the patient will present with findings of restrictive respiratory disease in addition to obstructive disease. Previously, it was thought that bullae represented positive pressure areas within the lung that compressed surrounding lung tissue. It is now appreciated that a bulla is actually a localized area of loss of structural support tissue in the lung with elastic recoil of surrounding parenchyma (Figure 1-15). The pressure in a bulla is actually the mean pressure in the surrounding alveoli averaged over the respiratory cycle. This means that during normal spontaneous ventilation, the intrabulla pressure is actually slightly negative in comparison to the surrounding parenchyma.[80] Whenever positive pressure ventilation is used, however, the pressure in a bulla will become positive in relation to the adjacent lung tissue, and the bulla will expand with the attendant risk of rupture, tension pneumothorax, and bronchopleural fistula. Positive pressure ventilation can be used safely in patients with bullae provided the airway pressures are kept low and there is adequate expertise and equipment immediately available to insert a chest tube and obtain lung isolation if necessary. Management of patients for bullectomy is discussed in Chapter 11.

FLOW LIMITATION

Severe COPD patients are often *flow limited* even during tidal volume expiration at rest.[81] Flow limitation is present in normal patients only during a forced expiratory maneuver (Figure 1-16). Flow limitation occurs when an equal pressure point (EPP) develops in the intrathoracic airways during expiration. During quiet expiration in the normal patient, the pressure in the lumina of the airways always exceeds the intrapleural pressure because of the upstream elastic recoil pressure that is transmitted from the alveoli. The effect of this elastic recoil pressure diminishes as air flows downstream in the airway. With a forced expiration, the intrapleural pressure may equal the intraluminal pressure at a certain point, the EPP, which then limits the expiratory flow. Thereafter, any increase in expiratory effort will not produce an increase in flow at that given lung volume.[82]

Flow limitation occurs particularly in emphysematous patients, who primarily have a problem with loss of lung elastic

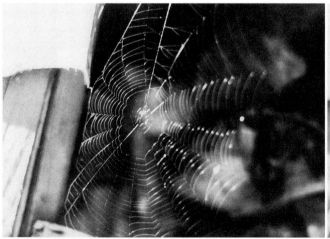 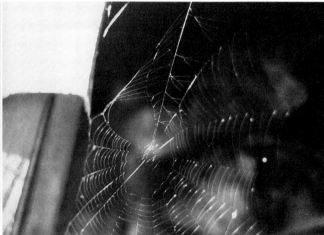

A   B

FIGURE 1-15 **A,** A spider's web is used as a lung model to demonstrate the pathophysiology of bullae. **B,** Breaking one septum of the spider's web causes a bulla to appear as elastic recoil pulls the web away from the area where structural support has been lost. Although the cells surrounding the bulla appear compressed, this is due only to redistribution of elastic forces. It is not positive pressure inside the bulla that causes this appearance of surrounding compression. (From Slinger P: Anesthesia for lung resection surgery. In Thys D (ed): *Textbook of cardiothoracic anesthesia,* New York, 2001, McGraw Hill.)

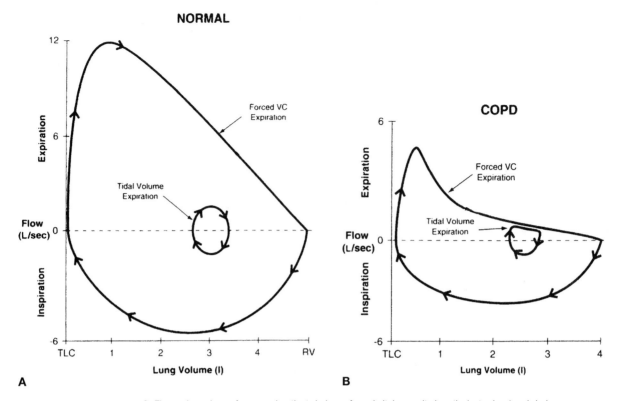

FIGURE 1-16 A, Flow-volume loop of a normal patient during a forced vital capacity breath *(outer loop)* and during tidal volume breathing *(inner loop)*. Note that in the lung volume range used for tidal volume breathing, the expiratory flow can be increased twofold or threefold before reaching the flow limit imposed by the forced vital capacity flow. Ventilation is mechanically most efficient in this tidal volume range. **B,** Flow-volume loops of a patient with moderate COPD during forced vital capacity *(outer loop)* and tidal volume *(inner loop)* breathing. Note the change in shape of the forced expiratory curve vs. the normal curve. Also note that tidal volume expiration is flow limited and that it is impossible for this patient to increase expiratory flows in the lung volume range used for normal tidal volume breathing. (From Slinger P: Anesthesia for lung resection surgery. In Thys D (ed): *Textbook of cardiothoracic anesthesia,* New York, 2001, McGraw Hill.)

recoil and have marked dyspnea on exertion. Flow limitation causes dyspnea because mechanoreceptors in the muscles of respiration, the thoracic cage, and in the airway distal to the EPP are stimulated. Any increase in the work of respiration will lead to increased dyspnea.[83] This variable mechanical compression of airways by overinflated alveoli is the primary cause of the airflow obstruction in emphysema. In the patients with predominantly emphysematous pathology (vs. those with bronchitic or asthmatic pathology), the FEV_1 is not as valid an indicator of the severity of disease.[84] This may explain why emphysematous patients frequently have an improvement of symptoms and plethysmographic respiratory function (decreased hyperinflation) from β-agonist bronchodilators without a change in FEV_1.[85]

Severely flow-limited patients are at risk for hemodynamic collapse with the application of positive pressure ventilation because of dynamic hyperinflation of the lungs.[86] Even the modest positive airway pressures associated with manual ventilation with a bag or mask at induction of anesthesia can lead to hypotension because these patients have no increased resistance to inspiration but rather a marked obstruction of expiration. In some of these patients, this phenomenon has contributed to the "Lazarus" syndrome, in which patients have recovered from a cardiac arrest only after resuscitation and positive pressure ventilation were discontinued.[87]

POSITIVE END-EXPIRATORY PRESSURE

Patients with severe COPD often breathe in a pattern that interrupts expiration before the alveolar pressure has fallen to atmospheric pressure. This incomplete expiration is due to a combination of factors that include flow limitation, increased work of respiration, and increased airway resistance. This interruption leads to an elevation of the end-expiratory lung volume above the FRC—even above the already increased FRC because of loss of lung elastic recoil. This positive end-expiratory pressure (PEEP) in the alveoli at rest has been termed *auto-PEEP* or *intrinsic-PEEP*.[88] During spontaneous respiration, the intrapleural pressure will have to be decreased to a level that counteracts auto-PEEP before inspiratory flow can begin. Thus COPD patients can have an increased inspiratory load added to their already increased expiratory load.

Auto-PEEP becomes even more important during mechanical ventilation. It is directly proportional to tidal volume and inversely proportional to expiratory time. The presence of auto-PEEP is not detected by the manometer of standard anesthesia ventilators. It can be measured by end-expiratory flow interruption, a feature available on the newer generation of intensive care ventilators. Auto-PEEP has been found to develop in most COPD patients during one-lung anesthesia.[89]

COMBINED CANCER AND EMPHYSEMA SURGERY

Although the predicted values for ppoFEV$_1$ are very useful for the anesthesiologist wishing to stratify a patient's perioperative risk, the actual postoperative FEV$_1$ that the patient reaches by 3 months after recovery from surgery usually exceeds the ppoFEV$_1$ as a result of compensatory hyperinflation of the residual lung. For lobectomies, the eventual FEV$_1$ will usually exceed the ppoFEV$_1$ by approximately 250 mL, and for pneumonectomies, the eventual FEV$_1$ exceeds the ppoFEV$_1$ by 500 mL.[90] This improvement can be particularly noticed in some emphysema patients who experience a *volume reduction* effect from their pulmonary resection for cancer. The combination of volume reduction surgery and/or bullectomy in addition to lung cancer surgery has been reported in emphysematous patients who previously would not have met minimal criteria for pulmonary resection because of their concurrent lung disease (Figure 1-1).[91] Although the numbers of patients reported to have undergone both surgeries is small, the expected improvements in postoperative pulmonary function have been seen, and the outcomes are encouraging. This positive outcome offers an extension of the standard indications for surgery in a small, well-selected group of patients.

Preoperative Therapy of COPD

There are four treatable complications of COPD that must be accurately detected and for which therapy must begin at the time of the initial prethoracotomy assessment. These are atelectasis, bronchospasm, respiratory tract infections, and pulmonary edema (Table 1-3). Atelectasis impairs local lung lymphocyte and macrophage function, predisposing the patient to infection.[92] Pulmonary edema can be very difficult to diagnose by auscultation in the presence of COPD and may present very abnormal radiologic distributions (unilateral, upper lobes, etc.).[93] Bronchial hyperreactivity may be a symptom of congestive heart failure or may represent an exacerbation of reversible airway obstruction.[94] All COPD patients should receive maximum bronchodilator therapy as guided by their symptoms. Only 20% to 25% of COPD patients will respond to corticosteroids. In a patient who is poorly controlled on sympathomimetic and anticholinergic bronchodilators, a trial of corticosteroids may be beneficial.[95] It is not clear whether corticosteroids are as beneficial in COPD as they are in asthma. Pharmacotherapy for reactive airway diseases is discussed in Chapter 6.

Physiotherapy

It has been shown clearly that patients with COPD have fewer postoperative pulmonary complications when a perioperative program of intensive chest physiotherapy is initiated prior to surgery.[96] It is uncertain whether this benefit applies to other pulmonary resection patients. Among the different modalities available (cough and deep breathing, incentive spirometry, PEEP, continuous positive airway pressure [CPAP]) there is no method that has been clearly proven to be superior to the others.[97] The important variable is the quantity of time spent with the patient and devoted to chest physiotherapy. Family members or nonphysiotherapy hospital staff can easily be trained to perform effective preoperative chest physiotherapy, and such therapy should be arranged at the time of the initial preoperative assessment. Even in the most severely afflicted COPD patient, it is possible to improve exercise tolerance with a physiotherapy program.[98] Little improvement is seen before 1 month. Among COPD patients, those with excessive sputum benefit the most from chest physiotherapy.[99]

A comprehensive program of pulmonary rehabilitation involving physiotherapy, exercise, nutrition, and education has been shown to consistently improve functional capacity for patients with severe COPD.[62,100] These programs are usually of several months' duration and are generally not an option in resections for malignancy (although for nonmalignant resections in severe COPD patients, rehabilitation should be considered). The benefits of short-term rehabilitation programs before malignancy resection have not been fully assessed.

Smoking

Pulmonary complications are decreased in thoracic surgical patients who are not smoking when compared with those who continue to smoke up until the time of surgery.[101] Patients having cardiac surgery, however, show no decrease in the incidence of respiratory complications unless smoking is discontinued for more than 8 weeks before surgery.[102] Carboxyhemoglobin concentrations decrease if smoking is stopped for longer than 12 hours.[103] It is extremely important for patients to avoid smoking after surgery. Smoking leads to a prolonged period of tissue hypoxemia. Wound tissue oxygen tension correlates with wound healing and resistance to infection.[104] The balance of the evidence suggests that thoracic surgical patients should be counseled to stop smoking and advised that the longer the period of cessation before surgery, the greater the reduction in risk for postoperative pulmonary complications.[105]

Primary Thoracic Tumors

The majority of patients presenting for major pulmonary surgery will have some type of malignancy. Because the different types of thoracic malignancy have different implications both for surgery and for anesthesia, it is useful for the anesthesiologist to have some knowledge of the presentation and biology of the more commonly encountered cancers. By far, the most common tumor is lung cancer. More than 200,000 new cases of lung cancer are diagnosed annually in North America, and more than 1.2 million are diagnosed annually worldwide. Lung cancer is currently the leading cause of cancer deaths in both sexes in North America subsequent to the peak incidence of smoking in the period 1960 to 1970 (Figure 1-17).[106,107]

TABLE 1-3

Concurrent Problems That Should Be Treated in COPD Patients Before Anesthesia

Problem	Method of Diagnosis
Bronchospasm	Auscultation
Atelectasis	Chest x-ray
Infection	History, sputum analysis
Pulmonary edema	Auscultation, chest x-ray

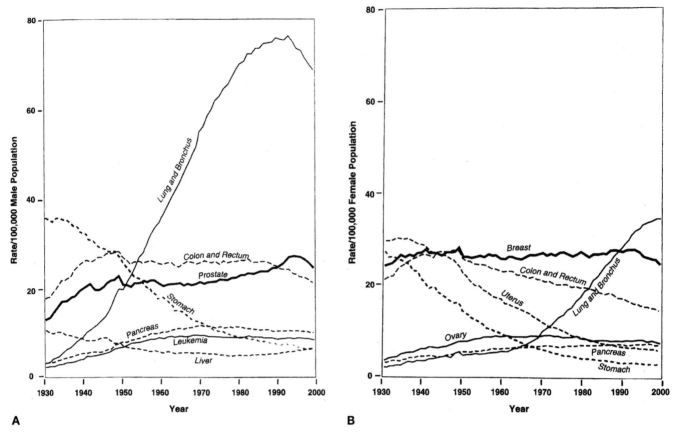

FIGURE 1-17 Age-adjusted mortality rates for men **(A)** and women **(B)** in the United States from 1930 to 1988. Respiratory malignancies have become the leading cause of cancer deaths in both sexes. (From Vital statistics of the United States: 1998. www.cancer.org.)

Because of biologic and therapeutic considerations, lung cancer is broadly divided into small cell lung cancer (SCLC) and non–small cell lung cancer (NSCLC), with about 75% to 80% of these tumors being NSCLC. Other less common and less aggressive tumors of the lung include the carcinoid tumors (typical and atypical) and adenoid cystic carcinoma. In comparison to lung cancer, primary pleural tumors are rare. These include the localized fibrous tumors of pleura (previously referred to as *benign mesotheliomas*) and malignant pleural mesothelioma (MPM). Asbestos exposure is implicated as a causative effect in up to 80% of MPM. A dose-response relationship is not always apparent, and even brief exposure can lead to the disease. An exposure history is often difficult to obtain because the latent period before clinical manifestation of the tumor might be as long as 40 to 50 years.

Tobacco smoke is responsible for approximately 90% of all lung cancers, and the epidemiology of lung cancer follows the epidemiology of cigarette smoking, with approximately a three-decade lag time.[106] Other environmental causes include asbestos and radon gas (a decay product of naturally occurring uranium), which act as cocarcinogens with tobacco smoke. For a pack-a-day cigarette smoker, the lifetime risk of lung cancer is approximately 1 in 14.[108] Assuming that current mortality patterns continue, cancer will surpass heart disease as the leading cause of death in North America in this decade.

Non–Small Cell (NSC) Carcinomas

This pathologically heterogenous group of tumors includes squamous cell carcinoma, adenocarcinoma, and large cell carcinoma, with several subtypes and combined tumors (Table 1-4). This represents the largest grouping of lung cancers and the vast majority of those that present for surgery. They are grouped together because the surgical therapy, and by inference the anesthetic implications with definitive surgical excision, depend on the stage of the cancer at diagnosis (Tables 1-5 and 1-6). Survival can approach 80% for Stage I lesions. Unfortunately, these represent a minority of potentially

---

TABLE 1-4

Frequency of Cell Types of Primary Lung Cancers

Histologic Type	Proportion
Adenocarcinoma	40%
Squamous cell	27%
Small cell	19%
Large cell	8%
Bronchoalveolar cell	4%
Mixed adeno/squamous	2%
Carcinoid	1%

From Feinstein MB, Bach PB: *Chest Surg Clin North Am* 10:653, 2000.

TABLE 1-5
International Staging System for Non–Small Cell Lung Cancer

TNM Classification	Tumor, Nodes, Metastases
Stage I	T_{1-2}, N_0, M_0
Stage II	T_{1-2}, N_1, M_0
Stage IIIa	T_{1-2}, N_2, M_0
	T_3, N_{0-1}, M_0
Stage IIIb	T_{1-4}, N_3, M_0
Stage IV	Any T, any N, M_1
T_1	Tumor <3 cm
T_2	Tumor >3 cm or visceral pleural invasion, or distal obstruction
T_3	Tumor extension to chest wall, diaphragm, mediastinal pleura or pericardium
T_4	Tumor extension to mediastinum, heart, great vessels, carina, or vertebra
N_1	Ipsilateral peribronchial or hilar nodes
N_2	Ipsilateral mediastinal or subcarinal nodes
N_3	Contralateral nodes, or ipsilateral scalene or supraclavicular nodes
M_1	Distant metastasis

resectable lesions. Overall 5-year survival with surgery approaches 40%. This seemingly low figure must be viewed in the light of an estimated 5-year survival without surgery of less than 10% and the overall survival rate of 13%.[109]

Although it is not always possible to be certain of the pathology of a given lung tumor preoperatively, many patients will have a known tissue diagnosis at the time of preanesthetic assessment on the basis of prior cytology, bronchoscopy, mediastinoscopy, or transthoracic needle aspiration. This is useful preoperative information for the anesthesiologist to obtain. Specific anesthetic implications for the various types of lung cancer are listed in Table 1-7.

SQUAMOUS CELL CARCINOMA

This is the subgroup of NSCLC most strongly linked to smoking. This type of tumor tends to grow to a large size and to metastasize less frequently than other types. Squamous cell carcinomas are more likely to attain large size before presentation and to be associated with the local effects of a large tumor mass with a dominant endobronchial component such as cavitation, fatal hemoptysis, obstructive pneumonia, superior vena cava syndrome, and involvement of the airway and pulmonary arteries. Hypercalcemia is specifically associated with squamous cell cancer, not resulting from bone metastases but rather because of elaboration of a parathyroid-like factor.

TABLE 1-6
Indications for Surgery in Non–Small Cell Lung Cancer

Stages I and II	Primary resection, no postoperative therapy
Stage IIIa	Induction chemoradiation therapy; resection in patients with stable or responding disease
Stage IIIb	Chemoradiation therapy; highly selective resection of T_4, N_0, M_0 tumors
Stage IV	Palliative therapy (exception: selected patients with resected isolated cerebral metastasis may undergo lung resection)

TABLE 1-7
Anesthetic Considerations for Various Types of Lung Cancer

Type	Considerations
Squamous cell	Central lesions (predominantly)
	Mass effects: obstruction, cavitation
	Hypercalcemia
Adenocarcinoma	Peripheral lesions
	Metastases (distant)
	Growth hormone, corticotropin
	Hypertrophic osteoarthropathy
Small cell	Central lesions (predominantly), few surgically treatable
	Paraneoplastic syndromes
	Lambert-Eaton syndrome
	Fast growth rate
	Early metastases
Carcinoid	Proximal, intrabronchial
	Benign (predominantly)
	No association with smoking
	5-year survival >90%
	Carcinoid syndrome (rarely)
Mesothelioma	Intraoperative hemorrhage
	Direct extension to diaphragm, pericardium, etc.

ADENOCARCINOMA

Adenocarcinoma is currently the most prevalent NSCLC in both sexes. These tumors tend to be peripheral and often metastasize early in their course, particularly to brain, bone, liver, and adrenals. A variety of paraneoplastic metabolic factors, such as growth hormone and corticotropin, can be secreted by adenocarcinomas. Hypertrophic pulmonary osteoarthropathy is particularly associated with adenocarcinoma.

BRONCHIOLOALVEOLAR CARCINOMA

Bronchioloalveolar carcinoma (BAC) is a subtype of adenocarcinoma that is not related to cigarette smoking. In its early stages, it lines the alveolar membrane with a thin layer of tumor cells without destroying the alveolar architecture. BAC can present as an isolated peripheral lesion, as multifocal disease (often in both lungs), or as panlobar disease (sometimes with production of enormous quantities of mucus). It is the tumor most often identified in low-dose CT scan screening studies and has more than a 90% 5-year survival rate if treated early. In more advanced stages, however, it behaves similarly to adenocarcinoma.

LARGE CELL UNDIFFERENTIATED CARCINOMA

Large cell undifferentiated carcinomas are the least common of the NSCLCs. They tend to present as large, often cavitating, peripheral tumors. Their rapid growth rate can lead to widespread metastases, similar to adenocarcinoma.

SMALL CELL LUNG CANCER

This tumor of neuroendocrine origin is considered metastatic on presentation and is usually regarded as a medical disease, not a surgical one.[110] The staging system differs from NSCLC and is divided simply into limited stage and extensive stage. Treatment of limited-stage SCLC with combination chemotherapy (etoposide/cisplatin or cyclophosphamide/doxorubicin/vincristine) yields a response in more than 80% of patients. In addition, these patients typically receive aggressive radiotherapy to the primary lung tumor and prophylactic cranial irradiation. Despite this initial response, the tumor invariably recurs and is quite resistant to further treatment. The overall survival rate is no better than 10%. Extensive-stage disease is treated with chemotherapy and palliative radiation as needed.

There are two situations in which surgery for SCLC might be considered. The rare instance in which a solitary pulmonary nodule is diagnosed as SCLC should be treated with surgical resection followed by chemotherapy.[111] Salvage resection of a residual mass after chemotherapy for limited-stage disease may offer long-term survival in selected cases.[112] Many of these patients will have a mixed SCLC/NSCLC in which the small cell component has responded to chemotherapy, and the non–small cell component is then resected.

Small cell tumors are more likely than other lung tumors to cause paraneoplastic syndromes as a result of the production of peptide hormones. The most common of these is hyponatremia, usually due to an inappropriate production of antidiuretic hormone (SIADH). Also commonly associated are Cushing's syndrome and hypercortisolism through ectopic production of adrenocorticotropic hormone (ACTH).

A well-known but rare neurologic paraneoplastic syndrome associated with small cell lung tumors is the Lambert-Eaton (also called Eaton-Lambert) myasthenic syndrome, caused by impaired release of acetylcholine from nerve terminals. This typically presents as proximal lower limb weakness and fatigability that may temporarily improve with exercise. The diagnosis is confirmed by electromyogram (EMG) showing increasing amplitude of unusual action potentials with high-frequency stimulation.[113] Similar to true myasthenia gravis patients, myasthenic syndrome patients are extremely sensitive to nondepolarizing muscle relaxants; however, they respond poorly to anticholinesterase reversal agents. Aminopyridine has been reported to be useful both as a maintenance medication and to reverse residual postoperative neuromuscular blockade in these patients.[114] Other treatments for the Eaton-Lambert syndrome include plasmapheresis, immunoglobulin, and guanidine.[115] It is important to realize that there may be sub-clinical involvement of the diaphragm and muscles of respiration.[116] Thoracic epidural analgesia has been used after thoracotomy in these patients without complication.[117] These patients' neuromuscular function may improve after resection of the lung cancer.

Carcinoid Tumors

Carcinoid tumors are usually benign tumors that form a spectrum of diseases, from SCLC as the most malignant to typical carcinoid as the most benign. Five-year survival after resection exceeds 90%.[118] Lymph node metastasis is not uncommon and does not impact the rate of survival. Systemic metastasis is rare, as is the carcinoid syndrome, which is caused by the ectopic synthesis of vasoactive mediators and is usually seen with carcinoid tumors of gut origin that have metastasized to the liver. Atypical carcinoid tumors are more aggressive. They often metastasize both regionally and systemically. Surgical resection is indicated for locoregional disease.

Carcinoid tumors can precipitate an intraoperative hemodynamic crisis or coronary artery spasm, even during broncho-scopic resection.[119] The anesthesiologist should be prepared to deal with severe hypotension that may not respond to the usual

vasoconstrictors and will require the use of the specific antagonists octreotide or somatostatin.[120]

Pleural Tumors

Localized fibrous tumors of pleura are usually large, space-occupying masses that are attached to visceral or parietal pleura by a well-defined stalk. They can be either benign or malignant histologically, but most are easily resected with good results. From an anesthetic perspective, about 15% of these patients have presenting symptoms of severe hypoglycemia, which resolves when the tumor is resected.

Malignant pleural mesotheliomas are strongly associated with exposure to asbestos fibers. Their incidence in Canada has almost doubled in the past 15 years. With the phasing out of asbestos-containing products and the long latent period between exposure and diagnosis, the peak incidence is not predicted for another 10 to 20 years. The tumor initially proliferates within the visceral and parietal pleura, typically forming a bloody effusion. Most patients have presenting symptoms of shortness of breath or dyspnea on exertion from this pleural effusion. Thoracentesis often relieves the symptoms but rarely provides a diagnosis. Pleural biopsy by video-assisted thoracoscopy is most efficient to secure a diagnosis, and talc poudrage is performed under the same anesthetic to treat the effusion.

Malignant pleural mesotheliomas respond poorly to any therapy, and the median survival rate is less than one year. In patients with very early-stage disease, extrapleural pneumonectomy may be considered, but it is difficult to know whether survival rate is improved thereby. Recently several groups have reported improved results from radiation, chemotherapy, and surgery. Extrapleural pneumonectomy is an extensive procedure that is rife with potential complications, both intraoperatively and postoperatively. Blood loss from the denuded chest wall or major vascular structures is always a risk. Complications related to resection of diaphragm and pericardium are additional risks beyond that of pneumonectomy.

At the time of initial assessment, cancer patients should be assessed for the "4 M's" associated with malignancy (Table 1-8): mass effects,[121] metabolic abnormalities, metastases,[122] and medications. The prior use of medications (such as bleomycin) that can exacerbate oxygen-induced pulmonary toxicity should be considered.[123-125] Recently, the authors saw

---

TABLE 1-8

Anesthetic Considerations in Lung Cancer Patients (the "4 Ms")

Mass effects	Obstructive pneumonia, lung abscess, SVC syndrome, tracheobronchial distortion, Pancoast's syndrome, recurrent laryngeal nerve or phrenic nerve paresis, chest wall or mediastinal extension
Metabolic effects	Lambert-Eaton syndrome, hypercalcemia, hyponatremia, Cushing's syndrome
Metastases	Particularly to brain, bone, liver, and adrenals
Medications	

several lung cancer patients who received preoperative chemotherapy with cisplatin and then developed an elevation of serum creatinine when they received postoperative NSAIDs. For this reason, NSAIDs are not given routinely to patients who have been treated recently with cisplatin.

Postoperative Analgesia

The strategy for postoperative analgesia should be developed and discussed with the patient during the initial preoperative assessment. Full discussion of postoperative analgesia is presented in Chapter 20. In terms of pain control, many techniques have been shown to be superior to the use of on-demand parenteral (intramuscular or intravenous) opioids alone.[126] These techniques include the addition of neuraxial blockade, intercostal/paravertebral blocks, interpleural local anesthetics, or NSAIDs to narcotic-based analgesia. However, only epidural techniques have been shown to consistently have the capability to decrease postthoracotomy respiratory complications.[127,128] It is becoming more evident that thoracic epidural analgesia is superior to lumbar epidural analgesia. This seems to be due to the synergy that local anesthetics have with opioids in producing neuraxial analgesia. Studies suggest that epidural local anesthetics increase segmental bioavailability of opioids in the cerebrospinal fluid and that they also increase the binding of opioids by spinal cord receptors.[129,130] Although lumbar epidural opioids can produce similar levels of postthoracotomy pain control at rest, only the segmental effects of thoracic epidural local anesthetic and opioid combinations can reliably produce increased analgesia with movement and increased respiratory function after a chest incision.[131,132] In patients with coronary artery disease, thoracic epidural local anesthetics seem to reduce myocardial oxygen demand and supply in mutual proportion.[133] This is unlike the effects of lumbar epidural local anesthetics, which can cause a fall in myocardial perfusion and oxygen supply as diastolic pressure falls but leave heart rate and oxygen demand unchanged. These changes have been shown to correlate with echocardiographic evidence of ischemia during lumbar epidural analgesia.[134]

It is at the time of initial preanesthetic assessment that the risks and benefits of the various forms of postthoracotomy analgesia should be explained to the patient. Potential contraindications to specific methods of analgesia, such as coagulation problems, sepsis, or neurologic disorders, should be determined. When it is not possible to place a thoracic epidural because of problems with patient consent or other contraindications, a reasonable second choice for analgesia is a paravertebral infusion of local anesthetic via a catheter placed intraoperatively in the open hemithorax by the surgeon.[135] This is combined with intravenous patient-controlled opioid analgesia and NSAIDs whenever possible.

If the patient is to receive prophylactic anticoagulants and the election is made to use epidural analgesia, appropriate timing of anticoagulant administration and neuraxial catheter placement need to be arranged. ASRA guidelines suggest an interval of 2 to 4 hours before or 1 hour after catheter placement for prophylactic heparin administration.[136] Low-molecular-weight heparin (LMWH) precautions are less clear; an interval of 12 to 24 hours before and 24 hours after catheter placement is recommended.

Premedication

Premedication should be discussed and ordered at the time of the initial preoperative visit. The most important aspect of preoperative medication is to avoid inadvertent withdrawal of those drugs that are taken for concurrent medical conditions (bronchodilators, antihypertensives, β-blockers, and so forth). For some types of thoracic surgery, such as esophageal reflux surgery, preoperative oral antacid and H_2-blockers are routinely ordered. Although there is some theoretical concern in giving patients who may be prone to bronchospasm an H_2-blocker without an H_1-blocker, this has not been a clinical problem, and H_2-blockers are frequently used in patients who have asthmatic symptoms triggered by chronic reflux. The authors do not routinely order preoperative sedation or analgesia for pulmonary resection patients. Mild sedation such as an intravenous short-acting benzodiazepine is often given immediately before placement of invasive monitoring catheters. In patients with copious secretions, an antisialagogue (such as glycopyrrolate) is useful to facilitate fiberoptic bronchoscopy for positioning of a double-lumen tube or bronchial blocker. To avoid an intramuscular injection, this can be given orally or intravenously immediately after placement of the intravenous catheter. It is a common practice to use short-term intravenous antibacterial prophylaxis (such as a cephalosporin) in thoracic surgical patients. If it is the local practice to administer these drugs before admission to the operating room, they will have to be ordered preoperatively. Consideration for those patients allergic to cephalosporins or penicillin will have to be made at the time of the initial preoperative visit.

Summary of the Initial Preoperative Assessment

The anesthetic considerations that should be addressed at the time of the initial preoperative assessment are summarized in Table 1-9. Patients need to be specifically assessed for risk factors associated with respiratory complications, which are the major cause of morbidity and mortality after thoracic surgery (Table 1-10). Risk factors that can be modified preoperatively are summarized in Table 1-11.

TABLE 1-9

Initial Preanesthetic Assessment for Thoracic Surgery

Patient type	Assessments
All patients	Assess exercise tolerance, estimate ppoFEV$_1$%, discuss postoperative analgesia, discontinue smoking
Patients with ppoFEV$_1$ < 40%	D$_{LCO}$, V̇/Q̇ scan, V̇o$_2$ max
Cancer patients	Consider the "4 Ms": mass effects, metabolic effects, metastases, medications
COPD patients	Arterial blood gas, physiotherapy, bronchodilators
Increased renal risk	Measure creatinine and BUN

TABLE 1-10
Risk Factors Associated with Postoperative Pulmonary Complications

PATIENT-ASSOCIATED RISKS

Established Risks

Smoking		
Obstructive lung disease		
		COPD
		Poorly controlled asthma
	Malnutrition	
	Respiratory tract infections	

Potential Risks

	Age
	Obesity
	Stable mild asthma

SURGERY-ASSOCIATED RISKS

Established Risks

	Surgery type	
		Thorax/upper abdomen > lower abdomen > peripheral
	Incision type	
		Thoracotomy > sternotomy
	Anesthesia	
		General > neuraxial/regional
	Duration of surgery	

Potential Risks

	Posterolateral thoracotomy >
	muscle-sparing thoracotomy > thoracoscopic

From Kempanien RR, Benditt JO: *Semin Thorac Cardiovasc Surg* 13:105, 2001.

Final Preoperative Assessment

The final preoperative anesthetic assessment for the majority of thoracic surgical patients is carried out immediately before admission of the patient to the operating room. At this time it is important to review the data from the initial prethoracotomy assessment (Table 1-9) and the results of tests ordered at that time. In addition, two other specific concerns affecting thoracic anesthesia need to be assessed: the potential for difficult lung isolation and the risk of desaturation during one-lung ventilation (Table 1-12).

Difficult Endobronchial Intubation

Anesthesiologists are familiar with clinical assessment of the upper airway for ease of endotracheal intubation. In a similar fashion, each thoracic surgical patient must be assessed for the ease of endobronchial intubation. At the time of the preoperative visit, there may be historic factors or physical findings that lead

TABLE 1-11
Probability for Preoperative Interventions to Reduce the Risk of Pulmonary Complications

Risk Factor	Intervention	Probability
Smoking	Cessation > 8 weeks	++++
	Cessation < 8 weeks	+
Exacerbation of COPD or asthma	Steroids, bronchodilators and delay elective surgery	++++
	Antibiotics indicated by sputum	+++
Stable COPD or asthma	Physiotherapy	++++
	Bronchodilators	+++
	Rehabilitation	++
Obesity	Physiotherapy	++++
	Weight loss	++
Malnutrition	Oral nutrition program	++

From Kempanien RR, Benditt JO: *Semin Thorac Cardiovasc Surg* 13:105, 2001.
++++, Multiple studies confirming; +++, both some data plus physiologic rationale supporting; ++, either some data or good physiologic rationale; +, limited data or physiologic rationale.

TABLE 1-12

Final Preanesthetic Assessment for Thoracic Surgery

1. Review initial assessment and test results
2. Assess difficulty of lung isolation: Examine chest x-ray and CT scan
3. Assess risk of hypoxemia during one-lung ventilation

to suspicion of difficult endobronchial intubation (e.g., previous radiotherapy, infection, or prior pulmonary or airway surgery). In addition, there may be a written bronchoscopy report with a detailed description of anatomic features. However, fiberoptic bronchoscopy is not totally reliable for estimating potential problems with endobronchial tube positioning.[137] The single most useful predictor of difficult endobronchial intubation is the plain chest x-ray (Figure 1-18).[1,138]

The anesthesiologist should view the chest images before induction of anesthesia, as neither the radiologist's nor the surgeon's report of the x-ray is made with the specific consideration of lung isolation in mind. A large portion of thoracic surgical patients will also have had a preoperative chest CT scan done. As anesthesiologists have learned to assess x-rays for potential lung-isolation difficulties, it is also worthwhile to learn to examine the CT scan. Distal airway problems not detectable on the plain chest film can sometimes be visualized on the CT scan: a side-to-side compression of the distal trachea (the so called "saber-sheath" trachea) can cause obstruction of the tracheal lumen of a left-sided double-lumen tube during

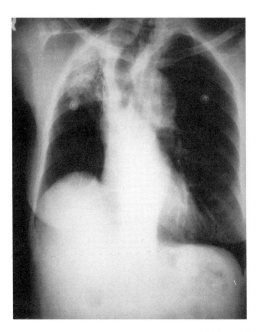

FIGURE 1-18 Preoperative chest x-ray of a 50-year-old female with a history of previous tuberculosis, right upper lobectomy, and recent hemoptysis presenting for right thoracotomy and possible completion pneumonectomy. The potential problems in positioning a left-sided, double-lumen tube in this patient are easily appreciated by viewing the x-ray but are not mentioned in the radiologist's report. The anesthesiologist must examine the chest image preoperatively to anticipate problems in lung isolation. (From Slinger PD, Johnston MR: *J Cardiothorac Vasc Anesth* 14:202, 2000.)

ventilation of the dependent lung for a left thoracotomy.[139] Similarly, extrinsic compression or intraluminal obstruction of a mainstem bronchus that can interfere with endobronchial tube placement may only be evident on the CT scan (Figure 1-19). The major factors in successful lower airway management are anticipation and preparation based on the preoperative assessment. Management of lung isolation in patients with difficult upper and lower airways is discussed in Chapter 8, and imaging of the airways appears in Chapter 2.

Prediction of Desaturation During One-Lung Ventilation

In the vast majority of cases, it is possible to determine those patients who are most at risk of desaturation during one-lung ventilation (OLV) for thoracic surgery. The factors that correlate with desaturation during OLV are listed in Table 1-13. Identification of those patients most likely to desaturate allows the anesthesiologist and surgeon to make a more informed decision about the use of intraoperative OLV. In patients at high risk of desaturation, prophylactic measures can be used during OLV to decrease this risk. The most useful prophylactic measure is the use of continuous positive airway pressure (CPAP), 2 to 5 cmH$_2$O of oxygen to the nonventilated lung.[140] Because this often tends to make the surgical exposure more difficult, it is worthwhile to quickly identify those patients who will require CPAP so that it can be discussed with the surgeon and instituted at the start of OLV.

The most important predictor of Pao$_2$ during OLV is the Pao$_2$ during two-lung ventilation. Although the preoperative Pao$_2$ correlates with the intraoperative OLV Pao$_2$, the strongest correlation is with the intraoperative Pao$_2$ during two-lung ventilation in the lateral position before OLV.[141] The proportion of perfusion or ventilation to the nonoperated lung on preoperative V̇/Q̇ scans also correlates with the Pao$_2$ during OLV.[142] If the operative lung has little perfusion preoperatively due to unilateral disease, the patient is unlikely to desaturate during OLV. The side of the thoracotomy has an effect on Pao$_2$ during OLV. Because the left lung is 10% smaller than the right, there is less shunt when the left lung is collapsed. In a series of patients, the mean Pao$_2$ during left thoracotomy was approximately 70 mmHg higher than during right thoracotomy.[143]

Finally, the degree of obstructive lung disease correlates in an inverse fashion with Pao$_2$ during OLV. Other factors being equal, patients with more severe airflow limitation on preoperative spirometry will tend to have a better Pao$_2$ during OLV than patients with normal spirometry.[144] The etiology of this

TABLE 1-13

Factors That Correlate with an Increased Risk of Desaturation During One-Lung Ventilation

1. High percentage of ventilation or perfusion to the operative lung on preoperative V̇/Q̇ scan
2. Poor Pao$_2$ during two-lung ventilation, particularly in the lateral position intraoperatively
3. Right-sided thoracotomy
4. Normal preoperative spirometry (FEV$_1$ or FVC) or restrictive lung disease
5. Supine position during one-lung ventilation

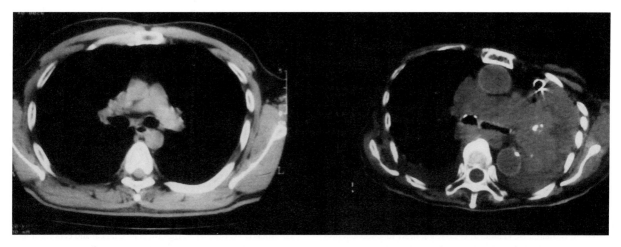

FIGURE 1-19 CT scans from just below the level of the carinal bifurcation. A normal patient is shown on the left. On the right is a 70-year-old female scheduled for thoracoscopic left lung biopsy. The patient has a left-sided lung tumor and effusion that compress the left mainstem bronchus. This bronchial compression was not evident on the chest x-ray. It may be difficult to place a left-sided, double-lumen tube in this patient. (From Slinger P: Anesthesia for lung resection surgery. In Thys D (ed): *Textbook of cardiothoracic anesthesia*, New York, 2001, McGraw Hill.)

seemingly paradoxical finding seems to be related to the development of auto-PEEP during OLV in the obstructed patients.[145] Patients with normal, healthy lungs with good elastic recoil and patients with increased elastic recoil (such as those with restrictive lung diseases) tend to benefit from applied PEEP during one-lung ventilation, while those with COPD do not.[146]

Assessment for Repeat Thoracic Surgery

Patients who survive lung cancer surgery form a high-risk cohort to have a recurrence of the original tumor or to develop a second primary tumor. The incidence of developing a second primary lung tumor is estimated at 2% per year.[147] The increased use by surgeons and oncologists of routine clinical surveillance programs after lung cancer surgery with screening chest x-rays should mean that more second primary lung tumors are detected early when they are still potentially resectable. The use of routine screening by low-dose spiral CT scans will probably increase the rate of early detection.[148] Patients who present for repeat thoracotomy should be assessed within the same framework as those who present for surgery for the first time. Predicted values for postoperative respiratory function based on the preoperative lung mechanics, parenchymal function, exercise tolerance, and the amount of functioning lung tissue resected should be calculated and used to identify patients at increased risk.

Summary

Because of recent advances in anesthesia and surgery, almost any patient with a resectable lung malignancy is now an operative candidate, given a full understanding of the risks and after appropriate investigation. Understanding and stratifying the perioperative risks allows the anesthesiologist to develop a systematic, focused approach to these patients, both at the time of

the initial contact and immediately before induction, which can be used to guide anesthetic management.

REFERENCES

1. Slinger PD, Johnston MR: Preoperative assessment for pulmonary resection, *J Cardiothorac Vasc Anesth* 14:202, 2000.
2. Johnston MR: Curable lung cancer, *Postgrad Med* 101:155, 1997.
3. Brusasco V, Ratto GB, Crimi P, et al: Lung function after upper sleeve lobectomy for bronchogenic carcinoma, *Scand J Thor Cardiovasc Surg* 22:73, 1988.
4. Nakahara K, Ohno K, Hashimoto J, et al: Prediction of postoperative respiratory failure in patients undergoing lung resection for cancer, *Ann Thorac Surg* 46:549, 1988.
5. Reilly J: Evidence-based preoperative evaluation of candidates for thoracotomy, *Chest* 116:474s, 1999.
6. Culver BH: Preoperative assessment of the thoracic surgery patient: pulmonary function testing, *Semin Thorac Cardiovasc Surg* 13:92, 2001.
7. Pierce RJ, Copland JM, Sharpek K, et al: Preoperative risk evaluation for lung cancer resection: predicted postoperative product as a predictor of surgical mortality, *Am J Resp Crit Care Med* 150:947, 1994.
8. Cerfolio RJ, Allen MS, Trastak VF, et al: Lung resection in patients with compromised pulmonary function, *Ann Thorac Surg* 62:348, 1996.
9. Slinger PD, Kruger M, McRae K, et al: The relation of the static compliance curve and positive end-expiratory pressure to oxygenation during one-lung ventilation, *Anesthesiology* 95:1096, 2001.
10. McKenna RJ, Fischel RJ, Brenner M, Gelb AF: Combined operations for lung volume reduction surgery and lung cancer, *Chest* 110:885, 1996.
11. Wang J, Olak J, Ferguson MK: Diffusing capacity predicts mortality but not long-term survival after resection for lung cancer, *J Thorac Cardiovasc Surg* 117:581, 1999.
12. Ferguson MK, Reeder LB, Mich R: Optimizing selection of patients for major lung resection, *J Thorac Cardiovasc Surg* 109:275, 1995.
13. Olsen GN, Bolton JWR, Weiman DS, Horning CA: Stair climbing as an exercise test to predict postoperative complications of lung resection, *Chest* 99:587, 1991.
14. Kinasewitz GT, Welsh MH: A simple method to assess postoperative risk, *Chest* 120:1057, 2001.
15. Weisman IM: Cardiopulmonary exercise testing in the preoperative assessment for lung resection surgery, *Semin Thorac Cardiovasc Surg* 13:116, 2001.
16. Walsh GL, Morice RC, Putnam JB, et al: Resection of lung cancer is justified in high-risk patients selected by oxygen consumption, *Ann Thorac Surg* 58:704, 1994.

17. Cahalin L, Pappagianapoulos P, Prevost S, et al: The relationship of the 6-min walk test to maximal oxygen consumption in transplant candidates with end-stage lung disease, *Chest* 108:452, 1995.
18. Ninan M, Sommers KE, Landranau RJ, et al: Standardized exercise oximetry predicts post-pneumonectomy outcome, *Ann Thorac Surg* 64:328, 1997.
19. Bollinger CT, Wyser C, Roser H, et al: Lung scanning and exercise testing for the prediction of postoperative performance in lung resection candidates at increased risk for complications, *Chest* 108:341, 1995.
20. Reed CR, Dorman BH, Spinale FGL: Mechanisms of right ventricular dysfunction after pulmonary resection, *Ann Thorac Surg* 62: 225, 1996.
21. Van Miegham W, Demedts M: Cardiopulmonary function after lobectomy or pneumonectomy for pulmonary neoplasm, *Respir Med* 83:199, 1989.
22. Vesselle H: Functional imaging before pulmonary resection, *Semin Thorac Cardiovasc Surg* 13:126, 2001.
23. Tisi GM: Preoperative evaluation of pulmonary function, *Am Rev Respir Dis* 119:293, 1979.
24. Lewis JW Jr, Bastanfar M, Gabriel F, et al: Right heart function and prediction of respiratory morbidity in patients undergoing pneumonectomy with moderately severe cardiopulmonary dysfunction, *J Thorac Cardiovasc Surg* 108:169, 1994.
25. Amar D, Burt M, Roistacher N, et al: Value of preoperative echocardiography in patients undergoing major lung resection, *Ann Thorac Surg* 61:516, 1996.
26. Neuman GG, Wiengarten AE, Abramowitz RM, et al: The anesthetic management of the patient with an anterior mediastinal mass, *Anesthesiology* 60:144, 1984.
27. Pullerits J, Holzman R: Anaesthesia for patients with mediastinal masses, *Can J Anaesth* 36:681, 1989.
28. Schamberger RC, Hozman RS, Griscom NT: Prospective evaluation by computed tomography and pulmonary function tests of children with mediastinal masses, *Surgery* 118:468, 1995.
29. Weisman IM: Cardiopulmonary exercise testing in the preoperative assessment for lung resection surgery, *Semin Thorac Cardiovasc Surg* 13:116, 2001.
30. Osaki T, Shirakusa T, Kodate M, et al: Surgical treatment of lung cancer in the octogenarian, *Ann Thorac Surg* 57:188, 1994.
31. Mizushima Y, Noto H, Sugiyama S,et al: Survival and prognosis after pneumonectomy in the elderly, *Ann Thorac Surg* 64:193, 1997.
32. Barry J, Mead K, Nadel EC, et al: Effect of smoking on the activity of ischemic heart disease, *JAMA* 261-398, 1989.
33. ACC/AHA Task Force on Practice Guidelines, *Anesth Analg* 82:854, 1996.
34. Von Knorring J, Leptantalo M, Lindgren L: Cardiac arrhythmias and myocardial ischemia after thoracotomy for lung cancer, *Ann Thorac Surg* 53:642, 1992.
35. Ghent WS, Olsen GN, Hornung CA, et al: Routinely performed multigated blood pool imaging (MUGA) as a predictor of postoperative complication of lung resection, *Chest* 105:1454, 1994.
36. Miller JI: Thallium imaging in preoperative evaluation of the pulmonary resection candidate, *Ann Thorac Surg* 1992;54:249, 1992.
37. Rao V, Todd TRS, Weisel RD, et al: Results of combined pulmonary resection and cardiac operation, *Ann Thorac Surg* 62:342, 1996.
38. Rao TKK, Jacob KH, El-Etr AA: Reinfarction following anesthesia in patients with myocardial infarction, *Anesthesiology* 59:499, 1983.
39. Kauza GI, Josepah J, Lee LR, et al: Catastrophic outcomes of noncardiac surgery soon after coronary stenting, *J Am Coll Cardiol* 35:1288, 2000.
40. Kim MH, Eagle KA: Cardiac risk assessment in noncardiac thoracic surgery, *Semin Thorac Cardiovasc Surg* 13:137, 2001.
41. Ritchie AJ, Bowe P, Gibbons JRP: Prophylactic digitalisation for thoracotomy: a reassessment, *Ann Thorac Surg* 50:86, 1990.
42. Amar D, Roistacher N, Burt M, et al: Clinical and echocardiographic correlates of symptomatic tachydysrhythmias after noncardiac thoracic surgery, *Chest* 108:349, 1995.
43. Ritchie AJ, Danton M, Gibbons JRP: Prophylactic digitalisation in pulmonary surgery, *Thorax* 47:41, 1992.
44. Krowka MJ, Pairolero PC, Trastek VF, et al: Surgical treatment of lung cancer in the octogenarian, *Ann Thorac Surg* 57:188, 1994.
45. Breyer RH, Zippe C, Pharr WF, et al: Thoracotomy in patients over age seventy years: ten-year experience, *J Thorac Cardiovasc Surg* 81:187, 1981.
46. Osaki T, Shirakusa T, Kodate M, et al: Surgical treatment of lung cancer in the octogenarian, *Ann Thorac Surg* 57:188, 1994.
47. Amar D, Roistacher N, Burt ME, et al: Effects of diltiazem versus digoxin on dysrhythmias and cardiac function after pneumonectomy, *Ann Thorac Surg* 63:1374, 1997.
48. Van Knorring J, Lepantalo M, Lindgren L, et al: Cardiac arrythmias and myocardial ischemia after thoracotomy for lung cancer, *Ann Thorac Surg* 53:642, 1992.
49. Boldt J, Muller M, Uphus D, et al: Cardiorespiratory changes in patients undergoing pulmonary resection using different anesthetic management techniques, *J Cardiothorac Vasc Anesth* 10:854, 1996.
50. Lewis JW, Bastanfar M, Gabriel F, et al: Right heart function and prediction of respiratory morbidity in patients undergoing pneumonectomy with moderately severe cardiopulmonary dysfunction, *J Thoracic Cardiovasc Surg* 108:164, 1994.
51. Okada M, Ota T, Okada M: Right ventricular dysfunction after major pulmonary resection, *J Thorac Cardiovasc Surg* 108:503, 1994.
52. Amar D, Burt ME, Roistacher N, et al: Value of perioperative Doppler echocardiography in patients undergoing major lung resection, *Ann Thorac Surg* 61:516, 1996.
53. Amar D, Roistacher N, Burt M, et al: Clinical and echocardiographic correlates of symptomatic tachydsyrythmias after non-cardiac thoracic surgery, *Chest* 108:349, 1995.
54. Entwistle MD, Roe PG, Sapsford DJ, et al: Patterns of oxygenation after thoracotomy, *Br J Anaesth* 67:704, 1991.
55. Kearney DJ, Lee TH, Reilly JJ, et al: Assessment of operative risk in patients undergoing lung resection, *Chest* 105:753, 1994.
56. Sekine Y, Kesler KA, Behnia M, et al: COPD may increase the incidence of refractory supraventricular arrhythmias following pulmonary resection for non-small cell lung cancer, *Chest* 120:1783, 2001.
57. Ritchie AJ, Danton M, Gibbons JRP: Prophylactic digitalisation in pulmonary surgery, *Thorax* 47:41, 1992.
58. Bayliff CD, Massel DR, Inculet RI, et al: Propranolol fro the prevention of postoperative arrhythmias in general thoracic surgery, *Ann Thorac Surg* 67:182: 1999.
59. Van Meighan W, Tits G, Denuyn CK, et al: Verapamil as prophylactic treatment for atrial fibrillation after lung operations, *Ann Thorac Surg* 61:1083, 1996.
60. Van Meigham W, Coolen L, Malysse I, et al: Amiodarone and the development of ARDS after lung surgery, *Chest* 105:1642, 1994.
61. Lindgren L, Lepantalo M, Von Knorring J, et al: Effect of verapamil on right ventricular pressure and atrial tachyarrhythmia after thoracotomy, *Br J Anaesth* 66:205, 1991.
62. Slinger P, Shennib H, Wilson S: Postthoracotomy pulmonary function: a comparison of epidural versus intravenous meperidine infusions, *J Cardiothorac Vasc Anesth* 9:128, 1995.
63. Staats PS, Panchal SJ: Pro: Thoracic epidural analgesia for treatment of angina, *J Cardiothorac Vasc Anesth* 11:105, 1997.
64. Saada M, Catoire P, Bonnet F, et al: Effect of thoracic epidural anesthesia combined with general anesthesia on segmental wall motion assessed by transesophageal echocardiography, *Anesth Analg* 75:329, 1992.
65. Backlund M, Laasonen L, Leptantalo M: Effect of oxygen on pulmonary hemodynamics and incidence of atrial fibrillation after noncardiac thoracic surgery, *J Cardiothorac Vasc Anesth* 12:421, 1998.
66. Oka T, Ozawa Y, Ohkubo Y: Thoracic epidural bupivacaine attenuates supraventricular tachyarrhythmias after pulmonary resection, *Anesth Analg* 93:253, 2001.
67. Golledge J, Goldstraw P: Renal impairment after thoracotomy: incidence, risk factors and significance, *Ann Thorac Surg* 58:524, 1994.
68. Slinger PD: Post-pneumonectomy pulmonary edema: is anesthesia to blame? *Curr Opin in Anesthesiol* 12:49, 1999.
69. American Thoracic Society: Standards for the diagnosis and care of patients with chronic obstructive pulmonary disease, *Am J Resp Critic Care Med* 152:78, 1995.
70. Parot S, Saunier C, Gauthier H, et al: Breathing pattern and hypercapnia in patients with obstructive pulmonary disease, *Am Rev Respir Dis* 121:985, 1980.
71. Aubier M, Murciano D, Milic-Emili J, et al: Effects of the administration of O_2 on ventilation and blood gases in patients with chronic obstructive pulmonary disease during acute respiratory failure, *Am Rev Respir Dis* 122:747, 1980.
72. Hanson CW III, Marshall BE, Frasch HF, et al: Causes of hypercarbia in patients with chronic obstructive pulmonary disease, *Crit Care Med* 24:23, 1996.
73. Douglas NJ, Flenley DC: Breathing during sleep in patients with obstructive lung disease, *Am Rev Respir Dis* 141:1055, 1990.

74. Douglas NJ, Calverley PMA, Leggett RJE, et al: Transient hypoxaemia during sleep in chronic bronchitics and emphysema, *Lancet* 1(8106):1, 1979.
75. Klinger JR, Hill NS: Right ventricular dysfunction in chronic obstructive pulmonary disease, *Chest* 99:715, 1991.
76. Schulman DS, Mathony RA: The right ventricle in pulmonary disease, *Cardiol Clin* 10:111, 1992.
77. Myles PE, Madder H, Morgan EB: Intraoperative cardiac arrest after unrecognized dynamic hyperinflation, *Br J Anaesth* 74:340, 1995.
78. MacNee W: Pathophysiology of cor pulmonale in chronic obstructive pulmonary disease, *Am J Resp Crit Care Med* 150:833, 1994.
79. Cote TR, Stroup DF, Dwyer DM, et al: Chronic obstructive pulmonary disease mortality, *Chest* 103:1194, 1993.
80. Morgan MDL, Edwards CW, Morris J, et al: Origin and behavior of emphysematous bullae, *Thorax* 44:533, 1989.
81. O'Donnell DE, Sami R, Anthonisen NR, et al: Effect of dynamic airway compression on breathing pattern and respiratory sensation in severe chronic obstructive pulomonary disease, *Am Rev Respir Dis* 135:912, 1987.
82. Slinger P: Anesthesia for patients with COPD, *Curr Rev Clin Anesth* 15:169, 1995.
83. Kanek R, Fahey PS, Vanderworf C: Oxygen cost of breathing, *Chest* 87:126, 1985.
84. Geld AF, Hogg JC, Muller NL: Contribution of emphysema and small airways in COPD, *Chest* 109:353, 1996.
85. Gimeno F, Postma DS, von Altena R: Plethysmographic parameters in the assessment of reversibility of airways obstruction in patients with clinical emphysema, *Chest* 104:467, 1993.
86. Myles PE, Madder H, Morgan EB: Intraoperative cardiac arrest after unrecognized dynamic hyperinflation, *Br J Anaesth* 74:340, 1995.
87. Ben-David B, Stonebraker VC, Hershman R, et al: Survival after failed intraoperative resuscitation: a case of "Lazarus syndrome," *Anesth Analg* 92:690, 2001.
88. Tobin MJ, Lodato RF: PEEP, auto-PEEP and waterfalls, *Chest* 96:449, 1989.
89. Slinger P, Hickey D: The interaction between applied PEEP and auto-PEEP during one-lung ventilation, *J Cardiothorac Vasc Anesth* 12:133, 1998.
90. Zehier B, Gross T, Kern J, et al: Predicting post-operative pulmonary function in patients undergoing lung resection, *Chest* 105:753, 1995.
91. DeMeester SR, Patterson GA, Sundareson RS, et al: Lobectomy combined with volume reduction for patients with lung cancer and advanced emphysema, *J Thorac Cardiovasc Surg* 115:681, 1998.
92. Nguyen DM, Mulder DS, Shennib H: Altered cellular immune function in atelectatic lung, *Ann Thorac Surg* 51:76: 1991.
93. Huglitz UF, Shapiro JH: Atypical pulmonary patterns of congestive failure in chronic lung disease, *Radiology* 93:995, 1969.
94. Susaki F, Ishizaki T, Mifune J, et al: Bronchial hyperresponsiveness in patients with chronic congestive heart failure, *Chest* 97:534, 1990.
95. Nisar M, Eoris JE, Pearson MG, et al: Acute bronchodilator trials in chronic obstructive pulmonary disease, *Am Rev Resp Dis* 146:555, 1992.
96. Warner DO: Preventing postoperative pulmonary complications, *Anesthesiology* 92:1467, 2000.
97. Stock MC, Downs JB, Gauer PK, et al: Prevention of postoperative pulmonary complications with CPAP, incentive spirometry and conservative therapy, *Chest* 87:151, 1985.
98. Niederman MS, Clemente P, Fein AM, et al: Benefits of a multidisciplinary pulmonary rehabilitation program, *Chest* 99:798, 1991.
99. Selsby D, Jones JG: Some physiological and clinical aspects of chest physiotherapy, *Br J Anaesth* 64:621, 1990.
100. Kesten S: Pulmonary rehabilitation and surgery for end-stage lung disease, *Clin Chest Med* 18:174, 1997.
101. Dales RE, Dionne G, Leech JA, et al: Preoperative prediction of pulmonary complications following thoracic surgery, *Chest* 104:155, 1993.
102. Warner MA, Diverti MB, Tinker JH: Preoperative cessation of smoking and pulmonary complications in coronary artery bypass surgery, *Anesthesiology* 60:383, 1994.
103. Akrawi W, Benumof JL: A pathophysiological basis for informed preoperative smoking cessation counseling, *J Cardiothorac Vasc Anesth* 11:629, 1997.
104. Jonsson K, Hunt TK, Mathes SJ: Oxygen as an isolated variable influences resistance to infection, *Ann Surg* 208:783, 1988.
105. Kempanien RR, Benditt JO: Evaluation and management of patients with pulmonary disease before thoracic and cardiovascular surgery, *Semin Thorac Cardiovasc Surg* 13:105, 2001.
106. Feinstein MB, Bach PB: Epidemiology of lung cancer, *Chest surgery clinics of North America* 10:653, 2000.
107. Vital statistics of the United States 1998. www.cancer.org.
108. Beckett WS: Epidemiology and etiology of lung cancer, *Clinics in Chest Medicine* 14:1, 1993.
109. Ishida T, Yano T, Maeda K, et al: Strategy for lymphadenectomy in lung cancer three centimeters or less in diameter, *Ann Thorac Surg* 50:708, 1990.
110. Johnson BE: Management of small cell lung cancer, 109. *Clin Chest Med* 14:173, 1993.
111. Ginsberg RJ: Operation for small cell lung cancer - where are we?, *Ann Thorac Surg* 49:692, 1990.
112. Sheppard FA, Ginsberg R, Patterson GA, et al: Is there ever a role for salvage operation in limited small-cell lung cancer, *J Thorac Cardiovasc Surg* 97:196, 1991.
113. Lambert EH, Elinquist D: Quantal components of end-plate potentials in the myasthenic syndrome, *Ann NY Acad Sci* 183:183, 1978.
114. Telford RJ, Holloway TE: The myasthenic syndrome: anesthesia in a patient treated with 3-4 diaminopyridine, *Br J Anaesth* 64:363, 1990.
115. Levin KH: Paraneoplastic neuromuscular syndromes, *Neurol Clin* 15:597, 1997.
116. Wilcox PG, Morrison NJ, Auzarut ARA, et al: Lambert-Eaton myasthenic syndrome involving the diaphragm, *Chest* 93:604, 1988.
117. Sakura S, Saito Y, Maeda M, et al: Epidural analgesia in Eaton-Lambert myasthenic syndrome, *Anaesthesia* 46:560, 1991.
118. Stamatis G, Freitag L, Gresichuchua D: Limited and radical resection for tracheal and bronchopulmonary carcinoid tumor, *Eur J Cardiothorac Surg* 4:527, 1990.
119. Metha AC, Rafanan AL, Bulkley R, et al: Coronary spasm and cardiac arrest during laser bronchoscopy, *Chest* 115:598, 1999.
120. Vaughan DJ, Brunner MD: Anesthesia for patients with the carcinoid syndrome, *Int Anesthesiol Clin* 35:129, 1997.
121. Gilron I, Scott WAC, Slinger P, et al: Contralateral lung soiling following laser resection of a bronchial tumor, *J Cardiothorac Vasc Anesth* 8:567, 1994.
122. Mueurs MF: Preoperative screening for metastases in lung cancer patients, *Thorax* 49:1, 1994.
123. Ingrassia TS III, Ryu JH, Trasek VF, et al: Oxygen-exacerbated bleomycin pulmonary toxicity, *Mayo Clin Proc* 66:173, 1991.
124. Van Miegham W, Collen L, Malysse I, et al: Amiodarone and the development of ARDS after lung surgery, *Chest* 105:1642, 1994.
125. Thompson CC, Bailey MK, Conroy JM, et al: Postoperative pulmonary toxicity associated with mitomycin-C therapy, *South Med J* 85:1257, 1992.
126. Kavanagh BP, Katz J, Sandler AN: Pain control after thoracic surgery: a review of current techniques, *Anesthesiology* 81:737, 1994.
127. Licker M, de Perrot M, Hohn L, et al: Perioperative mortality and major cardiopulmonary complications after lung surgery for non-small call carcinoma, *Eur J Cardiothorac Surg* 15:314, 1999.
128. Ballantyne JC, Carr DB, deFerranti S, et al: The comparative effects of postoperative analgesic therapies on pulmonary outcome: cumulative metaanalysis of randomized, controlled trials, *Anesth Analg* 86:598, 1998.
129. Hansdottir V, Woestenborghs R, Nordberg G: The pharmacokinetics of continuous epidural sufentanil and bupivacaine infusion after thoracotomy, *Anesth Analg* 83:401, 1996.
130. Tejwani GA, Rattan AK, Mcdonald JS: Role of spinal opioid receptors in the antinociceptive interactions between intrathecal morphine and bupivacaine, *Anesth Analg* 74:726, 1992.
131. Hansdottir V, Bake B, Nordberg G: The analgesic efficiency and adverse effects of continuous epidural sufentanil and bupivacaine infusion after thoracotomy, *Anesth Analg* 83:394, 1996.
132. Mourisse J, Hasenbos MAWM, Gielen MJM, et al: Epidural bupivacaine, sufentanil or the combination for post-thoracotomy pain, *Acta Anaesthesiol Scand* 36:70, 1992.
133. Saada M, Catoire P, Bonnet F, et al: Effect of thoracic epidural anesthesia combined with general anesthesia on segmental wall motion assessed by transesophageal echocardiography, *Anesth.Analg* 75:329, 1992.
134. Saada M, Duval AM, Bonnet F, et al: Abnormalities in myocardial wall motion during lumbar epidural anesthesia, *Anesth Analg* 71:26, 1989.
135. Karmakar MK: Thoracic paravertebral block, *Anesthesiology* 95:771, 2001.
136. Liu SS: ASRA consensus statements. Neuraxial analgesia and anticoagulation, *Reg Anesth* 23:s1, 1998.

137. Alliaume B, Coddens J. Deloof T: Reliability of auscultation in positioning of double-lumen endobronchial tubes, *Can J Anaesth* 39:687, 1992.

138. Saito S, Dohi S, Tajima K: Failure of double-lumen endobronchial tube placement: congenital tracheal stenosis in an adult, *Anesthesiology* 66:83, 1987.

139. Bayes J, Slater EM, Hadberg PS, et al: Obstruction of a double-lumen tube by a saber-sheath trachea, *Anesth Analg* 79:186, 1994.

140. Slinger P, Triolet W, Wilson J: Improving arterial oxygenation during one-lung ventilation, *Anesthesiology* 68:29, 1988.

141. Slinger P, Suissa S, Triolet W: Predicting arterial oxygenation during one-lung anaesthesia, *Can J Anaesth* 39:1030, 1992.

142. Hurford WE, Kokar AC, Strauss HW: The use of ventilation/perfusion lung scans to predict oxygenation during one-lung anesthesia, *Anesthesiology* 64:841, 1987.

143. Lewis JW, Serwin JP, Gabriel FS, et al: The utility of a double-lumen tube for one-lung ventilation in a variety of non-cardiac thoracic surgical procedures, *J Cardiothorac Vasc Anesth* 6:705, 1992.

144. Katz JA, Lavern RG, Fairley HB, et al: Pulmonary oxygen exchange during endobronchial anesthesia, effect of tidal volume and PEEP, *Anesthesiology* 56:164, 1982.

145. Myles PS: Auto-PEEP may improve oxygenation during one-lung ventilation, *Anesth Analg* 83:1131, 1996.

146. Slinger PD, Kruger M, McRae K, et al: The relation of the static compliance curve and positive end-expiratory pressure to oxygenation during one-lung ventilation, *Anesthesiology* 95:1096, 2001.

147. Johnkoski JA, Wood DE: Bronchogenic carcinoma: counterpoint. In Johnson FE, Virgo KS (eds): Cancer patient follow up, St. Louis,1997, Mosby.

148. Naunheim KS, Virgo KS: Postoperative surveillance following lung cancer resection, *Chest Surg Clin N Am* 11:213, 2001.

Radiology of the Chest

2

Richard L. Goldwin, MD, FACR
James C. Reed, MD, FACR

CHEST radiography plays an important role in the preoperative and postoperative evaluation of patients undergoing many types of surgery, not just thoracic surgery. Plain film chest radiography remains the most commonly performed imaging examination and the primary imaging technique for chest diagnosis in the United States.[1,2] Although the study of chest x-rays can be a lifelong endeavor, understanding certain basic principles will enable physicians to approach films in a systematic manner that reveals a great deal of useful information.[3]

In this chapter, the authors present some concepts regarding the formation of images, anatomy and pathophysiology as it relates to chest radiography, the role that perception plays in interpretation of films, and a logical approach to evaluating a film. The authors will show examples of major classes of disease that are evaluated with a chest film and how monitoring and life support devices should look—and more important, how they should *not* look. Some postoperative changes resulting from thoracic surgery will also be reviewed. Finally, the authors will demonstrate some examples of newer imaging technologies that may be seen in the operating room during surgery.

It is not sufficient to spot a possibly abnormal area on a film. Clinicians must follow a routine to evaluate a suspected abnormality and decide whether it is a normal variant or a problem that requires attention.[4] Perceptions of findings on a film are perhaps the most important part of the diagnostic process. Perception depends on multiple factors: the search pattern used, the viewing conditions, the experience of the observer, and even the threshold of visibility *(border)* of the presumed abnormal area. *Seeing* is based on the information content of the object, on its border, and on its radiographic density and conspicuity. *Perceiving* is based on the information content of the observer—on the interpreter's experience, and on his or her personal database of normal findings, variants, and usual and rare or abnormal findings related to the specific disease.[5]

Conditions in the operating room and intensive care unit are often less than optimal for obtaining or reading films. Additionally, clinicians are often caring for the sickest patients in the hospital, with the result that portable films become a technical compromise when compared with an upright examination done in a fixed radiographic room. Frequently, films are checked in a room where there is too much ambient light, or where more view boxes are lit than the one needed to view the films. Traffic and interruptions can also distract the reader. Fatigue also plays a part in the diagnostic process and can lead to errors.[6] When

radiologists have visitors in their department, they are often focusing solely on the films, almost ignoring the visitor's presence so as not to break their concentration. When asked questions, they continue to scan the film, looking for subtle clues that will answer the clinical question.

Image Production

One of the basic advantages of the chest x-ray is the natural contrast that air-filled lungs bring to a film. Although CT technology might offer better detail, the simplicity of the chest radiograph and the portability of standard x-ray equipment allow the gathering of useful information even at the patient's bedside. Of course, with every advantage comes a potential problem, and the superimposition of many structures—both natural and those added to help monitor the patient's condition—onto a thin sheet of plastic film or on a CRT where digital conversion has occurred, can add confusion to the interpretation of these images. X-rays produce images in relation to the amount of radiation that passes through the body part being examined. The image is created by fluorescence of certain rare-earth materials as a response to stimulation by ionizing radiation. This light, in turn, exposes the film in the classic case. More frequently, the images are captured on sensitized metal plates with photostimulable phosphors, which are then "read" by a laser beam and translated into a digital image (computed or digital radiography). These images can be viewed on a monitor or printed on a film. Normal structures, especially the interstitium, are accentuated on digital images whether viewed on a CRT or printed on film, and they require a different threshold of normal values.

Some tissues—for example, an air-filled lung—stop very little x-ray and appear near-black, while bone or metal lets little radiation pass and appear white. Those materials that are denser also tend to change the quality of the radiation on its passage through the body.

The beam's interaction with tissues causes secondary or scatter radiation, which degrades the image. The use of grids—parallel lead strips imbedded in a plastic matrix—has helped reduce the amount of scatter radiation. Faster, more sensitive film-screen combinations and digital receptors also produce better-quality radiographs.

The normal chest contains four radiographic densities that are easily identified—air, fat, water, and calcium and other metals (bones, granulomata, vascular calcifications, etc.)

24

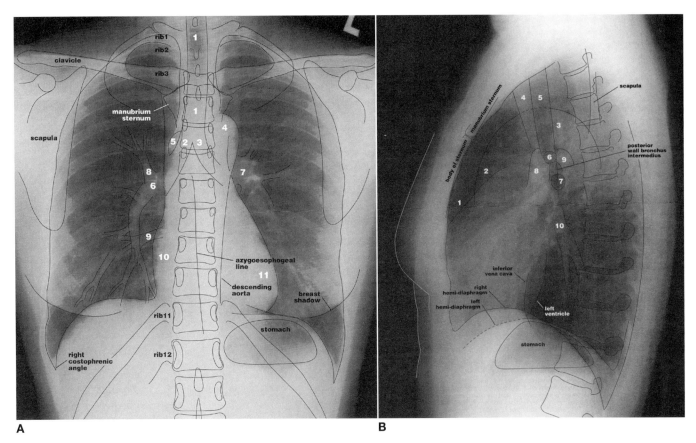

FIGURE 2-1 A, Normal anatomic structures viewed in a posterioranterior (PA) radiograph. A PA view showing trachea *(1)*, right main bronchus *(2)*, left main bronchus *(3)*, aortic "knob" or arch *(4)*, azygos vein emptying into superior vena cava *(5)*, right interlobar artery *(6)*, left pulmonary artery *(7)*, right upper lobe pulmonary artery (truncus anterior) *(8)*, right inferior pulmonary vein *(9)*, right atrium *(10)*, left ventricle *(11)*, and other structures as labeled. **B,** Normal anatomic structures viewed in a lateral radiograph. A lateral view showing pulmonary outflow tract *(1)*, ascending aorta *(2)*, aortic arch *(3)*, brachiocephalic vessels *(4)*, trachea *(5)*, right upper lobe bronchus *(6)*, left upper lobe bronchus *(7)*, right pulmonary artery *(8)*, left pulmonary artery *(9)*, confluence of pulmonary veins *(10)*, and other structures as labeled. (From Collins J, Stern EJ: *Chest radiology: the essentials*, Philadelphia, 1991, Lippincott Williams & Wilkins.)

(Figure 2-1).* The lungs, which are mostly air but do contain some water, blood vessels, bronchi, nerves, lymphatics, alveolar walls, and interstitial tissues, provide the natural contrast that is the basis of chest radiology. When evaluating a chest x-ray, the changes in these densities, which provide natural contrast, are what are observed. Whatever processes might influence the path of the beam and therefore alter the usual contrast between the lungs and other thoracic organs, are evaluated.

Radiologists traditionally speak of two signs—the *silhouette sign* and *summation*—that indicate that a change of tissue opacity is present on a film. Depending on which part or parts of the lung are involved, the result of this change in the absorption of x-rays is seen by the effect that it has on the normal structures of the lung. When a heart border, the surface of a hemidiaphragm, or the descending aorta cannot be seen, this is an indication that the usual amount of aerated lung no longer

touches that anatomic part. Sometimes this occurs because the alveolar spaces are wholly or partially filled with fluid—usually blood, pus, or water (edematous fluid)—or because the lung has collapsed and decreased the normal ratio of air and soft tissue. The end result in the latter case would be an increase in opacity, which is what the x-ray beam reveals as less of a difference in tissue opacity than would normally be expected. The heart border and the diaphragm are normally seen because of their interface with aerated lung. When the contiguous lung is not aerated, the opaque tissue of the affected lung blends visually with the soft tissue opacity of the heart, and the heart border is no longer visible. This is the *silhouette sign,* or more correctly, the loss of silhouette sign (Figure 2-2). *Summation,* on the other hand, is the result of superimposition of many layers of lung tissue, so that the final visual effect is that of a greater amount of tissue in the path of a particular part of the x-ray beam (Figure 2-3). This is seen when the opacity of fluid in the pleural space, interstitium, or even lung parenchyma is added (summated) on the normal structures of the lung.

---

*Please refer to Chapter 2 in the second edition of *Thoracic Anesthesia* for additional interstitial normal and abnormal x-rays.

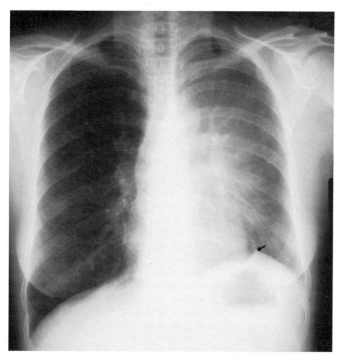

FIGURE 2-2 Silhouette sign. A PA radiograph of the chest with collapse of the upper lobe of the left lung demonstrates that most of the left border of the heart is not clearly seen when it is no longer surrounded by aerated lung (see also Figures 2-10 and 2-29, *E*). When the upper lobe collapses, it often produces a *juxtaphrenic peak* (see *arrow*), an area where the diaphragmatic pleura is pulled upward as a result of the volume loss.

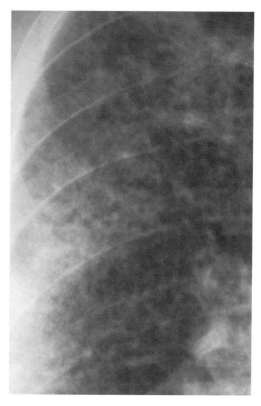

FIGURE 2-3 Summation sign. A PA radiograph showing a patient in mild heart failure, with a generalized increase in interstitial markings throughout the lungs. These represent fluid-filled interstitium that are usually not visible in the normal lung. Vascular structures are also not clearly seen, and the increase in fluid absorbs more x-ray than could the interstitium alone, adding (summating) the various absorbers of radiation.

Approaching the Film

As in most areas of medicine, adopting a routine will help avoid missed diagnoses (Tables 2-1 and 2-2). Although it is tempting to jump to the most obvious abnormality on a film, the discipline of checking all areas in a set pattern each time a new film is viewed should help minimize missed abnormalities. Some reviewers start at the periphery of the chest and work toward the center, whereas others search by organ system (e.g., bones first, followed by soft tissues of the thorax, heart, and mediastinal structures, and finally the lungs).[7] Research into search patterns over the years has shown that reviewers tend to look at only a small part of each film and do so in a random order. Looking at each film from two different perspectives—up close for detail and from a distance of 2 meters for an overall impression—can help identify abnormalities. Viewing from a distance might help the reviewer see subtle changes in opacity that signal abnormal areas on the film. When the reviewer is viewing on a monitor, the "up-close" review should include the use of magnification; otherwise, subtle abnormalities such as a small pneumothorax might remain nearly invisible.

Visual perception and optical illusions can play a role in perceiving adjacent opacities on a chest radiograph. Because each film represents multiple layers of tissue superimposed on each other, the eye can easily be fooled by following edges of various normal structures and being convinced that there are cysts or other abnormal structures on a normal study. *Mach bands*—often seen as black lines below breast shadows and for years thought to represent air—are a well-known and well-documented example of this optical phenomenon. The process of how mach bands come to exist is poorly understood, but it produces a fictitious difference in luminescence between similar opacities on a film, when in fact there is no area of density that can be measured with a densitometer between the similar opacities.[8]

The most important skill for evaluating a chest x-ray is knowledge of normal anatomic variants, specific patterns of pathologic changes, and the common signs of abnormal states. For instance, familiarity with the various positions of a possible azygous fissure can raise the suspicion that a paratracheal soft tissue opacity on the right is merely a consolidated accessory lobe rather than a mass or adenopathy. The ability to spot a right-sided aortic arch or even dextrocardia should alert the viewer to the possibility of other underlying cardiac malformations. Occasionally, a persistent left superior vena cava can alter the course that a pulmonary artery catheter (PAC) or pacing electrode takes from its point of insertion to its final resting place (Figure 2-4).

TABLE 2-1

Guidelines to Follow When Reading and Interpreting the Chest Radiograph

1. Both posteroanterior (PA) and lateral views should be examined when these are available. Unless pathology is seen on both views, it is not certain that the pathology is in the chest.
2. The right border of the heart is formed by the right atrium, and it is obscured by the medial segment of the right middle lobe processes. Disease limited to the lateral segment will not obscure the right heart border.
3. The left border of the heart is formed mainly by the left ventricle and is obscured by lingular processes of the left upper lobe.
4. The right side of the diaphragm is usually 1.5 to 2.0 cm higher than the left.
5. The diaphragm is obscured by processes of the lower lobe of the lung on frontal or lateral views, unless only the superior segment of a lower lobe is involved, in which case the diaphragm is clearly seen. If only a frontal view is available, disease in the posterior segment of the lower lobes might not affect the diaphragmatic contour.
6. From a lateral view, the major fissures of the lungs are seen as oblique lines extending from the anterior diaphragm to the upper thoracic spine and on to the level of the aortic arch.
7. The minor fissure of the lungs is on the right, separating the right upper lobe from the right middle lobe. It courses from the right hilum to the right lateral anterior chest wall and can be seen on both PA and lateral chest radiographs.
8. Hilar opacities are predominantly due to the presence of the pulmonary arteries and should be symmetric in size and opacity.
9. The aortic arch or "knob" is above the left hilum. There is the possibility of a right aortic arch variant and can indicate other abnormalities.
10. The trachea is midline but may be deviated to the right or forward from a tortuous aorta.
11. The costophrenic angles should be sharp on both views, except in patients with severe pulmonary emphysema.
12. With good inspiratory effort, the size of the heart on the PA radiograph is normally 50% or less of the widest diameter of the thoracic cage.
13. On a lateral view chest x-ray, right middle lobe and lingular processes of the lung are projected over the heart.
14. A young, healthy person can take a breath deep enough to inflate the lungs to the level of the tenth rib posteriorly (equivalent to the level of the sixth rib anteriorly).
15. Normal right and left lung opacification should be symmetric unless the patient is rotated. (The clavicles are used as a reference standard—if they are the same opacity, then the problem is in the lung, not in the film).
16. The stomach bubble is located under the left hemidiaphragm. *Situs inversus* may be present and must be considered.
17. The bones and soft tissues must be observed. The ribs should be compared from side to side.

Modified from Collins J, Stern EJ: *Chest radiology: the essentials,* Philadelphia, 1999, Lippincott Williams & Wilkins.

TABLE 2-2

Size and Opacity Ratios on the PA Chest Radiograph

SIZE RATIOS

Cardiothoracic	The heart diameter should less than half of the chest diameter. An easy way to evaluate this, assuming that the spine is straight and in the middle of the chest, is to see whether the heart to the right of the midline fits between the left border of the heart and the left ribs.
Aortopulmonary	The left pulmonary artery, as it passes over the left main bronchus, should be less than the width of the aortic knob. The aortic arch is approximately 3 cm above the carina in the adult until the aorta becomes tortuous. The left pulmonary artery is seen approximately 3 cm down the left main bronchus, then courses up and out at approximately 45 degrees.
Azygotracheal	The azygos vein, if visualized at the right tracheobronchial angle, should be no wider than approximately half the width of the trachea while its height should be no wider than the width of the trachea.
Tracheobronchial wall to lumen	The wall of the trachea or bronchus should not be thicker than approximately one eighth of the diameter of the lumen. The tracheal diameter should be equal on the PA and lateral views and should be less than the width of one vertebral body.
Right lower lobar artery to tracheal	The width of the artery of the right lower lobe should not be wider than the width of the tracheal lumen.
Hilar height	The left hilum should be approximately 2 cm higher than the right because the left pulmonary artery must pass above the left main bronchus.
Arteriobronchial	An artery and its accompanying bronchus should be of equal size (seen best "end-on").

OPACITIES

Cardiohepatic	The heart should be about half as opaque as the middle of the liver (it is about half as thick). This reference requires good exposure to be seen.
Intracardiac	The heart should have a similar degree of opacity on each side of the spine.
Intrahepatic	The top of the liver should be about half as opaque as the middle because it is about half as thick, provided that the diaphragm domes normally.
Right paratracheal-aortic	The opacity to the right of the trachea at the level of the aortic arch should never be as great or greater than the opacity of the aortic knob.
Hilar	The opacity of the two hila should be equal because they are composed of the same vascularity.

Modified from Collins J, Stern EJ: *Chest radiology: the essentials,* Philadelphia, 1999, Lippincott Williams & Wilkins.

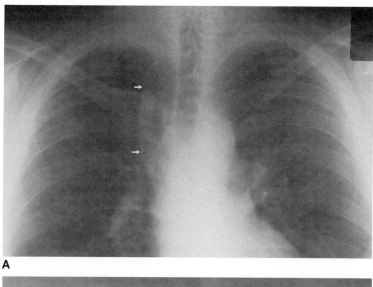

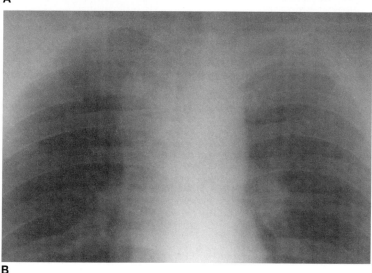

FIGURE 2-4 A, Normal variant (azygos lobe). A coned down portion of a normal PA chest radiograph demonstrating an azygos fissure (see *arrows*), which separates the most medial portion (the azygos lobe) from the remainder of the upper lobe of the right lung. An azygos lobe often reacts like a distinct segment of lung in response to various disease states. **B,** Normal variant (azygos lobe) with opacity. A PA film on the same patient now shows consolidation of this azygos lobe, which could be mistaken for a paratracheal mass if the presence of the lobe and its fissure was not known. The convex shape should not be mistaken for atelectasis of the upper lobe.

Continued

Chest Diseases on Radiographs

The basic, underlying change in the chest film that allows the detection and diagnosis of abnormalities is usually due to an alteration in lung opacity. This can be caused by technical factors, physiologic variations, or pathologic mechanisms.[9] Obviously, knowledge of the first two enables the reviewer to determine the significance of findings.

Diseases that affect the chest can usually be thought of as either those that make the film lighter (increase opacity) or those that make it darker (increase lucency). In simplest terms, what is being evaluated is whether there is more or less tissue (or water, or absorber) in the path of the beam.

Readers often speak of perceiving a *density* on a film; this is a confusing term. Density is the blackening seen on a film (not just on a chest x-ray) and indicates either too much radiation (overexposure) or an increase in the absolute amount or ratio of air in the path of the beam. What is usually meant is that there is opacity—an area of whitening—on the film, usually from an increase in water in the path of the beam, or from a decrease in the air/water ratio, or from too little x-radiation (underexposure).

There is a tendency to think of lung diseases that cause an increase in opacity as being either interstitial or alveolar. Although this is a significant distinction, it often does not take into account other important absorbers of x-rays in the chest wall or the pleural space as potential causes of this increase in opacity. When the summation of abnormal opacities is considered, we would expect that the opacity of pleural effusion might be inseparable from the opacity of consolidated lung, especially

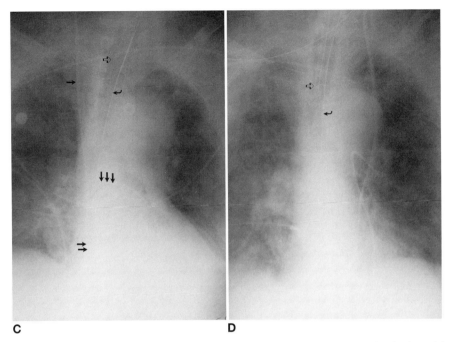

C   D

FIGURE 2-4 Cont'd C, Normal film (right superior vena cava). A pulmonary artery catheter placed using a right internal jugular approach following the superior vena cava (single arrow) to the right atrium (double arrows) and right main pulmonary artery (triple arrows). Note the position of the endotracheal tube (open arrow) and the nasogastric tube (curved arrow). **D,** Normal variant (persistent left superior vena cava). The same patient four days later with a new pulmonary artery catheter placed using a left internal jugular approach, following a persistent left superior vena cava to the left lower lobe pulmonary artery. Note again the endotracheal tube (open arrow) in good position near the level of the aortic arch, and the nasogastric tube (curved arrow) passing close to the aortic arch before swinging to the right around the left atrium (see also Figure 2-24, *A*).

on a film taken in a supine position. In such a case, fluid in the pleural space will spread out posteriorly to the lungs. The opacified lung and pleural opacity are summated, a phenomenon that might lead to an appearance of total opacification.

Those conditions that tend to increase opacity, those that increase lucency, specific postoperative changes related to major pulmonary surgery, and various life support and monitoring devices that are so much a part of most portable chest radiography are covered in the sections that follow.

Chest Diseases with Increased Opacity on Radiographs

Conditions that are marked by focal or global increases in the opacity on the film are first examined. In these cases, the normal structures that reviewers are trained to look for as part of the examination of a film are lost in this additional whiteness and are no longer visible. Conditions discussed include atelectasis, consolidation (usually pneumonia), pulmonary edema, pulmonary contusion and hemorrhage, aspiration, acute respiratory distress syndrome (ARDS), and, less frequently, pulmonary embolism with infarction.

ATELECTASIS

Atelectasis comes from the Greek meaning "imperfect expansion." Today, the term connotes "airlessness," or at least decreased air with volume loss. It usually appears on an x-ray as a focal opacity, although complete collapse of a lobe or lung can lead to a dramatic appearance because the heart border or diaphragm is no longer visible (Figure 2-5). Atelectasis is

usually classified by its etiology, recognizing four typical mechanisms:

1. Obstruction of some portion of the airway leading to resorption of the air in the terminal spaces
2. Displacement of lung by adjacent structures or fluid (passive or compressive atelectasis)
3. Deformity of the lung secondary to scarring (cicatrization atelectasis)
4. Loss of surfactant (most commonly due to hyaline membrane disease or to surfactant deficiency disorder in premature newborn infants)

Although acute atelectasis can occasionally result simply in an airless portion of lung, in most cases there is some fluid present, and in chronic cases there is also cellular debris, referred to as *obstructive pneumonitis*. Radiographically, however, there is no way to distinguish between fluid, cellular debris, and a small area of consolidation.[10]

There are only two direct radiological signs of atelectasis: an increase in the opacity of the lung and displacement of an interlobar fissure (in cases of at least segmental atelectasis). Often with small areas of linear, platelike, or subsegmental atelectasis, the acuity of the findings cannot be determined without prior films for comparison, and even then, ongoing changes can be seen for several days. Scarring has a more consistent appearance over a longer period of time. A number of secondary signs of atelectasis are also sought—approximation of the ribs on the affected side, displacement of mediastinal structures, elevation of the hemidiaphragm, compensatory overinflation, nonvisualization of the

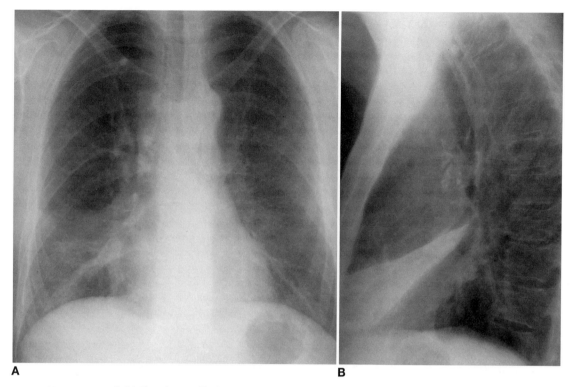

A   **B**

FIGURE 2-5 A, PA Chest image with right middle lobe atelectasis. There is a focal opacity with poorly defined margins in the lower right area of the chest that obscures the right border of the heart. The loss of the heart border has been described as a silhouette sign and indicates that the abnormality is anterior and, therefore, probably in the right middle lobe. **B,** Lateral chest image with right middle lobe atelectasis. This lateral image shows the opacity that was seen on the PA image as an anterior opacity. In contrast with the PA image, the opacity is well defined on the lateral image. The area of opacity is outlined by the horizontal and oblique fissures. The fissures are displaced and appear to be drawn together. This appearance indicates volume loss, which is the expected appearance of right middle lobe atelectasis.

interlobar artery, and the absence of air bronchograms—although these are not as consistent or reliable as the direct signs.[11]

Subsegmental atelectasis usually presents as seemingly random patches of increased opacity when a segment or a lobe is involved. There is a predictable pattern of collapse, in most cases resulting from the way the lungs are attached by bronchi and vascular structures at the hila.[12,13] For example, the right upper lobe swings upward toward the right side of the upper mediastinum (Figure 2-6); while the middle lobe pulls the minor fissure downward and the major fissure forward, obliterating the heart border because it is no longer outlined by air-containing lung. The lower lobes may cause loss of definition of the diaphragm on either the frontal or lateral film, depending on which segments are involved. The left upper lobe tends to collapse forward toward the chest wall, covering and obliterating the normal left border of the heart. The aortic knob, on the other hand, is accentuated by the expansion of the superior segment of the lower lobe, a situation known as *luftsichel* (Figure 2-7).

ALVEOLAR LUNG DISEASE

The second major cause of increased opacity on chest radiographs is alveolar lung disease (ALD), which is also called *air space disease,* although this term is really not accurate because atelectasis is also a disease state of the air spaces (with lack of air, rather than filling of the alveoli, being the problem). *Consolidation* is another term often substituted for ALD, although the meaning here is a bit more narrow, usually referring

to pneumonia. The causes of this alveolar filling are quite diverse, although they are usually thought of as being "blood, pus, or water," with cellular material (e.g., tumors or debris) and protein responsible for a very small percentage of the abnormal chest x-rays seen in clinical practice.[14]

Certain features are expected when a patient has one of these conditions: an acinar or terminal lobular shadow, coalescence of adjacent areas into more complete consolidation, unsharp margins, air bronchograms, distribution that usually respects the fissures, and the absence of atelectasis (Figure 2-8).[15,16]

Although the organism that is responsible for the disease is used to classify pneumonia pathologically, pneumonias are classified radiographically by anatomic distribution as bronchopneumonia, lobular pneumonia, lobar pneumonia, or interstitial pneumonia. In simple terms, pneumonia can be considered to be infected pulmonary edema, remembering that the initial response to the infection is the outpouring of edema fluid into the alveolar spaces, followed by the rapid multiplication of the microorganisms and, finally, invasion by polymorphonuclear leukocytes.[12] Each of these steps adds tissue (fluid, microbes, cells) in sufficient quantity to displace the air that usually makes up the majority of the volume of a lung, thereby changing the tissue properties and normal ability of x-rays to penetrate the lungs.

Pulmonary edema, on the other hand, is usually a more diffuse process, although patients can certainly have very

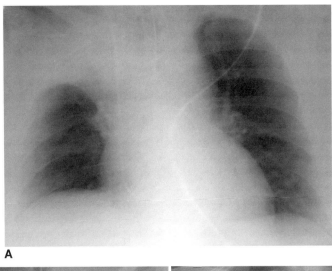

A

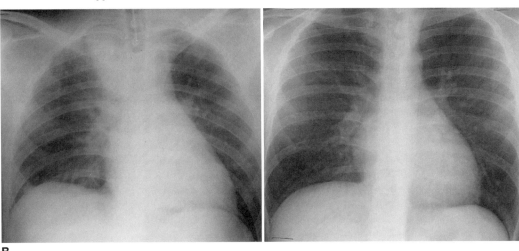

B

FIGURE 2-6 A, Right upper lobe atelectasis. This AP chest image demonstrates opacification of the right upper lobe with superior shift and bowing of the horizontal fissure. This is a typical appearance for right upper lobe atelectasis. **B,** Right upper lobe atelectasis. This AP chest (left image) demonstrates opacity in the medial aspect of the right upper chest obscuring the right mediastinal border. In contrast with the previous case, the minor fissure is not apparent. This could represent pneumonia or partial right upper lobe atelectasis. The follow-up examination (right image) taken 24 hours later shows the opacity to have completely resolved. This rapid clearing and the absence of clinical symptoms of pneumonia confirm the diagnosis of atelectasis.

extensive involvement from infection (Figure 2-9). *Edema* is defined as an excess of fluid in the extravascular compartment of the lung and usually results from one of two different mechanisms:

1. Hemodynamic, usually cardiogenic (from an imbalance of transmural pressures) or
2. What is usually termed *permeability edema*.

The term *permeability edema* is a misnomer because all capillaries are permeable. It is more correct to refer to this as an injury edema from alveolar wall damage.[17]

Heart failure is usually thought of when the term *pulmonary edema* is used, but there are many noncardiogenic causes. Congenital pulmonary venous obstruction and overhydration are closely related to cardiogenic edema, although in these cases the underlying cause is not a failing heart but rather an overload on the system. In contrast, drowning, renal failure, uremia, fat embolism, smoke, or chemical gas inhalation, and even aspiration pneumonia are forms of pulmonary edema, representing either a diffuse or focal chemical pneumonitis resulting from alveolar damage rather than from a true infection (Figure 2-10). Central nervous system injury can also lead to an edema-like picture, but there is disagreement about the actual mechanism. Often these less common forms of pulmonary edema are radiographically indistinguishable from one another without significant clinical information.

Ketai and Godwin have suggested that there should be four classes of pulmonary edema[18]:

1. Hydrostatic edema
2. ARDS—permeability edema caused by diffuse alveolar damage
3. Permeability edema without alveolar damage
4. Mixed hydrostatic and permeability edema

There is some overlap radiographically among these classes, and the diagnosis often depends on accurate clinical information.

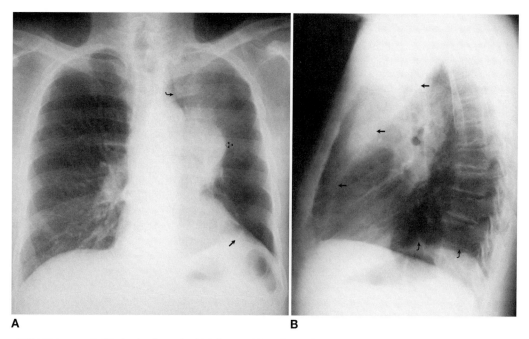

FIGURE 2-7 A, PA chest radiograph with left upper lobe collapse. PA film shows generalized increase in opacity of the left hemithorax, elevation of the left hemidiaphragm and soft tissue shadow projected over the left hilum (hilum overlay sign—*open arrow*), a small juxtaphrenic peak *(arrow),* and air from the hyperexpanded left lower lobe medial to the collapsed left upper lobe (luftsichel—*curved arrow*). **B,** Lateral radiograph with left upper lobe collapse. This view shows the collapsed upper lobe of the left lung as an opacity paralleling the inside of the anterior chest wall *(arrows)* and poor definition of the left hemidiaphragm *(curved arrows)* as a consequence of the uneven diaphragmatic contour resulting from the volume loss.

Ketai and Godwin point out that findings that are predominantly interstitial should predict a benign clinical course and rapid resolution.[18]

ARDS is a special form of acute lung injury that warrants separate mention, especially because it can involve many patients undergoing thoracic surgery, and, conversely, can delay such surgery. ARDS is a form of acute respiratory failure usually associated with serious injury. The failure is severe, progressive, and unremitting, attended by a degree of hypoxia that does not respond to simple O_2 therapy and that leads to considerable difficulty in ventilator management while trying to avoid barotrauma.[19] This syndrome is further complicated by a decrease in pulmonary compliance. In reality, ARDS is a clinical diagnosis with radiographic changes that are suggestive of or compatible with the condition, but not necessarily diagnostic of it. Radiographically, it appears as patchy, dependent pulmonary edema that does not significantly improve in the short term (Figure 2-11). The dependent distribution of the edema is best appreciated on CT scans, where the upper lobes (which are anterior) are less involved than the more dependent lower lobes.[20] Recently, it has been shown that placing these patients in a prone position for 2 hours twice a day will improve oxygenation, although the effect on survival is not known.[21] More recently, the observation that the heart primarily rests on the lower lobes when the patient is supine (and primarily on the sternum when prone) may provide a mechanical explanation for this distribution and also explain why atelectasis and consolidation more frequently involve the left lower lobe in hospitalized, nonmobile patients, especially after several days of bed rest.

INTERSTITIAL LUNG DISEASE

The next major cause of opacity on chest radiographs is a heterogenous group of disorders that primarily affect the supportive structures of the lung, including the alveolar wall, the interlobular septa, and the peribronchovascular tissues. There are usually four patterns, named according to the gross appearance: linear, reticular, nodular, and reticulonodular.[22] These may occur acutely, as in congestive heart failure (which represents the most common cause of acute interstitial change seen on chest films) or from a variety of infections, usually viral pneumonias or *Pneumocystis carinii* pneumonia (PCP) (Figure 2-12). More commonly, especially in the non–acutely ill, nonhospitalized patient, chronic changes come from a variety of granulomatous diseases, occupational exposure (in the cases of pneumoconiosis and some long-standing hypersensitivity pneumonias), chronic interstitial pneumonias. or, finally, neoplastic and proliferative disorders. Recognition that chronic problems are just that—chronic, not acute diseases (especially in the cases of linear and reticular interstitial patterns)—can be useful in evaluating which patients are candidates for surgery. End-stage scarring can result from a variety of diseases, including sarcoidosis, rheumatoid arthritis, scleroderma, and idiopathic pulmonary fibrosis. The radiologic appearance is most often a coarse reticular pattern (Figure 2-13). These conditions are often fatal, but the patients could be candidates for lung transplantation.

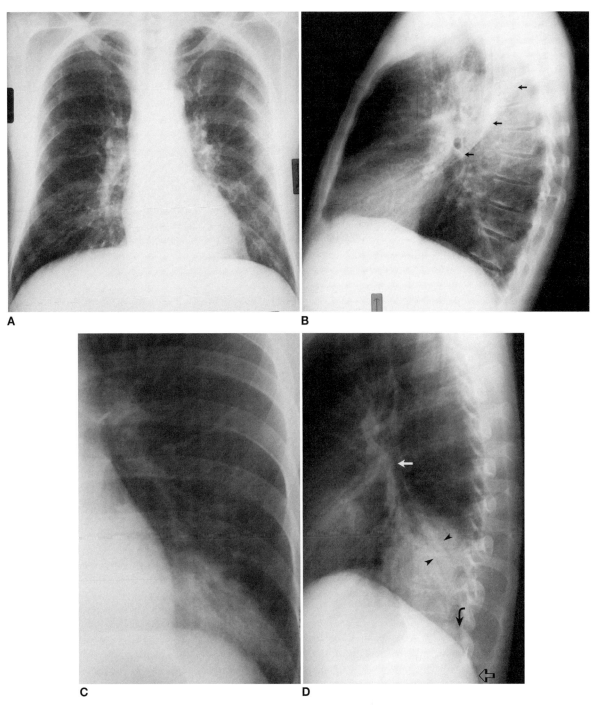

FIGURE 2-8 A, PA chest film with alveolar lung disease. PA radiograph shows a subtle area of alveolar lung disease in the left upper lobe. Notice the slight increase in opacity laterally opposite the left hilum. In this position it could easily be mistaken for the lower end of the scapula without the lateral film. **B,** Lateral chest radiograph with alveolar lung disease. On the lateral view, this area of alveolar filling is seen to best advantage as a slightly curved line *(arrows)* caused by the fluid-filled alveoli in the posterior segment of the upper lobe as they interface with the major fissure (and, therefore, with the air-containing lower lobe). Note the relative sharpness of the interface with the fissure and the less distinct other margin, indicating that not all of the alveolar spaces are equally filled. **C,** Left lower lobe consolidation (alveolar lung disease). This close-up PA film shows an irregular opacity overlying (but not obscuring) the left border of the heart and obscuring only a small portion of the left hemidiaphragm. **D,** Left lower lobe consolidation (alveolar lung disease). On the lateral radiograph the area of alveolar lung disease is seen deep within the left lower lobe. The dome of the diaphragm is readily visible on this film, which explains why it is also so apparent on the PA part of the study. Air bronchograms are seen as branching, tapering lucent *(black)* tubular structures *(arrowheads)* radiating from the hilum *(straight arrow)* toward the costophrenic angle *(curved arrow)* in this area of consolidation. Note how the right costophrenic angle *(open arrow)* shows the normal sharp appearance of its interface with normally aerated lung.

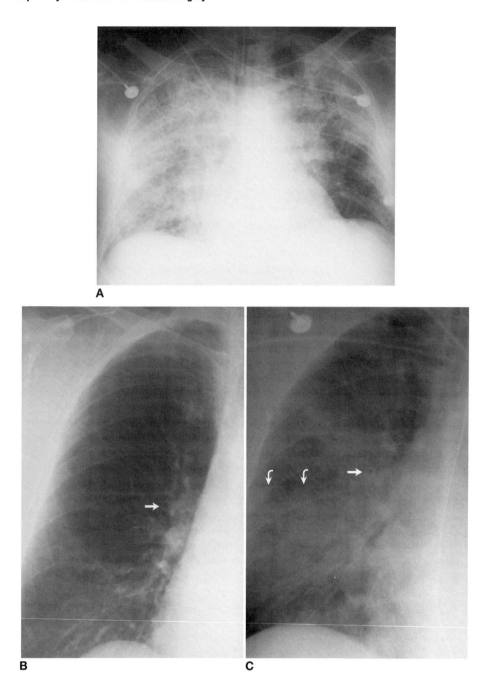

FIGURE 2-9 A, Pulmonary edema. This portable anteroposterior (AP) study shows diffuse, fluffy opacities through-out the lungs, especially in the upper zones. Note the poor definition of the right border of the heart (the silhouette sign). This is the same patient seen in Figure 2-3 about 12 hours after the interstitial edema had progressed to alveolar disease. **B,** Normal film. This patient's PA study shows the right upper lobe bronchus, which is seen on end with its cross section appearing as a ring *(straight arrow)*. This is of normal caliber. There is no fluid in the fissure *(curved arrows)*, and the heart and diaphragmatic contours are sharp. **C,** Pulmonary edema. On this PA film, note the marked increase in the thickness of the bronchial wall in the right upper lobe *(straight arrow)*, fluid in the minor fissure *(curved arrows)*, and loss of the normal heart silhouette at the apex and right atrium when compared to the earlier study (see Figure 2-9, *B*).

In terms of lung opacity, abnormally "hazy" lung parenchyma that does not obscure normal vascular or bronchial markings may also be seen. This "ground glass" opacification can be either interstitial or alveolar lung disease, or even a combination of the two. It is not always possible to differentiate between alveolar and interstitial disease.

Congestive heart failure presents in a number of ways, depending on the severity of the underlying cardiac condition and the stage in which it is seen. The fact that a chest x-ray represents only a fraction of a second in the life of a particular patient, and that there can be a significant discrepancy between the clinical and radiographic findings, is often overlooked.

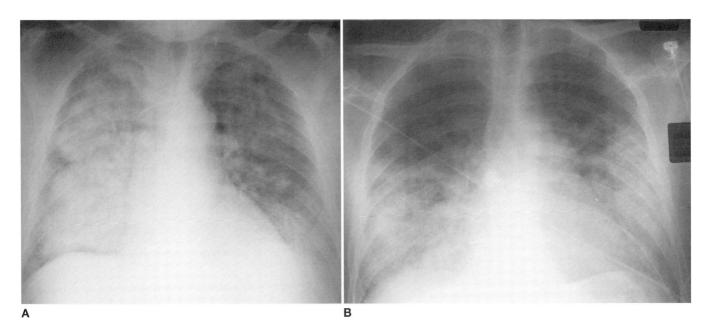

A   B

FIGURE 2-10 A, Noncardiogenic pulmonary edema. This AP film is of a patient with uremia. Note that the peripheral centimeter of lung is spared, yielding the "bat wing" or "butterfly" appearance. **B,** Noncardiogenic pulmonary edema. This patient experienced sudden respiratory difficulty with other clinical signs of fat emboli approximately 10 days after major trauma. Note how difficult it is to see the heart border and the right diaphragmatic surface, suggesting diffuse alveolar filling or edema. Neither this patient nor the one in *A* shows signs of pleural effusion. It is often difficult to distinguish among various etiologies of pulmonary edema without clinical information.

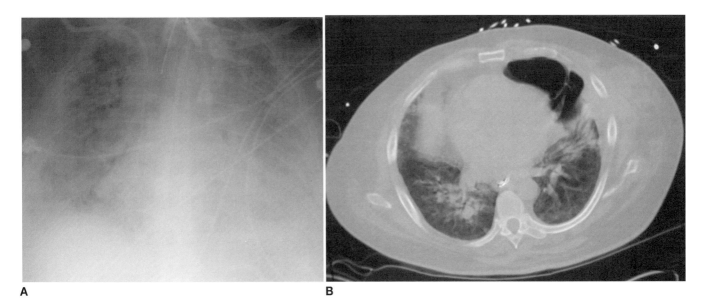

A   B

FIGURE 2-11 A, ARDS with interstitial emphysema. This portable AP image shows diffuse opacification of both lungs that could result from pulmonary edema, pneumonia, or ARDS. Making a precise differential diagnosis requires careful clinical correlation. Serial radiographs confirming that the air-space disease is stable for days and that cardiomegaly and pleural effusions are absent would support the diagnosis of ARDS. The observation that diffuse, bubbly, small lucent areas, such as those seen over the upper lung zones, are developing is suggestive of complicating interstitial emphysema. This results from high ventilator pressures and indicates that the patient is at risk for development of pneumomediastinum and pneumothorax. **B,** ARDS on CT scan. On this section, the dependent nature of the capillary injury edema is noted in both lungs, although it is more prominent on the right. Note the absence of any sign of interstitial involvement. The large lucent area in the left upper lobe is a cystic space that has developed as a result of barotrauma.

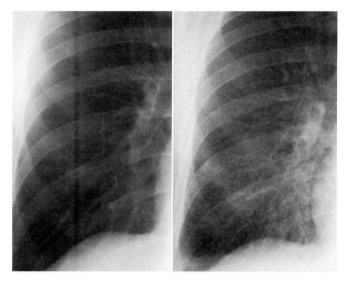

FIGURE 2-12 Acute mixed interstitial and alveolar disease. Normal PA chest film *(left image)* and a second PA film obtained at a time when *Pneumocystis carinii* pneumonia was diagnosed by culture *(right image)*. Clearly visible are the interstitial Kerley B lines near the costophrenic angles, as well as the diffuse nodular opacities that most likely represent alveolar involvement in the lower lung zones.

Evaluating pulmonary vascular redistribution is perhaps one of the more difficult tasks on portable films, as the supine position can accentuate the appearance of upper lobe vessels. It is only when there is a change on films of comparable technique that a valid comparison can be made.[23] More often, subtle interstitial edema (Kerley B lines) and small pleural effusions are the only signs of the cardiac dysfunction. There is no such finding as a Kerley B line. A single, centimeter-long line near the pleural surface is not indicative of edema in an interlobular septum; to be considered as a significant finding, there must be multiple lines, parallel to each other about 1 cm apart in the lower lung fields (Figure 2-14). Sometimes, the earliest sign is a vague increase in opacity surrounding the hila, the so-called *hilar haze*. In reality, this is peripheral edema similar to Kerley B lines seen near the costophrenic angles—the portion of the lung that surrounds the hilum is at the far end of the bronchial and vascular trees functionally, even if it is located in the center of the lung on a gross anatomic level. Because the radiograph presents a summation of shadows, this may represent peripheral edema anteriorly and posteriorly superimposed over the central hilar vessels. More advanced stages of congestive heart failure will take on an alveolar pattern as the fluid continues to leak from the vessels into the interstitium and finally into the air spaces.

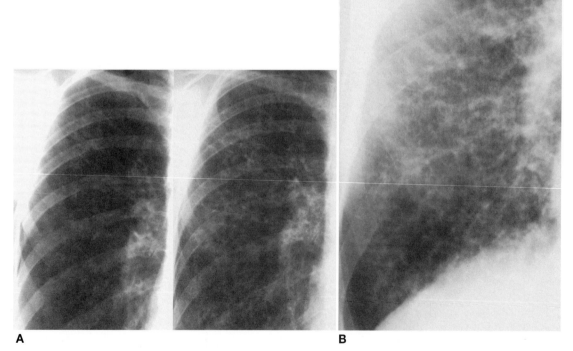

A   **B**

FIGURE 2-13 Chronic interstitial disease. **A,** The left side of the figure shows the right upper lung zone with fibrosis that had been present but had not changed significantly for a period of years. These linear and netlike (reticular) opacities are composed of scar tissue in the interstitium, the supportive portion of lung tissue. Although interstitial tissue is present in all patients, it is usually so fine that it cannot be detected on a standard radiograph. On the right side of the figure is a film obtained 5 years later showing that the abnormality of the interstitium film has progressed and thickened, and new areas have appeared. **B,** Severe pulmonary fibrosis. Severe fibrosis in a different patient, showing a reticular (netlike) pattern that is similar to the one seen in acute interstitial edema (see also Figure 2-3, *B*). This patient also had pleural scarring and calcification on the left lung with an appearance suggestive of possible asbestos exposure, which has a predilection for lower lobe distribution.

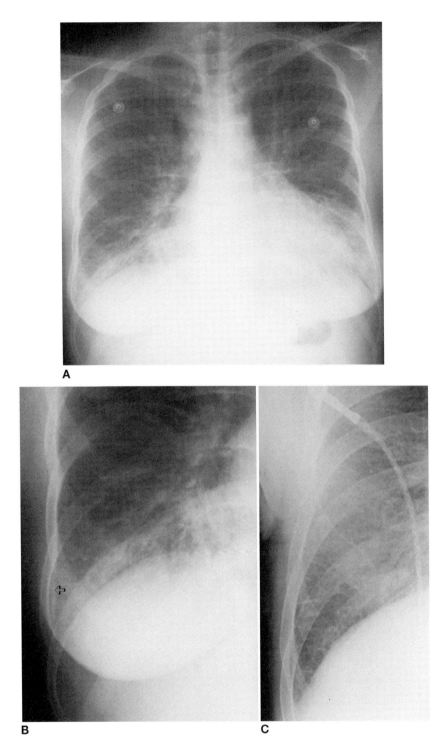

FIGURE 2-14 A, Pulmonary interstitial edema. The AP radiograph shows a patient with moderate interstitial pulmonary edema. In addition to the cardiomegaly, the vasculature visible in the upper lobes is more prominent than in a normal state. The cardiac borders and diaphragmatic contours are not as sharp as in a healthy patient, indicating increased fluid; in this case, the fluid is primarily in the interstitium. **B,** Pulmonary interstitial edema. Note on the close-up view the opacity paralleling the chest wall just above the costophrenic angle *(open arrow)*. This represents early subpleural effusion. At the same level, Kerley B lines are barely visible as short parallel lines near the periphery of the lung over the lower third of the field. **C,** Pulmonary interstitial edema. This close-up image of a different patient shows lines in the subpleural lateral aspect of the lungs caused by thickening of the interlobular septa. These lines are often described as Kerley B lines. In this case, the linear opacities are the result of interstitial edema.

PULMONARY NEOPLASM

Pulmonary neoplasia also present as opacities on films, although usually as more focal areas with varying contours than the other entities that have been covered. Smaller lesions may be very difficult to visualize, especially when these are overlying bones or other soft tissues. The portable bedside radiograph is rarely adequate for evaluation of pulmonary neoplasms. Even upright PA and lateral views of the chest are often inadequate for detection and evaluation of thoracic neoplasms, whereas CT is the standard for determining the extent and stage of a tumor.

PLEURAL EFFUSION

As mentioned previously, most classifications of lung disease refer to interstitial or alveolar disease. Although pleural effusion does not involve the lung parenchyma, it can be the source of a significant amount of absorbing material in the path of the x-ray beam, causing opacity on the films. Large pleural effusions, which cause significant passive atelectasis, are easy to spot, but small effusions can be overlooked easily, especially on portable films because the patients are almost always supine or semierect, and the fluid can collect either in a subpulmonic location or deep in the posterior costophrenic sulcus where it is hidden from view.[24] Most often, smaller effusions are seen as a veil-like opacity that is most pronounced at the base and tapers toward the lung apex. One feature that can help differentiate effusions from either ALDs or atelectasis is the reader's ability to still visualize the pulmonary vessels through this additional opacity, an indication that there is little change in the air content of the hemithorax. Also, on supine and semierect films, small amounts of fluid might not necessarily produce a curved meniscus at the costophrenic angle; instead, these small effusions can be recognized as a thin band of opacity paralleling the lower chest wall. Of course, if there are PA and lateral views of the chest, evaluation of small amounts of fluid becomes an easier task, with thickening of the major and minor fissures and blunting of the posterior sulcus by as little as 25 mL of fluid visible on the lateral view (Figure 2-15).

At times, the appearance of fluid in the fissures can lead to some confusing shadows on a frontal film, especially if the interlobar fissure is incomplete or there is some scarring from antecedent disease.[25] Loculated fluid—whether in the peripheral pleural space or the interlobar fissure—can present diagnostic challenges and might require a CT scan or ultrasound for precise localization. And, as with fluid in the alveolar space, it is often not possible to differentiate among simple effusion, pus, or blood.

PERICARDIAL EFFUSION

Small pericardial effusions are usually most accurately identified by means of echocardiography, although some fluid collections may be seen as an incidental finding on a CT scan. They should be suspected in any instance where there is significant pleural effusion that appears to be related to heart failure. In cases of larger effusions, the shape of the heart may become quite globular. Except for the temporal difference, it is difficult to differentiate this shape from dilated cardiomyopathy.

Chest Diseases with Increased Lucency on Radiographs

The conditions discussed in the following sections have in common either focal or generalized increase in the blackness of films that may also be described as *increased lucency*. In contrast to the variety of causes (infection, heart failure, trauma, volume loss) of those diseases with increased opacity, these diseases are linked by the presence of air in parts of the lung (or of the thoracic cage or cavity) where air is not a normal component. With the exception of emphysema and various air-containing cysts, most of these diseases are related to trauma.

EMPHYSEMA

Emphysema is characterized by a permanent increase in the air spaces distal to the terminal bronchiole beyond the normal size. There is destruction of tissue, leading to a loss of alveolar surface available to participate in air exchange, and, sometimes, severe displacement of the adjacent normal lung. Although emphysema is often used synonymously with chronic obstructive pulmonary disease (COPD), this broader term also includes chronic bronchitis, bronchiectasis, and asthma. In all of these situations, there is an increase in resistance to bronchial airflow. In reality, these represent both pathologic and clinical entities, all of which share some radiographic findings.[26,27]

Many of the cases of emphysema seen in adult patients are strongly associated with cigarette smoking. Other chronic insults to the lung parenchyma, such as work-related or environmentally-related exposure and α-1-antitrypsin deficiency, account for a minority of cases. Radiographically, changes in the lung parenchyma, chest wall, diaphragm, and the heart and great vessels are seen, often with significant adverse effects on the physiology of the circulation.

The most striking image that comes to mind in a patient with advanced emphysema is that of marked hyperinflation, with an increase in the AP diameter of the chest, flattening of the diaphragmatic surfaces (even to the point of inversion), and a generalized increase in the blackness of the film. However, patients with significant functional impairment can present with a chest x-ray that is considered essentially normal. The heart usually appears smaller than expected, and hilar vessels are often quite prominent. On closer inspection, the changes in the vascular pattern, with vessels attenuated (thinned) and spread apart, can be observed. Often areas of bullous destruction are noted, as are large, thin-walled air cysts, especially at the apices. These apical air spaces are easily recognized but may also be present in lungs that are otherwise normal (Figure 2-16).[28] Although a classic example of advanced emphysema is easy to spot, it is important to remember that some patients with significant functional obstruction can have a fairly normal-appearing chest x-ray, and high-resolution CT scanning may be needed to demonstrate the degree of abnormality. It is also important to remember that when there are other significant abnormalities of the underlying lung parenchyma, the radiographic appearances that depend on interaction of air-filled lung with fluids (blood, pus, or water) seen in common conditions might have a very different appearance. Pneumonia and heart failure, for instance, can be more difficult to image and diagnose accurately in patients with preexisting emphysema.

AIR CYSTS (BULLAE, BLEBS, AND PNEUMATOCELES)

Bullae were briefly mentioned in the context of their frequent presence in patients with emphysema. Although it is quite common to use the term *blebs* interchangeably with bullae, these two entities are very different from one another. Blebs are specifically blisterlike areas in the thickness of the pleura, not areas of destruction of lung. Blebs are not commonly seen

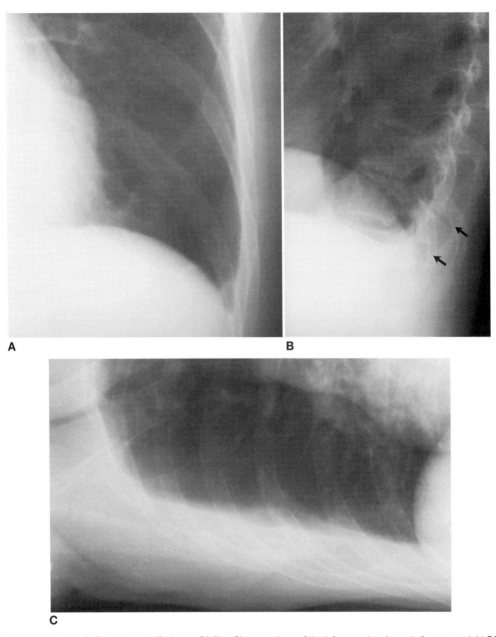

A   B

C

FIGURE 2-15 A, Small pleural effusion on PA film. Close-up views of the left costophrenic angle from an upright PA film show only minimal blunting of the costophrenic angle. **B,** Small pleural effusion on lateral film. On this close-up lateral view, the fluid deep in the costophrenic sulcus is more apparent as it displaces the pleura from the lower ribs *(straight arrows),* although the effusion is still apparently small enough not to cause a silhouette sign of the dome of the diaphragm on either the PA or lateral film. **C,** Small pleural effusion on decubitus film. On this film taken with the patient lying on his right side, there is evidence of significant free-flowing pleural fluid in that hemithorax. This suggests that a large portion of the fluid may have been subpulmonic in location on the upright films.

unless there is an associated pneumothorax, which allows the pleural surface of the lung to be clearly imaged.

A *pneumatocele* is a reversible cyst, which usually results from one of two insults to the lung, either in an area of pneumonia (usually of the *Staphylococcus aureus* variety) or following a laceration of lung tissue. Temporally, these should be easy to differentiate from the permanent destruction of a bulla, because a pneumatocele usually clears in about 6 weeks' time. The importance of a pneumatocele is its ability to cause a pneumothorax, especially if it is close to the surface of the lung. Pneumatoceles also cause difficulty in respirator management, as they can increase in size in the presence of positive pressure ventilation.

PNEUMOTHORAX

Pneumothorax is, simply put, the presence of air in the pleural space. It is frequently the result of trauma, even though at times the source of the air leak cannot readily be detected. The presence of air may be simple, as the only finding; or it can be complex, accompanied by fluid, in which case it is called a hydropneumothorax or hemopneumothorax (Figure 2-17). Depending on

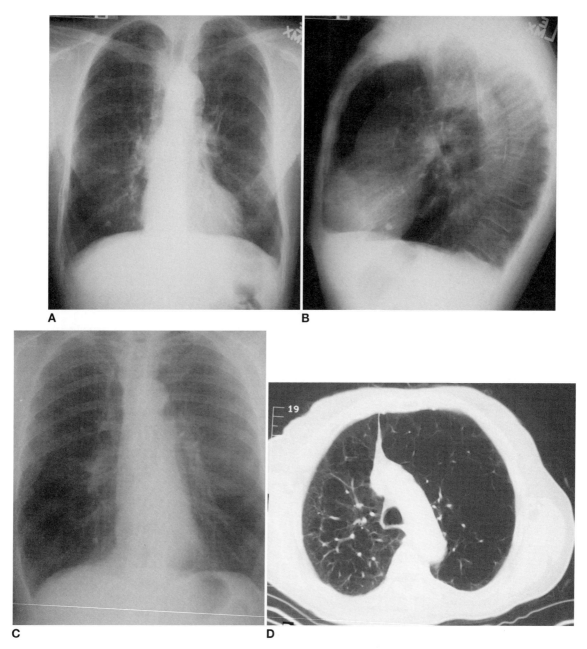

FIGURE 2-16 A, Emphysema. This PA image shows the lungs to be hyperinflated with loss of normal vascular markings, which causes a hyperlucent appearance. These findings are specific for emphysema, but the chest x-ray is not very sensitive for the diagnosis of emphysema. **B,** Emphysema. On the accompanying lateral film, the changes of hyperinflation are clearly seen, with flattening of the normal diaphragmatic curvature and an increased AP diameter of the thoracic cage. The retrosternal clear space is more spacious than in normal patients (see Figure 2-1, *B*). **C,** Emphysema. This PA film shows a heart that appears small in relation to the remainder of the thorax. There are other changes of hyperinflation with some flattening of the diaphragm, and there are also thin, stretched pulmonary vessels. **D,** Emphysema on a CT scan. This section of a CT scan at the level of the aortic arch *(arrow)* is from a different patient. The areas of tissue destruction are seen as dark spaces surrounded by thin residual lung on both sides, although the bullae on the left are larger than those on the right and the resulting hyperexpansion has shifted the mediastinal structures toward the right. The thin band of tissue reaching to the anterior chest wall represents the four layers of pleura (two parietal and two visceral) that form the anterior junction line. (Case courtesy Dr. Peter Hentzen.)

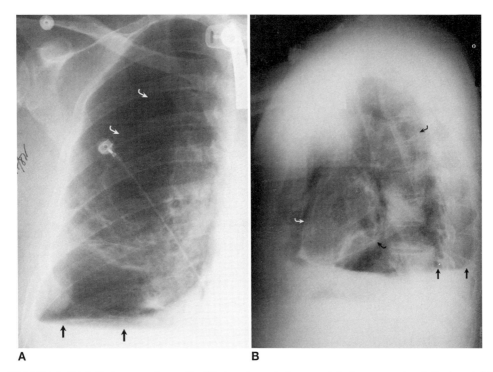

A   **B**

FIGURE 2-17 A, Hydropneumothorax. The PA view demonstrates several findings seen when both air and fluid occupy the pleural space. The air-fluid level *(straight arrows)* is clearly seen, as is the pleural stripe *(curved arrows)* outlined by air in the lung and the pleural space. **B,** Hydropneumothorax. The additional perspective afforded by the lateral view also demonstrates the extent of the air. In this case, pleural air *(curved arrows)* is clearly seen anterior, posterior, and beneath the lung, allowing the fluid in the pleural space to seek its own level *(straight arrow)* on an upright film or on decubitus films. Note how the lung has not completely collapsed around the hilum, as is often the case in patients without a history of trauma or significant inflammatory disease that could cause adhesions.

the amount of air that is present and its location, there may or may not be atelectasis of the underlying lung. In extreme cases, so-called *tension pneumothorax,* the air leak brings about significant displacement of the mediastinum and contralateral lung into the opposite hemithorax, causing significant functional compromise.

Pleural air is not always at the periphery of the thoracic cavity. Anterior air is quite common in those patients who are confined to bed and imaged with portable equipment. Posterior, subpulmonic, and medial collections are not rare.[29] The presence of prior lung disease, especially if it has resulted in adhesions, can radically alter the way a lung collapses away from the chest wall, leaving pockets of air in unusual locations. It is even possible to have lung markings all the way to the chest wall and still have a significant pneumothorax present if, for example, the upper lobe remains well expanded and the lower lobe pulls away from the chest wall collapsing toward the hilum (Figure 2-18).

Many clinicians ask for an estimation of the percentage of air, but without a CT scan and calculation of the area of air on each slice, it is not possible to obtain an accurate measure of a three-dimensional process on a two-dimensional image. If a measurement in centimeters is given at a particular point along the chest wall (usually where the air collection is greatest), this can be compared from day to day to evaluate any change in the pneumothorax.

Although visualization of a pleural line is very helpful, it might not always be possible. When seen, this line is the result

of air delineating both sides of the visceral pleura—from the inside by normally aerated lung and on the outside by the pleural air. The pleural line is best seen where the beam is tangential to the peripheral surface (even if this is medial). At times, the only clue to the presence of this air is an extraordinary sharpness to the cardiac or diaphragmatic silhouette, a clarity made possible because it is outlined by pure air and not by normal lung containing soft tissues in addition to the air—a sort of reverse silhouette sign.

PNEUMOMEDIASTINUM

Detection of air in the soft tissue space between the lungs can present a difficult diagnostic challenge, especially if only a small amount is present. The almost routine use of CT scan in cases of chest trauma has shown that it is not uncommon for air to be present in the mediastinum even when it cannot be demonstrated on plain film studies. The presence of this air, seen acutely in cases of injury to the tracheobronchial tree, peripheral airways, esophagus, or, even more significantly as the result of an abscess within the mediastinum, carries grave prognostic implication for the patient.[30]

If air is seen in the upper mediastinum or supraclavicular fossae, then diagnosis is usually not a problem. However, when there is air along the heart border on either side but not demonstrated clearly elsewhere, the differentiation between pneumomediastinum and medial pneumothorax might not be possible, the difference being whether the air is beneath the parietal pleura or between the pleural layers.

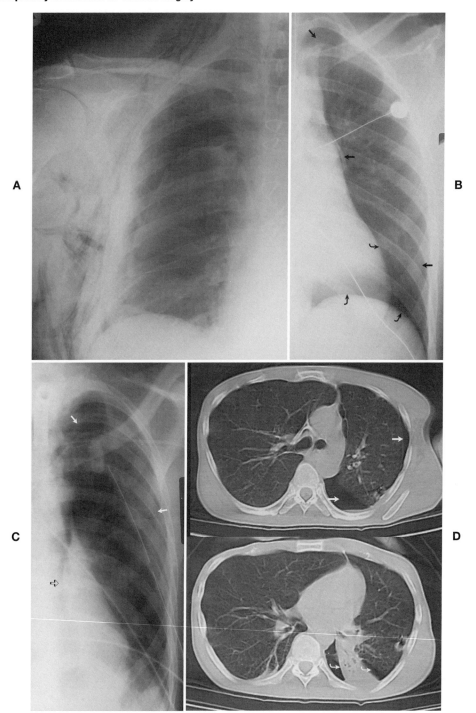

FIGURE 2-18 A, Pneumothorax. This PA computed radiograph (CR) shows a significant pneumothorax on the right, with much of the lung retracted toward the hilum following the breach of the pleura. Note on the CR how the pleural margin is easier to see than on the other films in this figure, and how much more of the normal vascular and interstitial structures are also more readily identified. This particular example also shows extensive subcutaneous emphysema, which is probably related to the leak that produced the pneumothorax. **B,** Medial and subpulmonic pneumothorax. This PA film shows a pneumothorax (pleural line is marked with *straight arrows*) that extends around the periphery of the lung to the apex and then can be seen medially near the heart border. Notice how sharp the heart border and diaphragm *(curved arrows)* appear because they are touched only by air and not by air-containing lung with blood and interstitial soft tissues in addition to the alveolar air. **C,** Posteromedial pneumothorax. PA film demonstrating a posteromedial pneumothorax *(open arrow)* in addition to more typical peripheral pleural air *(straight arrows)* seen at the apex and along the lateral chest wall. **D,** Posteromedial pneumothorax. Frames from a CT scan done the same day showing the pleural air peripherally *(top section—arrow)* and the loculated posteromedial collections *(lower section—curved arrows)* outlining a partially atelectatic lung. This air is represented by the lucent area near the spine on the standard radiograph **(C).** Note also the thoracostomy tube (which appears to be in the pleural space but is not communicating with the pneumothorax in this case) and air bronchograms in the partially atelectatic lung.

Pneumomediastinum, especially in those cases resulting from injury to the airways, can dissect downward through the posterior soft tissues into the retroperitoneum (and from there, even into the scrotum); more rarely, it can break into the peritoneal cavity, presenting as pneumoperitoneum. As in the case of pneumothorax, these mediastinal collections of air are often seen more easily on CT than on plain film examination. Pneumomediastinum must also be distinguished from pneumopericardium, in which air surrounds the inferior aspect of the heart rather than just the sides (Figure 2-19).

INTERSTITIAL AIR

A number of small, lucent areas in either one or both lungs are occasionally seen in premature infants being treated with positive end-expiratory pressure (PEEP) for surfactant deficiency disorder (formerly referred to as *hyaline membrane disease* or *respiratory distress syndrome*). As in these newborns, this pulmonary interstitial emphysema (PIE) can lead to other, more ominous extraalveolar collections, namely pneumomediastinum or pneumothorax. It is often difficult to identify PIE in adults unless the alveoli are filled with fluid (blood, pus, or water). In these cases it might have the cystic or circular appearance expected in infants but also present as streaky lucency in the peribronchial and perivascular spaces.[31]

SUBCUTANEOUS EMPHYSEMA

Air in the soft tissues outside the thoracic skeleton is almost always of traumatic origin. In rare cases, the presence of an abscess of the chest wall will present with gas in the soft tissues, although this is frequently bubbly in appearance rather than streaklike. Rib fractures, thoracostomy tubes, and penetrating injuries are frequently associated with this finding, usually close to the point of break in the skin or pleura initially, but eventually spreading a distance from this spot. Pneumomediastinum that breaks through into the supraclavicular fossa is also a fairly common finding. In longstanding leaks, the air can cover a significant expanse of the thorax, at times outlining individual bundles within the pectoralis and other chest wall muscles. When this air is projected over the lung fields, it can make it quite difficult to fully evaluate the underlying parenchyma.

Monitoring and Life Support Devices

A significant number of films are obtained on ICU and recovery room patients to evaluate newly placed vascular catheters, endotracheal tubes, or pleural drainage (thoracostomy or "chest") and mediastinal tubes. For each of these devices, there

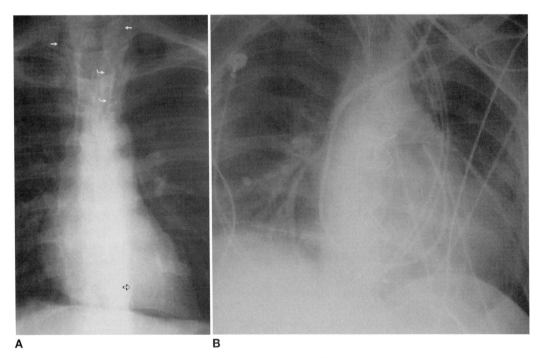

A   **B**

FIGURE 2-19 A, Pneumomediastinum. On this close-up view of a PA radiograph, streaky lucent lines are seen overlying the soft tissues of the neck *(straight arrows),* the upper mediastinum *(curved arrows),* and the paraspinal region *(open arrow),* representing air that has leaked from a small injury somewhere in the bronchial tree. Note also the sharp border of the left side of the heart, similar to that seen with a medial pneumothorax, and air beneath the heart on the right side. **B,** Pneumopericardium. Pneumomediastinum is a more common observation than pneumopericardium, but both can have the appearance of a lucent line surrounding the heart. The radiologic difference is that air surrounding the inferior aspect of the heart indicates that the most likely diagnosis is pneumopericardium. This PA image was taken following a heart-lung transplant. A thin opaque line is separated from the heart by a lucent area. The lucency extends completely around the inferior aspect of the heart. This appearance is the result of pneumopericardium, which is an infrequent but life-threatening complication.

are preferred locations within which the tip of these devices should be found for optimal functioning. The chest film serves not only to verify the position of the catheter or tube but also to detect possible complications related to inadvertent injury from placement of the device. There are many brands of these devices, and although the function of each type is similar, detailed differences in their specific appearance may vary.

Central Venous Pressure Catheters

Central venous pressure (CVP) catheters are used to administer large volumes of fluids or medications that need to be given centrally rather than via peripheral venous access.[32] At the same time, proximity to the heart and great vessels allow monitoring of intravascular volume and the efficiency of the pumping action of the heart. The peripheral route should not be used to administer some types of hyperalimentation products, antibiotics, chemotherapeutic agents, or cardiovascular drugs.

These catheters are usually placed either by a subclavian or internal jugular vein (IJV) approach. In the acutely ill patient, they are often placed percutaneously; in the more chronically ill, they may have a tunneled approach or implanted subcutaneous chamber that permits easy vascular access without the need for repeated venipuncture. These catheters are usually located in the superior vena cava between the level of the arch of the azygous vein and above the right atrium, although the precise location of the atriocaval junction can often be difficult to discern. They definitely should terminate central to the valves that are located near the end of the subclavian vein or the internal jugular vein. Those placed by a left IJV approach can present special challenges, as these catheters may enter the superior intercostal vein and follow the hemiazygous vein rather than the left subclavian vein into the superior vena cava. Occasionally, the presence of a persistent left superior vena cava is demonstrated by the course of these catheters along the left side of the spine. Care must be taken that these catheters are not placed with the tip in a location that would place them against the flow of blood (i.e., below the right atrium into the upper part of the inferior vena cava or the contralateral subclavian vein or even the IJV) (Figure 2-20). In cases in which the vena cava is obstructed, the tips of these catheters might not lie in the desired location, although there should be a suspicion that this is the case based on the contours of the mediastinum. The catheter's position can change with patient motion—especially flexion or extension of the neck—and the position should be carefully evaluated on any chest film taken on the patient, even if for other reasons. In addition to the multiple-lumen catheters usually seen, a simple vascular sheath that permits the placement or exchange of different catheters may be placed by either of these routes.

Although not a common type of malpositioning, placement of subclavian venous catheters in an artery may occur. It is not always possible to tell clinically by the color of the blood or its pulsations that an arterial catheter has been placed. Radiographically, the key is the course of the catheter, which tends to rise in a gentle curve above the medial end of the clavicle rather than parallel this structure and then cross to the left side of the spine, following the course of the aorta (Figure 2-20, *B*).

Central catheters inserted by a peripheral approach are also quite popular. The position of the tip of peripherally inserted catheters should be in the same area as a more centrally placed catheter, and the same potential for malpositioning (except for arterial placement) exists. With these catheters there is a fairly common tendency to be poorly positioned at or near the level of the axilla, with the catheters frequently directed into collateral veins, sometimes turning 180 degrees backward into the upper arm (Figure 2-20, *C* and *D*).

At times, a catheter might pass through the wall of the vein, in which case the tip is in the perivascular soft tissues. In these cases, infusion of intravenous fluids can lead to a widened mediastinum (Figure 2-21). This is usually quite easy to detect by careful comparison of preinsertion and postinsertion films. Because the subclavian vein lies close to the pleural surface of the lung, a pneumothorax might result, even when there is little or no difficulty with insertion of the catheter. Expiratory films are helpful to accentuate small pleural air collections.

Pulmonary Arterial Catheters

These catheters are most often placed by either an IJV or a subclavian vein approach. They measure pulmonary capillary wedge pressure, which gives a more accurate reflection of left atrial volume (and, therefore, left ventricular end-diastolic volume) than is possible with other central catheters. On rare occasions they may be inserted via the femoral venous route. The tip of one of these catheters should preferably be in the right or left main pulmonary artery, or occasionally in the interlobar artery on the right or the lower lobe artery on the left (Figure 2-22). A more central location is preferable. Care should be taken not to allow the catheter tip to "float" too far peripherally, where it could potentially occlude a smaller branch causing a pulmonary infarction, even if the balloon used to temporarily occlude the vessel for pressure measurement is not inflated. With these pulmonary arterial catheters, the main problem of malpositioning occurs if the catheter coils within the right atrium of the right ventricle, although the problems covered under CVP catheters apply as well.

Aortic Counterpulsation Balloon Pump

Aortic counterpulsation balloon pumps, which are used to improve the circulation of a failing heart, operate by rapidly inflating in the descending aorta during diastole. The tip, which is visible as the result of a small, radioopaque marker, should be at the level of the aortic arch, which would place it just distal to the left subclavian artery.

Transvenous Pacemakers and Implanted Defibrillators

These pacing leads are usually placed by one of the same routes used for pulmonary arterial catheters. The main difference is that for pacemakers and defibrillators, the tip should be within the apex of the right ventricle. This is usually clearly apparent on the AP film, but occasionally a lateral view is needed. Often, evaluation of the position of the electrode is done by electrocardiography.

Endotracheal Tubes

The major means of providing ventilatory support is through an endotracheal tube.[33] Because clinical evaluation of the

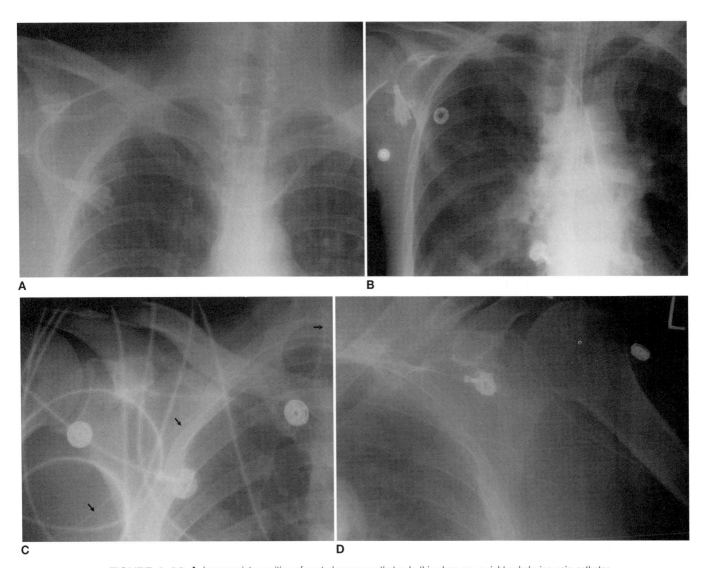

FIGURE 2-20 A, Inappropriate position of central venous catheter. In this close-up, a right subclavian vein catheter crosses the midline into the lower end of the left subclavian vein rather than downward into the superior vena cava. **B,** Inappropriate position of central venous catheter. PA film of the chest showing the result of an attempted insertion of a right subclavian vein catheter that is actually in the artery. Note the upward curve over the medial end of the clavicle (venous catheters should more closely parallel the lower margin of this bone) and its course toward the left side of the spine overlying the descending aorta. **C,** Inappropriate position of central venous catheter. This close-up view of the right side of the chest and neck shows a common occurrence when a central catheter is inserted through this area. The catheter can be followed from the axilla through the right subclavian vein and upward into the internal jugular vein *(arrows),* again against the flow of blood. **D,** Inappropriate position of central venous catheter. In this patient, a catheter was inserted on the left side and is coiled into a collateral vein at the level of the shoulder. Note also that the tip is coiled in a tight loop, creating a potential trap for platelets and the eventual possibility of formation of an embolus.

adequacy of the position of these tubes is sometimes unreliable, it is important to radiographically confirm the location of the tip of the tube and, by inference, of the balloon used to seal the airway. A radiopaque stripe in the wall of the tube aids in visualization. In a so-called *armored endotracheal tube,* a spring in the wall makes evaluation of the level easier, although the nonopaque portion of the tube may extend some distance below the coil, making estimation of the actual location of the tip difficult (Figure 2-23, *A*).

The position of a tube can change easily with flexion or extension of the neck, or even if the patient turns his or her head from one side to the other. In general, the tube should be located from 3 to 5 centimeters above the carina, a landmark that is often easily identified on portable films. If the carina is not easily identified, positioning of the tube at about the level of the aortic arch is a quick way to avoid the potential complications that come from bronchial intubation, which can often result in very rapid collapse of the contralateral lung (Figures 2-23, *B* and *C*). If the tip of the tube is high—well above the level of the medial end of the clavicles—then inflation of the balloon in the larynx is possible. Ideally the tube will be one half to two thirds of the diameter

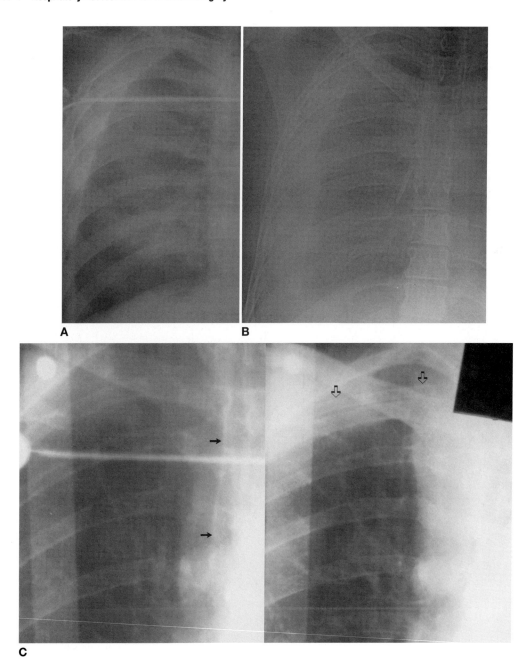

FIGURE 2-21 **A,** Central catheter with fluid in the pleural space. The end of the right subclavian central catheter projects over the mid-chest, indicating an extravascular location. The pleural effusion resulted from direct infusion of intravenous fluid into the pleural space. **B,** Central catheter with fluid in the pleural space. PA chest image shows the tip of a right subclavian catheter projecting over the right pulmonary artery. The tip is too lateral and inferior to be in the superior vena cava. The large pleural effusion resulted from infusion of intravenous fluid directly into the pleural space. **C,** Vascular sheath with fluid in the mediastinum. In this figure, on the original film obtained upon arrival at the hospital *(left image),* there is a normal contour to the right side of the mediastinum. Note the right paratracheal stripe *(straight arrows).* On the follow-up study 5 minutes later *(right image),* following insertion of a vascular sheath in the right subclavian vein *(open arrows),* note the widened indistinct margin of the mediastinum. The medial end of the sheath is directed a bit cephalad, indicating that it probably passed through the vein, and that fluid that was administered is not intravascular but rather is accumulating in the upper mediastinum.

of the trachea, and the inflated cuff will not bulge the tracheal wall.

Complications that rarely occur, even in times of difficult intubation, include perforation of the trachea, larynx, or even one of the pyriform sinuses. In these cases, the appearance of pneumomediastinum and difficulty with maintaining ventilation following intubation can be a valuable clue. Intubation of the esophagus is also a recognized complication, and radiographic diagnosis can be difficult on the AP film, although the addition of a lateral study can help.

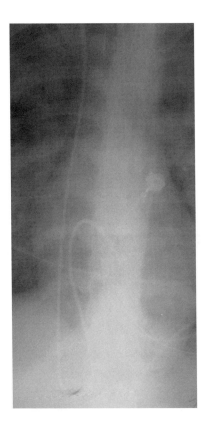

FIGURE 2-22 Abnormal pulmonary artery catheter position. This PA portable film shows a pulmonary artery catheter that apparently lodged in the apex of the right ventricle or beneath the papillary muscles and folded downward into the inferior vena cava as more catheter was introduced in an effort to place the tip in the usual location. The pulmonary edema seen was the result of an allergic reaction to paint, and it cleared rather quickly.

Double-Lumen Endobronchial Tubes

Double-lumen endobronchial tubes allow differential ventilation of each lung. The tip of each lumen is identified with a radioopaque marker. The main portion of the tube is placed in the lower trachea approximately 1 to 2 cm above the carina, with the bronchial extension inserted far enough into one of the main bronchi that the inflated cuff does not project across the carina and accidentally occlude the other bronchus (Figure 2-23, *D*). Care must be taken not to place the tube too far into the main bronchus, which could lead to the possible occlusion of the upper lobe bronchus, which, in turn, might result in atelectasis or hyperexpansion if the tip were directed into a smaller bronchial branch.

Tracheostomy Tubes

Tracheostomy tubes are used when longer-term ventilatory support will be needed, or in those patients who undergo neck surgery. These devices can be either plastic or metal and in either case are radiopaque and quite visible on films. The tip should be several centimeters above the carina. Tracheostomy tubes are not as sensitive to changes in position of the head and neck, and if it should become dislodged it is more readily apparent than is the case with an endotracheal tube. Complications with a tracheostomy are usually related to the

placement of the device, although they can become dislodged and lose effectiveness.

Nasogastric Tubes

Nasogastric tubes seem to be almost ubiquitous among patients in intensive care units. By clearing excess fluid, they are important for minimizing the possibility of aspiration and can also be used to deliver medications or nutritional support. Visualizing the course through the esophagus is aided by the presence of barium sulfate as a marker in the wall of most tubes. The course of the tube can be an indicator of significant shift of mediastinal structures or the presence of abnormal tissues such as blood or tumor (Figures 2-24). It is important to see that both the side port and the end hole of this tube are below the gastroesophageal junction, to minimize the possibility of reflux of gastric contents into the lower esophageal segment and subsequent aspiration. Dobbhoff tubes are a particular type of nasoenteric tube with weighted tips that aid in their passage through the stomach and into the duodenum (or even on to the jejunum). These tubes may have a stiffening wire used for insertion that also aids in visualization, but they do not have the opaque marker in the wall and may be more difficult to see, especially on films that are not taken with ideal technique.

The major concern with the placement of either of these types of enteric tubes is accidental intubation of one of the main bronchi, usually the right because of its more vertical orientation. It is especially important to confirm the location of the end of the tube before administration of medications, hyperalimentation products, or even water, as serious chemical pneumonitis can result from inadvertently placing these fluids in the lungs. Perforation of the upper airway or even the esophagus is fairly rare but shares many of the same findings seen with perforation by an endotracheal tube—pneumomediastinum or an unusual course of the tube (Figure 2-25).

Percutaneous gastrostomy tubes are not included in this discussion, as these are rarely seen on chest radiographs.

Pleural Drainage Catheters

The last life support device in common use that is discussed the pleural drainage catheter, usually referred to as a *chest tube* or *thoracostomy tube*. There are three main types used: the usual large-caliber tube (20 to 30 French), the small-caliber tube, and a pigtail catheter. Pigtail catheters are often used in the evacuation of viscous fluid collections.

The typical and most common tubes have a side hole and end hole in addition to an opaque marker similar to a nasogastric tube. These are also used as mediastinal drains in many cases of cardiac surgery. Smaller-caliber tubes are frequently used following minor surgery, such as after a percutaneous lung biopsy or placement of a central venous catheter that has resulted in a pneumothorax. Equipped with a one-way valve, these small-caliber tubes are ideal for short-term placement to manage minor air leaks. The pigtail catheters placed for drainage of thicker fluid collections have multiple side holes that help assure continued functioning even in the presence of material that can obstruct other types of tubes.

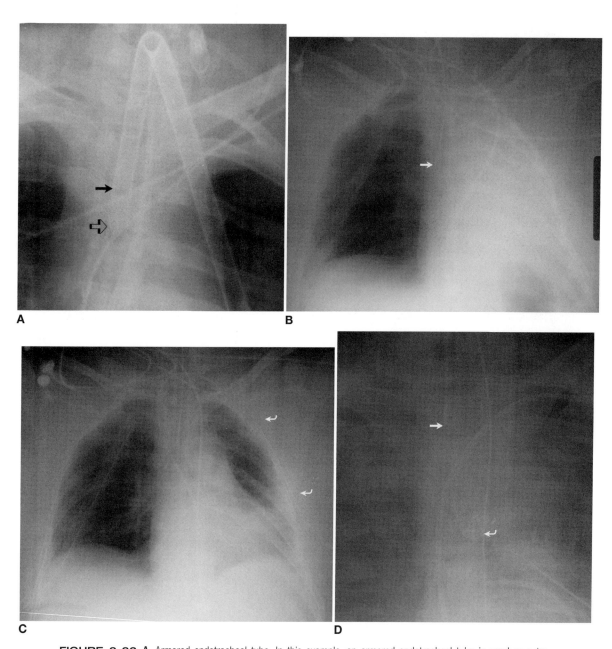

FIGURE 2-23 **A,** Armored endotracheal tube. In this example, an armored endotracheal tube is used as a tracheostomy tube, with the tip *(open arrow)* approximately 2 cm below the end of the coil *(straight arrow),* but still approximately 3 cm above the carina. **B,** Endotracheal tube obstructing the left main bronchus. This PA portable film shows an endotracheal tube in the right main bronchus *(straight arrow)* with collapse of the left lung, and a shift of the mediastinal structures to that side. The very opaque left hemithorax might be mistaken for a large pleural effusion or hemothorax, although in those cases the mediastinal structures should be shifted toward the opposite side. **C,** Endotracheal tube repositioned. Another film done 1 hour later shows the tube withdrawn to a normal position with subsequent reexpansion of the left lung and return of the heart to its usual position. Also note that a thoracostomy tube has been inserted on the left but is located outside the thoracic cage *(curved arrows).* **D,** Double-lumen endobronchial tube, properly located. A portable PA film shows a double-lumen endobronchial tube with the tracheal orifice *(straight arrow)* and bronchial extension in the left main bronchus *(curved arrow),* allowing differential ventilation in this postoperative patient.

The placement of these tubes is fraught with potential for malpositioning. Many tubes can be inadvertently placed either in the major fissure or the lung parenchyma. Depending on whether the mission is to drain pleural fluid or relieve a pneumothorax, positioning of the tube will alter the effectiveness of a particular device. At times, tubes can be inadvertently directed into the posterior costophrenic sulcus or subpulmonic space. To fully evaluate the position of a drain, AP and lateral films are very useful.[34] Although CT scans yield the greatest sensitivity for following the course of a tube through the thorax, they should be necessary only in rare cases. On the AP film, a tube that has been inserted low on the

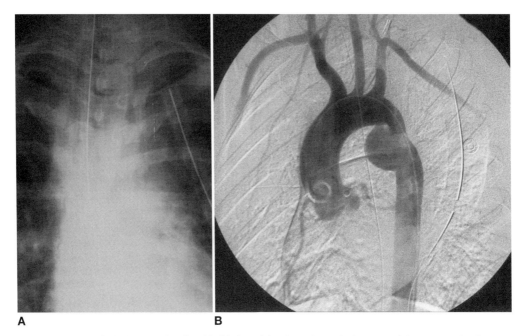

A   **B**

FIGURE 2-24 A, Aortic laceration. Portable PA view of the chest shows displacement of the nasogastric tube away from the aortic arch, suggesting mediastinal hematoma in this patient with significant trauma from a deceleration injury (see also Figure 2-4, C and D for comparison of the normal relation of the esophagus with a nasogastric tube and the aortic arch). Note also the pneumomediastinum. **B,** Aortic laceration. A single frame from the angiogram demonstrates the intimal tear of the descending aorta that was the source of the blood.

lateral wall should parallel the thoracic cage toward the apex. If it crosses the lung field or curves away from the chest wall, it is quite possibly in the interlobar fissure or the lung parenchyma, and in either location it is less effective, as it might not be communicating with the pleural space (Figure 2-26).

Specific Postoperative Changes From Thoracotomy

Segmental Resection

In some ways, resection of a segment of the lung will produce changes somewhat similar to segmental atelectasis, in that a portion of the lung is no longer present (rather than collapsed), and the remaining segments of the lobe, and other lobes on that side, will expand to fill the space. Although the increased opacity typical of atelectasis might not be present, there could be displacement of the interlobar fissure and elevation of the diaphragm. There might be displacement of the hilum. Often the most telling sign of the surgery is the presence of fine metallic sutures on the pleural surface at the site of resection and of a chest tube (and sometimes an osteotomy of a posterior portion of a rib). Initially, there may be changes related to the trauma of the surgery; that is, small nonspecific areas of opacity representing contusion or atelectasis, or even a small effusion (in the case of hemothorax). In spite of the breach in the pleural space, subcutaneous emphysema is not as common following surgery as in other forms of trauma, although persistent pneumothorax can be a vexing problem.

Lobectomy

Removal of an entire lobe will often lead to a greater initial deformity of the involved hemithorax and some shift of the midline structures. As in cases of atelectasis, there should be compensatory overinflation of the noninvolved lobes, which follows predictable patterns. Prior surgery or infection with resultant adhesions can slow or stop this process. Careful evaluation for the presence of atelectasis in the operated lung is important to prevent further complications, such as exudates or pneumonia. With a lobectomy there are often surgical clips at the hilum and sutures on the surface, as fissures are often not complete and the cut pleural surface must be sealed to prevent air leaks.

Pneumonectomy

Removal of an entire lung leads to more drastic radiographic changes that evolve with the passage of time. Initially, the affected side shows expected postoperative changes at the hilum and chest wall with a complete absence of lung tissue, leaving a very stark, air-filled cavity with extremely sharp margins of the heart and diaphragm. Immediate postoperative evaluation should also include the search for any significant shift in the position of normal mediastinal structures and signs of atelectasis in the remaining lung. Rapid mediastinal shift can signify the presence of an air leak with a "ball-valve" effect leading to a tension pneumothorax. There is usually some elevation of the hemidiaphragm and a shift of the heart and other midline structures toward the operated side as the remaining lung expands to take up some (though not all) of the space. Gradually, the hemithorax fills with fluid, showing a distinct air

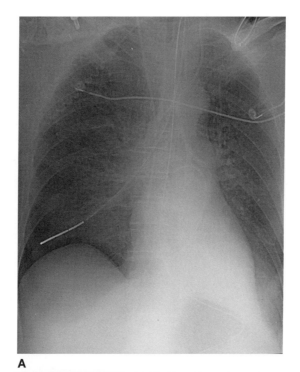

A

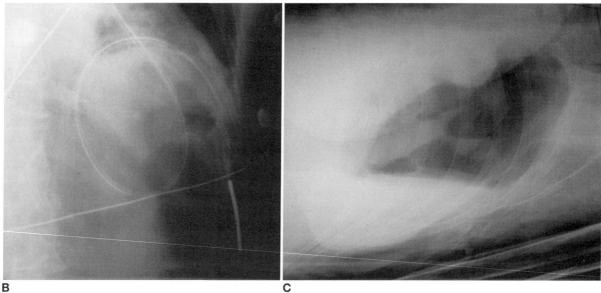

B   **C**

FIGURE 2-25 A, Feeding tube in right lower lobe with pneumothorax. The tube projected over the right lower lobe is a feeding tube that has been placed in the trachea and advanced into the right lower lobe bronchus. The lucent area in the right costophrenic angle is the result of an inferior pneumothorax. This indicates that the tube has perforated the bronchus, passed into the lung and entered the pleural space. This is a serious complication of feeding tube placement. It is possible that the pneumothorax might expand when the feeding tube is removed. **B,** Abdominal image with feeding tube looped in left pleural space. Coned view of the upper left quadrant of the abdomen shows a feeding tube that is looped with the tip in a position lateral to the expected location of the fundus of the stomach. The more proximal portion of the tube is lateral to the expected position of the esophagus. The tube is actually in the left lower lobe bronchus and has advanced into the pleural space. The large loop is in the posterior inferior pleural space. **C,** Feeding tube in left lower lobe with pneumothorax. Left side down lateral decubitus chest image shows multiple air-fluid levels and a large lucent space with no lung markings. The large opacity adjacent to the hilum is the collapsed left lung. The lucency and the air-fluid levels are the result of a loculated hydropneumothorax. The patient had a left pleural effusion before placement of the feeding tube, but the pneumothorax resulted from the perforation of the tube through the bronchus and lung into the pleural space. Rapid development of a large pneumothorax following the pleural placement or removal of a feeding tube from the pleural space can require urgent placement of a thoracostomy tube.

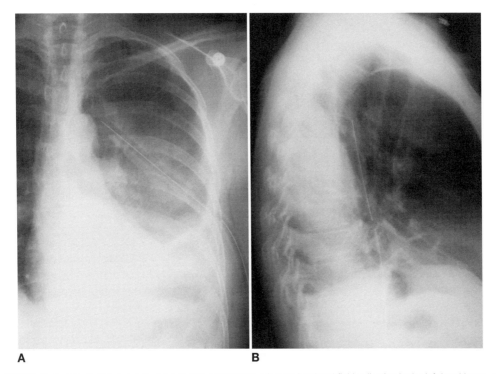

A   B

FIGURE 2-26 A, Thoracostomy tube. In this patient with a known loculated fluid collection in the left hemithorax, a PA film shows a thoracostomy tube projected over this opacity. Placement of the tube did not decrease the size of the collection compared to earlier studies. **B,** Thoracostomy tube. The lateral film shows that the tube is in the major fissure, displaced anteriorly by the mass effect of the fluid on the lower lobe or in the lung parenchyma but not in the pleural fluid collection. A lateral view in addition to the frontal film will frequently show the need to reposition a tube so that it is able to drain either the fluid or air that may be present in the pleural space.

fluid level if the patient is upright, or a more subtle increase in opacity if the patient is supine. Too rapid an accumulation of fluid can signify the presence of bleeding, although it may be seen with extrapleural thoracostomy or when the surgery involves lysis of adhesions. The fluid can remain for years, although much of the longer-term radiographic change is related to changes in the position of the heart and expansion of the remaining lung. On later films, at first glance it might seem that there is a large effusion causing the complete opacification of the hemithorax, but careful observation will reveal that the heart is shifted into and covered by this opacity rather than being displaced toward the opposite side, as would be the case with fluid.

Volume Reduction Surgery

Recently, surgery to reduce the size of bullae in an effort to improve the efficiency of the remaining lung tissue has taken its place in the treatment of emphysema. In practical terms, large bullous cysts behave just like any other space-occupying lesion to cause passive (compressive) atelectasis. These cysts can be eliminated, and then the reexpanded lung should be able to function closer to its ideal state. Evaluation of the postoperative state should be fairly straightforward, with staples and fine wire sutures indicating which part of the lung was restored. Although these findings can be quite subtle, if the preoperative films are available for comparison, the radiographic changes can be quite dramatic.

Video-Assisted Thoracic Surgery

More recently, video-assisted thoracic surgery (VATS) has enabled surgeons to sample and remove small, peripheral lesions that previously required more extensive surgery and a longer hospitalization. Depending on the extent of the biopsy or resection, changes similar to those for any other type of thoracic surgery may be seen, from an essentially normal film, to one or more vascular clips, to sutures indicating resection of a portion of the lung.

Other Imaging Techniques

Up to this point, this discussion has focused on traditional radiographs in the preoperative and postoperative phases. Newer imaging technology studies, however, will often accompany the patient to the operating room. Computed tomography (CT), magnetic resonance imaging (MRI), nuclear medicine (NM), and even ultrasound images quite frequently play a part in the preoperative evaluation of patients about to undergo thoracic surgery.

Computed Tomography

CT scans bear the closest relationship of these other imaging studies to plain film radiographs in that the source of the image is ionizing radiation, although with CT scans the image is seen through the "eyes" of a digital computer rather than by an analog or digital cassette. With the patient lying supine on the table, an x-ray tube with one to four rows of detectors (soon to be increased to 16 or 32 rows) directly opposite the tube spins around the patient, usually in less than 1 second, recording the amount of radiation absorbed (attenuated) by its passage through the body. Using mathematical formulas, these powerful computers create an image based on the differing tissue densities present, assigning shades of gray or a color in proportion to a particular tissue's ability to stop the x-ray beam—from very black (representing air) to very white (representing bone or metal), with water considered the midpoint. Fatty tissues have a negative attenuation coefficient and appear darker than pure fluid, and soft tissues (heart, muscle, lymph nodes, or tumor) have a mildly positive coefficient and so appear more toward the white end of the scale. These computer-based images offer two main advantages: the ability to discriminate tissue differences better than film alone, and the ability to view images in cross section, leaving only a limited thickness of body to view at a given time. And because CT scans are computer generated and stored, they can be "tuned" to highlight specific tissue types and can be viewed and filmed in multiple modes without additional radiation exposure to the patient. Three-dimensional reconstructions of these various data sets allow visualization of entire organs or structures in a manner closer to what is observed in the operating room. Virtual angiography, colonoscopy, or bronchoscopy further extends the preoperative evaluation of many disease states.

Although CT is usually considered for evaluating tumors, the procedure is also valuable for observing focal or diffuse parenchymal disease, bronchiectasis, emphysema, chest wall and mediastinal lesions, and pleural fluid collections, demonstrating their effect on the underlying lung tissue. It is commonly used in the postoperative patient to "see through" pleural effusion or through lungs that are too opaque with alveolar lung disease or atelectasis to be adequately visualized by standard radiographs, or to gain a better understanding of the position of drainage tubes that are not performing as expected. Today, rapid infusion contrast CT with a multidetector scanner is the examination of choice in many departments for evaluation of suspected pulmonary embolism. The main disadvantage in using CT in these cases is the difficulty encountered in moving critically ill patients to the radiology department (Figure 2-27).

Magnetic Resonance Imaging

MRI produces images that superficially appear similar to CT scans. These are also computer-generated images, usually in cross-sectional orientation but also with direct sagittal or coronal views, with tissues displayed in varying shades of black, white, and gray. The most significant difference is the source of

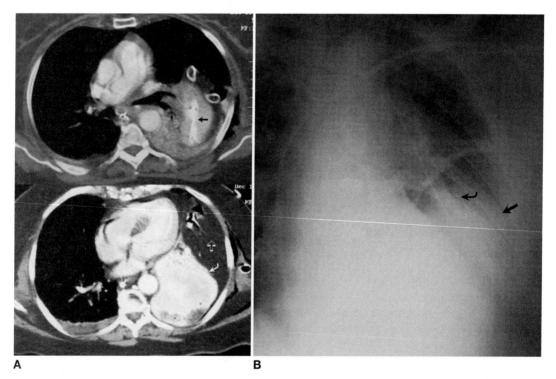

A   **B**

FIGURE 2-27 A, CT scan in a trauma patient. Two of more than 50 sections from this patient with diaphragmatic rupture show the fundus of the stomach with a nasogastric tube *(straight arrow on the top image)* and the contrast-filled stomach adjacent to the heart *(curved arrow on the bottom image)*. On this bottom image, the somewhat darker area anterior to the stomach *(open arrow)* represents abdominal fat that was herniated with the stomach through the defect created in the diaphragm. (Case courtesy Dr. Peter Hentzen.) **B,** Diaphragmatic rupture. This PA film in a different patient who also had a rupture of the diaphragm following trauma shows a similar opacity in the left lower hemithorax, corresponding to the body of the stomach (straight arrow) herniated through a defect in the diaphragm created as a result of trauma. The tip of the nasogastric tube is also seen *(curved arrow)*, but it could easily be mistaken for a second thoracostomy tube.

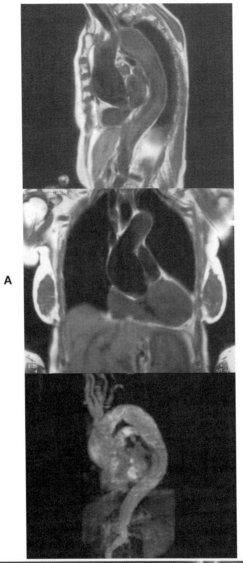

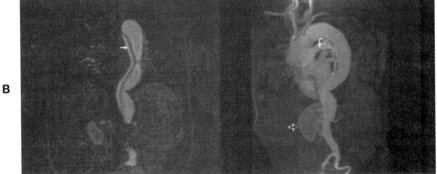

FIGURE 2-28 A, MRI of thorax showing aortic insufficiency. These three images demonstrate the way MRI allows reconstruction of data in several different ways. The top image shows a sagittal view of the thoracic aorta with dilatation at its root and tortuosity of the descending portion of the artery. The middle image (coronal) shows not only the dilated root but also origins of both carotid arteries and the left subclavian artery. A portion of the innominate artery is seen overlying the apex of the right lung. The bottom image shows just the root of the aorta and major vessels seen on the other views and the vertebral arteries. (Case courtesy Dr. Peter Hentzen.) **B,** MRI of thorax showing aortic dissection. The *left image* is a single coronal frame from a study that demonstrates an intimal flap from a dissection *(straight arrow)* originating just distal to the origin of the left subclavian artery and extending down into the abdominal aorta. The *right image* is a composite showing the full length of the aorta from its origin to the bifurcation. Also seen are the main and left pulmonary arteries *(curved arrow)* and even the right kidney *(open arrow).* (Case courtesy Dr. Peter Hentzen.)

the information used to produce the sections, not the method by which the computers reconstruct the data.

Instead of using ionizing radiation, MRI scans rely primarily on the evaluation of the amount of protons (water) in different tissues. The data are acquired by placing the patient in a powerful magnetic field and "interrogating" the body with radiowaves of a specific frequency, then listening for the response. By varying the frequency of the radiowave, the body can be imaged in multiple planes, not just in axial sections. Direct sagittal and coronal images enable the radiologist to evaluate involvement of mediastinal structures and the chest wall with greater clarity than what a CT scan offers. The lungs are not well imaged because they contain mostly air and little water. In the cases of apical masses, MRI can demonstrate extension into the chest wall or the brachial plexus. Again, powerful computers and programs extract information, giving almost lifelike renderings of the heart and the great vessels in the thorax, even though there is motion related to each heartbeat. MRI is helpful in imaging these structures in patients with allergy to x-ray contrast (Figure 2-28).

Ultrasound

Because air blocks the transmission of sound waves, ultrasound has limited use in the mostly air-filled thorax. Its chief use is in studying movement and anatomy of the heart (which can be accessed using small, parasternal transducers) and fluid collections at the periphery of the lung. Ultrasound technique is occasionally used to guide thoracentesis procedures for either diagnostic or therapeutic purposes.

Nuclear Medicine and Position Emission Tomography Scans

As the name implies, nuclear medicine depends on the administration of radioactive isotopes to image and evaluate specific physiologic and pathologic processes in the body. Depending on the isotope used, the administered agent will accumulate in specific parts of the body and can then be imaged using cameras that convert the radiant energy of the radiopharmaceutical first into light, then into an electronic pulse, and eventually into an image. For a number of years, the majority of nuclear medicine studies in the operating rooms of patients undergoing thoracic surgery were bone scans for evaluation of metastatic disease. Occasionally, lung scans—usually consisting of a ventilation scan (originally radioactive xenon, now aerosolized compounds with Tc99^m) followed by injection of a small amount of microaggregated albumin (MAA, also labeled with Tc99^m), the tiny particles of which lodge in the capillary bed at the periphery of the lung. The absence of activity (termed a "filling defect") can indicate the presence of an obstruction (embolus or tumor) upstream (Figure 2-29, *A* and *B*). These studies are rapidly being replaced by thin-section multiple-slice CT scans through the major vessels of the lung, using standard intravenous contrast to outline filling defects within the pulmonary arteries. These CT scans can usually be done with less delay than the nuclear medicine examinations, primarily because with nuclear medicine, there is the need to build in time for the preparation of the radiopharmaceuticals. The thin-section CT scans take less time to acquire the images, although review of the large number of sections obtained (up to 80) can take more time unless specific imaging stations or picture

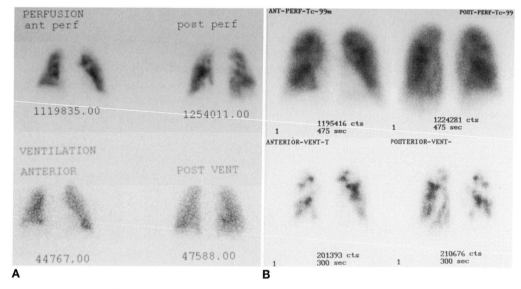

A   **B**

FIGURE 2-29 A, Nuclear medicine scan with pulmonary emboli. Limited views from a study show normal ventilation of both lungs *(bottom row)* following inhalation of technetium 99^m-labeled DTPA aerosol spray. Note the fairly uniform distribution of the activity in comparison to the patchy appearance of the perfusion images *(top row)* done a short time later following injection of 99^m-labeled microaggregated albumin (MAA). The very irregular appearance indicates numerous small emboli throughout the lungs. (Case courtesy Dr. Elliott Turbiner.) **B,** Nuclear medicine scan in a patient with asthma. On these ventilation images *(bottom row)*, the distribution of the inhaled radiopharmaceutical is quite uneven because of areas of air trapping, while the perfusion images *(top row)* are now homogenous, indicating good blood flow throughout the lungs. (Case courtesy Dr. Elliott Turbiner.)

Continued

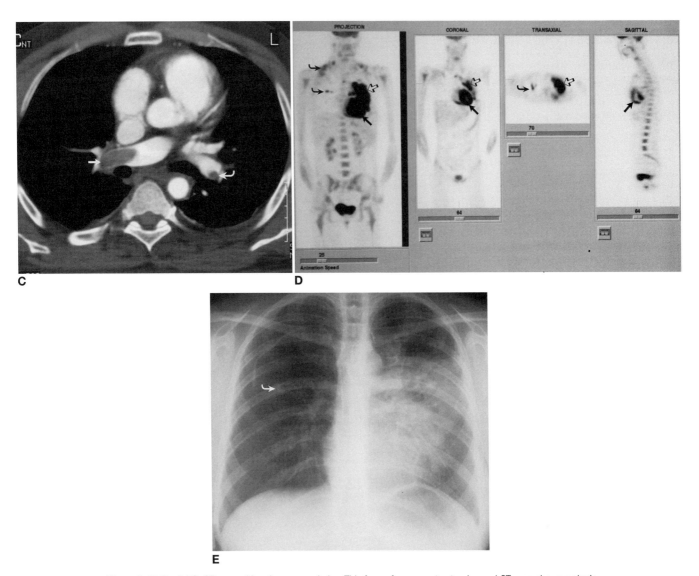

Figure 2-29 Cont'd C, CT scan with pulmonary embolus. This frame from a contrast-enhanced CT scan shows a single large embolus in the right main pulmonary artery *(straight arrow)* and a smaller clot in the left lower lobe pulmonary artery *(curved arrow).* These particular emboli would not have produced the pattern seen on the accompanying perfusion scan, but would probably have shown little or no activity in the right lung and possible segmental defects in the left lower lobe and elsewhere. (Case courtesy Dr. Peter Hentzen.) **D,** PET scan of lung tumor. The positron emission tomography (PET) scan obtained after administration of F^{18}-labeled deoxyglucose (FDG) shows, from left to right, a whole-body projection, a single coronal image, a single axial level, and a sagittal view. When these are viewed in real time, the whole body rotates, and the other planes are reviewed sequentially. The heart is the largest area of activity in the chest *(straight arrows),* with the primary tumor seen on the left *(open arrows)* and metastatic disease on the right *(curved arrows).* (Case courtesy Dr. Elliott Turbiner.) **E,** Chest radiograph of patient with lung tumor in Figure 2-29, *D* (PET scan). This PA film shows the extent of the tumor present in the left side of the chest, but it shows only one of the abnormal areas on the right *(curved arrow).* In this case, the tumor causes a silhouette sign with tumor (rather than alveolar lung disease or atelectasis) responsible for replacement of normally aerated lung at the left border of the heart.

archive communication system (PACS) monitors are used that allow the viewer to scroll through the sections (Figure 2-29, *C*).

The future of nuclear medicine in the thorax is through *positron emission tomography (PET)*, an evolving technology that uses radioactive tracers that are imaged in multiple planes and then displayed in three dimensions, showing areas of activity rather than specific anatomic structures. The current technology primarily relies on F^{18}-labeled deoxyglucose (FDG), which plays a central role in cellular metabolism and tends to concentrate in the heart, brain, and actively growing tissue (i.e., tumors) when the patient is kept at rest. PET-CT fusion scanners that overlay images from each technology, allowing identification of the anatomic point that is the source of the increased activity, are just entering clinical use at this time. FDG PET scans are very sensitive and specific for detection of lung cancer metastases and are increasingly used in lung cancer staging. Ongoing research with isotopes of carbon, oxygen and other elements will likely yield other significant imaging techniques in the future (Figure 2-29, *D* and *E*).

Summary

A disciplined and systematic approach to chest radiographs based on a solid foundation of understanding radiologic principles and techniques should enable even nonspecialists to feel comfortable in approaching these studies in either the preoperative or postoperative patient. Knowledge of normal anatomy and its variants, of usual patterns of atelectasis and alveolar consolidation, and of how changes in the underlying lung affect the radiograph, produce the common signs of abnormal states and greatly aid in the evaluation of patients undergoing anesthesia for thoracic surgery.

REFERENCES

1. Milne EN, Pistolesi M: *Reading the chest radiograph: a physiologic approach,* St. Louis, 1993, Mosby.
2. Proto AV: Conventional chest radiographs: anatomic understanding of newer observations, *Radiology* 183(3):593, 1992.
3. Proto AV: The chest radiograph: anatomic considerations, *Clin Chest Med* 5(2): 213, 19843. .
4. Kundel HL, La Follette PS: Visual search patterns and experience with radiologic images, *Radiology* 103:523, 1972.
5. Milne EN, Pistolesi M: *Reading the chest radiograph: a physiologic approach,* St. Louis, 1993, Mosby.
6. Fraser RS, Paré JA, Fraser RG, Paré PD: *Synopsis of diseases of the chest,* ed 2, Philadelphia, 1994, WB Saunders.
7. Freundlich IM, Bragg DG (eds): *A radiologic approach to diseases of the chest,* ed 2, Baltimore, 1997, Williams & Wilkins.
8. Lane EJ, Proto AV, Phillips TW: Mach bands and density perception, *Radiology* 121:9, 1976.
9. Fraser RS, Paré JA, Fraser RG, Paré PD: *Synopsis of diseases of the chest,* ed 2, Philadelphia, 1994, WB Saunders.
10. Fraser RS, Paré JA, Fraser RG, Paré PD: *Synopsis of diseases of the chest,* ed 2, Philadelphia, 1994, WB Saunders.
11. Fraser RS, Paré JA, Fraser RG, Paré PD: *Synopsis of diseases of the chest,* ed 2, Philadelphia, 1994, WB Saunders.
12. Groskin SA: *Heitzman's the lung, radiologic pathologic correlations,* ed 3, St. Louis, 1993, Mosby.
13. Proto AV, Tocino I: Radiographic manifestations of lobar collapse, *Semin Roentgenol* 15:117, 1980.
14. Collins J, Stern EJ: *Chest radiology, the essentials,* Philadelphia, 1999, Lippincott Williams & Wilkins.
15. Fraser RS, Paré JA, Fraser RG, Paré PD: *Synopsis of diseases of the chest,* ed 2, Philadelphia, 1994, WB Saunders.
16. Groskin SA: *Heitzman's the lung, radiologic pathologic correlations,* ed 3, St. Louis, 1993, Mosby.
17. Milne EN, Pistolesi M: *Reading the chest radiograph: a physiologic approach,* St. Louis, 1993, Mosby.
18. Ketai LH, Godwin JD: A new view of pulmonary edema and acute respiratory distress syndrome, *J Thorac Imaging* 13:147, 1998.
19. Tocino I: Chest imaging in the intensive care unit. In Freundlich IM, Bragg DG (eds): *A radiologic approach to diseases of the chest,* ed 2, Baltimore, 1997, Williams & Wilkins.
20. Greene R, Putnam C, Goodman L: Regional distribution of lung derangement in the adult respiratory distress syndrome. In Potchen EJ, Grainger R, Greene R (eds): *Pulmonary radiology, by members of the Fleischner Society,* Philadelphia, 1993, WB Saunders.
21. Gattoni L, Tognoni G, Pesenti A, et al: Effect of prone positioning on the survival of patients with acute respiratory failure, *N Engl J Med* 345:568, 2001.
22. Collins J, Stern EJ: *Chest radiology, the essentials,* Philadelphia, 1999, Lippincott, Williams & Wilkins.
23. Milne EN, Pistolesi M: *Reading the chest radiograph: a physiologic approach,* St. Louis, 1993, Mosby.
24. Fraser RS, Paré JA, Fraser RG, Paré PD: *Synopsis of diseases of the chest,* ed 2, Philadelphia, 1994, WB Saunders.
25. Proto AV, Ball JV Jr: The superolateral major fissures, *Am J Roentgen* 140:431, 1983.
26. Groskin SA: *Heitzman's the lung, radiologic pathologic correlations,* ed 3, St. Louis, 1993, Mosby.
27. Foster WL, Gimenez EI, Roubidoux MA, et al: The emphysemas: radiologic-pathologic correlations, *Radiographics* 13:311, 1993.
28. Groskin SA: *Heitzman's the lung, radiologic pathologic correlations,* ed 3, St. Louis, 1993, Mosby.
29. Tocino IM, Miller MH, Fairfax WR: Distribution of pneumothorax in the supine and semirecumbent critically ill adult, *Am J Roentgen,* 144:901, 1985.
30. Semenkovich JW, Freundlich IM: Abnormal thoracic air. In Freundlich IM, Bragg DG (eds): *A radiologic approach to diseases of the chest,* ed 2, Baltimore, 1997, Williams & Wilkins.
31. Semenkovich JW, Freundlich IM: Abnormal thoracic air. In Freundlich IM, Bragg DG (eds): *A radiologic approach to diseases of the chest,* ed 2, Baltimore, 1997, Williams & Wilkins.
32. Vail CM, Ravin CE: Cardiovascular monitoring devices. In Goodman LR, Putman CE (eds): *Critical care imaging,* ed 3, Philadelphia, 1993, WB Saunders.
33. Goodman LR: Pulmonary support and monitoring apparatus. In Goodman LR, Putman CE (eds): *Critical care imaging,* ed 3, Philadelphia, 1993, WB Saunders.
34. Goodman LR: Pulmonary support and monitoring apparatus. In Goodman LR, Putman CE (eds): *Critical care imaging,* ed 3, Philadelphia, 1993, WB Saunders.

Anatomy and Physiology of the Respiratory System and the Pulmonary Circulation

3

Thomas J. Gal, MD

F AMILIARITY with the anatomy and physiology of the respiratory system provides an essential framework for the safe and rational practice of anesthesiology. The uniqueness and complexity of the respiratory system are exemplified by its principal component, the lung. The lung must accept the entire cardiac output as it carries out its gas exchange and metabolic functions. This discussion will address three major areas, the behavior of all of which is altered during anesthesia:

1. Functional anatomy of the airways and respiratory muscles
2. Lung volumes
3. Pulmonary circulation and gas exchange

Functional Anatomy

Upper Airway Anatomy

The normal upper airway begins functionally at the nares or mouth and extends to the cricoid cartilage. As air passes through the nose, the very important functions of warming and humidification occur. The nose is the primary pathway for normal breathing unless obstruction by polyps or upper respiratory infection is present. During quiet breathing, the resistance to airflow through the nasal passages accounts for nearly two thirds of the total airway resistance.[1] The resistance through the nose is nearly twice that associated with mouth breathing. This explains why mouth breathing is used when high flow rates are necessary, as with exercise.

The next segment of the upper airway, the pharyngeal airway, extends from the posterior aspect of the nose down to the cricoid cartilage, where the passage continues as the esophagus. An upper area, the nasopharynx, is separated from the lower oropharynx by the tissue of the soft palate. The principal impediments to air passage through the nasopharynx are the prominent tonsillar lymphoid structures. The tongue is the principal source of oropharyngeal obstruction, usually because of decreased tone of the genioglossus muscle. The latter contracts to move the tongue forward during inspiration and thus acts as a pharyngeal dilator.

The most important segment of the upper airway is the larynx, which lies at the level of the third through sixth cervical vertebrae. It serves as the organ of phonation and as a valve to protect the lower airways from the contents of the alimentary tract. The structure consists of muscles, ligaments, and a framework of cartilages. These include the thyroid, cricoid, arytenoids, corniculates, and epiglottis. The epiglottis, a fibrous cartilage, has a mucous membrane covering that reflects as the glossoepiglottic fold onto the pharyngeal surface of the tongue. On either side of this fold are depressions called *valleculae*. These areas provide the site for placement of the curved Macintosh laryngoscope blade. The epiglottis projects into the pharynx and overhangs the laryngeal inlet; however, it is not absolutely essential for sealing off the airway during swallowing.

The laryngeal cavity extends from the epiglottis to the lower level of the cricoid cartilage. The inlet is formed by the epiglottis, which joins to the apex of the arytenoid cartilages on each side by the aryepiglottic folds. Inside the laryngeal cavity the vestibular folds, which are narrow bands of fibrous tissue on each side of the cavity, are first encountered. These extend from the anterolateral surface of each arytenoid to the angle of the thyroid, where the latter attaches to the epiglottis. These folds are referred to as the "false vocal cords" and are separated from the true vocal cords by the laryngeal sinus or ventricle. The true vocal cords are pale, white ligamentous structures that attach anteriorly to the angles of the thyroid and posteriorly to the arytenoids. The triangular fissure between these vocal cords is termed the *glottic opening;* it represents the narrowest segment of the laryngeal opening in adults. In small children (younger than 10 years old), the narrowest segment lies just below the vocal cords at the level of the cricoid ring. The mean length of the relaxed open glottis is about 23 mm in males and 17 mm in females. The glottic width is 6 to 9 mm but can be stretched to 12 mm. Thus the cross-sectional area of the relaxed glottis may be 60 to 100 mm^2.

The actions of the laryngeal muscles may be classified into three basic groups on the basis of their actions on the vocal cords:

1. Abductors
2. Adductors
3. Regulators of tension

The entire motor innervation to these muscles, as well as the sensory supply to the larynx, are supplied by two branches of the vagus nerve: the superior and recurrent laryngeal nerves. The latter supplies motor function to all but one of the laryngeal muscles and some sensory innervation to the subglottic mucosa. The superior laryngeal nerve provides most of the sensory innervation of the laryngeal area and innervates a single muscle, the cricothyroid, which serves largely as a tensor of the vocal cords.

UPPER AIRWAY FUNCTION

Upper Airway Protection. The pharynx, epiglottis, and vocal cords play a role in protecting the lower airway from aspiration of foreign bodies and secretions. Although the epiglottis covers the laryngeal inlet, it is not absolutely essential for airway protection.[2] Most vital in this protective function is the glottic closure reflex, which produces protective laryngeal closure during deglutition. The physiologic exaggeration of this reflex, laryngospasm, is counterproductive to respiration. Laryngospasm consists of prolonged, intense glottic closure in response to direct glottic or supraglottic stimulation from inhaled agents, secretions, or foreign bodies. Stimulation from the periosteum or celiac plexus or dilation of the rectum can also precipitate laryngospasm on a reflex basis.

An indispensable mechanism for expelling secretions and foreign bodies from the respiratory tract is the act of coughing. The major stages of a cough are characterized by three events. First, there is a deep inspiration to attain a high lung volume, which allows attainment of maximum expiratory flow rates. Next, a tight closure of the glottis occurs along with the contraction of the expiratory muscles. Intrapleural pressure rises above 100 cmH_2O, with the result that during the final or expiratory phase, a sudden expulsion of air occurs as the glottis opens. Glottic opening at the onset of the phase is associated with oscillation of tissue and gas, which results in the characteristic noise of a cough. Various physiologic aspects of cough have been observed with radiologic and endoscopic techniques. None is more important than the dramatic narrowing of the airway lumen that occurs. The physiologic significance of this reduced airway caliber is that the decreased cross-sectional area increases linear velocity of gas flow and improves cough effectiveness. Various estimates suggest that this dynamic compression decreases the cross-sectional area of the trachea and main bronchi to about 40% of their caliber during normal breathing and thus increases linear velocity two and a half times.[3]

Glottic closure is the one phase of cough that differentiates it from the other forced expiratory maneuvers and allows for greater development of pressures. Closure of the glottis is not crucial, however, to the development of high pressures and flow rates of a normal cough. This is well illustrated in patients who have undergone tracheal intubation or tracheostomy. The presence of the endotracheal tube, for example, does not lessen the buildup of peak pressure during coughing. But by preventing normal glottic closure, the tube allows flow to begin as soon as pressure begins to increase, and, in most cases, the tube allows flow to continue between cough bursts.[4] The normal timing of pressure and flow is altered such that cough resembles a normal forced expiration. Also, because the tube is noncollapsible, it does not permit the high velocities through the tracheal segment that it occupies. Secretions, therefore, are likely to accumulate in the area at the end of the tube unless subsequent coughs are begun from high lung volumes that allow high flow rates to be achieved.

Obstruction. Airway obstruction can be total or partial. Total obstruction is characterized by the lack of any air movement or breath sounds. In the face of ineffective breathing efforts, it is important that inexperienced persons not interpret any diaphragmatic tugging motions or retractive movements of the rib cage as respiration. Actual air movements must be perceived by feeling with the hand or placing the ear over the mouth. Recognition of obstruction depends on close observation and a high index of suspicion.

In the presence of partial obstruction, there is usually diminished tidal exchange, which is associated with retraction of the

upper chest and accompanied by a snoring sound (if the obstruction is nasopharyngeal) or by inspiratory stridor (if obstruction is near the area of the larynx). If inspiratory efforts are severe, the upper airway may undergo a dynamic inspiratory compression because of the marked pressure gradient in the upper airway.

Treatment of upper airway obstruction depends, for the most part, on whether the cause is soft tissue obstruction, tumor, foreign body, or laryngospasm. Most often, upper-airway obstruction is due to reduction of the space between the pharyngeal wall and the base of the tongue by relaxation of the tongue and jaw. The same picture of obstruction can occur with foreign bodies or even dentures. In the absence of a foreign body, airflow may be restored by preventing the mandible from falling backward. Forward motion is applied by placing the forefinger and second finger behind the angle of the mandible. The patient's neck can also be slightly extended to provide an optimal airway. The resultant changes in head position have been shown to modify upper airway resistance significantly.[5]

Oropharyngeal obstruction can also be overcome to some extent by increased oropharyngeal pressure from manual inflations with a breathing bag. One of the major concerns about manual inflation of the lungs without tracheal intubation is the potential for gastric insufflation with high inflation pressures. The relationship between pressure and gas entry into the stomach has been examined in unconscious paralyzed patients.[6] Lawes et al reported that gastric inflation rarely occurred when pressures lower than 15 to 20 cmH_2O were utilized. In general, pressures above such values were associated with excessively large delivered tidal volumes (more than 1 L).

In the awake individual, pharyngeal muscles oppose collapse of the upper airway. This force opposing collapse is lost with anesthesia or sedation. The tongue was once believed to be the major contributor to this airway obstruction. Boidin, however, demonstrated bronchoscopically that the obstruction was due to the epiglottis occluding the laryngeal opening.[7] He also showed that neck extension and anterior displacement of the mandible move the hyoid bone anteriorly to lift the epiglottis.

Lower Airways
TRACHEA

The lower airway begins with the trachea at the lower border of the cricoid cartilage. The trachea is a tubular structure that begins opposite the sixth cervical vertebra at the level of the thyroid cartilage. It is flattened posteriorly and supported along its 10- to 15-cm length by 16 to 20 horseshoe-shaped cartilaginous rings until it bifurcates into right and left main bronchi at the level of the fifth thoracic vertebra. The cross-sectional area of the trachea is considerably larger than that of the glottis and can be more than 150 mm^2 to 300 mm^2.

A number of receptors in the trachea are sensitive to mechanical and chemical stimuli. Slowly adapting stretch receptors are located in the trachealis muscle of the posterior tracheal wall. These are involved in regulating the rate and depth of breathing, but they also produce dilation of upper airways and the bronchi by decreasing vagal efferent activity. Other rapidly adapting irritant receptors lie all around the tracheal circumference. These are usually considered to be cough receptors, although their other reflex actions consist of bronchoconstriction. Studies of topical anesthesia in dogs suggest that the latter receptors are more readily blocked by local anesthetics than are the slowly adapting stretch receptors.[8]

These receptors in airway walls travel to the central nervous system via vagal afferents. The efferent parasympathetic pathways pass down the vagus nerve to synapses in ganglia within the airway walls. The postsynaptic membranes of these intramural ganglia contain nicotinic-cholinergic receptors (NC). These receptors are activated by acetylcholine (ACH). This activation can be modified by muscarinic receptors (M_1), which are present in these same autonomic ganglia. From this point, short postganglionic fibers pass to smooth muscle and submucosal glands in the airway. Presynaptic vesicles release ACH on stimulation to produce contraction of smooth muscle and mucus secretion via action on the postjunctional muscarinic (M_3) receptors. The further release of ACH is also attenuated by activation of prejunctional muscarinic (M_2) receptors on the short postganglionic fibers. These M_2 inhibitory receptors may serve to limit the degree of cholinergic bronchoconstriction by providing a negative feedback to ACH release.

These parasympathetic actions on the airways are opposed by sympathetic stimulation. Sympathetic stimulation appears to be entirely humoral in nature via the action of catecholamines, as actual sympathetic innervation of the airways remains to be demonstrated.

From a functional standpoint, it is important to note that the upper half of the trachea is extrathoracic, while the lower half resides within the thoracic cavity. This positioning creates differences in behavior during inspiration and expiration. The extrathoracic portion of the trachea, which is subject to the surrounding influence of atmospheric pressure, undergoes a slight decrease in caliber during inspiration and an increase during expiration. The intrathoracic portion, on the other hand, undergoes expansion during inspiration as the surrounding pleural pressure becomes more subambient (i.e., more negative). During expiration, however, the surrounding pleural pressure may diminish the tracheal caliber, especially in the face of increased expiratory effort as with obstruction.

CONDUCTING AIRWAYS

Physiologists use the classification of Weibel, which refers to the trachea as generation zero ("0") (Table 3-1).[9] The trachea bifurcates at the sternal angle, which usually lies at the level of the fourth thoracic vertebra. The two mainstem bronchi that arise from the trachea have a diameter approximately two-thirds that of the trachea, but they differ markedly from one another in length. The right bronchus is about 2.5 cm long, whereas the left extends about twice that length before branching into the next generation of airways, the lobar bronchi. The left bronchus also leaves the trachea at an angle of about 45 degrees from the latter's axis, while the right forms an angle of about one-half that with the trachea.

These second-generation lobar bronchi divide into segmental and then into subsegmental bronchi; with each airway generation, cartilaginous support progressively diminishes while total cross-sectional area increases. After 12 or more generations, the bronchioles are reached. These very small airways (less than 1-mm diameter) have no cartilage but only a great deal of smooth muscle. The smallest of the three or four generations of bronchioles are designated as the terminal bronchioles.

TABLE 3-1
Airway Generations

Airway Region	Generation	Number (2^x)
Trachea	0	1
Main bronchi	1	2
Lobar bronchi	2-3	4-8
Segmental bronchi	4	16
Small bronchi	5-11	32-2,000
Bronchioles		
Terminal bronchioles	12-14	4,000-16,000
Respiratory bronchioles	15-18	32,000-260,000
Alveolar ducts	19-22	520,000-4,000,000
Alveoli	23	8,000,000

2^x, Where x = generation number

These are the last component of the conducting airways (i.e., the portion of the tracheobronchial tree not directly involved in gas exchange).

RESPIRATORY AIRWAYS

The first portions of the tracheobronchial tree that allow direct gas exchange with the pulmonary circulation are the respiratory bronchioles (generation #15). These have intermittent saclike outpouchings. The next airway generation consists of the alveolar ducts, which have multiple sac-like openings whose final divisions terminate into alveolar clusters. The actual alveoli themselves are 100 to 300 μm in diameter. The interface with pulmonary capillaries facilitates exchange of oxygen (O_2) and carbon dioxide (CO_2) and consists of thin capillary epithelial layers, basement membrane, capillary endothelium, and a surfactant lining. The flat type I alveolar cells provide the surface for gas exchange, while the interspersed type II cells produce surfactant. Both of the epithelial cells form tight junctions that markedly restrict transport of fluids across them.

RESPIRATORY MUSCLES

Air moves in and out of the lungs as the thoracic cavity expands and decreases in size. This volume change is accomplished by the contraction of the respiratory muscles. Functionally, these are skeletal muscles whose prime task is to rhythmically displace the chest wall. There are three major muscle groups responsible for ventilation: the diaphragm, the intercostal muscles, and the accessory muscles. Although the functions of these muscles will be considered individually, it is most important to remember that they actually must work together in a coordinated fasion.[10]

Diaphragm. The diaphragm is a dome-shaped muscle that separates the thoracic cavity from the abdomen. The muscle is somewhat unique in that its fibers radiate from a central tendon to insert peripherally on the anterolateral aspects of the upper lumbar vertebrae (crural portion) and on the xiphoid and upper margins of the lower ribs (costal portion). The motor innervation originates from the phrenic nerve, which is formed by the combination of cervical roots III, IV, and V. Contraction of the diaphragm causes its dome to descend, thereby longitudinally expanding the chest. The attachments to costal margins also cause the lower ribs to rise and the chest to widen. This action of the diaphragm is responsible for about two-thirds of quiet resting ventilation. The normal excursion of the diaphragm during such quiet breathing is about 1.5 cm. As the dome descends to expand the thorax, the abdominal contents are displaced caudally. In this way, the fall in pleural pressure and accompanying lung expansion produce an increase in abdominal pressure and some outward protrusion of the abdominal wall.

Intercostal Muscles. The intercostal muscles are composed of two sheetlike layers that run between the ribs and receive their innervation from nerves that exit from the spinal cord at levels from the first to eleventh thoracic segments. The external intercostals and the parasternal portion of the internal intercostals produce an inspiratory action. Their contraction elevates the upper ribs to increase the anteroposterior dimensions of the chest in a pump-handle motion. The lower ribs are also raised to increase the transverse diameter of the thorax in a bucket-handle motion. Although these actions of the intercostals do not play a major role in normal resting ventilation, they are important in maintaining high levels of ventilation such as required by exercise.

Accessory Muscles. The accessory muscles contribute to inspiration by elevating and stabilizing the rib cage. The principal accessory muscles are the scalenes and sternocleidomastoids. The scalenes originate from the transverse processes of the lower five cervical vertebrae and receive innervation from the same spinal segments. The muscles slope caudally to insert on the first two ribs in such a way that contraction elevates and fixes the rib cage. Although this plays only a minor role in quiet breathing, the enlargement of the upper chest is important at high levels of ventilation. The second group of accessory muscles, the sternocleidomastoids, elevates the sternum and increases the longitudinal dimensions of the thorax. They are also only active at high levels of ventilation and assume great importance in disease states such as severe airway obstruction.

EXPIRATORY MUSCLES

In contrast to the active phase of inspiration, expiration is passive during quiet breathing and occurs because of the elastic recoil of the respiratory system. However, when high levels of ventilation are required or if air movement is impeded by airway obstruction, expiration must involve active muscle contraction. This is achieved in part by the internal intercostal muscles, which depress the ribs, but the major participants in active expiration are the abdominal muscles. These muscles, which comprise the ventrolateral abdominal wall, are innervated by the lower six thoracic and first lumbar nerves. They consist of the midline rectus abdominus and, laterally, the internal and external oblique and transversus abdominus.

These muscles act to displace the rib cage by pulling the lower ribs downward and inward. They also pull the abdominal wall inward and thus increase intraabdominal pressure. This higher pressure displaces the diaphragm cranially into the thorax, with a resultant increase in pleural pressure and a decrease in lung volume at the conclusion of expiration. In addition to their role as powerful muscles of expiration, the abdominal muscles are also important contributors to other respiratory activities, such as forced expiration and coughing and the nonrespiratory functions of defecation and parturition.

All measurements of pulmonary function that require patient effort are influenced by respiratory muscle strength. This can be evaluated specifically by measurements of maximal forced effort and can be measured with simple aneroid gauges.[11] The

inspiratory muscles are at their optimal length near residual volume. Thus, maximal inspiratory pressure (PI_{max}) is usually measured after a forced exhalation. Similarly, maximum expiratory pressure (PE_{max}) is measured at total lung capacity, when expiratory muscles are stretched to their optimum length by a full inspiration. Typical values for PI_{max} in healthy young males are approximately $-125\ cmH_2O$, whereas PE_{max} may be as high as $+200\ cmH_2O$.

Values for PE_{max} less than $+40\ cmH_2O$ suggest impaired coughing ability, whereas PI_{max} values of $-25\ cmH_2O$ or less indicate severe inability to take a deep breath. The latter value is often used as a criterion for extubation; however, observations in healthy volunteers during partial curarization suggest that this level of ventilatory ability does not ensure adequate upper airway integrity.[12]

Lung Volumes

To study the behavior of the respiratory system, it is useful to define its various dimensions. These are the subdivisions of gas volumes contained within the lungs during various breathing maneuvers. Although not the first to measure ventilatory volume, John Hutchinson is credited with inventing the spirometer, coining the term *vital capacity,* and defining the functional subdivisions of lung volumes.[13] The four major subdivisions of lung volume are as follows:

- Residual volume (RV)
- Tidal volume (VT)
- Expiratory reserve volume (ERV)
- Inspiratory reserve volume (IRV)

These four volumes can in turn be combined to form the following four capacities:

- Total lung capacity (TLC)
- Vital capacity (VC)
- Inspiratory capacity (IC)
- Functional residual capacity (FRC)

The relationships among these various lung volumes and capacities are defined in Table 3-2.

Physiologic Determinants

A young adult male of average height would be likely to have a TLC of about 6.5 L, of which 1.56 L is residual volume. Therefore vital capacity is about 5 L. Differences in lung volumes among individuals are largely a function of differences in body size (particularly height). Other determinants of TLC include the strength of the inspiratory muscles and elastic recoil properties of lung and chest wall. The magnitude of the RV is primarily influenced by expiratory muscle strength and the outward recoil of the chest wall. The limits of expiration may also be affected by dynamic airway closure, particularly with advancing age.[14] The volume at the end of the spontaneous exhalation during quiet breathing—the FRC—corresponds to the resting volume of the respiratory system. At this volume, airway pressure is zero, as a reflection of the balance between the opposing recoil pressures of the lung and chest wall.

The respiratory system and its component lung and chest wall are elastic structures; that is, they tend to regain their original size and configuration following deformation when deforming forces are removed. Both lung and chest wall have

TABLE 3-2

Lung Volumes and Capacities

Lung Volume and Capacity	Definition
Tidal volume (VT)	Air volume inspired and expired during quiet breathing
Residual volume (RV)	Volume remaining in the lungs after a maximal expiration
Expiratory reserve volume (ERV)	The volume of air that can be forcibly exhaled between the resting end-expiratory position and RV
Inspiratory reserve volume (IRV)	The volume of air that can be inspired with maximal effort over and above the normal resting end-inspiratory position of a tidal volume
Vital capacity (VC)	The amount of air that can be exhaled from the point of maximal inspiration to the point of maximal expiration
Total lung capacity (TLC)	Total volume of air in the lungs after a maximal inspiration. It is the sum of all subdivisions of lung volume
Functional residual capacity (FRC)	Amount of air in the lung at the end of a quiet exhalation. It is the sum of RV + ERV

their own positions of equilibrium. These are the volumes that they tend to assume in the absence of external forces acting upon them, and the volumes to which they continuously attempt to return when displaced. The equilibrium position of the lung is at or near RV (Figure 3-1, *A*). To sustain any volume in the lung above this, force must be applied to the lung, and the lung will recoil with an equal and opposite force. At all volumes above RV, the lung tends to recoil inward. The equilibrium position of the chest wall is at a relatively large volume, about 60% of vital capacity (Figure 3-1, *B*). To sustain any volume in the chest wall above this point, the chest wall must be actively enlarged by inspiratory muscle contraction, and at such large volumes it will tend to recoil inward in concert with the lung.

In the intact respiratory system, the lung and chest wall are coupled and work together. Behavior of the respiratory system is determined by the individual properties of the lung and chest wall. The equilibrium position of the respiratory system will be at that volume at which the tendency of the lung to recoil inward is balanced by the tendency of the chest wall to recoil outward. To sustain any volume in the respiratory system other than this resting volume, a force must be applied to displace both lung and chest wall. The recoil pressure of the respiratory system

(P_{rs}) that develops is the algebraic sum of the individual recoil pressure of the lung (P_L) and the chest wall (P_{cw}). Thus,

$$P_{rs} = P_L + P_{cw}$$

The volume at which Prs is zero is termed the *resting* or *relaxation volume* (V_{rx}) of the respiratory system (Figure 3-1, *C*). In normal persons during quiet breathing, the volume of the lung at the close of expiration (FRC) approximates this V_{rx}. Under certain circumstances, however, FRC may differ from V_{rx}. Static factors such as respiratory muscle tone, posture, and external forces may reduce end-expiratory lung volume, while dynamic mechanisms may increase it.

Postural alterations in the pressure-volume relationships of the respiratory system are largely accounted for by the influence of gravity on the abdomen, which behaves mechanically like a fluid-filled container. In the erect posture, the downward pull of gravity on the abdominal contents exerts an inspiratory action on the diaphragm. In contrast, the action on the rib cage is more expiratory in nature. In the supine posture, gravity also exerts a small expiratory action on the rib cage by pulling the ribs down and inward, but it has a marked expiratory action on the diaphragm and abdomen. The pressure-volume curve for the chest wall is thus shifted to the right (i.e., it produces less

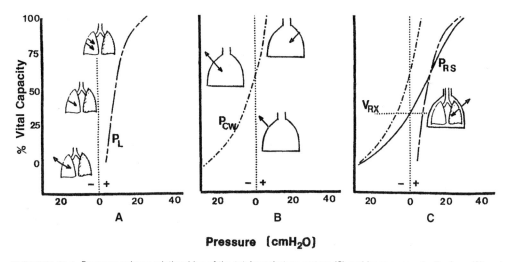

Pressure (cmH₂O)

FIGURE 3-1 Pressure-volume relationships of the total respiratory system **(C)** and its components, the lung **(A)** and chest wall **(B)**. *V_rx*, relaxation volume of the respiratory system (i.e., resting equilibrium volume); *P_L*, recoil pressure of the lung; *P_cw*, chest wall recoil pressure; *P_rs*, recoil pressure for the total respiratory system. (From Gal TJ: *Respiratory physiology in anesthetic practice*, Baltimore, 1991, Williams & Wilkins.)

opposition to the inward recoil of the lung). As a result, FRC in normal individuals decreases from about 50% to about 40% TLC in the supine position, and even further to about 30% of TLC in Trendelenburg position. Interestingly, these striking changes with posture do not appear to be manifest in patients with pulmonary emphysema. The enlarged FRC volume in such patients is relatively unaffected by body position.[15]

Adult humans and most of the larger terrestrial mammals with relatively stiff chest walls breathe near their Vrx, and FRC is approximately equal to Vrx or about 50% TLC. The single exception to this is the horse, which appears to breathe around its Vrx with active inspiratory and expiratory phases such that FRC is less than Vrx. This respiratory pattern is believed to minimize the high elastic work of breathing, associated with the horse's low chest wall compliance.[16]

During quiet breathing, ample time exists for passive emptying of the lungs. When ventilation must be increased (as with exercise) or when emptying is delayed because of obstruction to flow, the end-expiratory lung volume may be determined by a dynamic rather than a static equilibrium. In obstructive lung disease, for example, FRC is commonly increased. Although an increase in Vrx may result from decreased lung elastic recoil, factors such as expiratory flow limitation may result in an even higher, dynamically determined FRC.

The human newborn provides a particularly important example of a dynamically determined end-expiratory lung volume. The chest wall of infants and neonates is highly compliant (i.e., its outward recoil is exceedingly small). Although the inward recoil of the lungs is slightly less in infants than in the adult, the lungs are relatively stiff compared to the chest wall. The static balance of forces would predict an FRC at a very low lung volume (as low as 10% of TLC).[17] Because such a low lung volume seems incompatible with airway stability and adequate gas exchange, there is reason to suspect that the infant's dynamically determined FRC is substantially above the passive static Vrx. Indeed, it has been observed that the lung volume during apnea is lower than the usual end-expiratory level in neonates.[18]

Dynamic FRC is determined by the balance between two factors: the time available for expiration (TE) and the rate of lung emptying. The expiratory time (TE) is highly influenced by respiratory rates. In the neonate, the rapid breathing frequency results in a relatively short TE. The rate of lung emptying is governed by the expiratory time constant (τ), which can be most simply viewed as the product of resistance (R) and compliance (C). Neonates, because of the small size of the airways, have an increased R, and because of the mechanical properties of the rib cage, they have a highly compliant chest wall (increased C). Thus τ, which equals $R \times C$, is relatively prolonged. Whenever the ratio TE/τ is less than 3, dynamic FRC exceeds Vrx and airway pressure at end-expiration does not reach zero. Such appears to be the case in the human neonate. The transition from this dynamically maintained FRC appears to occur at about 1 year of age.[19] At this point in time, the end-expiratory level approximates Vrx, presumably because of changes in the mechanical properties of the lungs and chest wall as well as increases in TE.

In adults with prolonged expiratory times as a result of airway obstruction, incomplete expiration may occur during spontaneous or mechanical ventilation. The latter results in a phenomenon termed *dynamic hyperinflation,* which is associated with an increase in airway pressure above the normal zero value at the end of normal expiration. This is termed *intrinsic PEEP* and implies that the pulmonary end-expiratory pressure (PEEP) is a distending pressure responsible for the increased lung volume. Actually, the PEEP represents the recoil pressure of the respiratory system at the elevated lung volume. Thus PEEP is the result, not the cause, of the increased lung volume.

Closing Volume

The term *closing volume* describes the lung volume at which airways in dependent areas in the lung begin to close or, more precisely, cease contributing to the expired gas. This phenomenon presumably occurs because of gravity-dependent gradients in pleural pressure (Figure 3-2) during inspiration. These gradients serve to provide better ventilation of the smaller dependent airspaces. During expiration at or near RV, the lower portions of the lungs are subjected to pleural pressures in excess of airway pressures. Hence, these airways are prone to close or, more precisely, contribute little to the expired gas.

The closing volume (CV) test attempts to detect the lung volume at which this phenomenon occurs. The basic technique is to tag these dependent lung areas by giving them a concentration of a tracer gas that differs from the concentration in the areas that remain open near the close of expiration. As a subject inspires from RV to TLC, a concentration difference for the tracer gas is created between the top and the bottom of the lung as a result of differences in distribution of ventilation. During the subsequent slow exhalation, the changing concentration of tracer gas is plotted against lung volume on an X-Y recorder. Two methods utilize this principle to estimate CV: the bolus technique and the resident-gas technique.

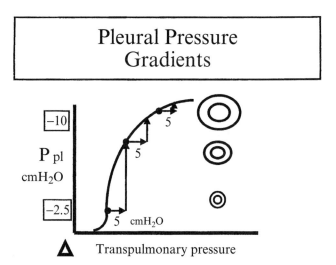

FIGURE 3-2 Plural pressure gradient increases down the lung in such a way that the dependent alveoli are small and nondependent ones are relatively large. A change in transpulmonary pressure of 5 cmH$_2$O produces a greater change in volume (or ventilation) of the small dependent air spaces because they lie on a relatively steeper portion of the compliance or pressure-volume curve. The larger nondependent alveoli lie on a flatter portion of the curve and thus undergo less volume change.

The bolus technique employs a bolus of tracer gas. Although xenon and argon were originally used, the easier availability of helium has made it most popular. The technique depends on the principle that a bolus of gas inspired at RV is preferentially distributed to the apical lung areas because small airways in dependent lung zones are far less patent at these low lung volumes. Therefore the preexpiratory concentration gradient created for the tracer gas results in the apical areas' containing most of the marker gas, whereas lower basilar areas contain very little.

The resident-gas technique also depends on the creation of a preexpiratory concentration gradient of marker gas from top to bottom of the lung. This technique differs from bolus technique, however, in two ways. First, the tracer gas for the resident-gas technique is the nitrogen already present or resident in the lungs. Second, in the resident-gas technique there is normally little difference in nitrogen concentration at TLC between the top and the bottom of the lung when a person is breathing air. For this reason, a preexpiratory concentration gradient is artificially created by the use of oxygen to dilute the nitrogen normally present in the lungs. The nitrogen in all alveoli is not equally diluted. At RV, the alveoli at the bottom of the lung are smaller than those at the top. At TLC, all alveoli reach essentially equal volumes. Thus, during inspiration from RV to TLC, the lower basal alveoli undergo almost one and a half times the volume change undergone by the upper or apical alveoli. As a result, the nitrogen in the lower zones is diluted more by the inspired oxygen than is the nitrogen in the upper zones. There is approximately a 2:1 concentration gradient for nitrogen between top and bottom of the lungs.

In normal subjects, the nitrogen concentration appearing at the mouth after inspiration of 100% oxygen changes gradually throughout the expiration. A typical trace displays four basic phases. The first three are familiar from Fowler's original single-breath nitrogen test. Phase I contains expired gas essentially free of marker, representing emptying from the dead space of the apparatus as well as of the conducting airways (anatomic dead space). Phase II consists of a rapid rise in the concentration of marker gas, which mixes with deadspace gas as alveolar emptying begins. Phase III, known as the *alveolar plateau,* is produced by the mixing of expired air with marker gas from all lung regions, each gas having a different concentration.

Near the end of expiration, another abrupt increase in tracer gas concentration occurs (phase IV). The point at which phase IV begins has been designated the CV because the dependent airways have presumably closed or, more correctly, they have essentially ceased contributing to the expired gas. At this point, the exhaled gas arises almost entirely from the upper lung zones, whose concentration of marker gas (in this case, nitrogen) was previously high. The CV is the difference in volume between the onset of phase IV and RV. Because it represents a portion of the VC maneuver, it is usually expressed as a percentage of VC (CV/VC percent). Most published values for CV in normal healthy subjects in the sitting position are between 15% and 20% of VC.

The terminology is confused by another term, *closing capacity* (CC). This term is used to designate the volume between the onset of phase IV and zero lung volume; it thus includes CV and RV. Because it is the absolute lung volume at which phase IV occurs, it is usually expressed as a percentage of TLC (CC/TLC %).

Although the onset of phase IV is usually taken to represent a unique volume at which actual closure of the small airways occurs, it appears that rather than closing off, the small airways might merely be emptying more slowly because of dynamic compression and the resultant increased resistance to flow. This impression is based on the evidence that phase IV occurs at the time the lungs reach flow limitation and continue to empty at a decreased rate despite increasing transpulmonary pressures. This same phenomenon occurs during the later portions of the NEFV curve. In fact, high expiratory flow rates, such as those characterizing the NEFV curve, can actually increase the lung volume at which phase IV occurs, presumably because of some dynamic airway compression. Thus to produce a satisfactory trace when measuring CV, expiration must be performed slowly (at about 0.5 L/sec). This rate can be ensured by introducing mechanical resistance into the breathing circuit.

Whether the mechanism is closure or compression, most observers have noted significantly increased values for CC in cigarette smokers when compared with nonsmokers of the same age. These findings have been cited as evidence of loss of elastic recoil, not of necessarily intrinsic small airway pathology. This same relationship between CC and lung elastic recoil is clearly demonstrated by the changes that occur with age. The progressive reduction in lung recoil and its associated tethering action on the bronchioles produce an increase in CC with advancing age; until age 65, CC exceeds the FRC (CC > FRC), even in seated individuals.[20] Young children who exhibit reduced values for lung elastic recoil likewise have increased closing capacities.[21] The smallest CC values occur in subjects during the late teens, when maximal values for static elastic recoil are observed.

Lung Volumes and Gas Exchange During Anesthesia
ALTERATIONS IN RESPIRATORY MECHANICS

General anesthesia affects the static (pressure-volume) and the dynamic (pressure-flow) behaviors of the respiratory system. These mechanical effects have interested clinicians and investigators because of their potential contribution to the impaired gas exchange so characteristic in anesthetized patients. Perhaps no facet of respiratory system behavior has received as much attention as the change in FRC. A decrease in FRC with induction of general anesthesia was first noted by Bergman.[22] Subsequent observations in supine anesthetized humans indicate that FRC is reduced by an average of about 500 mL, or 15% to 20% of the awake value. The decreased volume is similar in magnitude to that observed when subjects go from the erect to the recumbent position. The magnitude of FRC reduction also appears to be related to age and body habitus (i.e., weight-height ratio). In fact, morbidly obese patients demonstrate a much larger decrease in FRC, to about 50% of the preanesthetic values.[23]

Perhaps the most overlooked consequence of this reduced FRC relates to the effect on the size of the airways. The latter are large at high lung volume and small at low lung volume. These changes in airway caliber effect a passive change in

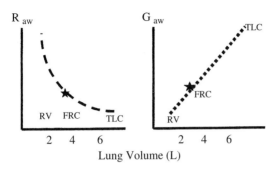

FIGURE 3-3 The hyperbolic relationship of airway resistance (Raw) to lung volume is contrasted with the linear relationship of its reciprocal airway conductance (G_{aw}). *RV*, Residual volume; *TLC*, total lung capacity; *FRC*, functional residual capacity.

airway resistance independent of active airway constriction. (Figure 3-3). This observation has led physiologists to use the relationship of airway resistance (or its reciprocal conductance) to lung volume when assessing bronchoconstriction or dilation.

The reduction in FRC occurs within a minute after induction of anesthesia,[24] is not progressive with time,[25] and is not further affected by addition of muscle paralysis.[25,26] A number of factors contribute to the FRC reduction, but the underlying mechanisms are complex and as yet not totally understood. Some of the possibilities include atelectasis, increased expiratory muscle activity, trapping of gas in distal airways, cephalad displacement of the diaphragm, decreased outward chest wall recoil, increasing lung recoil, and increases in thoracic blood volume.

Atelectasis may contribute to or result from the reduction of FRC. The rapid appearance of densities on computed tomography (CT) supports this possibility.[27] The prompt development of the densities and their lack of dependence on high inspired oxygen concentrations suggest that they may be due to compression of gas rather than to resorption.

Trapping of gas behind closed distal airways does not appear to be a major contributor to the decreased FRC because measurements of thoracic gas volume have demonstrated the FRC changes.[28] Furthermore, measurement of nitrogen washout, which measures only gas in contact with the open airways, gave results similar to those that measured total thoracic gas volume by body plethysmography.[26]

During rapid-eye-movement sleep and with halothane anesthesia, the tonic activity of the diaphragm decreases. Muller et al postulated that this reduced diaphragmatic tone was responsible for the FRC reduction with anesthesia.[29] The intercostal muscles appear to be even more sensitive to depression by volatile agents such as halothane.[30] This observation would make it attractive to hypothesize that the reduced tone of diaphragm and intercostals results in a reduced outward recoil of the chest wall. This process does not appear to progress further, as addition of neuromuscular blockade, which would be expected to further diminish muscle tone, produces no

additional changes in FRC. The absence of any additional effect with paralysis also argues against any role of increased tone of the expiratory (abdominal) muscles in determining the end-expiratory lung volume.

Another possible mechanism contributing to reduction of FRC involves a shift of blood from the limbs to the lung and abdomen. The blood in the lungs may have a twofold effect. First, lung congestion may decrease lung compliance and thus increase lung recoil. Second, the blood competes with air for intrathoracic volume. At the same time, an increase in abdominal blood volume can act to displace the diaphragm upward or the abdominal wall outward. A report by Hedenstierna et al suggested that the diaphragm was displaced cranially and that the decrease in thoracic volume of FRC is associated with a shift of blood from the thorax to the abdomen.[31] Others noted that changes in the volume of the rib cage affect the position of the diaphragm, and that intrathoracic fluid (blood) and gas contribute in varying amounts to reducing FRC in different subjects.[32] In the study just cited, thoracic gas volume was reduced considerably more than thoracic volume. This suggests that there is some increase in thoracic blood volume with induction of anesthesia.

Reduction in FRC with intravenous agents differs from the more dramatic effect of inhalation anesthetics. Thiopental and methohexital produced changes in nonintubated subjects that were similar to those associated with normal sleep.[24,33,34] In most cases, the decrement in FRC was less than 200 mL. The relatively small magnitude of change was attributed to maintenance of rib cage activity in contrast to the marked depression seen with agents such as halothane.[30] Another intravenous agent, ketamine, also appears to have a sparing action on intercostal muscle activity and is associated with a maintenance of FRC at awake levels in adults and children.[35,36] In the group associated with this study, the increased respiratory rates and prolonged passive lung emptying as illustrated by the τ were associated with an FRC greater than the static relaxation volume.[37] The authors speculated that the prolonged τ with ketamine anesthesia was the result of increases in respiratory system compliance (thus τ, the product of R × C, is increased). With halothane, on the other hand, τ is shortened, presumably because respiratory system compliance decreases.

In supine subjects the induction of general anesthesia reduces FRC to the extent that end-expiratory volume decreases close to the level of residual volume. This FRC may lie below the closing capacity (i.e., the volume associated with dependent airway closure or, more precisely, dynamic flow limitation). Early observations with halothane anesthesia suggested a correlation between the degree of impaired oxygenation and the reduction in FRC and led to the hypothesis that airway closure and atelectasis were the consequences of a reduced FRC.[38]

The degree of intrapulmonary shunting does appear to correlate with the reduction in FRC and with the degree of atelectasis demonstrated with CT in dependent lung regions.[39,40] It is thus tempting to attribute such atelectasis simply to the reduced FRC. A study in awake supine subjects with thoracoabdominal restriction, however, argues against this simple mechanism.[41] The restriction in these subjects reduced lung volume and altered pulmonary mechanics in a fashion similar to that seen with general anesthesia. The FRC decreased by more than 20% and was matched by a reduction of CC as measured by the resident gas (N_2) technique. No atelectasis was noted with CT scanning and $\dot{V}_A/\dot{Q}$ distribution, and arterial blood gases were unchanged from the control state. Thus, gas exchange in these awake subjects with chest restriction differed from gas exchange in anesthetized subjects, although both groups had some relative decrement in FRC. The authors concluded that the development of compression atelectasis in the anesthetized patients cannot be ascribed solely to a decrease in FRC, nor can the changes in pulmonary mechanics with restriction be attributed solely to the development of atelectasis.

The atelectasis that develops in the dependent lung regions of anesthetized subjects was seen to a similar extent, whether patients were anesthetized with inhalation agents (halothane, enflurane, or isoflurane) or with intravenous agents such as thiopental or propofol.[42,43] Quite interestingly, ketamine, which, unlike the other agents, did not reduce muscle tone or FRC, did not produce such atelectasis unless neuromuscular blockade was instituted.

The past decades have witnessed numerous attempts to reverse the atelectasis. These have included phrenic nerve stimulation to induce diaphragmatic tone and the application of PEEP.[44] The PEEP was effective in reducing atelectasis but not in reducing intrapulmonary shunt. It appears that the beneficial effects of PEEP on gas exchange in anesthetized subjects are limited to morbidly obese patients.[45]

The most effective means of reexpanding atelectatic areas was an inflation to total lung capacity that was sustained at an airway pressure of 40 cmH_2O for 10 seconds.[46] The benefits, unfortunately, are transient but can be extended for nearly 40 minutes if gas composition limits O_2 concentration to below 40% (balance N_2).[47]

ALTERED DISTRIBUTION OF VENTILATION

Ventilation is not normally uniform throughout the lung. The effects of gravity on the lung and the forces necessary to allow it to conform to the shape of the thorax result in a vertical gradient of pleural pressure. The pleural pressure acting on the upper (nondependent) areas of the lung is more subatmospheric (negative) than that acting on the lower (dependent) portions. As a result, the nondependent areas are more inflated than the dependent ones. The gradient of pleural pressure up and down the lung changes about 0.4 cmH_2O per each centimeter of lung height. Thus in a lung 30 cm high, a 7.5-cmH_2O pressure difference exists from apex to base. In the supine position, the dorsal areas become dependent. The height of the lungs is reduced by nearly one third, and thus the gravitational effect is somewhat diminished.

Although the nondependent lung areas are more distended at FRC, a given transpulmonary pressure generated during a normal breath produces a greater volume change or ventilation to the dependent areas. This is because of the rather sigmoid shape of the lung's pressure-volume curve (see Figure 3-2). The larger nondependent areas have a lower regional compliance (i.e., they lie on a less steep portion of the pressure-volume curve).

These regional differences in ventilation are important in matching ventilation to perfusion. The dependent or basal areas tend to be better perfused because of gravitational effects. Because the bases are also better ventilated, there is good

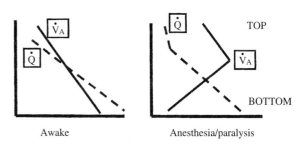

FIGURE 3-4 Diaphragmatic representation of the distribution of ventilation ($\dot{V}_A$) and perfusion ($\dot{Q}$) between nondependent *(top)* lung areas and dependent *(bottom)* areas. Note that $\dot{V}_A$ tends to be distributed more uniformly from top to bottom in the anesthetized paralyzed state.

matching of ventilation and perfusion (Figure 3-4). Higher ventilation and blood flow are delivered to the bases. In supine, anesthetized, paralyzed humans, the ventilation or distribution of inspired gas becomes more uniform from top to bottom lung areas (Figure 3-4), largely because basal lung units undergo further reduction in size to a point that reduces their regional compliance. Anesthetics, meanwhile, produce a decrease in pulmonary arterial pressure, which impedes perfusion of nondependent lung regions. Increased alveolar pressures with mechanical ventilation interfere further with perfusion of nondependent areas. Thus, dependent lung areas are well perfused but rather poorly ventilated. In contrast, nondependent areas receive more ventilation but considerably less perfusion.

In addition to changes in static lung mechanics, the overall $\dot{V}_A/\dot{Q}$ inhomogeneity may also be increased during anesthesia because of changes in dynamics (i.e., the pressure-flow relationships in the airways). The smooth muscle relaxation associated with anesthetics may be useful in preventing the increased bronchial tone associated with bronchospasm. Reductions in normal bronchomotor tone, however, may interfere with the normal $\dot{V}_A/\dot{Q}$ matching and thus impair gas exchange.[48]

Local decreases in alveolar CO_2 tension also tend to improve the normal $\dot{V}_A/\dot{Q}$ matching by producing local increases in bronchomotor tone. In a sense, this hypocapnic bronchoconstriction is analogous to hypoxic pulmonary vasoconstriction. Whether the inhalation anesthetics as a group block this bronchoconstriction induced by hypocapnia is not known. Thus far, only halothane has been shown to reduce this bronchoconstrictive effect of hypocapnia.[49,50]

Pulmonary Circulation

The pulmonary circulation has as its primary function the respiratory transport of mixed venous blood through the alveolar capillary bed to accomplish gas exchange. This requires mechanisms to regulate the volume and distribution of blood flow.

The gas exchange role of the pulmonary circulation is accompanied by the bronchial circulation, which arises from the aorta. The bronchial circulation provides nutritional support for the airways and blood vessels down to the level of the terminal bronchioles. These bronchial vessels supply important heat for humidification and warming of inspired air. Not all of the bronchial flow returns to the systemic veins; some enters the pulmonary veins and produces a small physiologic shunt.

Pressure-Flow Relationships

The pulmonary circulation resembles its systemic counterpart in that it has a pump, the right ventricle. It also has an exchange system (capillaries) interposed between the distributing system (pulmonary arteries and arterioles) and the collecting system (pulmonary veins). The pulmonary circulation differs from the systemic circuit because of the relatively low pressure within its very compliant vessels (Table 3-3). This low pressure occurs despite the fact that the lung receives a higher blood flow than any other organ because it must accept the entire cardiac output. Thus in contrast to the systemic circuit with its high pressure and high resistance, the pulmonary circulation may be characterized as a high-flow, low-pressure, low-resistance system. The high-flow, low-pressure relationship exists not only at rest but also during exercise. The pulmonary circuit can accommodate a three- to fourfold increase in cardiac output with only minimal increases in pulmonary artery pressure, largely because the thinner pulmonary vessels contain less smooth muscle and are more distensible than their systemic counterparts. The systemic vessels regulate blood flow to various organs, some of which lie above the level of the heart. The pulmonary vessels, on the other hand, must always accept the entire cardiac output.

Pulmonary arterial pressures may increase in the face of pulmonary vasoconstriction, destruction of pulmonary vasculature, or increases in downstream pressure because of decreased cardiac function. In such conditions, pulmonary vessels are no longer able to sufficiently recruit and distend to maintain the low-pressure, low-resistance system. Generally, a mean pulmonary artery pressure less than 25 mmHg is considered indicative of pulmonary hypertension. If the latter is allowed to progress, right ventricular hypertrophy and failure may ultimately result.

DISTRIBUTION OF PULMONARY BLOOD FLOW

Vessels in the lung are classified on the basis of how their resistance or caliber responds to the extravascular pressures of lung inflation. The response to lung inflation is largely a function of where the vessels lie within the lung parenchyma. The pulmonary arteries and veins within the lung parenchyma are surrounded by sheaths of connective tissue that serve as attachments for the alveolar walls. Thus, when the subatmos-

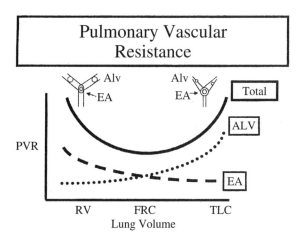

FIGURE 3-5 Effects of lung volume expansion on the caliber and resistance of the alveolar (ALV) and extraalveolar (EA) pulmonary vessels. Note that the net effect on total resistance (TOTAL) results in the lowest value at functional residual capacity (FRC). Values for total resistance increase toward residual volume (RV) and total lung capacity (TLC).

pheric pleural pressure acts on the outer surface of the lung to produce lung expansion, an outward radial traction is exerted on the vessel sheaths, increasing vessel diameter (Figure 3-5). Although the resistance of the extraalveolar vessels decreases with lung expansion, the alveolar vessels undergo compression and reduction in caliber, which increases their resistance. The net effect on both types of vessels results in a total pulmonary vascular resistance that is lowest at functional residual capacity (Figure 3-5) and increases toward both extremes of lung volume.

REGIONAL BLOOD FLOW STRATIFICATION

Within the lung, considerable inequality of blood flow exists. The use of radioactive xenon has demonstrated the topographic distribution of pulmonary blood flow. In the upright position, blood flow decreases linearly from the bottom to the top of the lung such that flow at the apex is minimal. This uneven distribution has been attributed to hydrostatic pressure differences within the blood vessels arising from the effects of gravity. Thus the low-pressure pulmonary circuit appears barely able to raise a column of blood to the lung apex. This somewhat simplistic gravity-oriented explanation has been challenged by Badeer, who attributes the decreased apical blood flow to increased vascular resistance.[51] The gravitational pressure at the apex significantly lowers the intravascular pressure (and hence the

---

TABLE 3-3

Hemodynamic Differences in Systemic and Pulmonary Circulations

Measurement Entity	Pulmonary Circulation	Systemicm Circulation
Arterial pressure, mmHg systolic/diastolic mean	25/8	125/80
Mean arterial pressure, mmHg	12	95
Mean capillary pressure, mmHg	5 (left)	2 (right)
Blood flow, L/min	5	5
Blood volume, mL	400-500	5000-6000
Vascular resistance, mmHg/L/min	1.4*	18.6*

*To convert to CGS units (dyne/sec/cm²), multiply by 80.

transmural pressure) of the highly compliant pulmonary vessels. As a result, these vessels collapse and increase their resistance to flow.

The distribution of pulmonary blood flow is chiefly governed by the distensibility of vessels and their transmural distending pressure. Because of the vertical gradient of pressure in this low-pressure system, several zones have been described in an effort to characterize the hemodynamic conditions that govern flow. West and colleagues have described these zones on the basis of the relationships among pressures in the pulmonary artery (P_{pa}), alveolus (P_{alv}), and pulmonary vein (P_v).[52] These relationships are summarized in Table 3-4.

In zone 1, which corresponds to the lung apices in the upright posture, alveolar pressure (P_{alv}) is greater than pulmonary artery (P_{pa}) and pulmonary venous (P_v) pressures. This results in a decreased transmural pressure and virtual collapse of these vessels, which receive very little or no blood flow. Farther down the lung in zone 2, the P_{pa} increases and exceeds P_{alv}, but P_{alv} still exceeds P_v. Resistance to blood flow in this zone is therefore governed by the difference between P_{pa} and P_{alv} and has been variously described as a *vascular waterfall* or a Starling resistor.

In zone 3, both P_{pa} and P_v exceed P_{alv}, and blood flow is determined by the more conventional arterial-to-venous-pressure gradient. This gradient is constant throughout zone 3 and suggests that blood flow is constant throughout this zone, rather than continuing to increase toward more dependent lung zones. In reality, however, blood flow does increase toward the bottom of zone 3 because the transmural or distending pressure across vessel walls increases due to increases in P_{pa} and P_v, while P_{alv} does not change. This progressive distending force serves to reduce resistance to blood flow through the vessels of zone 3. If other extrinsic factors are present to cause narrowing of these vessels, resistance to blood flow in these dependent regions may increase, and an additional area (zone 4) may exist in which the P_{pa}, P_v, and P_{alv} relationships are the same as in zone 3 but with decreased blood flow.

The zonal distribution of blood flow based on the relationships of P_{pa}, P_v, and P_{alv} provides a conceptual framework for understanding the nature of pulmonary blood flow distribution. However, these relationships do not account for all of the changes in blood flow distribution—for example, those associated with differing degrees of lung inflation. The vertical gradient of blood flow described in the zonal model is most pronounced at total lung capacity (i.e., after a maximal inspiration). After maximal expiration, the gradient is actually reversed to residual volume. Because relationships among P_{pa}, P_v, and P_{alv} remain relatively unchanged, other mechanical factors that affect vascular caliber must be invoked. These most likely represent changes in perivascular pressure and the influence of lung expansion on extraalveolar vessels.[53]

Pulmonary Vascular Resistance

The resistance to blood flow through the pulmonary circuit, pulmonary vascular resistance (PVR), is determined by the difference between the inflow pressure in the pulmonary artery (P_{pa}) and the outflow pressure or left atrial pressure (P_{la}). The ratio of this pressure drop across the pulmonary circuit to the total pulmonary blood flow (Q), or cardiac output, is defined as PVR. The calculation of PVR provides information about the state of the pulmonary vasculature. When PVR is increased, it is generally assumed, as with other vascular beds, that the pulmonary vessels are constricted. In the lung, however, the situation is more complex because of such factors as lung inflation, the collapsibility of vessels, and hydrostatic forces that alter the interpretations of PVR.

PARTITIONING OF PULMONARY VASCULAR RESISTANCE

A variety of techniques have been used to assess the distribution of pulmonary vascular resistance. There is still much uncertainty, however, about the relative partition of resistance among the vessels that make up the pulmonary circuit. Clinically, the measurement of pulmonary artery occlusion pressure (PAOP) has been used to estimate left atrial pressure and also pulmonary capillary pressure (P_c). These latter two pressures are only the same if postcapillary or venous resistance is negligible. Nevertheless, under most normal conditions this venous resistance may contribute about 40% of total PVR.

Total PVR can be calculated as

$$PVR = \frac{P_{pa} - PAOP}{CO}$$

where PAOP is an estimate of left atrial pressure, CO is cardiac output, and P_{pa} is mean pulmonary artery pressure.

This total PVR can in turn be divided into two components: a precapillary or pulmonary arterial resistance (R_a) and a postcapillary or venous resistance (R_v). These can be calculated as follows:

$$R_a = \frac{P_{pa} - P_c}{CO}$$

$$R_v = \frac{P_c - PAOP}{CO}$$

Although it is not possible to measure pulmonary capillary pressure (P_c) in intact animals or patients, Holloway et al have developed a technique that uses pulmonary artery occlusion curves to derive P_c and thus estimate the components of PVR.[54] The declining P_{pa} profile after balloon occlusion of a large pulmonary artery changes to a slower rate as blood spreads throughout the larger cross-sectional area of capillaries, veins, and left atrium. The inflection point from fast to slow is thought to represent P_c, and the difference between P_c and PAOP reflects the postcapillary or venous resistance (R_v). Although

---

TABLE 3-4

Regional Flow Zones of the Lung

Zone	Pressure Relationships	Vessel Behavior	Determinant of Flow
I	$P_{alv} > P_{pa} > P_v$	Collapse	Minimal flow
II	$P_{pa} > P_{alv} > P_v$	Starling resistor ("waterfall")	$P_{pa} - P_{alv}$
III	$P_{pa} > P_v > P_{alv}$	Distention	$P_{pa} - P_v$

From West JB, Dollery CT, Nairnark A: *J Appl Physiol* 19:713, 1964.

PAOP is often used clinically to estimate what is termed *pulmonary capillary wedge pressure*, PAOP is not a capillary pressure and so tends to underestimate P_c whenever PVR is increased as a result of changes in Rv.

FACTORS THAT ALTER PULMONARY VASCULAR RESISTANCE

Changes in PVR may be classified as active or passive. Active changes imply pulmonary vasoconstriction and presuppose that no passive changes have occurred. Table 3-5 lists some neurogenic, chemical, and humoral factors that actively alter pulmonary vascular resistance. For the most part, these vasoactive agents have similar effects on both systemic and pulmonary vessels. One of the most obvious exceptions, however, is histamine. This is a vasodilator in the systemic circuit, whereas in the pulmonary circulation it produces vasoconstriction. Also unique among the vasodilators are nitric oxide and prostaglandin E, both of which can be administered via inhalation to lessen systemic effects.

Passive changes in PVR imply that vessel caliber changes in response to factors such as lung mechanics or hemodynamics. Several such factors are also listed in Table 3-5. It is difficult to identify the precise contribution of each of the factors; many are interrelated, so a change in one effects a change in another (e.g., P_{la} and P_{pa}).

One remarkable characteristic of the low-pressure pulmonary circuit is its capacity to decrease PVR as pressure within the system (either venous or arterial) rises. Two mechanisms have been described to explain this: recruitment and distention. Recruitment reflects a reserve capacity of the capillary bed, which under normal conditions has some vessels essentially closed. As pressure increases, these vessels open, and blood flow is conducted through a vascular bed of greater cross-sectional area, thus lowering PVR. Most data indicate recruitment to be the primary mechanism for the decrease in PVR as pulmonary artery pressure increases above its normally low values. Further pressure increases result in distention of vessels that are open in response to the increase in perfusion. In this way, distention appears to contribute to the decrease in PVR associated with higher intravascular pressures.

Another unique feature of the pulmonary circulation is that vessels are exposed to different distending forces as lung volume expands and contracts above and below functional residual capacity (see Figure 3-5). As a result, the caliber and length of the vessels (and hence their resistance) are passively governed by changes in lung volume. At low lung volumes (below FRC) the extraalveolar vessels are compressed and offer increased resistance to flow, which diminishes as lung volume is increased. Although the extraalveolar vessels are maximally expanded at high lung volumes and offer low resistance to flow, alveolar vessels offer increased resistance because they become stretched and compressed.

Hypoxic Pulmonary Vasoconstriction

In the systemic vascular beds, hypoxia produces vasodilation to aid oxygen delivery and carbon dioxide removal. The pulmonary vessels, on the other hand, respond to acute hypoxia by constricting. This unique behavior in response to hypoxia is called hypoxic pulmonary vasoconstriction (HPV). This HPV response is an important compensatory mechanism that serves to divert flow away from hypoxic alveoli. Blood flow thus shifts from poorly ventilated alveoli to better-ventilated ones to match ventilation and perfusion and minimize arterial hypoxemia.

The physiologic manifestation of HPV depends heavily on the size of the lung area that is hypoxic. If the segment of hypoxic lung is small, HPV will result in diversion of flow away from the hypoxic area and little or no change in pulmonary artery pressure (Figure 3-6). If, on the other hand, the hypoxic area is very large (or more so if the alveolar hypoxia is diffuse and generalized), flow cannot be diverted, and the vasoconstriction results in an increased pulmonary arterial pressure (Figure 3-6). For flow diversion to occur, then, the hypoxic segment must constitute a small fraction of the total lung— flow diversion must be inversely related to the size of the hypoxic segment (Figure 3-4). The increases in pulmonary artery pressure are therefore directly related to the fraction of the total lung that is hypoxic. Thus the proportion of flow

---

TABLE 3-5

Factors That Alter Pulmonary Vascular Resistance

Increased PVR	Decreased PVR
ACTIVE	
Sympathetic stimulation	Isoproterenol
Hypoxia	Acetylcholine
Hypercapnia	Bradykinin
Acidemia	Prostaglandins (E_1, I_2)
Catecholamines	Theophylline
Histamine (H_1)	Nitric oxide
Serotonin	
Angiotensin II	
Prostaglandins (D_2, E_2, F_2, H_2)	
Substance P (tachykinins)	
PASSIVE	
Lung inflation or deflation from FRC	Increased cardiac output
Increased perivascular pressure	Increased P_{pa} and P_{la}
Increased blood viscosity	Increased pulmonary blood volume

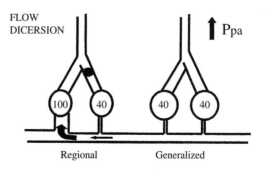

FIGURE 3-6 Changes in pulmonary artery pressure (P_{pa}) and diversion of blood flow are depicted for regional hypoxia and for diffuse or generalized hypoxia.

changes to pressure change decreases as the size of the hypoxic lung segment increases. This distinction between localized and the more generalized or diffuse hypoxia is essential to understanding the nature of HPV.

The major segment of the vascular system at which HPV occurs appears to be at the level of the precapillary arterioles (30 to 50 μm). These small muscular vessels are closely related to alveoli and are in an ideal position to respond to changes in alveolar oxygen concentration. Indeed, the most important stimulus to HPV appears to be the alveolar oxygen tension (Pao_2). Constriction occurs as Pao_2 decreases below normal, and the response reaches a maximum at about 30 mmHg. The oxygen tension in the mixed venous blood (Pvo_2) also plays a role in the HPV response. The Pvo_2 becomes increasingly important at very low levels of Pao_2 and in an atelectatic lung may be the only stimulus for HPV. At alveolar oxygen tensions of about 60 mmHg, Pvo_2 appears to have only a minor effect.

The HPV response is attenuated in a number of diverse clinical situations and by many classes of drugs (Table 3-6), the most notable of which are the anesthetic drugs. Intravenous drugs of most classes utilized in anesthesia (opioids, barbiturates, benzodiazepines, ketamine) do not appear to have a detectable effect on the HPV response. In vitro and in vivo experiments have shown that the pulmonary vasoconstrictive response to hypoxia is maintained at blood concentration of these drugs sufficient to produce analgesia and anesthesia.[55,56]

In vitro experiments utilizing isolated perfused lungs have generally shown that the halogenated inhalation agents in current use all inhibit HPV in a dose-related manner. In vitro observations with nitrous oxide also suggest that it produces little or no effect on HPV.[55] Studies in intact animals, however, suggest that 70% nitrous oxide moderately diminishes the HPV response.[56] The halogenated anesthetics also appear to antagonize the HPV response in intact animals and humans, but widely divergent results have been reported. The Marshals have provided a unifying concept for these findings based on the proportion of the lung that is made hypoxic.[57] They suggest that the differences in most previous studies arose from the size of the lung segment used. The larger the hypoxic segment studied, the less effective are the vasoconstriction and flow diversion away from the hypoxic site. The Marshals have also suggested that the antagonism of HPV by inhalation anesthetics may be obscured by other hemodynamic effects. The anesthetics depress myocardial function and produce a decrease in cardiac output. The latter is associated with decreased Pvo_2 and pulmonary artery pressures, both of which tend to intensify

HPV. Thus, unless such effects are considered, anesthetic actions on HPV might be subtle or misinterpreted.

The hypothesis that antagonism of HPV by inhalation anesthetics is important in the etiology of abnormal gas exchange during anesthesia is indeed an attractive one. Blunting of the HPV response, however, does not appear to account sufficiently for the impaired oxygenation observed. Inappropriately low Pao_2 values are often seen in patients breathing hyperoxic mixtures that would be expected to provide most, if not all, alveolar units with an oxygen tension far above that at which HPV comes into play. Therefore other factors, such as altered lung mechanics, might play a more significant role in the impaired gas exchange observed during general anesthesia (see Chapter 4).

REFERENCES

 1. Ferris BG, Mead J, Odie LH: Partitioning of respiratory flow resistance in man, *J Appl Physiol* 19:653, 1964.
 2. Proctor DF: The upper airway. II: Larynx and trachea, *Am Rev Respir Dis* 115:315, 1977.
 3. Macklem PT, Wilson NJ: Measurement of intrabronchial pressure in man, *J Appl Physiol* 20:653, 1965.
 4. Gal TJ: Effects of endotracheal intubation on normal cough performance, *Anesthesiology* 52:324, 1980.
 5. Liistro G, Stanescu D, Dooms G, et al: Head position modifies upper airway resistance in men, *J Appl Physiol* 64:1285, 1988.
 6. Lawes EG, Campbell I, Mercer D: Inflation pressure, gastric insufflation and rapid sequence induction, *Br J Anaesth* 59:315, 1987.
 7. Boidin MP: Airway patency in the unconscious patient, *Br J Anaesth* 57:306, 1985.
 8. Camporesi EM, Mortola JP, SantAmbrogia F, et al: Topical anesthesia of tracheal receptors, *J Appl Physiol* 47:1123, 1979.
 9. Weibel ER: *Morphometry of the human lung,* Berlin, 1963, Springer.
10. Detroyer A, Estenne M: Functional anatomy of the respiratory muscles, *Clin Chest Med* 9:175, 1988.
11. Black LF, Hyatt RE: Maximal respiratory pressures: normal values and relationship to age and sex, *Am Rev Respir Dis* 103:641, 1971.
12. Pavlin EG, Holle RH, Schoene RB: Recovery of airway protection compared with ventilation in humans after paralysis with curare, *Anesthesiology* 70:381, 1989.
13. Hess D: History of pulmonary function testing, *Respir Care* 34:427, 1989.
14. Leith DE, Mead JL: Mechanisms determining residual volume of the lungs in normal subjects, *J Appl Physiol* 23:221, 1967.
15. Tucker DH, Sieker HO: The effect of change in body position on lung volumes and intrapulmonary gas mixing in patients with obesity, heart failure and emphysema, *Am Rev Respir Dis* 85:787, 1960.
16. Koterba AM, Kosch PC, Beech J, Whitlock T: Breathing strategy of the adult horse *(Equus caballus)* at rest, *J Appl Physiol* 64:337, 1988.
17. Bryan AC, Wohl ME: Respiratory mechanics in children. In Macklem PT, Mead J (eds): *Handbook of physiology: the respiratory system,* Bethesda, 1986, American Physiological Society.
18. Olinsky A, Bryan MH, Bryan AC: Influence of lung inflation on respiratory control in neonates, *J Appl Physiol* 36:426, 1974.
19. Colin AA, Wohl MEB, Mead J, et al: Transition from dynamically maintained to relaxed end expiratory volume in human infants, *J Appl Physiol* 67:2107, 1989.
20. LeBlanc P, Ruff F, Milic-Emili J: Effects of age and body position on airway closure in man, *J Appl Physiol* 28:448, 1970.
21. Mansell A, Bryan C, Levinson H: Airway closure in children, *J Appl Physiol* 33:711, 1972.
22. Bergman NA: Distribution of inspired gas during anesthesia and artificial ventilation, *J Appl Physiol* 18:1085, 1963.
23. Damia G, Mascheroni D, Croci M, et al: Perioperative changes in functional residual capacity in morbidly obese patients, *Br J Anaesth* 60:574, 1988.
24. Bergman NA: Reduction in resting end-expiratory position of the respiratory system with induction of anesthesia and neuromuscular paralysis, *Anesthesiology* 57:14, 1982.
25. Hewlett AM, Hulands GH, Nunn JF, et al: Functional residual capacity during anesthesia. II: Spontaneous respiration, *Br J Anaesth* 46:486, 1974.

TABLE 3-6

Hypoxic Pulmonary Vasoconstriction (HPV): Drug Effects

Decreased HPV	Increased HPV
β-Adrenergic agonists	Almitrine
Calcium channel blockers	Cyclooxygenase inhibitors
Inhalation anesthetics	β-Blockers
Minoxidil	
Nitrosovasodilators	
Theophylline	

26. Westbrook PR, Stubbs SE, Sessler AD, et al: Effects of anesthesia and muscle paralysis on respiratory mechanics in normal man, *J Appl Physiol* 34:81, 1973.
27. Brismar B, Hedenstierna G, Lundquist H, et al: Pulmonary densities during anesthesia with muscular relaxation: a proposal of atelectasis, *Anesthesiology* 62:422, 1985.
28. Hedenstierna G, Lofstrom B, Lundh R: Thoracic gas volume and chest abdomen dimensions during anesthesia and muscle paralysis, *Anesthesiology* 55:499, 1981.
29. Muller N, Volgyesi G, Becker L, et al: Diaphragmatic muscle tone, *J Appl Physiol* 47:279, 1979.
30. Tusiewicz K, Bryan AC, Froese AB: Contributions of changing rib cage-diaphragm interactions to the ventilatory depression of halothane and anesthesia, *Anesthesiology* 47:327, 1977.
31. Hedenstierna G, Strandberg A, Brismar B, et al: Functional residual capacity, thoracoabdominal dimensions, and central blood volume during general anesthesia with muscle paralysis and mechanical ventilation, *Anesthesiology* 62:247, 1985.
32. Krayer S, Render K, Beck KC, et al: Quantification of thoracic volumes by three-dimensional imaging, *J Appl Physiol* 62:591, 1987.
33. Bickler PE, Dueck R, Prutow R: Effects of barbiturate anesthesia and functional residual capacity and rib cage/diaphragm contributions to ventilation, *Anesthesiology* 60:147, 1987.
34. Hudgel DQ, Devadatta P: Decrease in functional residual capacity during sleep in normal humans, *J Appl Physiol* 57:1319, 1984.
35. Mankikian B, Cantineau JP, Sartene R, et al: Ventilatory pattern and chest wall mechanics during ketamine anesthesia in humans, *Anesthesiology* 65:492, 1986.
36. Shulman D, Bearsmore CS, Aronson HG, et al: The effect of ketamine on functional residual capacity in young children, *Anesthesiology* 62:551, 1985.
37. Shuman D, Bar-yishay E, Beardsmore C, et al: Determinants of end-expiratory lung volume in young children during ketamine or halothane, *Anaesthesia* 66:636, 1987.
38. Hickey RF, Visick WD, Fairley HB: Effects of halothane anesthesia on functional residual capacity and alveolar-arterial oxygen tension difference, *Anesthesiology* 38:20, 1973.
39. Dueck R, Prutow RJ, Davies NHJ, et al: The lung volume at which shunting occurs with inhalation anesthesia, *Anesthesiology* 69:854, 1988.
40. Hedenstierna G, Tokics L, Strandberg A, et al: Correlation of gas exchange impairment to development of atelectasis during anesthesia and muscular paralysis, *Acta Anaesthesiol Scand* 30:183, 1986.
41. Tokics L, Hedenstierna G, Brismar BO, et al: Thoracoabdominal restriction in supine men: CT and lung function measurements, *J Appl Physiol* 64:599, 1988.
42. Hedenstierna G: Gas exchange during anaesthesia, *Br J Anaesth* 64:507, 1990.
43. Hedenstierna G, Tokics L, Lundquist H, et al: Phrenic nerve stimulation during halothane anesthesia, *Anesthesiology* 80:751, 1994.
44. Tokics L: Lung collapse and gas exchange during general anesthesia: effects of spontaneous breathing, muscle paralysis, and positive end-expiratory pressure, *Anesthesiology* 66:159, 1987.
45. Pelosi P, Ravagnan I, Guirati G, et al: Positive end expiratory pressure improves respiratory function in obese but not in normal subjects during anesthesia and paralysis, *Anesthesiology* 91:1221, 1999.
46. Rothen HU, Sporre B, Engberg G, et al: Re-expansion of atelectasis during general anesthesia: a computed tomography study, *Br J Anaesth* 71:788, 1993.
47. Rothen HU, Sporre B, Engberg G, et al: Influence of gas composition on recurrence of atelectasis after a reexpansion maneuver during general anesthesia, *Anesthesiology* 82:832, 1995.
48. Crawford ABH, Makowska M, Engel LA: Effect of bronchomotor tone on static mechanical properties of lung and ventilation distribution, *J Appl Physiol* 63:2278, 1987.
49. McAslan C, Mima M, Norden I, et al: Effects of halothane and methoxyflurane on pulmonary resistance gas flow during lung bypass, *Scand J Thorac Cardiovasc Surg* 5:193, 1971.
50. Coon RL, Kampine JP: Hypocapnic bronchoconstriction and inhalation anesthetics, *Anesthesiology* 43:635, 1975.
51. Badeer HS: Gravitational effects on the distribution of pulmonary blood flow: hemodynamic misconceptions, *Respiration* 43:408, 1982.
52. West JB, Dollery CT, Naimark A: Distribution of blood flow in isolated lung, relation to vascular and alveolar pressures, *J Appl Physiol* 19:713, 1964.
53. Hughes JMB, Glazier JB, Maloney JE, et al: Effect of lung volume on the distribution of pulmonary blood flow in man, *Respir Physiol* 4:58, 1968.
54. Holloway H, Perry M, Downey J, et al. Estimation of effective pulmonary capillary pressure in intact lungs, *J Appl Physiol* 54:846, 1983.
55. Bjertaines LJ: Hypoxia-induced vasoconstriction in isolated perfused lungs exposed to injectable or intravenous anesthetics, *Acta Anaesthesiol Scand* 21:133, 1977.
56. Benumof JL, Wahrenbrock EA: Local effects of anesthetics on regional hypoxic pulmonary vasoconstriction, *Anesthesiology* 43:525, 1975.
57. Marshall BE, Marshall C: Continuity of response to hypoxic pulmonary vasoconstriction, *J Appl Physiol* 49:189, 1980.

Physiology of the Lateral Decumitus Position, the Open Chest, and One-Lung Ventilation

4

Anastasios N. Triantafillou, MD

Jonathan L. Benumof, MD

Harish S. Lecamwasam, MD

IN the last 50 years, the development of reliable lung-isolation techniques, using devices such as double-lumen tubes and bronchial blockers, gave the impetus for extraordinary ground-breaking work in pulmonary physiology and, particularly, in the physiology of the lateral decubitus position (LDP) and one-lung ventilation (OLV). Most of this pioneering work is cited in this chapter. Thanks to this work, the understanding of LDP and OLV reached such a level of sophistication that surgery for thoracic disease became a reality and is now routine. The improved understanding of pathophysiologic changes that developed from this body of work also led to the improvement of skills for successfully managing patients undergoing thoracic surgery. As a result, today not only patients awaiting routine lung resections, but also those with end-stage lung disease (such as lung transplant recipients and candidates for lung-volume reduction surgery), can also be successfully managed. Despite improved knowledge, however, LDP, OLV, and prevention and treatment of hypoxemia under these conditions continue to present challenges to the anesthesiologist. Because of the significant pathophysiologic alterations that occur because of the interaction of general anesthesia and muscle paralysis, LDP, opening of the chest, and OLV, a review of these pathophysiologic changes is crucial for an understanding of these disturbances and their mutual interactions during thoracic anesthesia and surgery.

The first part of this chapter discusses each of these anesthetic and surgical effects on the distribution of ventilation ($\dot{V}$) and perfusion ($\dot{Q}$) and on the $\dot{V}/\dot{Q}$ relationship during two-lung ventilation. The second part of the chapter considers the physiologic consequences of spontaneous ventilation with an open chest; and, the third part considers the physiology of OLV.

PHYSIOLOGY OF THE LUNG RELATED TO POSITION

Upright Position

DISTRIBUTION OF PULMONARY PERFUSION

From a physiologic standpoint, the lung can be divided into four *zones*. Each zone has distinct characteristics related to its perfusion and ventilation and their matching. Explanations of these characteristics are provided in the text that follows.

Contraction of the right ventricle propels blood into the main pulmonary artery. Most of the kinetic energy of the blood in the main pulmonary artery is expended because the blood is climbing a vertical distance. The absolute pressure in the pulmonary artery (P_{pa}) decreases 1 cmH_2O for each centimeter traveled vertically up the lung (Figure 4-1). As the blood travels vertically, its energy is progressively diminished and at a height above the heart, P_{pa} becomes equal to atmospheric pressure (zero). At an even higher distance, the P_{pa} becomes negative.[1] In this region, alveolar pressure (P_A) equals atmospheric pressure and thus exceeds P_{pa} and pulmonary venous pressure (P_{pv}), which is naturally lower than Ppa. Because the pressure outside the vessels (P_A) is greater than the pressure inside the vessels, the vessels in this region of the lung are collapsed and there is no blood flow. This state characterizes zone 1, where $P_A > P_{pa} > P_{pv}$. Because there is no blood flow, no gas exchange is possible; therefore ventilation of the region is "wasted," and the region functions as alveolar deadspace. Little or no zone 1 exists in the lung under normal conditions. In conditions such as hypotension (decreased P_{pa}) or positive pressure ventilation (increased P_A), however, zone 1 lung may be greatly increased.

As blood travels below the level of the feet in the opposite direction, absolute P_{pa} becomes positive (higher than atmospheric pressure because of gravity). Therefore blood flow will occur only when P_{pa} exceeds P_A. At this vertical level within the lung, P_A also exceeds Ppv; therefore blood flow is determined by the $P_{pa} - P_A$ difference rather than by the conventional $P_{pa} - P_{pv}$ difference, and this characterizes the physiology of zone 2, where $P_{pa} > P_A > P_{pv}$.[2] The zone 2 relationship between blood flow and alveolar pressure has the same physical characteristics as a river waterfall flowing over a dam. The height of the upstream river (before reaching the dam) is equivalent to P_{pa}, and the height of the dam is equivalent to P_A. The rate of water flow over the dam is only proportional to the difference between the height of the upstream river and the dam ($P_{pa} - P_A$), and it does not matter how far below the dam the downstream riverbed (P_{pv}) is located. This phenomenon has various names, including the "waterfall," "Starling resistor," "weir," and "sluice" effect. Because mean P_{pa} increases down this region of the lung but mean P_A is relatively constant, the mean driving pressure ($P_{pa} - P_A$) increases linearly; therefore mean blood flow also increases linearly. It should be noted, however, that respiration and pulmonary blood flow are cyclic phenomena. Therefore the instantaneous values of P_{pa}, P_{pv}, and P_A change at any given time, and their relationships are dynamically determined by the phase lags between the cardiac and respiratory cycles. Consequently, a given point in zone 2 may

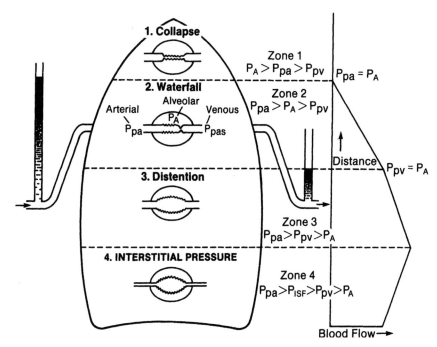

FIGURE 4-1 Schematic diagram showing the distribution of blood flow in the upright lung. In zone 1, alveolar pressure (P_A) exceeds pulmonary artery pressure (P_{pa}), and no flow occurs because the intraalveolar vessels are collapsed by the compressing alveolar pressure. In zone 2, arterial pressure exceeds alveolar pressure, but alveolar pressure exceeds venous pressure (P_{pv}). Flow in zone 2 is determined by the difference between arterial and alveolar pressure $(P_{pa} - P_A)$ and has been likened to an upstream river waterfall over a dam. Because P_{pa} increases down zone 2 and P_A remains constant, the perfusion pressure increases, and flow steadily increases down the zone. In zone 3, pulmonary venous pressure exceeds alveolar pressure, and flow is determined by the arterial-venous pressure difference $(P_{pa} - P_{pv})$, which is constant in this portion of the lung. However, the transmural pressure across the wall of the vessel increases down this zone so that the caliber of the vessels increases (resistance decreases); therefore flow increases. Finally, in zone 4, pulmonary interstitial pressure (P_{isf}) becomes positive and exceeds both pulmonary venous pressure and alveolar pressure. Consequently, flow in zone 4 is determined by the difference between arterial and interstitial pressure $(P_{pa} - P_{isf})$. (From West JB [ed]: *Regional differences in the lung*, San Diego, 1977, Academic Press.)

actually be in either a zone 1 or zone 3 condition, depending on the phase of the respiratory and cardiac cycles the subject is in at any given moment.

Still lower in the lung, there is a vertical level where P_{pv} becomes positive and exceeds P_A. In this region, zone 3, blood flow is governed by the pulmonary arteriovenous pressure difference $(P_{pa} - P_{pv})$; in this zone, intravascular pressures (P_{pa}, P_{pv}) exceed the P_A, the capillary systems are permanently open, and blood flow is continuous. In descending zone 3, gravity causes both absolute P_{pa} and P_{pv} to increase at the same rate so that the perfusion pressure $(P_{pa} - P_{pv})$ is unchanged. However, the pressure outside the vessels, namely, pleural pressure (P_{pl}), increases less than P_{pa} and P_{pv} so that the transmural distending pressures $(P_{pa} - P_{pl}$ and $P_{pv} - P_{pl})$ increase down zone 3, the vessel radii increase, vascular resistance decreases, and blood flow therefore increases further. These phenomena characterize zone 3, where $P_{pa} > P_{pv} > P_A$.

Finally, at a very low lung volume (i.e., the residual volume), the vascular resistance of extraalveolar vessels may increase, and the tethering action of the pulmonary tissue on the vessels may be lost. These circumstances may cause pulmonary interstitial pressure (P_{isf}) to increase and exceed PV, in extraalveolar vessel compression, increased extraalveolar vascular resistance, and decreased regional blood flow. For these reasons, zone 4 blood flow is governed by the arterio-interstitial pressure difference $(P_{pa} - P_{isf})$, which is less than the

$P_{pa} - P_{pv}$ difference; therefore zone 4 blood flow is less than zone 3 blood flow. These conditions characterize lung zone 4, where $P_{pa} > P_{isf} > P_{pv} > P_A$.

Similarly, in certain pathologic conditions, when intravascular pressures are elevated (e.g., in a volume-overloaded patient, in cases of a restricted and constricted pulmonary vascular bed, an extremely dependent lung [far below the vertical level of the left atrium], and in patients with pulmonary embolism and mitral stenosis), fluid may move out of the pulmonary vessels into the pulmonary interstitial compartment. As the fluid accumulates in the interstitial connective tissue around the large vessels and airways, peribronchial and periarteriolar edema fluid cuffs form. In this situation, the distribution of pulmonary blood flow may be altered significantly. The transuduated pulmonary interstitial fluid fills the pulmonary interstitial space and may eliminate the normally present negative and radially expanding interstitial tension (traction) on the extra-alveolar pulmonary vessels (Figure 4-2). The expansion of the pulmonary interstitial space by fluid causes P_{isf} to exceed P_{pv}.[3-6]

In summary, zone 4 is a region of the lung with decreased flow because of increased interstitial pressure and increased resistance of the extraalveolar vessels. It has been described in healthy humans.[7] It can also occur in certain conditions in which a large amount of fluid transudates into the pulmonary interstitial compartment.

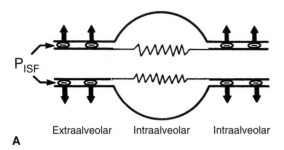

A   Extraalveolar   Intraalveolar   Intraalveolar

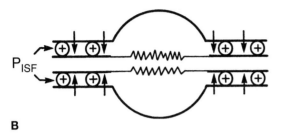

B

FIGURE 4-2 The effect of pulmonary interstitial fluid pressure (P_{isf}) on extra-alveolar vessels. In normal lungs **(A)**, a negative P_{isf} around the extraalveolar vessels tethers or keeps them open. When either pulmonary interstitial fluid accumulates or lung volume is extremely low, P_{isf} may become positive, exceed both pulmonary venous and alveolar pressures, and create a zone 4 **(B)** of the lung (where flow is proportional to the difference between pulmonary artery pressure and pulmonary interstitial pressure). (From Benumof JL: General respiratory physiology and respiratory function during anesthesia. In Benumof JL [ed]: *Anesthesia for thoracic surgery.* WB Saunders, 1987, Philadelphia.)

Consequently, as P_{pa} and P_{pv} increase, important changes take place in the pulmonary circulation, namely[8,9]:
1. Recruitment or opening of previously unperfused vessels
2. Distention or widening of previously perfused vessels
3. Transudation of fluid from very distended vessels.

Thus as mean P_{pa} increases, zone 1 arteries may become zone 2 arteries, and as mean P_{pv} increases, zone 2 veins may become zone 3 veins. The increases in both mean P_{pa} and P_{pv} distend zone 3 vessels according to their compliance and decrease the resistance to flow through them. Zone 3 vessels may become so distended that they leak fluid and become converted to zone 4 vessels. In general, recruitment is the principal change as P_{pa} and P_{pv} increase from low to moderate levels; distention is the principal change as P_{pa} and P_{pv} increase from moderate to high levels of vascular pressure; and, finally, transudation is the principal change when P_{pa} and P_{pv} increase from high to very high levels.

The gravitational model of pulmonary blood flow has been the traditional model according to which the effect of gravity governs the formation of the various zones of pulmonary blood flow distribution. Over the years, however, questions have been raised regarding inability of this model to explain certain phenomena—for example, decreased blood flow in midlung fields in the lateral position in awake or anesthetized humans or lack of significant alterations in lung blood flow under conditions of zero gravity.[10]

Single-photon emission computed tomography (SPECT) has been used by Hakin et al to study pulmonary blood flow in supine, awake humans.[11] The use of this technique revealed a new aspect in the traditional thinking of distribution of pulmonary blood flow. Using SPECT, a three-dimensional analysis of the pulmonary blood distribution is possible, as is an analysis of blood flow within horizontal slices of lung tissue. Scans revealed the well-known, gravity-dependent, top-to-bottom distribution of pulmonary blood flow and, in addition, revealed a strong pattern of a concentric, central-to-peripheral, "onion-like" distribution of flow. This pattern may indicate that the flow to a given area is also inversely proportional to that area's distance from the hilum. These observations do not disprove the traditional theory of vertical distribution of lung blood flow; however, they add a new center-to-periphery dimension to the understanding of blood flow distribution in the lung.

DISTRIBUTION OF VENTILATION

The pressure outside the lung—pleural pressure—also changes according to gravity. Thus, vertical P_{pl} differences bring about differences in regional alveolar volume, compliance, and ventilation. The vertical gradient of P_{pl} can best be understood by thinking of the lung as a plastic bag filled with semifluid contents. Without the presence of a supporting chest wall, the effect of gravity on the contents of the bag would be to cause the bag to assume a globular shape. In the presence of the supporting air-tight chest wall, the lung cannot assume a globular shape. The combination of gravity and the chest wall cause the fluid-filled bag (lung) to have a relatively more positive pressure at the bottom of the lung (where the lung is compressed against the chest wall) and a relatively more negative pressure at the top of the pleural space (where the lung pulls away from the chest wall) (Figure 4-3). The magnitude of this pressure gradient is determined by density of the lung. Because the lung is approximately one quarter of the density of water, the gradient of P_{pl} (in cmH_2O) is approximately one quarter of the height of the

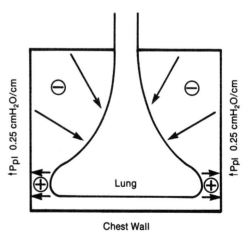

FIGURE 4-3 Schematic diagram of the lung within the chest wall showing the tendency of the lung to assume a globular shape because of the lung's viscoelastic nature. The tendency of the top of the lung to collapse inward creates a relatively negative pressure at the apex of the lung, and the tendency of the bottom of the lung to spread outward creates a relatively positive pressure at the base of the lung. Thus pleural pressure increases by 0.25 cmH_2O/cm of lung dependency. (From Benumof JL: Respiratory physiology and respiratory function during anesthesia. In Miller RD [ed]: *Anesthesia,* ed 3, New York, 1990, Churchill Livingstone.)

upright lung (30 cm). Thus, P_{pl} increases positively by 30/4 = 7.5 cmH_2O from the top to the bottom of the lung.[12]

Because P_A is the same throughout the lung, the Ppl gradient causes regional differences in transpulmonary distending pressures ($P_A - P_{pl}$). Because P_{pl} is most positive (least negative) in the dependent basilar lung regions, alveoli in these regions are more compressed and, therefore considerably smaller than superior, relatively non compressed apical alveoli (there is an approximately fourfold alveolar volume difference).[13] If the regional differences in alveolar volume are translated over to a pressure-volume curve for normal lung (Figure 4-4), the dependent small alveoli are on the midportion and the nondependent large alveoli are on the upper portion of the S-shaped curve. As the different regional slopes of the composite curve are equal to the different regional lung compliances, dependent alveoli are relatively compliant (steep slope) and nondependent alveoli are relatively noncompliant (flat slope). Thus the majority of the tidal volume is preferentially distributed to dependent alveoli because they expand more per unit of pressure change than do nondependent alveoli.

DISTRIBUTION OF THE VENTILATION-TO-PERFUSION RATIO

Figure 4-5 shows that both blood flow and ventilation (both on the left vertical axis) increase linearly with distance down the normal upright lung (horizontal axis, reverse polarity).[14] Because blood flow increases from a very low value and more rapidly than ventilation as distance down the lung increases, the ventilation-to-perfusion $\dot{V}/\dot{Q}$ ratio (right vertical axis) decreases rapidly at first, then more slowly.

The $\dot{V}_A/\dot{Q}$ ratio best expresses the amount of ventilation relative to perfusion in any given lung region. Thus alveoli at the base of the lung are somewhat overperfused in relation to their ventilation ($\dot{V}_A/\dot{Q}$ less than 1). Figure 4-6 shows the calculated ventilation ($\dot{V}_A$) and blood flow ($\dot{Q}$) in liters per minute, the $\dot{V}_A/\dot{Q}$ ratio, and the alveolar P_{O_2} and P_{CO_2} in mmHg for horizontal slices from the top (7% of lung volume), middle (11% of lung volume), and bottom (13% of lung volume) of the lung.[15] It can be seen that the Pa_{O_2} increases by more than 40 mmHg; from 89 mmHg at the base to 132 mmHg at the apex, while Pa_{CO_2} decreases by 14 mmHg; from 42 mmHg at the bottom to 28 mmHg at the top. Thus in keeping with the regional $\dot{V}_A/\dot{Q}$, the bottom of the lung is relatively hypoxic and hypercarbic compared with the top of the lung. Ventilation-to-perfusion inequalities have different effects on Pa_{CO_2} compared with Pa_{O_2}. Blood passing through underventilated alveoli tends to retain its CO_2 and does not take up enough O_2; blood traversing overventilated alveoli gives off an excessive amount of CO_2 but cannot take up a proportionately increased amount of O_2 owing to the flatness of the oxyhemoglobin dissociation curve in this region. Hence, a lung with uneven ventilation-to-perfusion relationships can eliminate CO_2 from the overventilated alveoli to compensate for the underventilated alveoli. Thus with uneven ventilation-to-perfusion relationships, PA_{CO_2}-to-Pa_{CO_2} gradients are small and PA_{O_2}-to-Pa_{O_2} gradients are usually large.

Lateral Decubitus Position: Distribution of Perfusion and Ventilation

AWAKE, CLOSED CHEST

Gravity causes a vertical gradient in the distribution of pulmonary blood flow in the lateral decubitus position for the same

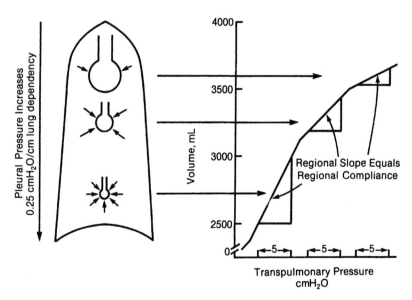

FIGURE 4-4 Pleural pressure increases by 0.25 cmH_2O with each centimeter down the lung. The increase in pleural pressure causes a fourfold decrease in alveolar volume. The caliber of the air passages also decreases as lung volume decreases. When regional alveolar volume is translated over to a regional transpulmonary pressure-alveolar volume curve, small alveoli are on a steep *(large slope)* portion of the curve, and large alveoli are on a flat *(small slope)* portion of the curve. Because the regional slope equals regional compliance, the dependent small alveoli normally receive the largest share of the tidal volume. Over the normal tidal volume range (lung volume increases by 500 mL from 2500 [normal FRC] to 3000 mL), the pressure-volume relationship is linear. Lung volume values in this diagram relate to the upright position. (From Benumof JL: Respiratory physiology and respiratory function during anesthesia. In Miller RD [ed]: *Anesthesia,* ed 3, New York, 1990, Churchill Livingstone.)

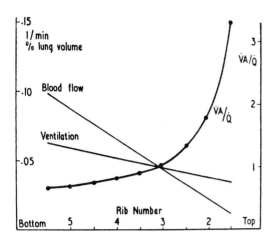

FIGURE 4-5 Distribution of ventilation and blood flow *(left vertical axis)* and the ventilation-to-perfusion ratio *(right vertical axis)* in a normal upright lung. Both blood flow and ventilation are expressed in liters per minute per percent alveolar volume and have been drawn as smoothed-out linear functions of vertical height. The *closed circles* mark the ventilation-to-perfusion ratios of horizontal lung slices (three of which are shown in Figure 4-6). A cardiac output of 6 L/min and a total minute ventilation of 5.1 L/min were assumed. (From West JB: *J Appl Physiol* 17:892, 1962.)

reason that it does in the upright position. Because the vertical hydrostatic gradient is lower in the LDP than in the upright position, there is ordinarily less zone 1 blood flow (in the nondependent lung) in the former position compared with the latter position (Figure 4-7). Nevertheless, blood flow to the dependent lung is still significantly greater than blood flow to the

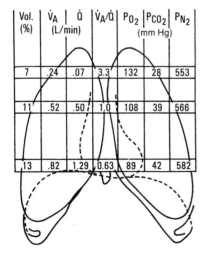

Vol. (%)	$\dot{V}_A$ (L/min)	$\dot{Q}$	$\dot{V}_A/\dot{Q}$	P_{O_2}	P_{CO_2}	P_{N_2}
					(mm Hg)	
7	.24	.07	3.3	132	28	553
11	.52	.50	1.0	108	39	566
13	.82	1.29	0.63	89	42	582

FIGURE 4-6 The ventilation-to-perfusion ratio ($\dot{V}_A/\dot{Q}$) and the regional composition of alveolar gas. Values for the regional flow ($\dot{Q}$), ventilation ($\dot{V}_A$), P_{O_2}, and P_{CO_2} are derived from Figure 4-5. P_{N_2} has been obtained by what remains from the total gas pressure (which, including water vapor, equals 760 mmHg). The volumes [vol. (%)] of the three lung slices are also shown. Compared with the top of the lung, the bottom of the lung has a low $\dot{V}_A/\dot{Q}$ ratio and is relatively hypoxic and hypercarbic. (From West JB: *J Appl Physiol* 17:892, 1962 and West JB: *Ventilation blood flow and gas exchange,* ed 4, Oxford, 1985, Blackwell Publications.)

nondependent lung. Consequently, when the right lung is nondependent, it should receive approximately 45% of the total blood flow, in contrast to the 55% of the total blood flow it receives in the upright and supine positions. When the left lung is nondependent, it should receive approximately 35% of the total blood flow, in contrast to the 45% of the total blood flow that it receives in the upright and supine positions.[16,17] Because gravity also causes a vertical gradient in pleural pressure (P_{pl}) (Figures 4-3 and 4-4) in the lateral decubitus position (as it does in the upright position, Figure 4-8, *A*), ventilation is relatively increased in the dependent lung compared with the nondependent lung (Figure 4-8, *B*). In addition, in the lateral decubitus position, the dome of the lower diaphragm is pushed higher into the chest than the dome of the upper diaphragm; therefore, the lower diaphragm is more sharply curved and has a higher preload than the upper diaphragm. As a result, the lower diaphragm is able to contract more efficiently during spontaneous respiration. Thus, in the lateral decubitus position in the awake patient, the lower lung is normally better ventilated than the upper lung, regardless of the side on which the patient is lying, although there remains a tendency toward greater ventilation of the larger right lung.[18] Because there is greater perfusion to the lower lung, the preferential ventilation to the lower lung is matched by its increased perfusion, so that the distribution of the $\dot{V}/\dot{Q}$ ratios of the two lungs is not greatly altered when the awake subject assumes the lateral decubitus position. Perfusion increases to a greater extent than does ventilation with lung dependency, so the $\dot{V}/\dot{Q}$ ratio decreases from nondependent to dependent lung (just as it does in upright and supine lungs).

ANESTHESIA, SPONTANEOUS VENTILATION, CLOSED CHEST

Comparing the awake state to the anesthetized state in the lateral decubitus position shows that there is no difference in the distribution of pulmonary blood flow between the dependent and nondependent lungs. In the anesthetized patient, the dependent lung continues to receive relatively more perfusion than the nondependent lung. The induction of general anesthesia, however, does cause significant changes in the distribution of ventilation between the two lungs.

In the anesthetized state, the majority of ventilation is switched from the dependent lung in the awake state to the nondependent lung when the patient is in the LDP (Figure 4-9).[19,20] The induction of general anesthesia usually causes a decrease in functional residual capacity (FRC), and both lungs share in the loss of lung volume. Because each lung occupies a different initial position on the pulmonary pressure-volume curve while the subject is awake, a general anesthesia-induced reduction in the FRC of each lung causes each lung to move to a lower but still different portion of the pressure-volume curve (Figure 4-9). The dependent lung moves from an initially steep part of the curve (with the subject awake) to a lower and flatter part of the curve (after anesthesia is induced), while the nondependent lung moves from an initially flat portion of the pressure-volume curve (with the subject awake) to a lower and steeper part of the curve (after anesthesia is induced). Thus, with the induction of general anesthesia, the lower lung moves to a less favorable (flat, noncompliant) portion and the upper lung to a more favorable (steep, compliant) portion of the pressure-volume curve.

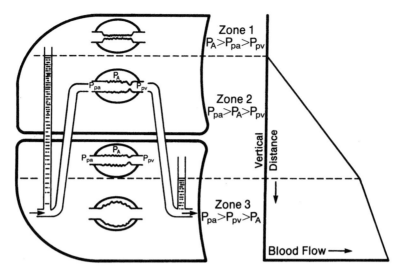

FIGURE 4-7 Schematic representation of the effects of gravity on the distribution of pulmonary blood flow in the lateral decubitus position. The vertical gradient in the lateral decubitus position is less than in the upright position. Consequently, there is less zone 1 and more zone 2 and 3 blood flow in the lateral decubitus position compared with the upright position. Nevertheless, pulmonary blood flow increases with lung dependency and is greater in the dependent lung than in the nondependent lung. P_A, Alveolar pressure; P_a, pulmonary artery pressure; P_v, pulmonary venous pressure. (From Benumof JL: Physiology of the open chest and one-lung ventilation. In Benumof JL [ed]: *Anesthesia for thoracic surgery*, Philadelphia, 1987, WB Saunders.)

ANESTHESIA, MUSCLE PARALYSIS, ARTIFICIAL VENTILATION, CLOSED CHEST

If the anesthetized patient in the lateral decubitus position is also paralyzed and artificially ventilated, the high curved diaphragm of the lower lung is no longer actively contracting and thus does not play a role in ventilation as it does in the awake state.[21] In addition, the mediastinum rests on the lower lung and physically impedes lower lung expansion; it also selectively further decreases lower lung FRC. The weight of the abdominal contents pushing cephalad against the diaphragm is greatest in the dependent lung, and this factor physically further impedes lower lung expansion and disproportionately decreases lower lung FRC. Finally, patient positioning (flexion, jackknife) may further compress the

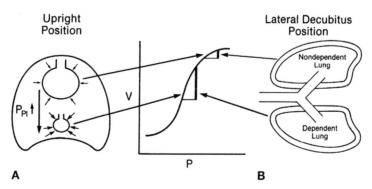

FIGURE 4-8 Pleural pressure *(P_{pl})* in the awake upright patient **(A)** is most positive in the dependent portion of the lung, and alveoli in this region are, therefore, most compressed and have the lowest volume. Pleural pressure is least positive (most negative) at the apex of the lung, and alveoli in this region are therefore least compressed and have the highest volume. When these regional differences in alveolar volume are translated in to a regional transpulmonary pressure-alveolar volume curve, the small dependent alveoli are on a steep *(large slope)* portion of the curve, and the large nondependent alveoli are on a flat *(small slope)* portion of the curve. In this diagram, regional slope equals regional compliance. Thus, for a given and equal change in transpulmonary pressure, the dependent part of the lung receives a much larger share of the tidal volume than close the nondependent lung. In the lateral decubitus position **(B)**, gravity also causes pleural pressure gradients and therefore, affects the distribution of ventilation similarly. The dependent lung lies on a relatively steep portion and the nondependent lung lies on a relatively flat portion of the pressure-volume curve. Thus in the lateral decubitus position, the dependent lung receives the majority of the tidal ventilation. *V*, Alveolar volume; *P*, transpulmonary pressure. (From Benumof JL: Physiology of the open chest and one-lung ventilation. In Benumof JL [ed]: *Anesthesia for thoracic surgery*, Philadelphia, 1987, WB Saunders.)

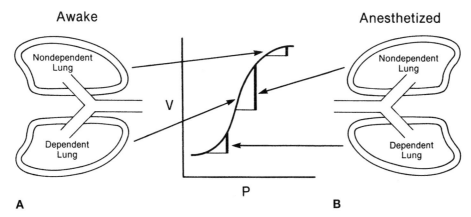

FIGURE 4-9 Schematic diagram showing the distribution of ventilation in the awake patient in the lateral decubitus position **(A)** and the distribution of ventilation in the anesthetized patient in the lateral decubitus position **(B)**. The induction of anesthesia has caused a loss of lung volume in both lungs, with the nondependent lung moving from a flat, noncompliant portion to a steep, compliant portion of the pressure-volume curve and the dependent lung moving from a steep, compliant part to a flat, noncompliant part of the pressure-volume curve. Thus the anesthetized patient in the lateral decubitus position has the majority of the tidal ventilation in the nondependent lung (where there is the least perfusion) and the minority of the tidal ventilation in the dependent lung (where there is the greatest perfusion). *V,* Alveolar volume; *P,* transpulmonary pressure. (From Benumof JL: Physiology of the open chest and one-lung ventilation. In Benumof JL [ed]: *Anesthesia for thoracic surgery,* Philadelphia, 1987, WB Saunders.)

dependent lung considerably. Opening the nondependent hemithorax during artificial ventilation causes a disproportionate preferential ventilation of the nondependent lung.

In summary, the anesthetized patient (with or without paralysis) in the lateral decubitus position and with a closed chest, has a nondependent lung that is well ventilated but poorly perfused and a dependent lung that is well perfused but poorly ventilated, resulting in maldistribution of blood flow and inequality of ventilation to perfusion. Later in this chapter, measures to counteract this imbalance are presented.

ANESTHESIA, OPEN CHEST

Compared with the condition of the anesthetized, closed-chest patient in the lateral decubitus position, opening the chest wall and pleural space alone does not ordinarily cause any further alteration in the distribution of pulmonary blood flow between the dependent and nondependent lungs. The dependent lung continues to receive relatively more perfusion than the nondependent lung. Opening the chest wall and pleural space in a patient who is simultaneously anesthetized, paralyzed, and ventilated, however, does have a significant impact on the distribution of ventilation, which may result in a further mismatching of ventilation with perfusion (Figure 4-10).[22] If the upper lung is no longer confined by the chest wall and the total effective compliance of that lung becomes equal to that of the lung parenchyma alone, it will be relatively free to expand and, consequently, be overventilated while remaining underperfused.

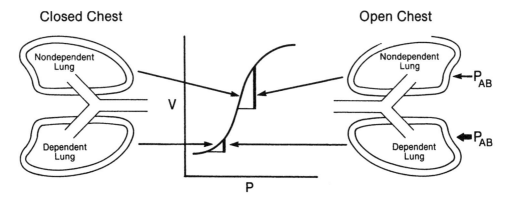

FIGURE 4-10 Schematic diagram of a patient in the lateral decubitus position, comparing the closed-chest anesthetized condition with the open-chest anesthetized and paralyzed condition. Opening the chest increases nondependent-lung compliance and reinforces or maintains the larger part of the tidal ventilation going to the nondependent lung. Paralysis also reinforces or maintains the larger part of tidal ventilation going to the nondependent lung because the pressure of the abdominal contents *(P$_{AB}$)* pressing against the upper diaphragm is minimal *(smaller arrow),* and it is therefore easier for positive-pressure ventilation to displace this lesser resisting dome of the diaphragm. *V,* Alveolar volume; *P,* transpulmonary pressure. (From Benumof JL: Physiology of the open chest and one-lung ventilation. In Benumof JL [ed]: *Anesthesia for thoracic surgery,* Philadelphia, 1987, WB Saunders.)

Conversely, the dependent lung may continue to be relatively noncompliant, poorly ventilated, and overperfused.[16] If expansion of the exposed lung is mechanically or externally restricted (via surgical retraction and compression), then ventilation will be diverted to the dependent, better-perfused lung.[23]

ANESTHESIA, MUSCLE PARALYSIS, ARTIFICIAL VENTILATION, OPEN CHEST

In the open-chest, anesthetized patient in the lateral decubitus position, the induction of paralysis alone does not cause any significant alteration in the distribution of pulmonary blood flow between the dependent and nondependent lungs. There are, however, strong theoretical and experimental considerations that indicate that paralysis might cause significant changes in the distribution of ventilation between the two lungs under these conditions.

In the supine and lateral decubitus positions, the weight of the abdominal contents pressing against the diaphragm is greatest on the dependent part of the diaphragm (posterior lung and lower lung, respectively) and least on the nondependent part of the diaphragm (anterior lung and upper lung, respectively) (see Figure 4-10). In the awake, spontaneously breathing patient, the weight of the abdominal contents acts as an increased preload on the diaphragm, which makes the largest excursion in the dependent portion and the smallest in the nondependent portion. This condition helps in directing the greatest amount of ventilation to where there is the most perfusion (dependent lung) and the least amount of ventilation where there is the least perfusion (nondependent lung). During paralysis and positive pressure ventilation, the diaphragm becomes passive and flaccid and, thus, it is displaced preferentially toward the nondependent area, where the resistance to passive diaphragmatic movement by the abdominal contents is least. Conversely, the diaphragm is minimally displaced in the dependent portion, where the resistance to passive diaphragmatic movement by the abdominal contents is greatest.[24] This is an unfavorable condition because the greatest amount of ventilation may occur where there is the least perfusion (nondependent lung), and the least amount of ventilation may occur where there is the greatest perfusion (dependent lung).

SUMMARY OF PHYSIOLOGY OF THE LATERAL DECUBITUS POSITION AND THE OPEN CHEST

The preceding section dealt with the pathophysiologic changes associated with the lateral decubitus position in the anesthetized, paralyzed patient with an open chest. Under such conditions, a considerable ventilation-perfusion mismatch may occur because of greater ventilation but less perfusion to the nondependent lung and less ventilation but more perfusion to the dependent lung. Gravitational effects primarily determine the distribution of blood flow. The relatively good ventilation of the upper lung is a result of its higher compliance resulting from the loss of the confines of the chest wall. The relatively poor ventilation of the dependent lung is due to the restriction caused by its compression by the mediastinum, abdominal contents, and suboptimal positioning effects and by loss of its volume (Figure 4-11). In addition, poor mucociliary clearance and atelectasis may cause further volume loss to the dependent lung.

A logical solution to this problem would be to apply positive end-expiratory pressure (PEEP) to the dependent lung.[25] A

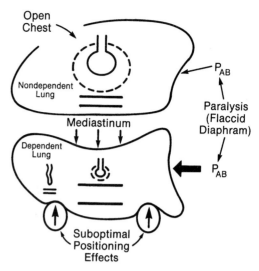

FIGURE 4-11 Schematic summary of ventilation-perfusion relationships in the anesthetized patient in the lateral decubitus position who has an open chest and is paralyzed and suboptimally positioned. The nondependent lung is well ventilated (as indicated by the *large dashed lines*) but poorly perfused (small perfusion vessel), while the dependent lung is poorly ventilated *(small dashed lines)* but well perfused (large perfusion vessel). In addition, the dependent lung may also develop an atelectatic shunt compartment (indicated on the left side of the lower lung) because of the circumferential compression of this lung. (See text for detailed explanation.) P_{AB}, Pressure of the abdominal contents. (From Benumof JL: Physiology of the open chest and one-lung ventilation. In Benumof JL [ed]: *Anesthesia for thoracic surgery,* Philadelphia, 1987, WB Saunders.)

more detailed discussion of the various measures to deal with the pitfalls associated with one-lung ventilation and TAE lateral position is presented later in this chapter.

PHYSIOLOGY OF THE OPEN CHEST WITH SPONTANEOUS VENTILATION

Mediastinal Shift

An examination of the physiology of the open chest during spontaneous ventilation reveals why controlled positive pressure ventilation is the only practical way to provide adequate gas exchange during thoracotomy.[26] In the spontaneously breathing, closed-chest patient in the lateral decubitus position, gravity causes the pleural pressure in the dependent hemithorax to be less negative than in the nondependent hemithorax (see Figures 4-3, 4-4, and 4-8), but there is still negative pressure in each hemithorax on each side of the mediastinum. In addition, the weight of the mediastinum causes some compression of the lower lung, which contributes to the pleural pressure gradient. With the nondependent hemithorax open, atmospheric pressure in that cavity exceeds the negative pleural pressure in the dependent hemithorax; this imbalance of pressure on the two sides of the mediastinum causes a further downward displacement of the mediastinum into the dependent thorax. During inspiration, the caudal movement of the dependent lung diaphragm increases the negative pressure in the dependent lung and causes still further displacement of the mediastinum into the dependent hemithorax. During expiration, as the dependent-lung diaphragm moves cephalad, the pressure in the

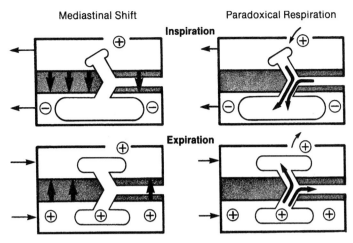

FIGURE 4-12 Schematic representation of mediastinal shift and paradoxical respiration in the spontaneously ventilating patient in the lateral decubitus position with an open chest. The open chest is always exposed to atmospheric pressure *(+)*. During inspiration, negative pressure *(–)* in the intact hemithorax causes the mediastinum to move vertically downward (mediastinal shift). In addition, during inspiration, movement of gas from the nondependent lung in the open hemithorax into the dependent lung in the closed hemithorax, and movement of air from the environment into the open hemithorax, cause the lung in the open hemithorax to collapse (paradoxical respiration). During expiration, relative positive pressure *(+)* in the closed hemithorax causes the mediastinum to move vertically upward (mediastinal shift). In addition, during expiration, the gas moves from the dependent lung to the nondependent lung and from the open hemithorax to the environment; consequently, the nondependent lung expands during expiration (paradoxical respiration). (From Benumof JL: Physiology of the open chest and one-lung ventilation. In Benumof JL [ed]: *Anesthesia for thoracic surgery*, Philadelphia, 1987, WB Saunders.)

dependent hemithorax becomes relatively positive, and the mediastinum is pushed upward out of the dependent hemithorax (Figure 4-12). Thus, the tidal volume in the dependent lung is decreased by an amount equal to the inspiratory displacement caused by mediastinal movement. This phenomenon is called *mediastinal shift* and is one mechanism that results in impaired ventilation in the open-chest, spontaneously breathing patient in the lateral decubitus position. The mediastinal shift can also cause circulatory changes (decreased venous return) and reflexes (sympathetic activation) that result in a clinical picture similar to shock: The patient is hypotensive, pale, and cold, with dilated pupils. Local anesthetic infiltration of the pulmonary plexus at the hilum and the vagus nerve can diminish these reflexes. More practically, controlled positive pressure ventilation abolishes these ventilatory and circulatory changes that are associated with mediastinal shift.

Paradoxical Respiration

When a pleural cavity is exposed to atmospheric pressure, the lung is no longer held open by negative intrapleural pressure, and it tends to collapse because of unopposed elastic recoil.[26] Thus the lung in an open chest is at least partially collapsed. It has long been observed during spontaneous ventilation with an open hemithorax that lung collapse is accentuated during inspiration and, conversely, that the lung expands during expiration. This reversal of lung movement with an open chest during respiration has been termed *paradoxical respiration*. The mechanism of paradoxical respiration is similar to that of mediastinal shift. During inspiration, the descent of the diaphragm on the side of the open hemithorax causes air from the environment to enter the pleural cavity on that side through the thoracotomy

opening and fill the space around the exposed lung. The descent of the hemidiaphragm on the closed side of the chest causes gas to enter the closed-chest lung in the normal manner. However, gas also enters the closed-chest lung (which has a relatively negative pressure) from the open-chest lung (which remains at atmospheric pressure); this results in further reduction in the size of the open-chest lung during inspiration. During expiration, the reverse occurs, with the collapsed, open-chest lung filling from the intact lung and air moving back out of the exposed hemithorax through the thoracotomy incision. The phenomenon of paradoxical respiration is illustrated in Figure 4-12. Paradoxical breathing is increased by a large thoracotomy and by increased airway resistance in the intact lung. Paradoxical respiration may be prevented either by manual collapse of the open-chest lung or, more commonly, by controlled positive pressure ventilation.

PHYSIOLOGY OF ONE-LUNG VENTILATION

Comparison of Arterial Oxygenation and CO₂ Elimination During Two-Lung Versus One-Lung Ventilation

As discussed previously, the matching of ventilation and perfusion is impaired during two-lung ventilation in an anesthetized, paralyzed, open-chest patient in the lateral decubitus position. The reason for the mismatching of ventilation and perfusion is two-fold: relatively good ventilation and poor perfusion of the nondependent lung, and relatively poor ventilation and good perfusion of the dependent lung (see Figrue 4-11). Despite the presence of nongravitational determinants of pulmonary blood flow as discussed previously, the blood flow gradient favoring the dependent lung during OLV is a result of gravity. The opening of the chest and muscle paralysis are the causes for the relatively better ventilation of the nondependent lung. The relatively poor ventilation of the dependent lung is a result of both the loss of lung volume with general anesthesia and the circumferential compression of lung tissue by the mediastinum, abdominal contents, and suboptimal positioning. In addition to this ventilation-perfusion mismatch, compression of the dependent lung also produces a shunt compartment from areas of atelectasis in this lung (see Figure 4-11). As a result of this worsened ventilation-perfusion mismatch and shunt, two-lung ventilation in an open-chest patient in the lateral decubitus position often results in an increased $P(A-a)O_2$ gradient and impaired oxygenation.

If the nondependent lung is also not ventilated (as is the case during one-lung ventilation), any blood flow to it also becomes shunt flow, in addition to the shunt flow that might exist in the dependent lung (Figure 4-13). Thus one-lung ventilation creates an additional obligatory right-to-left transpulmonary shunt through the nonventilated nondependent lung, as compared with two-lung ventilation in the lateral decubitus position. It can, therefore be predicted that one-lung ventilation, when compared with two-lung ventilation in the lateral decubitus position, results in a larger alveolar-to-arterial oxygen tension difference and lower PaO_2 given the identical inspired oxygen concentration (FIO_2), hemodynamic conditions, and metabolic state. This prediction is supported both by clinical experience and by studies that have compared arterial oxygenation during two-lung and one-lung ventilation under a wide variety of conditions.[27-40]

One-lung ventilation has much less of an effect on $PaCO_2$ than on the PaO_2. Blood flowing through relatively underventilated alveoli will retain more than a normal amount of CO_2 and not take up a normal amount of O_2. Because of the linear shape of the CO_2 dissociation curve over the physiologic range, however, blood flowing through relatively well-ventilated alveoli releases a proportionately greater amount of CO_2. Conversely, because of the flatness of the top end of the sigmoid-shaped oxygen-hemoglobin dissociation curve, the blood flowing through the same relatively well-ventilated alveoli is unable to take up a proportionately increased amount of O_2. Thus, during one-lung ventilation, the ventilated lung is typically able to eliminate sufficient CO_2 to compensate for the nonventilated lung and maintain a small $PACO_2$-to-$PaCO_2$ gradient. The ventilated lung is, however, unable to take up sufficient O_2 to compensate for the nonventilated lung, leading to an elevated PAO_2/PaO_2 gradient.

Ventilation and Perfusion Distribution During One-Lung Ventilation
THE NONDEPENDENT, NONVENTILATED LUNG

Passive mechanical and active vasoconstrictor mechanisms operate during one-lung ventilation to minimize blood flow to the nondependent, nonventilated lung, preventing the PaO_2 from decreasing as much as would be predicted by the distribution of blood flow during two-lung ventilation.

The passive mechanical mechanisms that decrease blood flow to the nondependent lung include gravity, surgical manipulation, and the severity of preexisting disease in the nondependent lung (see Figure 4-13). Gravity causes a vertical gradient in the distribution of pulmonary blood flow in the lateral decubitus position for the same reason that it does in the upright and supine positions (see Figure 4-7). Consequently, blood flow to the nondependent lung is less than blood flow to the dependent lung. This gravity component of blood flow reduction should be constant with respect to both time and magnitude. Surgical compression (directly compressing lung vessels) and retraction (causing kinking and tortuosity of lung vessels) of the nondependent lung may further passively reduce blood flow to the nondependent lung. Interruption (clamping or ligation) of the blood supply to the nondependent lung would greatly reduce or eliminate its blood flow and improve O_2 saturation.

The degree of disease in the nondependent lung is also a significant determinant of the amount of blood flow to the nonde-

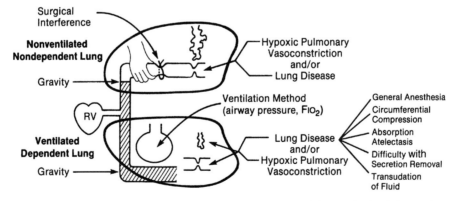

FIGURE 4-13 Schematic diagram showing the major determinants of blood flow distribution during one-lung ventilation. Blood flow to the nonventilated, nondependent lung is reduced by the force of gravity, surgical interference (compression, tying off of vessels), hypoxic pulmonary vasoconstriction, and/or lung disease (vascular obliteration, thrombosis). Blood flow to the ventilated, dependent lung is increased by gravity; however, dependent-lung blood flow and vascular resistance may be altered in either direction depending on the method of ventilation (amount of airway pressure, FIO_2, and the amount of dependent-lung disease and/ or hypoxic pulmonary vasoconstriction). Factors that may increase the amount of dependent lung disease intraoperatively are listed on the extreme right of the figure. (From Benumof JL: Physiology of the open chest and one-lung ventilation. In Benumof JL [ed]: *Anesthesia for thoracic surgery,* Philadelphia, 1987, WB Saunders.)

pendent lung. If the nondependent lung is severely diseased, there may be a fixed reduction to its blood flow preoperatively, and collapse of such a diseased lung might not cause much of an increase in shunt. Indeed, it has been shown prospectively that patients who have less than 45% of their pulmonary blood flow to their diseased lung are at significantly less risk for hypoxemia during one-lung ventilation.[41] It has been observed that administration of sodium nitroprusside or nitroglycerin—which should abolish hypoxic pulmonary vasoconstriction [HPV] to patients with chronic obstructive pulmonary disease, who have a fixed reduction in the cross-sectional area of their pulmonary vascular bed—does not cause an increase in shunt.[30] This observation supports the notion that a diseased pulmonary vasculature is incapable of developing HPV. Conversely, these drug agents have been shown to increase shunt in patients with acute regional lung disease who have an otherwise normal pulmonary vascular bed.[29] Therefore a greater degree of shunt through the nondependent lung during one-lung ventilation may be more likely to occur in patients who require thoracotomy for nonpulmonary disease.[30]

The most significant reduction in blood flow to the nondependent lung is caused by an active vasoconstrictor mechanism. The normal response of the pulmonary vasculature to atelectasis is an increase in pulmonary vascular resistance (in the atelectatic lung region); the increase in atelectatic lung pulmonary vascular resistance is thought to be due almost entirely to HPV.[31-33] This selective increase in atelectatic lung pulmonary vascular resistance diverts blood flow toward the remaining normoxic or hyperoxic lung. This diversion of blood flow minimizes the amount of shunt flow that occurs through the hypoxic lung. Figure 4-14 shows the theoretically expected effect of HPV on arterial oxygen tension (Pao_2) as the amount of lung that is made hypoxic increases.[34] Based upon this data, when very little of the lung is hypoxic (near 0%), the Pao_2 is

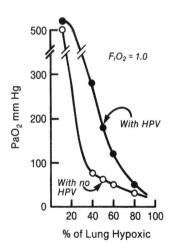

FIGURE 4-14 A model of the effect of hypoxic pulmonary vasoconstriction (HPV) on Pao_2 as a function of the percentage of lung that is hypoxic. The model assumes an Fio_2 of 1.0 and normal hemoglobin, cardiac output, and oxygen consumption. In the range of 30% to 70% of the lung being hypoxic, the normal expected amount of HPV can increase Pao_2 significantly. (From Benumof JL: Conventional and differential lung management of one-lung ventilation. In Benumof JL [ed]: *Anesthesia for thoracic surgery,* Philadelphia, 1987, WB Saunders.)

relatively insensitive to the degree of HPV because the shunt fraction is small. When most of the lung is hypoxic (near 100%), the Pao_2 is again relatively insensitive to the degree of HPV because there is no significant normoxic region to which the hypoxic region blood flow can be diverted. The greatest impact of HPV and therefore the largest degree of difference between the Pao_2 expected with a normal amount of HPV (a 50% blood flow reduction for a single lung) compared with when there is no HPV is seen when the percentage of lung that is hypoxic is intermediate (between 30% and 70%). This is the amount of lung that is typically hypoxic during one-lung ventilation. It is therefore not surprising that numerous clinical studies of one-lung ventilation have shown that the shunt through the nonventilated lung is usually 20% to 30% of the cardiac output as opposed to the 40% to 50% that might be expected if HPV were absent in the nonventilated lung.[27,30,35-40] Thus HPV is an autoregulatory mechanism that protects the Pao_2 by decreasing the amount of shunt flow that can occur through a hypoxic lung.

Figure 4-15 outlines the major determinants of the amount of atelectatic lung HPV that might occur during anesthesia. In the following discussion, the HPV issues or considerations are numbered as they are in Figure 4-15.

1. The distribution of alveolar hypoxia is probably not a determinant of the amount of HPV. All regions of the lung—either the basilar or dependent parts of the lungs (supine or upright) or discrete anatomic units such as a lobe or single lung—respond to alveolar hypoxia with vasoconstriction.[42]

2. As with low ventilation/perfusion ($\dot{V}/\dot{Q}$) ratios and nitrogen-ventilated lungs, it appears that the vast majority of blood flow reduction in an acutely atelectatic lung is due to HPV, not to passive mechanical factors such as vessel tortuosity.[31-33] This conclusion is based on the observation that reexpansion and ventilation of a collapsed lung with nitrogen (removing any mechanical factor) do not increase the blood flow to the lung, whereas ventilation with oxygen restores all of the blood flow to the precollapse values. This conclusion applies regardless of whether ventilation is spontaneous or with positive pressure, or whether the chest is open or closed.[32] A canine model has suggested that a small amount of additional subacute (more than 30 minutes) blood flow diminution may occur with atelectasis from mechanical compression of the blood vessels.[43] In humans, however, a prolonged unilateral hypoxic challenge during anesthesia has been shown to result in an immediate vasoconstrictor response with no further potentiation or diminution of the HPV response.[44]

3. Most systemic vasodilator drugs have been shown to either directly inhibit regional HPV or to have a clinical effect consistent with inhibition of regional HPV (i.e., decreasing Pao_2 and increasing shunt in patients with acute respiratory disease). The vasodilator drugs that have been shown to inhibit HPV or to have a clinical effect consistent with inhibition of HPV are nitroglycerin,[29,45-51] nitroprusside,[52-58] dobutamine,[59,60] several calcium antagonists,[61-66] and many β-agonists (isoproterenol, ritodrine, orciprenaline, salbutamol, adenosine triphosphatase, and glucagon).[59,65,67-73] Aminophylline and hydralazine may not decrease HPV.[74,75]

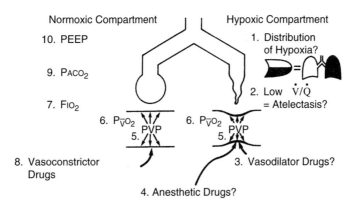

FIGURE 4-15 Diagram showing many of the components of the anesthetic experience that might determine the amount of regional HPV. The clockwise numbering of considerations corresponds to the order in which these considerations are discussed in the text. $\dot{V}/\dot{Q}$, Ventilation-to-perfusion ratio; *PVP*, pulmonary vascular pressure; $P_{\bar{v}}O_2$, mixed venous oxygen tension; F_{IO_2}, inspired oxygen tension; P_ACO_2, alveolar carbon dioxide tension; *PEEP*, positive end-expiratory pressure. (From Benumof JL, Alfery DD: Anesthesia for thoracic surgery. In Miller RD [ed]: *Anesthesia*, ed 3, New York, 1990, Churchill Livingstone.)

4. The effect of anesthetic drugs on regional HPV must be considered from both experimental (animal studies) and clinical (human one-lung ventilation studies) points of view, as discussed below.

a. *Effect of anesthetics on experimental hypoxic pulmonary vasoconstriction*—It would be undesirable if general anesthetics inhibited HPV in the nonventilated, nondependent lung. All of the inhalation and many of the intravenous anesthetics have been studied with regard to their effect on HPV. These studies have been referenced in great detail by Benumof.[76] The experimental preparations used may be divided into four basic categories: (1) in vitro; (2) in vivo–not intact (pump-perfused lungs, no systemic circulation or neural function); (3) in vivo–intact (normally perfused lungs, normal systemic circulation); and, (4) humans (volunteers or patients). According to this experimental preparation breakdown, it appears that the inhibition of HPV by halothane is a universal finding in the in vitro and in vivo–not intact preparations. In the more normal or physiologic in vivo-intact and human studies, however, halothane has caused no or only a very slight decrease in HPV response. Thus it appears that a fundamental property of halothane is its inhibition of HPV in experimental preparations, which can be controlled for other physiologic influences (e.g., pulmonary vascular pressure, cardiac output, mixed venous oxygen tension, CO_2 level, temperature) that can have an effect on the HPV response. In the more biologically complex in vivo–intact models, other factors seem to be involved that greatly diminish the inhibitory effect of halothane on HPV. Important methodologic differences exist between the in vitro and in vivo–not intact preparations and the in vivo–intact and human models that could account for the observed differences in halothane effect on HPV. The methodological differences include presence (or absence) of perfusion pulsations, perfusion fluid composition, size of the perfusion

circuit, baroreceptor influences, absence of bronchial blood flow (which abolishes all central and autonomic nervous activity in the lung), chemical influences (e.g., pH, PO_2), humoral influences (i.e., histamine and prostaglandin release from body tissues), lymph flow influences, unaccounted-for or uncontrolled changes in physiologic variables (such as cardiac output, mixed venous oxygen tension, and pulmonary vascular pressures, which might have directionally opposite effects on HPV), and, very importantly, the use of different species.

Although the number of studies involving halogenated drugs other than halothane (desflurane, isoflurane, sevoflurane, enflurane, and methoxyflurane) is relatively small, most of these anesthetics have demonstrated inhibition of HPV (at least in the in vitro models), although with mostly minimal clinically relevant effect. Nitrous oxide appears to cause a small, somewhat consistent inhibition of HPV. All intravenous anesthetics studied to date have no effect on HPV.

To summarize previous animal studies, it appears that a fundamental property of inhalation anesthetics is to decrease HPV. However, in intact animal preparations, some biologic or physiologic property seems to remove or greatly lessen the inhibitory effect of anesthetic drugs on HPV. It may be that the cause(s) of the difference in effect of anesthetic drugs on regional HPV from preparation to preparation, anesthetic to anesthetic, and species to species relate closely to the fundamental mechanism of HPV, which is still unknown.

b. *Effect of anesthetics on arterial oxygenation during clinical one-lung ventilation.* An often-made extrapolation of the much more numerous in vitro and in vivo–not intact HPV studies is that anesthetic drugs might impair arterial oxygenation during one-lung anesthesia by inhibiting HPV in the nonventilated lung. One of the previously cited studies on the effect of isoflurane on regional canine HPV was especially well controlled and showed that when all nonanesthetic drug variables that might change regional HPV are kept constant, isoflurane inhibits single-lung HPV in a dose-dependent manner.[77] Additionally, the study is valuable because the investigators offer an easily comprehensible quantitative summary of the relationship between dose of isoflurane administered and degree of inhibition of the single-lung canine HPV response. If the summary can be extrapolated or applied to the clinical one-lung ventilation situation (at least as an approximation), insights can be gained into what might be expected with regard to arterial oxygenation when such patients are anesthetized with isoflurane. To put this insight into clinical focus, it is necessary to first understand what should happen to blood flow, shunt flow, and arterial oxygenation, as a function of a normal amount of HPV, when two-lung ventilation is changed to one-lung ventilation in the lateral decubitus position. Once the stable one-lung ventilation condition has been described, it is then possible, using the data from the previously mentioned study, to see how isoflurane administration would affect the one-lung ventilation blood flow distribution, shunt flow, and arterial oxygen tension.

(i) Two-lung ventilation: blood flow distribution—Gravity causes a vertical gradient in the distribution of pulmonary blood flow in the lateral decubitus position for the same reason that it does in the upright position (see Figure 4-7). Based on Figure 4-7 and the previous discussion, the average two-lung ventilation distribution of blood flow of in the lateral decubitus position would consist of 40% of total blood flow perfusing the nondependent lung and 60% of total blood flow perfusing the dependent lung (Figure 4-16, left side of figure).

(ii) One-lung ventilation: blood flow distribution, shunt flow, and arterial oxygen tension—When the nondependent lung is not ventilated (made atelectatic), HPV in the nondependent lung increases nondependent lung pulmonary vascular resistance and decreases nondependent lung blood flow. In the absence of any confounding or inhibiting factors to the HPV response, a single-lung HPV response should decrease the blood flow to that lung by 50%.[34] Consequently, the nondependent lung should be able to reduce its blood flow from 40% to 20% of total blood flow, and the nondependent-to-dependent lung blood flow ratio during one-lung ventilation should be 20% to 80% (see Figure 4-16, *middle*).

All the blood flow to the nonventilated nondependent lung is shunt flow; therefore, one-lung ventilation creates an obligatory right-to-left transpulmonary shunt flow that was not present during two-lung ventilation. If no shunt existed during two-lung ventilation conditions (ignoring the normal 1% to 3% shunt flow because of the bronchial, pleural, and thebesian circulations), it would be expected that the ideal total shunt flow during one-lung ventilation (i.e., with intact HPV) would be a minimal 20% of total blood flow. With normal hemodynamic and metabolic states, the arterial oxygen tension should be approximately 280 mmHg.[78] Other, much more complicated models have been constructed to describe what to expect in terms of shunt during one-lung ventilation when varying degrees of shunt exist during two-lung ventilation.[79]

(iii) Effect of isoflurane on the one-lung ventilation blood flow distribution, shunt flow, and arterial oxygen tension—Domino et al found that the percentage inhibition of regional HPV response was equal to 22.8 (percentage of alveolar isoflurane) minus 5.3 (see Figure 4-16, *top equation*).[77] The top

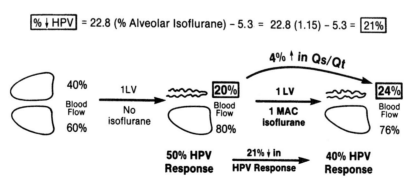

$$\boxed{\% \downarrow HPV} = 22.8 \,(\% \text{ Alveolar Isoflurane}) - 5.3 = 22.8\,(1.15) - 5.3 = \boxed{21\%}$$

FIGURE 4-16 Schematic diagram showing the effect of 1 MAC isoflurane anesthesia on shunt during one-lung ventilation (1 LV) of normal lungs. The two-lung ventilation nondependent/dependent lung blood flow ratio is 40%/60% *(left side)*. When two-lung ventilation is converted to one-lung ventilation (as indicated by atelectasis of the nondependent lung), the HPV response decreases the blood flow to the nondependent lung by 50%, so that the nondependent/-dependent lung blood flow ratio is now 20%/80% *(middle)*. According to the data of Domino et al, administration of 1 MAC isoflurane anesthesia should cause a 21% decrease in the HPV response, which would decrease the 50% blood flow reduction to a 40% blood flow reduction in the HPV response.[77] Consequently, the nondependent/dependent lung blood flow ratio would now become 24%/76%, representing a 4% increase in the total shunt across the lungs *(right side)*. (From Benumof JL: *Anesthesiology* 64:419, 1986.)

equation and right side of Figure 4-16 show that one minimum alveolar concentration (MAC) isoflurane anesthesia would inhibit the nondependent lung HPV response by approximately 21%, which would decrease the nondependent lung HPV response from a 50% to a 40% blood flow reduction in the nondependent lung. This, in turn, would increase nondependent lung blood flow from 20 to 24% of total blood flow, causing shunt to increase by 4% of the cardiac output and PaO_2 to decrease a moderate amount to 205 mmHg ($FIO_2 = 1.0$). A decrease in PaO_2 and an increase in shunt of this magnitude are small and may not be detectable given the usual accuracy of clinical methodology. In fact, in clinical one-lung ventilation studies involving intravenously anesthetized patients with this level of shunting, administration of 1 MAC isoflurane (and halothane) anesthesia during stable one-lung ventilation conditions caused no detectable decrease in PaO_2.[35,80] In one of these clinical studies, stable one-lung ventilation conditions in the lateral decubitus position were established in patients who were anesthetized with only intravenous drugs.[35] While stable one-lung ventilation was maintained, inhalation anesthetics were administered (halothane and isoflurane end-tidal concentrations were more than 1 MAC for at least 15 minutes) and then discontinued (halothane and isoflurane end-tidal concentrations decreased to near zero). In the other study, steady-state OLV conditions in the lateral decubitus position were established in patients who were anesthetized with only inhalation drugs (halothane and isoflurane end-tidal concentrations were more than 1 MAC for more than 40 minutes).[80] While one-lung ventilation was continued, inhalation anesthesia was then discontinued, and intravenous anesthesia was administered (halothane and isoflurane end-tidal concentrations decreased to near zero). There was no significant difference in PaO_2 during inhalation anesthesia with either halothane or isoflurane compared with intravenous anesthesia during one-lung ventilation in either of the two experimental sequences. In addition, there were no significant changes in physiologic variables—such as cardiac output, pulmonary vascular pressure, and mixed venous oxygen tension—that might secondarily alter nondependent lung HPV. Thus, irrespective of whether inhalation anesthesia is administered before or after intravenous anesthesia during one-lung ventilation, inhalation anesthesia does not appear to further impair arterial oxygenation. These findings are consistent with the interpretation that 1 MAC halothane and isoflurane in patients with a moderate level of shunting does not inhibit HPV enough to cause a significant decrease in PaO_2 during OLV in the lateral decubitus position. Almost identical results have been obtained during one-lung ventilation of volunteers with

nitrogen (while the other lung was ventilated with 100% O_2) who were alternately anesthetized with isoflurane and intravenous drugs and enflurane and intravenous drugs.[81,82] Desflurane and sevoflurane have similarly been shown to typically not cause clinically significant impairment in oxygenation in both intact animal models and humans.[83–87] The commonly used intravenous anesthetics, such as propofol, are believed not to have any inhibitory effects on HPV.[88,89] Given such apparent sparing of HPV by intravenous anesthetic agents as compared with their inhalation counterparts (despite evidence that their clinical effects with regard to causing hypoxia are minimal), it may be argued that total intravenous anesthesia (TIVA) could be a preferable anesthetic option for patients at high risk for significant hypoxia when undergoing surgery with OLV.

5. The HPV response is maximal when pulmonary vascular pressure is normal and is decreased by either high or low pulmonary vascular pressure. The mechanism for high pulmonary vascular pressure inhibition of HPV is simple: the pulmonary circulation is poorly endowed with smooth muscle and cannot constrict against an increased vascular pressure.[90–92] The mechanism for low pulmonary vascular pressure inhibition of HPV is more complex. For this to occur, the hypoxic compartment must be atelectatic. Under these circumstances, when pulmonary vascular pressure decreases, it is possible for part of the ventilated lung (but not the atelectatic lung) to be in a zone 1 condition (alveolar pressure increases relative to pulmonary artery pressure) and to experience a disproportionate increase in pulmonary vascular resistance, which would divert blood flow back over to the atelectatic lung, thereby inhibiting atelectatic lung HPV.[93]

6. The HPV response is also maximal when the mixed venous oxygen tension ($P\bar{v}O_2$) is normal and is decreased by either high or low $P\bar{v}O_2$. The mechanism for high $P\bar{v}O_2$ inhibition of HPV is presumably due to reverse diffusion of oxygen, causing the oxygen tension of either the vessels, interstitial or alveolar spaces, or all of these to be increased above the HPV threshold.[94] That is, if enough oxygen can reach some receptor in the small arteriole-capillary-alveolar area, then the vessels will not vasoconstrict. The mechanism for low $P\bar{v}O_2$ inhibition of HPV is a result of the low $P\bar{v}O_2$ decreasing alveolar oxygen tension in the normoxic compartment down to a level sufficient to induce HPV in the supposedly "normoxic" lung.[95,96] The HPV in the "normoxic" lung competes against and offsets the HPV in the originally hypoxic lung and results in no blood flow diversion away from the more obviously hypoxic lung.

7. Selectively decreasing the FIO_2 in the normoxic compartment (from 1.0 to 0.5–0.3) causes an increase in the vascular tone of the normoxic lung, thereby decreasing blood flow diversion from the hypoxic lung to the normoxic lung.[92,96]

8. Vasoconstrictor drugs (dopamine, epinephrine, phenylephrine) appear to constrict normoxic lung vessels preferentially and therefore to disproportionately increase vascular resistance in the normoxic lung.[54,64,70,90] The

increase in normoxic lung vascular resistance decreases normoxic lung blood flow and increases atelectatic lung blood flow. The HPV-inhibiting effect of vasoconstrictor drugs is similar to decreasing FIO_2 in the normoxic lung.

9. The interaction between the $PaCO_2$ and HPV is complex. Hypocapnia has been thought to directly inhibit regional HPV, and hypercapnia has been considered to directly enhance regional HPV.[91,97] Furthermore, during OLV, hypocapnia can only be produced by hyperventilation of the one lung. This hyperventilation requires an increased ventilated lung airway pressure, which may cause increased ventilated lung pulmonary vascular resistance (given the U-shaped curve describing the pulmonary vascular resistance vs. lung volume), which in turn may divert blood flow back into the hypoxic lung, further inhibiting HPV. Hypercapnia during OLV also seems to act as a vasoconstrictor and selectively increases ventilated lung pulmonary vascular resistance (diverting blood flow to the nonventilated lung), inhibiting HPV. Hypercapnia is also typically caused by hypoventilation of the ventilated lung, which greatly increases the risk of developing low $\dot{V}/\dot{Q}$ and atelectatic regions in the dependent lung, further exacerbating the alveolar-arterial oxygen gradient. Therefore, despite its direct effects on HPV, hypercapnia can worsen oxygenation. It should, however, be noted that hypoventilation of the dependent lung can theoretically decrease ventilated lung airway pressure, leading to a decrease in ventilated lung pulmonary vascular resistance and enhancement of HPV in the nonventilated lung (the converse of what can be expected with hyperventilation and increased pressures).

10. The effects of changes in airway pressure due to PEEP and tidal volume changes are discussed in detail in the section on the methods used to ventilate the dependent lung. In brief, selective application of PEEP to the normoxic ventilated lung only can selectively increase pulmonary vascular resistance in the ventilated lung and shunt blood flow back into the hypoxic nonventilated lung (i.e., decrease nonventilated lung HPV) and worsen oxygenation.[98,99] Conversely, it was recently shown that PEEP can improve oxygenation if application of PEEP moves the end-expiratory pressure to the lower inflection point of the static lung compliance curve.[100] In this particular study, application of 5 cmH_2O PEEP to the dependent lung improved oxygenation in only 6 out of 42 individuals. The individuals who benefited from application of extrinsic PEEP were those who had a lower PaO_2, during two-lung ventilation and a lower intrinsic PEEP.

As will also be discussed, high-frequency ventilation of the gas exchanging lung can be associated with a low airway pressure, an enhancement of HPV in the collapsed lung, and improved oxygenation during one-lung ventilation.[101]

11. A combined anesthetic technique involving a general anesthetic and a thoracic epidural has become the standard of anesthetic care for patients undergoing thoracotomy. It is important to consider the effects of epidural anesthesia on HPV, given that epidural anesthesia has been shown to alter FRC and that it can alter blood flow via its effects on the autonomic system. It has been shown in an analysis of pressure-flow relations in a canine model, however, that thoracic epidural anesthesia has no significant effect on pulmonary vascular tone and may in fact enhance HPV.[102]

12. Finally, there is some evidence that certain types of infections (which may cause atelectasis), particularly granulomatous and pneumococcal infections, may inhibit HPV.[103,104]

THE DEPENDENT, VENTILATED LUNG. The dependent lung usually has an increased amount of blood flow because of both passive gravitational effects and active, nondependent lung vasoconstrictor effects (see Figure 4-13, *lower panel*). However, the dependent lung may also have a hypoxic compartment (areas of low $\dot{V}/\dot{Q}$ ratio and atelectasis) that was present preoperatively or that developed intraoperatively. The dependent lung hypoxic compartment may develop intraoperatively for several reasons. First, regardless of position, general anesthesia is associated with a decrease in lung volume and with atelectasis as the relaxation volume exceeds the closing capacity. Additionally, in the lateral decubitus position, the ventilated dependent lung is compressed by the mediastinum from above, by the abdominal contents from a caudal direction, and by suboptimal positioning effects (rolls, packs, chest supports) pushing in from the dependent side and axilla (see Figure 4-13).[17,21,24,105]

Absorption atelectasis can also occur in regions of the dependent lung that have low $\dot{V}/\dot{Q}$ ratios when they are exposed to a high inspired oxygen concentration.[106,107] Retained secretions can lead to mucous plugging and to the development of poorly ventilated and/or atelectatic areas in the dependent lung. Finally, maintaining the lateral decubitus position for prolonged periods of time may cause fluid to transude into the dependent lung (which may be vertically below the left atrium), causing a further decrease in lung volume and increased airway closure.[108]

The development of a low $\dot{V}/\dot{Q}$ ratio and/or atelectatic areas in the dependent lung will increase vascular resistance in the dependent lung because of dependent lung HPV, decreasing dependent lung blood flow, and increasing nondependent lung blood flow.[42,105,109,110] Stated differently, the pulmonary vascular resistance in the ventilated compartment of the lung determines the ability of the ventilated (and supposedly normoxic) lung to accept redistributed blood flow from the hypoxic lung. Clinical conditions that are independent of specific dependent lung disease, but which may still increase dependent lung vascular resistance in a dose-dependent manner, are a decreasing inspired oxygen tension in the dependent lung (from 1.0 to 0.5-0.3) and a decreasing temperature (from 40° to 30° C).[92,96,110,111]

MISCELLANEOUS CAUSES OF HYPOXEMIA DURING ONE-LUNG VENTILATION

Still other factors contribute to hypoxemia during one-lung ventilation. Malfunction of the dependent lung airway lumen (blockage by secretions) and malposition of the double-lumen endotracheal tube are, from experience, the most common causes of an increased $P(A-a)O_2$ and hypoxemia. Hypoxemia resulting from mechanical failure of the oxygen supply system or the anesthesia machine is a recognized hazard of any kind of anesthesia. Gross hypoventilation of the dependent lung can be a major cause of hypoxemia. Resorption of residual oxygen from the clamped nonventilated lung is time dependent and accounts for a gradual increase in shunt and decrease in PaO_2 after one-lung ventilation is initiated.[108] With all other anesthetic and surgical factors constant, anything that decreases the $P\overline{v}O_2$ (decreased cardiac output, increased oxygen consumption via excessive sympathetic nervous system stimulation, hyperthermia, or shivering) will cause an increased $P(A\text{-}a)O_2$.[112,113]

Management of One-Lung Ventilation
CONVENTIONAL MANAGEMENT

The proper initial conventional management of one-lung ventilation is based logically on the preceding determinants of blood flow distribution during one-lung ventilation. Because induction of one-lung ventilation incurs a risk of systemic hypoxemia, it is extremely important that dependent lung ventilation, as it affects these determinants, be optimally managed. This section considers the usual management of OLV in terms of the most appropriate FIO_2, tidal volume, and respiratory rate that should be used. While consideration of these parameters remains paramount, it is important to remember that the approach to hypoxia during OLV should always begin with an assessment of proper endotracheal tube placement and endotracheal tube patency.

Inspired Oxygen Concentration. Although the theoretical possibilities of absorption atelectasis and oxygen toxicity exist, the benefits of ventilating the dependent lung with 100% O_2 far exceed the risks. A high FIO_2 in the single ventilated lung may critically increase the PaO_2 from arrhythmogenic and life-threatening levels to safer levels. In addition, a high FIO_2 in the dependent lung causes vasodilation and increases the dependent lungs capability of accepting blood flow redistribution from non-dependent lung HPV.[92] Oxygen toxicity typically does not occur during the limited operative period, and absorption atelectasis in the dependent lung also becomes unlikely given typical one-lung ventilatory strategies (intermittent positive pressure ventilation with or without low-level PEEP).[107,114]

Tidal Volume. Classically, it has been recommended that the dependent lung be ventilated with a tidal volume of approximately 10 to 12 mL/kg. This recommendation is based upon data showing that: tidal volumes between 8 to 15 mL/kg produced no significant change in transpulmonary shunt or oxygenation during OLV[38,115]; tidal volumes less than 8 mL/kg can cause atelectasis; and tidal volumes greater than 15 mL/kg can increase dependent-lung airway vascular resistance and decrease nondependent-lung HPV[98,109,116] A tidal volume of 10 to 12 mL/kg was considered "preferred" because it lay in the middle of the range of tidal volumes suggested by the data just discussed. It should be kept in mind, however, that tidal volumes even within the recommended 10 to 12 mL/kg range can be inappropriately high for selected patients and can result in lung injury. This phenomenon of volume-related lung injury is termed *volutrauma*.[117,118] Whether mechanical ventilator-associated lung injury is a result of volutrauma, barotrauma (lung injury because of excessive pressure), or a combination of the two remains indeterminate.[119] Therefore if mechanical ventilation during OLV with a tidal volume of 10 to 12 mL/kg causes lung hyperinflation, excessive airway pressure, or both, the tidal volume should be lowered (after mechanical causes, e.g., tube malfunction, have been ruled out) and other measures to maintain adequate oxygenation and ventilation should be instituted.

Respiratory Rate. Traditionally, the respiratory rate during OLV was adjusted to maintain a $PaCO_2$ of 40 mmHg. Because tidal volumes during OLV are typically reduced (to lower the risk of volutrauma and barotrauma to the ventilated lung), the maintenance of "normal" minute ventilation often requires supranormal respiratory rates. And because the CO_2 dissociation curve over the physiologic range is linear, this unchanged minute ventilation results in normocapnia despite the ventilation-perfusion mismatches associated with OLV.[109,120-122] Although elevated respiratory rates can maintain normocapnia, they can also be associated with dynamic air trapping and hyperinflation in patients with increased airway resistance. Indeed, over the last decade, the importance of maintaining normocapnia has been brought under scrutiny with the advent of controlled mechanical hypoventilation—called permissive hypocapnia— a ventilatory strategy in which limitation of pulmonary hyperinflation is given priority over maintaining normocapnia. Permissive hypercapnia was first proposed in the mechanical ventilation of asthma patients and is now commonly used in the ventilation of patients with a variety of pathologies including acute respiratory distress syndrome (ARDS) and lung volume reduction surgery.[123-125] As a detailed discussion of permissive hypercapnia is beyond the scope of this chapter, the interested reader is directed to the numerous excellent reviews of this topic that have appeared in the recent medical literature.[126-128] One of the lingering controversies related to permissive hypercapnia concerns the maximum level of respiratory acidosis that can be considered safe in patients who are critically ill. While $PaCO_2$ levels exceeding 100 mmHg with a corresponding pH less than 7.0 have been reported in the literature, most authorities would not recommend routinely tolerating pH less than 7.2 given the potential deleterious effects of the acidosis.[129] The effects of hypercapnia on the nondependent lung HPV should also be taken into consideration when initiating permissive hypercapnia.

Hypocapnia should also be avoided because the dependent lung hyperventilation typically required to produce systemic hypocapnia may excessively increase dependent-lung vascular resistance and divert blood to the nonventilated lung, worsening its HPV. Furthermore, hypocapnia may directly inhibit HPV in the nondependent lung.[91,97]

Once OLV is initiated, ventilation and arterial oxygenation are monitored by use of frequent arterial blood gases, end-tidal carbon dioxide concentration, and pulse oximetry. If either ventilation or oxygenation following optimization of the FIO_2, tidal volume, and respiratory rate is inadequate, then one or more of the differential lung management techniques described next should be considered.

Differential Lung Management
SELECTIVE DEPENDENT-LUNG PEEP

Because the ventilated dependent lung often has a decreased lung volume during OLV (Figures 4-11, 4-13, and 4-17, *A*) for the numerous reasons discussed previously, it is not surprising that several attempts have been made to improve oxygenation by selectively treating the ventilated lung with PEEP.[17-21,40,115,116] An accepted risk of selective dependent-lung PEEP is that the PEEP-induced increase in lung volume will cause compression of the dependent-lung intra-alveolar vessels and increase

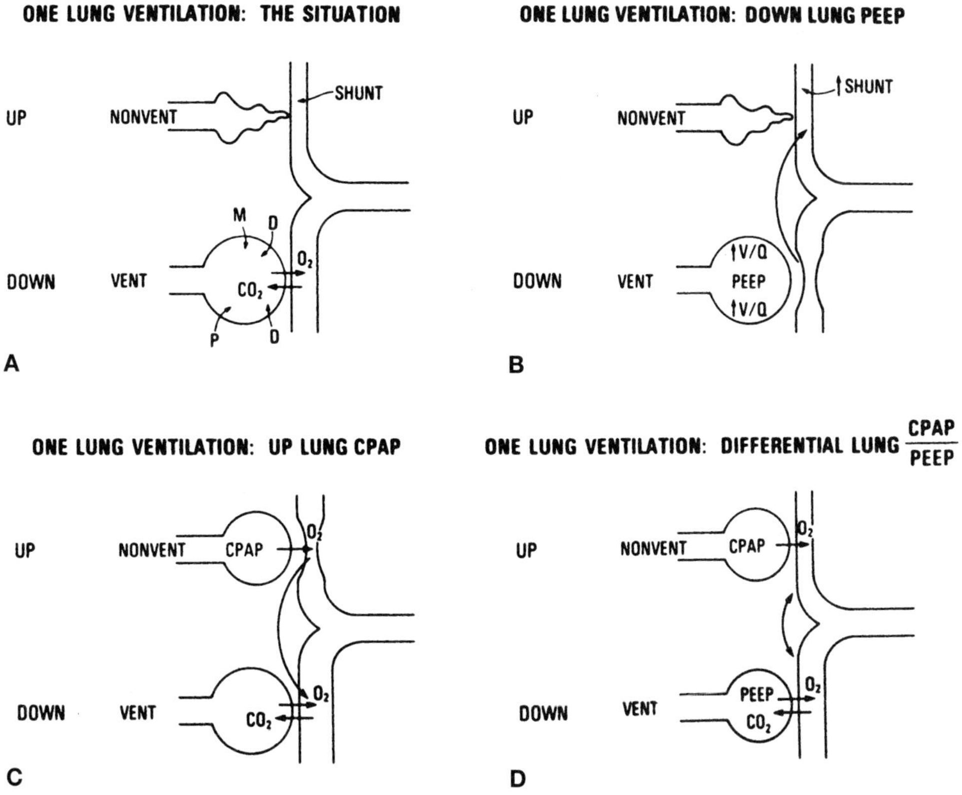

ONE LUNG VENTILATION: THE SITUATION

ONE LUNG VENTILATION: DOWN LUNG PEEP

ONE LUNG VENTILATION: UP LUNG CPAP

ONE LUNG VENTILATION: DIFFERENTIAL LUNG $\frac{CPAP}{PEEP}$

FIGURE 4-17 A four-part schematic diagram showing the effects of various differential lung management approaches. **A,** The one-lung ventilation situation. The dependent lung *(DOWN)* is ventilated *(VENT)* but is compressed by the weight of the mediastinum *(M)* from above, the pressure of the abdominal contents against the diaphragm *(D)*, and by positioning effects of rolls, packs, and shoulder supports *(P)*. The nondependent lung *(UP)* is nonventilated *(NONVENT)* and blood flow through this lung is shunt flow. **B,** The dependent lung has been selectively treated with PEEP, which improves ventilation-to-perfusion *(V̇/Q̇)* relationships in the dependent lung but also increases dependent-lung vascular resistance; this diverts blood to, and thereby increases shunt flow through, the nonventilated lung. **C,** Selective application of continuous positive airway pressure *(CPAP)* to the nondependent lung permits oxygen uptake from this lung. Even if the CPAP causes an increase in vascular resistance and diverts blood flow to the dependent lung, the diverted blood flow can still participate in gas exchange in the ventilated dependent lung. Consequently, selective nondependent-lung CPAP can greatly increase Pao_2. **D,** With differential lung CPAP (nondependent lung)/PEEP (dependent lung), it does not matter where the blood flow goes, as both lungs can participate in O_2 uptake. With this latter one-lung ventilation pattern, Pao_2 can be restored to levels near those achieved by two-lung ventilation. (From Benumof JL, Alfery DD: Anesthesia for thoracic surgery. In Miller RD [ed]: *Anesthesia,* ed 3, New York, 1990, Churchill Livingstone.)

dependent-lung pulmonary vascular resistance, diverting blood flow away from the ventilated lung to the nonventilated lung (Figure 4-17, *B*), increasing the shunt and decreasing the Pao_2. The fact that increases in both PEEP and tidal volume in the dependent ventilated lung have an additive effect in decreasing Pao_2 during OLV greatly supports the one ventilated lung volume vs. vascular resistance hypothesis.[98,115] Therefore the effect of dependent-lung PEEP on arterial oxygenation is a trade-off between the positive effect of increasing dependent-lung functional residual capacity (FRC) and V̇/Q̇ ratio and the negative effect of increasing dependent lung vascular resistance and shunting blood flow to the nonventilated lung. Not surprisingly, therefore, the various OLV-PEEP studies have included patients who have had an increase, no change, or a decrease in oxygenation.[39,115,130-133] It may be expected that in patients with a very diseased dependent lung (low lung volume and V̇/Q̇ ratio), the positive effect of selective dependent-lung

PEEP (increased lung volume and increased V̇/Q̇ ratio) might outweigh the negative effects of selective dependent-lung PEEP (shunting of blood flow to the nonventilated, nondependent lung); whereas in patients with a normal dependent lung, the negative effects of dependent-lung PEEP would outweigh the benefits. In one study in which 10 cmH$_2$O of PEEP was selectively applied to the dependent lung, the Pao_2 increased in those patients with an initial Pao_2 of less than 80 mmHg (Fio_2 = 0.5), whereas Pao_2 decreased or remained constant in patients with an initial Pao_2 higher than 80 mmHg (Fio_2 = 0.5).[130] Presumably, in the patients with Pao_2 lower than 80 mmHg (Fio_2 = 0.5), the dependent lung had a low FRC (had low V̇/Q̇ ratio and atelectatic regions) and, therefore, the positive effect of increased dependent-lung volume predominated over the negative effect of shunting blood flow to the nonventilated lung. Conversely, the patients with the higher Pao_2 presumably had a dependent lung with an adequate FRC and V̇/Q̇ ratio, and the negative effect of shunting blood flow to the nonventilated lung predominated over the positive effect of increased dependent-lung volume. Although none of these studies described a dose (ventilated-lung PEEP)-response (PaO$_2$, QS/QT value) relationship, it seems reasonable to postulate that the therapeutic margin of using PEEP to increase PaO$_2$ during OLV is quite narrow. This possibility of a narrow therapeutic window for the application of PEEP is corroborated by a recent study showing that PEEP improved oxygenation in patients undergoing OLV if the PEEP induced the end-expiratory pressure to increase to the lower inflection point of the lung static pressure-volume relationship.[100] The effect of PEEP to the dependent lung during OLV has also been shown to be dependent on the level of preexisting intrinsic PEEP (auto-PEEP).[134] In fact, it has been shown that external PEEP can improve oxygenation if the external PEEP is added to a patient with intrinsic PEEP such that the external PEEP equals the internal PEEP. This beneficial effect of PEEP was lost when the external PEEP exceeded the intrinsic PEEP by 5 mmHg.[135] PEEP applied just to the dependent ventilated lung may be delivered by the same anesthesia machine apparatus that is ordinarily used to deliver PEEP to the whole lung. There are indications that high tidal volumes, variations in the inspiratory-to-expiratory ratio, and intermittent manual hyperventilation of the dependent lung are not beneficial in increasing PaO$_2$ during OLV.[132]

SELECTIVE NONDEPENDENT LUNG CONTINUOUS POSITIVE AIRWAY PRESSURE (CPAP)

Low levels of positive pressure can be applied selectively to just the nonventilated, nondependent lung. Because under these conditions the nonventilated lung is only slightly, but constantly, distended by oxygen, an appropriate term for this ventilatory arrangement is *nonventilated-lung continuous positive airway pressure* (CPAP). In the early 1980s, two reports, one based on human study and one on dogs, showed that the application of CPAP (without tidal ventilation) to only the nonventilated lung significantly increased oxygenation.[136,137] The latter study was performed with the dogs in the lateral decubitus position and showed that low levels of CPAP (5 to 10 cmH$_2$O) to the nonventilated, nondependent lung greatly increased PaO$_2$ and decreased shunt, while blood flow to the nonventilated lung remained unchanged. That this improvement in oxygenation is from improved oxygen transfer and not from diversion of blood flow to the dependent lung was shown by demonstrating no improvement in oxygenation when CPAP was applied with nitrogen. In humans, it has been shown that the institution of 10 cmH$_2$O of nondependent-lung CPAP significantly improved oxygenation without a significant hemodynamic effect.[138,139] Therefore low levels of CPAP appear to facilitate oxygen transfer in the nondependent lung (see Figure 4-17, *C*) without significantly affecting its pulmonary vasculature. Clinical studies have further shown that the application of 5 to 10 cmH$_2$O of CPAP does not interfere with the performance of surgery and may, in fact, facilitate intralobar dissection.[136,138,140] The lack of surgical interference is not surprising given that the 5 to 10 cmH$_2$O CPAP should cause an increase in nondependent lung volume of only 50 to 100 mL, assuming a typical collapsed lung compliance of 10 mL/cmH$_2$O.

Interestingly, a canine model has shown that a nondependent-lung CPAP of 15 cmH$_2$O caused changes in PaO$_2$ and shunt similar to that from CPAP of 5 to 10 cmH$_2$O.[137] With the CPAP of 15 cmH$_2$O, however; blood flow to the nonventilated, nondependent lung decreased significantly. Therefore high levels of nonventilated-lung CPAP (more than 15 cmH$_2$O) appear to act by permitting oxygen uptake in the nonventilated lung as well as by causing blood flow diversion to the ventilated lung, where both oxygen and carbon dioxide exchange can take place (Figure 4-17, *C*). Because low levels of nonventilated-lung CPAP appear as efficacious as high levels and have less surgical interference and fewer hemodynamic implications, it is reasonable to start with low levels of nonventilated CPAP when it is indicated.

Clinical studies have consistently shown that 5 to 10 cmH$_2$O of nondependent-lung CPAP will significantly increase PaO$_2$ during OLV.[136,138,141-143] Therefore it can be argued that the single most efficacious maneuver to increase PaO$_2$ during OLV— that is, after appropriate DLT positioning and patency as well as optimization of FIO$_2$, tidal volume and respiratory rate—is the application of 5 to 10 cmH$_2$O CPAP to the nondependent lung.[144,145] From experience, low levels of nonventilated-lung CPAP can correct severe hypoxemia (PaO$_2$ less than 50 mmHg) more than 95% of the time. This nondependent-lung CPAP, however, must be applied to the nondependent lung during the deflation phase of a large tidal volume through a patent, properly placed endotracheal tube so that the deflating lung can lock into a CPAP level with uniform expansion and avoid the need to overcome critical opening pressures of airways and alveoli.

In both the human and canine studies, oxygen insufflation, at zero airway pressure, did not consistently improve PaO$_2$ and shunt.[136,137] This result is likely due to the inability of zero transbronchial airway pressure to maintain airway patency and overcome critical alveolar opening pressures. Although one study in human patients has concluded that insufflation of O$_2$ at zero airway pressure does increase PaO$_2$, the study is difficult to interpret because the patients did not serve as their own controls.[146]

Several selective nondependent-lung CPAP systems that are easy to assemble have been described.[133,141-143] All of these nondependent-lung CPAP systems have three features in common (Figure 4-18).

1. First, they have a source of oxygen to flow into the nonventilated lung.
2. Second, they have some type of restrictive mechanism (hand-screw valve, pop-off valve, weight-loaded valve) to retard the egress of oxygen from the nonventilated lung so that the nonventilated lung faces a constant distending pressure.
3. Third, they have a manometer that will measure the distending pressure.

If the nondependent-lung CPAP system has a reservoir bag included (which is highly desirable), the reservoir bag will reflect the amount of CPAP (by distention). This reservoir bag will also facilitate intermittent positive pressure ventilation of the nondependent lung as needed.

DIFFERENTIAL LUNG PEEP/CPAP

In theory, and based on the foregoing considerations, it appears that the ideal way to improve oxygenation during OLV is by applying differential lung PEEP/CPAP (see Figure

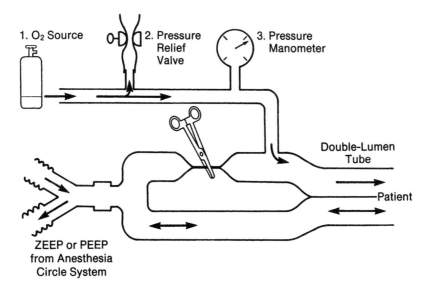

FIGURE 4-18 The three essential components of a nondependent-lung continuous positive airway pressure (CPAP) system consist of *(1)* an oxygen source, *(2)* a pressure relief valve, and *(3)* a pressure manometer to measure the CPAP. The CPAP is created by the free flow of oxygen into the lung versus the restricted outflow of oxygen from the lung by the pressure relief valve. It is also very desirable to have a reservoir bag somewhere in-line in the CPAP system. *ZEEP,* Zero end-expiratory pressure; *PEEP,* positive end-expiratory pressure. (From Benumof JL: Conventional and differential lung management of one-lung ventilation. In Benumof JL [ed]: *Anesthesia for thoracic surgery,* Philadelphia, 1987, WB Saunders.)

4-17, *D*). In this situation, the ventilated (dependent) lung is given PEEP in an effort to improve ventilated lung volume and ventilation-perfusion relationships. Simultaneously, the non-ventilated (nondependent) lung receives CPAP in an attempt to improve oxygenation of the blood perfusing this lung. Therefore, with differential lung PEEP/CPAP, it should not matter where the blood flow goes nearly as much as during simple OLV; wherever blood flows (to either ventilated or non-ventilated lung), it should be able to participate in some gas exchange with alveoli that are expanded with oxygen. In support of this hypothesis, arterial oxygenation has been shown to increase significantly in patients during thoracotomy in the lateral decubitus position (using two-lung ventilation) when PEEP was added to the ventilated dependent lung, while the nondependent lung was being ventilated at zero end-expiratory pressure (ZEEP).[25] In patients undergoing thoracotomy and OLV, arterial oxygenation was unchanged by the application of 10 cmH$_2$O of dependent-lung PEEP alone (consistent with an equal positive/negative effect trade-off). It was significantly improved by 10 cmH$_2$O of nondependent-lung CPAP alone and was further, and even more significantly, increased by use of 10 cmH$_2$O of nondependent-lung CPAP and 10 cmH$_2$O of dependent-lung PEEP together (differential lung PEEP/CPAP ventilation). The use of 10 cmH$_2$O of nondependent-lung CPAP with 10 cmH$_2$O of dependent-lung PEEP has also been shown to cause only small, clinically insignificant hemodynamic effects.[130,131] It should be noted, however, that some investigators have not been able to reproduce the benefit of differential PEEP/CPAP over CPAP alone during OLV.[144] There are now multiple reports of significant increases in oxygenation obtained with the application of differential lung ventilation and PEEP (either PEEP/PEEP, PEEP/CPAP, or CPAP/CPAP)

through double-lumen endotracheal tubes to patients in the intensive care unit with acute respiratory failure because of predominantly unilateral lung disease.[147] In all cases, conventional two-lung therapy (mechanical ventilation, PEEP, CPAP) had been administered via a standard single-lumen tube and had either failed to improve or actually decreased oxygenation. In most cases, the amount of PEEP initially administered to each lung was inversely proportional to the compliance of each lung; ideally, this PEEP arrangement should result in equal FRC in each lung. In some cases, the amount of PEEP that each lung received was later adjusted and titrated in an effort to find a differential lung-PEEP combination that resulted in the lowest right-to-left transpulmonary shunt.

HIGH-FREQUENCY VENTILATION (HFV)

High-frequency ventilation of the nondependent lung has been used for the management of hypoxia during OLV.[148-151] Clinical studies have shown that HFV and conventional OLV result in similar Pao$_2$ and Paco$_2$ levels.

Note, however, that a comparison of HFV vs. CPAP applied at the identical airway pressure to the nondependent lung during OLV has also shown that HFV was superior to CPAP in improving oxygenation.[150] The smaller tidal volumes and airway pressures associated with HFV will also typically cause less air leak through open airways or bronchopleural fistulae. Regardless, CPAP is more commonly used than HFV for the treatment of hypoxia during OLV because of the following:

1. CPAP has been clearly shown to increase Pao$_2$ during OLV to a degree comparable to that from HFV.
2. CPAP and HFV have been shown to equivalently eliminate CO$_2$.
3. The mechanical institution of CPAP is significantly simpler than HFV.

The reader interested in learning more about HFV is directed to the many excellent reviews of this topic available in the medical literature.[152,153]

INHALED NITRIC OXIDE (iNO)

Because iNO has been shown to decrease pulmonary vascular resistance in a variety of models, it is reasonable to speculate that it might be able to improve oxygenation during OLV by diverting blood to the dependent, ventilated lung. The results of studies investigating the benefits of iNO during OLV have been mixed. In a study of 15 patients, 9 receiving iNO reported improved oxygenation.[154] A number of investgators have shown that iNO during OLV (up to 40 ppm) might decrease pulmonary artery pressure but did not significantly improve oxygenation.[155-158] A recent clinical trial, however, showed that although iNO does not improve oxygenation in patients with normal pulmonary arterial pressures undergoing OLV, it can improve oxygenation in patients with pulmonary hypertension who are undergoing OLV and are hypoxemic.[159] As a more detailed discussion of iNO is beyond the scope of this chapter, the interested reader is directcd to one of the many excellent reviews of iNO available in the medical literature.[160] Almitrine bimesylate, a peripheral chemoreceptor agonist that can increase HPV, has recently been evaluated in conjunction with iNO during OLV.[161,162] In these studies, it appears that the combination of almitrine and iNO optimized oxygenation to the extent that patients receiving the combination therapy had almost no change in their PaO_2 with induction of OLV. Almitrine can be associated with peripheral neuropathy, and therefore it is not available for clinical use. Other agents (such as phenylephrine) that can be combined with iNO for similar effect are currently under investigation.[163]

RECOMMENDED COMBINED CONVENTIONAL AND DIFFERENTIAL MANAGEMENT

Table 4-1 summarizes the recommended plan for obtaining satisfactory arterial oxygenation during one-lung anesthesia. First, proper position of the double-lumen endotracheal tube and endotracheal tube patency must be confirmed during two-lung ventilation. Two-lung ventilation should typically be maintained as long as possible (usually until the pleura is opened). When OLV is commenced, the FIO_2 should initially be set to 1.0. The FIO_2 can be decreased gradually if oxygenation

is adequate, keeping in mind the effects of decreasing the FIO_2 on the vascular resistance of the ventilated lung. Tidal volume can be set initially at 8 to 10 mL/kg and adjusted according to the resulting airway pressures and hemodynamics. The respiratory rate can be initially adjusted to target a $PaCO_2$ of 40 mmHg. If maintenance of normocapnia results in air trapping, dynamic hyperinflation and hemodynamic instability, the respiratory rate, tidal volume, and the inspiratory/expiratory time ratio should be adjusted appropriately and the target should be reset (permissive hypercapnia).

If severe hypoxemia persists following this initial conventional approach, malposition or obstruction of the DLT must again be ruled out. Proper tube position and tube patency at this stage are best confirmed using fiberoptic bronchoscopy. It should always be remembered that a disposable DLT can be malpositioned at any time because of surgical manipulations or even gravity alone, and it can malfunction even if it had previously been functioning perfectly. The common cause is migration of the tube outward. When this occurs, the distal (bronchial) cuff can migrate into the trachea, ride on the carina, and cause serious inability for proper lung isolation or even seriously impair ventilation on the whole. If the DLT is correctly positioned and patent, and if the patient's hemodynamic status is satisfactory, simple tidal volume and respiratory rate adjustments can be attempted. If these simple maneuvers do not resolve the problem quickly, 5 to 10 cmH$_2$O of CPAP can be applied to the nondependent lung. Nondependent-lung CPAP should be applied during the deflation phase of a large tidal volume breath in order to overcome critical opening pressures in the atelectatic lung. If oxygenation does not improve with nondependent-lung CPAP (which it does in the majority of cases), 5 to 10 cmH$_2$O of PEEP can be applied to the ventilated dependent lung. If this dependent-lung PEEP does not improve oxygenation, the nondependent-lung CPAP can be increased to 10 to 15 cmH$_2$O while the dependent-lung PEEP is maintained at 5 to 10 cmH$_2$O. If arterial oxygenation is still not satisfactory, the nondependent-lung CPAP level should be matched with an equal amount of dependent-lung PEEP. In this way, differential lung PEEP/CPAP can be modulated to find the maximum compliance, minimum right-to-left transpulmonary shunt, and the

TABLE 4-1

Recommended Combined Conventional and Differential Lung Management

1. Confirm proper position of double-lumen endotracheal tube and tube patency.
2. Maintain two-lung ventilation until the pleura is opened.
3. Initial "conventional" one-lung ventilation
   - FIO_2 = 1.0
   - TV = 8-10 mL/kg and adjusted according to airway pressure.
   - RR to initially target a $PaCO_2$ of 40 mmHg, adjusted according to presence of dynamic hyperinflation. Watch hemodynamic status.
4. Modified one-lung ventilation for hypoxemia
   - Recheck endotracheal tube position and patency using fiberoptic bronchoscopy.
   - Nondependent-lung CPAP of 5-10 mmHg.
   - Dependent-lung PEEP at 5-10 mmHg if CPAP to nondependent lung fails to treat hypoxemia.
   - Adjust dependent-lung PEEP to match nondependent-lung CPAP, watching for hemodynamic instability.
   - Consider intermittent positive-pressure ventilation of nondependent lung.
   - Consider high-frequency ventilation of nondependent lung.
   - Consider inhaled nitric oxide if hypoxia coexists with pulmonary hypertension.
   - Consider early clamping of pulmonary artery of operative lung during pneumonectomy.

optimal end-expiratory pressure for each lung and for the patient as a whole.

If severe hypoxemia persists following the application of differential lung PEEP/CPAP (which would be extremely rare), the nondependent lung can be ventilated intermittently with positive pressure with oxygen. Of course, such a process would require absolute surgical cooperation. High-frequency ventilation of the nondependent lung can also be considered. If the patient has pulmonary hypertension, inhaled nitric oxide can also be considered. It should also be kept in mind that most of the ventilation-perfusion imbalance—during a pneumonectomy, in particular—can be eliminated by the early tightening of a ligature around the pulmonary artery of the nonventilated lung. Indeed, clamping the pulmonary artery to a collapsed lung functionally resects the entire lung and restores the PaO_2 to a level not significantly different from that of two-lung ventilation or postpneumonectomy OLV. Of course, it should be remembered that some patients may not tolerate such abrupt diversion of the entire blood flow into the nonoperative lung and may develop pulmonary hypertension and hemodynamic instability (right venticular heart dysfunction).

Acknowledgment

The authors would like to express our deepest gratitude to Dr. Jonathan L. Benumof for his pioneer work in this field, over the span of many years. His work has given us the knowledge to improve our clinical skills. Also, we would like to express our appreciation to him for giving us the opportunity to update and coauthor this chapter.

REFERENCES

1. West JB, Dollery CT, Naimark A: Distribution of blood flow in isolated lung: relation to vascular and alveolar pressures, *J Appl Physiol* 19:713, 1964.
2. Permutt S, Bromberger-Barnea B, Bane HN: Alveolar pressure, pulmonary venous pressure and the vascular waterfall, *Med Thorac* 19:239, 1962.
3. West JB, Dollery CT, Heard BE: Increased pulmonary vascular resistance in the dependent zone of the isolated dog lung caused by perivascular edema, *Circ Res* 17:191, 1965.
4. West JB (ed): *Regional differences in the lung,* San Diego, 1977, Academic Press.
5. Hughes JMB, Glazier JB, Maloney JE, et al: Effect of lung volume on the distribution of pulmonary blood flow in man, *Respir Physiol* 4:58, 1968.
6. Hughes JM, Glazier JB, Maloney JE, et al: Effect of extra-alveolar vessels on the distribution of pulmonary blood flow in the dog, *J Appl Physiol* 25:701, 1968.
7. Landmark SJ, Knopp TJ, Rehder K, Sessler AD: Regional pulmonary perfusion and $\dot{V}/\dot{Q}$ in awake and anesthetized-paralyzed man, *J Appl Physiol* 43:993, 1977.
8. Permutt S, Caldini P, Maseri A, et al: Recruitment versus distensibility in the pulmonary vascular bed. In Fishman AP, Hecht H (eds): *The pulmonary circulation and interstitial space,* Chicago, 1969, University of Chicago.
9. Maseri A, Caldini P, Harward P, et al: Determinants of pulmonary vascular volume: recruitment versus distensibility, *Circ Res* 31:218, 1972.
10. Stone HL, Warren BH, and Wagner H: The distribution of pulmonary blood flow in human subjects during zero gravity, *Proc Advisory Group Aerosp Res Develop Conf* 2:139, 1965.
11. Hakim TS, Lisbona R, Dean GW: Gravity-independent inequality in pulmonary blood flow in humans, *J Appl Physiol* 63:1114, 1987.
12. Hoppin FG, Jr, Green ID, Mead J: Distribution of pleural surface pressure, *J Appl Physiol* 27:863, 1969.
13. Milic-Emili J, Henderson JAM, Dolovich MB, et al: Regional distribution of inspired gas in the lung, *J Appl Physiol* 21:749, 1966.
14. West JB: *Ventilation/blood flow and gas exchange,* ed 2, Oxford, 1970, Blackwell Scientific.
15. West JB: Regional differences in gas exchange in the lung of erect man, *J Appl Physiol* 17:892, 1962.
16. Wulff KE, Aulin I: The regional lung function in the lateral decubitus position during anesthesia and operation, *Acta Anaesthesiol Scand* 16:195, 1972.
17. Rehder K, Wenthe FM, Sessler AD: Function of each lung during mechanical ventilation with ZEEP and with PEEP in man anesthetized with thiopental-meperidine, *Anesthesiology* 39:597, 1973.
18. Svanberg L: Influence of posture on lung volumes, ventilation and circulation in normals, *Scand J Clin Lab Invest,* 9:1, 1957.
19. Rehder K, Sessler AD: Function of each lung in spontaneously breathing man anesthetized with thiopental-meperidine, *Anesthesiology* 38:320, 1973.
20. Potgieter SV: Atelectasis: its evolution during upper urinary tract surgery, *Br J Anaesth* 31:472, 1959.
21. Rehder K, Hatch DJ, Sessler AD, Folwer WS: The function of each lung of anesthetized and paralyzed man during mechanical ventilation, *Anesthesiology* 37:1626, 1972.
22. Nunn JF: The distribution of inspired gas during thoracic surgery, *Ann R Coll Surg Engl* 28:223, 1961.
23. Werner O, Malmkvist G, Beckman A, et al: Gas exchange and haemodynamics during thoractomy, *Br J Anaesth* 56:1343, 1984.
24. Froese AB, Bryan CA: Effects of anesthesia and paralysis on diaphragmatic mechanics in man, *Anesthesiology* 41:242, 1974.
25. Brown DR, Kafer ER, Roberson VO, et al: Improved oxygenation during thoracotomy with selective PEEP to the dependent lung, *Anesth Analg* 56:26, 1977.
26. Tarhan S, Moffitt EA: Principles of thoracic anesthesia, *Surg Clin North Am* 53:813, 1973.
27. Tarhan S, Lungborg RO: Carlens endobronchial catheter versus regular endotracheal tube during thoracic surgery: a comparison of blood gas tensions and pulmonary shunting, *Can Anaesth Soc J* 18:594, 1971.
28. Casthely PA, Lear F, Cottrell JE, Lear E: Intrapulmonary shunting during induced hypotension, *Anesth Analg* 61:231, 1982.
29. Benumof JL: Hypoxic pulmonary vasoconstriction and sodium nitroprusside infusion, *Anesthesiology* 50:481, 1979.
30. Kerr JH, Smith AC, Prys-Roberts C, et al: Observations during endobronchial anesthesia II: Oxygenation. *Br J Anaesth* 46:84, 1974.
31. Benumof JL: Mechanism of decreased blood flow to atelectatic lung, *J Appl Physiol* 46:1047, 1978 30.
32. Pirlo AF, Benumof JL, Trousdale FR: Atelectatic lung lobe blood flow: open vs. closed chest, positive pressure vs. spontaneous ventilation, *J Appl Physiol* 50:1022, 1981.
33. Bjertnaes LJ, Mundal R, Hauge A, et al: Vascular resistance in atelectatic lungs: effect of inhalation anesthetics, *Acta Anaesthesiol Scand* 24:109, 1980.
34. Marshall BE, Marshall C: Continuity of response to hypoxic pulmonary vasoconstriction, *J Appl Physiol* 59:189, 1980.
35. Rogers SN, Benumof JL: Halothane and isoflurane do not decrease P_aO_2 during one-lung ventilation in intravenously anesthetized patients, *Anesth Analg* 64:946, 1985.
36. Torda TA, McCulloch CH, O'Brien HD, et al: Pulmonary venous admixture during one-lung anesthesia: the effect of inhaled oxygen tension and respiration rate, *Anaesthesia* 29:272, 1974.
37. Khanom T, Branthwaite MA: Arterial oxygenation during one-lung anesthesia (1): a study in man, *Anaesthesia* 28:132, 1973.
38. Flacke JW, Thompson DS, Read RC: Influence of tidal volume and pulmonary artery occlusion on arterial oxygenation during endobronchial anesthesia, *South Med J* 69:619, 1976.
39. Tarhan S, Lundborg RO: Effects of increased expiratory pressure on blood gas tensions and pulmonary shunting during thoracotomy with use of the Carlens catheter, *Can Anaesth Soc J* 17:4, 1970.
40. Fiser WP, Friday CD, Read RC: Changes in arterial oxygenation and pulmonary shunt during thoracotomy with endobronchial anesthesia, *J Thorac Cardiovasc Surg* 83:523, 1982.
41. Hurford, WE, Kolker, AC, Strauss, WH: The use of ventilation/perfusion scans to predict oxygenation during one-lung anesthesia, *Anesthesiology* 67: 841, 1987.
42. Prefaut CH, Engel LA: Vertical distribution of perfusion and inspired gas in supine man, *Respir Physiol* 43:209, 1981.
43. Glasser SA, Domino KB, Lindgren L, et al: Pulmonary pressure and flow during atelectasis, *Anesthesiology* 57:A504, 1982.

44. Carlsson AJ, Bindslev L. Santesson J, et al: Hypoxic pulmonary vasoconstriction in the human lung: the effect of prolonged unilateral hypoxic challenge during anesthesia, *Acta Anaesthesiol Scand* 29:346, 1985.
45. Hill NS, Antman EM, Green LH, Alpert JS: Intravenous nitroglycerin: a review of pharmacology, therapeutic effects and indications, *Chest* 79:69, 1981.
46. Colley PS, Cheney FW, Hlastala MP: Pulmonary gas exchange effects of nitroglycerin in canine edematous lungs, *Anesthesiology* 55:114, 1981.
47. Chick TW, Kochukoshy KN, Matsumoto S, Leach JK: The effect of nitroglycerin on gas exchange, hemodynamics and oxygen transport in patients with chronic obstructive pulmonary disease, *Am J Med Sci* 276:105, 1978.
48. Kadowitz PJ, Nandiwada P, Grueter CA, et al: Pulmonary vasodilator responses to nitroprusside and nitroglycerin in the dog, *J Clin Invest* 67:893, 1981.
49. Anjou-Lindskog E, Broman L, Holmgren A: Effects of nitroglycerin on central hemodynamics and $\dot{V}_A/\dot{Q}$ distribution early after coronary bypass surgery, *Acta Anaesthesiol Scand* 26:489, 1982.
50. Kochukoshy KN, Chick TW, Jenne JW: The effect of nitroglycerin on gas exchange in chronic obstructive pulmonary disease, *Am Rev Respir Dis* 111:177, 1975.
51. Holmgren A, Anjou E, Broman L, Lundberg S: Influence of nitroglycerin on central hemodynamics and $\dot{V}_A/\dot{Q}_c$ of the lungs in the postoperative period after coronary bypass surgery, *Acta Med Scand* S562:135, 1982.
52. Parsons GH, Leventhal JP, Hansen MM, Goldstein JD: Effect of sodium nitroprusside on hypoxic pulmonary vasoconstriction in the dog, *J Appl Physiol* 51:288, 1981.
53. Sivak ED, Gray BA, McCurdy TH, Phillips AK: Pulmonary vascular response to nitroprusside in dogs. *Circ Res* 45:360, 1979.
54. Hill AB, Sykes MK, Reyes A: Hypoxic pulmonary vasoconstrictor response in dogs during and after sodium nitroprusside infusion, *Anesthesiology* 50:484, 1979.
55. Colley PS, Cheney FW, Hlastala MP: Ventilation-perfusion and gas exchange effects of nitroprusside in dogs with normal and edematous lungs, *Anesthesiology* 50:489, 1979.
56. Colley PS, Cheney FW: Sodium nitroprusside increases Q_s/Q_t in dogs with regional atelectasis, *Anesthesiology* 47:338, 1977.
57. Wildsmith JAW, Drummond GB, Macrae WR: Blood gas changes during induced hypotension with sodium nitroprusside, *Br J Anaesth* 47:1205, 1975.
58. Veltzer JL, Doto JO, Jacoby J: Depressed arterial oxygenation during sodium nitroprusside administration for intraoperative hypertension, *Anesth Analg* 55:880, 1976.
59. Furman WR, Summer WR, Kennedy PP, Silvester JT: Comparison of the effects of dobutamine, dopamine and isoproterenol on hypoxic pulmonary vasoconstriction in the pig, *Crit Care Med* 10:371, 1982.
60. McFarlane PA, Mortimer AJ, Ryder WA, et al: Effects of dopamine and dobutamine on the distribution of pulmonary blood flow during lobar ventilation hypoxia and lobar collapse in dogs, *Eur J Clin Invest* 15:53, 1985.
61. Bishop MJ, Cheney FW: Minoxidil and nifedipine inhibit hypoxic pulmonary vasoconstriction, *J Cardiovasc Pharmacol* 5:184, 1983.
62. Tucker A, McMurtry IF, Grover RF, et al: Attenuation of hypoxic pulmonary vasoconstriction by verapamil in intact dogs, *Proc Soc Exp Biol Med* 151:611, 1976.
63. Simonneau J, Escourrou P, Duroux P, Lockhart A: Inhibition of hypoxic pulmonary vasoconstriction by nifedipine, *N Engl J Med* 304:1582, 1981.
64. Redding GJ, Tuck R, Escourrou P: Nifedipine attenuates hypoxic pulmonary vasoconstriction in awake piglets, *Am Rev Respir Dis* 129:785, 1984.
65. McMurtry IF, Davidson AB, Reeves TJ, Grover RF: Inhibition of hypoxic pulmonary vasoconstriction by calcium antagonists in isolated rat lungs, *Circ Res* 38:99, 1976.
66. Brown SE, Linden GS, King RR, et al: Effect of verapamil on pulmonary haemodynamics during hypoxaemia at rest, and during exercise in patients with chronic obstructive pulmonary disease, *Thorax* 38:840, 1983.
67. Ward CF, Benumof JL, Wahrenbrock EA: Inhibition of hypoxic pulmonary vasoconstriction by vasoactive drugs, *Abstracts of Scientific Papers, 1976 Annual Meeting,* American Society of Anesthesiology, 1976.
68. Johansen I, Benumof JL: Reduction of hypoxia-induced pulmonary artery hypertension by vasodilator drugs, *Am Rev Respir Dis* 199:375, 1979.
69. Conover WB, Benumof JL, Key TC: Ritodrine inhibition of hypoxic pulmonary vasoconstriction, *Am J Obstet Gynecol* 146:652, 1983.
70. Marin JLB, Orchard C, Chakrabarti MK, Sykes MK: Depression of hypoxic pulmonary vasoconstriction in the dog by dopamine and isoprenaline, *Br J Anaesth* 51:303, 1979.
71. Reyes A, Sykes MK, Chakrabarti MK, et al: Effect of orciprenaline on hypoxic pulmonary vasoconstriction in dogs, *Respiration* 38:185, 1979.
72. Reyes A, Sykes MK, Chakrabarti MK, et al: The effect of salbutamol on hypoxic pulmonary vasoconstriction in dogs, *Bull Eur Physiopathol Respir* 14:741, 1978.
73. Rubin LJ, Lazar JD: Nonadrenergic effects of isoproterenol in dogs with hypoxic pulmonary vasoconstriction: possible role of prostaglandins, *J Clin Invest* 71:1366, 1983.
74. Benumof JL, Trousdale FR: Aminophylline does not inhibit canine hypoxic pulmonary vasoconstriction, *Am Rev Respir Dis* 126:1017, 1982.
75. Bishop MJ, Kennard S, Artman LD, Cheney FW: Hydralazine does not inhibit canine hypoxic pulmonary vasoconstriction, *Am Rev Respir Dis* 128:998, 1983.
76. Benumof JL: Choice of anesthetic drugs and techniques. In Benumof JL (ed), *Anesthesia for thoracic surgery.* Philadelphia, 1987, WB Saunders.
77. Domino KB, Borowec L, Alexander CM, et al: Influence of isoflurane on hypoxic pulmonary vasoconstriction in dogs, *Anesthesiology* 64:423, 1986.
78. Lawler PGP, Nunn JF: A reassessment of the validity of the iso-shunt graph, *Br J Anaesth* 56:1325, 1984.
79. Benumof JL: Special physiology of the lateral decubitus position, the open chest, and one-lung ventilation. In Benumof JL (ed), *Anesthesia for thoracic surgery,* Philadelphia 1987, WB Saunders.
80. Benumof JL, Augustine SD, Gibbins J: Halothane and isoflurane only slightly impair arterial oxygenation during one-lung ventilation in patients undergoing thoracotomy, *Anesthesiology* 67:910-915, 1987.
81. Carlsson AJ, Bindslev L, Hedenstierna G: Hypoxic pulmonary vasoconstriction in the lung, *Anesthesiology* 66:312, 1987.
82. Carlsson AJ, Hedenstierna G, Bindslev L: Hypoxia-induced vasoconstriction in human lung exposed to enflurane anaesthesia, *Acta Anaesthesiol Scand* 31:5762, 1987.
83. Schwarzkopf K, Schreiber T, Bauer R, et al: The effects of increasing concentrations of isoflurane and desflurane on pulmonary perfusion and systemic oxygenation during one-lung ventilation in pigs, *Anesth Analg* 93:1434, 2001.
84. Karzai W, Haberstroh J, Priebe HJ: The effect of increasing oxygen concentrations on systemic oxygenation during one-lung ventilation in pigs, *Anesth Analg* 89:215, 1999.
85. Wang JY, Russell GN, Page RD, et al: Pennefather: a comparison of the effects of desflurane and isoflurane on arterial oxygenation during one-lung ventilation, *Anesthesia* 55:167, 2000.
86. Beck DH, Doepfmer UR, Sinemus C, et al: Effects of sevoflurane and propofol on pulmonary shunt fraction during one-lung ventilation for thoracic surgery, *Br J Anaesth* 86:38, 2001.
87. Wang JY, Russell GN, Page RD, et al: Comparison of the effects of sevoflurane and isoflurane on arterial oxygenation during one-lung ventilation, *Br J Anaesth* 81:850, 1998.
88. Abe K, Shimizu T, Takashina M, et al: The effects of propofol, isoflurane and sevoflurane on oxygenation and shunt fraction during one-lung ventilation, *Anesth Analg* 87:1164, 1998.
89. Kellow N, Scott AD, White SA, Feneck RO: Comparison of the effects of propofol and isoflurane anesthesia on right ventricular function and shunt fraction during thoracic surgery, *Br J Anaesth* 75:578, 1995.
90. Gardaz JP, McFarlane PA, Madgwick RG, et al: Effect of dopamine, increased cardiac output and increased pulmonary artery pressure on hypoxic pulmonary vasoconstriction, *Br J Anaesth* 55:238, 1983.
91. Benumof JL, Wahrenbrock EA: Blunted hypoxic pulmonary vasoconstriction by increased lung vascular pressures, *J Appl Physiol* 38:846, 1975.
92. Scanlon TS, Benumof JL, Wahrenbrock EA, Nelson WL: Hypoxic pulmonary vasoconstriction and the ratio of hypoxic lung to perfused normoxic lung, *Anesthesiology* 49:177, 1978.
93. Colley PS, Cheney FW, Butler J: Mechanism of change in pulmonary shunt flow with hemorrhage, *J Appl Physiol* 42:196, 1977.
94. Domino KB, Glasser SA, Wetstein L, et al: Influence of $P\bar{v}O_2$ on blood flow to atelectatic lung, *Anesthesiology* 57:A471, 1982.
95. Benumof JL, Pirlo AF, Trousdale FR: Inhibition of hypoxic pulmonary vasoconstriction by decreased P_vO_2, a new indirect mechanism, *J Appl Physiol* 51:871, 1981.
96. Pease RD, Benumof JL: P_AO_2 and P_vO_2 interaction on hypoxic pulmonary vasoconstriction, *J Appl Physiol* 53:134, 1982.
97. Benumof JL, Mathers JM, Wahrenbrock EA: Cyclic hypoxic pulmonary vasoconstriction induced by concomitant carbon dioxide changes, *J Appl Physiol* 41:4664, 1976.
98. Benumof JL, Rogers SN, Moyce PR, et al: Hypoxic pulmonary vasoconstriction and regional and whole-lung PEEP in the dog, *Anesthesiology* 51:503, 1979.

99. Benumof JL: One-lung ventilation and hypoxic pulmonary vasoconstriction: implications for anesthetic management, *Anesth Analg* 64:821, 1985.
100. Slinger PD, Kruger M, McRae K, Winton T: Relation of the static compliance curve and positive end-expiratory pressure to oxygenation during one-lung ventilation, *Anesthesiology* 95:1096, 2001.
101. Hall SM, Chapleau M, Cairo J, et al: Effect of high-frequency positive pressure ventilation on halothane ablation of hypoxic pulmonary vasoconstriction, *Crit Care Med* 13:641, 1985.
102. Ishibi Y, Shiokawa Y, Umeda T, et al: The effect of thoracic epidural anesthesia on hypoxic pulmonary vasoconstriction in dogs: an analysis of the pressure-flow curve, *Anesth Analg* 82: 1049, 1996.
103. Irwin RS, Martinez-Gonzalez-Rio H, Thomas HM III, Fritts HW Jr: The effect of granulomatous pulmonary disease in dogs on the response of the pulmonary circulation to hypoxia *J Clin Invest* 60:1258, 1977.
104. Light RB, Mink SN, Wood LDH: Pathophysiology of gas exchange and pulmonary perfusion in pneumococcal lobar pneumonia in dogs, *J Appl Physiol* 50:524, 1981.
105. Craig JOC, Bromley LL, Williams R: Thoracotomy and contralateral lung: a study of the changes occurring in the dependent and contralateral lung during and after thoracotomy in the lateral decubitus position, *Thorax* 17:9, 1962.
106. Benumof JL: General respiratory physiology and respiratory function during anesthesia. 39-103. In ed *Anesthesia for thoracic surgery,* Philadelphia, 1987, WB Saunders.
107. Dantzker DR, Wagner PD, West JB: Instability of lung units with low V/Q ratios during O_2 breathing, *J Appl Physiol* 38:886, 1975.
108. Ray JF III, Yost L, Moallem S, et al: Immobility, hypoxemia and pulmonary arteriovenous shunting, *Arch Surg* 109:537, 1974.
109. Kerr JH: Physiological aspects of one-lung (endobronchial) anesthesia, *Int Anesthesiol Clin* 10:61, 1972.
110. Johansen I, Benumof JL: Flow distribution in abnormal lung as a function of F_IO_2, abstracted, *Anesthesiology* 51:369, 1979.
111. Benumof JL, Wahrenbrock EA: Dependency of hypoxic pulmonary vasoconstriction on temperature, *J Appl Physiol* 72:56, 1977.
112. Kelman GF, Nunn JF, Prys-Roberts C, et al: The influence of the cardiac output on arterial oxygenation: a theoretical study, *Br J Anaesth* 39:450, 1967.
113. Prys-Roberts C: The metabolic regulation of circulatory transport: scientific foundations of anesthesia. In Scurr C, Feldman S (eds): St. Louis, 1982, Mosby.
114. Winter PM, Smith G: The toxicity of oxygen. Anesthesiology 37:210-241, 1972.
115. Katz JA, Laverne RG, Fairley HB, Thomas AN: Pulmonary oxygen exchange during endobronchial anesthesia: effects of tidal volume and PEEP, *Anesthesiology* 56:164, 1982.
116. Finley TN, Hill TR, Bonica JJ: Effect of intrapleural pressure on pulmonary shunt to atelectatic dog lung, *Am J Physiol* 205:1187, 1963.
117. Dreyfuss D, Soler P, Basset G, Saumon G: High inflation pressure pulmonary edema: respective effects of high airway pressure, high tidal volume, and positive end-expiratory pressure, *Am Rev Respir Dis* 137:1159, 1988.
118. Carlton DP, Cummings JJ, Scheerer RG, et al: Lung overexpansion increases pulmonary microvascular protein permeability in young lambs, *J Appl Physiol* 69:577, 1990.
119. Chao DC. Scheinhorn DJ: Barotrauma vs volutrauma [Letter], *Chest.* 109(4):1127, 1996.
120. Bachand RR, Audet J, Meloche R, et al: Physiological changes associated with unilateral pulmonary ventilation during operations on one lung, *Can Anaesth Soc J* 22:659, 1975.
121. Kerr J, Smith AC, Prys-Roberts C, et al: Observations during endobronchial anaesthesia. I. Ventilation and carbon dioxide clearance, *Br J Anaesth* 45:159, 1973.
122. Hatch D: Ventilation and arterial oxygenation during thoracic surgery, *Thorax* 21:310, 1996.
123. Menitove SM, Goldring RM: Combined ventilator and bicarbonate strategy in the management of status asthmaticus, *Am J Med* 74:898, 1983.
124. Darioli R, Perret C: Mechanical controlled hypoventilation in status asthmaticus, *Am Rev Respir Dis* 129:387, 1984.
125. Triantafillou AN: Anesthetic management for bilateral volume reduction surgery. In Cox JL, Cooper JD (eds): *Seminars in thoracic and cardiovascular Surgery: volume reduction surgery for emphysema,* Philadelphia, 1996, WB Saunders.
126. Bigatello LM. Patroniti N. Sangalli F: Permissive hypercapnia, *Curr Opin Crit Car* 7:34, 2001.
127. Hirvela ER: Advances in the management of acute respiratory distress syndrome: protective ventilation, *Archives Surg* 135:126, 2000.
128. Laffey JG, Kavanagh BP: Carbon dioxide and the critically ill: too little of a good thing? *Lancet* 354:1283, 1999.
129. Goldstein B, Shannon DC, Todres ID: Supercarbia in children: clinical course and outcome, *Crit Car Med* 18:166, 1990.
130. Cohen E, Thys DM, Eisenkraft JB, Kaplan JA: PEEP during one-lung anesthesia improves oxygenation in patients with low arterial P_aO_2, *Anesth Analg* 64:201, 1985.
131. Cohen E, Eisenkraft JB: Positive end-expiratory pressure during one-lung ventilation improves oxygenation in patients with low arterial tensions, *J Cardiothor Vasc Anesth* 10:578, 1996.
132. Khanam T, Branthwaite, MA: Arterial oxygenation during one-lung anesthesia (2), *Anaesthesia* 23:280, 1973.
133. Aalto-Setala M, Heinonen J, Salorinne Y: Cardiorespiratory function during thoracic anesthesia: comparison of two-lung ventilation and one-lung ventilation with and without PEEP, *Acta Anaesthesiol Scand* 19:287, 1975.
134. Slinger PD, Hickey DR: The interaction between applied PEEP and auto-PEEP during one-lung ventilation, *J Cardiothor Vasc Anesth* 12:133, 1998.
135. Inomata S, Nishikawa T, Saito S, Kihara S: Best PEEP during one-lung ventilation, *Br J Anaesth* 78:754, 1997.
136. Capan IM, Turndorf H, Chandrakant P, et al: Optimization of arterial oxygenation during one-lung anesthesia, *Anesth Analg* 59:847, 1980.
137. Alfery DD, Benumof JL, Trousdale FR: Improving oxygenation during one-lung ventilation: the effects of PEEP and blood flow restriction to the nonventilated lung, *Anesthesiology* 55:381, 1981.
138. Cohen E, Eisenkraft JB, Thys DM, Kaplan JA: Oxygenation and hemodynamic changes during one-lung ventilation: effects of $CPAP_{10}$, $PEEP_{10}$ and $CPAP_{10}/PEEP_{10}$, *J Cardiothorac Anesth* 2:34, 1988.
139. Cohen E, Thys DM, Eisenkraft JB, et al: Effect of CPAP and PEEP during one-lung anesthesia: left versus right thoracotomies, *Anesthesiology* 63:A564, 1985.
140. Merridew CG, Jones RDM: Non-dependent lung CPAP (5 cmH_2O) with oxygen during ketamine, halothane or isoflurane anesthesia and one-lung ventilation, *Anesthesiology* 63:A567, 1985.
141. Thiagarajah S, Job C, Rao A: A device for applying CPAP to the nonventilated upper lung during one-lung ventilation. I, *Anesthesiology* 60:253, 1984.
142. Hannenberg AA, Satwicz PR, Pienes RS, Jr, O'Brien JC: A device for applying CPAP to the nonventilated upper lung during one-lung ventilation. II, *Anesthesiology* 60:254, 1984.
143. Brown DL, Davis RS: A simple device for oxygen insufflation with continuous positive airway pressure during one-lung ventilation, *Anesthesiology* 61:481, 1984.
144. Fujiwara M, Abe K, Mashimo T: The effect of positive end-expiratory pressure and continuous positive airway pressure on the oxygenation and shunt fraction during one-lung ventilation with propofol anesthesia, *J Clin Anesth* 13:473, 2001.
145. Hogue CW Jr: Effectiveness of low levels of nonventilated lung continuous positive airway pressure in improving arterial oxygenation during one-lung ventilation, *Anesth Analg* 79:364, 1994.
146. Rees DI, Wansbrough SR: One-lung anesthesia: percent shunt and arterial oxygen tension during continuous insufflation of oxygen to the nonventilated lung, *Anesth Analg* 61:507, 1982.
147. Benumof JL: Conventional and differential lung management of one-lung ventilation. In Benumof JL (ed) *Anesthesia for thoracic surgery,* Philadelphia, 1987, WB Saunders.
148. den Hoed PT, Leendertse-Verloop K, Bruining HA, Bonjer HJ: Comparison of one-lung ventilation and high-frequency ventilation in thoracoscopic surgery, *Eur J Surg* 165:1031, 1999.
149. Nakatsuka M: 1988: Unilateral high-frequency jet ventilation during one-lung ventilation for thoracotomy, *Ann Thorac Surg* 59:1610, 1995.
150. Godet G, Bertrand M, Rouby JJ: High-frequency jet ventilation vs continuous positive airway pressure for differential lung ventilation in patients undergoing resection of thoracoabdominal aortic aneurysm, *Acta Anaesthes Scand* 38:562, 1994.
151. Nakatsuka M, Wetstein L, Keenan RL: Unilateral high-frequency jet ventilation during one-lung ventilation for thoracotomy, *Ann Thorac Surg* 59:1610, 1995.
152. Krishnan JA, Brower RG: High-frequency ventilation for acute lung injury and ARDS, *Chest* 118(3):795, 2000.
153. Charney J, Hamid RK: Pediatric ventilation outside the operating room, *Anesth Clin North Am* 19(2):399, 2001.

154. Booth, J: Effect of unilateral inhaled NO during selective ventilation in anesthetized humans, *Anesthesiology* 81A:1457, 1994.
155. Rich GF, Lowson SM, Johns RA: et al: Inhaled nitric oxide selectively decreases pulmonary vascular resistance without impairing oxygenation during one-lung ventilation in patients undergoing cardiac surgery, *Anesthesiology* 80:57; 1994.
156. Wilson WC, Kapelanski DP, Benumof JL: Inhaled nitric oxide (40 ppm) during one-lung ventilation, in the lateral decubitus position, does not decrease pulmonary vascular resistance or improve oxygenation in normal patients, *J Cardiothor Vasc Anesth* 11:172, 1997.
157. Fradj K, Samain E, Delefosse D: Placebo-controlled study of inhaled nitric oxide to treat hypoxaemia during one-lung ventilation, *Br J Anaesth* 82:208, 1999.
158. Schwarzkopf K, Klein U, Schreiber T, et al: Oxygenation during one-lung ventilation: the effects of inhaled nitric oxide and increasing levels of inspired fraction of oxygen, *Anesth Analg* 92:842, 2001.
159. DellaRocca GD, Passariello M, Coccia C, et al: Inhaled nitric oxide administration during one-lung ventilation in patients undergoing thoracic surgery, *J Cardiothor Vasc Anesth* 15:218, 2001.
160. Steudel WS, Hurford WM, Zapol WM: Inhaled nitric oxide: basic biology and clinical applications, *Anesthesiology* 91:1090, 2000.
161. Moutafis M, Liu N, Dalibon N, et al: The effects of inhaled nitric oxide and its combination with intravenous almitrine on P_aO_2 during one-lung ventilation in patients undergoing thoracoscopic procedures, *Anesth Analg.* 85:1130, 1997.
162. Moutafis M, Liu N, Dalibon A, et al: Improving oxygenation during bronchopulmonary lavage using nitric oxide and almitrine infusion, *Anesth Analg* 89:302, 1999.
163. Doering EB, Hanson CW, Reily D: Improvement in oxygenation by phenylephrine and nitric oxide in patients with adult respiratory distress syndrome, *Anesthesiology* 87:18, 1997.
164. Benumof JL: Respiratory physiology and respiratory function during anesthesia. In Miller RD (ed): *Anesthesia,* ed 3, New York, 1990, Churchill Livingstone.
165. West JB: *Ventilation blood flow and gas exchange*, ed 4, Oxford, 1985, Blackwell.
166. Benumof JL: Physiology of the open chest and one-lung ventilation. In *Anesthesia for thoracic surgery*, Philadelphia, 1987, WB Saunders.
167. Benumof JL: Conventional and differential lung management of one-lung ventilation. In Benumof JL (ed): *Anesthesia for thoracic surgery,* Philadelphia, 1987, WB Saunders.
168. Benumof JL, Alfery DD: Anesthesia for thoracic surgery. In Miller RD (ed): *Anesthesia,* ed 3, New York, 1990, Churchill Livingstone.
169. Benumof JL: Isoflurane anesthesia and arterial oxygenation during one-lung ventilation, *Anesthesiology* 64:419, 1986.

Metabolic and Hormonal Functions of the Lung

5

Rajiv M. Jhaveri, MD

Roger A. Johns, MD

Introduction and Overview

Once viewed as an organ involved solely in gas exchange, the lung is now regarded as an active metabolic organ that plays an important role in maintaining cardiovascular homeostasis. The anatomic location of the lungs makes this possible, as it ensures that the lungs receive the entire cardiac output. Therefore, the lungs are in an optimal position to actively modulate the chemical composition of the blood. This may be achieved via the removal, metabolism, or activation of a wide variety of substances present in the circulation (e.g., norepinephrine, 5-hydroxytryptamine, angiotensin II, bradykinin). In addition, vasoactive (e.g., endothelium-derived relaxing factor [EDRF], eicosanoids) and immunoregulatory substances (e.g., eicosanoids, adenine nucleotides) are released into the vasculature, where they elicit localized or systemic effects. Table 5-1 lists some of the compounds that are either acted upon by or released from the lungs.

Metabolic and Secretory Components of the Lung

The lung contains at least 40 different cell types derived from the foregut epithelium and the surrounding mesenchyma. Only a small proportion of these cell types are primarily involved with the metabolic and hormonal characteristics of this organ. These include the type II pneumocytes, neuroendocrine cells, Clara cells, mast cells, and the vascular endothelial cells.

VASCULAR ENDOTHELIUM

The vascular endothelium comprises approximately 30% of the cellular composition of the human lung parenchyma (Table 5-2).[1] These cells are responsible for a major portion of the metabolic activity of the lungs and also fulfill important secretory functions. The pulmonary endothelial cells are joined by tight intracellular junctions and form a continuous lining of the pulmonary vasculature.[2,3] Endothelial lining of larger pulmonary vessels displays prominent gap junctions; however, the capillaries are devoid of gap junctions.[4] This monolayer of cells acts as part of a physical barrier (the alveolar-capillary membrane) between the blood and the outside environment and also functions in the transport of water, solutes, and respiratory gases.[2] The pulmonary endothelium is unique mainly by virtue of its extensive surface area, the fact that it is exposed to the entire cardiac output, and its anatomic location in the circulatory system.

The metabolic function of the pulmonary endothelium depends on the interplay among blood flow, transit time, perfusion, and surface area. The human pulmonary capillary bed is the largest capillary bed in the body, estimated to have a total surface area at rest of 50 to 70 m^2, which, at 75% total lung capacity, may expand to 90 m^2.[5] In addition, the surface of the pulmonary endothelial cells is covered by many projections (Figure 5-1) and invaginations (caveolae; Figure 5-2) which serve to further increase the total surface area. The total perfused endothelial surface area (and therefore the total surface area available for metabolism) is under active control. Physiologic and pathophysiologic changes in pulmonary arterial pressure can lead to recruitment of portions of the pulmonary vasculature, which are normally poorly perfused. Endothelial uptake and surface metabolism of blood-borne substances are influenced by transit time; therefore changes in the rate of blood flow (which affects transit time) directly influence metabolism. The pulmonary capillary blood flow can increase from 4 L/min at rest to 40 L/min during exercise.

In particular, the pulmonary endothelium removes compounds such as norepinephrine and 5-hydroxytryptamine (5-HT) from the blood, synthesizes and releases vasoactive agents such as prostacyclin (PGI_2) and nitric oxide, and metabolizes other compounds such as the adenine nucleotides.[6-11] The pulmonary endothelium also converts inactive peptides to metabolites with vasoactive properties (e.g., angiotensin I to angiotensin II); conversely, vasoactive peptides such as bradykinin are inactivated.[12,13] In addition to these activities, the endothelium is involved in the metabolism of xenobiotics (foreign substances including drugs and environmental pollutants) via several metabolic enzyme systems, which include the cytochrome P-450 monooxygenases.[14,15] The pulmonary cytochrome P-450 monooxygenase system may also be important in producing endogenous vasoactive compounds.[16]

CLARA CELLS

Clara cells are nonciliated, columnar cells that line the terminal bronchioles and may project into the airway lumen. These are nonmucous, nonserous secretory cells that have a high level of metabolic activity, as demonstrated by cytochemical and ultrastructural studies.[17] The secretory functions of the Clara cell are poorly understood, and they have been variously suggested to secrete pulmonary surfactant, components of the bronchiolar periciliary fluid, cholesterol, and carbohydrates.[18] Clara cells act as progenitor cells for bronchial epithelial cells and are responsible for regeneration of the epithelial lining after injury.[19] Furthermore, through secretion of Clara cell 10-kDa (CC10) protein, these cells have been shown to protect the respiratory tract against inflammation and oxidative injury.

TABLE 5-1

Handling of Biologically Active Compounds by the Lung

Compounds selectively cleared and/or metabolized

Norepinephrine
5-Hydroxytryptamine (5-HT, serotonin)
Adenosine triphosphate (ATP)
Adenosine diphosphate (ADP)
Adenosine monophosphate (AMP)
Adenosine
Bradykinin
Angiotensin I (converted to angiotensin II)
Atrial natriuretic peptides
Prostaglandins E_1, E_2, and $F_{2\alpha}$
Morphine
Steroids

Compounds unaffected by the lung

Epinephrine
Dopamine
Isoproterenol
Angiotensin II
Substance P
Oxytocin
Vasopressin
Eledoisin
Bombesin
Vasoactive intestinal peptide (VIP)
Gastrin
Prostaglandin A_1, A_2, and I_2 (prostacyclin)
Thromboxane A_2

Compounds released from the lung

Adenosine
Prostaglandin I_2, E, and F
Endothelium-derived relaxing factor (EDRF), NO
Leukotriene A_4, B_4, C_4, D_4, and E_4
Histamine
5-HT
Heparin
Plasminogen activator

TABLE 5-2

Cellular Composition of Alveolar Region of Human Lung

Cell Type	Cells (n× 10^6)	% of Total Lung Cells
Interstitial cells	84	36
Endothelial cells	68	30
Alveolar type II cells	37	16
Macrophages	23	9
Alveolar type I cells	19	8

From Crapo JD, Barry BE, Gehr P, et al: *Am Rev Respir Dis* 125:332, 1982.

Clara cells secrete a number of different proteins, the major protein being Clara cell 10-kDa protein (also known as Clara cell 16-kDa protein, Clara cell secretory protein, polychlorinated biphenyl binding protein, urinary protein 1, human protein 1, or uteroglobin). Although high constitutive levels of CC10 protein are present in the bronchoalveolar fluid, its primary physiologic role is poorly understood. Cigarette smoking reduces the number of Clara cells in the lungs, leading to reduced production of CC10 protein in the bronchoalveolar fluid as well as in the serum.[23,24] The expression of CC10 protein is decreased in human non–small cell lung tumors, suggesting that it may contribute to tumor suppression.[25] CC10 protein also plays an important role in modulating airway inflammatory reaction by influencing the production and/or activity of phospholipase A_2, proinflammatory cytokines, and chemokines.[26-29] Increased levels of CC10 protein are demonstrated in survivors with acute lung injury compared to those in nonsurvivors.[26]

NEUROENDOCRINE CELLS AND NEUROENDOCRINE BODIES

Neuroendocrine cells—also known as K cells or Kultschitzky-like cells—are specialized basal epithelial cells of the lung that are derived from an endocrine cell line referred to

There is substantial evidence to suggest that these cells represent a primary site of cytochrome P-450–dependent metabolism in the lung. Cytochrome P-450 isozymes have been localized in Clara cells, and these cells have been demonstrated to exhibit cytochrome P-450–like metabolic activity.[20-22] The cytochrome P-450 monooxygenase system provides a major route for the oxidative metabolism of xenobiotics. This pathway, although being primarily involved in detoxification, can also lead to the formation of metabolites that are more toxic than the parent compound. Therefore the Clara cell, while being an important pulmonary site for the inactivation of xenobiotics, may also be the initial site of parenchymal injury induced by the metabolic activation of certain agents of environmental (e.g., paraquat, carbon tetrachloride) or clinical (e.g., bleomycin) origin. In addition, the ability of Clara cells to metabolize exogenous substances may indicate that these cells are an important site for the metabolic activation of certain carcinogens.

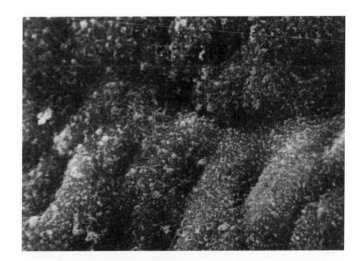

FIGURE 5-1 Scanning electron photomicrograph demonstrating surface projections of pulmonary endothelial cells (× 2.500). (From Tracey WR, Bend JR, Hamilton JT, Paterson NAM: *J Pharmacol Exp Ther* 250:1097, 1989.)

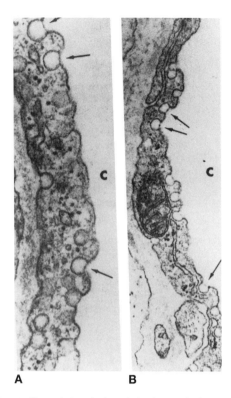

FIGURE 5-2 Transmission electron photomicrograph demonstrating caveolae in pulmonary capillary endothelial cells. *C* represents the capillary lumen. The liminal stoma of the caveola is spanned by a delicate membrane composed of a single lamella *(arrows)* in contrast to the bilamellar cell and caveolae membranes. **A,** × 68,000; **B,** × 44,000. (From Ryan US, Ryan JW: Correlations between the fine structure of the alveolar-capillary unit and its metabolic activities. In Bakhle YS, Vane JR [eds]: *Metabolic functions of the lung,* New York, 1977, Marcel Dekker.)

as APUD (amine precursor, uptake, and decarboxylation). These cells are found alone or in groups, when they are referred to as neuroendocrine bodies, and are localized most frequently in subsegmental bronchi, primarily at or near bifurcation points and at the sites of transition from terminal bronchioles to respiratory bronchioles.[18,30] Nonmyelinated afferent and efferent nerve endings are found in close synaptic contact with clusters of neuroendocrine cells (>3).[31] In humans and in other species, neuroendocrine cells and bodies are most prevalent in the fetal lung and decrease with age in adults.[18,30,31]

Neuroendocrine cells are believed to contain the peptides bombesin, leuenkephalin, somatostatin, and calcitonin, as well as 5-HT and catecholamines.[32-37] In addition, neuroendocrine bodies (but not neuroendocrine cells) stain positive for acetylcholinesterase.[31] Interestingly, the same neuroendocrine cells may contain all the different neuropeptides and amines. It is unclear, however, whether neuroendocrine cells serve primarily a paracrine (i.e., exerting local effects) or an endocrine (i.e., exerting systemic effects) function. Because these cells are predominantly located at the bifurcations of the airways, it has been suggested that they may serve as chemoreceptors, sensitive to the changes in the intraluminal environment and responding by releasing bioactive substances. For example, airway hypoxia (but not arterial hypoxemia) causes neuroendocrine cell degranulation and release of 5-HT.[30,38,39]

Lauweryns et al suggested that the neuroendocrine cells may be involved in maintaining hypoxic pulmonary vasoconstriction during intrauterine life.[39]

The neuroendocrine cells are suspected to be involved in several pulmonary disorders. For example, the neuroendocrine cells are the sites of origin of smallcell lung carcinomas and of carcinoid tumors of the lung, both of which may produce abnormal quantities of the chemical mediators produced by the neuroendocrine cells.[18,37] Exposure to hypoxia elicits neuroendocrine cell degranulation, and various other environmental stimuli, such as nitrogen dioxide and asbestos, are able to induce neuroendocrine cell proliferation.[40-44] Excessive production of bombesin-like peptides by neuroendocrine cells may be responsible for the development of bronchopulmonary dysplasia.[45]

TYPE II PNEUMOCYTES

In comparison to the type I cells, the type II pneumocytes are smaller and more cuboidal in shape. They are located predominantly at the corners of alveoli and comprise 60% of the alveolar epithelial cells by number; however, they provide only 4% of the alveolar epithelial surface area.[46]

Type II pneumocytes are the well-known primary source of pulmonary surfactant synthesis and secretion. The surfactant, which covers the entire alveolar surface, is stored in the lamellar bodies within the alveolar cells.[47] The main component of the pulmonary surfactant is dipalmitoylphosphatidylcholine, which is responsible for reducing surface tension at the air-liquid interface, thereby preventing alveolar collapse at end-expiration.[48] Besides the phospholipid, surfactant also contains 4 different proteins—two hydrophilic proteins (SP-A and SP-D) and two hydrophobic proteins (SP-B and SP-C). SP-A is the most abundant of these proteins. Genes for SP-A are expressed not only in the type II pneumocytes, but also in Clara cells and airway submucosal gland cells.[49] Recent evidence suggests that SP-A is actually not directly responsible for the surface tension reduction by surfactant.[50] The most important functions of SP-A appear to be providing innate (nonspecific) immunity and protecting the lung against microbial infections. SP-A–deficient mice exhibit increased susceptibility to pulmonary infections with group B streptococci, pseudomonas, and *Pneumocystis carinii.*[51] In addition, SP-A is essential for the formation of tubular myelin, increasing the rate of adsorption of surfactant phospholipids to a surface, and preventing inactivation of surfactant by alveolar proteins.[52,53] SP-B is largely responsible for the reduction in surface tension by increasing 150-fold the rate of adsorption of phospholipids to the air-water interface.[49] It is indispensable for the lung function and survival of the newborn. SP-B may also possess anti-inflammatory activity and protect against oxygen-induced pulmonary toxicity.[54,55] SP-C is produced exclusively by the type II pneumocytes. Its in vivo function is unclear, although it reduces surface tension in in vitro experiments.[56] SP-C also stabilizes the surface activity of the surfactant film during inflation and deflation of the lungs.[49] SP-D, produced by both the type II pneumocytes and the Clara cells, is believed to provide innate immunity and is also important in the regulation of surfactant turnover and metabolism.[57,58]

Type II pneumocyte cells are capable of dividing following epithelial injury and may be the progenitor of both type I and

98 PART II Respiratory Physiology and Pharmacology

type II pneumocytes.[59] Thus they may be involved in the repair of the damaged alveolar epithelium and in restoring normal cellular architecture and lung function.[60] The presence of a cytochrome P-450 monooxygenase system suggests that the type II pneumocytes may also be responsible for the metabolism of xenobiotics.[21,22] Type II cells also have the ability to rapidly and actively transport large amounts of water and sodium across the plasma membrane.[61,62] In this respect, they could have an important role to play in keeping alveoli free of edema.

MAST CELLS

Mast cells develop from bone marrow–derived progenitor cells and mature and differentiate in the peripheral tissues. In the respiratory tract, they are found in the airway lumen, in the submucosa, in the connective tissue surrounding small airways and blood vessels, and beneath the pleura.[63] Two subsets of mast cells have been described—the mucosal type (MMC) and the connective tissue type (CTMC)—based on their location, morphology, staining properties, chemical content, and response to chemical agents and drugs.[64] These cells contain an immense repertoire of bioactive compounds (Table 5-3). Mast cells play a key role in immune surveillance and host defense by activating innate and acquired immune reactions and through phagocytosis.[63,65-67] Mast cells are intricately involved in generating a complex inflammatory response when exposed to a variety of stimuli, including antigens, superoxides, complement proteins, neuropeptides, and lipoproteins. Mast cells, along with T cells, produce the cytokine pool, which modulates

airway smooth muscle tone and vascular permeability and induces many of the changes observed in inflammatory diseases. Allergic inflammatory diseases such as asthma, rhinitis, urticaria, and anaphylaxis involve mast cell activation and degranulation. Mast cells also play a role in the development of fibrosis and may be implicated in such fibrotic diseases as sarcoidosis, farmer's lung disease, cryptogenic fibrosing alveolitis, and histiocytosis.[68]

Types of Metabolic Processes Within the Lung

Several different processes are responsible for the metabolic functions of the lung. These include metabolism of humoral substances at the cell surface, specific uptake mechanisms for humoral substances (which may be followed by intracellular metabolism), and synthesis and release of vasoactive compounds. These processes may apply to some or all of the metabolically active pulmonary cell types, but they are most important in the pulmonary endothelium, which is in intimate contact with the blood passing through the pulmonary circulation. A brief overview of these processes is given here; a more specific discussion relating to the metabolism of various compounds can be found later in this chapter.

METABOLISM OF HUMORAL SUBSTANCES AT THE CELL SURFACE

Several enzymes associated with the luminal plasma membrane of the pulmonary endothelial cells are responsible for the metabolism of the adenine nucleotides, bradykinin, and angiotensin I. The enzymes that handle the adenine nucleotides—ATPase, ADPase, and 5'-nucleotidase—appear to reside solely in the endothelial caveolae.[69-71] On the other hand, angiotensin converting enzyme (ACE), carboxypeptidase N, and carbonic anhydrase appear to be less restricted in their distribution, having been localized both in the caveolae and on the endothelial projections (Figure 5-3).[72,73] A well-known class of drugs used in the treatment of hypertension, the ACE inhibitors (e.g., captopril, enalapril, lisinopril) prevent the conversion of angiotensin I to angiotensin II (and the inactivation of bradykinin) by ACE.

SPECIFIC UPTAKE MECHANISMS FOR HUMORAL SUBSTANCES THAT UNDERGO SUBSEQUENT INTRACELLULAR METABOLISM

Norepinephrine (but not epinephrine or isoproterenol) and 5-HT are the compounds primarily handled via this pathway. Approximately 65% of 5-HT, a substance produced in a vast array of mammalian cells, is cleared during a single passage through the lungs.[74] Because 5-HT is lipid insoluble, it requires carrier-mediated transport for its uptake by the pulmonary endothelium.[74] Norepinephrine is a polar molecule that does not rapidly diffuse through lipoprotein membranes, which is why it also requires carrier-mediated transport for its uptake. The active transport mechanisms of both compounds are saturable and energy dependent, require Na-K ATPase, and are influenced by temperature.[74,75] The sites of 5-HT and norepinephrine uptake are distinct, however, as neither amine inhibits the uptake of the other.[76] Uptake of norepinephrine occurs mainly in the precapillary and postcapillary vessels and the pulmonary veins, whereas 5-HT uptake is confined primarily to the arterioles and capillaries.[77-79] The uptake process is blocked by cocaine, chlorpromazine, tricyclic antidepressants (e.g., imipramine, desipramine, amitriptyline), certain steroids (e.g., estradiol and corticosterone), anoxia, hyperoxia, and hypothermia.[12,75] Anesthetic

---

TABLE 5-3
Mast Cell–Derived Mediators

Preformed and rapidly released mediators

Histamine
Eosinophil chemotactic factor
Neutrophil chemotactic factor
Kininogenase
Arylsulfatase A
Exoglycosidases
5-HT

Mediators generated de novo

Superoxide radical
Leukotrienes C, D, and E
Prostaglandins
Thromboxanes
Hydroxyeicosatetraenoic acids
Hydroperoxyeicosatetraenoic acids
Prostaglandin-generating factor
Platelet-activating factor (PAF)
Adenosine

Granule-associated mediators

Heparin
Tryptase
Chymotrypsin
Arylsulfatase B

From Friedman MM, Kaliner MA: *Am Rev Respir Dis* 135:1157, 1987 and Marom Z, Casale TB: *Ann Allergy* 50:367, 1983.

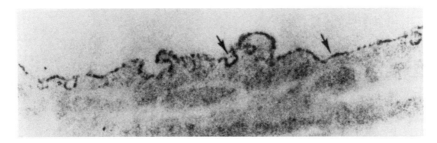

FIGURE 5-3 Immunocytochemical localization of angiotensin-converting enzyme in pulmonary endothelial cells. The reaction product is localized on the luminal surface of the endothelial cells *(arrows)* (× 81,000). (From Ryan JW, Ryan US: *Fed Proc* 36:2683, 1977.)

gases (nitrous oxide, halothane) can partially reduce norepinephrine uptake, and exposure to environmental agents such as paraquat and monocrotaline results in decreased 5-HT extraction.[75] In fact, in various experimental models, 5-HT and/or norepinephrine extraction is used as a sensitive index of endothelial functional integrity.[80]

Once within the endothelial cell, norepinephrine and 5-HT are deaminated by monoamine oxidase (MAO); 5-HT is converted to 5-hydroxyindoleacetic acid, and norepinephrine is further metabolized by catechol-*O*-methyltransferase (COMT) (see Figure 5-10).[12] The characteristics of the uptake process itself are similar to those for the accumulation of 5-HT and norepinephrine by nerve endings and synaptosomes (uptake 1, neuronal), but this process also shares characteristics with uptake 2 (extraneuronal)—the subsequent intracellular metabolism by MAO and COMT.[75]

Adenosine, produced at the endothelial surface by metabolism of ADP, is taken up by the endothelial cells and metabolized within the cell. Part of adenosine is broken down to inosine; the rest is incorporated into intracellular AMP, ADP, and ATP. Dipyridamole has been shown to inhibit the cellular uptake of adenosine.[81]

Prostaglandins of the E and F series—specifically PGE_1, PGE_2, and $PGF_{2\alpha}$—are largely cleared during a single passage through pulmonary circulation. In contrast, PGA, PGB, and PGI_2 (prostacyclin) remain essentially unchanged during transit through the lung. Prostaglandins are taken up by the endothelial cells by an active mechanism and metabolized by 15-hydroxyPG dehydrogenase.[74,82]

Some steroids—notably cortisone, cortisol, and some androgens—are also taken up by the lungs. Interestingly, cortisone is converted to the more potent cortisol in the lungs.[83] 11 β-Hydroxysteroid dehydrogenase type II ($11\beta HSD_2$), which catalyzes reversible conversion of cortisol to the inactive compound cortisone, has been demonstrated in the bronchial epithelial cells in fetal lungs (but not in the alveoli), throughout the course of lung development.[84] Glucocorticoid receptors in the bronchial epithelial cells may be the target for the antiinflammatory effects of inhaled steroids.[85]

SYNTHESIS AND RELEASE OF COMPOUNDS

The lung can be described as an endocrine organ by virtue of the fact that humoral agents are released from or produced within the lung, which may then act on distant parts of the body—in particular, on the cardiovascular system. Examples of these humoral compounds are PGI_2 and angiotensin II. The lung is also an important shock organ in humans, as indicated by the vast repertoire of potent vasoactive compounds released from the lung during anaphylaxis, which include 5-HT, histamine, thromboxane, leukotrienes, platelet-activating factor and kinins. The lung also regulates its own circulation through the release of locally acting substances such as NO, EDHF, adenosine, and endothelium-derived contracting factors (EDCF).

Processing and Action of Specific Factors
Eicosanoids

The term *eicosanoids* refers to a group of compounds derived from the metabolism of arachidonic acid (icosatetraenoic acid), a component of membrane lipids. These compounds are continuously produced at a low rate, as membrane lipids are constantly being turned over under normal basal metabolic conditions. Over and above its constitutive production, arachidonic acid is also released in response to a variety of biological or mechanical stimuli. Arachidonic acid is present in its esterified form in the cell membrane and is released following the activation of phospholipase A_2 or the sequential action of phospholipase C and diacylglycerol lipase. After release from its glycerol backbone, arachidonic acid can be metabolized via three major pathways: the cyclooxygenase pathway (producing prostaglandins, thromboxane and prostacyclin), the lipoxygenase pathway (producing the leukotrienes, midchain hydroxyicosatetraenoic acids [HETEs] and lipoxins), or the cytochrome P-450 monooxygenase pathway (producing midchain and ω-terminal HETEs and *cis*-epoxyeicosatrienoic acids [EETs]) (Figure 5-4). Metabolites arising from these pathways are biologically active and elicit responses that include dilation or constriction of pulmonary vessels and bronchi and regulation of pulmonary immune responses. Several of the cell types found within the lungs contain the full complement of enzymes required for the synthesis of these metabolites, as well as those enzymes necessary for their subsequent inactivation. Thus the lung is capable of finely regulating the levels of various eicosanoids in the cardiovascular system and may even use these compounds as a means of regulating its own perfusion.

In addition to its enzymatic metabolism, arachidonic acid is also subject to nonenzymic peroxidation, either in its free form or while still esterified to the lipid membrane. This nonenzymatic pathway leads to the production of isoprostanes that have effects on virtually every cell type found in the lungs.[86]

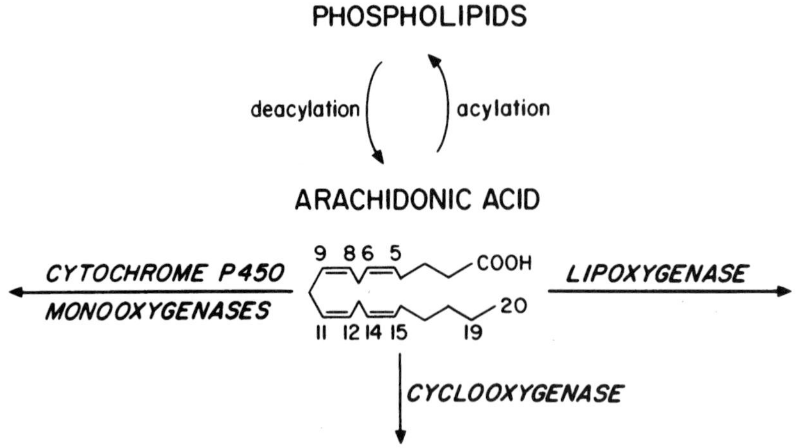

FIGURE 5-4 Metabolic pathways for the metabolism of arachidonic acid to eicosanoids. (From Johns RA, Peach MJ: Metabolism of arachidonic acid and release of endothelium-derived relaxing factors. In Vanhouttte PM (ed): *Relaxing and contracting factors,* Clifton NJ, 1988, Humana.)

CYCLOOXYGENASE PATHWAY

The metabolism of arachidonic acid via cyclooxygenase results in the formation of the cyclic endoperoxides PGG_2 and PGH_2 (Figure 5-5). The endoperoxides are highly unstable and are further metabolized to the relatively more stable prostaglandins (such as PGD_2, PGE_2 and $PGF_{2\alpha}$), as well as to thromboxane A_2 (TXA_2) and prostacyclin (PGI_2). This group of eicosanoids has potent, varied, and often opposing actions in both the pulmonary vasculature and airways, including eliciting vasoconstriction (TXA_2, $PGF_{2\alpha}$, PGE_2, PGD_2) or vasodilation (PGI_2, PGE_1), promoting (TXA_2) or inhibiting platelet aggregation (PGI_2), or causing bronchoconstriction ($PGF_{2\alpha}$, PGD_2, TXA_2) or bronchodilation (PGE_2, PGI_2).[87-90] Furthermore, PGE_2 has an antiinflammatory effect in the lung, and PGI_2 is a potent inhibitor of platelet aggregation, whereas $PGF_{2\alpha}$ and TXA_2 promote platelet aggregation.[91,92]

Probably the most important pulmonary cell type responsible for the synthesis and release of cyclooxygenase products is

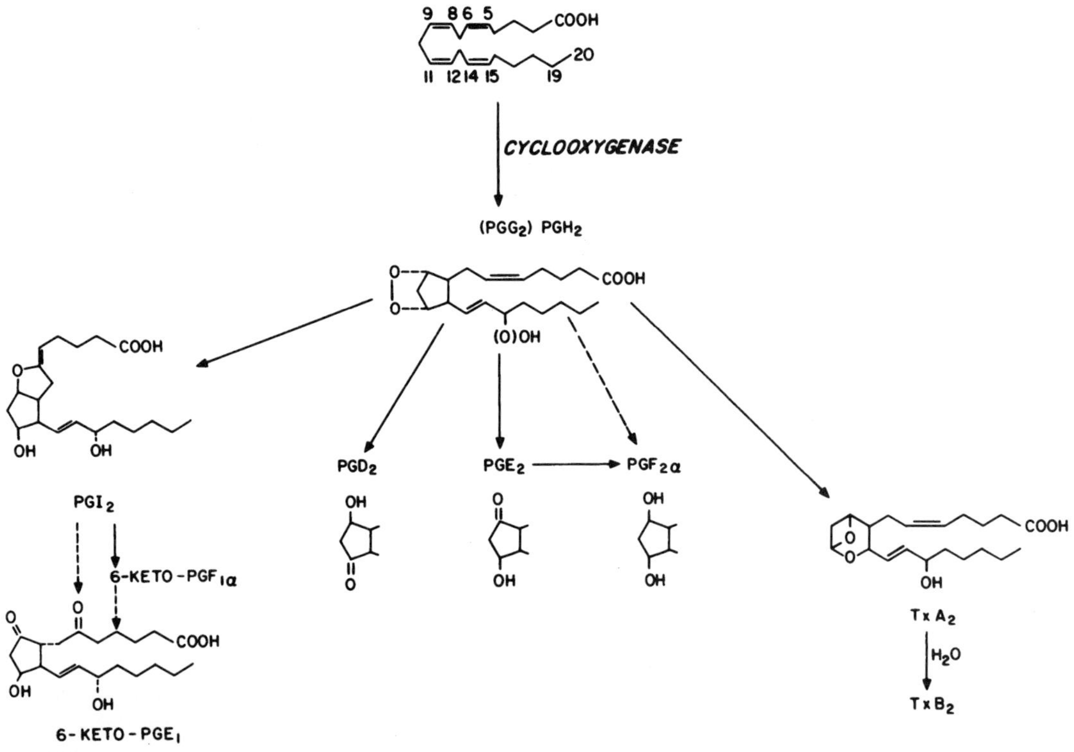

FIGURE 5-5 The cyclooxygenase pathway for arachidonate metabolism. (From Johns RA, Peach MJ: Metabolism of arachidonic acid and release of endothelium-derived relaxing factors. In Vanhouttte PM (ed): *Relaxing and contracting factors,* Clifton NJ, 1988, Humana.)

the endothelium. All of the major prostaglandins have been demonstrated in endothelial cell culture preparations using chromatographic and/or prostaglandin bioassays; however, the endothelium primarily produces PGI_2.[10] PGI_2 is continuously released from the lung, and it is known that PGI_2 production can be upregulated via increases in blood flow and shear stress, leading to subsequent pulmonary vasodilation.[93,94] Increasing the rate of respiration can also increase the release of both PGI_2 and TXA_2, PGI_2 release being preferentially increased over that of TXA_2.[95] This increase in PGI_2 release may in fact be due to respiration-induced alterations in pulmonary hemodynamics (i.e., local blood flows and shear stresses). Under varying experimental conditions, human lungs have been demonstrated to produce PGI_2, PGD_2, PGE_1, PGE_2, and $PGF_2\alpha$.[96,97]

Cyclooxygenase metabolites are handled by the lung via a combination of an active, carrier-mediated transport process and intracellular metabolism.[97,98] Ferreira and Vane were the first to study the metabolism of prostaglandins in the pulmonary circulation in vivo.[99] These investigators found that more than 90% of PGE_1, PGE_2, or $PGF_{2\alpha}$ was removed on one passage through the lung. On the other hand, PGA_1 and PGA_2, as well as PGI_2, survive passage through the pulmonary circulation essentially unchanged.[100,101] The survival of PGA_1 and pulmonary extraction of PGE_1 have been confirmed in the human lung.[102] Although it is unclear whether the lung is able to extract TXA_2 from the pulmonary circulation, this compound is highly unstable and is believed to be hydrolytically inactivated to TXB_2 while still in the circulation.[96] Nevertheless, TXB_2 is subject to pulmonary extraction, albeit via a mechanism that may be distinct from that responsible for the uptake of prostaglandins, as PGE_1, PGE_2, and $PGF_{2\alpha}$ do not prevent its uptake.[103] It is clear that within the closely related group of cyclooxygenase products, only certain members are subject to the selective uptake mechanisms of the lung. Following their removal from the pulmonary circulation, the prostaglandins are metabolized and inactivated intracellularly; however, the pulmonary cell types responsible for this inactivation have yet to be elucidated.

LIPOXYGENASE PATHWAY

Metabolism of membrane-derived arachidonic acid by lipoxygenase enzymes leads to the production of leukotrienes and lipoxins (Figures 5-6 and 5-7).

Leukotrienes. Cytosolic, perinuclear 5-lipoxygenase interacts with a docking protein on the plasma membrane, 5-lipoxygenase activating protein (FLAP) when cytosolic calcium levels rise.[104] This complex then acts on arachidonic acid to form 5-HPETE, which is then acted upon by a dehydrase to yield the unstable intermediate, leukotriene (LT) A_4 (see Figure 5-6). Leukotriene A_4 may then be converted to LTB_4 by the enzyme LTA_4 hydrolase, or via a second pathway to the cysteinyl leukotrienes LTC_4, LTD_4, and LTE_4 (historically known as the slow-reacting substance of anaphylaxis, SRS-A).

The leukotrienes are important regulators of immune function within the lung, as well as potent activators of airway and vascular smooth muscle. Unlike the prostaglandin family, whose members have opposing actions on bronchomotor and pulmonary vascular tone, leukotrienes have exclusively proinflammatory action. Leukotriene B_4 is both chemotactic and chemokinetic for leukocytes (particularly for neutrophils)

and is also able to elicit neutrophil degranulation.[89,98,105] LTB_4 does not affect bronchial tone or induce smooth muscle cell proliferation in the airway.[106] Cysteinyl leukotrienes C_4 and D_4 induce profound changes in the pulmonary vasculature, including an increase in vascular permeability.[105] These compounds are potent constrictors of both the pulmonary arteries and veins, although they appear to preferentially constrict the pulmonary veins.[107-110] The leukotrienes have been suggested to play a role in various pulmonary syndromes such as the acute respiratory distress syndrome (ARDS), hypoxic pulmonary vasoconstriction (HPV), and persistent pulmonary hypertension of the neonate.[111-114] Furthermore, LTC_4, LTD_4, and LTE_4 induce bronchoconstriction and increase endothelial membrane permeability leading to airway edema and increased mucus production, indicating that these compounds are important mediators in asthma.[115-117] Specific cysteinyl leukotriene antagonists and 5-lipoxygenase inhibitors have been developed as effective therapeutic agents for asthma.

Initial reports indicated that leukotrienes were released from the lung in response to hypoxia, and a role for leukotrienes in hypoxic pulmonary vasoconstriction was suggested.[118] Others have reported that decreased oxygen tensions inhibit leukotriene release.[109,119,120] It appears that leukotrienes, especially the cysteinyl leukotrienes, may have a modulatory but not an obligatory role in HPV.[121] Leukotriene release from lung parenchyma has also been demonstrated following antigen challenge.[119,120,122]

Leukotrienes are released from most inflammatory cells present in, or recruited to, the airways in response to a variety of stimuli. LTB_4 is produced by monocytes, alveolar macrophages, and neutrophils. Eosinophils, basophils, mast cells, and alveolar macrophages produce cysteinyl leukotrienes. LTC_4 is produced by platelets and vascular endothelium from LTA_4 derived from the circulating neutrophils.[123,124]

The leukotrienes do not appear to be subject to an active uptake mechanism comparable to the one that removes prostaglandins from the pulmonary circulation. Human lung tissue primarily converts LTC_4 to LTD_4, whereas pulmonary neutrophils are a likely site of inactivation of LTB_4 and LTC_4.[125-127] LTB_4 is inactivated by successive steps involving hydroxylation, carboxylation of C20, and subsequent β-oxidation.[128] Cysteinyl leukotrienes are degraded extracellularly by myeloperoxidases to form sulfoxides.[129] A more complete discussion of the metabolism of the leukotrienes can be found in Garcia et al, Hammarstrom et al, Drazen and Austin, and Bray.[105,130-132]

Lipoxins. The lipoxins (LxA_4 and its positional isomer LxB_4) are a class of arachidonic acid metabolites formed by the sequential actions of 15- and 5-lipoxygenases (LO), or 5- and 12-lipoxygenases (see Figure 5-7).[133] In the presence of cytokines, aspirin inhibits prostanoid production by the endothelium and promotes production of 15(R)HETE from arachidonic acid, which may then be converted to 15-epi-LXA_4 or 15-epi-LXB_4 in neutrophils. These 15-R-enantiomers of LXA_4 and LXB_4 are known as aspirin-triggered lipoxins (ATLs) and possess similar bioactivity to the native lipoxins but are more potent.[134] 15-LO is found abundantly in alveolar macrophages, monocytes, eosinophils, and epithelial cells, whereas 5-LO is found in neutrophils and monocytes, and 12-LO is found in

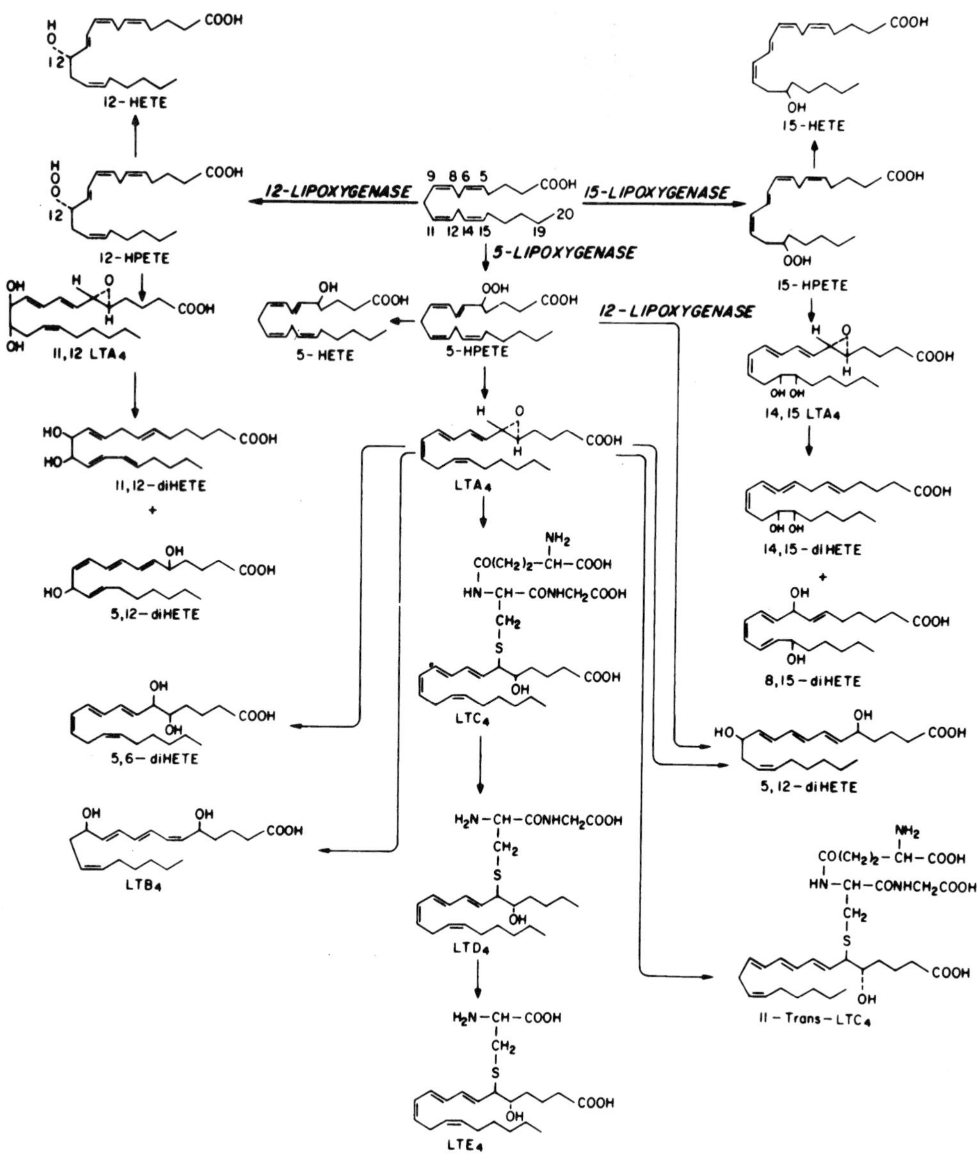

FIGURE 5-6 The lipoxygenase pathway for arachidonate metabolism. (From Johns RA, Peach MJ: Metabolism of arachidonic acid and release of endothelium-derived relaxing factors. In Vanhouttte PM (ed): *Relaxing and contracting factors,* Clifton NJ, 1988, Humana.)

platelets; thus, lipoxin generation requires trascellular and cell-to-cell interactions. For example, 15-HPETE generated in the respiratory epithelial cells may be converted to LXA_4 and LXB_4 in the neutrophils, where 5-LO is abundantly available.

Lipoxins possess antiinflammatory properties and serve to counterbalance the proinflammatory effects of leukotrienes. In fact, leukotriene biosynthesis is blocked at the 5-LO level during lipoxin production.[133] Lipoxins inhibit neutrophil and eosinophil chemotaxis, transmigration, and adhesion at inflammation sites and also inhibit neutrophil adhesion to epithelial and endothelial cell surfaces.[135-137] They also inhibit natural killer cell activation, thus preventing cytotoxicity. Lipoxins stimulate chemotaxis of monocytes. Furthermore, lipoxins exert potent vasodilatory effects on both aorta and pulmonary artery. The vasodilation is endothelium dependent and may be

mediated by stimulating release of prostacyclin or nitric oxide by the endothelial cells.[138,139] The lipoxins are short-lived, being taken up by the circulating monocytes and dehydrogenated to the inactive metabolite, 15-oxi-lipoxin.[133]

CYTOCHROME P-450 MONOOXYGENASE PATHWAY

Cytochrome P-450–dependent metabolism of arachidonic acid can proceed via one of three major pathways to form several different types of hydroxyeicosatetraenoic or dihydroxyeicosatetraenoic acids (HETEs and di-HETEs, respectively) or unstable epoxyeicosatetraenoic acids (EETs) (Figure 5-8). These metabolites are present in a number of organ systems in the body, including the liver, kidneys, cerebral and coronary vasculature, gastrointestinal tract, and lungs.[140] Isoforms of cytochrome P-450 (CYP) enzymes in the lung are expressed either constitutively in the lung or are induced by xenobiotics. The CYPA4 subfamily is

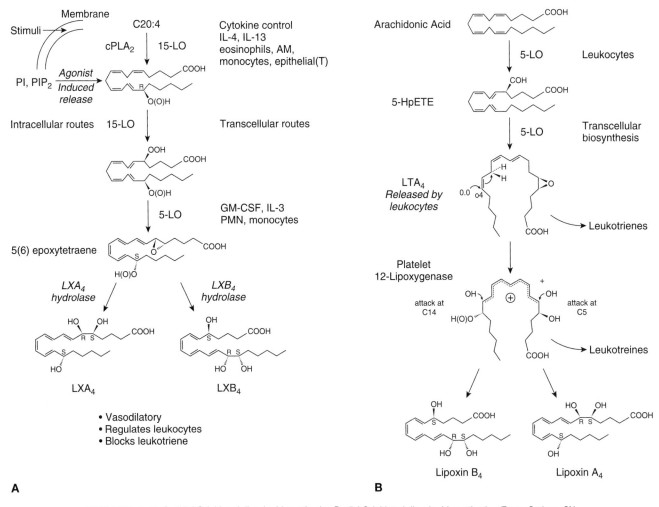

FIGURE 5-7 A, 15-LO-initiated lipoxin biosynthesis. **B,** 5-LO-initiated lipoxin biosynthesis. (From Serhan CN: *Prostaglandins* 53:107, 1997.)

located in the peripheral lung microsomes and produces 20-HETE. The CYP2J subfamily is found in both ciliated and non-ciliated airway epithelial cells, bronchial and vascular smooth muscle cells, and endothelium and alveolar macrophages.[140,141] Numerous other isoforms of CYP enzymes have been detected in the lungs, although their cellular location remains to be elucidated.

The HETEs and EETs are involved in regulating the bronchomotor and pulmonary vascular tone; 5-, 6-, 11-, 12-EETs and 20-HETE produce bronchodilation by hyperpolarizing resting membrane potential.[142-144] These EETs and 20-HETE also reduce pulmonary vascular tone.[140,144] These eicosanoids may also play a role in numerous other activities, such as anti-inflammatory actions, prevention of platelet aggregation, and a protective effect against endothelial reperfusion injury. Furthermore, 20-HETE is believed to be one of the factors that modulates acute hypoxic pulmonary vasoconstriction. EETs may also be involved in modulating airway smooth muscle tone, inflammatory reaction, and composition of alveolar fluid. There is an excellent review by Jacobs et al providing a more detailed discussion of these proposed functions of HETEs and EETs in the lung.[140]

The role of pulmonary cytochrome P-450 in the metabolism of xenobiotics is discussed in Section III of this book.

PLATELET ACTIVATING FACTOR (PAF)

PAF is a family of structurally related acetylated phospholipids that has biologic activities similar to those associated with acute allergic and inflammatory reactions; the family has a wide range of pathophysiologic effects upon the lung. PAF is not an eicosanoid but is included here because, like the eicosanoids, it is released from membrane phospholipids by phospholipase A_2. It causes pulmonary hypertension, increased airway resistance, decreased dynamic compliance, airway hyperreactivity, edema, and pulmonary inflammatory cell accumulation in both experimental animals and humans.[145] PAF has been proposed as an important mediator in chronic obstructive airway disease and asthma.[146]

Peptides

A wide variety of bioactive peptides have been found to be present in the lung (Table 5-4). These substances are not unique to the pulmonary circulation but are also present in several other organ systems, particularly the nervous system and gastrointestinal tract. It is not surprising that the lung contains

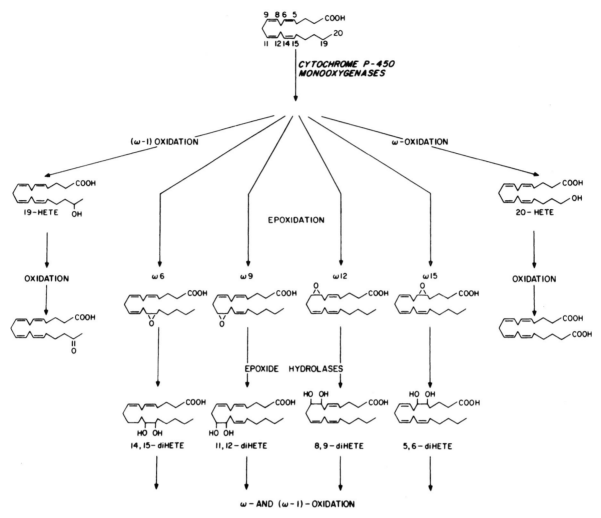

FIGURE 5-8 The cytochrome P-450 pathway for arachidonate metabolism. (From Johns RA, Peach MJ: Metabolism of arachidonic acid and release of endothelium-derived relaxing factors. In Vanhouttte PM (ed): *Relaxing and contracting factors,* Clifton NJ, 1988, Humana.)

TABLE 5-4

Bioactive Peptides in the Lung

Angiotensin II
Bradykinin
Substance P
Vasoactive intestinal peptide (VIP)
Neuropeptide Y
Atrial natriuretic peptides
Bombesin-like peptide
Cholecystokinin
Enkephalins
Eosinophil-chemotactic peptides
Neurotensin
Spasmogenic lung peptide
Eledoisin
Adrenocorticotrophic hormone (ACTH)
Somatostatin

several peptides also found in the upper gastrointestinal tract, as the lung is derived from the embryonic foregut.[147] Those peptides of more defined physiologic or clinical importance are discussed in the sections that follow.

ADRENOCORTICOTROPHIC HORMONE (ACTH)

ACTH has been found in normal lung and in increased amounts in bronchial tumors and in lung from chronic smokers.[148-151] Intrapulmonary ACTH may play an important role in lung maturation. Hypophysectomized fetal sheep have a decreased surfactant production and delayed pulmonary maturation even following administration of exogenous cortisol. The administration of exogenous ACTH, however, increases surfactant biosynthesis and enhances pulmonary compliance, implying an effect independent of corticosteroids.[152] ACTH has also been shown to inhibit ACE and may play a role in regulating angiotensin metabolism in the lung.[153]

ANGIOTENSIN

Angiotensin I is converted to its active form, angiotensin II, during a single passage through the pulmonary circulation.[154] This conversion is due to angiotensin-converting enzyme (ACE), a carboxypeptidase located within the caveolae intracellulare (pinocytic vesicles) and on the projections of the endothelial cells lining the pulmonary vasculature (Figure 5-9).[155] Although 20% of angiotensin I will be converted to angiotensin II in a single pass through the pulmonary circulation, angiotensin II is not metabolized within the lung but is allowed to pass freely to the systemic circulation.[154] Angiotensin II has multiple effects on the cardiovascular system including vaso-constriction, smooth muscle cell proliferation, myocardial hypertrophy, and altered ventricular remodeling.[156] It also stimulates nonosmotic release of arginine vasopressin, promoting renal water retention and increased thirst. The renin-angiotensin system plays an important role in the pathophysiology of congestive heart failure. This fact is underscored by the improvement in survival with angiotensin-converting enzyme inhibitor (ACEI) and angiotensin-receptor blocker classes of drugs in a broad spectrum of patients with congestive heart failure and left ventricular dysfunction.[157-161] Angiotensin II in the local circulation may directly contribute to regional blood flow regulation by activating angiotensin type I receptors and producing vasoconstriction of both the muscular large arteries and the resistance vessels. This may explain the increased production of angiotensin II in the hypoxic lung.[162,163] Inhibition of angiotensin-converting enzyme reduces pulmonary artery pressure and vascular resistance.[164] Stimulation of angiotensin receptors on the endothelial cells also induces the release of nitric oxide and prostacyclin.[165-167] More recently, Wang et al noted that angiotensinogen and angiotensin II are synthesized and expressed by myofibroblasts from human fibrotic lung.[168] Based on these findings and similar findings by other investigators, the role of locally produced angiotensin II as a regulator of apoptosis of pulmonary endothelial cells and in pulmonary fibrosis has been suggested.[169]

BRADYKININ

Bradykinin, a nonapeptide, is produced in the lungs (as in the rest of the body) through metabolism of plasma and tissue kininogens. Bradykinin is also inactivated in the lung by the same dipeptidyl carboxypeptidase, angiotensin-converting enzyme (see Figure 5-9) that is responsible for the conversion of angiotensin I to angiotensin II.[12,13] Bradykinin is a potent endothelium-dependent vasodilator of the pulmonary circulation. If the endothelium is damaged or destroyed, bradykinin manifests itself as a potent vasoconstrictor.[170] In addition, bradykinin stimulates the metabolism of arachidonic acid in pulmonary endothelial cells, causing the release of a variety of vasoactive eicosanoids.[10,171,172] Bradykinin constricts bronchial smooth muscle in asthmatic subjects, yet it has minimal effect on isolated bronchial smooth muscle.[173]

ATRIAL NATRIURETIC PEPTIDE

Atrial natriuretic peptide (ANP) is mainly produced by the atrial myocytes in response to atrial stretch (e.g., during heart failure) and links the heart, the kidneys, the adrenals, the blood vessels, and the brain in a complex hormonal system related to circulating blood volume and blood pressure homeostasis.[174,175] Its primary physiologic function seems to be prevention of sodium and fluid overload and hypertension.[177] Although the cardiac atria are the main source of circulating ANP, significant amounts of prohormone and the active form of ANP are also detected in human lung tissue.[177] ANP gene expression is found in pulmonary veins, as well as in pneumocytes.[178] Thus, lungs appear to be an important source of extracardiac ANP production. Pulmonary production of ANP is stimulated by glucocorticoids, hypoxia, thyroid hormones, and water overload, on the other hand, it is inhibited by dehydration.[178] Lung is an important site of clearance of circulating ANP, with 20% to 25% of ANP being removed during a single passage through the lungs.[179]

Although ANP produces varied and complex biological responses, its precise role in health or disease is still unclear. ANP is a potent endothelium-independent pulmonary vasodilator, with greater effect on pulmonary arteries than on the pulmonary veins.[180,181] In humans, ANP has only a weak bronchodilator effect, especially in the presence of bronchospasm, as in asthmatic patients.[182,183] ANP appears to increase capillary permeability in

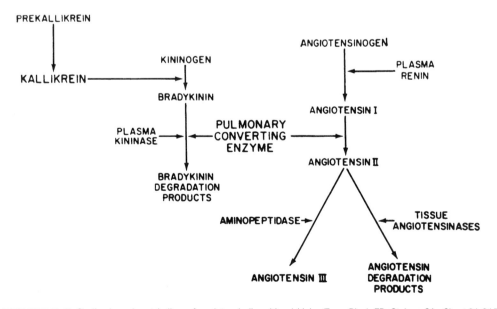

FIGURE 5-9 Synthesis and metabolism of angiotensin II and bradykinin. (From Block ER, Stalcup SA: *Chest* 81:215, 1982.)

the lung, inducing leakage of both water and proteins into the alveolar space.[184,185] On the other hand, ANP seems to protect against oxidant-induced increases in endothelial permeability.[186] ANP suppresses the renin-angiotensin-aldosterone system at three separate sites; it suppresses renin release, reduces ACE activity and blocks aldosterone secretion from the adrenal glands, thus promoting renal natriuresis and diuresis.[187] ANP also has been shown to decrease the hypoxic pulmonary vasoconstrictor response.[188] Increased ANP secretion has been demonstrated in a variety of disease states characterized by hypoxia and pulmonary hypertension; however, the role and significance of elevated ANP levels in these conditions remain to be elucidated.[189-191]

VASOACTIVE INTESTINAL PEPTIDE. The biologic activity of vasoactive intestinal peptide (VIP) was discovered in the lung prior to its isolation and chemical identification from the intestine.[192,193] Nerve fibers and nerve terminals containing VIP are present in several structures of the lung, including the tracheobronchial tree, bronchial and pulmonary blood vessels, bronchial smooth muscle, and bronchial submucosal glands. Many of these nerve fibers originate from microganglia within the lung, providing a source of intrinsic innervation of pulmonary structures.[194,195] VIP has also been found in mast cells of the lung.[196] VIP is a potent pulmonary vasodilator, as well as a relaxant of airway smooth muscle.[197-199] Its bronchodilatory effect is independent of adrenergic and cholinergic receptors or of cyclooxygenase activity.[200] Decreased biologic activity of VIP may be a contributing factor to the pathogenesis of cystic fibrosis and bronchial asthma.[194,195,201-203] VIP also reduces or prevents acute lung injury in experimental models of acute respiratory distress syndrome (ARDS) by modulating apoptotic cell death in alveolar epithelial cells and endothelial cells.[204,205]

ENDOTHELINS

Endothelins are 21-amino acid peptides produced by the endothelial cells and smooth muscle cells, mainly in response to hypoxia, ischemia, and shear stress. Endothelins and their precursors have also been found in airway epithelial cells and submucosal glands.[206] These are potent vasoconstrictors with a slow onset of action and are believed to have an important role in regulation of basal vasomotor tone. Of the three isoforms of endothelins (ET-1,2,3), ET-1 is the most common in man. ET-1 acts locally as a paracrine factor. Although ET-1 is not stored in lungs, it is produced within minutes in response to stimuli. The half-life of the mRNA is approximately 15 to 20 minutes, and that of ET-1 is 4 to 7 minutes.[207] ET-1 does not cross cell membranes but acts via endothelin receptors, ET_A, ET_B, and ET_C; 80% of ET-1 is cleared from the lungs during a single passage.[208] In diseases such as primary pulmonary hypertension and acute respiratory distress syndrome, impaired clearance of endothelins has been implicated.[209,210]

Endothelin receptors ET_A are predominantly vasoconstrictors and are most numerous in large pulmonary vessels. In contrast, ET_B receptors mediate vasodilatation in the peripheral resistance vessels by stimulating release of PGI_2 and nitric oxide.[211] Pulmonary vascular response to endothelins may depend on the baseline vascular tone.[211,212] In the presence of normal vascular tone, endothelins produce vasoconstriction. In the presence of increased vascular resistance, however, endothelin infusion initially causes vasodilatation, which is then followed by vasoconstriction. Endothelins increase bronchial

blood flow and increase vascular permeability causing airway edema.[213,214] ET-1 causes bronchoconstriction via ET_B receptors in both asthmatics and nonasthmatics.[215] Endothelins may play a role in an array of pulmonary diseases, including acute lung injury, acute and chronic lung infections, asthma, pulmonary hypertension, and ischemia-reperfusion injury.[211]

CYTOKINES AND CHEMOKINES

Cytokines are a group of small extracellular signaling proteins produced by a number of both resident and inflammatory cell types, including endothelial cells, epithelial cells, monocytes, eosinophils, activated macrophages, T-helper (Th) cells, and platelets. Members of the cytokine family play an integral role in the maintenance and coordination of the inflammatory response in chronic inflammatory pulmonary conditions such as asthma.[216] Cytokines cause activation of the target cells, proliferation, chemotaxis, immunomodulation, growth and cell differentiation, and apoptosis. In addition, they may stimulate release of the same or other cytokines.[217] Because of their ability to stimulate production of other cytokines, and because different cytokines possess overlapping functions, the role of individual cytokines in inflammatory conditions is difficult to ascertain. Chung and Barnes grouped the various cytokines as follows[217]:

- Lymphokines: Interleukin (IL) -2, IL-3, IL-4, IL-5, IL-13, IL-15, IL-16, IL-17
- Proinflammatory cytokines: IL-1, tumor necrosis factor (TNF), IL-6, IL-11, GM-CSF, SCF
- Antiinflammatory cytokines: IL-10, IL-1ra, IFN-γ, IL-12, IL-18
- Chemotactic cytokines (chemokines): RANTES, MCP-1, MCP-2, MCP-3,MCP-4, MCP-5, MIP-1α, eotaxin, IL-8.
- Growth factors: PDGF, TGF-β, FGF, EGF, IGF

Cytokines produce their biological effects by binding to a number of receptor families on the cell surface. Although they act primarily in a paracrine fashion, they are also capable of functioning as endocrine or autocrine mediators. They are involved in the development of atopy and chronic inflammatory states with release of mediators such as histamine and cysteinyl leukotrienes, airway remodeling, bronchoconstriction, and bronchial hyperresponsiveness. Chemokines are chemotactic cytokines. More than 40 chemokines have been identified. They mediate their effects through specific G-protein–coupled receptors and cause leucocyte recruitment and activation, smooth muscle proliferation, and regulation of fibrogenesis. They also play an important role in development and maintenance of airway hyperreactivity. A detailed discussion of the biological activities of individual cytokines is beyond the scope of this chapter. The reader is referred, however, to excellent reviews by Barnes et al, Chung and Barnes, and Blease et al.[216-218]

SUMMARY OF PHYSIOLOGIC ACTIONS OF PEPTIDES IN THE LUNG

Several of the peptides occurring in the lungs have vasoactive and bronchoconstrictive properties. Angiotensin II, spasmogenic lung peptide, substance P, and bombesin are pulmonary vasoconstrictors, while VIP and ANP are potent pulmonary vasodilators.[194,195,219-221] Bombesin, substance P, cholecystokinin, and spasmogenic lung peptide all induce bronchoconstriction.[194,220] Activated complement C5a is capable of increasing pulmonary microvascular permeability and may be important in mediating pulmonary edema in a variety of disease states.[147,222] Substances P and VIP also stimulate bronchial secretion, while bombesin and ACTH have been strongly implicated in the regulation of normal growth and development of the fetal lung.[151] Kinins may be generated by lung tissues during IgE-mediated allergic responses. Eosinophil and granulocyte-stimulating chemotactic peptides and kinins are mediators of anaphylaxis and acute inflammation.[151,223]

In conclusion, a multitude of bioactive peptides have been localized in the lung. These compounds are both constrictors and dilators of vascular and bronchial smooth muscle and are capable of influencing pulmonary vascular permeability and inflammatory responses within the lung. The exact role of these agents in normal pulmonary homeostasis continues to be studied.

Other Nonpeptide Substances

CATECHOLAMINES

As discussed earlier, the pulmonary endothelium is responsible for both the uptake and the inactivation of norepinephrine. More than 30% of this catecholamine is removed from the venous blood in a single passage through the lungs.[37] The carrier-mediated uptake is saturable, sodium-dependent, and temperature-dependent.[13,75,224,225] The specificity of this uptake process is demonstrated by the inability of the lung to remove epinephrine or dopamine from the circulation; isoprenaline is also not affected by this uptake mechanism.[12,37,75,224] Once within the endothelial cell, norepinephrine is metabolized via MAO and COMT to inactive metabolites (Figure 5-10).[12,66,75] Several different drugs can significantly reduce the pulmonary removal and/or metabolism of norepinephrine. These drugs include estradiol and corticosterone, imipramine, cocaine, halothane, and nitrous oxide.[12,75,226] In addition to the obvious autonomic neuronal sources of norepinephrine within the lung,

the neuroendocrine cells of the tracheobronchial tree are another source of catecholamine production.[37]

5-HYDROXYTRYPTAMINE

Enterochromaffin cells of the gastrointestinal mucosa are the main source of 5-HT. Smaller amounts of 5-HT are also released from mast cells, pulmonary neuroendocrine cells, and neuroepithelial bodies.[227,228] Both neuroendocrine cells and mast cells represent pulmonary sources of 5-HT.[37,63,66] Most of the 5-HT is taken up by platelets in the portal circulation. The small amounts of 5-HT that escape the portal circulation and reach the pulmonary circulation are cleared via endothelium-dependent mechanisms.[6,13,75,225] These mechanisms reflect a primary process of uptake rather than enzymatic degradation (Figure 5-11) and are virtually identical to those responsible for norepinephrine extraction. 5-HT is also taken up by pulmonary smooth muscle cells in vitro.[229] Unlike norepinephrine, however, 5-HT is essentially completely removed from the circulation (by as much as 98%) during one passage through the lung.[12,37,224] In addition, although the mechanisms of norepinephrine and 5-HT uptake are comparable, the sites of uptake appear to be different, as suggested by the inability of each amine to inhibit the uptake of the other.[225,226] 5-HT uptake is inhibited by cocaine, chlorpromazine, and tricyclic antidepressants (imipramine, amitriptyline).[12,75]

HISTAMINE

Histamine differs from norepinephrine and 5-HT in that histamine is not removed from the pulmonary circulation to any appreciable degree.[75,224] The lack of pulmonary metabolism of histamine apparently reflects the absence of an uptake mechanism, as pulmonary homogenates are quite capable of inactivating histamine.[12,75,224] Given that pulmonary mast cells

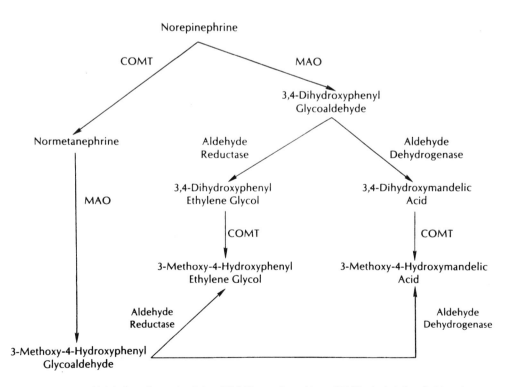

FIGURE 5-10 Metabolism of norepinephrine. *MAO,* Monoamine oxidase; *COMT,* catechol-*O*-methyl transferase.

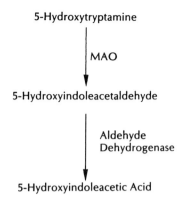

5-Hydroxytryptamine

MAO

5-Hydroxyindoleacetaldehyde

Aldehyde
Dehydrogenase

5-Hydroxyindoleacetic Acid

FIGURE 5-11 Metabolism of serotonin (5-HT). *MAO,* Monoamine oxidase.

contain significant stores of this agent, the absence of a pulmonary uptake mechanism for histamine may have important pathophysiologic consequences arising from the resulting vulnerability of the airways and pulmonary vessels to endogenously released histamine.

ADENINE NUCLEOTIDES

Adenine nucleotides (adenosine triphosphate, ATP; adenosine diphosphate, ADP; adenosine monophosphate, AMP) are substantially (40% to 90%) removed from the pulmonary circulation during one passage through the lung.[6,12,37,230] Cellular uptake is not required because these compounds are metabolized at the pulmonary endothelial surface by 5′-nucleotidase and ATPase localized in the endothelial caveolae.[6,69,70,230] Adenosine, which is produced during the degradation of the adenine nucleotides, is taken up by the endothelial cells via a saturable process that is inhibited by dipyridamole.[231] Once within the endothelial cell, adenosine may subsequently be utilized in the formation of intracellular nucleotides, primarily ATP.[230] This metabolic pathway also represents the conversion of endothelium-dependent vasodilators (ATP, ADP) to endothelium-independent vasodilators (AMP, adenosine); therefore, it is capable of regulating the extracellular concentration of these agents as well as the associated biological responses. Not only does the endothelium efficiently remove adenosine and adenine nucleotides from the circulation; it may also release adenosine after exposure to hypoxia (and various other stimuli), which could explain the increase in pulmonary adenosine levels observed during acute alveolar hypoxia.[230,232,233]

ACETYLCHOLINE

Acetylcholine is a potent, endothelium-dependent pulmonary vasodilator and is mentioned here due to the fact that clinical administration of this compound or its analogs may have potential benefits in conditions in which pulmonary hypertension is a problem. However, the physiologic pulmonary actions of this compound are restricted to sites of neuronal release, as it is rapidly degraded by synaptic acetylcholinesterase, and any acetylcholine that might enter the vasculature is equally rapidly degraded by blood-borne cholinesterases.[224] A more comprehensive review of the pharmacologic effects of acetylcholine on the pulmonary circulation can be found in a review by Peach et al.[234]

Endothelium-Derived Relaxing, Hyperpolarizing and Contracting Factors

NITRIC OXIDE

In 1980, Furchgott and Zawadzki observed that intact endothelium was obligatory for producing relaxation of strips of rabbit aorta by acetylcholine and other muscarinic agonists.[235] The relaxing substance produced by the endothelium was later labeled endothelium-derived relaxing factor (EDRF).[236] In 1987, Ignarro et al and Furchgott independently noted closely similar properties of nitric oxide and EDRF and suggested that EDRF and NO were either the same or some closely related radicals.[237] Over the next few years, several investigators using a variety of techniques established that NO was indeed the endothelial factor responsible for the vasodilatory properties.[238-240]

It is now known that vascular relaxation is dependent on mechanisms that are either endothelium dependent or independent. Sodium nitroprusside, a functional analog of NO, acts as NO donor to stimulate guanylyl cyclase and produce cGMP in the vascular smooth muscle causing vasorelaxation.[241] The many agents that require a functionally intact endothelium to produce vascular relaxation include several potent vasodilators present in the pulmonary circulation such as bradykinin, histamine, substance P, VIP, ATP, ADP, thrombin, calcitonin gene-related peptide, arachidonic acid, and trypsin. In addition, several contractile agents including norepinephrine, 5-HT, and vasopressin cause release of NO from the endothelium to modulate their direct contractile actions on the vascular smooth muscle.[16,234,242-246]

NO is a highly reactive free radical with an unpaired electron. It is produced by oxygen-dependent oxidation of L-arginine, catalyzed by the heme-containing enzyme NO synthase (Figure 5-12). NO synthase (NOS) exists in three isoforms. Isoform I is expressed constitutively, mainly in central and peripheral neurons, and is known as neuronal NOS (nNOS). It is also detected in the lung in epithelial and vascular smooth muscle cells. It is activated by a calcium-calmodulin complex. Synthesis of isoform II, also known as inducible NOS (iNOS), is upregulated by inflammatory mediators such as tumor necrosis factor, interleukin-I, and endotoxin. Once expressed, its production proceeds at a high rate independent of intracellular concentrations of free calcium ion. The third isoform, known as endothelial NOS (eNOS), is also expressed constitutively in the endothelial cells in a calcium-calmodulin dependent fashion. Its production is modulated by shear force on the endothelial cells.

NO produces vasodilatation by activating soluble guanylyl cyclase, leading to increased levels of cyclic GMP (cGMP) in the target cells. cGMP is capable of producing vascular relaxation by several mechanisms.[10,247-251] NO is also able to produce pulmonary vasodilatation by cGMP-independent mechanisms, including activation of Ca^{++}-dependent K^+ channels and regulation of angiotensin II receptors.[252,253] At higher concentrations, NO can readily react with oxygen and superoxides, producing peroxynitrite that can produce the toxic hydroxyl radical. NO is short-lived, with a biological half-life of 2 to 30 seconds. It rapidly binds to hemoglobin with an affinity 1500 times greater than that of carbon monoxide and forms nitrosylhemoglobin. Both oxyhemoglobin and

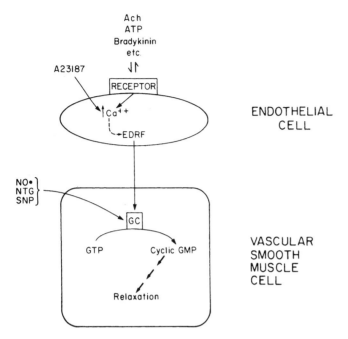

FIGURE 5-12 Synthesis and mechanism of action of nitric oxide. Agents that release NO directly (e.g., the calcium ionophore, A23187) or through endothelial cell receptors (e.g., *ACH*, acetylcholine; *ATP*, adenosine triphosphate, bradykinin) elicit an increase in intracellular calcium that correlates with NO release. NO is transferred to the vascular smooth muscle, where it activates soluble guanylate cyclase *(GC)*. GC causes an increase in cyclic GMP, which subsequently leads to vascular relaxation.

deoxyhemoglobin are able to bind NO. Methemoglobin is formed from the NO-hemoglobin complexes. This rapid and avid binding to hemoglobin is the basis for the selective nature of the pulmonary vasodilator action of NO therapeutically administered by inhalation. NO binds to and is inactivated by hemoglobin before it can reach the systemic circulation.

In humans, NOS is expressed in pulmonary vasculature as well as in the alveolar cells and the airway. Furthermore, NOS is also present in macrophages, mast cells, neutrophils, autonomic neurons, fibroblasts, smooth muscle cells, platelets, endothelial cells, and epithelial cells.[254] In the cells, NOS is widely distributed in the nucleus, Golgi apparatus, mitochondria, plasma membrane, and endoplasmic reticulum.[255] Thus NO is likely to be involved in a number of different physiologic and pathophysiologic processes in the lung.

NO is a potent pulmonary vasodilator, relaxing the precapillary resistance vessels to a greater degree than the large capacitance vessels.[256,257] Although there is a significant basal production of NO by the endothelial cells, NO is only modestly expressed in the pulmonary resistance vessels in normal lung and, therefore it appears to play only a limited role in maintaining low basal tone in the pulmonary vasculature.[258] On the other hand, it plays a central role in modulating the response to pulmonary vasoconstrictor stimuli such as hypoxia and to bioactive compounds like angiotensin II, endothelin-I, or thromboxane. NOS expression is markedly upregulated in pulmonary resistance vessels in response to hypoxia or inflammation. Decreased expression of NOS and reduced production of NO have been demonstrated in patients with primary and secondary pulmonary hypertension, although whether it is a

primary or secondary effect of the disease remains to be elucidated. In other studies, NO production has been shown to be increased in pulmonary hypertension.

Circulating platelets are also capable of producing NO. NO released from both the endothelial cells and platelets inhibits platelet aggregation, inhibits platelet recruitment by the platelet thrombus, and breaks up preformed platelet aggregates.[259-261] Thus NO, along with other agents such as prostacyclin, participates in prevention of endothelial thrombus formation. In addition to its influence on platelet activity, NO also inhibits leukocyte adhesion and prevents smooth muscle cell migration and proliferation. NO production by inhibitory nonadrenergic, noncholinergic neurons modulates bronchomotor tone. Thus NO influences vascular, airway, and inflammatory events in the lungs.

The role of NO in modulating a number of events in the pathogenesis of acute lung injury, ischemia-reperfusion injury, and acute respiratory distress syndrome is under intense investigation. The ability of endogenous or exogenous inhaled NO to reduce leukocyte adhesion and activation, reduce production of inflammatory mediators in ARDS patients, and prevent microvascular thrombosis by its effects on platelet function may be responsible for the reduction in lung injury. NO is also believed to have antioxidant properties, providing cytoprotection against oxidant-induced lung injury.

EDHF

It is now recognized that vasodilators such as acetylcholine and bradykinin produce endothelium-dependent vasorelaxation of vascular smooth muscle in both systemic and pulmonary vessels even after inhibition of NOS and prostacyclin dependent pathways with L-NAME and indomethacin.[262,263] This vasorelaxation involves hyperpolarization of vascular smooth muscle cell membrane caused by activation of calcium-sensitive potassium channels, and the putative transmitter has been called the endothelium-dependent hyperpolarizing factor (EDHF).[264] Myoendothelial gap junctions, which facilitate exchange of second messengers and the conduction of electrical signals between cells, may also play a role in hyperpolarization of the vascular smooth muscle cell.[265] Although the precise nature of EDHF has not been determined, epoxide products of the cytochrome P-450–arachidonic acid system have been suggested to be responsible for the hyperpolarizing response.[266,267] Although the presence of an endothelium-dependent, NO-independent hyperpolarizing factor is not in doubt, its role in regulation of vascular tone is not yet understood.

ENDOTHELIUM-DERIVED CONTRACTING FACTORS

In addition to the vasorelaxing factors, endothelium also releases a number of factors that induce contraction of the vascular smooth muscle: endothelins and a number of products of the cyclooxygenase pathway, such as thromboxane A_2 and prostaglandins D_2, E_2, and $F_{2\alpha}$. These substances have been discussed previously in this chapter.

Another important metabolic function of the endothelium is its ability to modulate cell growth within the vessel wall.[268-270] In its basal state, the endothelium produces heparin-like factors that inhibit smooth muscle proliferation.[271] When the endothelial cell is replicating or injured, it produces a variety of growth factors (e.g., platelet-derived growth factor and epidermal growth factor) and stops producing antiproliferative factors.[268,272]

This production of growth factors and inhibition of antiprolif-erative factors may play a role in the hypertrophy and hyper-plasia of the vasculature in conditions such as chronic hyperoxia, hypoxia, and lung injury.[234]

Metabolism of Xenobiotics

Because of the lungs' unique position that exposes them to the external environment, as well as to the total cardiac output, the lungs are involved in the uptake, accumulation, and/or metab-olism of both blood-borne and environmental xenobiotics. Venous drainage from the entire body perfuses the alveolar-capillary unit. The thin and apposed epithelial-endothelial cel-lular structure of the alveolar-capillary unit provides an enormous surface area to the air on one side and to the blood on the other.

A wide variety of drugs and chemicals is actively taken up and/or metabolized by the lungs. Lipophilic compounds and inhaled gases, such as tobacco smoke constituents, anesthetic gases, organic solvents, and some of the inhaled bronchodilator drugs, diffuse along their concentration gradient across the phospholipid membrane. On the other hand, hydrophilic com-pounds such as xanthines and mannitol require transcellular transport before their metabolism. Similarly, a vast array of blood-borne chemicals are removed by the lung either via sim-ple diffusion or by active transport mechanisms. Numerous metabolic enzyme systems have been detected within the lung (Table 5-5) and provide the means for metabolism of these sub-stances. Some of the substances filtered by the lung are highly accumulated in the lung, where they have a potential for pro-ducing pulmonary toxicity.

The most studied and perhaps most important route of metabolism is via the family of cytochrome P-450 monooxy-genase enzymes. The lung is known to be a rich source of at least three different isozymes of cytochrome P-450.[273-275] Consequently, the lung is actively involved with xenobiotic metabolism. As was mentioned earlier, several pulmonary cell types are rich sources of cytochrome P-450 enzymes or cytochrome P-450-like activity—namely, the Clara cell, the type II pneumocyte, and the endothelium.[14,15,20-22] In addi-tion, the medial layer of the pulmonary vasculature may also contain a functional cytochrome P-450 system, if it is assumed that the data obtained from systemic vessels can be extrapo-lated to the pulmonary vasculature.[276,277] Therefore the lung

TABLE 5-5

Metabolic Enzyme Pathways Present in Lung

Cytochrome P-450 mixed function oxygenase
Amine oxidase
Glutathione-S-epoxide transferase
Glutathione-S-aryl transferase
Epoxide hydrolase
Glucuronyl transferase
Nitro reductase
Sulfotransferase
N-Methyltransferase

From Philpot RM, Anderson MW, Eling TE: Uptake, accumulation, and metabolism of chemicals by the lung. In Bakhle YS, Vane JR (eds): *Metabolic functions of the lung,* New York, 1977, Marcel Dekker.

has the capacity to metabolize xenobiotics presented to it by either the atmospheric environment (via the Clara cell and the type II pneumocytes) or the blood (via the endothelium). Although both cytochrome P-450 and NADPH cytochrome P-450 reductase are present in Clara cells and type II pneu-mocytes, NADPH cytochrome P-450 reductase has not been localized to endothelial cells.[14] Thus it is possible that this enzyme system may be nonfunctional in the endothelium. In contrast, however, cytochrome P-450–dependent monooxy-genase activity has been reported in isolated endothelial cells.[278,279]

Isozymes of cytochrome P-450 may be involved in protec-tive mechanisms within the lung and, conversely, may also play a role in the development of pulmonary toxicity arising from the metabolism of xenobiotics. For example, Mansour and col-leagues recently demonstrated that induction of certain pul-monary cytochrome P-450 isozymes led to a reduction in the pathophysiologic changes induced by exposure to hyper-oxia.[280,281] On the other hand, although the cytochrome P-450 system generally produces metabolites that are less toxic than the parent compounds, the pulmonary damage induced by agents such as paraquat, nitrofurantoin, mitomycin C, benzo(a)pyrene, and 4-ipomeanol reflects the cytochrome P-450–dependent production of toxic metabolites.[6,282] A great deal of further investigation is required in order to clarify the understanding of the potential physiologic and pathophysiologic roles of the cytochrome P-450 monooxygenase system of the lung.

Many of the drugs known to be metabolized by the lung are of interest to the anesthesiologist (Table 5-6). These include sympathomimetics, antihistamines, morphine-like analgesics, tricyclic antidepressants, and local anesthetics. The metabolism of some of these drugs leads to the production of metabolites associated with lung injury (Table 5-7).

There is evidence that a few of these agents (amphetamine, metaraminol, isoprenaline) are taken up by specific carrier-mediated uptake mechanisms, but for most drugs, uptake is nonspecific. To be effectively removed, these compounds have certain common physicochemical properties. Most are basic amines with a pKa greater than 8, and all are lipophilic. These drugs also often possess a charged cationic group at physio-logic pH.[6] The cationic component of these amines is attracted to the multiple anionic domains on the endothelial cell mem-brane; thereafter, the lipophilic component facilitates entry into the cell.[283,284]

Bupivacaine and lidocaine are two lipophilic basic amines that undergo extensive pulmonary uptake on passage through the pulmonary circulation. Rothstein et al observed an 81% extraction of bupivacaine on a single pass through the rabbit pulmonary circulation in vivo.[285] Similar results have been observed with lidocaine.[286-288] Propranolol is another hydrophobic amine with local anesthetic properties that is taken up by the lung in a manner similar to lidocaine and bupi-vacaine.[6] The uptake of all of these agents is decreased by a reduction in temperature.[289] The uptake of propranolol appears to be saturable, as first-pass uptake is markedly decreased in patients regularly taking this drug.[290]

Several narcotic agents used in anesthesia are also lipophilic basic amines. Roerig et al studied the first-pass uptake of fen-tanyl, meperidine and morphine in patients before elective

TABLE 5-6

Xenobiotics Metabolized by the Lung

Drug	Reference
Amphetamine	Anderson MW, Orton TC, Pickett RD, Eling TE: The accumulation of amines in the isolated perfused rabbit lung, *J Pharmacol Exp Ther* 189:456, 1974.
	Bend JR, Serabjit-Singh CJ, Philpot RM: The pulmonary uptake, accumulation, and metabolism of xenobiotics, *Ann Rev Pharmacol Toxicol* 25:97, 1985.
Metaraminol	Davila T, Davila D: Uptake and release of 3H-metaraminol by rat lung. The influence of various drugs, *Archs Int Pharmacodyn* 215:336, 1975.
	Junod AF: Uptake, metabolism and efflux of 14C-5-hydroxytryptamine in isolated, perfused rat lungs, *J Pharmacol Exp Ther* 183:341, 1972.
	Alabaster VA, Bakhle YS: The removal of noradrenaline in the pulmonary circulation of rat isolated lungs, *Br J Pharmacol* 40:468, 1983.
Isoprenaline	Briant RH, Blackwell EW, Williams FM, et al: The metabolism of sympathomimetic bronchodilator drugs by the isolated perfused dog lung, *Xenobiotica* 3:787, 1973.
Chlorphenteramine	Minchin RF, Madsen BW, Ilett KF: Effect of desmethylimipramine on the kinetics of chlorophenteramine accumulation in isolated perfused rat lung, *J Pharmacol Exp Ther* 211:514, 1979.
Chlorpromazine	Bend JR, Serabjit-Singh CJ, Philpot RM: The pulmonary uptake, accumulation, and metabolism of xenobiotics, *Ann Rev Pharmacol Toxicol* 25:97, 1985.
Diphenhydramine	Bend JR, Serabjit-Singh CJ, Philpot RM: The pulmonary uptake, accumulation, and metabolism of xenobiotics, *Ann Rev Pharmacol Toxicol* 25:97, 1985.
Imipramine	Junod AF: Accumulation of 14C-imipramine in isolated perfused rat lungs, *J Phrmacol Exp Ther* 183:182, 1972.
Mescaline	Roth RA, Roth JA, Gillis CN: Disposition of 14C-mescaline by rabbit lung, *J Pharmacol Exp Ther* 200:394, 1977.
Methadone	Wilson AGE, Law FCP, Eling TE, Anderson MW: Uptake, metabolism and efflux of methadone in 'Single Pass' isolated rabbit lungs, *J Pharmacol Exp Ther* 199:360, 1976.
Fentanyl	Roerig DL, Kotrly KJ, Vucins EJ, et al: First pass uptake of fentanyl, meperidine, and morphine in the human lung, *Anesthesiology* 67:466, 1987.
Meperidine	Roerig DL, Kotrly KJ, Vucins EJ, et al: First pass uptake of fentanyl, meperidine, and morphine in the human lung, *Anesthesiology* 67:466, 1987.
Propranolol	Geddes DM, Nesbitt K, Traill T, Blackburn JP: First pass uptake of 14C-propranolol by the lung, *Thorax* 34:810, 1979.
Bupivacaine	Rothstein R, Cole JS, Pitt BR: Pulmonary extraction of [3H]bupivacaine: modification by dose, propranolol and interaction with [14C]5-hydroxytryptamine, *J Pharmacol Exp Ther* 240:410, 1987.
Lidocaine	Post C, Andersson RGG, Ryrfeldt A, Nilsson E: Transport and binding of lidocaine by lung slices and perfused lungs of rats, *Acta Pharmacol Toxicol* 43:156, 1978.

surgery.[291] They found rapid uptake of fentanyl and meperidine, but no significant uptake of morphine. These differential effects can be explained by the physicochemical differences between these basic amines. Fentanyl and meperidine are orders of magnitude more lipid soluble than morphine. Morphine is also a less basic amine (pKa = 7.9) when compared with fentanyl (pKa = 8.4) and meperidine (pKa = 8.5). This extensive uptake of fentanyl and meperidine clearly has a major effect on the peak concentrations of these drugs seen by other organ systems.

Certain anesthetic agents also have been shown to inhibit lung metabolism. Halothane and nitrous oxide decrease 5-HT and norepinephrine uptake by pulmonary endothelial cells in a competitive and rapidly reversible manner.[292-295] Halothane and pentobarbital inhibit the synthesis of lung proteins, and ketamine has been shown to competitively and reversibly inhibit lung 5-HT metabolism.[296-298]

Physiologic and Pathophysiologic Implications
Hypoxic Pulmonary Vasoconstriction

The tone in pulmonary resistance vessels is altered in order to closely match lung ventilation with perfusion. The pulmonary vessels differ from systemic vessels in that in lungs, pulmonary vasoconstriction occurs in response to alveolar hypoxia, whereas in the systemic circulation, vasorelaxation is the usual response to local hypoxia. This response of pulmonary vessels to hypoxia has been termed *hypoxic pulmonary vasoconstriction* (HPV) and was first described by Euler and Liljestrand in 1946.[299] Although HPV in response to acute hypoxia helps to divert blood away from the poorly ventilated areas of the lung, exposure to chronic hypoxia as in chronic lung disease results in sustained pulmonary vasoconstriction, vascular remodeling, pulmonary hypertension, and eventually right ventricular heart failure and death. The mechanisms of

TABLE 5-7

Metabolized Xenobiotics Associated with Lung Injury

Drug	Reference
Bleomycin	Catane R, Schwade JG, Turrisi At, et al: Pulmonary toxicity after radiation and bleomycin: a review, *Int J Radiat Oncol Biol Phys* 5:1513-1518, 1979.
Nitrofurantoin	Boyd MR, Stiko AW, Sasme HA: Metabolic activation of nitrofurantoin-possible implications for circinogenesis, *Biochem Pharmacol* 28:601-606, 1979.
Mitomycin C	Jarasch ED, Bruder G, Heid HW: Significance of xanthine oxidase in capillary endothelial cells, *Acta Physiol Scand* (Suppl) 548:39-46, 1986.
Paraquat	Smith LL: The identification of an accumulation system for diamines and polyamines into the lung and its relevance for paraquat toxicity, *Arch Toxicol* 5:1-14(Suppl), 1982.
Carbon tetrachloride	Mihm FG: Nonrespiratory functions of the lung. In *40th Annual Refresher Course Lectures and Clinical Update Program.* Chicago, 1989, American Society of Anesthesiologists.

hypoxic pulmonary vasoconstriction remain poorly understood. Response to hypoxia has been demonstrated in isolated pulmonary arterial rings denuded of endothelium, as well as in isolated pulmonary artery smooth muscle cell.[300,301] Thus it appears that endothelium is not necessary for inducing pulmonary vasoconstriction and that the pulmonary arterial smooth muscle cell has intrinsic capacity to sense and react to hypoxia. However, endothelium does modulate HPV through release of endothelium-derived contracting factors (EDCFs), NO, and EDHF. Experimental evidence suggests that hypoxia inhibits the production and/or release of NO from the endothelium, thereby leading to pulmonary vasoconstriction.[302,303] Loss of basal NO production in pathologic situations in which the endothelium is damaged may also lead to augmented HPV.[304] More recently, closure of voltage-gated potassium (Kv) channels in response to acute hypoxia has been demonstrated.[305] Potassium currents through these channels are mainly responsible for maintenance of the resting membrane potential in pulmonary arterial smooth muscle cells. Change in membrane potential resulting from closure of Kv channel allows opening of the voltage-dependent calcium channels (VDCC), resulting in an influx of calcium into the cells.[306] Increase in intracellular calcium concentrations causes contraction of the arterial smooth muscle cells and the development of HPV.

Acute Lung Injury and Acute Respiratory Distress Syndrome

Acute lung injury (ALI) and its extreme manifestation, acute respiratory distress syndrome (ARDS), result from direct insult to the lung, as well as in the setting of a systemic process such as sepsis, severe trauma, or acute pancreatitis. The clinical picture is characterized by the acute onset of bilateral pulmonary infiltrates in the absence of left atrial hypertension, and hypoxemia. The characteristic exudation of protein-rich edema fluid into the air spaces is a consequence of damage to the vascular endothelium leading to increased capillary permeability.[307] However, epithelial injury also plays a critical role in the development of and recovery from ALI. Indeed, the extent of epithelial injury is a predictor of outcome after ALI and ARDS.[308] Damage to the alveolar epithelium contributes to the disease process in a number of ways. Disruption of the epithelial barrier may allow alveolar flooding. Injury to the type II pneumocytes causes impaired clearance of alveolar edema fluid, decreased production and turnover of surfactant, and impairment of innate immunity leading to increased susceptibility to bacterial infections. Furthermore, as discussed previously, type II pneumocytes are important for cellular repair after injury, and severe damage to these cells may lead to disorganized or insufficient epithelial repair and fibrosis.[309]

Sequestration and activation of neutrophils in the pulmonary vasculature is the hallmark of ALI and ARDS (Figure 5-13). The cytokine network, and particularly the "early-response cytokines" (IL-1β, TNFα, and CXC group of chemokines) are involved in the initial recruitment of the neutrophils.[310] Activation of the sequestered neutrophils mainly involves adhesion molecules, IL-8, and platelet activating factor.[309] An inflammatory response involving a complex balance between proinflammatory and antiinflammatory cytokines leads to the endothelial and epithelial injury and alterations in the complex

metabolic activities of the lung. Arachidonate metabolites may also contribute to these events through direct actions causing vascular and bronchial constriction or dilation, endothelial cell damage, and increases in microvascular permeability. In addition, eicosanoids may have indirect effects through the stimulation of complement, leukocytes, and platelets.[311] Leukotrienes may contribute to acute lung injury through their actions of chemotaxis, increased permeability, and pulmonary vasoconstriction.[111,112,114] This can result in increases in the amounts of prostaglandins, thromboxanes, leukotrienes, platelet activating factor, activated complement, thrombin, and oxygen-derived free radicals.[312] The quantities of other factors derived from the endothelium, including EDRF and endothelin, may be markedly reduced or enhanced. Conversely, some metabolic products of the lung may help to modulate or prevent lung injury.[307] Vasoactive intestinal peptide is an endogenous bronchodilator and vasodilator that may counteract the effects of leukotrienes and other bronchoconstrictors during lung injury. Prostacyclin, in addition to being a strong relaxant of vascular smooth muscle and an inhibitor of thromboxane generation, also inhibits polymorphonuclear leukocyte aggregation, lysosomal enzyme release, and platelet aggregation. In several experimental studies of acute lung injury, prostacyclin has been shown to prevent the development of pulmonary vascular permeability and pulmonary hypertension and to exert a stabilizing activity on polymorphonuclear leukocytes.[313] The production of leukotrienes and their subsequent effects of vasoconstriction and increased pulmonary vascular permeability are also inhibited.[313] The pathophysiologic role of these biochemicals in acute lung injury has been reviewed.[220,310,314]

The acute phase of injury is followed by a reparative phase in which alveolar type II cells replicate to replace damaged alveolar type I cells, with subsequent inflammatory cell infiltration and fibrosis.[312,315,316] The pulmonary vasculature exhibits structural changes with loss of precapillary units and hypertrophy of vascular smooth muscle.[312,317]

Pulmonary Embolism

Several aspects of pulmonary metabolism contribute to the response of the lung to thromboembolism. The activation of fibrinolysis and an increase in prostacyclin formation help to decrease the effects of emboli and maintain normal ventilation-perfusion balance. Other factors such as neutrophil chemotoxins, adherence-inducing agents, and oxygen-derived free radicals may be detrimental. The production of the superoxide radical from activated leukocytes, for example, may directly inactivate EDRF and damage the endothelium, thereby contributing to pulmonary hypertension. The balance between the varied metabolic effects during pulmonary embolism determines the degree to which pulmonary vascular resistance will increase, as well as the development of lung vascular injury and tissue edema.[318]

Asthma

Asthma is a complex syndrome with several phenotypes, characterized by airway inflammation, bronchial hyperresponsiveness, and reversible airflow obstruction. Inflammatory changes are observed throughout the central and peripheral airways, even in patients with mild disease and in those with intermittent

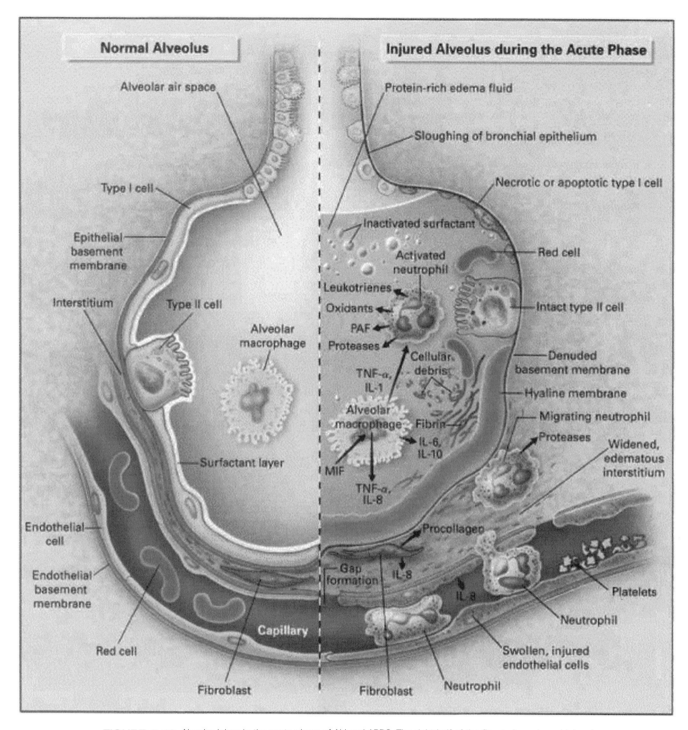

FIGURE 5-13 Alveolar injury in the acute phase of ALI and ARDS. The right half of the figure shows bronchial and epithelial cell sloughing, exudation of edema fluid, and formation of a hyaline membrane. Sequestration of neutrophils in the pulmonary vasculature and their migration into the air space is seen. Type I alveolar cell is injured; however, the type II cell is spared in the initial stage. Secretion of cytokines, interleukins and TNF_α by alveolar macrophages leads to chemotaxis and activation of the neutrophils. A variety of mediators—including proinflammatory and antiinflammatory cytokines, eicosanoids, proteases, and oxidants—are generated to produce the inflammatory response. (From Wave LB, Matthaw MA: *N Engl J Med* 342(18):1334, 2000.)

disease.[319,320] In response to antigen exposure, a number of inflammatory cells, including mast cells, eosinophils, and T-lymphocytes infiltrate mucosa and submucosa. These cells are involved in the production and release of a vast array of inflammatory mediators. In addition, structural cells of the airway, such as epithelial cells, endothelial cells, fibroblasts, and airway smooth muscle cells are known to change their phenotype to produce mediators such as adhesion molecules, endothelin, NOS, cytokines , and chemokines in response to a variety of biologic stimuli.[321,322] The lymphocytes, and in particular the CD4+ T-helper (Th) lymphocytes, are primarily responsible for orchestrating the inflammatory response in asthma. The Th2 phenotype has been recovered from bronchoalveolar fluid as well as from airway biopsies of asthmatics. These cells produce a number of cytokines, including interleukins (IL) 4, 5, 9, and 13—the so-called Th2 cytokines. Airway eosinophilia and IgE production are induced, and an inflammatory response ensues. Cysteinyl leukotrienes as well as IL-5 are released from activated eosinophils. As mentioned above, cysteinyl leukotrienes induce bronchoconstriction and increase endothelial membrane permeability, leading to airway edema and increased mucus production. Chemokines produced by inflammatory as well as structural cells also play a role in recruiting the inflammatory mediators.

In addition to airway inflammation, bronchial hyperresponsiveness is also a major characteristic of asthma. Furthermore, airway remodeling is observed in chronic asthma and is related to the severity of the disease. Several mediators including TGFβ, IL-1, and IL-6 induce both hypertrophy and hyperplasia of the airway smooth muscle cells.[323,324] Increase in airway wall thickness is also associated with epithelial damage, basement thickening, an increase in the bronchial capillary bed, airway edema, and goblet cell hyperplasia.[325]

Steroid therapy in asthma results in a reduction of CD4+ Th2 cells in the airways and a decrease in mRNA for IL-4, IL-5, and IL-13.[326] Reduction in airway inflammation and symptomatic improvement are achieved by a reduction in the production of cytokines, chemokines, and cell adhesion molecules. More recently, antileukotriene (anti-LT) agents have shown beneficial effect against many types of asthma. There are two general classes of anti-LT drugs: those that inhibit leukotriene synthesis, and cysteinyl-leukotriene receptor blocking agents. Zileuton prevents LT synthesis by blocking 5-lipoxygenase enzyme and is useful in the treatment of exercise-, cold-air, and aspirin-induced asthma.[327-329] Zafirlukast (Accolate) and Montelukast (Singulair) are the leukotriene receptor-blocking drugs available in the United States.

Markers of Pulmonary Disease Processes

The understanding of pulmonary metabolism has been applied to an evaluation of pulmonary endothelial function in vivo. Indicator dilution techniques have been used to assess 5-HT, PGE_1, or norepinephrine uptake in normal individuals and in patients with pulmonary disease. Observed decreases in uptake or clearance of these substances by the lungs have proven to be early indicators of pulmonary endothelial cell dysfunction, an initial derangement of many types of lung injury.[330,331]

In recent years, there has been an interest in the analysis of exhaled breath constituents as markers of inflammation and oxidative stress in the lungs.[332] Exhaled nitric oxide has been widely studied in a variety of disease processes. Increased levels of exhaled NO are detected in normal individuals with subclinical asthma, as well as in asthmatic patients. Exhaled NO may be used as an early warning of impending asthmatic exacerbation, as the levels rise early. Exhaled NO levels are rapidly reduced by inhaled corticosteroids and so may be useful in monitoring response to treatment. Low levels of exhaled NO are found in some pulmonary diseases (COPD, chronic bronchitis, cystic fibrosis, Kartagener's syndrome), while increased levels are detected in other diseases (bronchiectasis, fibrosing alveolitis, sarcoidosis, lung cancer). Exhaled NO levels are decreased in patients with primary pulmonary hypertension and increase with inhaled prostacyclin treatment. Kaneko et al demonstrated an inverse correlation of biochemical reaction products of NO with pulmonary artery pressures in primary pulmonary hypertension.[333] Exhaled NO levels are reduced in the perioperative period after lung transplantation. Serial measurements of exhaled NO may be useful in early detection of obliterative bronchiolitis or acute rejection. In ARDS, the NO production is upregulated, but the consumption of NO by oxygen-free radicals leads to low exhaled levels of NO.

Exhaled carbon monoxide (CO) has also been studied as a marker of disease processes. Elevated levels of exhaled CO are detected in stable asthma, bronchiectasis, cystic fibrosis, interstitial pulmonary fibrosis, scleroderma, and allergic rhinitis. A wide variety of other markers such as hydrocarbons, prostanoids, leukotrienes, isoprostanes, cytokines, vasoactive amines, ammonia, and so on, have been studied in many pulmonary diseases. Further long-term clinical studies will help realize the enormous potential of the exhaled breath analysis as a noninvasive diagnostic and monitoring tool in many lung diseases.

Summary

Beyond its respiratory functions, the lung has important and wide-ranging metabolic and hormonal activity. It is the site of production, activation, and metabolism of multiple agents including eicosanoids, peptides, and amines as well as endothelium-derived dilating and constricting factors (EDRF, EDCF, EDHF, endothelins). These autacoids and hormones have multiple functions both within and outside the lung. Included among them are potent vascular and bronchial dilators and constrictors, immunoregulators, modulators of vascular growth and hypertrophy, activators and inhibitors of platelet aggregation, and mediators of permeability. The lungs are also capable of affecting the disposition of a number of exogenous compounds and drugs by extracting and/or metabolizing these substances during their passage through the pulmonary vasculature. These agents contribute to the normal pulmonary vascular tone and the ability of the pulmonary vasculature to accommodate changes in flow in response to physiologic and pathophysiologic stimuli.

REFERENCES

1. Crapo JD, Barry BE, Gehr P, et al: Cell number and cell characteristics of the normal human lung, *Am Rev Respir Dis* 125:332, 1982.

2. Simionescu M: Cell organization of the alveolar-capillary unit: structural-functional correlations. In Said SI (ed): *The pulmonary circulation and acute lung injury,* Mount Kisco, NY, 1985, Futura Publishing.

3. Smith U, Ryan JW: Electron microscopy of endothelial and epithelial components of the lungs: correlations of structure and function. *Fed Proc* 32:1957, 1973.

4. Ryan JW, Ryan US: Metabolic functions of the pulmonary vascular endothelium, *Adv Vet Sci Comp Med* 26:79, 1982.

5. Weibel ER, Gomez DM: The architecture of the human lung, *Science* 137:577, 1962.

6. Ryan US, Grantham CJ: Metabolism of endogenous and xenobiotic substances by pulmonary vascular endothelial cells, *Pharmacol Ther* 42:235, 1989.

7. Johns RA, Izzo NJ, Milner PJ, et al: Use of cultured cells to study the relationship between arachidonic acid and endothelium-derived relaxing factor, *Am J Med Sci* 31:287, 1988.

8. van Grondelle A, Worthen GS, Ellis D, et al: Altering hydrodynamic variables influences PGI2 production by isolated lungs and endothelial cells, *J Appl Physiol* 57:388, 1984.

9. Gryglewski RJ, Korbut R, Dietkiewicz A: Generation of prostacyclin by lungs in vivo and its release into the arterial circulation, *Nature* 273:765, 1978.

10. Johns RA, Peach MJ: Parabromophenacyl bromide inhibits endothelium-dependent arterial relaxation and cyclic GMP accumulation by effects produced exclusively in the smooth muscle, *J Pharmacol Exp Ther* 244:859, 1988.

11. Ignarro LJ, Buga GM, Chaudhuri G: EDRF generation and release from perfused bovine pulmonary artery and vein, *Eur J Pharmacol* 149:79, 1988.

12. Said SI: Metabolic functions of the pulmonary circulation, *Circ Res* 50:325, 1982.

13. Ryan JW, Ryan US: Pulmonary endothelial cells, *Fed Proc* 36:2683, 1977.

14. Serabjit-Singh CJ, Nishio SJ, Philpot RM, Plopper CG: The distribution of cytochrome P-450 monooxygenase in cells of the rabbit lung: an ultra-structural immunocytochemical characterization, *Mol Pharmacol* 33:279, 1988.

15. Dees JH, Masters BSS, Muller-Eberhard U, Johnson EF: Effect of 2,3,7,8-tetrachlorodibenzo-*p*-dioxin and phenobarbital on the occurrence and distribution of four cytochrome P-450 isozymes in rabbit kidney, lung and liver, *Cancer Res* 42:1423, 1982.

16. Johns RA, Peach MJ: Metabolism of arachidonic acid and release of endothelium-derived relaxing factors. In Vanhouttte PM (ed): *Relaxing and contracting factors,* Clifton, NJ, 1988, Humana.

17. Widdicombe JG, Pack RJ: The Clara cell, *Eur J Respir Dis* 63:202, 1982.

18. Gail DB, Lenfant CJM: Cells of the lung: biology and clinical implications, *Am Rev Respir Dis* 127:366, 1983.

19. Hook GE, Brody AR, Cameron GS, et al: Repopulation of denuded tracheas by Clara cells isolated from the lungs of rabbits, *Exp Lung Res* 12(4):311, 1987.

20. Serabjit-Singh CJ, Wolf CR, Philpot RM, Plopper CG: Cytochrome P-450: localization in rabbit lung, *Science* 207:1469, 1980.

21. Devereux TR, Serabjit-Singh CJ, Slaughter SR, et al: Identification of cytochrome P-450 isozymes in nonciliated bronchiolar epithelial (Clara) and alveolar type II cells isolated from rabbit lung, *Exp Lung Res* 2:221, 1981.

22. Devereux TR, Fouts JR: Xenobiotic metabolism by alveolar type II cells isolated from rabbit lung, *Biochem Pharmacol* 30:1231, 1981.

23. Shijubo N, Itoh Y, Yamaguchi T, et al: Serum and BAL Clara cell 10 kDa protein (CC10) levels and CC10-positive bronchiolar cells are decreased in smokers, *Eur Respir J* 10(5):8, 1997.

24. Andersson O, Cassel TN, Skold CM, et al: Clara cell secretory protein. Levels in BAL fluid after smoking cessation, *Chest* 118(1):180, 2000.

25. Linnoila RI, Szabo E, DeMayo F, et al: The role of CC10 in pulmonary carcinogenesis: from a marker to tumor suppression, *Ann N Y Acad Sci* 923:249, 2000.

26. Jorens PG, Sibille Y, Goulding NJ, et al: Potential role of Clara cell protein, an endogenous phospholipase A2 inhibitor, in acute lung injury, *Eur Respir J* 8(10):1647, 1995.

27. Lesur O, Bernard A, Arsalane K, et al: Clara cell protein (CC-16) induces a phospholipase A2-mediated inhibition of fibroblast migration in vitro, *Am J Respir Crit Care Med* 152(1):290, 1995.

28. Singh G, Katyal SL: Clara cell proteins, *Ann N Y Acad Sci* 923:43, 2000.

29. Cowan MJ, Huang X, Yao XL, Shelhamer JH: Tumor necrosis factor alpha stimulation of human Clara cell secretory protein production by human airway epithelial cells, *Ann N Y Acad Sci* 923:193, 2000.

30. Scheuermann DW: Morphology and cytochemistry of the endocrine epithelial system in the lung, *Int Rev Cytol* 106:35, 1987.

31. Cutz E: Neuroendocrine cells of the lung. An overview of morphologic characteristics and development, *Exp Lung Res* 3(3-4):185, 1982.

32. Wharton J, Polak JM, Bloom SR, et al: Bombesin-like immunoreactivity in the lung, *Nature* 273:769, 1978.

33. Cutz E, Chan W, Track NS: Bombesin, calcitonin, and leu-enkephalin immunoreactivity in endocrine cells of human lung, *Experientia* 37:765, 1981.

34. Dayer AM, Rademakers A, DeMey J, Will JA: Serotonin, bombesin, and somatostatin-like immunoreactivity in neuroepithelial bodies (NEBs) of rhesus monkey fetal lung, *Fed Proc* 43:880, 1984.

35. Becker KL, Monaghan KG, Silva OL: Immunocytochemical localization of calcitonin in Kulchitsky cells of human lung, *Arch Pathol Lab Med* 104:196, 1980.

36. Hage E, Hage J, Juel G: Endocrine-like cells of the pulmonary epithelium of the human adult lung, *Cell Tissue Res* 178:39, 1977.

37. Mihm FG: Non-respiratory functions of the lung. In American Society of Anesthesiologists (ed): *40th annual refresher course lectures and clinical update program,* Chicago, 1989, Lecture 155.

38. Youngson C, Nurse C, Yeger H. Cutz E: Oxygen sensing in airway chemoreceptors, *Nature* 365(6442):153, 1993.

39. Lauweryns JM, Cokelaere M: Hypoxia-sensitive neuro-epithelial bodies: Intrapulmonary secretory neuroreceptors, modulated by the CNS, *Z Zellforsch Mikrosk Anat* 145(4):521, 1973.

40. Bonikos DS, Bensch KG: Endocrine cells of bronchial and bronchiolar epithelium, *Am J Med* 63:765, 1977.

41. Becker KL, Silva OL: Hypothesis: the bronchial Kulchitsky (K) cell as a source of humoral biologic activity, *Med Hypotheses* 7:943, 1981.

42. Keith IM, Will JA: Hypoxia and the neonatal rabbit lung: neuroendocrine cell numbers, 5-HT fluorescence intensity, and the relationship to arterial thickness, *Thorax* 36:767, 1981.

43. Kleinerman J, Marchevsky AM, Thornton J: Quantitative studies of APUD cells in airways of rats, *Am Rev Respir Dis* 124:458, 1981.

44. Johnson NF, Wagner JC, Wills HA: Endocrine cell proliferation in the rat lung following asbestos inhalation, *Lung* 158:221, 1980.

45. Sunday ME, Yoder BA, Cuttitta F, et al: Bombesin-like peptide mediates lung injury in a baboon model of bronchopulmonary dysplasia, *J Clin Invest* 102(3):584, 1998.

46. Crapo JD, Young SL, Fram EK, Pinkerton KE, Barry BE, Crapo RO: Morphometric characteristics of cells in the alveolar region of mammalian lungs, *Am Rev Respir Dis* 128:S42, 1983.

47. Askin FB, Kuhn C: The cellular origin of pulmonary surfactant, *Lab Invest* 25:260, 1971.

48. van Rozendaal BA, van Golde LM, Haagsman HP: Localization and functions of SP-A and SP-D at mucosal surfaces, *Pediatr Pathol Mol Med* 20:319, 2001.

49. Griese M. Pulmonary surfactant in health and human lung diseases: state of the art, *Eur Respir J* 13(6):1455, 1999.

50. Korfhagen TR, Bruno MD, Ross GF, et al:. Altered surfactant function and structure in SP-A gene targeted mice, *Proc Natl Acad Sci USA* 93(18):9594, 1996.

51. LeVine AM, Kurak KE, Bruno MD, et al: Surfactant protein-A-deficient mice are susceptible to *Pseudomonas aeruginosa* infection, *Am J Respir Cell Mol Biol* 19(4):700, 1998.

52. Phelps DS: Surfactant regulation of host defense function in the lung: a question of balance, *Pediatr Pathol and Mol Med* 20(4):269, 2001.

53. Casals C: Role of surfactant protein A (SP-A)/lipid interactions for SP-A functions in the lung, *Pediatr Pathol Mol Med* 20:249, 2001.

54. Miles PR, Bowman L, Rao KM, et al: Pulmonary surfactant inhibits LPS-induced nitric oxide production by alveolar macrophages, *Am J Physiol* 276:L186, 1999.

55. Tokeida K, Ikegami M, Wert SE, et al: Surfactant protein B corrects oxygen-induced pulmonary dysfunction in heterozygous surfactant protein B-deficient mice, *Pediatr Res* 46:708, 1999.

56. Weaver TE, Conkright JJ: Function of surfactant proteins B and C, *Annu Rev Physiol* 63:555, 200l.

57. Crouch E. Wright JR: Surfactant proteins A and D and pulmonary host defense, *Annu Rev Physiol* 63:521, 2001.

58. Hawgood S, Poulain FR: The pulmonary collectins and surfactant metabolism, *Annu Rev Physiol* 63:495, 2001.

59. Uhal BD. Kpsjo O. Trie AL, et al: Fibroblasts isolated after fibrotic lung injury induce apoptosis of alveolar epithelial cells in vitro, *Am J Physiol* 269:L819, 1995.

60. Sutherland LM, Edwards YS, Murray AW: Alveolar type II cell apoptosis, *Comp Biochem Physiol A Mol Integr Physiol* 129:267, 2001.

61. Jones GS, Miles PR, Lantz RC, et al: Ionic content and regulation of cellular volume in rat alveolar type II cells, *J Appl Physiol Respir Environ Exercise Physiol* 53:258, 1982.

62. Goodman BE. Fleischer RS, Crandall ED: Evidence for active Na⁺ transport by cultured monolayers of pulmonary alveolar epithelial cells, *Amer J Physiol* 245:C78, 1983.

63. Friedman MM, Kaliner MA: Symposium on mast cells and asthma: human mast cells and asthma, *Am Rev Respir Dis* 135:1157, 1987.

64. Okuda M: Functional heterogeneity of airway mast cells, *Allergy* 54:S57, 1999.

65. Wasserman SI: The lung mast cell: its physiology and potential relevance to defense of the lung, *Environ Health Perspect* 35:153, 1980.

66. Marom Z, Casale TB: Mast cells and their mediators, *Ann Allergy* 50:367, 1983.

67. Krishnaswamy G, Kelley J, Johnson D, et al: The human mast cell: functions in physiology and disease, *Front Biosci* 6:D1109, 2001.

68. Pesci A, Bertorelli G, Gabrielli M, Olivieri D: Mast cells in fibrotic lung disorders, *Chest* 103(4):989, 1993.

69. Ryan JW, Smith U: Metabolism of adenosine 5'-monophosphate during circulation through the lungs, *Trans Assoc Am Physicians* 84:297, 1971.

70. Smith U, Ryan JW: Pinocytolic vesicles of the pulmonary endothelial cells, *Chest* 59:125, 1971.

71. Smith U, Ryan JW: Electron microscopy of endothelial and epithelial components of the lungs: correlations of structure and function, *Fed Proc* 32:1957, 1973.

72. Ryan US, Frokjaer-Jensen J: Pulmonary endothelium and processing of plasma solutes: structure and function. In Said, Vane J (eds): *The pulmonary circulation and acute lung injury,* Mount Kisco, NY, 1985, Futura Publishing.

73. Ryan US, Ryan JW: Cell biology of pulmonary endothelium, *Circulation* 70(5 Pl-2):46, 1984.

74. Fishman AP, Pietra GG: Handling of bioactive materials by the lung, *N Engl J Med* 291:953, 1974.

75. Junod AF: 5-hydroxytryptamine and other amines in the lungs. In Fishman AP, Fisher AB (eds): *Handbook of physiology, section 3, the respiratory system, vol I, circulation and nonrespiratory functions,* Bethesda MD, 1985, American Physiological Society.

76. Alabaster VA, Bakhle YS: Removal of 5-hydroxytryptamine in the pulmonary circulation of rat isolated lungs, *Br J Pharmacol* 40:468, 1970.

77. Nicholas TE, Strum JM, Angelo LS, Junod AF: Site and mechanism of uptake of 3H-1-norepinephrine by isolated perfused rat lungs, *Circ Res* 35:670, 1974.

78. Strum JM, Junod AF: Radioautographic demonstration of 5-hydroxytryptamine-3H uptake by pulmonary endothelial cells, *J Cell Biol* 54:456, 1972.

79. Fisher AB, Pietra GG: Comparison of serotonin uptake from the alveolar and capillary spaces of isolated rat lung, *Am Rev Respir Dis* 123:74, 1981.

80. Block ER, Stalcup SA: Today's practice of cardiopulmonary medicine: metabolic functions of the lung—of what clinical relevance? *Chest* 81:215, 1982.

81. Ryan US, Ryan JW, Crutchley DJ: The pulmonary endothelial surface, *Fed Proc* 44:2603, 1985.

82. Piper PJ, Vane JR, Wyllie JH: Inactivation of prostaglandins by the lungs, *Nature* 225:600, 1970.

83. Torday JS, Olson EB Jr: First NL: Production of cortisol from cortisone by the isolated, perfused fetal rabbit lung, *Steroids* 27(6):869, 1976.

84. Suzuki T, Sasano H, Suzuki S, et al: 11Beta-hydroxysteroid dehydrogenase type 2 in human lung: possible regulator of mineralocorticoid action, *J Clin Endocrinol Metab* 83(11):4022, 1998.

85. LeVan TD, Babin EA, Yamamura HI, Bloom JW: Pharmacological characterization of glucocorticoid receptors in primary human bronchial epithelial cells, *Biochem Pharmacol* 57(9):1003, 1999.

86. Janssen LJ: Isoprostanes: an overview and putative roles in pulmonary pathophysiology, *Am J Physiol Lung Cell Mol Physiol* 280:L1067, 2001.

87. Hanley SP: Prostaglandins and the lung, *Lung* 164:65, 1986.

88. Kadowitz PJ, Spannhake EW, Hyman AL: Prostaglandins evoke a whole variety of responses in the lung, *Environ Health Perspect* 35:181, 1980.

89. Kadowitz PJ, Lippton HL, McNamara DB, et al: Action and metabolism of prostaglandins in the pulmonary circulation. In Oates JA (ed), *Prostaglandins and the cardiovascular system,* New York, 1982, Raven Press.

90. Ogletree ML: Pharmacology of prostaglandins in the pulmonary microcirculation, *Ann N Y Acad Sci* 384:191, 1982.

91. Pavord ID, Wong CS, Williams J, Tattersfield AE: Effect of inhaled prostaglandin E₂ on allergen-induced asthma, *Am Rev Respir Dis* 143:87, 1993.

92. Hyman AL, Mathe AA, Lippton HL, Kadowitz, PJ: Prostaglandins and the lung, *Med Clin North Am* 65:789, 1981.

93. Frangos JA, Eskin SG, McIntire LV, Ives CL: Flow effects on prostacyclin production by cultured human endothelial cells, *Science* 227:1477, 1985.

94. Reeves JT, van Grondelle A, Voelkel NF, et al: Prostacyclin production and lung endothelial cell shear-stress, *Prog Clin Biol Res* 136:125, 1983.

95. Korbut R, Boyd J, Eling T: Respiratory movements alter the generation of prostacyclin and thromboxane A2 in isolated rat lung: The influence of arachidonic acid pathway inhibitors on the ratio between pulmonary PGI2 and TXA2, *Prostaglandins* 21:491, 1981.

96. Robinson C, Hardy CC, Holgate ST: Pulmonary synthesis, release, and metabolism of prostaglandins, *J Allergy Clin Immunol* 76:265, 1985.

97. Eling TE, Ally AI: Pulmonary biosynthesis and metabolism of prostaglandins and related substances, *Environ Health Perspect* 55:159, 1984.

98. Bakhle YS, Ferreira SH: Lung metabolism of eicosanoids: prostaglandins, prostacyclin, thromboxane, and leukotrienes. In Fishman AP and Fisher AB (eds): *Handbook of physiology, section 3: the respiratory system vol I, circulation and nonrespiratory functions,* Bethesda MD, 1985, American Physiological Society.

99. Ferreira SH, Vane JR: Prostaglandins: their disappearance from and release into the circulation, *Nature* 216:868, 1967.

100. McGiff JC, Terragno NA, Strand JC, et al: Selective passage of prostaglandins across the lung, *Nature* 223:742, 1969.

101. Dusting GJ, Moncada S, Vane JR: Recirculation of prostacyclin (PGI2) in the dog, *Br J Pharmacol* 64:315, 1978.

102. Hammond GL, Cronau LH, Whitaker D, Gillis CN: Fate of prostaglandins E₁ and A₁ in the human pulmonary circulation, *Surgery* 81:716, 1977.

103. Hoult JRS, Robinson C: Selective inhibition of thromboxane B2 accumulation and metabolism in perfused guineapig lung, *Br J Pharmacol* 78:85, 1983.

104. Brady HR, Serhan CN: Lipoxins: putative braking signals in host defense, inflammation and hypersensitivity, *Curr Opin Nephrol Hypertens* 5:20, 1996.

105. Garcia JGN, Noonan TC, Jubiz W, Malik AB: Leukotrienes and the pulmonary microcirculation, *Am Rev Respir Dis* 136:161, 1987.

106. Nicosia S, Capra V, Rovati GE: Leukotrienes as mediators of asthma, *Pulm Pharmacol Ther* 14:3, 2001.

107. Hand JM, Will JA, Buckner CK: Effects of leukotrienes on isolated guinea pig pulmonary arteries, *Eur J Pharmacol* 76:439, 1981.

108. Ohtaka H, Tsang JY, Foster A, et al: Comparative effects of leukotrienes on porcine pulmonary circulation in vitro and in vivo, *J Appl Physiol* 63(2):582, 1987.

109. Tracey WR, Bend JR, Hamilton JT, Paterson NAM: Role of lipoxygenase, cyclooxygenase and cytochrome P-450 metabolites in contractions of isolated guinea pig pulmonary venules induced by hypoxia and anoxia, *J Pharmacol Exp Ther* 250:1097, 1989.

110. Schellenberg RR, Foster A: Differential activity of luekotrienes upon human pulmonary vein and artery, *Prostaglandins* 27:475, 1984.

111. Editorial review: Adult respiratory distress syndrome, *Lancet* 1(8476):301, 1986.

112. Stephenson AH, Lonigro AJ, Hyers TM, et al: Increased concentrations of leukotrienes in bronchoalveolar lavage fluid of patients with ARDS or at risk for ARDS, *Am Rev Respir Dis* 138:714, 1988.

113. Voelkel NF: Mechanisms of hypoxic pulmonary vasoconstriction, *Am Rev Respir Dis* 133:1186, 1986.

114. Stenmark KR, James SL, Voelkel NF, et al: Leukotriene C4 and D4 in neonates with hypoxemia and pulmonary hypertension, *N Engl J Med* 309:77, 1983.

115. Dahlen SE, Hedqvist P, Hammarstrom S, Samuelsson B: Leukotrienes are potent constrictors of human bronchi, *Nature* 288:484, 1980.

116. Adelroth E, Morris MM, Hargreave FE, O'Byrne PM: Airway responsiveness to leukotrienes C4 and D4 and to methacholine in patients with asthma and normal controls, *N Engl J Med* 315:480, 1986.

117. Wenzel SE: Arachidonic acid metabolites: mediators of inflammation in asthma, *Pharmacotherapy* 17:3S, 1997.

118. Morganroth ML, Stenmark KR, Zirrolli JA, et al: Leukotriene C4 production during hypoxic pulmonary vasoconstriction in isolated rat lungs, *Prostaglandins* 28:867, 1984.

119. Paterson NAM: Influence of hypoxia on histamine and leukotriene release from dispersed porcine lung cells, *J Appl Physiol* 61:1790, 1986.

120. Peters SP, Lichtenstein LM, Adkinson NF JR: Mediator release from human lung under conditions of reduced oxygen tension, *J Pharmacol Exp Ther* 238:8, 1986.

121. Pearl RG, Prielipp RC: Leukotriene synthesis inhibition and receptor blockade do not inhibit hypoxic pulmonary vasoconstriction in sheep, *Anesth Analg* 72(2):169, 1991.

122. Undem BJ, Pickett WC, Lichtenstein LM, Adams GK III: The effect of indomethacin on immunologic release of histamine and sulfidopeptide leukotrienes from human bronchus and lung parenchyma, *Am Rev Respir Dis* 136:1183, 1987.

123. Maclouf JA, Murphy RC: Transcellular metabolism of neutrophil-derived leukotriene A4 by human platelets. A potential cellular source of leukotriene C4, *J Biol Chem* 263:174, 1988.

124. Maclouf J, Murphy RC, Henson PM: Transcellular sulfidopeptide leukotriene biosynthetic capacity of vascular cells, *Blood* 74(2):703, 1989.

125. Aharony D, Dobson PT, Krell RD: In vitro metabolism of [3H]-peptide leukotrienes in human and ferret lung: A comparison with the guinea pig, *Biochem Biophys Res Commun* 131:892, 1985.

126. Brom J, Konig W, Stuning M, et al: Characterization of leukotriene B4-omega-hydroxylase activity within human polymorphonuclear granulocytes, *Scand J Immunol* 25:283, 1987.

127. Lee CW, Lewis RA, Corey EJ, et al: Oxidative inactivation of leukotriene C4 by stimulated human polymorphonuclear leukocytes, *Proc Natl Acad Sci USA* 79:4166, 1982.

128. Keppler D, Huber M, Baumer T, et al: Metabolic inactivation of leukotrienes. In Webber G (ed): *Advances in enzyme regulation,* Oxford, 1989, Pergamon Press.

129. Lewis RA, Austen KF: The biologically active leukotrines, *J Clin Invest* 73:889, 1984.

130. Hammarstrom S, Orning L, Bernstrom K: Metabolism of leukotrienes, *Mol Cell Biochem* 69:7, 1985.

131. Drazen JM, Austen KF: Leukotrienes and airway responses, *Am Rev Resp Dis* 136:985, 1987.

132. Bray MA: Leukotrienes in inflammation, *Agents Actions* 19:87, 1986.

133. Serhan CN: Lipoxins and novel aspirin-triggered 15-epi-lipoxins (ATL): a jungle of cell-cell interactions or a therapeutic opportunity? *Prostaglandins* 53:107, 1997.

134. McMahon B, Mitchell S, Brady HR, Godson C: Lipoxins: revelations on resolutions, *Trends Pharmacol Sci* 22:391, 2001.

135. Soyombo O, Spur BW, Lee TH: Effects of lipoxin A4 on chemotaxis and degranulation of human eosinophils stimulated by platelet-activating factor and N-formyl L-methionyl-L-leucyl-L-phenylalanine, *Allergy* 49:230, 1994.

136. Colgan SP, Serhan CN, Parkos CA, et al: Lipoxin A4 modulates transmigration of human neutrophils across intestinal epithelial monolayers, *J Clin Invest* 92:75, 1993

137. Raud J, Palmertz U, Dahlen SE, Hedqvist P: Lipoxins inhibit microvascular inflammatory actions of leukotriene B4, *Adv Exp Med Biol* 314:185, 1991.

138. Brezinski ME, Gimbrone MA Jr, Nicolaou KC, Serhan CN: Lipoxins stimulate prostacyclin generation by human endothelial cells, *FEBS Lett* 245(1-2):167, 1989.

139. Bratt J, Gyllenhammar H: The role of nitric oxide in lipoxin A4-induced polymorphonuclear neutrophil-dependent cytotoxicity to human vascular endothelium in vitro, *Arthritis Rheu* 38:768, 1995.

140. Jacobs ER, Zeldin DC: The lung HETEs (and EETs) up, *Am J Physiol Heart Circ Physiol* 280:H1, 2001.

141. Zeldin DC, Foley J, Ma J, et al: CYP2J subfamily P450s in the lung: expression, localization, and potential functional significance, *Mol Pharmacol* 50:1111, 1996.

142. Salvail D, Dumoulin M, Rousseau E: Direct modulation of tracheal Cl⁻ channel activity by 5,6- and 11, 12-EET, *Am J Physiol* 275(3):L423, 1998.

143. Zeldin DC, Plitman JD, Kobayashi J, et al: The rabbit pulmonary cytochrome P450 arachidonic acid metabolic pathway: characterization and significance, *J Clin Invest* 95(5):2150, 1995.

144. Birks EK, Bousamra M, Presberg K, et al: Human pulmonary arteries dilate to 20HETE, and endogenous eicosanoid of lung tissue, *Am J Physiol* 272(5):L823, 1997.

145. McManus LM, Deavers SI: Platelet activating factor in pulmonary pathobiology, *Clin Chest Med* 10:107, 1989.

146. Page CP: The role of platelet-activating factor in asthma, *J Allerg Clin Immunol* 81:144, 1988.

147. Said SI: Peptides, endothelium and pulmonary vascular reactivity, *Chest* 88(4 Suppl):207S, 1985.

148. Clements JA, Funder JW, Tracy K, et al: Adrenocorticotropin, β-endorphin, and β-lipotropin in normal thyroid and lung: possible implications for ectopic hormone secretion, *Endocrinology* 111:2097, 1982.

149. Gerwitz G, Yalow RS: Ectopic ACTH production in carcinoma of the lung, *J Clin Invest* 53:1022, 1974.

150. Yalow RS, Eastridge CE, Higgins G, et al: Plasma and tumor ACTH in carcinoma of the lung, *Cancer* 44:1789, 1979.

151. Dey RD, Said SI: Lung peptides and the pulmonary circulation. In Said SI (ed): *The pulmonary circulation and acute lung injury,* New York, 1985, Futura Publishing.

152. Liggins GC, Kitterman JA, Campos GA, Clements JA: Pulmonary maturation in the hypophysectomized ovine fetus: differential responses to adrenocorticotropin and cortisol, *J Dev Physiol* 3:1, 1981.

153. Verma PS, Miller RL, Taylor RE, et al: Inhibition of canine lung angiotensin converting enzyme by ACTH and structurally related peptides, *Biochem Biophys Res Commun* 104:1484, 1982.

154. Ryan JW, Stewart JM, Leary WP, Ledingham JG: Metabolism of angiotensin I in the pulmonary circulation, *Biochem J* 120:221, 1970.

155. Ryan JW, Smith U: A rapid, simple method for isolating pinocytotic vesicles and plasma membrane of lung, *Biochim Biophys Acta* 249:177, 1971.

156. Lee MA, Bohm M, Paul M, Ganten D: Tissue renin-angiotensin systems: Their role in cardiovascular disease, *Circulation* 87:IV7, 1993.

157. The Consensus Trial Study Group: Effects of enalapril on mortality in severe congestive heart failure, results of the cooperative North Scandinavian Enalapril survival study (CONSENSUS), *N Engl J Med* 316(23):1429, 1987.

158. The SOLVD investigators: Effect of enalapril on survival in patients with reduced left ventricular ejection fractions and congestive heart failure, *N Engl J Med* 325:293, 1991.

159. The SOLVD Investigators: Effect of enalapril on mortality and the development of heart failure in asymptomatic patients with reduced left ventricular ejection fractions, *N Engl J Med* 327:685, 1992.

160. Cohn JN, Johnson G, Ziesche S, et al: A comparison of enalapril with hydralazine-isosorbide dinitrate in the treatment of chronic congestive heart failure, *N Engl J Med* 325(5):303, 1991.

161. Hall D, Zeitler H, Rudolph W: Counteraction of the vasodilator effects of enalapril by aspirin in severe heart failure, *J Am Coll Cardiol* 20:1549, 1992.

162. Allison DJ, Clay T: Angiotensin II release from the hypoxic lobe of the intact dog lung, *J Physiol* 260:32P, 1976.

163. Berkov S: Hypoxic pulmonary vasoconstriction in the rat: the necessary role of angiotensin II, *Circ Res* 35:256, 1974.

164. Niarchos AP, Roberts AJ, Laragh JH: Effects of the converting enzyme inhibitor (SQ 20881) on the pulmonary circulation in man, *Am J Med* 67:785, 1979.

165. Seyedi N, Xu X, Nasjletti A, Hintze TH: Coronary kinin generation mediates nitric oxide release after angiotensin receptor stimulation, *Hypertension* 26:164, 1995.

166. Gryglewski RJ, Splawinski J, Korbut R: Endogenous mechanisms that regulate prostacyclin release, *Adv Prostaglandin Thromboxane Leukot Res* 7:777, 1980.

167. Lin L, Nasjletti A. Role of endothelium-derived prostanoid in angiotensin-induced vasoconstriction, *Hypertension* 18(2):158, 1991.

168. Wang R, Zagariya A, Ibarra-Sunga O: Angiotensin II induces apoptosis in human and rat alveolar epithelial cells, *Am J Physiol* 276:L885, 1991.

169. Filippatos G, Tilak M, Pinillos H, Uhal BD: Regulation of apoptosis by angiotensin II in the heart and lungs, *Intl J Mol Med* 7:273, 2001.

170. Chand N, Altura BM: Acetylcholine and bradykinin relax intrapulmonary arteries by acting on endothelial cells: role in lung vascular diseases, *Science* 213:1376, 1981.

171. Vargaftig BB, Dao Hai N: Selective inhibition by mepacrine of the release of "rabbit aorta contracting substance" evoked by the administration of bradykinin, *J Pharm Pharmacol* 24:159, 1972.

172. Barst RJ, Stalcup SA, Mellins RB: Bradykinin-induced changes in circulating prostanoids in unanesthetized sheep, *Fed Proc* 42:302, 1983.

173. Farmer SG: Role of kinins in airway disease, *Immunopharmacology* 22:1, 1991.

174. Lang RE, Tholken H, Ganten D, et al: Atrial natriuretic factor: a circulating hormone stimulated by volume loading, *Nature* 314:264, 1985.

175. Needleman P, Greenwald JE: Atriopeptin: A cardiac hormone intimately involved in fluid, electrolyte, and blood-pressure homeostasis, *N Engl J Med* 314:828, 1986.

176. Nicholls MG: Minisymposium: the natriuretic peptide hormones: Introduction, editorial and historical review, *J Int Med* 235:507, 1994.

177. Sirois P, Gutkowska J: Atrial natriuretic factor immunoreactivity in human fetal lung tissue and perfusates, *Hypertension* 11(S1):162, 1988.

178. Di Nardo P, Peruzzi G. Physiology and pathophysiology of atrial natriuretic factor in lungs, *Can J Cardiol* 8(5):503, 1992.

179. Turrin M, Gillis CN: Removal of atrial natriuretic peptide by perfused rabbit lungs in situ, *Biochem Biophys Res Commun* 140:868, 1986.

180. Numan NA, Gillespie MN, Altiere RJ: Pulmonary vasorelaxant activity of atrial peptides, *Pulm Pharmacol* 3:29, 1990.

181. Ignarro LJ, Wood KS, Harbison RG, Kadowitz PJ: Atriopeptin II relaxes and elevated cGMP in bovine pulmonary artery but not vein, *J Appl Physiol* 60:1128, 1986.

182. Fernandes LB, Preuss JM, Goldie RG: Epithelial modulation of the relaxant activity of atriopeptins in rat and guinea pig tracheal smooth muscle, *Eur J Pharmacol* 212(2-3):187, 1992.

183. Hulks G, Jardine A, Connell JM, Thomson NC: Bronchodilator effect of atrial natriuretic peptide in asthma, *BMJ* 299(6707):1081, 1989.

184. Almeida FA, Suzuki M, Maack T: Atrial natriuretic factor increases hematocrit and decreases plasma volume in nephrectomized rats, *Life Sci* 39:1193, 1986.

185. Valentin JP, Ribstein J. Mimran A: Effect of nicardipine and atriopeptin on transcapillary shift of fluid and proteins, *Am J Physiol* 257:174, 1989.

186. Lofton CE, Baron DA, Heffner JE, et al: Atrial natriuretic peptide inhibits oxidant-induced increases in endothelial permeability, *J Mol Cell Cardiol* 23:919, 1991.

187. Struthers AD: Ten years of natriuretic peptide research: a new dawn for their diagnostic and therapeutic use? *BMJ* 308:1015, 1994.

188. Rogers TK, Thompson JS, Morice AH: Inhibition of hypoxic pulmonary vasoconstriction in isolated rat resistance arteries by atrial natriuretic peptide, *Eur Respir J* 10(9):2061, 1997.

189. Adnot S, Andrivet P, Chabrier PE, et al: Plasma levels of atrial natriuretic factor, renin activity, and aldosterone in patients with chronic obstructive pulmonary disease, *Am Rev Respir Dis* 141:1178, 1990.

190. Burghuber OC, Hartter E, Weissel M, et al: Raised circulating plasma levels of atrial natriuretic peptide in adolescent and adult patients with cyctic fibrosis and pulmonary artery hypertension, *Lung* 169:291, 1991.

191. Kawashima A, Kubo K, Hirai K, et al: Plasma levels of atrial natriuretic peptide under acute hypoxia in normal subjects, *Respir Physiol* 76(1):79, 1989.

192. Said SI, Mutt V: Potent peripheral and splanchnic vasodilator peptide from normal gut, *Nature* 224(235):863, 1970.

193. Said SI, Mutt V: Polypeptide with broad biological activity: isolation from small intestine, *Science* 169:1217, 1970.

194. Said SI: Vasoactive peptides and the pulmonary circulation, *Ann N Y Acad Sci* 384:207, 1982.

195. Said SI: Vasoactive peptides in the lung, with special reference to vasoactive intestinal peptide, *Exp Lung Res* 3:343, 1982.

196. Cutz E, Chan W, Track NS, et al: Release of vasoactive intestinal polypeptide in mast cells by histamine liberators, *Nature* 275:661, 1978.

197. Hamasaki Y, Saga T, Mojarad M, Said SI: VIP counteracts leukotriene D4-induced contractions of guinea pig trachea lung and pulmonary artery, *Trans Assoc Am Physicians* 96:406, 1983.

198. Mojarad M, Said SI: Vasoactive intestinal peptide (VIP) dilates pulmonary vessels in anesthetized cats, *Am Rev Respir Dis* 123:239, 1981.

199. Diamond L, Szarek JL, Gillespie MN, Altiere RJ: In vivo bronchodilator activity of VIP in the cat, *Am Rev Respir Dis* 128:827, 1983.

200. Hand JM, Laravuso RB, Will JA. Relaxation of isolated guinea pig trachea, bronchi and pulmonary arteries produced by vasoactive intestinal peptide (VIP), *Eur J Pharmacol* 98(2):279, 1984.

201. Matsuzaki Y, Hamasaki Y, Said SI: Vasoactive intestinal peptide: a possible transmitter of nonadrenergic relaxation of guinea pig airways, *Science* 210:1252, 1980.

202. Said SI: Influence of neuropeptides on airway smooth muscle, *Am Rev Respir Dis* 136:552, 1987.

203. Said SI: Vasoactive intestinal peptide: a brief review, *J Endocrinol Invest* 9:191, 1986.

204. Said SI, Dickman, KG: Pathways of inflammation and cell death in the lung: modulation by vasoactive intestinal peptide, *Regul Pept* 93:21, 2000.

205. Said SI, Dickman K, Dey RD, et al: Glutamate toxicity in the lung and neuronal cells: prevention or attenuation by VIP and PACAP, *Ann N Y Acad Sci* 865:226, 1998.

206. Marciniak SJ, Plumpton C, Barker PJ, et al: Localization of immunoreactive endothelin and proendothelin in the human lung, *Pulm Pharmacol* 5:175, 1992.

207. Inoue A, Yanagisawa M, Takuwa Y, et al: The human preproendothelin-l gene: complete nucleotide sequence and regulation of expression, *J Biol Chem* 264:14954, 1989.

208. de Nucci G, Thomas R, D'Orleans-Juste P, et al: Pressor effects of circulating endothelin are limited by its removal in the pulmonary circulation and by the release of prostacyclin and endothelium-derived relaxing factor, *Proc Natl Acad Sci USA* 85(24):9797, 1988.

209. Dupuis J, Cernacek P, Tardif JC, et al: Reduced pulmonary clearance of endothelin-1 in pulmonary hypertension, *Am Heart J* 135:614, 1998.

210. Druml W, Steltzer H, Waldhausl W, et al: Endothelin-1 in adult respiratory distress syndrome, *Am Rev Respir Dis* 148:1169, 1993.

211. Boscoe MJ, Goodwin AT, Amrani M, Yacoub MH: Endothelins and the lung, *Intl J Biochem Cell Biol* 32:41, 2000.

212. MacLean MR, Mackenzie JF, Docherty CC: Heterogeneity of endothelin-B receptors in rabbit pumonary resistance arteries, *J Cardiovasc Pharmacol* 31:S115, 1998.

213. Matran R, Alving K, Hemsen A, Lundberg JM: Endothelin-1 increases airway mucosa blood flow in the pig, *Agents Actions* S31:237, 1990.

214. Filep JG, Sirois MG, Foldes-Filep E, et al: Enhancement by endothelin-1 of microvascular permeability via the activation of ETA receptors, *Br J Pharmacol* 109:880, 1993.

215. Goldie RG, Henry PJ, Knott PG, et al: Endothelin-1 receptor density, distribution, and function in human isolated asthmatic airways, *Am J Respir Crit Care Med* 152:1653, 1995.

216. Barnes PJ, Chung KF, Page CP: Inflammatory mediators of asthma: an update, *Pharmacol Rev* 50:515, 1998.

217. Chung KF, Barnes PJ: Cytokines in asthma, *Thorax* 54:825, 1999.

218. Blease K, Lukacs NW, Hogaboam CM, Kunkel SL: Chemokines and their role in airway hyper-reactivity, *Respr Res* 1:54, 2000.

219. Kulik TJ, Johnson DE, Elde RP, Lock JE: Pulmonary vascular effects of bombesin and gastrin-releasing peptide in conscious newborn lambs, *J Appl Physiol* 55:1093, 1983.

220. Said SI: Peptides and lipids as mediators of acute lung injury. In Lenfant C, Zapol WR, Falke KJ (eds): *Acute respiratory failure, lung biology in health and disease series,* New York, 1984, Marcel Dekker.

221. Worthen GS, Tanaka DT, Gumbay RS, et al: Substance P causes pulmonary vasoconstriction in rabbits, *Am Rev Respir Dis* 129:A337, 1984.

222. O'Brodovich HM, Stalcup SA, Pang LM, Lipset JS: Bradykinin production and increased pulmonary endothelial permeability during acute respiratory failure in unanesthetized sheep, *J Clin Invest* 67:514, 1981.

223. Desai U, Kruetzer DL, Showell H, et al: Acute inflammatory pulmonary reactions induced by chemotactic factors, *Am J Pathol* 96:71, 1979.

224. Vane JR: Metabolic activities of the lung, *Excerpta Medica* 78:1, 1980.

225. Hechtman HB, Shepro D: Lung metabolism and systemic organ function, *Circ Shock* 9:457, 1982.

226. Gillis CN: Metabolism of vasoactive hormones by lung, *Anesthesiology* 39:626, 1973.

227. Kobayashi Y, Amenta F: Neurotransmitter receptors in the pulmonary circulation with particular emphasis on pulmonary endothelium, *J Auton Pharmacol* 14(2):137, 1994.

228. MacLean MR, Herve P, Eddahibi S, Adnot S: 5-Hydroxytryptamine and the pulmonary circulation: receptors, transporters and relevance to pulmonary arterial hypertension, *Br J Pharmacol* 131(2), 2000.

229. Lee SL, Wang WW, Moore BJ, Fanburg BL: Dual effect of serotonin on growth of bovine pulmonary artery smooth muscle cells in culture, *Circ Res* 68(5):1362, 1991.

230. Pearson JD, Gordon JL: Nucleotide metabolism by endothelium, *Ann Rev Physiol* 47:617, 1985.

231. Fitzgerald GA: Dipyridamole, *N Engl J Med* 316:1247, 1987.

232. Shryock JC, Rubio R, Berne RM: Release of adenosine from pig aortic endothelial cells during hypoxia and metabolic inhibition, *Am J Physiol* 254:H223, 1988.

233. Mentzer RM Jr, Rubio R, Berne RM: Release of adenosine by hypoxic canine lung tissue and its possible role in pulmonary circulation, *Am J Physiol* 229:1625, 1975.

234. Peach MJ, Johns RA, Rose Jr CE: The potential role of interactions between endothelium and smooth muscle in pulmonary vascular physiology and pathophysiology. In Weir EK, Reeves JT (eds): *Pulmonary vascular physiology and pathophysiology,* New York, 1989, Marcel Dekker.

235. Furchgott RF, Zawadzki JV: The obligatory role of endothelial cells in the relaxation of arterial smooth muscle by acetylcholine, *Nature* 288:373, 1980.

236. Cherry PD, Furchgott RF, Zawadzki JV, Jothianandan D: Role of endothelial cells in relaxation of isolated arteries by bradykinin, *Proc Natl Acad Sci USA* 79(6):2106, 1982.

237. Ignarro LJ, Buga GM, Wood KS, et al: Endothelium-derived relaxing factor produced and released from artery and vein is nitric oxide, *Proc Natl Acad Sci USA* 84(24)9265, 1987.

238. Ignarro IJ, Buga GM, Wood KS, et al: Endothelium-derived relaxing factor produced and released from artery and vein is nitric oxide, *Proc Nat Acad Sci* l84:9265, 1987.
239. Palmer RM, Ferrige AG, Moncada S: Nitric oxide release accounts for the biological activity of endothelium-derived relaxing factor, *Nature* 327:524, 1987.
240. Kelm M, Feelisch M, Spahr R, et al: Quantitative and kinetic characterization of nitric oxide and EDRF released from cultured endothelial cells, *Biochem Biophys Res Commun* 154:236, 1988.
241. Ignarro IJ, Ross G, Tillisch J: Pharmacology of endothelium-derived nitric oxide and nitrovasodilators, *West J Med* 154:51, 1991.
242. Furchgott RF: Role of endothelium in response of vascular smooth muscle, *Circ Res* 53:557, 1983.
243. Furchgott RF: The role of the endothelium in the responses of vascular smooth muscle to drugs, *Annu Rev Pharmacol Toxicol* 24:175, 1984.
244. Peach MJ, Loeb AL, Singer HA, Saye JA: Endothelium-derived relaxing factor, *Hypertension* 7:194, 1985.
245. Peach MJ, Singer HA, Loeb AL: Mechanisms of endothelium-dependent vascular smooth muscle relaxation, *Biochem Pharmacol* 34:1867, 1985.
246. Busse R, Trogisch G, Bassenge E: The role of endothelium in the control of vascular tone, *Basic Res Cardiol* 80:475, 1985.
247. Holzmann S: Endothelium-induced relaxation by acetylcholine associated with larger rises in cyclic GMP in coronary arterial strips, *J Cyclic Nucl Res* 8:409, 1982.
248. Rapoport R, Murad F: Endothelium-dependent and nitrovasodilator-induced relaxation of vascular smooth muscle: role of cyclic GMP, *J Cyclic Nucleotide Protein Phosphor Res* 9:281, 1983.
249. Furchgott R, Jothianandan D: Relation of cyclic GMP levels to endothelium-dependent relaxation by acetylcholine in rabbit aorta, *Fed Proc* 42:619, 1983.
250. Ignarro LJ, Kadowitz PJ: The pharmacological and physiological role of cyclic GMP in vascular smooth muscle relaxation, *Ann Rev Pharmacol Toxicol* 25:171, 1985.
251. Hampl V, Herget J: Role of nitric oxide in the pathogenesis of chronic pulmonary hypertension, *Physiol Rev* 80:1337, 2000.
252. Bolotina VM, Najibi S, Palacino JJ, et al: Nitric oxide directly activates calcium-dependent potassium channels in vascular smooth muscle, *Nature* 368:850, 1994.
253. Hernandez I, Carbonell LF, Quesada T, Fenoy FJ: Role of angiotensin II in modulating the hemodynamic effects of nitric oxide synthesis inhibition, *Am J Physiol* 277:R104, 1999.
254. Hart CM: Nitric oxide in adult lung disease, *Chest* 115(5):1407, 1999.
255. Michel T, Feron O: Nitric oxide syntheses: which, where, how, and why? *J Clin Invest* 100(9):2146, 1997.
256. Roos CM, Rich GF, Uncles DR, et al: Sites of vasodilation by inhaled nitric oxide vs. sodium nitroprusside in endothelin-constricted isolated rat lungs, *J Appli Physiol* 77:51, 1994.
257. Ferrario I, Amin HM, Sugimori K, et al: Site of action of endogenous nitric oxide on pulmonary vasculature in rats, *Pflugers Arch* 432:523, 996.
258. Dupuis J. Langleben D, Stewart DJ: Pulmonary hypertension. In Rubanyi GM (ed): *Pathophysiology and clinical applications of nitric oxide*, 1999, Harwood Academic Publishers.
259. Radomski MW, Palmer RM, Moncada S: An L-arginine/nitric oxide pathway present in human platelets regulates aggregation, *Proc Natl Acad Sci USA* 87(13):5193, 1990.
260. Freedman JE, Loscalzo J, Barnard MR, et al: Nitric oxide released from activated platelets inhibits platelet recruitment, *J Clin Invest* 100(2):350, 1997.
261. Radomski MW, Palmer RM, Moncada S: The anti-aggregating properties of vascular endothelium: interactions between prostacyclin and nitric oxide, *Br J Pharmacol* 92:639, 1987.
262. Feletou M, Vanhoutte PM: Endothelium-dependent hyperpolarization of canine coronary smooth muscle, *Br J Pharmacol* 93:5515, 1988.
263. Chen G, Yamamoto Y, Miwa K, Suzuki H: Hyperpolarization of arterial smooth muscle induced by endothelial humoral substances, *Am J Physiol* 260:H1888, 1991.
264. Fulton D, MuGiff JC, Quilley J: Role of K+ channels in the vasodilator response to bradykinin in the rat heart, *Br J Pharmacol* 113:954, 1994.
265. Quilley H, Fulton D, McGiff JC: Hyperpolarizing factors, *Biochem Pharmacol* 54:1059, 1997.
266. Campbell WB, Gebremedhin D, Pratt PF, Harder DR: Identification of epoxyeicosatrienoic acids as endothelium-derived hyperpolarizing factors, *Circ Res* 78(3):415, 1996.
267. Bauersachs J, Hecker M, Busse R: Display of the characteristics of endothelium-derived hyperpolarizing factor by a cytochrome P450-derived arachidonic acid metabolite in the coronary microcirculation, *Br J Pharmacol* 113:1548, 1994.
268. DiCorleto PE: Cultured endothelial cells produce multiple growth factors for connective tissue cells, *Exp Cell Res* 153:167, 1984.
269. Campbell JH, Campbell GR: Endothelial cell influences on vascular smooth muscle phenotype, *Ann Rev Physiol* 48:295, 1986.
270. Clowes AW, Karnovsky MJ: Suppression by heparin of smooth muscle cell proliferation in injured arteries, *Nature* 265:625, 1977.
271. Castellot JJ, Rosenberg RD, Kamovsky MJ: Endothelium, heparin, and the regulation of cell growth. In Jaffe E (ed): *Biology of endothelial cells*, Boston, 1984, Martinus Nijihoff.
272. DiCorleto PE, Gajdusec CM, Schwartz SM, Ross R: Biochemical properties of the endothelium-derived growth factor: comparison to other growth factors, *J Cell Physiol* 114:339, 1983.
273. Domin BA, Serabjit-Singh CJ, Vanderslice RR, et al: Tissue and cellular differences in the expression of cytochrome P-450 isozymes. In Paton W, Mitchell J, Turner P (eds): *Proc IUPHAR, 9th international congress of pharmacology*, London, 1984, Macmillan.
274. Vanderslice RR, Domin BA, Carver GT, Philpot RM: Species-dependent expression and induction of homologues of rabbit cytochrome P-450 isozyme 5 in liver and lung, *Mol Pharmacol* 31:320, 1987.
275. Bend JR, Hook GER, Easterling RE, et al: A comparative study of the hepatic and pulmonary microsomal mixed-function oxidase systems in the rabbit, *J Pharmacol Exp Ther* 183:206, 1972.
276. Juchau MR, Bond JA, Benditt EP: Aryl 4-monooxygenase and cytochrome P-450 in the aorta: possible role in atherosclerosis, *Proc Natl Acad Sci USA* 73:3723, 1976.
277. Serabjit-Singh CJ, Bend JR, Philpot RM: Cytochrome P-450 monooxygenase system: localization in smooth muscle of rabbit aorta, *Mol Pharmacol* 28:72, 1985.
278. Abraham NG, Pinto A, Mullane KM, et al: Presence of cytochrome P-450-dependent monooxygenase in internal cells of the hog aorta, *Hypertension* 7:899, 1985.
279. Baird WM, Chemerys R, Grinspan JB, et al: Benzo(a)pyrene metabolism in bovine aortic endothelial and bovine lung fibroblast-like cell cultures, *Cancer Res* 40:1781, 1980.
280. Mansour H, Levacher M, Azoulay-Dupuis E, et al: Genetic differences in response to pulmonary cytochrome P-450 inducers and oxygen toxicity, *J Appl Physiol* 64:1376, 1988.
281. Mansour H, Brun-Pascaud M, Marquetty C, et al: Protection of rat from oxygen toxicity by inducers of cytochrome P-450 system, *Am Rev Respir Dis* 137:688, 1988.
282. Serabjit-Singh CJ, Wolf CR, Philpot RM: Cytochrome P-450: localization in rabbit lung, *Science* 207:1469, 1980.
283. Simionescu M, Simionescu N: Endothelial surface domains in pulmonary alveolar capillaries. In Ryan US (ed): *Pulmonary endothelium in health and disease*, New York, 1987, Marcel Dekker.
284. Pietra GG, Sampson P, Lanken PN, et al: Transcapillary movement of cationized ferritin in the isolated perfused rat lung, *Lab Invest* 49:54, 1983.
285. Rothstein R, Cole JS, Pitt BR: Pulmonary extraction of [3H]bupivacaine: modification by dose, propranolol and interaction with [14C]5-hydroxytryptamine, *J Pharmacol Exp Ther* 240:410, 1987.
286. Post C, Andersson RGG, Ryrfeldt A, Nilsson E: Transport and binding of lidocaine by lung slices and perfused lungs of rats, *Acta Pharmacol Toxicol* 43:156, 1978.
287. Jorfeldt L, Lewis DH, Lofstrom JB, Post C: Lung uptake of lidocaine in healthy volunteers, *Acta Anaesth Scand* 23:567, 1979.
288. Jorfeldt L, Lewis DH, Lofstrom JB, Post C: Lung uptake of lidocaine in man as influenced by anaesthesia, mepivacaine infusion or lung insufficiency, *Acta Anaesth Scand* 27:5, 1983.
289. Dollery CT, Junod AF: Concentration of (±)-propranolol in isolated perfused lungs of rat, *Br J Pharmacol* 57:67, 1976.
290. Geddes DM, Nesbitt K, Traill T, Blackburn JP: First pass uptake of 14C-propranolol by the lung, *Thorax* 34:810, 1979.
291. Roerig DL, Kotrly KJ, Vucins EJ, et al: First pass uptake of fentanyl, meperidine, and morphine in the human lung, *Anesthesiology* 67:466, 1987.
292. Bakhle YS, Block AJ: Effects of halothane on pulmonary inactivation of noradrenaline and prostaglandin E2 in anesthetized dogs, *Clin Sci Mol Med* 50:87, 1976.
293. Cook DR, Brandon BW: Enflurane, halothane, and isoflurane inhibit removal of 5-hydroxytryptamine from the pulmonary circulation, *Anesth Analg* 61:671, 1982.

294. Naito H, Gillis CN: Effects of halothane and nitrous oxide on removal of norepinephrine from the pulmonary circulation, *Anesthesiology* 39:575, 1973.

295. Watkins CA, Wartell SA, Rannels DER: Effect of halothane on metabolism of 5-hydroxytryptamine by rat lungs perfused in situ, *Biochem J* 210:157, 1983.

296. Rannels DER, Roake GM, Watkins CA: Additive effects of pentobarbital and halothane to inhibit synthesis of lung proteins, *Anesthesiology* 57:87, 1982.

297. Rannels DE, Christopherson R, Watkins CA: Reversible inhibition of protein synthesis in lungs by halothane, *Biochem J* 210:379, 1983.

298. Martin DC, Carr AM, Livingston RR, Watkins CA: Effects of ketamine and fentanyl on lung metabolism in perfused rat lungs, *Am J Physiol* 257:E379, 1989.

299. Von Euler US, Liljestrand G: Observations on the pulmonary arterial blood pressure in the cat, *Acta Physiol Scand* 12:301, 1946.

300. Madden JA, Dawson CA, Harder DR: Hypoxia-induced activation in small isolated pulmonary arteries from the cat, *J Appl Physiol* 59:113, 1985.

301. Murray TR, Chen L, Marshall BE, Macarak EJ: Hypoxic contraction of cultured pulmonary vascular smooth muscle cells, *Am J Respir Cell Mol Biol* 3:457, 1990.

302. Johns RA, Linden JM, Peach MJ: Endothelium-dependent relaxation and cyclic GMP accumulation in rabbit pulmonary artery are selectively impaired by hypoxia, *Circ Res* 65:1508, 1989.

303. Brashers VL, Peach MJ, Rose CE Jr: Augmentation of hypoxic pulmonary vasoconstriction in the isolated perfused rat lung by in vitro antagonists of endothelium-dependent relaxation, *J Clin Invest* 82:1495, 1988.

304. Tracey WR, Hamilton JT, Craig ID, Paterson NAM: Effect of endothelial injury on the responses of isolated guinea pig pulmonary venules to reduced oxygen tension, *Am Rev Respir Dis* 140:68, 1989.

305. Yuan XJ, Wang J, Juhaszova M, et al: Molecular basis and function of voltage-gated K^+ channels in pulmonary arterial smooth muscle cells, *Am J Physiol* 274:L621, 1998.

306. Yuan XJ: Voltage-gated K+currents regulate resting membrane potential and (Ca^{2+})i in pulmonary arterial myocytes, *Circ Res* 77:370, 1995.

307. Pugin J, Verghese G, Wildmer M-C, et al: The alveolar space is the site of intense inflammatory and profibrotic reactions in the early phase of acute respiratory distress syndrome, *Crit Care Med* 159(Suppl):A694, 1999.

308. Matthay MA, Wiener-Kronish JP Intact epithelial barrier function is critical for the resolution of alveolar edema in humans, *Am Rev Respir Dis* 142:1250, 1990.

309. Ware LB, Matthay MA: The acute respiratory distress syndrome, *N Engl J Med* 342(18):1334, 2000.

310. Strieter RM, Kunkel SL, Keane MP, Standiford TJ: Chemokines in lung injury, *Chest* 116(1):103S, 1999.

311. Snapper JR, Brigham KL: Arachidonate products as mediators of diffuse lung injury. In Said SI (ed): *The pulmonary circulation and acute lung injury,* Mt. Kisko NY, 1985, Futura Publishing.

312. Said SI: The pulmonary circulation and acute lung injury: introduction and overview. In Said SI (ed): *The pulmonary circulation and acute lung injury,* Mt. Kisco NY, 1985, Futura Publishing.

313. Hirose T: Prostacyclin as a modulator of acute lung injury. In Said SI (ed): *The pulmonary circulation and acute lung injury,* Mt. Kisko NY, 1985, Futura Publishing.

314. Martin TR: Lung cytokines and ARDS, *Chest* 116(1):2S, 1999.

315. Rinaldo JE, Rogers RM: Adult respiratory distress syndrome: changing concepts of lung injury and repair, *N Engl J Med* 206:900, 1982.

316. Bitterman PB: Pathogenesis of fibrosis in acute lung injury, *Am J Med* 92:39S, 1992.

317. Jones R, Zapol WM, Reid L: Progressive and regressive structural changes in rat pulmonary arteries during recovery from prolonged hyperoxia, *Am Rev Respir Dis* 125:227, 1982.

318. Malik AB, Johnson A: Role of humoral mediators in the pulmonary vascular response to pulmonary embolism. In Weir EK, Reeves JT (eds): *Pulmonary vascular physiology and pathophysiology, lung biology in health and disease,* New York, 1989, Marcel Dekker.

319. Haley KJ, Sunday ME, Wiggs BR, et al: Inflammatory cell distribution within and along asthmatic airways, *Am J Resp Crit Care Med* 158:565, 1998.

320. Kraft M, Djukanovic R: Alveolar tissue inflammation in asthma, *Am J Resp Crit Care Med* 154:1505, 1996.

321. Barnes PJ, Page C: Mediators of asthma: a new series, *Pulm Pharmacol Ther* 14:1, 2001.

322. Vignola AM, Gagliardo R, et al: New evidence of inflammation in asthma, *Thorax* 55(Suppl2):S59, 2000.

323. Cohen MD, Ciocca V, Panettieri RA: TGF-beta 1 modulates human airway smooth-muscle cell proliferation induced by mitogens, *Am J Respir Cell Mol Biol* 16(1):85, 1997.

324. De S, Zelazny ET, Souhrada JF, Guhrada M: IL-1 beta and IL-6 induce hyperplasia and hypertrophy of cultured guinea pig airway smooth muscle cells, *J Appl Physiol* 78(4):1555, 1995.

325. Brusasco V, Crimi E., Pellegrino R: Airway hyperresponsiveness in asthma: not just a matter of airway inflammation, *Thorax* 53(11):992, 1998.

326. Ray A, Cohn L: The cells and GATA-3 in asthma: new insights into the regulation of airway inflammation, *J Clin Invest* 104(8):985, 1999.

327. Meltzer SS, Hasday JD, Cohn J, et al: Inhibition of exercise-induced bronchospasm by zileuton: a 5-lipoxygenase inhibitor, *Am J Respir Crit Care Med* 153(3):931, 1996.

328. Israel E, Dermarkarian R, Rosenberg M, et al: The effects of a 5-lipoxygenase inhibitor on astham induced by cold, dry air, *N Engl J Med* 323:1740, 1990.

329. Israel E, Fischer AR, Rosenberg MA, et al: The pivotal role of 5-lipoxygenase products in the reaction of aspirin-sensitive asthmatics to aspirin, *Am Rev Respir Dis* 148:1447, 1993.

330. Pitt BR, Lister G: Interpretation of metabolic function of the lung. Influence of perfusion, kinetics, and injury, *Clin Chest Med* 10:1, 1989.

331. Dawson CA, Roerig DL, Linehan JH: Evaluation of endothelial injury in the human lung, *Clin Chest Med* 10:13, 1989.

332. Kharitonov SA, Barnes PJ: Exhaled markers of pulmonary disease, *Am J Respir Crit Care* Med 163:1693-1722, 2001.

333. Kaneko FT, Arroliga AC, Dweik RA, et al: Biochemical reaction products of nitric oxide as quantitative markers of primary pulmonary hypertension. *Am J Respir Crit Care Med* 1998;158:917-923.

Respiratory Pharmacology

6

Peter J. Papadakos, MD, FCCM, FCCP
Burkhard Lachmann, MD, PhD

THE lung contains a large surface area where both medications and gases can be absorbed and carry out their functions. Many patients who present for thoracic surgery are concurrently taking medications that modulate their lung function. Over the past decade, the development of pharmacologic agents that not only modulate bronchodilation and bronchoconstriction but also affect lung function and gas exchange in respiratory failure has accelerated significantly. These therapeutic agents and aerosols have greatly added to the understanding of how the lung functions during both normal and pathologic states.

Clinicians face challenges daily from patients with complex lung diseases who present for elective and emergency surgery and care. The importance of a rapid, complete workup that includes a comprehensive history and physical examination, an arterial blood gas test, and other specific tests cannot be overemphasized. All too often, patients receive care without the proper information being collected first. The preoperative and postoperative courses of treatment in patients with pulmonary diseases will be facilitated if a pulmonary diagnosis and the severity of pulmonary dysfunction are established prior to the start of surgery. It is wise to record at least one blood gas test preoperatively and to collect measurements of lung volumes and flow rates to ascertain the degree of functional impairment and baseline pulmonary function. Clinicians must also become expert in the actions and indications of many drugs and treatment modalities that act on the physiology of the lung. With proper use of pharmacologic substances and early intervention, outcomes in the care of both baseline disease states and acute lung diseases can be improved.

Airway Structure and Function

A basic review of the anatomy and physiology of the lung will aid in the understanding of pharmacologic actions on that organ. Gas enters the thorax via the mouth, nose, or artificial airway and then passes into the trachea, which divides into the right and left mainstem bronchi. The airways continue to branch, and each division results in two daughter branches that are unequal in diameter, length, and takeoff.[1] The primary function of these airways is to conduct gases to the gas-exchange zones. With each additional generation, cross-sectional surface area increases, leading to a reduction in airflow resistance as gases move to the periphery and mass flow of gases is facilitated. In respiratory bronchioles and alveolar ducts, gas

diffusion is more important than mass flow and is facilitated by the large cross-sectional area present (Chapter 3).

The airway wall consists of layers of mucosa and smooth muscle enveloped by a connective tissue sleeve. Bronchi and small bronchi within the airway wall contain cartilage, whereas bronchioles do not. Respiratory bronchioles contain alveoli that increase in number with each generation, with the result that only alveoli line the alveolar ducts and sacs. In the bronchi, the mucosal layer contains tall ciliated epithelial cells as well as mucus-producing glands, goblet cells, and Clara cells.[2] In the periphery of the lung, the mucosal layer thins, and ciliated cells become more cuboidal. In the bronchioles, glands disappear, and goblet cells decrease in number and finally disappear as the number of Clara cells increases. The Clara cells decrease in number and also finally disappear within respiratory bronchioles and alveolar ducts, which are lined with epithelial cells.[3]

The smooth muscle layer is continuous from the trachea to the alveolar ducts. Smooth muscle bundles encircle the airways in an oblique course, and contraction of the smooth muscle results in both narrowing and shortening of the airway. In the alveolar ducts, the smooth muscle bundles occur in the alveolar entrance rings.[1]

Pulmonary blood from the right and left pulmonary arteries follows the mainstem bronchi into the lung parenchyma. Both the arteries and the bronchi then follow the branching pattern to the level of the respiratory bronchiole, constituting about 17 to 23 generations. The arteries give rise to arteriolar and capillary networks within the walls of the alveolar ducts and alveoli.[4] These vessels produce a massive surface area; whereas the pulmonary arteries and arterioles comprise a surface area of about 2.5 m^2, the capillary surface area is estimated at 50 to 150 m^2. This large surface area makes it possible for drugs to be absorbed into the circulation.

Airway caliber and tone are regulated by the parasympathetic and sympathetic divisions of the autonomic nervous system.[5,6] The vagally mediated mechanisms of the parasympathetic nervous system are the primary determinants of normal bronchomotor tone and bronchial submucosal gland secretion.[5,7] When vagal efferent nerves are stimulated, the neurotransmitter acetylcholine is released from the presynaptic nerve terminal. Acetylcholine then diffuses through the synaptic cleft and binds to muscarinic cholinergic receptors found throughout the respiratory tree. Stimulation of these cholinergic receptors results in an increase in the intracellular levels of

121

guanosine monophosphate (cGMP) in the cytoplasm.[7] The acetylcholine receptors are located in or are adjacent to the submucosal glands, mast cells, and smooth muscle of the respiratory epithelium.[5,6,8] Stimulation of these acetylcholine receptors in the lung triggers bronchoconstriction, a decrease in airway caliber, activation of mast cell degranulation, and an increase in glandular secretion.[9]

The direct innervation of the respiratory tree by the sympathetic nervous system is sparse; nevertheless, the smooth muscle cells of the bronchi, especially those located in the small airways, are well populated with noninnervated β_2-adrenergic receptors.[10]

β_1-Adrenergic receptors are also present in the lung but have only a minimal role in lung physiology. β_2-Adrenergic receptors are stimulated by adrenergic agonists, both endogenous (e.g., the presynaptic neurotransmitter norepinephrine, or epinephrine released by the adrenal medulla) and exogenous (pharmacologic agents). Such stimulation results in activation of membrane-bound adenylate cyclase to catalyze the conversion of adenosine triphosphate to cyclic adenosine monophosphate (cAMP).[11] An activation of an enzymatic cascade then occurs, resulting in bronchodilation and, possibly, in increased secretion of mucus.

α-Adrenergic receptors are also found in the lung.[8] Stimulation of these receptors, which are located predominantly in the bronchial and vascular smooth muscle and submucosal glands, causes bronchoconstriction and increased mucous secretion. In the lung, α_2-receptors are located on the postsynaptic nerve terminal, although they are also located presynaptically elsewhere in the body. Presynaptic α_2-receptors regulate the release of norepinephrine from the presynaptic nerve terminal.[12]

A third nonadrenergic, noncholinergic (NANC) system of the lung has been demonstrated in the airways all the way to the small bronchi.[13] A major component of this system appears to be the principal inhibitor system in human airways, causing bronchodilation when stimulated. The neurotransmitter that is involved is a vasoactive intestinal polypeptide that is more potent than isoproterenol.[14] There is also an excitatory component to the NANC system, probably mediated by a peptide—substance P—which, when stimulated, causes bronchoconstriction. The exact function of the NANC system remains as yet unelucidated.

Various endogenous substances—for example, histamine, prostaglandins, platelet activating factor, bradykinin, and various leukotrienes—have inflammatory effects on smooth muscle tone and have been documented to cause bronchoconstriction.[15]

The alveolar macrophages, when stimulated by systemic inflammatory responses (SIRS), modulate a cascade that releases various leukotrienes and cytokines, which act both locally and in the systemic circulation.[16] In the past decade, it has also been discovered that the alveolar surfactant system may be involved in protecting the lung against its own mediators (e.g., angiotensin II) and in protecting the cardiocirculatory system against mediators and cytokines produced by the lung.[17] Surfactant may also act to prevent the transmigration of bacteria from the lung into the systemic circulation.

Bronchodilators and Bronchoactive Drugs

Bronchodilator drugs are categorized according to their three types of actions:
1. *Direct respiratory smooth muscle relaxants*—including theophylline and related salts
2. *β-Adrenergic agonists*—isoetharine isoproterenol, epinephrine, metaproterenol, albuterol, terbutaline, bitolterol, and pirbuterol
3. *Anticholinergics*—atropine, glycopyrrolate, and ipratropium

The sites of action of bronchodilator drugs are depicted in Figure 6-1, which was summarized by Kelly.[18]

Direct Respiratory Smooth Muscle Relaxants: Theophylline

Theophylline, a naturally occurring methylxanthine closely related to caffeine and found in tea, has been used to treat bronchospasm for more than 100 years.[19] At one time it was the most widely used drug in the treatment of reactive airway disease; but because of conflicting reports of efficacy and safety, use of theophylline in the treatment of acute bronchospasm remains controversial.[20] Still, theophylline has become one of the most extensively prescribed drugs in the world for the treatment of reversible airway obstruction. The development of methods to monitor serum theophylline concentrations in patients has contributed to the safe and effective clinical use of this drug.

PHARMACOLOGY

The exact mechanism by which theophylline exerts its pharmacologic effect is not completely clear.[21] It is well established that theophylline competitively inhibits the activity of cytoplasmic phosphodiesterases, the enzymes that catalyze the degradation of cAMP to 5′-AMP.[22] Previously, this was thought to be the primary mechanism of action; however, the in vitro doses used to achieve phosphodiesterase inhibition appear to be too high to achieve clinically.[23]

In guinea pig and dog tracheal muscle preparations, theophylline levels achievable in humans had no effect on cAMP or cGMP but did increase calcium ion uptake and redistribution, consistent with a decrease of myoplasmic calcium ion and calcium sequestration in the mitrochondrium.[24] Other postulated mechanisms of action include prostaglandin inhibition, indirect β-adrenergic stimulation via release of catecholamines, and increased binding of cAMP to cAMP-binding protein.[24-26] Adenosine receptor antagonism has been proposed as the primary mediator of the pharmacologic and therapeutic actions of methylxanthines; however, the exact cellular mechanisms underlying bronchial smooth muscle relaxation have yet to be elucidated.

Regardless of its mechanism of action, theophylline is a direct bronchial smooth muscle relaxant. If bronchospasm is not present, its effects on airflow and respiratory mechanics are minimal. The drug also acts by decreasing mucosal edema and reducing the production of excessive secretions.[27] Other effects of theophylline include direct augmentation of myocardial inotropy and chronotropy; stimulation of respiratory muscle contractility; dilation of the coronary, pulmonary, renal, and systemic arterioles and veins; diuresis; stimulation of

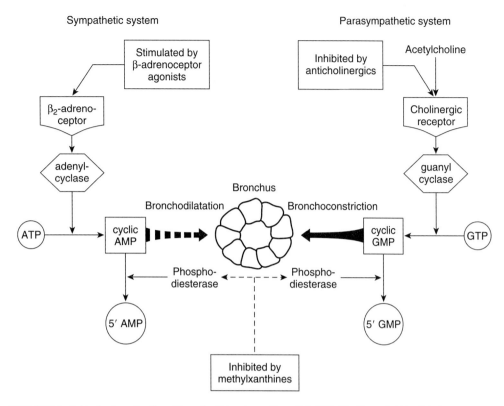

FIGURE 6-1 Mechanism of action of bronchodilator drugs. (From Kelly HW: *Clin Pharm* 3:385, 1984.)

epinephrine and norepinephrine synthesis and release by the adrenal medulla; stimulation of the medullary respiratory center; and decreased cerebral blood flow. In normal patients, theophylline causes a chronotropic effect, a decrease in coronary artery blood flow, an increase in myocardial oxygen extraction, and a decrease in left ventricular ejection time.[28] In patients with chronic obstructive pulmonary disease and cor pulmonale, increases in heart rate, stroke volume, and cardiac output and decreases in right ventricular end-diastolic pressure, left ventricular end-diastolic pressure, wedge pressure, and systemic vascular resistance can occur.[28]

SIDE EFFECTS

The most common side effects of theophylline are on the gastrointestinal tract and include nausea, vomiting, and anorexia.[29] Adverse gastrointestinal effects associated with oral use can be minimized by administering the drug with food. Central nervous system effects include headache, irritability, restlessness, nervousness, dizziness, and seizures.[20] Theophylline-induced seizures are often unresponsive to standard anticonvulsive therapy; the mortality rate is in the range of 50%.[30] Theophylline can cause a number of cardiovascular side effects that are often poorly tolerated by critically ill patients. These include palpitations and arrhythmias such as tachycardia, extrasystoles, multifocal atrial tachycardia, and ventricular arrhythmias. Other cardiovascular effects can include hypotension and circulatory collapse. Rapid intravenous injection of aminophylline and theophylline may increase the incidence of side effects; for this reason, slow intravenous titration or the use of an infusion pump is suggested. Cardiac arrest may fol-

low the rapid bolus dosage of aminophylline. Other side effects may include dizziness, palpitations, flushing, hypotension, and profound bradycardia.

An important point to consider is the pharmacologic preparation of theophylline. Prior to 1983, the only parenteral form of theophylline was aminophylline. Aminophylline is theophylline compounded with ethylenediamine, which confers water solubility to the insoluble theophylline molecule and contributes to the respiratory and cardiac stimulant effects of theophylline. Also of great importance is that ethylenediamine can induce hypersensitivity reactions characterized by urticaria, generalized pruritus, angioedema, and bronchospasm.[29]

PHARMACOKINETICS

Theophylline is manufactured as a variety of salts for oral, rectal, and parenteral administration. Rectal use of theophylline mixtures is no longer recommended due to their erratic absorption by this route. Liquid and plain tablet forms of theophylline are rapidly and completely absorbed.[31] Slow release preparations now dominate the market. The intravenous forms of theophylline are limited primarily to hospitalized patients and emergency use.

The pharmacokinetics of theophylline are well described. Once absorbed, the drug is distributed rapidly throughout the body fluids, more rapidly in the extracellular than in the intracellular fluids.[29] Theophylline binds to serum proteins (principally albumin), with its bound rate varying from 50% to 60%; the percentage bound increases proportionally with serum pH. Theophylline can pass freely into the breast milk and crosses the placenta. Theophylline achieves a volume of distribution of 0.3 to 0.7 L/kg in children and adults.[29] Oral standard non–time release preparations yield a peak serum level within 1 to 2 hours after administration. In contrast, extended-release and slow-release tablets release theophylline over a longer period of time; peak levels are reached approximately four hours after administration.

Administration of theophylline by intravenous infusion produces the highest and most rapidly achieved peak serum concentration. In healthy, nonsmoking adults, a standard 5 mg/kg infusion over a 30-minute period produces an average peak serum concentration of 10 μg/mL.[29]

Hepatic metabolism of theophylline occurs via the cytochrome P-450 system, which is also its principal method of elimination. Approximately 10% of the drug is eliminated unaltered through the kidney. Metabolism can be affected by the ingestion of other drugs. The half-life is increased in patients using cimetidine, ranitidine, erythromycin, allopurinol, propranolol, mexiletine, oral contraceptives, quinolones, verapamil, and diltiazem. Disease states—especially liver disease—can also affect and lengthen the half-life of theophylline. Patients who smoke either cigarettes or marijuana have a much shorter average elimination half-life, in the range of 4 to 5 hours. In contrast, patients with congestive heart failure, cor pulmonale, chronic obstructive pulmonary disease, or liver disease have a markedly prolonged elimination half-life—more than 12 hours in some cases.[29]

Great care must be taken in the administration of theophylline because of its low therapeutic ratio; but with close monitoring of blood levels, the drug can be given safely. Using caution, there should be few cardiovascular side affects and no convulsions or deaths. Theophylline endured a bad reputation in the 1970s and 1980s before the advent of rational dosage schedules and widespread monitoring.

A therapeutic range for theophylline in the range of 10 to 30 μg/mL is cited frequently. Most patients do not require levels in excess of 25 μg/mL to obtain adequate bronchodilation. Marked interpatient and intrapatient variability exist for dose-response curves. Therefore, the ideal way to use the drug is to titrate serum levels to the optimal drug level for achieving maximum bronchodilation.

The primary clinical use of theophylline is in the prevention of bronchospasm in patients with hyperactive airway disease. No theophylline products are currently used for the initial treatment of acute bronchospasm. Rather, they are used as second-line drugs if an inhaled β-adrenergic agonist gives a less than optimal effect. In such patients, 5 mg/kg of theophylline is administered as a loading dose over a 30-minute period if they have not received the drug within the past 24 hours. In patients already taking theophylline, the loading dose is lowered by half. Subsequent intravenous infusions are administered to the point of clinical effect with very close monitoring. The majority of patients now taking theophylline are being treated prophylactically for chronic bronchospasm. As newer agents have been introduced, the use of this classic drug has fallen.

β-Adrenergic Receptor Agonists

The introduction of inhaled β_2-agonists has greatly improved the care of patients with pulmonary diseases. The β_2-agonists are the most effective bronchodilators available. They have

now gained widespread use both in maintenance therapy and in acute care of patients.

β_2-Adrenergic receptor stimulation activates adenyl cyclase, which produces an increase in intracellular cyclic AMP. This in turn decreases unbound intracellular calcium, producing smooth muscle relaxation, mast cell membrane stabilization, and skeletal muscle stimulation.[32] β_2-Adrenergic stimulation also activates Na+→K+ ATPase (which produces gluconeogenesis) and enhances insulin secretion, producing a mild to moderate decrease in serum potassium concentration by driving potassium intracellularly. All β-adrenergic receptor agonists act by binding β_1 and β_2 cell membrane receptors. This action induces a relaxation of bronchial and vascular smooth muscle. These agents may also induce increased mucociliary transport of respiratory secretions. Stimulation of the β-adrenergic receptors also affects mast cells and inhibits the release of the mediators of bronchospasm, such as histamine and the slow-reacting substance of anaphylaxis. Sympathomimetic bronchodilators have been used widely for many years to induce bronchodilation. Figure 6-2 displays the structures of the sympathomimetic drugs.

EPINEPHRINE

Epinephrine is a naturally occurring catecholamine that is synthesized, stored, and released from the adrenal medulla and certain adrenergic nerve terminals. Because of its broad stimulation of adrenergic receptors, epinephrine is the drug of choice in systemic hypersensitivity reactions and is usually given in a subcutaneous dose of 0.3 to 1.0 mL of a 1:1000 aqueous solution. Similar doses can be used to treat acute bronchospasm. Subcutaneous epinephrine (0.3 to 0.5 mL of a 1:1000 aqueous solution) can be used for acute wheezing. It is an excellent drug and appears to have no more cardiovascular side effects than subcutaneous terbutaline, but it has a shorter duration of action than terbutaline (1 to 2 hours, compared with 2 to 4 hours).[33] The usual way to deliver epinephrine in its racemic form is by metered dose inhaler (MDI) or in solution delivered by a nebulizer.

In many cases, epinephrine is still used to break highly resistant bronchospasm. Norepinephrine, a weak β_2-agonist, has little utility in the treatment of airway and lung disease.

ISOPROTERENOL AND ISOETHARINE

Isoproterenol is the most potent β_1- and β_2-agonist. It is currently available either in a MDI or as a solution for use in a hand-held or gas-powered nebulizer; because of its cardiovascular effects, however, its use has been largely replaced by more specific agents.

Isoetharine has one-tenth the potency of isoproterenol and has a duration of action of up to 3 hours. It is available as an MDI or in solution for use in a nebulizer. The aerosolized dose is 0.25 to 0.5 mL diluted in 1 mL of sterile water or saline, or 0.68 mg (two puffs) from an MDI. It too has been replaced by more selective β_2-agonists.

TERBUTALINE

Terbutaline is a slightly less potent bronchodilator than isoproterenol but has far fewer cardiovascular side effects, with a duration of action up to 6 or 7 hours orally or by aerosol. Given subcutaneously, the incidence of cardiovascular side effects is similar to that of epinephrine, even though the duration of bronchodilation is longer.[33] Terbutaline is also given orally, in which case the dosage ranges from 1.25 to 5.0 mg every 6 hours.

The MDI dose of terbutaline is 200 μg/puff, and the usual dosage is two puffs every 4 to 6 hours. The injectable form of terbutaline can be nebulized by being diluted to a total volume of 2 to 3 mL by sterile water or saline. The usual dose is 1 mg every 4 to 6 hours. It is a very popular drug.

ALBUTEROL (SALBUTAMOL)

Albuterol is the most commonly used agent. It has the fewest cardiovascular side effects of all the sympathomimetic bronchodilators. Orally or by aerosol, its peak action occurs within 2 hours, and its duration of action is up to 6 hours.[32]

Oral doses for albuterol range from 1 to 8 mg every 6 hours for the standard, short-acting preparation, to 4 to 8 mg every 12 hours for the sustained-release preparation. Clinical studies have shown similar improvements in pulmonary function with the sustained-release preparations given every 12 hours, as compared with the standard product given four times daily.[34-36]

The MDI dose is 0.18 mg (two puffs) every 4 hours. The nebulizer dose is up to 3.0 mg. The frequency of administration depends on the severity of bronchospasm and wheezing and varies from every ½ to 1 hour for acute, severe asthma, to every 4 to 6 hours for stable airway disease.

PIRBUTEROL

Pirbuterol is a relatively selective β-agonist, but it does demonstrate both bronchodilator and cardiovascular effects.[37] Pirbuterol was nine times more selective for pulmonary tissue than albuterol and 1520 times more selective than isoproterenol.

The onset of pirbuterol activity occurs 5 minutes after aerosol administration and within 1 hour after oral administration. The peak activity for aerosol use is 30 minutes and 1 hour for oral use. The activity is equipotent to that of albuterol. The lowest doses that apparently produce maximum bronchodilation are 0.4 mg by aerosol and 15 mg of the oral preparation.[38]

The usual MDI dose is two inhalations (200 μg/puff) up to every 4 hours. The recommended oral dosage of pirbuterol is 10 to 15 mg three to four times per day. The complication profile is similar to other β_2-agonists; however, the neuromuscular side effects of pirbuterol are more marked than the cardiovascular side effects.

METAPROTERENOL

This agent was the first synthetic noncatecholamine bronchodilator introduced into clinical practice in the United States. It has a duration of action of up to 4 hours. Metaproterenol was also the first oral agent introduced. It has fewer cardiovascular effects than isoproterenol but is a weak bronchodilator. Oral doses of 5 to 20 mg can be used every 4 to 6 hours. The major side effects are neuromuscular (shakiness, tremor, cramps) or cardiovascular (tachycardia). Peak effect usually occurs within 1 to 2 hours. It is also delivered by MDI and as a solution for nebulization. The usual MDI dose is 1.3 mg (two puffs) given as needed up to every 3 to 4 hours at the onset of wheezing. The usual aerosolized dose is 10 to 15 mg (0.2 to 0.3 mL) diluted to 2 to 3 mL with sterile water or saline given every 3 to 4 hours.

LONG-ACTING AGENTS. The introduction of long-acting, inhaled β_2-agonists has been a major therapeutic development over the last few years and has led to a fundamental reappraisal of β-agonist use in asthma management.[34] Salmeterol

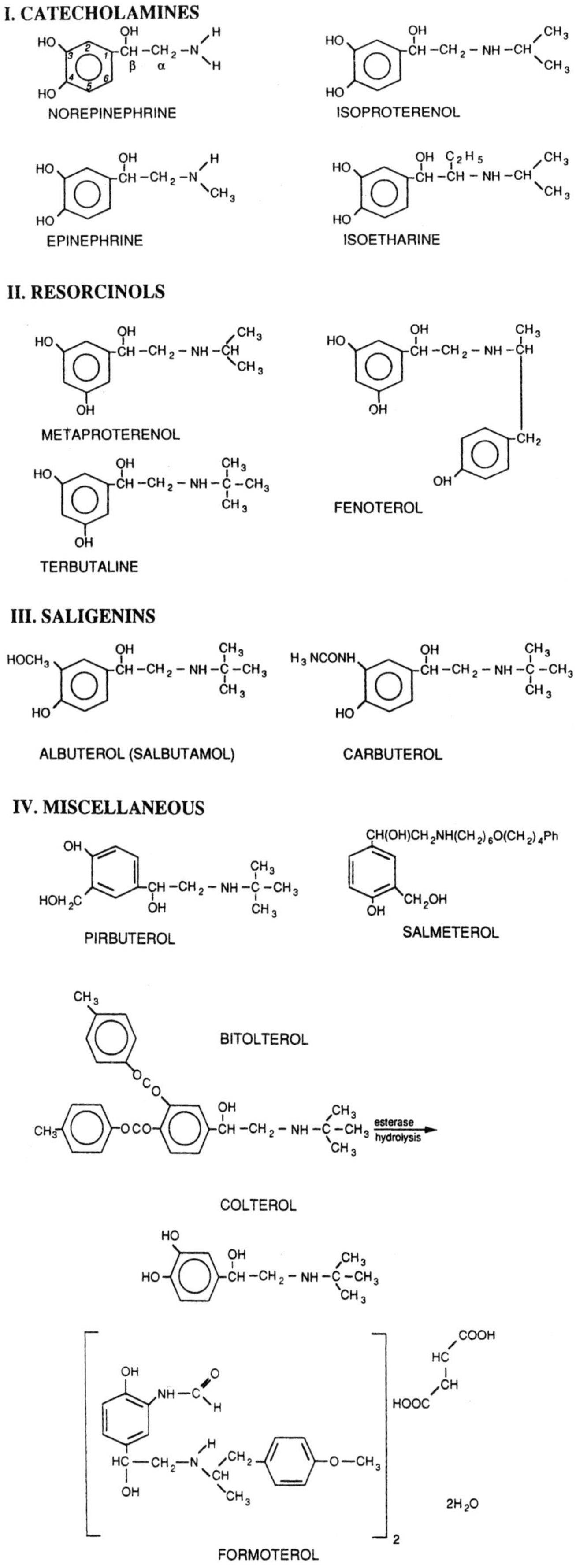

FIGURE 6-2 The structures of sympathomimetic drugs.

and formoterol are highly selective β_2-agonists with a bronchodilating effect lasting for at least 12 hours after a single inhalation.[35,36]

Salmeterol is the result of a specific program to achieve prolonged duration of action by molecular modification of the short-acting β_2-agonist salbutamol (albuterol).[35] Formoterol, a formanilide substituted phenoethanolamine, was serendipitously found to be long-acting when given by inhalation.[36] Sufficient drug remains available in the aqueous biophase to allow immediate interaction with the active side of the receptor, accounting for the rapid onset of action. Formation of a depot within the plasmalemma seems to require high topical concentrations of formoterol in the bronchi. This finding may explain why inhaled formoterol has a longer duration of action than when given orally, as the inhaled route achieves higher topical concentrations in the periciliary fluid of the bronchi.[39]

In addition to their differences in molecular structure, formoterol and salmeterol also have distinct pharmacologic features. As reflected in the routinely advocated dose for human use, formoterol has a higher potency than salmeterol.[40] Comparative studies in healthy volunteers indicate that formoterol and salmeterol cause side effects dose-dependently with a potency ratio of approximately 5:1.[41] This is very similar to their difference in bronchodilator potency in asthmatics. A few case reports have been published showing a significantly stronger bronchodilating effect with formoterol than with salmeterol in severe asthma.[42,43] In a larger comparative study with patients with persistent severe asthma, however, no differences were observed in the bronchodilating effect of these agents.[42] Also, chronic treatment with salmeterol does not hamper the bronchodilating effects of salbutamol in the acute phase in the emergency room.

Over the past 5 years, long-acting inhaled β_2-agonists have gained acceptance as the preferred form of "add-on" treatment in persistent asthma. Combining these agents with inhaled glucocorticosteroids is the future of asthma care. In the majority of patients, adding long-acting agents improves both lung function and symptoms.

Anticholinergics

The anticholinergic agents have been used in the treatment of asthma for several hundred years in the form of stramonium herbal preparations.[44] Anticholinergic bronchodilators are competitive inhibitors of muscarinic receptors. Unlike β_2-agonists and theophylline, they are not functional antagonists; they produce bronchodilation only in cholinergic-mediated bronchoconstriction. Normal bronchial tone is maintained through parasympathetic innervation of the airways via the vagus nerve. A number of well-known triggers of asthma and bronchospasm (histamine, prostaglandins, sulfur dioxide, allergens) produce bronchoconstriction.[44] Studies of asthmatics consistently demonstrate that anticholinergics are effective bronchodilators, though not as potent as β_2-agonists.

The most commonly used agent is ipratropium bromide, a quaternary ammonium derivative (Figure 6-3). Ipratropium bromide consistently produces a 10% to 20% improvement in FEV_1 over β_2-agonists alone in acute, severe bronchospasm.[45] Of note, however, is a significant variability in patient response, with some patients obtaining substantially greater

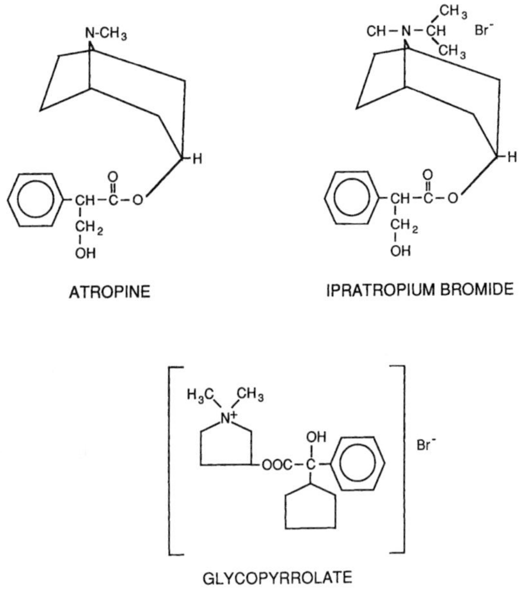

FIGURE 6-3 The structures of anticholinergic drugs.

(40% to 80%) improvement and others showing little or no improvement. This agent has also been shown not to improve outcome in chronic asthma when compared with the use of β_2-agonists alone.[46]

The anticholinergics that are currently available are nonselective muscarinic receptor blockers. Theoretically, blockade of inhibitory muscarinic receptors could result in an increased release of acetylcholine, which might overcome the block on smooth muscle receptors. Understanding this mechanism might explain why some patients, paradoxically, have experienced bronchoconstriction from nebulized anticholinergics. Only the quaternary ammonium derivative ipratropium bromide should be used because it has the advantage of poor absorption across mucosae and the blood-brain barrier. Anticholinergic agents yield only negligible systemic effects but do exert a prolonged, desired local effect (i.e., bronchodilation). They also have no effect on mucociliary clearance.[44] These agents have a duration of action of four to eight hours. Both intensity and duration of action are dose dependent. Time to maximal bronchodilation is considerably slower for anticholinergics than for aerosolized, short-acting β_2-agonists: 2 hours vs. 30 minutes. This difference, however, is of little clinical consequence because even with the slower-acting anticholinergics, limited bronchodilation is seen within 30 seconds, 50% of maximum response occurs within 3 minutes, and 80% of maximum response is reached within 30 minutes.[44]

In summary, the role of anticholinergics in the treatment of bronchospasm and asthma is limited. They are not currently recommended for the long-term control of these disease processes.[46]

Cromolyn Sodium and Nedocromil Sodium

Cromolyn sodium has been used for the prophylactic treatment of asthma for more than 20 years. A new, related agent, nedocromil sodium, a pyranoquinoline dicarboxylic acid, has been available in the United States only for the past 5 years (Figure 6-4).[46] The exact mechanism of action for these agents is still unknown. These drugs have minor differences in activity, however. The principal differences appear to be in potency, with 4 mg of nedocromil sodium by MDI equivalent to 20 mg of cromolyn sodium by spinhaler.[47] Both drugs produce mast-cell-membrane stabilization. Both agents inhibit in vitro activation of human neutrophils, macrophages, and eosinophils.[44,47] They also inhibit neurally mediated bronchoconstriction through C-fiber sensory nerve stimulation in the airways.[47] They do not, however, produce any bronchodilatory effects.

Both cromolyn sodium and nedocromil sodium are effective by inhalation only and are available as MDIs; cromolyn is also available as a nebulizer solution. They are not bioavailable orally, but the portion of the drug that reaches the lung is completely absorbed.[44] Absorption from the airway is slower than elimination (hours vs. minutes). Both the intensity and the duration of protection against various challenges are dose dependent.[47]

These two drugs have a highly nontoxic profile. The common side effects—cough and wheezing, bad taste, and headache, especially for nedrocromil sodium—have been reported following inhalation of each. Furthermore, the taste of nedocromil sodium is so unpleasant that for about 20% of patients for whom it is indicated, it precludes them from taking the drug. Cromolyn sodium has the best nontoxic profile of any compound to treat bronchospasm and asthma, with adverse effects occurring in fewer than one in 10,000 patients.[48]

Cromolyn sodium and nedocromil sodium are indicated for the prophylaxis of mild asthma in both children and adults, regardless of the etiology. They are particularly effective for allergic asthmatics on a seasonal basis or just before an acute exposure (such as entering a home where there are pets, etc.). These drugs can be used in combination with β_2-agonists in patients with severe symptoms. Their efficacy is directly related to the degree of deposition in the lung. These compounds, therefore, do not work during active bronchospasm. Patients should initially receive cromolyn or nedocromil four times daily; after stabilization, the frequency may be reduced to two times daily.

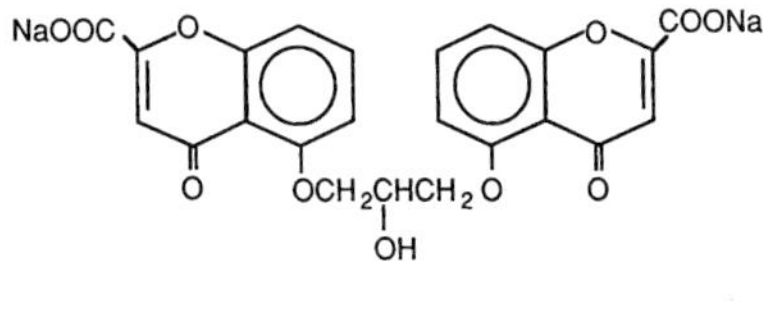

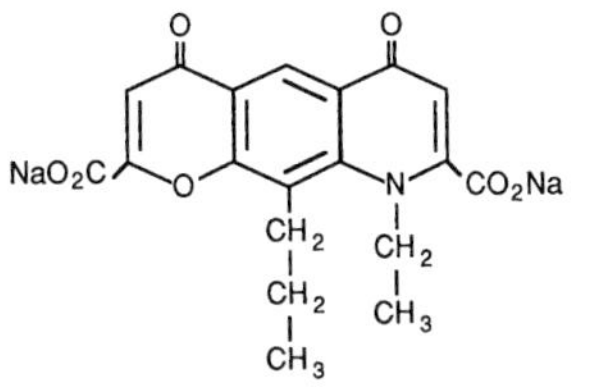

CROMOLYN SODIUM

NEDOCROMIL SODIUM

FIGURE 6-4 The structures of cromolyn sodium and nedocromil sodium.

Leukotriene Modifiers

The treatment agents most recently approved over the past 5 years address a new therapeutic pathway. They act by blocking the leukotriene receptors, inhibiting the action of cysteinyl leukotrienes (LTC$_4$, LTD$_4$, and LTE$_4$),[49] These medications are zafirlukast (Accolate), montelukast (Singulair), and zileuton (Zyflo). Leukotrienes are proinflammatory modulators increasing microvascular permeability and airway edema, thus producing bronchoconstriction.

Zafirlukast has been shown to improve pulmonary function, increase FEV$_1$, and reduce symptoms and bronchodilator medication requirements in patients.[50] At doses of 20 mg twice daily, zafirlukast has been shown to reduce airway responses to inhaled allergens, platelet-activating factor, and exercise. Adverse effects are minimal, although experience with this medication is limited. Rare cases of hepatotoxicity and eosinophilic vasculitis have been reported. Taking this medication with food may impair absorption, and zafirlukast interacts with warfarin, resulting in a prolonged prothrombin time.

Zileuton directly inhibits 5-1 ipozygenase, whereas other drugs in development bind to and prevent translocation of 5-lipoxygenase-activating protein.[49] Zileuton reduces bronchoconstriction caused by allergens, exercise, aspirin, and cold, dry air.[49] Doses of 600 mg four times daily reduce symptoms and bronchodilator requirements and improve pulmonary function. Zileuton may produce elevated liver enzymes, so patients need to be closely monitored. This drug also affects hepatic isozymes and therefore also increases blood concentrations of warfarin and theophylline.[46]

Neither zafirlukast nor zileuton completely attenuated induced bronchospasm in several challenge models.[49] These new agents show great promise, but their place in the scheme of asthma management is still in evolution. National Asthma Education and Prevention Program (NAEPP) guidelines suggest that these compounds may be used as alternatives to low-dose inhaled steroids in mild persistent asthma. They also have the advantage that they are oral medications, so patient compliance may be greater than with inhaled medications.

Magnesium Sulfate

Intravenous magnesium sulfate (MgSO$_4$) has been advocated for severe asthmatics who exhibit a suboptimal response to inhaled β_2-agonists. However, these initial trials did not use adequate doses of inhaled β_2-agonists, and bronchodilation from MgSO$_4$ was only modest and did not exceed the β_2-agonist response.[46]

Glucocorticoid Therapy

The most important treatment agents for bronchospasm and asthma are the inhaled corticosteroids. Actions of this class of compounds include the following[51]:
1. Increasing the number of β_2-adrenergic receptors and improving the responsiveness of β_2-adrenergic receptors to stimulation
2. Reducing mucous production and hypersecretion
3. Inhibiting the inflammatory response

The antiinflammatory effects of possible benefit in asthma include the following:

1. Decreasing the synthesis and release of several proinflammatory cytokines such as IL-1, IL-3, IL-4, IL-5, IL-6, IL-8, and GM-CSF
2. Reducing inflammatory cell activation recruitment and infiltration
3. Decreasing vascular permeability

Systemic Glucocorticoid Therapy

In severe acute asthma (status asthmaticus), the standard of care is treatment with systemic glucocorticoids combined with frequent administration of inhaled β_2-agonists.[46] Glucocorticoids can be administered by the parenteral route (methylprednisolone sodium succinate, hydrocortisone sodium succinate) or, alternatively, by the oral route (prednisone, methylprednisolone), either of which provides a rapid onset of action and a systemic effect (Figure 6-5).[52]

The glucocorticoids used in asthma are compared in Table 6-1. Recommended dosages for acute asthma are listed in Table 6-2. There is no difference in response between intravenous and oral administration of steroids.[52] Evidence suggests that divided doses should be used initially. Following resolution of symptoms (decrease in obstruction achievement of >50% of predicted normal FEV_1, which generally occurs within the first 48 hours), the steroid dose is reduced to one or two doses orally.[52] The duration of treatment is dependent on the responses of individual patients and on their history of past responses to these drugs. Tapering the dose after treatment is recommended, as in other cases of steroid use, to prevent adrenal insufficiency.

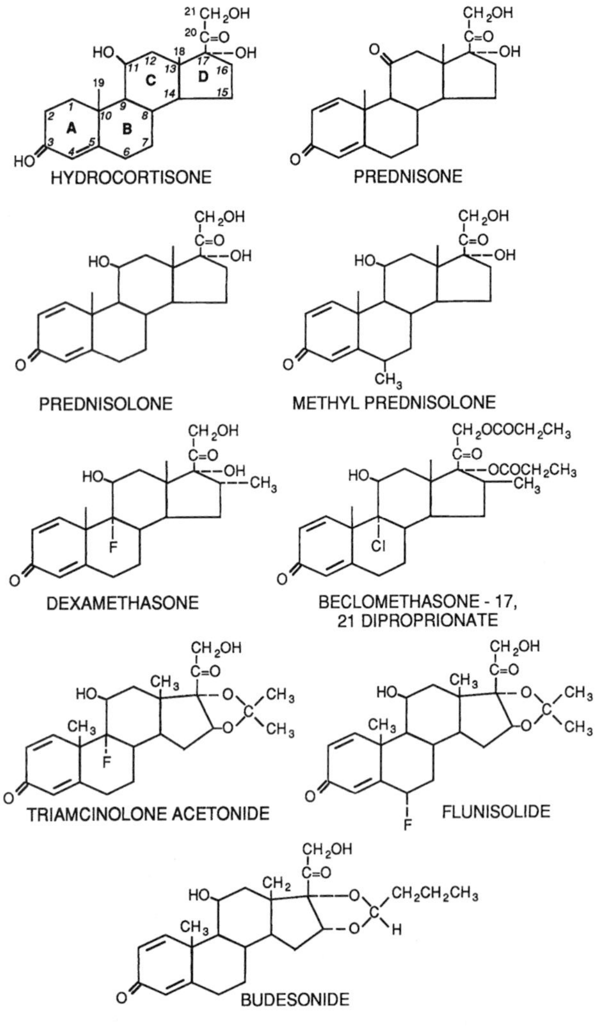

Systemic glucocorticoids are also recommended for the treatment of impending episodes of severe bronchospasm that are unresponsive to bronchodilator therapy.[46] Prednisone, 1 to 2 mg/kg daily (up to 40 to 60 mg daily), is administered orally in two divided doses for 3 to 10 days.[46] If an adequate response is not achieved, administration of prednisone three times daily may be worthwhile.

The balance between symptom control and toxicity must always be in the forefront. Because short-term (1 to 2 weeks) administration of high-dose steroids (1 to 2 mg/kg daily of prednisone) does not produce serious toxicities, the ideal is to administer the glucocorticoids in a short "burst" and then maintain the patient on appropriate long-term control therapy with extended periods between systemic glucocorticoid treatment.[46]

Extended use may affect adrenal cortisol release. Suppression of the hypothalamic-pituitary-adrenal axis, however, is short-lived (1 to 3 days) and readily reversible following short bursts (10 days or fewer) of pharmacologic doses.[52] Therefore, in patients who require chronic systemic glucocorticoids for control of disease, the lowest possible dose needed to control symptoms should be used. An accepted method to decrease toxicity is to use alternate-day therapy or to use inhaled glucocorticoids.

Inhaled Glucocorticoids

The advent of inhaled steroids represents the most significant breakthrough in the treatment of bronchoconstriction. These are now considered to be first-line therapy. As with all steroid use, the risk of systemic complications is less likely in low-to-moderate doses. Inhaled glucocorticoids demonstrate a favorable topical systemic potency ratio but are far from benign. If an "ideal" glucocorticoid were developed, it would have a high degree of topical potency, minimal systemic absorption of active drug, and minimal local or systemic side effects. No such agent is available.

The inhaled glucocorticoids have substantial topical antiinflammatory effects and are either poorly absorbed or metabolized to less active substances once absorbed.[53] The systemic effects vary from agent to agent. Aerosol delivery of the preparations varies from 10% to 30%, which can make a difference in both topical potency and systemic activity.[54] The delivery system can therefore make a significant difference when comparable doses are involved.[46]

Optimal dosing of inhaled steroids has not been studied thoroughly, but most patients may be controlled with twice-daily dosing. Investigations, however, have demonstrated an improved asthma response with decreased systemic effects by giving the same total daily dose in four divided doses daily instead of twice daily.[46]

There is an apparent additive effect when long-acting β-agonists and inhaled glucocorticoids are used together in

FIGURE 6-5 The structures of commonly used corticosteroids.

TABLE 6-1

Glucocorticoid Comparison Chart

SYSTEMIC ADMINISTRATION	RELATIVE ANTIINFLAMMATORY POTENCY	RELATIVE SODIUM-RETAINING POTENCY	DURATION OF BIOLOGIC ACTIVITY (HOURS)	PLASMA ELIMINATION HALF-LIFE (HOURS)
Hydrocortisone	1	1.0	8-12	1.5-2.0
Prednisone	4	0.8	12-36	2.5-3.5
Methylprednisolone	5	0.5	12-36	3.3
Dexamethasone	25	0	36-54	3-4-4-0

AEROSOL	TOPICAL POTENCY	RECEPTOR-BINDING	RECEPTOR COMPLEX	ORAL BIOAVAILABILITY (%)
Flunisolide (FLU)	330	1.8	3.5	21
Triamcinolone acetonide (TAA)	330	3.6	3.9	10.6
Beclomethasone dipropionate (BDP)	600	13.5	7.5	20
Budesonide (BUD)	980	9.4	5.1	11
Fluticasone propionate (FP)	1200	18	10.5	<1

patient management. One possible explanation is that steroids are antiinflammatory, whereas the smooth muscle-relaxing effect of long-acting β-agonists results in prolonged bronchodilation and bronchoprotection. It can be assumed that the combination of both pharmacologic activities is clinically beneficial.

Nitric Oxide

Nitric oxide (NO), in its role as an endothelial-derived relaxing factor, has been recognized as an important endogenous mediator for smooth-muscle relaxation.[50,55] Therefore, exogenously administered, inhaled NO might be expected to cause vasodilation in well-aerated areas of the lung with no systemic hemodynamic effects. Inhaled NO-induced vasodilation of pulmonary vessels should increase blood flow to well-ventilated areas of the lung and preferentially shunt blood away from poorly ventilated areas.[56]

Several years ago, there was interest in the use of NO in the treatment of acute respiratory distress syndrome (ARDS). Early studies showed some promise.[57] But in a large multicentered study, no change in mortality was noted.[55] That same study did, however, show that NO was well-tolerated and that it improved oxygenation over the first 4 hours of treatment when compared with placebo. The complex nature of ARDS and cytokine modulation may have led to the failure of NO to affect mortality. NO is still used in several centers as a bridge therapy when traditional support therapy for ARDS is failing.

Nitric oxide does have a place in some neonatal centers. It lowers the need for extracorporeal membrane oxygenation in neonatal respiratory failure.[58] The drug also plays a role in the treatment of neonatal pulmonary hypertension.[58,59] NO can increase oxygenation and decrease pulmonary arterial pressure

in some patients. The studies that obtained these results, however, have typically involved few patients, examined only the acute physiologic changes associated with administration of inhaled NO, and lacked concurrent placebo groups.

Further examination of using NO along with more advanced modes of mechanical ventilation that do not add to cytokine load may lead to better outcomes in long-term survival. More controlled trials must be designed in which only one aspect of the acute process and the reaction of specific tissues to NO are studied.

Surfactant

Surfactant has been known since 1959, when Avery and Mead published direct evidence linking absence of a surface-active material in the lung to that of a substance that actively changes the surface tension of the alveoli of the lung.[60] This substance was later named *pulmonary surfactant*. Pulmonary surfactant is a complex of phospholipids (80% to 90%), neutral lipids (5% to 10%), and at least four specific surfactant-proteins (5% to 10%) (SP-A, SP-B, SP-C, and SP-D), lying as a layer at the air-liquid interface in the alveoli and small airways, and having the effect of lowering surface tension.[61,62] Surfactant is synthesized by the alveolar type II cells and secreted into alveolar spaces.[62]

One possible additional function of bronchial surfactant, which to date has not been studied, is its masking of receptors on smooth muscle with respect to substances that induce contraction and lead to airway obstruction. If this function is valid, it means that lack of this surfactant may be possibly involved in asthma.[63] It has also been demonstrated that surfactant plays a role in the lung's defense against infection.[64] Surfactant, and in particular SP-A, enhances the antibacterial and antiviral

TABLE 6-2

Corticosteroids

Medications	Dosages (Adults)	Comments
Prednisone Methylprednisolone Prednisolone	120-180 mg in 3 or 4 divided doses for 48 hr, then 60-80 mg daily until PEF reaches 70% of personal best.	For outpatient "burst" use 1-2 mg/kg daily (maximum dose of 60 mg) for 3-7 days. It is unnecessary to taper following the course.

defense mechanisms of alveolar macrophages. Surfactant might also be involved in protecting the lung from lung-released mediators (e.g., angiotension II) and in protecting the cardiopulmonary system against mediators produced by the lung.[17,66]

Disturbances of the surfactant system can result from various factors. The most common of these is damage to the alveolar-capillary membrane, which leads to high-permeability edema with washout dilution of the surfactant and/or inactivation of the surfactant by plasma components such as fibrinogen, albumin, globulin, and transferred hemoglobin and cell membrane lipids. Also, surfactant can be easily depleted by the cyclic opening and closing of alveoli during mechanical ventilation. Disturbed synthesis, storage, or release of surfactant is secondary to direct injury of type II cells.[65,66] The diminished amount of surfactant in mechanical ventilation may play an important role in respiratory failure in ARDS.

A diminished amount of pulmonary surfactant has far-reaching consequences for lung function. Independent of cause, decreased surfactant function can lead directly or indirectly to one or more of the following:

1. Decreased pulmonary compliance
2. Decreased functional residual capacity
3. Atelectasis and an increase of the functional right-to-left shunt
4. Decreased gas exchange and respiratory acidosis
5. Hypoxemia with anaerobic metabolism and metabolic acidosis
6. Pulmonary edema with further inactivation of surfactant by plasma constituents

Surfactant replacement therapy has been used in preterm infants for 20 years with great success.[67] The rate of mortality has fallen, as clinicians are better able to deliver surfactant to these preterm infants. After birth, these infants can have their respiratory distress prevented or its severity reduced by the intratracheal administration of synthetic or natural surfactants. Synthetic (lecithin, tyloxapol, hexadecanol) or natural (fortified extract of cow lung) surfactant has also been administered repeatedly during the course of this disease process.

Ongoing research in surfactant replacement therapy in adults has not yet led to a decrease in mortality. Several formulations are under investigation, along with systems to deliver the agent into the adult lung. There are multiple technical problems in the delivery of surfactant into the adult lung in ARDS that have yet to be overcome. Also, the maturity of the immune system may also play a role in the lack of positive outcomes in adult studies. New formulations that are currently under development may lead to more positive results in the adult population.

Summary

Many agents are now available to maximize pulmonary function in multiple disease states. The physicians who care for these patients should be expert in the pharmacology of these drugs, from the older agents such as theophylline and atropine to the long-acting β_2-agonists and leukotriene modulators.

Physicians should also be familiar with the newer aerosol delivery systems. Aerosol delivery of drugs for asthma has the advantage of being site-specific. For example, inhalation of short-acting β_2-agonist provides more rapid bronchodilation than with oral agents. The various devices used to generate therapeutic aerosols include MDIs, jet nebulizers (JNS), ultrasonic nebulizers, and dry powder inhalers (DPIs). The single most important device factor determining the site of aerosol deposition is particle size. Anesthesiologists should also review the ability to deliver these drugs down an endotracheal tube. Important determinants of aerosol deposition in ventilator-supported patients include the delivery system, particle size, characteristics of the ventilator circuit, ventilator mode, and patient-related factors. An evaluation of these determinants on a patient-by-patient basis should dictate the development of a treatment plan for each high-risk patient before bronchospasm has a chance to occur.

REFERENCES

1. Weibel ER, Taylor CR: Design and structure of the human lung. In Fishman AP (ed): *Pulmonary diseases and disorders,* ed 2, New York, 1988, McGraw-Hill.
2. Breeze RG, Wheelden EB: The cells of the pulmonary airways, *Am Rev Respir Dis* 116:705, 1977.
3. Cauldwell FW, Siebert RG, Lininger RE, et al: Anatomic study of 150 human cadavers, *Surg Gynecol Obstet* 86: 395, 1948.
4. Jerome EH: Pulmonary circulation. In Hemmings IT, Hopkins P (eds): *Foundations of anesthesia: basic and clinical sciences,* London, 2000, Mosby.
5. Barnes PJ: State of the art: neural control of the human airways in health and disease, *Am Rev Respir Dis* 134:1289, 1986.
6. Barnes PJ: New concepts in the pathogenesis of bronchial hyperresponsiveness and asthma, *J Allergy Clin Immunol* 83:1013, 1989.
7. Gross NJ, Skorodin MS: The place of anticholinergic agents in the treatment of airway obstruction, *Immunol Allergy Pact* 7:224, 1986.
8. Richardson JB, Farguson CC: Neuromuscular structure and function in the airways, *Fed Proc* 38:202, 1979.
9. Boushey HA, Holtzman MJ, Shellar JR, et al: State of the art: bronchial hyperactivity, *Am Rev Respir Dis* 121:389, 1980.
10. Theodore AL, Beer DJ: Pharmacotherapy of chronic obstructive pulmonary disease, *Clin Chest Med* 7:657, 1986.
11. Lefkowitz RJ: Clinical physics of adrenoreceptor regulation, *Am J Physiol* 243:E43, 1982.
12. Seligman M, Chernow B: Use of adrenergic agents in the critically ill patient, *Hosp Formol* 223:348, 1987.
13. Richardson JO: Non-adrenergic inhibitory innervation of the lung, *Lung* 159:315, 1982.
14. Barnes PJ: Neural control of human airways in health and disease, *Am Rev Respir Dis* 134:1286, 1986.
15. Burgess C, Crane J, Pearce N, Beasley R: β_2-Agonists and New Zealand asthma mortality, *Lancet* 337:982, 1991.
16. Villar J, Petty TL, Slutsky AS: ARDS in its middle age: what have we learned? *Appl Cardiopulm Pathophys* 7:167, 1998.
17. So KL, Gommers D, Lachmann B: Bronchoalveolar surfactant system and intratracheal adrenaline, *Lancet* 341:120, 1993.
18. Kelly HW: Controversies in asthma therapy with theophylline and the β_2-adrenergic agents, *Clin Pharm* 3:386, 1984.
19. McFadden ER: Clinical use of β-adrenergic agonists, *J Allergy Clin Immunol* 76:352, 1985.
20. McFadden ER Jr: Methylxanthines in the treatment of asthma: the rise, the fall, and the possible rise again (editorial), *Ann Intern Med* 115:323, 1991.
21. Gora-Harper ML: *The injectable drug reference, society of critical care medicine,* Princeton NJ, 1998, Bioscientific Resources.
22. Weinberger M, Hendeles L: Slow-release theophylline: rationale and basis for product selection, *N Engl J Med* 308:76, 1983.
23. Persson CGA: Overview of effects of theophylline, *J Allergy Clin Immunol* 78:780, 1986.
24. Horrobin DF, Manku MS, Franks DJ, et al: Methylxanthine phosphodiesterase inhibitors behave as prostaglandin antagonists in a perfuse rat mesenteric artery preparation, *Prostaglandins* 13:33, 1977.

25. Murphy CM, Coonce SL, Simon PA: Treatment of asthma in children, *Clin Pharm* 10:685, 1992.
26. Miech RP, Niedzwick JG, Smith TR: Effect of theophylline on the binding of 26. C-AMP to soluble protein from tracheal smooth muscle, *Biochem Pharmacol* 3687, 1979.
27. Hendeles L, Weinberger M: Theophylline: a state of the art review, *Pharmacotherapy* 3:2, 1983.
28. Parker JO, Kelkar K, West RS: Hemodynamic effects of aminophylline in cor pulmonale, *Circulation* 38:17, 1966.
29. McEvoy GK: Theophylline. In McEvoy GK (ed): *AHFS drug information 1993,* Bethesda MD, 1993, American Society of Hospital Pharmacists.
30. Bergstrand H: Phosphodiesterase inhibition and theophylline, *Eur J Respir Dis* 61(S109):37, 1980.
31. Weinberger M, Hendeles L, Bighley L: Relationships of product formulation to absorption of oral theophylline, *N Engl J Med* 299:852, 1978.
32. Nelson HS: β-adrenergic bronchodilations, *N Engl J Med* 333:449, 1995.
33. Amory DW, Burnham SC, Cheney FW, Jr: Comparison of the cardiopulmonary effects of subcutaneously administered epinephrine and terbutaline in patients with reversible airway obstruction, *Chest* 67:279, 1975.
34. Kips JC, Pauwels RA: Long-acting inhaled β$_2$-agonist therapy in asthma, *Am J Respir Crit Care Med* 164:923, 2001.
35. Ullman A, Suedmyr N: Salmeterol, a new long-acting inhaled β$_2$-adrenoceptor agonist: comparison with solbutamol in adult asthmatic patients, *Thorax* 43:674, 1988.
36. Lofdahl CG, Suedmyr N: Formoterol fomarate, a new β$_2$-adrenoceptor agonist: acute studies of selectivity and duration of effect after inhaled and oral administration, *Allergy* 44:264, 1989.
37. Moore PF, Constantine JW, Barth WE: Pirbuterol selective β$_2$-adrenergic bronchodilator, *J Pharmacol Exp Ther* 207:410, 1978.
38. Littner MR, Tashkin DP, Culvarese B, Raotista M: Bronchial and cardiovascular effects of increasing doses of pirbuterol acetate aerosol in asthma, *Ann Allergy* 48:141, 1982.
39. Anderson GP, Linden A, Rabe KF: Why are long-acting β-adrenoceptor agonists long-acting? *Eur Resp J* 7:569, 1994.
40. Kallstrom BL, Sjoberg J, Waldeck B: The interaction between salmeterol and β$_2$-adrenoceptor agonists with higher efficacy on guinea pig trachea and human bronchus in vitro, *Br J Pharmacol* 113:687, 1994.
41. Guhan AR, Cooper S, Oborne J, et al: Systemic effects of formoterol and salmeterol: a dose-response comparison in healthy subjects, *Thorax* 55:650, 2000.
42. Nightingale JA, Rogers DF, Barnes PJ: Comparison of the effects of salmeterol and formoterol in patients with severe asthma. *Am J Resp Crit Car Med* 161:A190, 2000.
43. Noppen M, Vincken W: Bronchodilating effect of formoterol but not of salmeterol in two asthmatic patients, *Respiration* 67:112, 2000 (letter).
44. Weiss EB, Stein M, (eds): *Bronchial asthma: mechanisms and therapeutics,* ed 3, Boston, 1993, Little Brown.
45. Kelly HW, Murphy S: Should anticholinergics be used in acute severe asthma? *Ann Pharmacother* 24:409, 1990.
46. NHLBI, *National asthma education and prevention program, expert panel report 2: guidelines for diagnosis and management of asthma,* NIH Publication No. 97-4051, Bethesda, Md 1997, US Department of Health and Human Services.
47. Wasserman SI (ed): Nedocrimil sodium: a pyranoquinoline anti-inflammatory agent for the treatment of asthma, *J Allergy Clin Immunol* 92(S):143, 1993.
48. Murphy S, Kelly HW: Cromolyn sodium: a review of mechanisms and clinical use in asthma, *Drug Intel Clin Pharm* 21:22, 1987.
49. Hendeles L, Scheife RT (eds): New frontiers in asthma therapy: leukotriene receptor antagonists and 5-lipoxygenase inhibitors, *Pharmacotherapy* 17:1S, 1997.
50. Spector SL, Smith LJ, Glass M: Effects of six weeks of therapy with oral doses of ICI 204, 219, a leukotriene D$_4$ receptor antagonist, *Crit Care Med* 150:618, 1994.
51. Baraniuk JN (ed): Steroids in asthma: molecular mechanisms of glucocorticoid actions, *J Allergy Clin Immunol* 97(Suppl):141, 1996.
52. Kelly HW, Murphy S: Corticosteroids for acute severe asthma, *Ann Pharmacother* 25:72, 1991.
53. Barnes PJ: Inhaled glucocorticoids for asthma, *N Engl J Med* 332:868, 1995.
54. Kelly HW: Comparison of inhaled corticosteroids, *Am Pharmacother* 32:220, 1998.
55. Dellinger RP, Zimmerman JL, Taylor RW, et al: Inhaled nitric oxide in patients with acute respiratory distress syndrome: results of a randomized phase II trial, *Crit Care Med* 26:15, 1998.
56. Moncada S, Palmer RMJ, Higgs HA: Nitric oxide: physiology, pathophysiology and pharmacology, *Pharmacol Rev* 43:109, 1991.
57. Rossaint R, Falke KJ, López F, et al: Inhaled nitric oxide for the adult respiratory distress syndrome, *N Engl J Med* 328:399, 1993.
58. The Neonatal Inhaled Nitric Oxide Study Group: Inhaled nitric oxide in full-term and nearly full-term infants with hypoxic respiratory failure, *N Engl J Med* 336:597, 1997.
59. Roberts JD, Polaner DM, Lang P, et al: Inhaled nitric oxide in persistent pulmonary hypertension of the newborn, *Lancet* 340:819,
60. Avery MA, Mead J: Surface properties in relation to atelectasis and hyaline membrane disease. *Am J Dis Child* 97:517, 1959.
61. Lachmann B, Winsel K, Reutgen H: Der anti-atelektase-faktor der lunge, *I Z Erkr Atm* 137:267, 1972.
62. van Golde LMG, Batenburg JJ, Robertson B: The pulmonary surfactant system: biochemical aspects and functional significance, *Physiol Rev* 68:374, 1988.
63. Lachmann B, Becher G: Protective effect of lung surfactant on allergic bronchial constriction in guinea pigs, *Am Rev Resp Dis* 133:A118, 1986.
64. Van Iwaarden F: Surfactant and pulmonary defense system. In Robertson B, Van Golde LMG, Battenburg JJ (eds): *Pulmonary surfactant,* Amsterdam, 1992, Elsevier.
65. Verbrugge SJC, Lachmann B: Mechanisms of ventilation-induced lung injury and its prevention: role of surfactant, *Appl Cardiopul Pathophys* 7:173, 1998.
66. Papadakos PJ: Artificial ventilation. In Hemmings H, Hopkins P (eds): *Foundations of anesthesia: basic clinical sciences,* London, 2000, Mosby.
67. Tobin N: Asthma, airway biology and nasal disorders in AJRCCM, 2001, *Am J Resp Crit Care Med* 165:598, 2002.

Intraoperative Management for Thoracotomy

Katherine P. Grichnik, MD

William McIvor, MD

Peter D. Slinger, MD, FRCPC

THE number of patients presenting for pulmonary resection has been increasing steadily as indications for surgery have broadened and as the ability to care for patients with severe pulmonary dysfunction has improved. Patients are presenting with advanced respiratory disease states and multiple comorbid conditions. The management of such high-risk patients presenting for thoracotomy can be difficult and challenging. It is important to plan carefully for the preoperative, intraoperative, and postoperative anesthetic care of these patients. This chapter discusses anesthetic management just before surgery, intraoperative anesthetic considerations, potential intraoperative complications, and immediate postoperative concerns.

Anesthetic Management Just Before Surgery

Monitoring Choices

Patients undergoing thoracotomy often have significant concomitant pathophysiology. Surgical procedures requiring thoracotomy can threaten patients' abilities to oxygenate, ventilate, and maintain adequate blood pressure. Several studies have indicated that physicians and anesthesiologists can influence patients' long-term outcomes by guarding, optimizing, or manipulating patient physiology.[1-6] To facilitate appropriate, timely intraoperative management decisions, clinicians need accurate, accessible information about their patients' physiologic states. Intraoperative monitoring helps provide insight into those states during thoracotomy.

HEART RATE MONITORING

Preservation of an acceptable cardiac output (CO) depends in part upon maintaining heart rate within given physical limits. Bradycardia can be detrimental, as cardiac ventricles have finite compliance. Therefore, with profound bradycardia, neither end-diastolic volume nor stroke volume can increase sufficiently to maintain an adequate CO. The potential decrement in CO may be particularly pronounced in patients with ventricular diastolic dysfunction, which can result from chronic systemic or pulmonary hypertension. Because of abnormal compliance, these ventricles cannot alter stroke volumes easily. These concerns emphasize the need to maintain heart rate within circumscribed limits.

Conversely, tachycardia limits the time in diastole and, therefore the amount of time in a ventricular filling phase. With a fast enough heart rate, any patient's CO may fall as a result of decreased stroke volume. Tachycardia, with the attendant increase in myocardial oxygen (O_2) demand, also poses the risk of myocardial ischemia. Hence there is a need for an accurate assessment of the patient's heart rate during thoracotomy.

Several monitors can survey heart rate during thoracic procedures:

1. *Electrocardiography (ECG)*—Leads II and V_5 are routinely monitored intraoperatively. The electrocardiogram monitor counts the QRS complexes and displays this as heart rate. ECG monitors may interpret intraoperative electrical interference generated by electrocautery as QRS waves, which can lead to an inaccurate heart rate display. Redundant monitors aid in the confirmation of the actual heart rate.

2. *Pulse oximeters*—These determine O_2 saturation of arterial blood only if there is inflow and egress of blood across their light path (i.e., a pulse). These instruments use plethysmography to determine the presence of arterial pulsations, and thus heart rate. Electrical interference does not independently affect the heart rate determined by pulse oximetry.

3. *Invasive arterial waveforms*—Waveforms from either the pulmonary or systemic circulation display and quantify the patient's blood pressure and heart rate.

4. *Finger on the pulse*—Intraoperatively, externally applied monitoring devices do not interfere with the anesthesiologist's ability to conduct an ongoing physical examination. It is important to recognize that the basic tenets of physical examination always apply.

HEART RHYTHM MONITORING

The loss of coordinated atrial-ventricular contraction decreases CO. When the late diastolic contribution of atrial contraction is lost, ventricular end-diastolic and stroke volumes decrease. These decrements are, again, particularly exaggerated in patients with impaired ventricular diastolic function. The ECG is primarily used to determine heart rhythm, although redundancy in this monitoring modality also exists. Limb lead II displays large positive deflections (P-waves) as the atria depolarize. It prominently displays the morphology of the P-wave and its relationship to the QRS complex. Lead II is thus most commonly examined to determine the patient's cardiac rhythm.

The limitations of ECG rhythm monitoring are the same as for heart rate monitoring: Electrocautery-generated electrical interference can obscure the heart rhythm on ECG monitors. The shape, or absence, of pulse oximeter or intraarterial waveforms reflects the patient's CO. Therefore changes in invasive arterial or pulse oximetry waveforms can confirm a deleterious change in heart rhythm.

BLOOD PRESSURE MONITORING

Systemic arterial blood pressure is monitored intraoperatively to reflect intravascular conditions relating to blood flow. Noninvasive blood pressure (NIBP) monitoring is performed during each anesthetic. However, the tenuous nature of the thoracic surgical patient's physiology, and the potential for acute decreases in blood pressure associated with operating in the chest, require the use of invasive intraarterial catheters to measure blood pressure directly and continuously.

NIBP monitoring commonly employs automated blood pressure cuffs, which measure blood pressure at user-prescribed intervals. Frequently applied to the upper extremity, they measure pressure in the brachial artery by sensing the oscillations resulting from arterial pulsations. Low CO, improper cuff size, and motion artifact can cause inaccurate blood pressure determinations from the noninvasive technique.

Invasive blood pressure monitoring is achieved through cannulation of the radial or femoral arteries to measure systemic blood pressure directly and continuously. Errant measurements can result from faults within the system (inaccurate zeroing or other technical issues) and/or from proximal occlusion (either internal or external) of the cannulated artery.

ARTERIAL OXYGEN SATURATION

Arterial O_2 saturation is one of the primary determinants of arterial O_2 content, and it is routinely measured intraoperatively. This can be accomplished both invasively and noninvasively.

Pulse oximeters measure arterial O_2 saturation by emitting two wavelengths of light across a tissue bed. Oxygenated hemoglobin maximally absorbs the ultraviolet wavelength (990 nanometers); the infrared wavelength (660 nanometers) is maximally absorbed by deoxygenated hemoglobin. The pulse oximeter emits these wavelengths many times per second, essentially palpating the light absorbance of arterial inflow into the tissue bed. The pulse oximeter measures a ratio of absorption of these wavelengths, and, by applying a manufacturer's algorithm to the derived number, the oximeter determines the oxygen saturation of the arterial blood.

Direct assessment of arterial saturation can be accomplished by sampling arterial blood from the cannulated radial or femoral artery. Patients undergoing thoracotomy often have preexisting pulmonary disease that sometimes limits their ability to oxygenate or ventilate perioperatively. Clinicians measure blood gases to confirm arterial oxygen saturation, measure the partial pressure of oxygen (Pao_2), and determine the adequacy of ventilation as demonstrated by the partial pressure of carbon dioxide ($Paco_2$).

VENTILATION

End-tidal carbon dioxide ($Etco_2$) is analyzed in exhaled gases. $Etco_2$ provides information about respiratory and cardiac physiology as well as the breathing system being used to ventilate the patient. Because of deadspace volume, a gradient exists between the $Etco_2$ and the $Paco_2$. There is increased deadspace associated with chronic obstructive pulmonary disease (COPD). Thus, $Etco_2$ determinations may need to be calibrated with blood gases to determine the adequacy of ventilation. Changes in the capnogram waveform can indicate acute exacerbations of bronchospasm, circuit disconnections, malfunctioning endotracheal tubes or circle-system valves, or exhausted CO_2 absorbent.

CARDIAC OUTPUT

Cardiac output (CO) is another essential component of tissue O_2 delivery. In many patients, indirect estimates of CO (blood pressure, capnography, arterial and pulse oximeter waveforms, and peripheral pulses) provide sufficient reassuring information about the adequacy of CO perioperatively. Patients undergoing thoracotomy are at risk for severe and acute decreases in CO because of preexisting pathologies, new onset of myocardial dysfunction, or complications associated with operating in the thorax. Thus, monitors that directly measure CO are often employed to aid in the management of these patients' hemodynamics.

Capnography can be used to estimate CO. Carbon dioxide is present in the exhaled gases only if there is pulmonary blood flow delivering it to the alveoli. Decreases in $Etco_2$ can result from inadequate CO from pulmonary embolism, pneumothorax, pericardial tamponade, or malignant arrhythmias.

Pulmonary artery catheters (PACs) measure CO via the thermodilution technique. A bolus of fluid, colder than body temperature, is injected into the right atrium. A thermistor at the distal tip of the PAC senses the decrease and return of baseline pulmonary artery blood temperature associated with the negative-calorie bolus. The change in temperature is plotted against time, and the area described by the curve is used to determine right ventricular output. Numerous problems associated with this thermodilution dilution cardiac output (TDCO) technique have been described. Inaccurate bolus volumes, tricuspid regurgitation, and the timing of injection of the cold bolus during the respiratory cycle all can cause inaccurate CO determinations based on this technique.[7,8] Segal et al reported the accuracy of intermittent TDCO ranging from ±3% to 30%.[9]

PACs also allow measurement of central venous, pulmonary artery, and pulmonary artery occlusion pressures. These pressures are affected by changes in ventricular compliance, intrathoracic pressure, methods of ventilation, and extreme changes in preload and afterload.[10,11] Therefore they might not always offer accurate estimates of right and left ventricular preload during or after thoracic surgery.

Some types of PACs have the potential to pace the heart, deliver medications to the central circulation, and continuously measure and display CO and mixed venous oxygen saturation (Svo_2). Complications associated with PAC use include pulmonary artery rupture, sequelae associated with central venous cannulation, and catheter breakage or shearing off in the circulation and acting as a pulmonary artery embolus.[12-15] Connors et al reported increased mortality and increased utilization of resources in intensive care unit (ICU) patients managed with PACs.[16] Consensus panels have commented on the use of PACs.[17,18] Data from PAC use have been scrutinized using the methodologies of evidence-based medicine, outcome studies, and meta-analysis studies, attempting to better define the role of PACs in perioperative patient care.[19-21]

PACs remain commonly used perioperatively to manage patients' hemodynamics. Studies using data derived from PACs in a prescribed manner showed improved outcome in specific patients.[2,4,22] Even opponents of PAC use recognize its indication in certain patient populations.[23]

TRANSESOPHAGEAL ECHOCARDIOGRAPHY

Transesophageal echocardiography (TEE) allows anesthesiologists to observe the heart directly during an operation. Real-time values for left ventricular CO, end-diastolic volume, and the fractional area change (a measure of ventricular performance akin to ejection fraction) can be determined using TEE.[24-26] TEE as a quantitative monitor of CO and preload is limited because the necessary cardiac views are not available in all patients; the labor-intensive nature of the determinations also limits the anesthesiologist's ability to attend to the patient. TEE provides an excellent, continuous qualitative estimate of CO and preload, however. It may be especially useful in the absence of a PAC to determine CO. In addition to its uses for assessing ventricular function and volume, TEE offers several other monitoring capabilities, discussed in the sections of this chapter pertaining to lung transplantation.

TEE images may be difficult to assess when the patient is in the lateral position. Interpretation of waveforms from a pulmonary artery catheter may likewise be difficult in the lateral position; in both cases, trends and changes from baseline may be monitored. TEE may be useful in searching for intracardiac metastasis or neoplasms (a finding that would preclude pulmonary resection) or as an evaluation tool for a mediastinal mass. For example, a middle mediastinal mass diagnosed preoperatively was found intraoperatively by TEE to be a pulmonary vein aneurysm.[27]

The main limitations of TEE are as follows:

- It requires advanced training and practice in order to become proficient.
- The equipment needed to perform the examination is expensive and requires maintenance.
- TEE is poorly tolerated in conscious patients.

TEE is contraindicated in patients who have esophageal disease (fresh suture lines, interruption, stricture, or diverticulum) and in those who have undergone esophageal surgery. It is relatively contraindicated in patients with esophageal varices, though it has been used successfully during liver transplantation.[28,29]

PULMONARY COMPLIANCE

The term *pulmonary compliance* describes the distensibility of the lung parenchyma and chest wall. Clinically, it is the expiratory tidal volume divided by the difference between airway pressures at the beginning and at the end of exhalation. The unit of measurement is milliliters of air ventilated per centimeter of water pressure needed to move that amount of air.

Acute airway obstruction or bronchospasm can result in acute changes in pulmonary compliance during thoracotomy. Malpositioned double-lumen endotracheal tubes can cause airway obstruction or bronchospasm, as can pulmonary embolism, inadequate anesthesia, or pneumothorax. Pulmonary compliance is surveyed perioperatively via capnography and spirometry.

Capnograms have a characteristic square waveform pattern because of the uniform release of alveolar gas from the normal mechanically ventilated lung. A sharply upward-sloping waveform appears in a patient with chronic or acute obstruction of alveolar emptying.

Spirometry can be assessed with some anesthesia machines that measure and display pressure-volume and flow-volume loops during mechanical ventilation. Inspecting these loops can indicate changes in lung compliance, misplaced endotracheal or endobronchial tubes, and ventilator system faults.

END-ORGAN OXYGEN BALANCE

As discussed previously, evidence exists to indicate that anesthesiologists can have a positive impact on patients' long-term survival by ensuring adequate O_2 delivery to tissues. Two indices of end-organ O_2 balance that are monitored and treated perioperatively are myocardial ischemia and Svo_2.

Clinicians traditionally use the ECG to diagnose myocardial ischemia. Myocardial ischemia classically presents with horizontal or downsloping ST-segment depression, occurring 60 to 80 msec after the J-point. Other ECG signs of myocardial ischemia include inverted T waves, changes in cardiac rhythm, and ectopic atrial or ventricular beats.

London et al compared standard intraoperative ECG monitoring with 12-lead electrocardiograms and found only 80% of the ischemic episodes were noted in leads II and V_5.[30] ST-segment depression is obscured in patients with left bundle-branch blocks, paced ventricular rhythms, and during electrocautery-generated electrical interference. Bandwidth settings of intraoperative monitoring ECG also affect the sensitivity and specificity of the monitor.[31] The V_5 lead may not be possible to monitor during a left-sided thoracotomy.

TEE may also be used to monitor for cardiac ischemia. It has been shown that regional wall motion abnormalities (RWMA) precede ECG evidence of myocardial ischemia by several minutes.[32-34] Because no true gold standard for myocardial ischemia detection exists, it is difficult to ascribe sensitivity and specificity to myocardial ischemia monitoring via TEE. The development of new RWMA intraoperatively, however, may be associated with increased risk of perioperative myocardial infarction and sudden death. The American Society of Anesthesiologists and the Society of Cardiovascular Anesthesiologists formed a task force on TEE to make recommendations on its uses.[35] They noted that increased risk of myocardial ischemia or infarction during the perioperative period was a category II indication for TEE (category II indications are supported by weaker evidence and expert consensus but may be useful in improving clinical outcomes).

TEE as an intraoperative monitor of myocardial ischemia suffers from some of the same limitations as its use as a hemodynamic monitor. For example, TEE is unavailable during induction and emergence. Further to make the diagnosis of ischemia with TEE, the clinician must focus on the cardiac images, which distracts him or her from other intraoperative management tasks. Judging changes in regional wall motion is subjective and less quantifiable than changes noted with ST segments.

MIXED VENOUS OXYGEN SATURATION (SVO_2)

Svo_2 is determined by measuring the O_2 saturation of pulmonary artery blood. Svo_2 reflects the difference between total body O_2 delivery and extraction. Sampling blood from the distal pulmonary artery port of any PAC and measuring its O_2 saturation with a gas laboratory oximeter determines the Svo_2. Some PACs use spectroscopy to measure and continuously display Svo_2. Normal Svo_2 value is about 70%. Significant decreases result from increased O_2 extraction (light anesthesia, patient shivering, or hypermetabolic states) or decreased O_2 delivery (fall in Sao_2, CO, or hemoglobin concentrations). A Finnish study demonstrated decreased ICU stays and in-hospital morbidity in patients in whom Svo_2 was maintained at greater than 70%.[36]

BISPECTRAL INDEX MONITORING

The data from a two-channel electroencephalograph (EEG) can be analyzed and modified to present the EEG data as a nomogram between 1 and 100. This *bispectral index* (BIS) monitor has been validated as a useful indicator of anesthetic depth, with a value of 100 corresponding to a fully awake state and a value of 0 corresponding to an isoelectric EEG.[37,38] The obvious advantage of a BIS monitor in thoracic surgery is assurance of adequate anesthetic depth when an anesthetic may consist of smaller amounts of opioids, benzodiazepines, and inhalation agents than might be used in a healthier population of patients. The BIS is especially useful for titration of the anesthetic just before emergence to allow for a more rapid awakening.[39]

SPECIALIZED THORACOTOMY: MONITORING CONSIDERATIONS FOR LUNG TRANSPLANTATION SURGERY

The basic monitors for lung transplantation surgery include ECG monitoring, NIBP measurements, and pulse oximetry (see Chapter 14). The severe nature of lung transplant patients' pathophysiology may dictate placement of two intraarterial catheters for proper and accurate blood pressure monitoring. A femoral artery catheter can be placed to measure central aortic pressure continuously, while a radial artery can be cannulated to sample blood gases and other laboratory data.

PACs serve several purposes in thoracotomy for lung transplantation. In addition to measuring estimates of right and left ventricular preload, some PACs can continuously measure and display CO and/or Svo_2. Decreased pulmonary artery O_2 saturation could serve as a helpful early warning of inadequate O_2 delivery in these compromised patients who are undergoing a challenging procedure. To facilitate the pulmonary artery surgical anastomosis, the catheter may need to be pulled out of the right or left pulmonary artery to the main pulmonary artery. As with other thoracotomies, TEE is useful to estimate left ventricular end-diastolic volume, monitor for myocardial ischemia, and assess ventricular function. TEE has still other specific uses during lung transplantation. It is helpful for examination of the intra-atrial septum intraoperatively to rule out defects, which could lead to perioperative intracardiac shunting. The mitral and tricuspid valves can be examined to determine the presence and degree of regurgitation. The right ventricle can be visualized during pulmonary artery cross-clamping for signs of dilation and decreased systolic function. Intracardiac emboli, such as air, can also be seen on TEE; the aorta and pulmonary artery are examined to help facilitate the surgery. Finally, the patency of pulmonary venous anastomoses with the left atrium can be assessed with color and pulse-wave Doppler modalities.

Preoperative Sedation

Invasive monitoring catheters and regional anesthetics may be placed preoperatively before the patient receives a general anesthetic. During this time, sedation is often given to patients to increase comfort and cooperation. Patients with severe pulmonary disease, however, should be given sedation sparingly. Such patients may have baseline carbon dioxide (CO_2) retention and limited respiratory reserve, either of which would make them highly susceptible to small amounts of sedatives.

Further, residual sedative effect may create difficulty with emergence from anesthesia at the end of the operation.

Gross et al examined the effect of midazolam on changes in minute ventilation in response to hypercapnea in patients with and without COPD.[40] The two curves in Figure 7-1 represent a plot of the slopes of the minute-to-minute CO_2 response curves after midazolam administration. Both groups had a diminished minute ventilation response to hypercapnea under the influence of midazolam. The patients with COPD, however, had a more profound fall in the minute ventilation response to hypercapnea with midazolam than did normal patients; in the COPD patients, this response also persisted for a longer time. Thus, caution is indicated when sedatives are considered for patients with COPD. One approach is to avoid benzodiazepines and use small amounts of propofol (which has little subsequent effect on emergence) during invasive monitor placement.

Rationale for Regional Analgesia for Thoracic Surgery

Regional anesthesia can and should be considered where appropriate. It is usually initiated in the preoperative period when the patient is awake, able to cooperate, and able to move appropriately for positioning. Regional anesthesia can be used as part of a balanced anesthesia technique with general anesthesia or as a sole anesthetic and is discussed in the sections pertaining to intraoperative considerations.

Regional techniques (e.g., epidural, intercostal, paravertebral blocks) can allow for sparing of intraoperative opioid use and minimization of inhalation agents, leading to a more rapid emergence. In developing a strategy for postoperative analgesia, consideration should be given to the expected duration of chest tube drainage and/or the anticipated intensity of postsurgical pain (see Chapter 20). Epidural analgesia is especially effective for procedures that are expected to require more

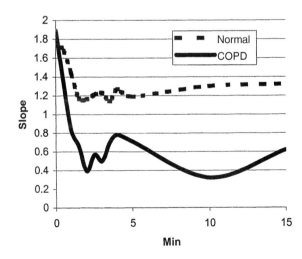

FIGURE 7-1 The slope of the fall in the minute ventilation response to carbon dioxide after midazolam administration over time. *Slope,* Difference in minute ventilation between normocapnea and hypercapnea divided by the difference in carbon dioxide tensions; *min,* minutes. At time *0,* midazolam was administered. (From Gross JB, Zebrowski ME, Carel WD, et al: *Anesthesiology* 58:540, 1983.)

than one day of analgesia and procedures in which delayed return of gastrointestinal function would prevent administration of oral analgesics.[41,42] The site of the epidural may also affect the amount of analgesic used. In general, placement of the epidural close to the dermatomal level of the surgical incision can increase the efficacy of the analgesics administered. Epidurally administered local anesthetic can minimize both the need for systemic opioids and their respiratory depressant effects; it has been suggested that the combination of local anesthetic and opioids for epidural or spinal analgesia is most effective.[43,44] Paravertebral blocks and intrathecal opioids are most commonly used as single-administration techniques and are especially useful for procedures that are not expected to require more than 12 to 24 hours of intense analgesia.[45-48] Paravertebral blocks have the advantage of providing unilateral analgesia with local anesthetic, thus avoiding narcotics and minimizing the hypotensive effects of a sympathectomy. Single administration paravertebral blocks provide effective analgesia for only 12 to 18 hours, however; catheter techniques have been advocated for longer analgesia.[49-51] Similarly, intercostal analgesia techniques are usually single-administration techniques, designed to last from 6 to 12 hours (although intercostal catheters can be used for a longer duration of analgesia).[52-54] Intrathecal opioids have been shown to be effective for control of postthoracotomy pain.[55] The optimal technique for postoperative analgesia in the patient with severe pulmonary disease has yet to be determined because of the lack of randomized, double-blinded, placebo-controlled prospective clinical trials.

In spite of its widespread use, thoracic epidural analgesia (TEA) has been criticized for use in patients with severe pulmonary disease as a result of the potential effects on bronchial tone and possible respiratory muscle weakness. Gruber et al examined 12 patients with severe emphysema presenting for lung volume reduction surgery (Table 7-1).[56] Patterns of breathing, gas exchange parameters, and ventilatory mechanics were established at baseline before the induction of anesthesia. TEA with bupivacaine was then established and confirmed; the patterns of breathing, gas exchange parameters, and ventilatory mechanics were measured again. Among the findings were that both tidal volume and peak inspiratory flow rate increased, while resistance to ventilation fell. It can be concluded that not only did the establishment of TEA not impair pulmonary function in patients with severe emphysema, but it also may even improve patterns of respiration.

Two analyses of multiple studies support the use of regional analgesia to preserve pulmonary function in the perioperative period. Richardson et al examined 55 studies using epidural analgesia, paravertebral or extrapleural analgesia, intercostal block, cryoablation, intrapleural analgesia, and transcutaneous nerve stimulation.[57] These authors found that paravertebral blockade preserved spirometric function to 75% of the preoperative values, whereas intercostal blockade and epidural analgesia preserved spirometric function to 52% and 47%, respectively, of their preoperative values. No assessment or comparison to intravenous analgesia was made.

In a more rigorous meta-analysis, Ballantyne et al examined 65 studies using epidural analgesia, intercostal blockade, local wound infiltration, and interpleural and intravenous analgesia

TABLE 7-1

Patterns of Breathing, Gas Exchange, and Ventilatory Mechanics Before and After Thoracic Epidural Analgesia with Bupivacaine

Variable	Pre-TEA	Post-TEA	P value
V_E (L)	7.5 ± 2.6	8.7 ± 2.1	0.04
V_T (L)	0.46 ± 0.16	0.53 ± 0.14	0.003 *
R_f (b/m)	16 ± 3	17 ± 3	0.63
T_I/T_{tot}	0.39 ± 0.04	0.39 ± 0.05	0.84
Pao_2 (mmHg)	69 ± 17	68 ± 9	0.79
$Paco_2$ (mmHg)	39 ± 4	38 ± 5	0.04
PIRF (L/s)	0.48 ± 0.17	0.55 ± 0.14	0.02 *
PEFR (L/s)	0.38 ± 0.17	0.40 ± 0.09	0.78
R_L (cmH$_2$O/L/sec)	20.7 ± 9.9	16.6 ± 8.1	0.02 *
PEEP$_{idyn}$ (cmH$_2$O)	4.8 ± 3.6	4.7 ± 3.9	0.67
WOB (J/L)	1.5 ± 0.5	1.5 ± 0.6	0.79
ΔP_{es} (cmH$_2$O)	16.5 ± 4.8	16.9 ± 6.9	0.82
MIP (cmH$_2$O)	81.7 ± 25.5	76.8 ± 32	0.52

From Gruber, EM, Tschernko EM, Kritzinger M, et al: *Anesth Analg* 92:1015, 2001.
TEA, thoracic epidural analgesia; V_E, minute ventilation; V_T, tidal volume; R_f, respiratory frequency; T_I/T_{tot}, duration of inspiration /duration of total cycle; *Pao$_2$*, partial pressure for oxygen; *Paco$_2$*, partial pressure for carbon dioxide; *PIRF,* peak inspiratory flow rate; *PERF,* peak expiratory flow rate; R_L, pulmonary resistance; *PEEP$_{idyn}$*, dynamic intrinsic positive end-expiratory pressure; *WOB,* work of breaking; ΔP_{es}, maximal change in esophageal pressure during an entire respiratory cycle; *MIP,* maximum inspiratory pressure; *L,* liters; *b/m,* breaths per minute; *mmHg,* millimeters of mercury; *L/sec,* liters per second; *cmH$_2$O/L/sec,* centimeters of water pressure per liter per second; *cmH$_2$O,* centimeters of water pressure; *J/L,* joules per liter. *Data presented in terms of mean ± SD.*

compared with systemic opioid analgesia for the more relevant outcomes of incidence of atelectasis, pulmonary infections, pulmonary complications, and postoperative Pao$_2$.[58] Secondarily, these authors examined spirometric function. Epidural opioid analgesia was found to reduce the incidence of atelectasis, whereas epidural local anesthetic/analgesia decreased the incidence of pulmonary infections and pulmonary complications and resulted in a greater postoperative Pao$_2$. In contrast to Richardson et al, there appeared to be no difference in spirometric function with any of the therapies. It can be concluded from these analyses that regional analgesic techniques can improve pulmonary outcomes perioperatively when compared with conventional intravenous analgesia. It has been suggested that the recent trend of improved outcome in high-risk thoracic patients following pulmonary resection seems to be related to the use of epidural analgesia.[59] Thoracic epidural bupivacaine has also been shown to attenuate supraventricular tachyarrhythmias after pulmonary resection when compared with epidural morphine alone.[60]

Intraoperative Anesthetic Considerations

An Overview of the Surgical Procedure

The anesthesiologist must understand and anticipate the conduct of the surgical procedure. A brief review of a typical thoracic surgical procedure is presented with a discussion of the pertinent anesthetic considerations to follow. A review of concerns for specific surgical procedures is presented in Chapter 12.

Initially, it is important to ensure the correct operative side, both for patient safety as well as for correct placement of regional analgesic techniques (paravertebral blocks) and/or for monitoring placement (internal jugular cannulation, placement of the arterial catheter in an accessible arm).

After induction of anesthesia and endotracheal intubation, the patient will be turned for positioning. This is usually a full lateral position but may be supine or only partially lateral. After appropriate surgical preparation and draping, an incision will be made, usually a posterolateral incision from the anterior axillary line toward the posterior 5th intercostal space. This incision may vary with the site of pathology within the thorax. After dissection through the muscle layers, the surgeon will prepare to enter the pleural space via a rib resection or through an intercostal space. The surgeon and the anesthesiologist should communicate before this event to ensure that the operative lung has been deflated to prevent unintended injury or bleeding. After entering the pleural space, the adequacy of lung deflation can be assessed. Inadequate deflation may be due to endotracheal tube malposition after patient positioning, intrinsic pulmonary disease, and/or pleural adhesions. The surgeon and the anesthesiologist can then determine the steps necessary to assure adequate operating conditions. These may include repositioning the endobronchial tube, a short period of bilateral lung deflation just before a bronchial blocker inflation, gentle suctioning of the deflated lung lumen, or lysis of pleural adhesions.

Specific procedures have specific intraoperative considerations as discussed elsewhere. There is, however, an unpredictable risk of blood loss for every thoracic surgical procedure; adequate intravenous access and the availability of blood products should be ensured. Deviations from the surgical plan should be communicated immediately to allow the anesthesiologist to prepare for potential problems with volume loss, oxygenation, and/or ventilation.

At the end of the procedure and before reinflation of the operative lung, the appropriate lumen of the endobronchial tube should be suctioned to clear secretions and blood. With surgical observation, the pulmonary suture line should be tested by compressing the anesthesia machine reservoir bag, applying 20 to 40 cmH_2O pressure to the airway. After chest tube placement, the chest will be closed. To avoid paradoxical respiration and possible mediastinal shift, the patient should not be allowed to breathe spontaneously until pleural closure and attachment of the chest tubes to the pleural drainage system have been achieved. If extubation is planned, it may be done in the lateral or supine position.

Respiratory Physiology During Thoracic Procedures

There are multiple physiologic principles that must be considered when choosing an anesthetic regimen, as many anesthetic and hemodynamic agents affect lung function, oxygenation, and ventilation. These principles, which will be discussed next, include the following:
1. Lung volume alterations
2. Changes in airways resistance
3. Effects on hypoxic pulmonary vasoconstriction
4. Depression of ventilatory control mechanisms (see Chapter 3)

LUNG VOLUME ALTERATIONS
Pulmonary volumes, including functional residual capacity (FRC), closing capacity (CC), and residual volume (RV), may all change with the administration of anesthesia. Best studied is FRC, which is reduced soon after the induction of anesthesia and is independent of spontaneous (vs. controlled) mechanical ventilation.[61-64] Proposed etiologies include atelectasis, increased expiratory muscle activity, gas trapped in distal airways, diaphragmatic displacement, decreased outward chest wall recoil, increased elastic lung recoil, and increased thoracic blood volume. Anesthetic agents affect this phenomenon variably, with the volatile anesthetic agents causing dramatic reductions in FRC when compared with intravenous anesthetic agents. It has been stated that anesthetic agents cause similar reductions in CC and FRC such that the relationship between the two volumes is unchanged.[65] Other studies have shown differences in the magnitude of change of FRC, CC, and RV with anesthesia and muscle relaxation and that the awake relationships are not maintained (Figure 7-2).[66] This concept is important to consider in the event of hypoxemia, as airway closure and atelectasis can occur when CC exceeds end-expiratory lung volumes.

CHANGES IN AIRWAYS RESISTANCE
Dramatic changes in airway's resistance can occur with the induction of anesthesia and intubation of the trachea. Most

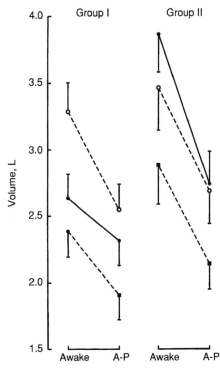

FIGURE 7-2 Changes in the relationships of lung volumes with anesthesia and muscle relaxation. Values: mean ± SE of functional residual capacity (FRC), closing capacity (CC), and residual volume (RV) for group I (12 patients whose FRC was greater than CC while awake) and for group II (11 patients whose FRC was less than CC while awake). FRC and CC were reduced when the patients were anesthetized and paralyzed. (A-P). In group I, FRC decreased more than CC; in group II, CC decreased more than FRC. (From Juno P, March HM, Knopp TJ, Rehdar KL: *J Appl Physiol* 44:238, 1978.)

studies have documented an increase in resistance, thought to be caused by changes in gas viscosity and density, airway caliber, and bronchomotor tone.[67-69] The physical properties of the inhaled anesthetic gases may not be as important as the changes in airway caliber (in part because of the reduction in FRC) and the changes in bronchomotor tone mediated by the autonomic nervous system and chemical messengers. There are multiple stimulants for increases in airway resistance. Mechanical causes include the effect of intubation on the airways, surgical manipulation, mucus plugging, and the physical properties of the endotracheal tube.[70] Chemical mediators include hypocapnea, histamine, leukotrienes, bradykinin, and prostaglandin F_2 alpha.[71] Sympathetic nervous system effects include vagally mediated bronchial smooth muscle constriction and adrenergically mediated β- and α-receptor effects. Patients also often present for thoracotomy with increased airway resistance at baseline and so are more susceptible to bronchoconstriction. In conjunction with all of these considerations, anesthetic agents have variable effects on airway caliber and bronchomotor tone, as outlined for the individual drugs (see below). In general, inhalation agents are beneficial and decrease bronchial tone, whereas many intravenous agents may release histamine and precipitate bronchoconstriction. It may be more important to ensure an adequate depth of anesthesia before instrumentation of the airway than to be concerned about the propensity of a particular agent to release histamine; use of a monitor such as the BIS can facilitate this goal.

HYPOXIC PULMONARY VASOCONSTRICTION

Hypoxic pulmonary vasoconstriction (HPV) was first identified in 1946, when Von Euler and Liljestrand suggested that local pulmonary vascular beds respond to regional hypoxia (resulting from low inspired oxygen or atelectasis) with vaso-constriction as a mechanism for redistributing pulmonary blood flow to more well-ventilated areas of the lung.[72] HPV is a unique response of the pulmonary vascular system and is most pronounced in the precapillary arterioles. HPV is now recognized to occur during one-lung ventilation (OLV), resulting in the limitation of hypoxia to a greater degree than would be expected without its occurrence (Figure 7-3).[73] This regulation of the distribution of ventilation-to-perfusion ratios by HPV contributes to both the efficiency of gas exchange and to pulmonary hemodynamics.[74] Such regulation by HPV opposes the vasodilatory effect that hypoxia has in systemic blood vessels and vascular smooth muscle (see Chapters 3 and 4).

HPV is also recognized as a critical factor in many serious medical conditions, including persistent pulmonary hypertension of the newborn, acute respiratory distress syndrome, chronic lung disease, and high-altitude sickness.[75-77] HPV is a local response that results in pulmonary artery pressure and blood flow diversion, the proportion of which occurs according to the amount of lung rendered hypoxic.[78] A complex set of factors influence the HPV response. First, the amount of lung affected is important. Small segments of hypoxic lung result in greater flow diversion than increased pulmonary artery pressure, whereas larger segments of hypoxic lung result in greater increases in pulmonary artery pressures when compared with flow diversion.[79,80] Further, small segments of hypoxic lung favor the Pao_2 as the main stimulus for HPV, whereas large segments of hypoxic lung favor the partial pressure of venous oxygen (Pvo_2) as the main stimulus.[81] Second, the primary inciting event may be important, as HPV may be provoked by primary hypoxia or by atelectasis resulting in hypoxia. When the lung is hypoxic due to ventilation with a low Fio_2, Pao_2 is the main stimulus for HPV, whereas HPV provoked by lung

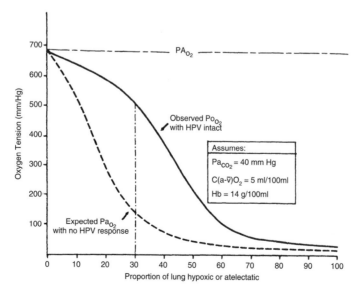

FIGURE 7-3 One-lung ventilation and hypoxic pulmonary vasoconstriction (HPV). The dashed line of this graph illustrates the expected partial pressure of oxygen in dogs in response to an increasing proportion of lung hypoxia or atelectasis under normocapnea. The non-dashed line illustrates the actual observed Pao_2. The higher than predicted Pao_2 can be attributed to a hypoxic pulmonary ventilatory response in the hypoxic or atelectatic lung, which limits perfusion to that lung segment. (From McMurty IF: *J Appl Physiol* 56:375, 1984.)

hypoxia because of atelectasis appears to be stimulated by Pv_{O_2}. The HPV response has been demonstrated to be maximal during the first 15 minutes of a hypoxic challenge and is not potentiated by repeated challenges.[82]

The mechanisms mediating HPV are less well understood but appear to alter the balance of vasodilatory and vasoconstrictive compounds locally. The etiology and modulation of HPV are variably thought to be due to the following[83-86]:

1. A direct pulmonary vascular smooth muscle cell response involving voltage-dependent potassium channels
2. Mediators that inhibit prostaglandin synthesis, enhance leukotriene synthesis, or alter calcium channel pathways
3. Changes in nitric oxide production that enhance vasoconstriction

Potential humoral agents include endothelin, angiotensin II, nitric oxide, and adrenomodulin (see Chapter 5).[87,88]

Physiologic factors may also affect HPV. Increases in CO lead to increases in pulmonary perfusion, which can inhibit HPV.[89] Intermittent hypoxia has been shown to variably increase or decrease the HPV response.[90,91] Hyperoxia has no effect on pulmonary vascular resistance, however.[92] Surgical manipulation may variably limit the HPV response, the magnitude of which is related to individual thromboxane and prostaglandin mediator release.[93-94]

The potential significance and importance of HPV as a homeostatic mechanism are most appreciated in thoracic anesthesia, in which obligatory atelectasis and unilateral lung hypoxia are introduced during OLV. Normally, collapse of the nonventilated, nondependent lung results in activation of reflex HPV. HPV is an important concept to understand because many of the anesthetic agents and drugs used to modulate hemodynamics affect the magnitude of the HPV response. The individual agents are addressed in following sections.

DEPRESSION OF VENTILATORY CONTROL

The control of ventilation is neurologically mediated, extremely complex, and requires coordination between the central and peripheral nervous systems. The inhalation anesthetics, opioids, and sedative agents all act to depress the central nervous system to achieve loss of awareness and analgesia. The common side effect is depression of ventilatory control. The response to CO_2 is a good indication of respiratory depression. The normal response to increases in Pa_{CO_2} is to increase minute ventilation in nonanesthetized, spontaneously breathing adults, called the CO_2 response curve (Figure 7-4).[95] In general, opioids and inhalation agents depress the ventilatory response to CO_2 (Figure 7-5).[96] Opioids characteristically decrease ventilatory rate with an increased tidal volume. In contrast, volatile agents and barbiturates depress tidal volume and increase respiratory rate.[97] Painful stimuli (such as a surgical incision) may reverse the respiratory depressant effects of agents used for anesthetic care, a phenomenon that is demonstrable when no neuromuscular blockade is used. It appears that the ventilatory response to low levels of O_2 is less sensitive than to hypercarbia. With alveolar CO_2 held constant at 40 mmHg, the effect of changing alveolar O_2 concentration on ventilation is shown in Figure 7-6.[98] The respiratory effects of agents used for anesthesia are usually unimportant intraoperatively, when ventilation is artificially controlled. It is most desirable, however, to use anesthetic agents that have minimal residual effects on

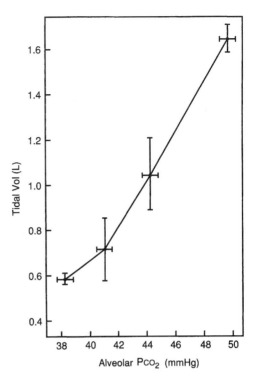

FIGURE 7-4 Carbon dioxide response curve. Spontaneous ventilation, depicted here as tidal volume, increases linearly as alveolar CO_2 rises when healthy, nonanesthetized subjects breathe increasing amounts of CO_2. (From Lambertsen CJ: *Anesthesiology* 21:642, 1960.)

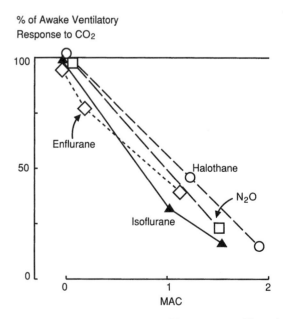

FIGURE 7-5 The ventilatory response to CO_2 was measured in awake volunteers breathing enflurane, halothane, isoflurane, and nitrous oxide. All inhalation anesthetics depress the ventilatory response to increases in CO_2 in a dose-dependent manner. (From Eger EI II: *Isoflurane (Forane): a compendium and reference*, ed 2, Madison, Wis, 1985, Anaquest.)

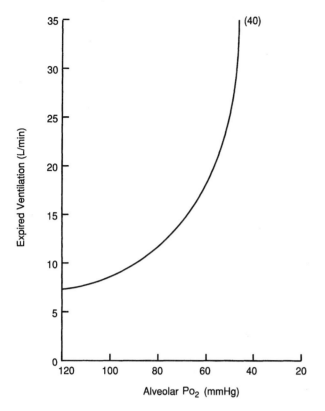

FIGURE 7-6 The ventilatory response to low levels of oxygen is less sensitive than to rises in carbon dioxide. With alveolar CO_2 held constant at 40 mmHg, the effect of changing alveolar oxygen concentration on expired ventilation is shown.

ventilation; most patients after pulmonary surgery are already at risk of respiratory depression and/or failure resulting from the mechanical consequences of the operation and underlying pathologic conditions. The respiratory depressant effects of individual agents are discussed in the sections that follow.

Anesthetic Agents for Thoracic Procedures

VOLATILE ANESTHETIC AGENTS. The choice of the volatile anesthetic agent for use during thoracic surgery is an individual one, dependent on desired effects (such as rapid emergence), availability, cost, and personal preference (Table 7-2). Historically, halothane is the best-studied volatile agent, but it is no longer in widespread use. In general, volatile agents decrease FRC through decreasing chest wall recoil, bronchodilation, inhibition of HPV, and blunting the ventilatory response to hypoxia.[99] Volatile anesthetics may also reduce airway resistance by both direct effects on airway smooth muscle and reductions in reflex neural activity.

In comparison with volatile agents, intravenous anesthetic agents have little direct effect on HPV. The clinical significance of these effects is questionable, however, as conflicting results have been obtained when comparing inhalation agents with one another and with intravenous techniques.[78,100-104] Benumof et al demonstrated the differences between inhalation and intravenous anesthetics in a study on 12 patients undergoing thoracic surgery (Figure 7-7).[100] Patients received isoflurane or halothane with an inspired O_2 concentration of 100 for 60 min-

utes with two-lung ventilation. OLV was then instituted for 40 minutes, after which the inhalation agent was discontinued and the intravenous anesthetic started. After 40 to 60 minutes of OLV with intravenous anesthetics, two-lung ventilation was reinstated with the intravenous technique. The study showed that Pao_2 was significantly less during inhalation anesthesia when compared with intravenous anesthesia. Interpretation of the study is somewhat complicated, however, by the effects of surgically induced lung trauma and the variability of individual HPV responses. Overall, it may be concluded that the clinical effect of inhalation agents is small, but that the HPV response of an individual may be more sensitive to the type of anesthetic administered. This may be due in part to other effects of volatile agents, such as depression of cardiac output with subsequent decrease in Pvo_2—a known stimulus for HPV.[105]

Isoflurane and enflurane are similar in having mild cardiovascular effects, causing bronchodilation, and inhibiting HPV.[106-108] In a dog model, HPV inhibition by isoflurane was independent of CO and Pvo_2, and enflurane at 1 minimum alveolar concentration (MAC) was found to inhibit HPV by 21.5% during OLV.[109,110]

Sevoflurane and desflurane are volatile agents with rapid onset and offset because of favorable blood gas coefficients. They are potent bronchodilators but can inhibit HPV.[111,112] The HPV effect of sevoflurane is noted at higher concentrations and thus may not be clinically relevant. Beck et al found that propofol (thought not to inhibit HPV) and sevoflurane were not significantly different with respect to changes in shunt fraction in the lateral position under OLV.[113] Clinical data suggest that desflurane may preserve arterial oxygenation to a greater extent than isoflurane during anesthesia and OLV, suggesting that desflurane has a smaller effect on HPV than isoflurane.[114]

At a similar MAC, enflurane and isoflurane depress ventilation to a greater degree than do sevoflurane and desflurane.[115-119] Postoperatively, it is important to note that the ventilatory response to hypoxemia may be impaired by tiny amounts of volatile agents (0.05 to 0.1 MAC)—something that is especially crucial to remember in patients with advanced pulmonary disease.[120] With respect to postoperative ventilatory depression, the elimination characteristics of sevoflurane and desflurane should confer a significant advantage for use in patients undergoing thoracotomy.

Nitrous oxide is an inorganic compound that is used in combination with other inhalation or intravenous anesthetics. Nitrous oxide can depress HPV independently and causes sympathetic nervous system activation, in part mediated by increases in circulating norepinephrine.[121-124] Nitrous oxide does depress the ventilatory drive to hypoxia with little effect on the CO_2 response curve unless it is used with volatile anesthetics, in which case it contributes to respiratory depression.[125,126] In a thoracic patient who is ill-equipped to compensate for it, this blunted respiratory drive may lead to postoperative diffusion hypoxia. Further, the intraoperative need for the ability to change anesthetic depth while maintaining high inspired oxygen concentrations limits the use of nitrous oxide during OLV.[127] It is noteworthy that nitrous oxide supports combustion almost as well as O_2 does—a concern for any thoracic surgical procedure that might involve the use of a laser. Nitrous oxide can also expand in a closed gas space within diseased lungs.

TABLE 7-2
Properties of Selected Anesthetic Agents Used for Thoracotomy

Anesthetic	Desirable	Undesirable
Volatile agents	Permits use of high FiO_2 Bronchodilation	Inhibit HPV Myocardial depression Diminishe airway reflexes Readily eliminated
Nitrous oxide	Readily eliminated Small HPV effect	Reduce FiO_2
Opioids	Little HPV effect Little myocardial depression Provide postoperative analgesia	Not a complete anesthetic Potential respiratory depression postoperatively Potential histamine release with some agents Variable elimination
Ketamine	Decreased airway irritability Little HPV effect Improved cardiovascular stability with hypovolemia	Myocardial ischemia Emergence delirium
Thiopental, Etomidate, Propofol	Little HPV effect	Potential histamine release and subsequent bronchospasm with some agents Potential hypotension, tachycardia, bradycardia Adrenocortical suppression with etomidate
Muscle relaxants	Facilitate endotracheal intubation and mechanical ventilation Enhance surgical exposure	Postoperative muscle weakness with inadequate reversal or elimination of effect Need for use of reversal agents with most muscle relaxants Potential for histamine release and subsequent bronchospasm with some agents
Cholinesterase inhibitors Local anesthetics	Reverse muscle relaxation Reduce airway reflexes Perioperative pain control Reduction of neuroendocrine responses with some regional anesthesia techniques	Possible acetylcholine-mediated bronchospasm Narrow therapeutic window Potential seizures, myocardial depression, and arrhythmias

HPV, Hypoxic pulmonary constriction.

INDUCTION AND SEDATIVE AGENTS

Intravenous anesthetic agents have little effect on HPV but may mediate a decrease in FRC through increases in lung elastic recoil.[64] These agents have variable postoperative effects on bronchial tone and control of ventilation.

Propofol is an anesthetic agent characterized by a rapid onset and offset, allowing a rapid return of the patient's ability to cooperate and potentially be extubated. Propofol is often used for induction and maintenance of anesthesia in patients undergoing thoracic procedures. Total intravenous anesthesia with propofol has been compared to inhalation anesthesia for thoracotomy and found to cause comparatively less impairment of postoperative lung function.[128] Propofol has been reported to either not influence HPV or actually potentiate HPV; however, clinically, no difference in intraoperative PaO_2 was demonstrated when a total intravenous anesthetic technique with propofol was compared with volatile anesthetics.[110,129-131] Propofol has been reported to cause histamine release in vitro but has been shown to have an incidence of histamine release in allergic patients similar to that of a midazolam-ketamine anesthetic when hydroxyzine is used as premedication.[132,133]

Thiopental is the most commonly used agent for the induction of anesthesia. At higher concentrations, it can cause histamine release in vitro.[132] Thiopental has been associated with bronchospasm in asthmatic patients, although inadequate depth of anesthesia cannot be excluded as a potential cause of bronchospasm.

Etomidate rarely causes histamine release and has been advocated for use in patients who are at risk for bronchocon-

striction on induction of anesthesia.[134,135] Ketamine is an agent with bronchodilatory but secretory properties and has been used for the treatment of asthma. When used in higher concentrations, however, it has been shown to provoke histamine release in vitro.[132] Ketamine does not appear to affect HPV.[129]

Midazolam is the most commonly used benzodiazepine. Midazolam has a shorter half-life than diazepam, thus conferring an advantage for use in thoracic surgery. Diazepam and midazolam cause similar decreases in tidal volume with an increased respiratory rate.[136] Both agents decrease hypoxic ventilatory drive.[137,138] Flumazenil, a benzodiazepine reversal agent, was only partially effective in reversing the respiratory effect of diazepam.[138] Midazolam can cause histamine release in lung tissue in vitro.[132]

OPIOIDS

Opioids are usually necessary to ablate pain during and after pulmonary surgery. The effects on pulmonary function vary depending on the particular agent, the timing of administration, the total dose, the route of administration, and coexisting pathology. All of the opioids cause respiratory depression; however, the magnitude of this effect depends on the type of opioid receptor that each individual drug stimulates.[139] For example, some opioids (such as morphine and fentanyl as pure μ-receptor agonists) exert effects on only one opioid receptor; thus the respiratory depression induced by these drugs can be due only to μ-related respiratory effects. Other opioids affect different opioid receptors or are agonist-antagonist agents that may have a ceiling effect for respiratory depression.[139] Timing of administration of opioids may determine their postoperative

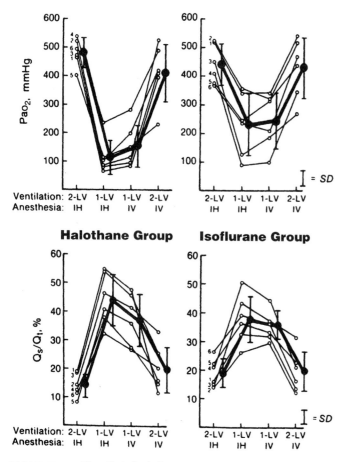

FIGURE 7-7 The effect of volatile anesthetic agents on the HPV response to OLV. During inhalation anesthesia, one-lung ventilation (1-LV) produced large reductions in Pao₂ and increases in shunt. Elimination of halothane (IH) and use of intravenous (IV) anesthesia during one-lung ventilation produced an increase in Pao₂ of 39 mmHg and a decrease in shunt by 7% of cardiac output. These effects were smaller when switching from isoflurane to intravenous anesthesia. Individual patient data are shown to demonstrate the considerable variability encountered clinically. *2-LV,* Two lung ventilation. (From Benumof J et al: *Anesthesiology* 82:940, 1995.)

effects—opioids administered late in the operation have a more profound effect than those administered early, as determined by the elimination half-life of each agent. The site of administration also affects the duration and timing of respiratory depression; intravenous opioids take effect within minutes, whereas regionally administered opioids may have delayed postoperative effects ranging from 1 to 2 hours (fentanyl, sufentanil) to six to 24 hours (morphine).[140-143] It is noteworthy that concomitant administration of additional parenteral opioids or other sedatives potentiate the respiratory depressive effects of regionally administered opioids. Only the commonly used opioids for thoracic surgery are considered here.

Fentanyl is often used as a part of a balanced anesthetic technique. It has little effect on HPV.[144,145] Fentanyl has been shown to cause increased lung and total respiratory system resistance with intravenous administration.[146,147] Clinically,

however, fentanyl appears to have insignificant effects on bronchomotor tone and does not cause histamine release. Fentanyl is not only used intravenously but also is often combined with local anesthetics for use in epidural analgesia. Nonetheless, the pharmacologic properties of fentanyl seem to be similar whether it is administered epidurally or intravenously.[148] The advantage of epidural administration is placement of the opioid close to the site of action at the spinal cord, therefore necessitating a much smaller dose. Sufentanil and alfentanil are similar to fentanyl with respect to the respiratory effects, but they have different potencies and durations of action.[145,147]

Morphine is the gold standard to which all other opioids are compared. It has minimal effects on HPV.[145,149] Morphine is thought to increase airway resistance. This effect may be mediated by histamine release, as the increase in airway resistance after morphine is administered can be blocked by pretreatment with an antihistamine drug.[150] Morphine may be protective, however, in that it has also been shown to inhibit the vagally mediated component of bronchoconstriction.[151] The histamine release caused by morphine may also mediate its venodilatory properties, which are important in the treatment of pulmonary edema, as venodilation can be inhibited by pretreatment with antihistamine agents.[152] Morphine may also have pulmonary volume effects, as FRC can be reduced by a single dose of intramuscular morphine.[153] Morphine can be used epidurally or intrathecally to achieve pain control after thoracotomy.[154,155] The doses used in these modes of administration are much smaller than those used intravenously: Epidural morphine is used in doses of 1 to 5 mg, and intrathecal morphine is used in doses of 0.2 to 0.8 mg.

Hydromorphone is an opioid with lipid solubility properties and a duration of action intermediate between fentanyl and morphine.[156,157] The physiologic effects on the respiratory system are those of a pure opioid μ-agonist. Hydromorphone can be used effectively for thoracic surgery either intravenously or as part of a regional technique. When used as an epidural analgesic, it has a duration of action of 4 to 12 hours.[158,159] A loading dose may be from 0.1 to 0.4 mg followed by an epidural infusion of 0.02 to 0.15 mg/hr.

Meperidine is a less commonly used opioid. It can cause histamine release, bronchoconstriction, and myocardial depression, making it less desirable than some other opioid agents for pulmonary surgery.[160-162]

NEUROMUSCULAR BLOCKADE AGENTS

Most neuromuscular relaxants do not have significant effects on lung volumes or HPV, other than effects introduced by muscle relaxation in contrast to a direct drug effect. Muscle relaxants can alter bronchomotor tone through histamine release or by interacting with muscarinic receptors as structural analogs of acetylcholine.[163] It is noteworthy that the intrinsic effects of a particular muscle relaxant may not be as important as inadequate muscle relaxant reversal or residual effects of a muscle relaxant, which cause postoperative difficulty with hypoventilation. Patients with pulmonary disease are usually exquisitely sensitive to small decrements of muscle function; assurance of fully recovered muscle tone is necessary for successful extubation after thoracotomy. Thus the choice of agent may be dictated by the need for rapid tracheal intubation, the anticipated duration of surgery, and the ease of reversibility, rather than by the effects on respiratory physiology (except for histamine and possible cholinergic effects).

Rocuronium, vecuronium, and cisatracurium have minimal cardiovascular or respiratory system effects.[164,165] Rocuronium has a more rapid onset time than vecuronium and is thus a useful drug for rapid tracheal intubation.[166] Vecuronium and cisatracurium are purported to be devoid of histamine release properties, although one investigator found evidence for abnormal histamine levels without hemodynamic consequences in patients treated with 0.25 mg/kg of cisatracurium.[167-169] Cisatracurium is useful in patients with both liver and renal dysfunction because it is metabolized independently of renal and hepatic system involvement. Rocuronium, vecuronium, and cisatracurium are considered intermediate-acting agents.

Pancuronium is a longer-acting agent and may stimulate the sympathetic nervous system to cause a tachycardia.[170] This drug has minimal histamine-releasing effects but may potentiate vagally mediated bronchoconstriction.[170,171]

Succinylcholine is the most commonly used drug for a rapid-sequence intubation and confers excellent intubating conditions for double-lumen endotracheal tube placement. Succinylcholine results in minimal release of histamine but can cause anaphylactoid reactions and anaphylaxis in patients sensitized and allergic to this compound.[132,168,172-174] Side effects of bradycardia and fasciculation leading to postoperative muscle pain should be anticipated.

Mivacurium is a very short-acting neuromuscular blocking agent, metabolized by plasma cholinesterase. It may be useful as an infusion for short procedures which may end quickly or unexpectedly. Mivacurium has been shown to release histamine, however, with possible hemodynamic consequences.[175] These effects may be diminished by antihistamine agent premedication.[176]

Reversal of neuromuscular blockade is usually achieved by administration of neostigmine, pyridostigmine, or edrophonium. Anticholinesterase agents can provoke airway constriction by inhibiting the destruction of endogenous acetylcholine.[163] It is important to use an anticholinergic agent with these drugs to attenuate increases in airway resistance, although it has been shown that reversal of neuromuscular blockade with neostigmine and atropine or glycopyrrolate can still result in significant increases in airway resistance.[177]

LOCAL ANESTHETICS

Local anesthetics are often used for regional analgesia and/or anesthesia during thoracotomy. In addition to improved pain control, benefits of regional anesthetics include suppression of the neuroendocrine stress response, a positive effect on postoperative nitrogen balance, potential improvement in postoperative myocardial O_2 supply and demand balance, potential reduction in cardiac ischemia, and improvement in pulmonary function.[56-58,178-181] Increased ventilatory responses to CO_2 have been noted with low doses of local anesthetics; these are thought to be due to a central effect from intravenous administration or absorption of regionally administered local anesthetics.[182-185] It is postulated that the local anesthetic agents may depress inhibitory pathways, leading to unopposed excitatory activity with stimulation of ventilation.[186-188] At higher blood concentrations of local anesthetics, central nervous system

depression occurs, such that the ventilatory response to isocapnic hypoxia is significantly depressed at a blood level of 3.6 μg/mL of lidocaine.[189]

The effects of local anesthetics on nerve function and muscle tone must also be considered. Few ventilatory effects of regional anesthesia should be apparent unless intercostal or phrenic nerve function is impaired.[190-192] Similarly, high thoracic epidural blockade may impair efferent and afferent pathways for the intercostal nerve roots, thus compromising rib cage function.[193]

Lidocaine is a commonly used agent, both intravenously and in regional techniques. Intravenous administration is purported to depress airway reflexes, which may lead to bronchospasm; thus, it may be useful during induction in patients with poor cardiac function who might not otherwise tolerate higher doses of other induction agents. Lidocaine can be nebulized and given intratracheally to achieve the same effect. Lidocaine is also used with efficacy for neural blockade in epidural catheters. In the hypovolemic patient, however, a bolus dose of as little as 3 mL of 2% lidocaine via a thoracic epidural catheter can result in profound hypotension. Fractionated dosing is therefore encouraged.

Bupivacaine and ropivacaine are longer-acting local anesthetic agents that are used only for infiltrative and regional anesthesia techniques.[194] These agents are used effectively in small doses or as infusions to block nerve conduction. Bupivacaine has a narrower therapeutic concentration range than ropivacaine.[195,196] However, both can result in malignant cardiac arrhythmias. The respiratory function effects are similar to those of lidocaine.

HEMODYNAMIC AGENTS

Vasodilators such as sodium nitroprusside (SNP) and nitroglycerin (NTG) have traditionally been thought to blunt the HPV response, but this concept has been challenged, as some studies have shown no change in shunt fraction or oxygenation with SNP administration during thoracotomy.[197-201] Hydralazine does not affect HPV in dogs.[202] $PGF_{2\alpha}$ is a potent pulmonary vasoconstrictor that inhibits HPV only when injected into the atelectatic lung pulmonary artery; systemic administration has little effect.[93,203] Dopamine and dobutamine may inhibit HPV indirectly by increasing CO and Pv_{O_2}.[204,205]

Nitric oxide (NO) is an inhaled pulmonary vascular dilator that acts locally in well-ventilated areas of lung. As such, it can inhibit an HPV response; however, the combination of almitrine bimesylate (which potentiates HPV by causing nonspecific pulmonary vasoconstriction) and NO (to locally vasodilated well-ventilated lung segments) has been shown to increase Pa_{O_2} during OLV for thoracoscopic procedures.[206] Others have tried phenylephrine to augment HPV.[207] In 50% of the patients who responded, the addition of NO further increased Pa_{O_2} (see Chapter 6).

ADJUVANT MEDICATIONS

Bronchodilators are very useful during thoracotomy for both preventing and treating bronchospasm. Albuterol has been shown to reduce airway resistance when used in patients anesthetized with isoflurane.[208] Antimuscarinic agents, such as ipratropium bromide, cause bronchodilation by inhibiting parasympathetically mediated bronchoconstriction and may be used perioperatively to prevent and treat bronchospasm.

It is also important to consider the role of prevention of post-operative nausea and vomiting in thoracic surgical patients. The concern is not only for patient comfort but also for the goal of preventing incision dehiscence and/or rupture of pulmonary blebs from forceful vomiting efforts. Droperidol is a dopamine antagonist, but it has been suggested that droperidol can reverse serotonin-induced small airway constriction via antagonism of serotonin receptors in the airway.[209] Droperidol has been used successfully to treat status asthmaticus, however.[210] It is worth noting that droperidol does cause sedation marked by decreases in tidal volume and minute ventilation.[211] Ondansetron is a peripherally active antagonist of the serotonin receptor 5-HT3 and is marketed for prevention of vagally mediated emesis.[212] As such, it should have a salutary effect on pulmonary function, although this has not been widely investigated; one researcher found no effect of a selective 5-HT3 receptor antagonist on lung compliance and lung resistance changes provoked by 5-hydroxytryptamine.[213]

Nonsteroidal antiinflammatory medications (NSAIDs) are alleged to produce analgesia without opioid-related side effects. They therefore comprise a powerful adjunctive therapy for use in thoracic anesthesia to limit the side effects of opioids. Ketorolac is the most commonly used NSAID; it is especially useful in combination with epidural analgesia to augment analgesia for areas of the body not treated by the epidural infusion spread.[214] An example is pain from an apical chest tube placement, which may be referred to the ipsilateral shoulder. Ketorolac has been shown to decrease the postoperative requirements for opioid analgesics.[215]

THORACIC EPIDURAL ANALGESIA

The use of thoracic epidural analgesia (TEA) has been advocated for multiple reasons including improved postoperative pain control, the ability to use smaller doses of intraoperative opioids, intravenous anesthetic agents, and/or inhalation anesthetic agents resulting in more rapid emergence, and improved perioperative pulmonary outcomes. Ishibe et al found that TEA had no influence on HPV and may actually have increased flow diversion from a hypoxic lobe to improve arterial oxygenation in dogs.[216] This effect was attributed to decreased Pvo_2 and a lower CO caused by the TEA. One group, however, found that a combined general (GA) and TEA technique resulted in lower Pao_2 values and higher shunt fractions than the GA-only technique.[217] The authors, in part, attributed this effect to a greater depression of HPV as a result of a sympathectomy and/or absorption of systemic local anesthetics in the TEA-with-GA group.

CHOICES OF ANESTHETIC AGENTS FOR THORACOTOMY— SUMMARY

After pulmonary surgery, early extubation and rapid return of consciousness with good respiratory function are the predominant goals. The particular combination of anesthetic agents used to achieve intraoperative anesthesia consistent with these goals is probably not as important as the skill with which they are administered. This skill includes knowledge of the individual's underlying pathology, baseline pulmonary function, comorbid disease states, and the type and extent of surgery that is planned. Further, individual responses to drugs used for anesthesia vary widely, requiring the anesthesiologist to use each agent with caution. Some have claimed improved

pulmonary function with a total intravenous anesthetic technique (as compared with a volatile anesthesia-based technique).[128] It is more practical, however, to use volatile agents unless the patient demonstrates an abnormally large inhibition of HPV. A combined anesthetic of smaller doses of benzodiazepines, opioids (intravenously or regionally), and volatile agents can achieve the goal of effective anesthesia while minimizing the side effects of each agent.

Anesthetic Induction

Induction must be undertaken carefully when general anesthesia with endotracheal intubation is necessary for the procedure. An extended period of time breathing 100% O_2 (preoxygenation or denitrogenation) must be considered. Samian et al reported that patients with COPD take 9 to 10 minutes to achieve an end-tidal fractional O_2 concentration of 90% after breathing 100% O_2, whereas patients with normal lung function take only 2 to 3 minutes (Figure 7-8).[218] This is most likely because of ventilation perfusion and diffusion abnormalities in patients with severe emphysema.

Care should be taken to avoid induction agents that could increase the likelihood of bronchospasm. Olssen et al reported that patients with a history of COPD have a 10-fold increased risk of bronchospasm under anesthesia compared to patients without emphysema.[219] The patient should be well anesthetized prior to endotracheal intubation.

Induction is also a time fraught with the risk of hemodynamic instability. Severe hypotension may occur, and cardiac arrest has been reported.[220-225] Multiple reasons for this instability are outlined in Table 7-3. It is extremely important to avoid excessive ventilation immediately after induction—a circumstance that can occur with mask ventilation or when confirming endotracheal tube placement. Overventilation can lead to breath stacking, dynamic pulmonary hyperinflation (DPH), and auto-positive end-expiratory pressure (PEEP) with hemodynamic compromise and possible barotrauma. Hypoventilation with the ventilator timing set for a prolonged expiratory phase after induction may be advantageous until the degree of pulmonary dysfunction under anesthesia can be determined. Although it is often difficult to eliminate CO_2 in these patients during one-lung ventilation, hypercarbia in the absence of severe acidosis and hypoxia can be tolerated.[226]

Positioning

The majority of thoracic procedures are performed in the lateral position (most often the lateral decubitus position), but depending on the surgical technique, a supine, semisupine, or semiprone lateral position may be used. These positions have specific implications for the anesthesiologist that arise only rarely in cardiac or vascular anesthesia.

It is awkward to induce anesthesia in the lateral position. Thus, monitors will be placed, anesthesia will usually be induced in the supine position, and the anesthetized patient will then be repositioned for surgery. It is possible to induce anesthesia in the lateral position, which may be indicated infrequently with unilateral lung diseases (such as bronchiectasis or hemoptysis) until lung isolation can be achieved. Even these patients, however, will then have to be repositioned and the diseased lung turned to the nondependent side.

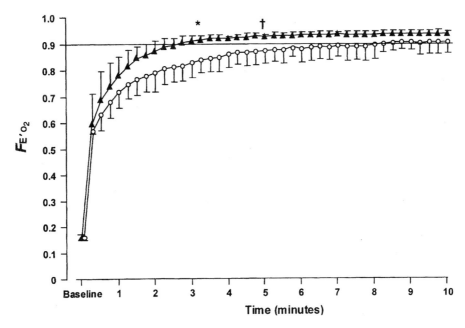

FIGURE 7-8 End-tidal oxygraphy over time in patients with and without chronic obstructive pulmonary disease (COPD). $F_E'O_2$, End-tidal fractional oxygen concentration, ▲, patients without COPD, **o**, patients with COPD. (From Samian E, Farah E, Delefosse D, et al: *Anaesthesia* 55:841, 2000.)

Because of the loss of venous vascular tone in the anesthetized patient, it is not uncommon to observe hypotension when turning the patient to or from the lateral position. This can occur at the beginning or end of the case and is more marked in patients who have a degree of intravascular volume depletion and those with sympathetic blockade from epidural local anesthesia. The anesthesiologist must always be observant for hemodynamic changes secondary to repositioning the patient.

All catheters and monitors will have to be secured during a position change and their function reassessed after repositioning. The anesthesiologist should take responsibility for the head, neck, and airway during position change and must be in charge of the operating team to direct repositioning. It is useful to make an initial "head-to-toe" survey of the patient after induction and intubation, checking oxygenation, ventilation, hemodynamics, catheters, monitors, and potential nerve injuries. This survey must then be repeated after repositioning. It is nearly impossible to avoid some movement of a double-lumen tube or bronchial blocker during repositioning.[227] Certainly the patient's head, neck, and endobronchial tube should be turned en bloc with the patient's thoracolumbar spine. However, the margin of error in positioning endobronchial tubes or blockers is often so narrow that even very small movements can have significant clinical implications.[228,229] The carina and mediastinum may shift independently with repositioning, leading to distal malplacement of a previously well-positioned tube.[230] Endobronchial tube/blocker position and the adequacy of ventilation must be rechecked by auscultation and fiberoptic bronchoscopy after patient repositioning. Access for additional intravascular catheters will be more difficult after the patient has been repositioned; this should be anticipated and all catheters placed, whenever possible, with the patient supine.

There is a specific set of nerve and vascular injuries related to the lateral position that must be understood and appreciated. The brachial plexus is the site of the majority of intraoperative nerve injuries related to the lateral position.[231] These are basically of two varieties: The majority of incidences are compression injuries of the brachial plexus of the dependent arm, but there is also significant risk of stretch injuries to the brachial plexus of the nondependent arm. The brachial plexus is fixed at two points: proximally by the transverse process of the cervical vertebrae and distally by the axillary fascia. This two-point fixation plus the extreme mobility of neighboring skeletal and muscular structures make the brachial plexus extremely liable to injury (Table 7-4). The patient should be positioned with padding under the dependent thorax (Figure 7-9) to keep the weight of the upper body off the dependent arm brachial plexus. This padding will exacerbate the pressure on the brachial plexus, however, if it migrates superiorly into the axilla.

TABLE 7-3

Postulated Mechanisms for Hypotension in Patients with Severe Emphysema During Induction of Anesthesia

Dynamic pulmonary hyperinflation (DPH)
Positive pressure ventilation
Application of extrinsic positive end-expiratory pressure
Pneumothorax
Vasodilatation from induction anesthetic agents
Sympathetic blockade from regional anesthesia
Hypovolemia
Myocardial ischemia

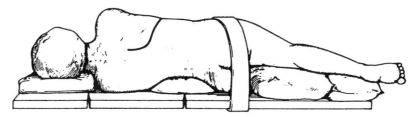

FIGURE 7-9 Padding under the dependent thorax. Typical positioning of a patient in the lateral decubitus position for thoracotomy seen from behind. It is useful for the anesthesiologist to survey the anesthetized patient from this perspective before draping to ensure that there is no lateral flexion of the cervical spine, which can be very difficult to appreciate from the head of the operating table. Note also padding of the dependent thorax and the nondependent leg. (From Pearson FG (ed): *Thoracic surgery*, New York, 1995, Churchill Livingstone.)

The brachial plexus of the nondependent arm is most at risk if it is suspended from an arm support or "ether screen"(Figure 7-10).[231] Traction on the brachial plexus in these situations is particularly likely to occur if the patient's trunk accidentally slips towards a semiprone or semisupine position after fixation of the nondependent arm. Vascular compression of the nondependent arm in this situation is also possible, and it is useful to monitor pulse oximetry in the nondependent hand to observe for this. The arm should not be abducted beyond 90 degrees and should not be extended posteriorly beyond the neutral position nor flexed anteriorly greater than 90 degrees. Fortunately, the majority of these nerve injuries resolve spontaneously over a period of months.

Anterior flexion of the arm at the shoulder (circumduction) across the chest or lateral flexion of the neck toward the opposite side can cause a traction injury of the suprascapular nerve.[232] This causes a deep, poorly circumscribed pain of posterior and lateral aspects of the shoulder and may be responsible for some cases of postthoracotomy shoulder pain.

It is very easy after repositioning the patient in the lateral decubitus position to cause excessive lateral flexion of the cervical spine because of improper positioning of the patient's head. This malpositioning, which exacerbates brachial plexus traction, can cause a "whiplash" syndrome and can be difficult to appreciate from the head of the operating table, particularly after the surgical drapes have been placed. It is useful for the anesthesiologist to survey the patient from the side of the table immediately after turning to ensure that the entire vertebral column is properly aligned.

The dependent leg should be flexed slightly, with padding under the knee to protect the peroneal nerve lateral to the proximal head of the fibula. The nondependent leg is placed in a neutral extended position, and padding is placed between it and the dependent leg. The dependent leg must be observed for vascular compression. Excessively tight strapping at the hip level can compress the sciatic nerve of the nondependent leg.

Other sites particularly liable for neurovascular injury in the lateral position are the dependent ear pinna and eye. A "head-to-toe" protocol to monitor for possible neurovascular injuries related to the lateral decubitus position is presented in Table 7-5.

Paraplegia has been reported as a complication of thoracotomy, but its incidence has been related to surgical trauma and not to positioning. Potential causes of paraplegia related to thoracotomy include damage to spinal branches of the intercostal arteries, creation of a communication between the epidural and

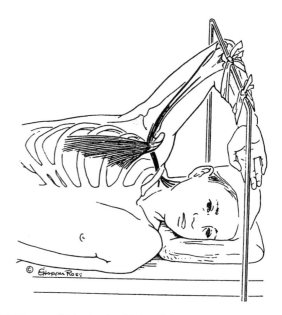

FIGURE 7-10 Bilateral malpositioning of the arms in the lateral decubitus position. The dependent arm is directly under the thorax with the potential for vascular compression and injury to the brachial plexus. The nondependent arm is hyperextended and fixed to an anesthetic screen. This causes traction of the brachial plexus as it passes under the clavicle and the tendon of the pectoralis minor muscle. (From Britt BA, Gordon RA: *Can Anaesth Soc J* 11:51, 1964.)

TABLE 7-4	
The Brachial Plexus Extremely Liable to Injury	
Location/type of injury	**Cause of injury**
Dependent arm (compression injuries)	Arm directly under thorax
	Pressure on clavicle into retroclavicular space
	Cervical rib
	Caudal migration of thorax padding into the axilla*
Nondependent arm (stretch injuries)	Lateral flexion of cervical spine
	Excessive abduction of arm (>90%)
	Semiprone or semisupine repositioning after arm fixed to a support

*Unfortunately this padding under the thorax is misnamed an "axillary roll" in some institutions. This padding absolutely should NOT be placed in the axilla.

TABLE 7-5

A "Head-to-Toe" Protocol to Monitor for Possible Neurovascular Injuries Related to the Lateral Decubitus Position

Area to be surveyed	Special considerations
Dependent eye	
Dependent ear pinna	
Dependent arm	Brachial plexus
	Circulation
*Nondependent arm	Brachial plexus
	Circulation
Dependent and nondependent suprascapular nerve	
Nondependent leg sciatic nerve	
Dependent leg	Peroneal nerve
	Circulation

*Neurovascular injuries of the nondependent arm are more likely to occur if the arm is suspended or held in an independently positioned armrest.

pleural spaces, and accidental intradural placement of hemostatic gauze to control bleeding from the deep-posterior end of the incision.[233] Because epidural hematoma is a possible complication of neuraxial analgesia, the anesthesiologist should be aware of these other potential causes of spinal cord injury from thoracotomy incisions.

Choices of Ventilation

The properties of the ventilator used may influence the intraoperative course of the patient. A volume-controlled ventilator, such as is found on many anesthesia machines, delivers a preset volume without regard for the pressure necessary to deliver that volume. Use of a pressure-limited ventilator can be considered and has been advocated in the literature.[234] The advantages of this approach are that if auto-PEEP or breath stacking should occur, the ventilator senses the accumulating pressure and responds by reducing the volume of the next breath; an alarm for low minute ventilation alerts the anesthesiologist if this phenomenon compromises minute ventilation. A "best inspiratory pressure level" can be sought by adjusting the pressure support settings and the duration of inspiratory-to-expiratory phases—minute ventilation can be assessed by evaluating the tidal volumes and the set ventilator rate. Newer anesthesia machines may allow the choice of pressure-control ventilation, although the pressure-support mode for augmentation of spontaneous ventilation is rarely available. If the routine operating room ventilator does not possess the required technology for pressure-limited and/or pressure-support ventilation, the use of a freestanding ICU ventilator with a total intravenous anesthesia technique may be required. Strict attention must always be paid to the peak and mean airway pressures, as these are surrogate measures for retained volume in the lungs. Flow volume loops are available on selected ventilators; these can display breath stacking directly by observation of continued expiratory flow at the point of starting the next inspiration.

A patient at risk for incomplete exhalation (as in cases of severe emphysema, asthma, dynamic intrinsic thoracic obstruction) might benefit from decreasing the inspiratory time with subsequent prolongation of the exhalation time. This strategy has been shown to reduce pulmonary hyperinflation with intrinsic PEEP.[235] In extreme settings, intermittent disconnection from the ventilator might be required to allow expiration of trapped pulmonary gas.

Most thoracic surgical procedures require controlled ventilation, especially with the need for OLV. Occasionally, however, spontaneous respiration may be the ventilatory strategy of choice, such as for procedures to treat or diagnose an anterior mediastinal mass. This is a situation in which the option of pressure support of spontaneous respiratory efforts may be advantageous to prevent atelectasis, hypoxia, and/or hypercarbia.

Use of Regional Anesthesia as the Sole Anesthetic for Thoracotomy

Historically, epidural anesthesia has been successfully used as a primary anesthetic for thoracic operations in spontaneously breathing patients.[236] This technique has regained favor and is especially useful in patients for whom general anesthesia and/or mechanical ventilation would pose an additional risk. The limits of using TEA as a sole anesthetic and the innervation of the thoracic structures are important to understand when considering the use of this technique. One consideration is that the operative position is lateral or partially lateral. The patient must be able to cooperate and tolerate single-lung spontaneous ventilation that is solely dependent on diaphragmatic mechanics. Should a patient develop dyspnea or should an intraoperative emergency occur, intubation of the patient would have to take place in the lateral position. Further, the contralateral airway is not protected from spillage of blood or other secretions from the operative lung. Knowledge of which structures are effectively anesthetized by thoracic epidural blockade is equally important (Table 7-6). Intercostal nerves innervate the chest wall, parietal pleura, and the peripheral diaphragm; the anterior and posterior pulmonary plexuses (both vagal and sympathetic fibers) innervate the lungs, visceral pleura, and pericardium; and the phrenic nerve innervates the mediastinal pleura, as well as the upper and lower surfaces of the central diaphragm.[237-241] The sympathetic fibers emerge from thoracic level 1 to thoracic level 5 and can be blocked, but the vagal fibers and the phrenic nerve will not be affected by TEA. Thus, potentially, sensation from parts of the lung, visceral pleura, diaphragm, and pericardium will not be affected by thoracic epidural blockade. This technique should be considered for procedures on structures that can be effectively anesthetized with TEA with or without supplementation by local anesthetic infiltration from the operative field.

TABLE 7-6

Innervation of Thoracic Structures

Nerve innervation	Structure innervated
Intercostal nerves	Chest wall, parietal pleural, peripheral diaphragm
Anterior and posterior pulmonary plexuses (vagal and sympathetic fibers)	Lungs, visceral pleura, pericardium
Phrenic nerve	Mediastinal pleura, upper and lower surfaces of the central diaphragm, pericardium

Williams et al reported the use of TEA as the sole anesthetic for repair of a bronchopleural fistula, which developed after a right pneumonectomy.[242] A thoracoscopy, small rib resection, and limited thoracotomy for a rib resection were accomplished successfully with a thoracic epidural catheter placed at thoracic level 7 to 8 to achieve anesthesia of thoracic 2 to 10 dermatomes. Similarly, Kempen used a thoracic epidural combined with an interpleural block for pleurodesis in a patient with recurrent pneumothorax, and Mukaida et al reported the sole use of TEA in four high-risk patients undergoing video-assisted thoracic surgery.[243,244] Pertinent to thoracic surgical procedures, coronary artery bypass grafting has also been performed under TEA through a left anterior thoracotomy.[245] The authors note that the patient felt localized pain at the proximal end of the left internal mammary artery dissection (which was treated with local infiltration of lidocaine) and felt referred shoulder pain with pericardial dissection (which was similarly treated by bathing the pleural space with lidocaine). All of the authors who report using this technique for intrathoracic procedures claim great patient satisfaction with avoidance of intubation and superior perioperative pain control.

Intraoperative Management of Fluids

The lung appears to be highly sensitive to injury and may accumulate interstitial fluid. This appears to occur more readily when lung tissue has been manipulated in the course of an operation, but it can also occur when the site of the operation is distant from the lungs. Certain operations—pneumonectomy, some thoracotomies, and even fewer thoracoscopies—are more prone to result in postoperative pulmonary edema. Therefore, the amount and type of fluids used during the course of thoracic procedures have been the subject of much debate.

The first issue is the role of intravenous (IV) colloid vs. crystalloid fluids. Among the benefits proposed for colloid solutions are slower and perhaps more limited translocation of the fluid from the intravascular (IVC) compartment to the extravascular space (EVC).[246,247] Improved tissue microperfusion with reduced endothelial swelling (resulting in improved tissue oxygen tension) has been proposed as another benefit.[248] Other studies, however, not only do not find a clinical difference in outcome between crystalloid and colloid use but also have found increased long-term mortality with colloid use in septic patients.[249-250] Ernst et al found that colloid agents, once translocated to the EVC space, actually increased the volume of that space in excess of the amount of colloid given in septic patients.[247] Others found that colloid administration can promote lung water retention in burn patients.[251]

A second issue is the amount of fluid to administer. In a review of the literature on post–lung resection pulmonary edema (to follow), the total *volume* of fluid seems to be a critical contributory (but not necessarily causative) factor for post–lung resection pulmonary edema. Perioperative fluid loading could aggravate primary mechanisms and patient risk factors by increasing cardiac output, pulmonary artery pressures, and the net filtration pressure across the pulmonary capillary bed, thus increasing the risk of fluid translocation to the pulmonary interstitial space. Rather than administer fluids to a preset determination based on the number of hours since oral intake and to replace insensible losses (as for other types of

surgical procedures), the following method should be considered. It can be proposed that a combination of crystalloid and colloid IV fluids be used for patients during thoracic surgery to attempt prevention of post–lung resection pulmonary edema. A minimal amount of crystalloid intravenous fluid can be administered initially with the understanding that much of this fluid will translocate to the EVC space. It is helpful to predetermine a set volume that is felt to be safe for a particular patient's risk of post–lung resection pulmonary edema; 1 to 2 L is a common recommendation. Further fluids can be administered as colloids to replace intravascular volume when necessary, as a lower total fluid volume is needed to replace those operative losses. The total amount of IV fluid to be given can be guided by indices of adequate volume status, such as urine output and central venous pressure. Decreases in blood pressure alone do not necessarily need to be treated with fluid boluses because positional changes and vasoactive agents can be used to support hemodynamics if urine output and CVP are adequate.

The decision to transfuse blood products is also controversial. It can be argued that a patient at risk of hypoxemia as a result of severe pulmonary disease should maintain a higher hemoglobin count than a patient with normal lungs. The absolute hemoglobin count that is considered safe, however, is unknown. It would seem prudent to transfuse blood below a hemoglobin of 7 g/dL to preserve oxygenation, with the goal of stable hemodynamics and respiratory parameters, especially during OLV. An argument in favor of transfusion is that blood is a colloid that should not significantly translocate to the interstitial space. Arguments against liberal transfusion criteria include the known infectious risks, the immunosuppressive effects of transfusion, and the association of transfusion with poorer outcomes.[252-254] The use of blood products such as fresh frozen plasma, platelets, and cryoprecipitate should be guided by indices of coagulation abnormalities such as abnormal laboratory parameters and/or diffuse microvascular bleeding noted in the operative field. To avoid a dilutional coagulopathy, transfusion of these products must be considered once 5 to 10 units of packed red cells have been administered.

Emergence

The first decision about emergence is whether to allow a particular patient to emerge from anesthesia at all. Emergence from anesthesia may be complicated by problems such as bronchospasm, laryngospasm, and the adverse consequences of respiratory efforts that are not synchronous with the ventilator during this period of time (risking damage to marginally viable lung tissue resulting in persistent air leaks). Further, perioperative respiratory depression may lead to reintubation early in the postoperative period. However, patients left intubated after thoracic surgery have been reported to have a higher mortality rate and a prolonged hospital stay.[255]

The first consideration for evaluating the appropriateness of extubation is an evaluation of the patient's muscle strength. Patients with pulmonary disease are exquisitely sensitive to neuromuscular blockade. Thus a patient must have recovered from intraoperative neuromuscular blockade sufficiently to allow the neuromuscular blockade reversal agents to work. Full reversal of neuromuscular blockade is recommended because of increased reliance of patients with pulmonary disease on secondary muscles of respiration. With adequate muscle tone, extubation and spontaneous ventilation can improve hemodynamic parameters and minimize DPH and should decrease stress on pulmonary suture lines.

The next consideration is whether the patient is hemodynamically stable and warm. Increased oxygen consumption requirements resulting from hemodynamic instability and/or hypothermia with shivering can place a patient with marginal respiratory function at risk. For these reasons, adequate volume administration, stable blood pressure, and heart rate and rhythm compatible with normal hemodynamics should be achieved before extubation. Although the absolute temperature at which a patient should remain intubated and sedated is unknown, it would be prudent to consider postoperative ventilation in patients with body temperatures lower than 35° C. A patient who is at risk for a coagulopathy may need to be even warmer to consider emergence.

A third consideration is to control airway reflexes with extubation to avoid "bucking" in an attempt to minimize postoperative air leaks. Some have suggested that the laryngeal mask might be useful for maintaining intraoperative pulmonary function, as it provokes less respiratory irritation than do endotracheal tubes.[256] Although laryngeal mask use is not feasible for thoracotomy and the achievement of OLV, this approach may be considered at the end of a thoracic surgery to improve the chance of extubation in a bronchospastic patient.

A fourth consideration is the adequacy of analgesia. Postoperative analgesia should have been planned in advance, with adequate analgesia augmenting the probability of a successful extubation. Adequate inspiratory and expiratory muscle function must be ensured when a regional analgesic technique using local anesthetics has been administered. The use of opioids as the only analgesic (intravenously, spinally or epidurally) may lead to hypoventilation and severe hypercarbia in the postoperative period—thus, combining opioids with nonopioid medications may be optimal.

The pathophysiology of severe chronic obstructive pulmonary disease (COPD) suggests that the duration of emergence from anesthesia may be slower than for patients without emphysema. As previously noted, volatile agents in concentrations as low as 0.1 MAC can depress the ventilatory response to hypoxia, and the effect is more profound in patients with emphysema.[257,258] Patients with COPD have a higher volume of deadspace, both when awake and when under GA; the $Paco_2$ is also significantly higher for spontaneously breathing patients under GA.[40] Preoperative medications such as midazolam may have a prolonged and profound effect on minute ventilation, especially in response to elevations in $Paco_2$.[40] Therefore it can be expected that the emphysematous patient may take a prolonged time to return to full wakefulness and adequate respiratory function. Vigilance during this time period is essential to avoid hypercarbia and respiratory failure.

A patient in a high-risk category for postoperative respiratory failure based on preoperative evaluation may derive the greatest benefit from a staged approach to emergence and extubation.[259] Such an approach may include establishment of effective thoracic epidural analgesia even for minimally invasive procedures, as well as planned postoperative mechanical ventilation.

Potential Intraoperative Complications

Hypoxia

Hypoxia during thoracic surgical procedures is a common problem. Patients often present with intrinsic pulmonary disease upon which OLV is superimposed. A complex set of interactions among inspired O_2 tension, shunt, HPV, intrinsic and extrinsic PEEP, and alveolar ventilation determine the resultant intraoperative PaO_2. A study by Katz et al demonstrated the acute fall in PaO_2 with OLV followed by a slower, persistent fall in PaO_2 over time (Figure 7-11).[260] Multiple mechanisms contribute to hypoxemia and its limitation. An extensive discussion of OLV is presented in Chapter 4.

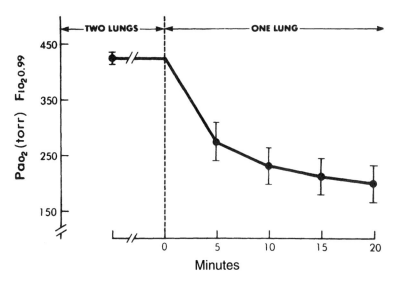

FIGURE 7-11 Arterial oxygen partial pressure with one-lung ventilation, showing the fall of arterial oxygen pressure over time after the institution of one-lung ventilation in the lateral position. Note the acute decrease followed by a more gradual decrease in Pao_2. (From Katz JA, Laverene RG, Fairley B, et al: *Anesthesiology* 56:164, 1982.)

Briefly, OLV imposes an obligatory shunt with an initial loss of approximately 50% of the ventilatory capacity of the pulmonary system. Factors that allow patients to tolerate OLV include a high F_{IO_2} and adequate alveolar ventilation. Further, under ideal conditions, HPV works quickly to limit perfusion to the atelectatic lung, with the result that the shunt effect is limited to about 20% to 30% of the total blood flow.[261] Thus, many patients can tolerate OLV for extended periods. When considering intraoperative causes for hypoxia, clinicians first must check the inspired O_2 concentration and ensure ventilation through a properly located endotracheal tube. Second, the effects of volatile agents and/or vasodilatory agents on the HPV response must be considered (see Table 7-2). Other causes of a reduced HPV response could be surgical positioning and manipulation.[91]

Treatment for hypoxemia includes the application of continuous positive airway pressure to the operative lung, extrinsic PEEP to the nonoperative lung, intermittent reinflation of the operative lung, and mechanical occlusion of blood flow to the operative lung (such as clamping the pulmonary artery).

Dynamic Pulmonary Hyperinflation and Auto-PEEP

Some of the most frequent intraoperative problems are due to dynamic pulmonary hyperinflation (DPH) and auto-PEEP, which can lead to progressive increases in end-expiratory volume and pressure within the lungs (Figure 7-12).[262-264] These conditions, which are common in patients with emphysema undergoing mechanical ventilation, can be aggravated by overventilation, inappropriate inspiration or expiration settings, high-resistance endotracheal tubes, the application of external PEEP, and/or use of a volume-controlled ventilator without alarms for increasing baseline pressure levels.[262,263] DPH and auto-PEEP may be particularly problematic with OLV because the entire ventilatory demand is placed on a single dependent, diseased lung. Hemodynamic consequences include impaired venous return, a tamponade-like effect on the right ventricle from hyperinflated lungs, compression of the alveolar blood vessels by elevated intraalveolar pressures, and right ventricle dysfunction contributing to left ventricle dysfunction.[264]

Unfortunately, the development of DPH or auto-PEEP has been called "occult," as standard anesthesia machines or most ICU ventilatory monitors do not detect it readily.[222] DPH or auto-PEEP may be an underappreciated cause of cardiac arrest because of electromechanical dissociation.[221-224] Ideally, an expiratory flowmeter can be used to monitor for DPH, especially for the purpose of constructing intraoperative flow-volume loops.[265] Knowledge of the physiology of emphysema and vigilance may be the best methods to detect the accumulation of trapped pulmonary volume. Upon recognition of this problem, the patient should be disconnected from the ventilator immediately and allowed to exhale. Depending on the amount of trapped air, this may take many seconds or several minutes. Hemodynamic parameters should improve with exhalation, but resuscitative medications may be necessary as well.

Ducros et al illustrated the problem of auto-PEEP and air trapping under two-lung supine, two-lung lateral, and OLV lateral conditions (Figure 7-13).[266] Patients with mild emphysema displayed minimal air trapping and developed auto-PEEP only with OLV, and patients with restrictive lung disease demonstrated little air trapping or auto-PEEP in all positions. Patients with severe emphysema, however, demonstrated high levels of auto-PEEP while supine with two-lung ventilation, which increased with OLV; they also maintained high levels of trapped air. Thus, pulmonary air trapping must be suspected in patients with mild or moderate obstructive lung disease during OLV and in those with severe COPD upon initiation of mechanical ventilation.

Barotrauma

Barotrauma can occur as the result of a sustained increase in intramural airway pressure secondary to alveolar overdistention. Unfortunately, alveolar volume is imperfectly related to alveolar pressure and is not easily measurable. In the setting of severe lung disease, attention to and minimization of airway pressures during mechanical ventilation continue to be means of preventing barotrauma.

The risk of barotrauma increases with high intrapleural pressure, increased expiratory resistance because of endotracheal tubes (especially dual-lumen tubes), increased resistance with coughing or "bucking" against the ventilator, and inappropriate

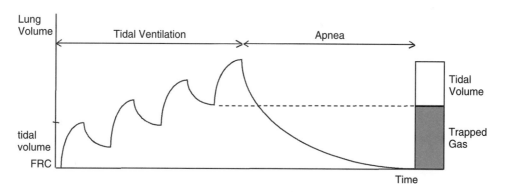

FIGURE 7-12 The development of dynamic pulmonary hyperinflation during mechanical ventilation and a representation of lung deflation during apnea. *FRC,* Functional residual capacity. (From Myles PS, Ryder IG, Weeks AM, et al: *J Cardiothorac Vasc Anesth* 11:100, 1997.)

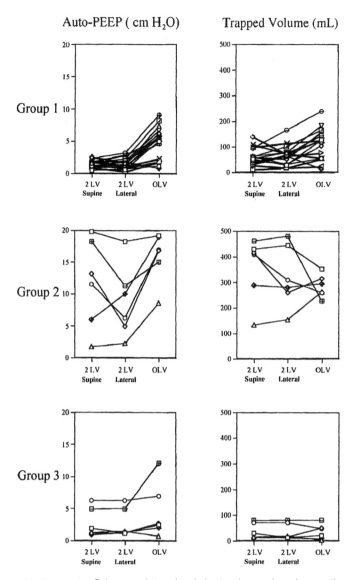

Auto-PEEP (cm H$_2$O)   Trapped Volume (mL)

Group 1

Group 2

Group 3

FIGURE 7-13 Pulmonary air trapping during two-lung and one-lung ventilation. In this study, patients were divided into three groups. *Group 1* consisted of routine thoracic surgery patients with mild obstructive airway disease; *group 2* consisted of patients for lung transplant with severe obstructive airway disease (severe emphysema); and *group 3* consisted of patients for lung transplant with severe restrictive pulmonary disease (pulmonary fibrosis). Auto-PEEP and milliliters (mL) of trapped air volume were measured during three surgical patient positions: two-lung supine, two-lung lateral, and one-lung lateral (OLV). Patients with mild obstructive airway disease only developed auto-PEEP with OLV and displayed only minimal air trapping. Patients with restrictive lung disease generated minimal amounts of auto-PEEP and trapped air. However, patients with severe emphysema had high levels of auto-PEEP after induction of anesthesia, and auto-PEEP increased with OLV; these patients also maintained high levels of trapped air. (From Ducros L, Moutafis M, Castelain MH, et al: *J Cardiothorac Vasc Anesth* 13:35, 1999.)

levels of extrinsic PEEP. The hemodynamic effects of barotrauma are similar to DPH but also include mediastinal shift toward the nontraumatized lung and a postulated negative inotropic effect. Further, increased inflation pressures in the nontraumatized lung can occur while it is being compressed by the volume of gas in the contralateral interpleural space.

Avoidance of barotrauma may be aided by the use of muscle relaxants, intermittent disconnection from the ventilator, long expiratory-to-inspiratory phase times, and vigilance in this high-risk patient population. Amato et al have shown improved outcomes in patients with acute respiratory distress syndrome in the ICU using a "lung-protective strategy," which included limiting peak and plateau inspiratory pressures.[267]

Barotrauma in the form of a pneumothorax can occur in the contralateral dependent lung during thoracic procedures; it can quickly become a tension pneumothorax with positive pressure ventilation.[268] Emergent treatment should include resuscitative vasoactive medications as necessary, and relief of intrapleural pressure through many methods, from needle placement to tube thoracostomy. It may be necessary to turn a patient with an open incision from a lateral to a supine position for adequate resuscitation. Barotrauma can also manifest as pneumomediastinum, pneumoperitoneum, and subcutaneous emphysema.

Hemorrhage

Hemorrhage is an ever-present danger with any surgical procedure, but it is especially a possibility in thoracic surgery, during which the great vessels are in proximity to the area of surgery. Clinicians must therefore be prepared for acute, rapid blood loss at any time during the procedure. It is prudent to be prepared with large-bore IV access and to have a blood sample screened in the blood bank. Larger or more difficult resections may mandate cross-match of packed red cells.

Adjacent Organ Injury

Organs in proximity to the lungs may be compromised during thoracic surgery. Cardiac irritation or compression with brief hemodynamic deterioration and/or arrhythmias is relatively common. Good communication between the surgeon and anesthesiologist will prevent overreaction but will also facilitate limiting the amount of time during which the patient's condition is unstable. Ensurance of normal electrolyte and acid-base status during surgery should allow the patient to tolerate cardiac manipulation as necessary. Atrial fibrillation is common after thoracic procedures, but it can occur intraoperatively as well. Early cardioversion may be the most efficacious treatment. Rarely is cardiac ischemia provoked by the surgical procedure per se. However, a patient with severe coronary artery disease may become ischemic intraoperatively because of the stress of the surgical procedure. Appropriate monitoring and attention to control of hemodynamic parameters should allow early detection and lessen the probability of serious intraoperative consequences.

Other organs and structures that may be compromised or injured include the esophagus, trachea, thoracic duct, phrenic nerve, and the recurrent laryngeal nerve. Injuries to these structures may not be apparent until after the procedure has been completed (see Chapter 17).

Immediate Postoperative Management
The Role of ICU Care

Whether patients are intubated or extubated, a period of postoperative ICU care or intensive postanesthetic care unit observation is indicated for patients who have undergone a thoracic surgical procedure. This period may be as short as that required to ensure adequate pulmonary function postoperatively, assess the chest radiograph, optimize analgesia, and assess any issues related to the operation. The ICU observation period can be lengthened as required to address any of the foregoing considerations if conditions are abnormal. ICU care should always be used for the patient with preexisting severe pulmonary dysfunction, as thoracic procedures themselves can increase that dysfunction (reduction in FRC, depression of respiratory drive, impaired mechanics of ventilation, impaired gas exchange), even in healthy patients.[269]

Immediate postoperative concerns include confirmation of adequate respiratory function, especially ventilation. It is not uncommon for patients to have a mild respiratory acidosis; this should improve over the first postoperative hours. Absence of a significant pneumothorax and significant pulmonary edema must also be confirmed. The chest tubes must be functioning properly with the correct amount of suction or water seal for a particular operation. It is especially important to ensure the patency and lack of kinking of the tubes. Analgesia should be optimized before transfer to a ward where the staff is less able to address significant pain issues. Should parenteral and/or epidural opioids be administered, care must be taken to monitor respiratory function meticulously because patients with severe pulmonary dysfunction are uniquely susceptible to CO_2 retention from the ventilatory depressant effects of the opioids. Supplemental analgesics devoid of respiratory depression (such as ketorolac) should be considered if appropriate. A blood count and electrolytes should be checked if major intraoperative volume shifts occurred. Although it is uncommon to find significant renal impairment in the immediate postoperative period, attention should be paid to ensurance of adequate urine output, as many thoracic patients have received a smaller total volume of fluid intraoperatively than other types of surgical patients.

PULMONARY EDEMA

Perioperative pulmonary edema, although it is usually not an immediate postoperative problem, is a pertinent concern for anesthesiologists.[270,271] Most of the descriptive information known about this syndrome of post–lung resection pulmonary edema is from studies of postpneumonectomy patients.[270-272] It has an incidence of 2% to 4% after pneumonectomies (incidence of right-lung edema higher than for left) and 1% after lobectomies, and its incidence is estimated at 0.1% to 0.2% after thoracoscopic surgery. Radiologic signs may appear before symptoms, which occur on postoperative days 2 to 4. There is a high mortality rate (30% to 50%), and the syndrome is resistant to treatment. Post–lung resection pulmonary edema can occur with normal pulmonary capillary wedge pressure (PCWP), although the measurement of PCWP may be misleading post-pneumonectomy.[270,273,274] The physiology of post–lung resection pulmonary edema is unclear. Some authors have implicated the volume of fluid given to the patient in the operative and immediate postoperative period. This belief is based on a number of small studies. Zeldin et al examined 10 patients with postpneumonectomy pulmonary edema but had adequate fluid data on only 40% of the patients.[275] They concluded that postpneumonectomy pulmonary edema was associated with a right pneumonectomy, a large operative fluid load, and an

increased postoperative urine output. Verheijen-Breemharr, Parquin et al and Mathru and Blakeman supported Zeldin's findings.[276-278]

The pathophysiology of pulmonary edema, however, may not entirely rest on the fluid balance. In two other studies, no correlation with perioperative fluid load was found.[272,279] Alvarez et al found that pneumonectomy patients with postoperative pulmonary edema had a net mean perioperative fluid intake of 1.4 L.[280]

If fluid loading is not the only causative factor, what are the possible mechanisms (Table 7-7)?[281-283] Disruption of the lymphatic system after lung and lymph node resection may lead to a decreased ability of the lung to absorb interstitial fluid. With lung resection, the blood flow to the remaining lung increases proportionally, leading to relatively increased pulmonary capillary perfusion pressure and, potentially, to edema resulting from hydrostatic pressure. A pulmonary panendothelial injury may also occur with lung deflation and reinflation during pulmonary resection. Additionally, hyperinflation of the remaining lung tissue, especially in the dependent lung during surgery or in the remaining lung after pneumonectomy, can lead to capillary endothelial damage with subsequent loss of the ability to prevent fluid accumulation in the lung tissue. Cytokine activation, relative oxygen toxicity with oxidative stress, and an ischemia/reperfusion injury during surgery have also been suggested. Further, microembolization of particulate matter such as fat, bone, or blood clots may occur.

Risk factors for post–lung resection pulmonary edema include a larger resection (shunting more of the cardiac output to the remaining lung tissue), difficult intraoperative ventilation (possibly by causing more pulmonary endothelial damage in the remaining lung tissue), prior radiation and/or chemotherapy, and resection of highly perfused lung tissue identified on preoperative ventilation perfusion scan (again shunting proportionally more blood flow to remaining lung tissue). It would seem prudent to manage fluids conservatively during surgery, as was discussed for patients considered to be at high risk of post–lung resection pulmonary edema. Postoperatively, fluid administration can be guided by central venous pressure and urine output.

Summary

Caring for the patient who is undergoing a thoracotomy can be very challenging. Immediate preoperative, intraoperative, and immediate postoperative considerations have been addressed. As always, patient pathophysiology, anesthesiologist judgment,

---

TABLE 7-7

Postulated Mechanisms for the Formation of Post–Lung Resection Pulmonary Edema

Lymphatic disruption
Increased pulmonary capillary perfusion pressure
Lung hyperinflation–capillary endothelial damage
Cytokine activation
Relative oxygen toxicity
Ischemia/reperfusion injury
Microembolization

and individual patient reaction to OLV, anesthetics, and intraoperative events will dictate the actual course. Knowledge of anticipated events and potential problems may prevent or limit intraoperative morbidity.

REFERENCES

1. Shoemaker WC, Montgomery ES, Kaplan E, Elwyn DH: Physiologic patterns in surviving and nonsurviving shock patients. Use of sequential cardiorespiratory parameters in defining criteria for therapeutic goals and early warning of death, *Arch Surg* 106:630, 1973.
2. Shoemaker WC, Appel PL, Kram H, et al: Prospective trial of supranormal values of survivors as therapeutic goals in high-risk patients, *Chest* 94:1176, 1988.
3. Fleming A, Bishop M, Shoemaker W, et al: Prospective trial of supranormal values as goals of resuscitation in severe trauma, *Arch Surg* 127:1175, 1992.
4. Boyd O, Grounds RM, Bennett ED: A randomized clinical trial of the effects of deliberate perioperative increase of oxygen delivery on mortality in high-risk surgical patients, *JAMA* 270:2699, 1993.
5. Bishop MH, Shoemaker WC, Appel PL, et al: Prospective, randomized trial of survivor values of cardiac index, oxygen delivery, and oxygen consumption as resuscitation endpoints in severe trauma, *J Trauma* 38:780, 1995.
6. Wilson J, Woods I, Fawcett J, et al: Reducing the risk of major elective surgery: randomized controlled trial of preoperative optimization of oxygen delivery, *BMJ* 318:1099, 1999.
7. Martin R, Ramsay, JG: Cardiac output technologies, *Int Anesthesiol Clin* 34:79, 1996.
8. Jansen JRC, Schreuder JJ, Bogaard JM, et al: Thermodilution technique for measurement of cardiac output during artificial ventilation, *J Appl Physiol* 50:584, 1981.
9. Segal J, Pearl RG, Ford AJ Jr, et al: Instantaneous and continuous cardiac output obtained with a Doppler pulmonary artery catheter, *J Am Coll Cardiol* 13:1382, 1989.
10. Tuman KJ, Carroll GC, Ivankovich AD: Pitfalls in interpretation of pulmonary artery catheter data, *J Cardiothorac Vasc Anesth* 3:625, 1989.
11. Fontes ML, Bellows W, Ngo L, et al: Assessment of ventricular function in critically ill patients: limitations of pulmonary artery catheterization, *J Cardiothorac Vasc Anesth* 13:521, 1999.
12. Slung HB, Scher KS: Complications of the Swan-Ganz catheter, *World J Surg* 8:76, 1984.
13. Dalen JE, Bone RC: Is it time to pull the pulmonary artery catheter? *JAMA* 276:916, 1996.
14. Schwartz AJ, Conahan TJ III: Pulmonary artery catheters: there are still concerns with their routine use, *J Cardiothorac Vasc Anesth* 92:727, 1987.
15. Robin ED: Death by pulmonary artery flow-directed catheter: time for a moratorium? *Chest* 92:727, 1987 (editorial).
16. Connors AF, Speroff T, Dawson NV: The effectiveness of right heart catheterization in the initial care of critically ill patients, *JAMA* 276:889, 1996.
17. Pulmonary Artery Catheter Consensus Conference Participants: Pulmonary artery consensus conference: consensus statement, *Crit Care Med* 25:910, 1997.
18. Mueller HS, Chatterjee K, Davis KB, et al: ACC expert consensus document. Present use of bedside right heart catheterization in patients with cardiac disease, *J Am Coll Cardiol* 32:840, 1998.
19. Cooper AB, Doig GS, Sibbald WJ: Pulmonary artery catheters in the critically ill. An overview using the methodology of evidence-based medicine, *Crit Care Clin* 12:777, 1996.
20. Tuman KJ, Roizen MF: Outcome assessment and pulmonary artery catheterization: why does the debate continue? *Anesth Analg* 84:1, 1997.
21. Ivanov R, Allen J, Calvin, JE: The incidence of major morbidity in critically ill patients managed with pulmonary artery catheters: a meta-analysis, *Crit Care Med* 28:615, 2000.
22. Tuchschmidt J, Fried J, Astiz M, et al: Elevation of cardiac output and oxygen delivery improves outcome in septic shock, *Chest* 102:216, 1992.
23. Prielipp RC, Morell R: Con: swan song for the Swan-Ganz? *APSF newslet,* 1997.
24. Darmon PL, Hillel Z, Mogtader A, et al: Cardiac output by transesophageal echocardiography using continuous wave Doppler across the aortic valve, *Anesthesiology* 18:796, 1994.
25. Harpole DH, Clements FN, Quill T, et al: Right and left ventricular performance during and after abdominal aortic aneurysm repair, *Ann Surg* 20:356, 1989.
26. Cahalan MK, Ionescu P, Melton HE, et al: Automated real-time analysis of intraoperative transesophageal echocardiograms, *Anesthesiology* 78:477, 1993.
27. DeBoer DA, Margolis ML, Livornese D, et al: Pulmonary venous aneurysm presenting as a middle mediastinal mass, *Ann Thorac Surg* 61:1261, 1996.
28. Sarier KK, Konstadt SN: Echocardiography for the anesthesiologist, *Int Anesthesiol Clin* 34:57, 1996.
29. Ellis JE, Lichtor JL, Feinstein SB, et al: Right heart dysfunction, pulmonary embolism, and paradoxical embolization during liver transplantation, *Anesth Analg* 68:777, 1989.
30. London MJ, Hollenberg M, Wong MG, et al: Intraoperative myocardial ischemia: localization by continuous 12-lead electrocardiography, *Anesthesiology* 69:232, 1988.
31. Steinbrook RA, Goldman DB, Mark JB, et al: How to best monitor for detection of myocardial ischemia? *Anesthesiology* 74:1171, 1991.
32. Tennant R, Wiggers CJ: The effect of coronary occlusion on myocardial contraction, *Am J Physiol* 112:351, 1935.
33. Battler A, Froelicher VF, Gallagher KP, et al: Dissociation between regional myocardial dysfunction and ECG changes during ischemia in the conscious dog, *Circulation* 62:735, 1980.
34. Hauser AM, Gangadharan V, Ramos RG, et al: Sequence of mechanical electrocardiographic and clinical effects of repeated coronary artery occlusion in human beings: echocardiographic observations during coronary angioplasty, *J Am Coll Cardiol* 5:193, 1985.
35. Thys D, Abel M, Bollew B, et al: Practice guidelines for perioperative transesophageal echocardiography: a report by the American Society of Anesthesiologists and the Society of Cardiovascular Anesthesiologists task force on transesophageal echocardiography, *Anesthesiology* 4:986, 1996.
36. Polonen P, Ruokonen E, Hippelainen M, et al: A prospective, randomized study of goal-oriented hemodynamic therapy in cardiac surgical patients, *Anesth Analg* 90:1052, 2000.
37. Glass PSA, Bloom M, Kearse L, et al: Bispectral analysis measures sedation and memory effects of propofol, midazolam, isoflurane, and alfentanil in healthy volunteers, *Anesthesiology* 86:836, 1997.
38. Lui J, Singh H, White PF: Electroencephalographic bispectral index correlates with intraoperative recall and depth of propofol-induced sedation, *Anesth Analg* 84:185, 1997.
39. Gan TJ, Glass PS, Windsor A, et al: Bispectral index monitoring allows faster emergence and improved recovery from propofol, alfentanil, and nitrous oxide anesthesia, *Anesthesiology.* 87:808, 1997.
40. Gross JB, Zebrowski ME, Carel WD, et al: Time course of ventilatory depression after thiopental and midazolam in normal subjects and in patients with chronic obstructive pulmonary disease, *Anesthesiology* 58:540, 1983.
41. Liu S, Carpenter RL, Neal JM: Epidural anesthesia and analgesia: their role in postoperative outcome, *Anesthesiology* 82:1474, 1995.
42. Cicala RS, Voeller GR, Fox T, et al: Epidural analgesia in thoracic trauma: effects of lumbar morphine and thoracic bupivacaine on pulmonary function, *Crit Care Med* 18:229, 1990.
43. Hansdottir V, Woestenborghs R, Nordberg G: The cerebrospinal fluid and plasma pharmcokinetics of sufentanil after thoracic or lumbar epidural administration, *Anesth Analg* 80:724, 1995.
44. Tejwani GA, Rattan AK, McDonald JS: Role of spinal opioid receptors in the antinociceptive interactions between intrathecal morphine and bupivacaine, *Anesth Analg* 74:726, 1992.
45. Cook TM, Riley RH: Analgesia following thoracotomy: a survey of Australian practice, *Anaesth Intens Care* 25:520, 1997.
46. Catala E, Casas JI, Unzueta MC, et al: Continuous infusion is superior to bolus doses with thoracic paravertebral blocks after thoracotomies, *J Cardiothorac Vasc Anesth* 10:58, 1996.
47. Gilbert J, Hultman J: Thoracic paravertebral blockade: a method of pain control, *Acta Anaesthsiol Scand* 33:142, 1989.
48. Liu N, Kuhlman G, Dalibon N, et al: A randomized, double-blinded comparison of intrathecal morphine, sufentanil and their combination versus IV morphine patient-controlled analgesia for post-thoracotomy pain, *Anesth Analg* 92:31, 2001.
49. Eng J. Sabanathan S: Post-thoracotomy analgesia, *J Royal Col Surg Edinburgh* 38:62, 1993.
50. Karmakar MK, Booker PD, Franks R: Bilateral continuous paravertebral block used for postoperative analgesia in an infant having bilateral thoracotomy, *Paed Anaesth* 7:469, 1997.

51. Bimston DN, McGee JP, Liptay MJ, et al: Continuous paravertebral extrapleural infusion for post-thoracotomy pain management, *Surgery* 126:650, 1999.
52. Doyle E, Bowler GM, Pre-emptive effect of multimodal analgesia in thoracic surgery, *Brit J Anaesth* 80:147, 1998.
53. Kaiser AM, Zollinger A, De Lorenzi D, et al: Prospective, randomized comparison of extrapleural versus epidural analgesia for post-thoracotomy pain, *Ann Thorac Surg* 66:367, 1998.
54. Barron DJ, Tolan MJ, Lea RE: A randomized controlled trial of continuous extrapleural analgesia post-thoracotomy: efficacy and choice of local anaesthetic, *Eur J Anaesth* 16:236, 1999.
55. Neustein SM, Cohen E: Intrathecal morphine during thoracotomy II. Effect on postoperative meperidine requirements and pulmonary function tests, *J Cardiothorac Vasc Anesth* 7:157, 1993.
56. Gruber, EM, Tschernko EM, Kritzinger M, et al: The effects of thoracic epidural analgesia with bupivacaine 0.25% on ventilatory mechanics in patients with severe chronic obstructive pulmonary disease, *Anesth Analg* 92:1015, 2001.
57. Richardson J, Sabanthan S, Shah R: Post-thoracotomy spirometric function: the effect of analgesia, *J Cardiovasc Surg* 40:445, 1999.
58. Ballantyne JC, Carr DB, deFerranti S, et al: The comparative effects of postoperative analgesic therapies on pulmonary outcome: cumulative meta-analyses of randomized controlled trials, *Anesth Analg* 86:598, 1998.
59. Cerfolio RJ, Allen MS, Trastek VF, et al: Lung resection in patients with compromised pulmonary function, *Ann Thorac Surg* 62:348, 1996.
60. Oka T, Ozawa Y, Ohkubo Y: Thoracic epidural bupivacaine attenuates supraventricular tachydysrhythmias after pulmonary resection, *Anesth Analg* 93:253, 2001.
61. Rehdar K, Sessler AD: Function of each lung in spontaneously breathing man anesthetized with thiopental-meperidine, *Anesthesiology* 38:320, 1973.
62. Froese AB, Bryan AC: Effects of anesthesia and paralysis on diaphragmatic mechanics in man, *Anesthesiology* 42:242, 1974.
63. Don HF, Wahba M, Cuadrado L, et al: The effects of anesthesia and 100 percent oxygen on the functional residual capacity of the lungs, *Anesthesiology* 32:521, 1970.
64. Westbrook PR, Stubbs SE, Sessler AD, et al: Effects of anesthesia and muscle paralysis on respiratory mechanics in normal man, *J Appl Physiol* 34:81, 1973.
65. Bergman NA, Ties YK: Contribution of the closure of pulmonary units to imposed oxygenation during anesthesia, *Anesthesiology* 59:395, 1983.
66. Juno P, March HM, Knopp TJ, Rehdar KL Closing capacity in awake and anesthetized-paralyzed man, *J Appl Physiol* 44:238, 1978.
67. Rehder K, Sessler AD, Marsh HM: General anesthesia and the lung, *Am Rev Respir Dis* 112:541, 1975.
68. Hedenstierna G, McCarthy G: Mechanics of breathing, gas distribution, and functional residual capacity at different frequencies of respiration during spontaneous and artificial ventilation, *Br J Anaesth* 57:706, 1975.
69. Dohi S, Gold MI: Pulmonary mechanics during general anesthesia. The influence of mechanical irritation on the airway, *Br J Anaesth* 51:205, 1979.
70. Rock P, Freed AN, Nyhan DP, et al: Thoracotomy increases peripheral airway tone and reactivity, *Am J Respir Crit Care Med* 151:1047, 1995.
71. Mehr EH, Lindeman KS: Effects of halothane, propofol and thiopental on peripheral airway reactivity, *Anesthesiology* 79:290, 1993.
72. Von Euler US, Lijestrand G: Observation on the pulmonary arterial blood pressure in the cat, *Acta Physiol Scand* 21:301, 1946.
73. McMurty IF: Angiotensin is not required for hypoxic constriction in salt-solution perfused rat lungs, *J Appl Physiol* 56:375, 1984.
74. Marshall BF, Marshall C, Frasch F, et al: Role of hypoxic pulmonary vasoconstriction in pulmonary gas exchange and blood flow distribution. I. Physiologic concepts, *Intensive Care Med* 20:291, 1994.
75. Zapol WM, Snider MT: Pulmonary hypertension in severe acute respiratory failure, *N Engl J Med* 296:476, 1976.
76. Harris P, Segal N, Bishop JM: The relationship between pressure and flow in the pulmonary circulation in normal subjects and in patients with chronic bronchitis and mitral stenosis, *Cardiovasc Res* 2:73, 1968.
77. Wagner PD, Gale GE, Moon RE, et al: Pulmonary gas exchange in humans at sea level and simulated altitude, *J Appl Physiol* 60:260, 1983.
78. Eisenkraft JB: Hypoxic pulmonary vasoconstriction, *Curr Opin Anaesth* 12:43, 1999.
79. Marshall BF, Marshall C, Benumof J, et al: Hypoxic pulmonary vasoconstriction in dogs : effects of lung segment size and oxygen tension, *J Appl Physiol* 51:1543, 1981.
80. Zasslow MA, Benumof JL, Trousdale FR: Hypoxic pulmonary vasoconstriction and the size of the hypoxic compartment, *J Appl Physiol* 53:626, 1982.
81. Domino KB, Wetstein L, Glasser SA: Influence of mixed venous oxygen tension (Pvo$_2$) on blood flow to atelectatic lung, *Anesthesiology* 59:428, 1983.
82. Bindslev L, Jolin A, Hedenstierna G, et al: Hypoxic pulmonary vasoconstriction in the human lung: effect of repeated hypoxic challenges during anesthesia, *Anesthesiology* 62:621, 1985.
83. Liu J, Ding Y, White PF, et al: Effects of ketorolac on postoperative analgesia and ventilatory function after laparoscopic cholecystectomy, *Anesth Analg* 76:1061, 1993.
84. Naeije R, Brimioulle S: Physiology in medicine: importance of hypoxic pulmonary vasoconstriction in maintaining arterial oxygenation during acute respiratory failure, *Crit Care Med* 5:67, 2001.
85. Lennon PF, Murray PA: Attenuated hypoxic pulmonary vasoconstriction during isoflurane anesthesia is abolished by cyclooxygenase inhibition in chronically instrumented dogs, *Anesthesiology* 91:760, 1999.
86. Kjaeve J, Bjertnaes LJ: Interaction of verapamil and halogenated inhalational anesthetics on hypoxic pulmonary vasoconstriction, *Acta Anaesthesiol Scand* 33:193, 1989.
87. Dumas JP, Bardou M, Goirand F, Dumas M: Hypoxic pulmonary vasoconstriction, *Gen Pharmacol* 33:289, 1999.
88. Wilkins MR, Zhao L, Al-Tubuly R: The regulation of pulmonary vascular tone, *Br J Clin Pharm* 42:127, 1996.
89. Domino KB, Eisenstein BL, Tran T, et al: Increased pulmonary perfusion worsens ventilation-perfusion matching, *Anesthesiology* 79:817, 1993.
90. Benumof J: Intermittent hypoxia increases lobar hypoxic pulmonary vasoconstriction, *Anesthesiology* 58:399, 1983.
91. Chen L, Miller FL, Williams JJ, et al: Hypoxic pulmonary vasoconstriction is not potentiated by repeated intermittent hypoxia in closed chest dogs, *Anesthesiology* 63:608, 1985.
92. Hambraeus-Jonzon K, Bindslev L, Millgard AJ, et al: Hypoxic pulmonary vasoconstriction in human lungs, *Anesthesiology* 86:308, 1997.
93. Chen L, Miller FL, Malmkvist G, et al: Intravenous PGF$_2$-α infusion does not enhance hypoxic pulmonary vasoconstriction during canine one-lung hypoxia, *Anesthesiology* 68:226, 1988.
94. Amira T, Matsuura M, Shiramatso T, et al: Synthesis of prostaglandins TXA$_2$ and PGI$_2$ during one-lung anesthesia, *Prostaglandins* 34:668, 1987.
95. Lambertsen CJ: Carbon dioxide and respiration in acid-base homeostasis, *Anesthesiology* 21:642, 1960.
96. Eger EI II: Isoflurane (Forane): a compendium and reference, ed 2, Madison, Wis 1985, Anaquest.
97. Munsson ES, Larson CP, Babad AA, et al: The effects of halothane, fluroxene and cyclopropane on ventilation: a comparative study in man, *Anesthesiology* 27:716, 1966.
98. Comroe JH Jr: The peripheral chemoreceptors. In Fenn WO, Rahn H (eds): *Handbook of physiology*, 1964.
99. Sjogren D, Lindahl SGE, Sollevi A: Ventilatory responses to acute and sustained hypoxia during isoflurane anesthesia, *Anesth Analg* 86:403, 1998.
100. Benumof JL, Augustine SD, Gibbons JA: Halothane and isoflurane only slightly impair arterial oxygenation during one-lung ventilation in patients undergoing thoracotomy, *Anesthesiology* 67:910, 1987.
101. Slinger P, Scott WAC: Arterial oxygenation during one-lung ventilation: a comparison of enflurane and isoflurane, *Anesthesiology* 82:940, 1995.
102. Karzai W, Haberstroh J, Preibe HJ: Effects of desflurane and propofol on arterial oxygenation during one-lung ventilation in the pig, *Acta Anaesthesiol Scand* 42:648, 1998.
103. Kellow NH, Scott AD, White SA, et al: Comparison of the effects of propofol and isoflurane anesthesia on right ventricular function and shunt fraction during thoracic surgery, *Br J Anaesth* 75:578, 1995.
104. Shimizu T, Abe K, Kinouchi K, et al: Arterial oxygenation during one-lung ventilation, *Can J Anaesth* 44:1162, 1997.
105. Rees DK, Gaines GY: One-lung anesthesia: a comparison of pulmonary gas exchange during anesthesia with ketamine or enflurane, *Anesth Analg* 63:521, 1984.
106. Choi JH, Rooke GA, Wu SC, et al: Reduction in postintubation respiratory resistance by isoflurane and albuterol, *Can J Anaesth* 44:717, 1997.
107. Bjertnaes LJ: Hypoxia-induced vasoconstriction in isolated perfused lungs exposed to injectable or inhalational anesthetics, *Acta Anaesthiol Scand* 21:133, 1977.
108. Marshall C, Lindgren L, Marshall BF: Effects of halothane, enflurane and isoflurane on hypoxic pulmonary vasoconstriction in rat lung in vitro, *Anesthesiology* 61:304, 1984.

109. Mathers J, Benumof JL, Wahrenbrock EA: General anesthetics and regional hypoxic pulmonary vasoconstriction, *Anesthesiology* 46:111, 1977.
110. Spies C, Zaune U, Pauli MH, et al: A comparison of enflurane and propofol in thoracic surgery, *Anaesthetist* 40(1):14, 1991.
111. Liu R, Ueda M, Okazaki N, et al: Role of potassium channels in isoflurane and sevoflurane-induced attenutation of hypoxic pulmonary vasoconstriction in isolated perfused rabbit lungs, *Anesthesiology* 95:939, 2001.
112. Loer SA; Scheeren TWL; Tarnow J: Desflurane inhibits hypoxic pulmonary vasoconstriction in isolated rabbit lungs, *Anesthesiology* 83:552, 1995.
113. Beck DH, Doepfmer UR, Sinemus C, et al: Effects of sevoflurane and propofol on pulmonary shunt fraction during one-lung ventilation for thoracic surgery, *Br J Anaesth* 86:38, 2001.
114. Pagel PS, Fu JJL, Damask MC, et al: Desflurane and isoflurane produce similar alterations in systemic and pulmonary hemodynamics and arterial oxygenation in patients undergoing one-lung ventilation during thoracotomy, *Anesth Analg* 87:800, 1998.
115. Calverley RK, Smith NT, Jones CW, et al: Ventilatory and cardiovascular effects of enflurane anesthesia during spontaneous ventilation in man, *Anesth Analg* 57:610, 1978.
116. Cromwell TH, Stevens WC, Eger EI, et al: The cardiovascular effects of compound 469 (Forane) during spontaneous ventilation and CO_2 challenge in man, *Anesthesiology* 35:17, 1971.
117. Wallin RF, Regan BM, Napoli MD, et al: Sevoflurane: a new inhalational anesthestic agent, *Anesth Analg* 54:758, 1975.
118. Green WB: The ventilatory effects of sevoflurane, *Anesth Analg* 81:S23, 1995.
119. Eger EI II: New inhaled anesthetics, *Anesthesiology* 80:906, 1994.
120. Hirshman CA, McCullough RH, Cohen PJ: Depression of hypoxic ventilation response by halothane, enflurane and isoflurane in dogs, *Br J Anaesth* 49:957, 1977.
121. Hurtig JB, Tait AR, Loh L, et al: Reduction of hypoxic pulmonary vasoconstriction by nitrous oxide administration in the isolated perfused cat lung, *Can Anaesth Soc J* 24:540, 1977.
122. Bindslev L, Cannon D, Sykes MK: Reversal of nitrous oxide-induced depression of hypoxic pulmonary vasoconstriction by lignocaine hydrochloride during collapse and ventilation hypoxia of the left lower lobe, *Br J Anaesth* 58:451, 1986.
123. Zhang C, Davies MF, Guo TZ, et al: The analgesic action of nitrous oxide is dependent on the release of norepinephrine in the dorsal horn of the spinal cord, *Anesthesiology* 91:1401, 1999.
124. Ebert TJ, Kampine JP: Nitrous oxide augments sympathetic outflow: direct evidence from human peroneal nerve recordings, *Anesth Analg* 69:444, 1989.
125. Yacoub O, Doell D, Kryger MH, et al: Depression of hypoxic ventilatory response by nitrous oxide, *Anesthesiology* 45:385, 1976.
126. Hornbein TF, Martin WE, Bonica JJ, et al: Nitrous oxide effects on the circulatory and ventilatory responses to halothane, *Anesthesiology* 31:250, 1969.
127. Liu EH, Gillbe CE, Watson AC: Anaesthetic management of patients undergoing lung volume reduction surgery for treatment of severe emphysema, *Anaesth Intens Care* 27:459, 1999.
128. Speicher A, Jessberger J, Braun R, et al: Postoperative pulmonary function after lung surgery: total intravenous anesthesia with propofol in comparison to balanced anesthesia with isoflurane, *Anaesthetist* 44:265, 1995.
129. Nakayama M, Murray PA: Ketamine preserves and propofol potentiates hypoxic pulmonary vasoconstriction compared with the conscious state in chronically instrumented dogs, *Anesthesiology* 91:760, 1999.
130. Van Keer L, Van Aken H, Vandermeersch E, et al: Propofol does not inhibit hypoxic pulmonary vasoconstriction in humans, *J Clin Anesth* 1:284, 1989.
131. Yondov D, Kounev V, Ivanov O, et al: A comparative study of the effect of halothane, isoflurane and propofol on partial arterial oxygen pressure during one-lung ventilation in thoracic surgery, *Folia Med* 41:45, 1999.
132. Marone G, Stellato C, Mastronardi P, et al: Mechanisms of activation of human mast cells and basophils by general anesthetic drugs, *Ann Fr Anesth Reanim* 12:116, 1993.
133. Kimura K, Adachi M, Kubo K: Histamine release during the induction of anesthesia with propofol in allergic patients: a comparison with the induction of anesthesia using midazolam-ketamine, *Inflamm Res* 48:582, 1999.
134. Guldager H, Sondergaard I, Jensen FM, et al: Basophil histamine release in asthma patients after in vitro provocation with althesin and etomidate, *Acta Anaesthsiol Scand* 29:352, 1985.
135. Watkins J: Etomidate: An "immunologically safe" aesthetic agent, *Anaesthesia* 38:34, 1983.
136. Berggren L, Eriksson I, Mollenholt P, et al: Changes in respiratory pattern after repeated doses of diazepam and midazolam in healthy subjects, *Acta Anaesthesiol Scand* 31:381, 1987.
137. Alexander CM, Gross JB: Sedative does of midazolam depress hypoxic ventilatory responses in humans, *Anesth Analg* 67:377, 1988.
138. Mora CT, Torjman M, White PF: Effects of diazepam and flumazenil on sedation and hypoxic ventilatory drive, *Anesth Analg* 68:473, 1989.
139. Shook JE, Watkins WD, Camporesi EM: Differential roles of opioid receptors in respiration, respiratory disease, and opiate-induced respiratory depression, *Am Rev Respir Dis* 142:895, 1990.
140. Ahuja BR, Strunin L: Respiratory effects of epidural fentanyl: changes in end-tidal CO_2 and respiratory rate following single doses and continuous infusion of epidural fentanyl, *Anaesthesia* 40:949, 1985.
141. Renaud B, Brichant JF, Clergue F, et al: Ventilatory effects of continuous epidural infusion of fentanyl, *Anesth Analg* 67:971, 1988.
142. Sandler AN, Chovaz P, Whiting W: Respiratory depression following epidural morphine: a clinical study, *Can Anaesth Soc J* 33:542, 1986.
143. Knill RL, Clement JL, Thompson WR: Epidural morphine causes delayed and prolonged ventilatory depression, *Can Anaesth Soc J* 28:537, 1981.
144. Bjertnaes L, Hauge A, Kriz M: Hypoxia-induced pulmonary vasoconstriction: effects of fentanyl following different routes of administration, *Acta Anaesthesiol Scand* 24:53, 1980.
145. Ellmauer S, Dick W, Otto S, et al: Different opioids in patients at cardiovascular risk. Comparison of central and peripheral hemodynamic adverse effects, *Anaesthetist* 43:743, 1994.
146. Cohendy R, Lefrant JY, Laracine M, et al: Effect of fentanyl on ventilatory resistances during barbiturate general anesthesia, *Br J Anaesth* 69:595, 1992.
147. Ruiz-Neto PP, Auler JO Jr: Respiratory mechanical properties during fentanyl and alfentanil anaesthesia, *Can J Anaesth* 39:458, 1992.
148. Sandler AN, Stringer D, Panos L, et al: A randomized, double-blind comparison of lumbar epidural and intravenous fentanyl infusions for post-thoracotomy pain relief: analgesic, pharmacokinetic, and respiratory effects, *Anesthesiology* 77:626, 1992.
149. Gibbs JM, Johnson H: Lack of effect of morphine and buprenorphine on hypoxic pulmonary vasoconstriction in the isolated perfused cat lung and the perfused lobe of the dog lung, *Br J Anaesth* 50:1197, 1978.
150. Ohya M, Taguchi H, Mima M, et al: Effects of morphine, buprenorphine and butorphanol on airway dynamics of the rabbit, *Masui* 42:498, 1993.
151. Eschenbacher WL, Bethel RA, Boushey HA, et al: Morphine sulfate inhibits bronchoconstriction in subjects with mild asthma whose responses are inhibited by atropine, *Am Rev Respir Dis* 130:363, 1984.
152. Grossman M, Abiose A, Tangphago O, et al: Morphine-induced venodilation in humans, *Clin Pharmacol Ther* 60:554, 1996.
153. Tantucci C, Paoletti F, Bruni B, et al: Acute respiratory effects of sublingual buprenorphine: comparison with intramuscular morphine, *Int J Clin Pharmacol Ther* 30:202, 1992.
154. Grant GJ, Zakowski M, Ramanathan S, et al: Thoracic versus lumbar administration of epidural morphine for postoperative analgesia after thoracotomy, *Reg Anesth* 18:351, 1993.
155. Neustein SM, Cohen E: Intrathecal morphine during thoracotomy. I. Effect on postoperative meperidine requirements and pulmonary function tests, *J Cardiothorac Vasc Anesth* 7:157, 1993.
156. Roy SD, Flynn GL: Solubility and related physiochemical properties of narcotic analgesics, *Pharm Res* 5:580, 1988.
157. Bernards CM, Hill HF: Physical and chemical properties of drug molecules governing their diffusion through the spinal meninges, *Anesthesiology* 72:750, 1992.
158. Brodsky JB, Chaplan SR, Brose WG, et al: Continuous epidural hydromorphone for post-thoracotomy pain relief, *Ann Thorac Surg* 50:888, 1990.
159. Singh H, Bossard RF, White PF, et al: Effects of ketorolac versus bupivacaine coadministration during patient-controlled hydromorphone epidural analgesia after thoracotomy procedures, *Anesth Anal* 84:564, 1997.
160. Finer BL, Partington MW: Pethidine and the triple response, *Br Med J* 1:431, 1953.
161. Shermano I, Wendel H: Effects of meperidine hydrochloride and morphine sulfate on the lung capacity of intact dogs, *J Pharmacol Exp Ther* 149:379, 1965.

162. Bowdle TA: Adverse effects of opioid agonists and agonist-antagonists in anaesthesia, *Drug Saf* 19:173, 1998.

163. Burwell DR, Jones JG: The airways and anaesthesia. II. pathophysiology, 51:943, 1996.

164. Donati F: Neuromuscular blocking drugs for the new millennium: current practice, future trends—comparative pharmacology of neuromuscular blocking drugs, *Anesth Analg* 90:S2, 2000.

165. Reich DL, Mulier J, Viby-Mogensen J, et al: Comparison of the cardiovascular effects of cisatracurium and vecuronium in patients with coronary artery disease, *Can J Anaesth* 45:794, 1998.

166. Lin PL, Liu CC, Fan SC, et al: Comparison of neuromuscular action of rocuronium, a new steroidal non depolarizing agent, with vecuronium, *Acta Anaesthsiol Scan* 35:127, 1997.

167. Doenicke A, Soukup J, Hoernecke R, et al: The lack of histamine release with cisatracurium: a double-blind comparison with vecuronium, *Anesth Analg* 84:623, 1997.

168. Moss J: Muscle relaxants and histamine release, *Acta Anaesthesiol Scand* 106:7, 1995.

169. Doenicke AW, Czeslick E, Moss J, et al: Onset time, endotracheal intubating conditions and plasma histamine after cisatracurium and vecuronium administration, *Anesth Analg* 87:434, 1998.

170. Brinkmann M, Gunnicker M, Freund U, et al: Histamine plasma concentration and cardiovascular effects of nondepolarizing muscle relaxants: comparison of atracurium, vecuronium, pancuronium and pipecuronium in coronary surgical patients at risk. *Anasthesiol Intensivmed Notfallmed Schmerzther* 33:362, 1998.

171. Vettermann J, Beck KC, Lindahl SGE, et al: Actions of enflurane, isoflurane, vecuronium,atracurium and pancuronium on pulmonary resistance in dogs, *Anesthesiology* 74:325, 1991.

172. Galletly DC: Comparative cutaneous histamine release by neuromuscular blocking agents, *Anaesth Intens Care* 14:365, 1986.

173. Assem ES, Ezeamuzie IC, Suxamethonium-induced histamine release from the heart of naive and suxamethonium-sensitized guinea pigs: evidence suggesting spontaneous sensitization in naive animals, and relevance to anaphylactoid reactions in man, *Agents Actions* 27:146, 1989.

174. Didier A, Benzarti M, Senft M, et al: Allergy to suxamethonium: persisting abnormalities in skin tests, specific IgE antibodies and leucocyte histamine release, *Clin Allergy* 17:385, 1987.

175. Loan PB, Elliott P, Mirakhur RK, et al: Comparison of the haemodynamic effects of mivacurium and atracurium during fentanyl anesthesia, *Br J Anaesth* 74:330, 1995.

176. Mayer M, Doenicke A, Nebauer AE, et al: Pharmacodynamics and clinical adverse effects of mivacurium: the effects of oral premedication with H1/H2 antagonists, *Anaesthetist* 42:592, 1992.

177. Hammond J, Wright D, Sale J: Pattern of change of bronchomotor tone following reversal of neuromuscular blockade, *Br J Anaesth* 55:955, 1983.

178. Scheinin B, Scheinin R, Asantila R, et al: Sympathoadrenal and pituitary hormone responses during and immediately after thoracic surgery—modulation by four different pain treatments, *Acta Anaesthesiol Scand* 31:762, 1987.

179. Wattwil M, Sundberg A, Arvill A, et al: Circulatory changes during high thoracic epidural anesthesia: influence of sympathetic block and of systemic effect of local anaesthetic, *Acta Anaesthesiol Scand* 29:849, 1985.

180. Blomberg S, Emanuelsson H, Ricksten SE: Thoracic epidural anesthesia and central hemodynamics in patients with unstable angina pectoris, *Anesthesiology* 69:558, 1989.

181. Blomberg S, Emanuelsson H, Kvist H, et al: Effects of thoracic epidural anesthesia on coronary arteries and arterioles in patients with coronary artery disease, *Anesthesiology* 73:840, 1990.

182. Gross JB, Caldwell CB, Shaw LM, et al: The effect of lidocaine on the ventilatory response to carbon dioxide, *Anesthesiology* 59:521, 1983.

183. Labaille T, Clerque F, Samii K, et al: Ventilatory response to CO_2 following intravenous and epidural lidocaine, *Anesthesiology* 63:179, 1985.

184. Steinbrook RA, Concepcion M, Topoulos GP: Ventilatory responses to hypercapnea during bupivacaine spinal anesthesia, *Anesth Analg* 67:247, 1988.

185. Steinbrook RA, Topulous GP, Concepcion M: Ventilatory responses to hypercapnea during tetracaine spinal anesthesia, *J Clin Anesth* 1:75, 1988.

186. Mori J, Fukuda T: Effects of thalamic stimulation on the reticular neuron activities and their modifications by lidocaine and pentobarbital, *Jpn J Pharmacol* 21:641, 1971.

187. Gross JB, Caldwell CB, Shaw LM, et al: The effect of lidocaine infusion on the ventilatory response to hypoxia, *Anesthesiology* 61:662, 1984.

188. Steen P, Michenfelder J: Neurotoxicity of anesthetics, *Anesthesiology* 50:437, 1979.

189. Gross JB, Caldwell CB, Shaw LM, et al: The effect of lidocaine infusion on the ventilatory response to hypoxia, *Anesthesiology* 61:662, 1984.

190. Takasaki M, Takahashi T: Respiratory function during cervical and thoracic extradural analgesia in patients with normal lungs, *Br J Anaesth* 52:1271, 1980.

191. Moir DD: Ventilatory function during epidural analgesia, *Br J Anaesth* 35:3, 1963.

192. Sjogren S, Weight B: Respiratory changes during continuous epidural blockade, *Acta Anaesthesiol Scand* 16:27, 1980.

193. Kochi T, Sako S, Nishino T, et al: Effect of high thoracic extradural anaesthesia on ventilatory response to hypercapnea in normal volunteers, *Br J Anaesth* 62:363, 1989.

194. Thomas JM, Schug SA: Recent advances in the pharmacokinetics of local anaesthetics: long-acting amide enantiomers and continuous infusions, *Clin Pharmacokinet* 36:67, 1999.

195. Mather LE, Chang DH: Cardiotoxicity with modern local anaesthetics: is there a safer choice? *Drugs* 61:333, 2001.

196. Markham A, Faulds D: Ropivacaine. A review of its pharmacology and therapeutic use in regional anaesthesia, *Drugs* 52:429, 1996.

197. Colley PS, Cheney FW: Sodium nitroprusside increases Q_S/Q_T in dogs with regional atelectasis, *Anesthesiology* 47:338, 1977.

198. Hill AB, Sykes MK, Reves A: A hypoxic pulmonary vasoconstriction response in dogs during and after infusion of sodium nitroprusside, *Anesthesiology* 50:484, 1979.

199. D'Oliveira M, Sykes MK, Chakrabarti MK, et al: Depression of hypoxic pulmonary vasoconstriction by sodium nitroprusside and nitroglycerin, *Br J Anaesth* 53:11, 1981.

200. Miller JR, Benumof JL, Trousdale FR: Combined effects of sodium nitroprusside and propranolol on hypoxic pulmonary vasoconstriction, *Anesthesiology* 57:267, 1982.

201. Friedlander M, Sandler A, Kavanagh B, et al: Is hypoxic pulmonary vasoconstriction important during single-lung ventilation in the lateral decubitus position? *Can J Anaesth* 41:26-30, 1994.

202. Bishop MJ, Kennard S, Artman LD, et al: Hydralazine does not inhibit canine hypoxic pulmonary vasoconstriction, *Am Rev Respir Dis* 128:998, 1983.

203. Scherer RW, Vigfusson G, Hultsch E, et al.: Prostaglandin f_2 alpha improves oxygen tension and reduces venous admixture during one-lung ventilation in anesthetized paralyzed dogs, *Anesthesiology* 62:23, 1985.

204. Gardaz JP, McFarlane PA, Sykes M: Mechanisms by which dopamine alters blood flow distribution during lobar collapse in dogs, *J Appl Physiol* 60:959, 1986.

205. McFarlane PA, Mortimer AJ, Ryder WA, et al: Effects of dopamine and dobutamine on the distribution of pulmonary blood flow during lobar ventilation in hypoxia and lobar collapse in dogs, *Eur J Clin Invest* 15:53, 1985.

206. Moutafis M, Liu N, Dalibon N, et al: The effects of inhaled nitric oxide and its combination with intravenous almitrine on PaO_2 during one-lung ventilation in patients undergoing thoracoscopic procedures, *Anesth Analg* 85:1130, 1997.

207. Doering EB, Hanson CW, Reily DJ, et al: Improvement in oxygenation by phenylephrine and nitric oxide in patients with adult respiratory distress syndrome, *Anesthesiology* 87:18, 1997.

208. Choi JH, Rooke GA, Wu SC, et al: Reduction in postintubation respiratory resistance by isoflurane and albuterol, *Can J Anaesth* 44:717, 1997.

209. Nakaoji T, Ochiai R, Takeda J, et al: The effect of droperidol and sevoflurane on serotonin-induced bronchoconstriction in dog, *Masui* 45:698, 1996.

210. Prezant DJ, Aldrich TK: Intravenous droperidol for the treatment of status asthmaticus, *Crit Care Med* 16:96, 1988.

211. Soroker D, Barzilay E, Konichezky S, et al: Respiratory function following premedication with droperidol or diazepam, *Anesth Anal* 57:695, 1978.

212. Faris PL, Kim SW, Meller WH, et al: Effect of decreasing afferent vagal activity with ondansetron on symptoms of bulimia nervosa: a randomized, double-blind trial, *Lancet* 355:792, 2000.

213. Yoshioka M, Goda Y, Togashi H, et al: Pharmacological characterization of 5-hydroxytryptamine-induced apnea in the rat, *J Pharmacol Exper Ther* 260:917, 1992.

214. Burgess FW, Anderson M, Colonna D, et al: Ipsilateral shoulder pain following thoracic surgery, *Anesthesiology* 78:365, 1993.

215. Liu J, Ding Y, White PF, et al: Effects of ketorolac on postoperative analgesia and ventilatory function after laparoscopic cholecystectomy, *Anesth Analg* 76:1061, 1993.

216. Ishibe Y, Shiokawa Y, Umeda T, et al: The effect of thoracic epidural anesthesia on hypoxic pulmonary vasoconstriction in dogs: an analysis of pressure-flow curve, *Anesth Analg* 82:1049, 1996.
217. Garutti I, Quintana B, Olmedilla L, et al: Arterial oxygenation during one-lung ventilation: combined versus general anesthesia, *Anesth Analg* 88:494, 1999.
218. Samian E, Farah E, Delefosse D, et al: End-tidal oxygraphy during pre-oxygenation in patients with severe diffuse emphysema, *Anaesthesia* 55:841, 2000.
219. Olssen GL: Bronchospasm during anesthesia: a computer aided incidence study of 136,929 patients, *Acta Anaesthesiol Scand* 31:244, 1987.
220. Lapinsky SE, Leung RS: Auto-PEEP and electromechanical dissociation, *New Engl J Med* 335:674, 1996.
221. Rosengarten PL, Tuxen DV, Dziukas L, et al: Circulatory arrest induced by intermittent positive pressure ventilation in a patient with severe asthma, *Anaesth Intens Care* 19:118, 1991.
222. Rogers PL, Schlichtig R, Miro A, et al: Auto-PEEP during CPR: an "occult" cause of electromechanical dissociation? *Chest* 99:492, 1991.
223. Martens P, Vandekerckhove Y, Mullie A: Restoration of spontaneous circulation after cessation of cardiopulmonary resuscitation, *Lancet* 341:841, 1993.
224. Sprung J, Hunter K, Barnas GM, et al: Abdominal distention is not always a sign of esophageal intubation: cardiac arrest due to "auto-PEEP," *Anesth Analg* 78:801, 1994.
225. Connery LE, Deignan MJ, Gujer MW, et al: Cardiovascular collapse associated with extreme iatrogenic PEEPi in patients with obstructive airways disease, *Br J Anaesth* 83:493, 1999.
226. Slinger P, Blundell PE, Metcalf IR: Management of massive grain aspiration, *Anesthesiology* 87:993, 1997.
227. Desiderio DP, Burt M, Kolker AC, et al: The effects of endobronchial cuff inflation on double-lumen endobronchial tube movement after lateral decubitus positioning, *J Cardiothorac Vasc Anesth* 11:595, 1997.
228. Klein U, Karzai W, Bloos F, et al: Role of fiberoptic bronchoscopy in conjunction with the use of double-lumen tubes for thoracic anesthesia, *Anesthesiology* 88:346, 1998.
229. Benumof JL, Partridge BL, Salvatierra C, et al: Margin of safety in positioning modern double-lumen endotracheal tubes, *Anesthesiology* 67:729, 1987.
230. Benumof JL, Harwood I, Pendleton S: Major obstruction of the right mainstem bronchus caused by placement of a right axillary roll, *J Cardiothorac Vasc Anesth* 7:200, 1993.
231. Britt BA, Gordon RA: Peripheral nerve injuries associated with anaesthesia, *Can Anaesth Soc J* 11:51, 1964.
232. Lawson NW: The lateral decubitus position. In Marton JT (ed), *Positioning in anesthesia and surgery,* ed 2, Philadelphia, 1987, WB Saunders.
233. Walker WE: Paraplegia associated with thoracotomy, *Ann Thorac Surg* 50:178, 1990.
234. Tugrul M, Camci E, Karadeniz H, et al: Comparison of volume-controlled with pressure-controlled ventilation during one-lung anaesthesia, *Br J Anaesth* 79:306, 1997.
235. Laghi F, Segal J, Choe WK, et al: Effect of imposed inflation time on respiratory frequency and hyperinflation in patients with chronic obstructive pulmonary disease, *Am J Respir Crit Care Med* 163:1365, 2001.
236. Crawford OB, Ottosen P, Buckingham WW, et al: Peridural anesthesia in thoracic surgery: a review of 677 cases, *Anesthesiology* 12:73, 1951.
237. Eisenkraft JB, Cohen E, Neustein SML: Anesthesia for thoracic surgery. In Barash PG, Cullen BF, Stoelting RK (eds): *Clinical anesthesia,* ed 3, Philadelphia, 1997, Lippincott-Raven.
238. Plummer S, Hartley M, Vaughan RS: Anaesthesia for telescopic procedures in the thorax, *Br J Anaesth* 80:223, 1998.
239. Fine PG, Rosenberg J: Functional neuroanatomy, regional anesthesia and analgesia. In Brown DL (ed): Philadelphia, 1996, WB Saunders.
240. Akesson EJ, Loeb JA, Wilson-Pauwels L. In McAllister L, Winters R, Heoltzel LE (eds): *Thompson's core textbook of anatomy,* ed 2, Philadelphia, 1990, Lippincott.
241. Moore KL. In Satterfield TS (ed): *Clinically oriented anatomy,* ed 3, Baltimore, 1992, Williams and Wilkins.
242. Williams A, Kay J: Thoracic epidural anesthesia for thoracoscopy, rib resection, and thoracotomy in a patient with a bronchopleural fistula post-pneumonectomy, *Anesthesiology* 92:1482, 2000.
243. Kempen PM: Complete analgesia during pleurodesis under thoracic epidural anesthesia, *Am Surg* 64:755, 1998.
244. Mukaida T, Andou A, Date H, et al: Thoracoscopic operation for secondary pneumothorax under local and epidural anesthesia in high-risk patients, *Ann Thorac Surg* 65:924, 1998.
245. Anderson MB, Kwong KF, Furst AJ, et al: Thoracic epidural anesthesia for coronary bypass via left anterior thoracotomy in the conscious patient, *Eur J Cardiothorac Surg* 20:415, 2001.
246. Vaupshas HJ, Levy M: Distribution of saline following acute volume loading: postural effects, *Clin Invest Med* 13:165, 1990.
247. Ernest D, Belzberg AS, Dodeck PM: Distribution of normal saline and 5% albumin infusions in septic patients, *Crit Care Med* 27:46, 1999.
248. Lang K, Boldt J, Suttner S, et al: Colloids versus crystalloids and tissue oxygen tension in patients undergoing major abdominal surgery, *Anesth Analg* 93:405, 2001.
249. Boldt J: The good, the bad, and the ugly: should we completely banish human albumin from our intensive care units? *Anesth Analg* 91:887, 2000.
250. Schierhout G, Roberts I: Fluid resuscitation with colloid or crystalloid solutions in critically ill patients: a systemic review of randomized trials, *BMJ* 316:961, 1998.
251. Goodwin CW, Dorethy J, Lam V, et al: Randomized trial of efficacy of crystalloid and colloid resuscitation on hemodynamic response and lung water following thermal injury, *Ann Surg* 197:520, 1983.
252. Klein HG: Will blood transfusion ever be safe enough? *Transfus Med* 11:122, 2001.
253. Claas FH, Roelen DL, van Rood JJ, et al: Modulation of the alloimmune response by blood transfusions, *Transfus Clin Biol* 8:315, 2001.
254. Leal-Noval SR, Rincon-Ferrari MD, Garcia-Curiel A, et al: Transfusion of blood components and postoperative infection in patients undergoing cardiac surgery, *Chest* 119:1461, 2001.
255. Desiderio D, Downey R: Critical issue in early extubation and hospital discharge in thoracic oncology surgery, *J Cardiothorac Vasc Anesth* 12(suppl 2):3-6, 1998.
256. Berry A, Brimacombe J, Keller C, et al: Pulmonary airway resistance with the endotracheal tube versus laryngeal mask airway in paralyzed anesthetized adult patients, *Anesthesiology* 90:395, 1999.
257. Knill R, Manninen P, Clement J: Ventilation and chemoreflexes during enflurane sedation and anesthesia in man, *Can Anaesth Soc J* 26:353, 1979.
258. Pietak S, Weening CS, Hickey RF, et al: Anesthetic effects on ventilation in patients with chronic obstructive pulmonary disease, *Anesthesiology* 42:160, 1975.
259. Slinger PD, Johnston MR: Preoperative assessment for pulmonary resection, *J Cardiothorac Vasc Anesth* 14:202, 2000.
260. Katz JA, Laverene RG, Fairley B, et al: Pulmonary oxygen exchange during endobronchial anesthesia: effect of tidal volume and PEEP, *Anesthesiology* 56:164, 1982.
261. Benumof JL: Special physiology of the lateral decubitus position, the open chest and one-lung ventilation. In Benumof JL (ed): *Anesthesia for thoracic surgery,* Philadelphia, 1987, WB Saunders.
262. Slinger PD, Leiuk L: Flow resistances of disposable double-lumen, single-lumen and univent tubes, *J Cardiothorac Vasc Anesth* 12:142, 1998.
263. Slinger P, Hickey DR: The interaction between applied PEEP and auto-PEEP during one-lung ventilation, *J Cardiothorac Vasc Anesth* 12:133, 1998.
264. Myles PS, Ryder IG, Weeks AM, et al: Diagnosis and management of dynamic hyperinflation during lung transplantation, *J Cardiothorac Vasc Anesth* 11:100, 1997.
265. Bardoczky G, d'Hollander A, Cappello M, et al: Interrupted expiratory flow on automatically constructed flow-volume curves may determine the presence of intrinsic positive end-expiratory pressure during one-lung ventilation, *Anesth Analg* 86:880, 1998.
266. Ducros L, Moutafis M, Castelain MH, et al: Pulmonary air trapping and one-lung ventilation, *J Cardiothorac Vasc Anesth* 13:35, 1999.
267. Amato MB, Barbas CS, Medeiros DM., et al: Effect of a protective-ventilation strategy on mortality in the acute respiratory distress syndrome, *New Engl J Med* 338:347, 1998.
268. Keller CA, Naunheim KS: Perioperative management of lung reduction patients, *Clin Chest Med* 18:285, 1997.
269. Nunn JF: Effects of anaesthesia on respiration, *Br J Anaesth* 65:54, 1990.
270. Slinger PD: Perioperative fluid management for thoracic surgery: the puzzle of postpneumonectomy pulmonary edema, *J Cardiothorac Vasc Anesth* 9:442, 1995.
271. Krasna MJ, Deshmukh S, McLaughlin JS: Complications of thoracoscopy, *Ann Thorac Surg* 61:1066, 1996.

272. Waller DA, Gebitekin C, Saunders NR, et al: Noncardiogenic pulmonary edema complicating lung resection, *Ann Thorac Surg* 55:140, 1993.

273. Jordan S, Mitchell JA, Quinlan GJ, et al: The pathogenesis of lung injury following pulmonary resection, *Eur Respir J* 15:790, 2000.

274. Wittnick C, Trudel J, Zidulka A, et al: Misleading "pulmonary wedge pressure" after pneumonectomy: its importance in postoperative fluid therapy, *Ann Thorac Surg* 42:192, 1986.

275. Zeldin RA, Normandin D, Landtwing D, et al: Postpneumonectomy pulmonary edema, *J Thorac Cardiovasc Surg* 87:359, 1984.

276. Verheijen-Breemharr L, Bogaard JM, van den Berg B: Noncardiogenic pulmonary edema complicating lung resection, *Ann Thorac Surg* 43:323, 1988.

277. Parquin F, Marchal M, Meehiri S, et al: Postpneumonectomy pulmonary edema: analysis and risk factors, *Eur J Cardiothorac Surg* 10:929, 1996.

278. Mathru M, Blakeman BP: Don't drown the "down" lung, *Chest* 103:1644, 1993.

279. Turnage WS, Lunn JJ: Postpneumonectomy pulmonary edema: a retrospective analysis of associated variables, *Chest* 103:1646, 1993.

280. Alvarez JM, Bairstow BM, Tang C, et al: post–lung resection pulmonary edema: a case for aggressive management, *J Cardiothorac Vasc Anesth* 12:199, 1998.

281. Satur CM, Gupta NK: Postpneumonectomy pulmonary edema or microembolism? *Ann Thorac Surg* 57:523, 1994.

282. Deslauriers J, Aucoin A, Gregoire J: Postpneumonectomy pulmonary edema, *Chest Surg Clin NA* 8:611, 1998.

283. Lases EC, Duurkens VA, Gerristen WB, et al: Oxidative stress after lung resection therapy: a pilot study 117:999, 2000.

Lung Separation Techniques

8

Javier H. Campos, MD

LUNG separation techniques are required in thoracic, esophageal, vascular, and nonthoracic surgical operations and in the management of critically ill patients who require differential lung ventilation. The primary objective of this technique is to selectively interrupt ventilation to one lung *(total lung collapse)* or to a portion of a lung *(selective lobar collapse)*. This chapter discusses the current use of double-lumen tube technology (left- and right-sided double-lumen endotracheal tubes [DLT]), bronchial blocking technology (Fogarty occlusion catheters, single-lumen endotracheal tube with enclosed bronchial blocker [Univent]), and the use of a wire-guided endobronchial blocker (WEB) to achieve lung separation.

More than 50 years ago, Carlens introduced the first practicable method of lung separation to facilitate lung surgery or prevent contamination of the contralateral lung while maintaining one-lung ventilation (OLV).[1] This DLT had two lumens—one endotracheal and one endobronchial—and a carinal hook to facilitate placement. Robertshaw later introduced a modification of the DLT.[2] Today, all DLTs in the United States are made of polyvinylchloride, are disposable, and have high-volume, low-pressure cuffs. Although the modern DLT is very effective, some argue that the large circumferential diameter makes it difficult to pass through the oral cavity and larynx, and that an alternative should, therefore, be sought.

In 1981, Ginsberg introduced a new method for OLV using a bronchial blocking technology (Fogarty occlusion catheter) by advancing the Fogarty through a single-lumen endotracheal tube.[3] The limitation of this device was that no channel opening was present for air evacuation or oxygen insufflation. In 1982, Inoue et al reported a new device for OLV based on the concept of using a single-lumen endotracheal tube with an enclosed bronchial blocker (Univent) so that when OLV is no longer needed, the tube can be left in situ.[4] One of the modifications of this bronchial blocker was the suction channel included in the center to facilitate suction or oxygen insufflation. Although this tube does solve some of the problems associated with DLTs, it does not resolve the issue of circumferential diameter—the enclosed channel for the bronchial blocker makes the outer diameter of the tube quite large. In 1999, Arndt et al introduced the use of a wire-guided endobronchial blocker (WEB), which consists of a single bronchial blocker that is hollow in the center and is advanced through a standard single-lumen endotracheal tube.[5]

Although these different tubes are designed to achieve OLV, there is no randomized trial demonstrating one to be superior over the others during elective thoracic surgical cases. Each device might have some advantages over the others in specific situations, however. Table 8-1 outlines six areas in which lung separation is required.

Double-Lumen Technology for Lung Separation

Double-lumen endotracheal tubes are the most commonly used tubes for lung separation.[6] These tubes are designed to isolate, selectively ventilate, and/or collapse the right or left lung. In the United States, all contemporary DLTs are plastic and disposable. The anatomic differences between the right and left mainstem bronchi determine the differences in design. Four manufacturers currently design DLTs: Mallinckrodt (St. Louis, Mo.), Portex (Keene, N.H.), Sheridan (Argyle, N.Y.), and Rüsch (Duluth, Ga.). The sizes that have been available over the years include 35F, 37F, 39F, and 41F (F is French measurement). Newer left- or right-sided sizes have been introduced recently—the 26F, 28F, and 32F sizes made by Rüsch and Sheridan and the 28F by Mallinckrodt. Mallinckrodt has made some recent modifications, reincorporating a bevel in the left-sided BronchoCath tubes. This change was prompted by a perceived difficulty in intubating the left mainstem bronchus with the BronchoCath tubes without a bevel at the bronchial tip.[7]

Left-Sided Double-Lumen Endotracheal Tube

SELECTING THE PROPER SIZE. A common problem found with the left-sided DLT is the lack of uniformity and the lack of objective guidelines for choosing a properly sized DLT. A left-sided DLT that is too small requires a large endobronchial cuff volume, which might increase the chances of malposition. Also, a small-sized DLT does not readily allow for adult fiberoptic bronchoscope access. A properly sized DLT is the one in which the main body of the tube passes atraumatically through the glottis and advances easily within the trachea, and the bronchial component passes into the intended bronchus without difficulty. Furthermore, an air leak should be present when the endobronchial cuff is fully deflated.

Selecting the proper size DLT is very important because there are increasing reports of complications related to the use of undersized DLTs. Sivalingan et al reported a tension pneumothorax and pneumomediastinum after a chest radiograph showed that the endobronchial tip of a smaller-than-predicted DLT had migrated too far into the left lower bronchus, and the whole tidal volume was delivered preferentially into a single lobe.[8]

TABLE 8-1

Indications for Lung Separation

THORACIC SURGERY
Lung Surgery

Thoracoscopy
Lobectomy, segmentectomy, pneumonectomy
Lung transplantation

Lung Isolation

Lung abscess

Bronchial Surgery

Intraluminal tumors, sleeve surgery, bronchopleural fistula

Pleural surgery

Pleurectomy, pleurodesis, decortication

SURGERY ON GREAT VESSELS, HEART, AND PERICARDIUM

Heart

Transmyocardial laser revascularization
Reoperation thoracotomy approach, robotic surgery

Thoracic Aorta

Descending thoracic aortic aneurysm

Pulmonary artery

Rupture—hemorrhage, embolectomy

Pericardium

Biopsy, pericardiectomy, pericardial window*

ESOPHAGEAL SURGERY
Esophagogastrectomy

NONTHORACIC SURGICAL PROCEDURES

Orthopedic Procedures

Spine surgery (thoracic column)

NONSURGICAL PROCEDURES
Pulmonary alveolar proteinosis

Pulmonary lavage

VENTILATORY MODALITIES
Differential lung ventilation
Positive end-expiratory pressure ventilation

*Thoracoscopic approach
From Campos JH: *Anesth Clin North Am* 19:455, 2001.

Multiple studies have been reported, including different radiographic measurements to determine the proper size of a left-sided DLT. Brodsky et al had reported that a direct measurement of the diameter of the tracheal width from edge to edge at the interclavicular plane from the preoperative posteroanterior chest radiograph can be used as a guide to help predict which left-sided DLT to select for each patient.[9] Their study led

to a 90% increase in the use of larger tubes (i.e., a left-sided 41F DLT in men and 39F and 41F DLTs in women). Chow et al, however, using the same methodology as Brodsky et al, found these sizes to be less reliable in the Asian patient population[10]; this result was presumably due to their shorter statures. In the Chow study, the predicted tube for female patients was originally an oversized left-sided DLT (i.e., a tight fit when the endobronchial lumen was passed into the bronchus when the cuff was fully deflated). In this study, the overall positive predictive value for predicting the proper size of a left-sided DLT was 77% for males and 45% for females. Considering different patient populations when applying the tracheal width method of estimation, it is possible that for patients of shorter stature this method might have a limited use, and that an alternative predictive method should be sought. The other method that can be considered when selecting a left-sided DLT is based on measurements of left mainstem bronchial diameter from a computer tomography (CT) scan.[11] This technique avoids overlying soft tissues, which can make the bronchus difficult to identify on the chest radiograph. The CT scan also identifies the bronchial wall, facilitating the measurement of bronchial diameter and detection of bronchial anatomic anomalies. The circumferential diameter of the entrance of the main bronchus is measured with calipers by an experienced radiologist. For this method to be reliable, the bronchial diameter of the DLT tip must be known, but at the present time this measurement is not included in the manufacturer's package insert. A properly sized left-sided DLT should have a bronchial tip 1 to 2 mm smaller than the patient's left bronchus to allow for the additional space occupied by the deflated bronchial cuff. The chest radiograph and/or the CT scan of the chest can objectively guide the size choice for a left DLT for individual patients in whom bronchial anatomy might be anomalous. A conversion table is recommended based on measurements of tracheal width from chest radiographs, bronchial width measurements based on CT scanning of the chest, and the predicted DLT tube size (Table 8-2).

TABLE 8-2

Conversion Measurements of Tracheal Width Based on Chest Radiograph and Bronchial Diameter Measurements, CT Scan of the Chest, and the Predicted Left-Sided Double-Lumen Endotracheal Tube Size

Measured Tracheal Width (mm)	Measured Bronchial Diameter (mm)	Left-sided DLT (F)
≥ 18	≥12	41
≥ 16	12	39
≥ 15	11	37
≥ 14	10	35
≥ 12.5	<10	32
≥ 11	NA	28
NA	NA	26

From Brodsky JB, Macario A, Mark JBD: *Anesth Analg* 82:861, 1996; Hannallah M, Benumof JL, Silverman PM, et al: *J Cardiothorac Vasc Anesth* 11:168, 1997; Fitzmaurice BG, Brodsky JB: *J Cardiothorac Vasc Anesth* 13:322, 1999.
NA, Not applicable; has not been investigated.

CONFIRMATION OF PLACEMENT AND POSITION OF LEFT-SIDED DOUBLE-LUMEN ENDOTRACHEAL TUBES. Techniques used for placement and positioning of left-sided DLTs have remained unchanged over the years. In the "blind" technique, the tube is passed after direct laryngoscopy and then turned 90 degrees counterclockwise after both cuffs have passed the vocal cords. It is then advanced until slight resistance is felt, which might indicate that the endobronchial lumen of the tube had entered the bronchus; or the tube can be advanced until the depth of insertion in relationship to the teeth is approximately 29 cm for either males or females if the patient's height is an average of 170 cm.[12] Recent studies have suggested that to increase the accuracy of placement, the stylet should be kept in the DLT until the endobronchial lumen is in the bronchus.[13] When the stylet was retained, the DLT was placed correctly 60% of the time, compared with only 17% accuracy if the stylet was removed. However, leaving the stylet in the tube as it is advanced may increase the rate of placement-related complications.

The second technique commonly used for tube placement is the fiberoptic-guided technique, which is performed after the endobronchial tip of the DLT is passed into the patient's trachea. The fiberoptic bronchoscope (FOB) is passed down the endobronchial lumen, and the tip of the DLT is directed into the left mainstem bronchus.

At the present time, no study has been done to demonstrate superiority of either the blind or the fiberoptic-guided technique during placement of these tubes. The advantage of the fiberoptic-guided technique is that the tracheal carina is identified and the left bronchus is visualized before advancing the tube so that the correct side is identified and the FOB and tube are advanced to the target bronchus. A 3.5- or 4.2-mm OD (outer diameter) bronchoscope will fit through a 35 to 41F DLT, whereas a 2.4-mm OD bronchoscope should be used for a 26F to 32F DLT.

Defining the proper placement and optimal position of the DLT is a challenging task. Although various methods of achieving this have been studied, only two are clinically relevant: auscultation and fiberoptic bronchoscopy.

AUSCULTATION VERSUS FIBEROPTIC BRONCHOSCOPY FOR CONFIRMATION OF LEFT-SIDED DOUBLE-LUMEN ENDOTRACHEAL TUBE PLACEMENT. Auscultation is one of the methods used to assess the position of DLTs. After the DLT is inserted, both the tracheal and the endobronchial cuffs are inflated to seal leaks. The endobronchial cuff usually requires 2 mL or a maximum of 3 mL of air to achieve a seal. The disposable connector of the DLT is then attached to the anesthesia breathing circuit. Auscultation and chest wall movements on bilateral ventilation are determined first. Then, upon clamping the endobronchial lumen limb adapter, if the endobronchial tip of a left-sided DLT is within the left bronchus, breath sounds should be absent in the left side of the chest. Finally, upon clamping the limb of the endotracheal lumen adapter and ventilating through the endobronchial lumen, breath sounds should be absent from the right side of the chest.

To determine the validity of auscultation for confirming DLT position by fiberoptic bronchoscopy, one study showed that auscultation alone is unreliable as an indicator of proper DLT placement. When an FOB was used, it resulted in 78% of left-sided DLTs and 83% of right-sided DLTs having to be repositioned.[14] In a second and larger study in which 200 patients were intubated by the blind method with a left- or right-sided DLT, followed by confirmation with an FOB, more than one-third of the DLTs required repositioning.[15] In Klein et al's study, malposition was defined as occurring when the DLT had to be moved more than 0.5 cm to correct its position with the aid of the FOB.[15] This indicates that fiberoptic bronchoscopy is recommended when positioning DLTs. The advantages of an FOB are the ability to guide the endobronchial lumen into the bronchus, the ability to correct intraoperative malpositions, and the ability to remove secretions through the suction channel.[15] The "margin of safety" on the endobronchial view is defined as the length of the mainstem bronchus where a correctly positioned DLT can be moved and still be correctly positioned without causing obstruction of any conducting airway. The average margin of safety in positioning a left-sided DLT from Mallinckrodt is 19 mm.[16] Visualization of the endobronchial cuff edge and of the distal tip of the endobronchial lumen is used to make this measurement.

FIBEROPTIC BRONCHOSCOPY AND LEFT-SIDED DOUBLE-LUMEN ENDOTRACHEAL TUBES. The best method for confirmation of a proper DLT placement in the tracheobronchial tree is by flexible fiberoptic bronchoscopy. In a standard approach, the tracheal lumen should be examined to ensure that there is no bronchial cuff herniation.[17] This is achieved by viewing the right mainstem bronchus and the right upper-lobe bronchus and, to the left below the carina, by visualizing the endobronchial cuff (seen in blue) 2 mm into the bronchus (Figure 8-1). The next step of the examination is made through the endobronchial lumen to check for patency of the tube. The tip of the endobronchial orifice must be identified to avoid distal impaction and partial occlusion of the left upper or lower bronchi (Figure 8-2). The average margin of safety in positioning left-sided double-lumen endotracheal tubes ranges from 16 to 19 mm.[16] The blue edge of the endobronchial cuff is visualized below the tracheal carina, 2 to 3 mm inside the left bronchus, and the endobronchial lumen tip is above the bronchial bifurcation so that the DLT can be moved without occluding a conducting airway. This confirmation of DLT positioning should be performed in the supine position first and then, after repositioning, in the lateral decubitus position. BronchoCath tubes from Mallinckrodt have a line encircling the tube, which is radio-opaque. This line is proximal to the bronchial cuff and can be useful while positioning a left-sided DLT. The line is 4 cm from the distal tip of the endobronchial lumen. This marker reflects white during fiberoptic visualization and, when positioned slightly above the carina, it should provide the necessary margin of safety for positioning into the left mainstem bronchus. The average length of the left mainstem bronchus is 5.0 cm for female and 5.5 cm for male patients, respectively.

The left-sided DLT is the most suitable tube for lung separation for the vast majority of elective thoracic surgical procedures. Benumof et al demonstrated that left-sided DLTs have a greater margin of safety and should be the tubes of choice in the majority of cases where OLV is needed, regardless of the surgical side.[16] The authors of this study pointed out, however, that in many instances a left-sided DLT cannot be placed and that a right-sided DLT is the only alternative.

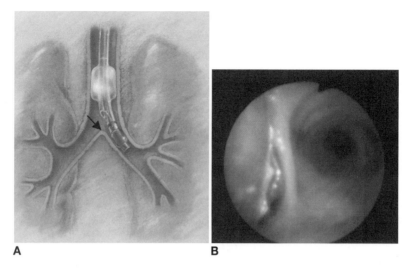

FIGURE 8-1 A, The optimal position of a left-sided DLT within the trachea. The *arrow* shows where the tip of the bronchoscope identifies tracheal carina. **B,** Optimal position of a left-sided DLT when the fiberoptic bronchoscope is passed through the tracheal lumen. The blue edge of the endobronchial cuff is seen 2 mm inside the left bronchus. (See also Color Plate 1.)

Right-Sided Double-Lumen Endotracheal Tubes

In the adult patient, the trachea bifurcates at the level of the fifth thoracic vertebra, forming the carina and the right and left mainstem bronchi. The left mainstem bronchus has a secondary bifurcation at a distance of 5 cm from the carina. The right mainstem bronchus is shorter than the left bronchus because the right upper-lobe bronchus originates at a distance of 1.5 to 2 cm from the carina. In 1 of 250 otherwise normal subjects, the right upper-lobe bronchus arises directly from the trachea.[18] Because of the relatively short length of the right mainstem bronchus, techniques employing right endobronchial intubation must take into account the location and potential for obstruction of the orifice of the right upper-lobe bronchus. In fact, the principal argument against the use of a right-sided DLT has been the low margin of safety in its

positioning and the high incidence of right upper-lobe collapse and obstruction.[19]

There are, however, clinical situations in which it may be preferable to avoid manipulation and intubation of the left main bronchus. For example, an exophytic lesion may compress the left bronchus or create a ball-valve effect that would obstruct the left lumen of the DLT. Other scenarios in which a left-sided DLT might not be appropriate include the following:

- An intraluminal tumor near the left main bronchus
- A left bronchial stent
- Left lung transplantation
- A descending thoracic aortic aneurysm compressing the left bronchus
- A left-sided pneumonectomy

During left pneumonectomy, the presence of a left-sided DLT in the left bronchus increases the risk for displacement during

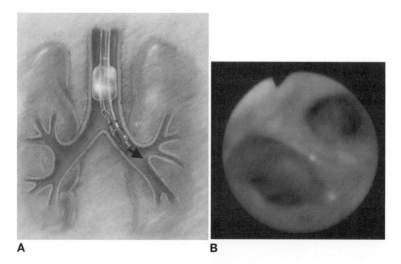

FIGURE 8-2 A, The optimal position of a left-sided DLT within the trachea. The *arrow* indicates where the tip of the fiberoptic bronchoscope emerges. **B,** A clear view of the bronchial bifurcation (left upper and lower bronchi). When the left-sided DLT is in the optimal position, the fiberoptic bronchoscope is being advanced through the endobronchial lumen. The left upper lobe orifice is on the left, and the left lower lobe is on the right. (See also Color Plate 2.)

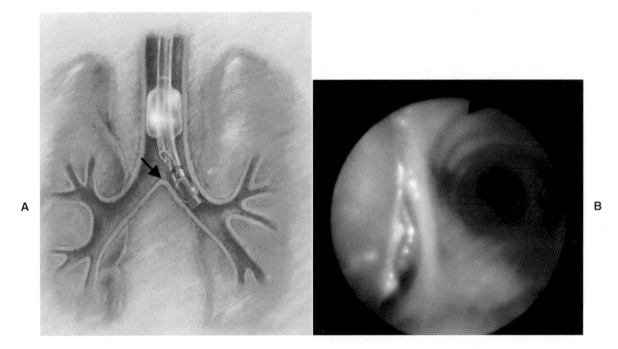

COLOR PLATE 1 A, The optimal position of a left-sided DLT within the trachea. The arrow shows where the tip of the bronchoscope identifies tracheal carina. **B,** Optimal position of a left-sided DLT when the fiberoptic bronchoscope is passed through the tracheal lumen. The blue edge of the endobronchial cuff is seen 2 mm inside the left bronchus.

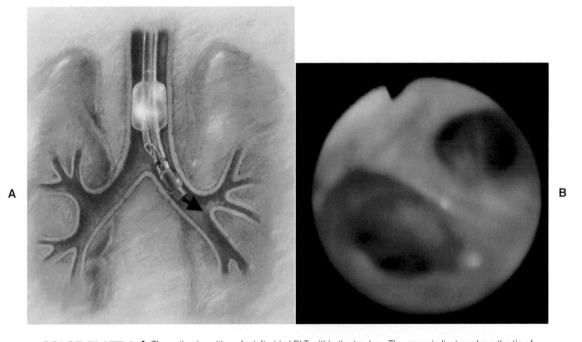

COLOR PLATE 2 A, The optimal position of a left-sided DLT within the trachea. The arrow indicates where the tip of the fiberoptic bronchoscope emerges. **B,** A clear view of the bronchial bifurcation (left upper and lower bronchi). When the left-sided DLT is in the optimal position, the fiberoptic bronchoscope is being advanced through the endobronchial lumen. The left upper lobe orifice is on the left, and the left lower lobe is on the right.

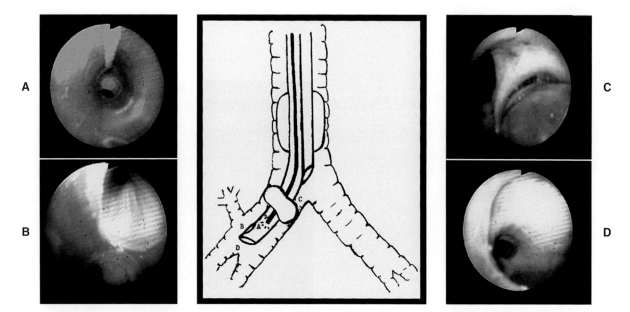

COLOR PLATE 3 Shows a fiberoptic bronchoscopic exam for a right-sided DLT. **A,** A white-line marker when the bronchoscope is passed through the endobronchial lumen. **B,** The slot of the endobronchial lumen properly aligned within the entrance of the right upper bronchus. **C,** The edge of the endobronchial cuff around the entrance of the right mainstem bronchus when the bronchoscope is passed through the tracheal lumen. **D,** Part of the bronchus intermedius when the bronchoscope is advanced through the distal portion of the endobronchial lumen.

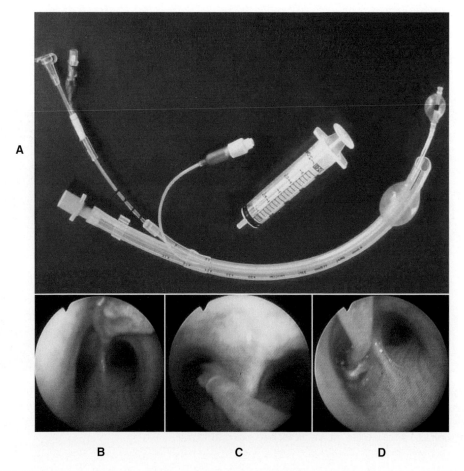

COLOR PLATE 4 A, The Univent tube. **B,** A bronchoscopic view of the deflated bronchial blocker while it is being advanced near the entrance of the tracheal carina. **C,** The bronchial blocker after entering the left mainstem bronchus. **D,** A proper and optimal position of the bronchial blocker of the Univent into the left bronchus.

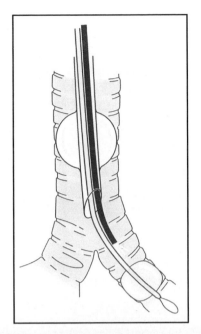

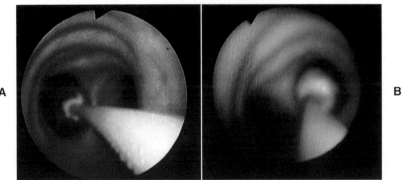

COLOR PLATE 5 The fiberoptic bronchoscope for the wire-guided endobronchial blocker. **A,** Left-sided placement. **B,** Right-sided placement.

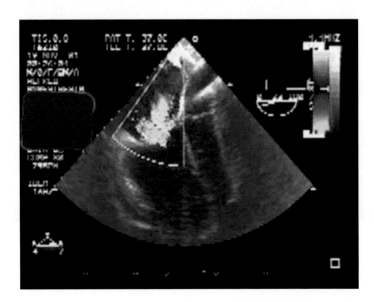

COLOR PLATE 6 Acute right ventricular failure and severe tricuspid regurgitation. Midesophageal four-chamber view.

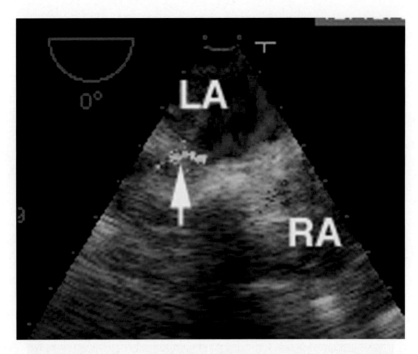

COLOR PLATE 7 Color Doppler echocardiography showing a mosaic pattern of right lower pulmonary vein inflow *(arrows)* where it enters the left atrium *(LA)* and revealing severe obstruction of its anastomosis. (From Huang YC, Cheng YJ, Lin YH, et al: *Anesth Analg* 91:558, 2000.)

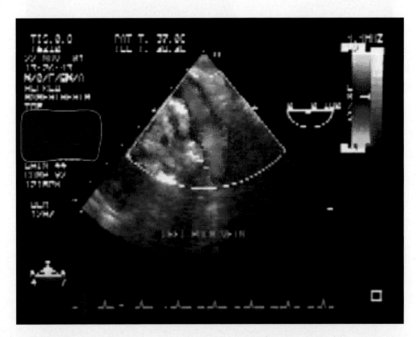

COLOR PLATE 8 Color Doppler echocardiography of an acceptable left upper pulmonary vein anastomosis with pulmonary transplantation.

TABLE 8-3

Indications for Right-Sided Double-Lumen Endotracheal Tubes

Exophytic tumor that compresses the left mainstem bronchus
Intraluminal tumor near entrance of the left mainstem bronchus
Left-sided pneumonectomy
Left-lung transplantation
Left-sided tracheobronchial disruption
Left mainstem bronchus stent already in place
Descending thoracic aortic aneurysm with distorted left mainstem bronchus anatomy
Sharp angle on the left mainstem bronchus

From Campos JH, Gomez MN: *J Cardiothorac Vasc Anesth* 17:246, 2002.

retraction, prevents surgical access to the entire ipsilateral bronchial tree, or limits the surgeon when palpating the left hilum during OLV, resulting in the need for frequent manipulation of the tube. During a left pneumonectomy, the endobronchial lumen must be withdrawn into the trachea before stapling the left main bronchus. If a right-sided DLT is used for left pneumonectomy, the risk of contamination or loss of seal is decreased because the right-sided DLT does not need to be withdrawn. Table 8-3 shows the indications for a right-sided DLT.[20]

Although the design of right-sided DLTs varies among manufacturers, all have an extra slot in the endobronchial port that varies in size to allow ventilation through the right upper-lobe bronchus and, if well aligned, prevents unnecessary obstruction. Figure 8-3 displays two different designs of right-sided double-lumen endotracheal tubes. An early study reported high incidences of obstruction and right upper-lobe collapse when right-sided DLTs were used.[19] In a study by McKenna et al, two

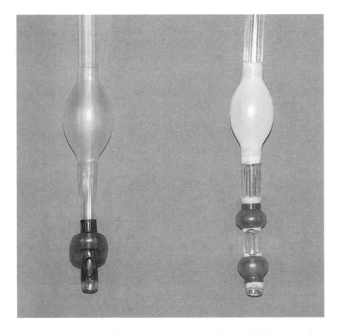

FIGURE 8-3 Two different designs of right-sided double-lumen endotracheal tubes. To the left is the Mallinckrodt BronchoCath, which shows the pear shape of the endobronchial cuff when it is fully inflated. To the right is the Sheridan right-sided DLT Sher-I–Bronch, which shows two balloons in the endobronchial cuff when they are fully inflated.

groups of patients were evaluated.[19] One group was assigned to receive a polyvinylchloride right-sided DLT manufactured by Mallinckrodt, and the second group was assigned to receive a red rubber Robertshaw (Leylland) nondisposable right-sided DLT. The results showed that 90% of the patients assigned to the red rubber tubes had bronchoscopically confirmed patency of the right upper-lobe bronchus. This was probably a result of the larger 20-mm diameter of the ventilation slot for ventilating the right upper bronchus. In contrast, the study group that received the polyvinylchloride disposable DLTs had to be discontinued in 9 out of 20 patients because a higher incidence (89%) of right upper-lobe obstruction was seen. This was presumed to be due to the smaller size of the ventilation slot (11 mm). One of the limitations of this study was that FOB confirmation of the right-sided DLT was not employed routinely after lateral decubitus positioning. Despite a lower margin of safety, two recent studies using improved placement techniques and better-designed right-sided DLTs have shown that there is no increased risk for right upper-lobe obstruction for left- or right-sided thoracic surgery.[21,22]

In a recent study, Campos et al reported very good results in patients requiring OLV for left-sided thoracic surgery when right-sided DLTs were used, compared with the use of modified left-sided DLTs.[22] In this study, the incidence of right upper-lobe collapse was assessed intraoperatively by a chest radiograph, which showed no collapse of the right upper lobe in any patient who received a right-sided DLT. The main difference from previous studies is that in this study, an FOB was used for guidance and positioning of the right-sided DLT during the supine and lateral decubitus positions.[19,22]

CONFIRMATION OF THE PLACEMENT AND POSITIONING OF RIGHT-SIDED DOUBLE-LUMEN ENDOTRACHEAL TUBES. Based on clinical research, the following technique is suggested for placement and positioning of right-sided double-lumen endotracheal tubes.[21,22] First, the right-sided DLT is introduced into the glottis using direct laryngoscopy. After the endobronchial tip has passed the vocal cords, the stylet is removed, and the tube is advanced and then rotated 90 degrees toward the right. Then the FOB guidance technique is used to advance the fiberscope into the endobronchial lumen. The tracheal carina and origins of the right upper bronchus and bronchus intermedius are identified. Next, fiberoptic bronchoscopy is used to guide the tube into the right mainstem bronchus. The white-line marker on the inner surface of the endobronchial lumen is identified distal to the right upper-lobe ventilation slot. To align the slot of the tube and the upper-lobe bronchus, a rotational movement of the DLT is necessary. The FOB is passed through the slot, and alignment with the origin of the right upper-lobe bronchus is assessed. After this, the FOB is passed through the tracheal lumen, and the blue bronchial cuff is positioned at the origin of the right mainstem bronchus below the level of the tracheal carina, where the blue edge of the bronchial balloon is seen when this is fully inflated (usually 2 to 5 mm below the carina in the right mainstem bronchus). Finally, the view through the distal end of the endobronchial lumen should show the bronchus intermedius. The FOB examination should be performed with the patient in both the supine and the lateral decubitus positions. Figure 8-4 shows step-by-step placement of the right-sided double-lumen endotracheal tube with the FOB technique.

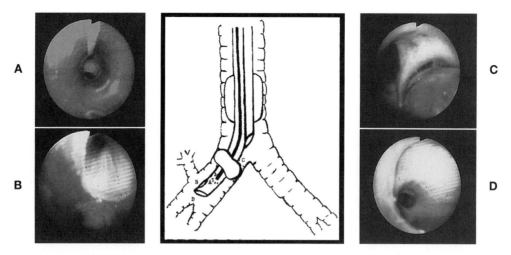

FIGURE 8-4 Fiberoptic bronchoscopic exam for a right-sided DLT. **A,** A white-line marker when the bronchoscope is passed through the endobronchial lumen. **B,** The slot of the endobronchial lumen properly aligned within the entrance of the right upper bronchus. **C,** The edge of the endobronchial cuff around the entrance of the right mainstem bronchus when the bronchoscope is passed through the tracheal lumen. **D,** Part of the bronchus intermedius when the bronchoscope is advanced through the distal portion of the endobronchial lumen. (See also Color Plate 3.)

Use of Double-Lumen Endotracheal Tubes in Patients with a Difficult Airway

Placement of a DLT in a patient who presents with a difficult airway is a challenging task. In general, the increased outside diameter of the DLT makes it relatively harder to place into a hole of any given size when compared with a conventional endotracheal tube of the same size. Also, the increased overall rigidity of the DLT might impair optimal shaping of the tube. The following techniques can be used when facing a patient who presents with a difficult airway without distorted anatomy.

The safest approach to secure an airway is by an awake oral intubation. Patane et al reported the use of awake fiberoptic bronchoscopy during placement of a DLT in a patient with a difficult airway[23]. The second alternative is to intubate the patient with a single-lumen endotracheal tube during awake oral intubation. Once the intubation is performed, an airway guide is passed through the single-lumen endotracheal tube. Available airway guides include commercial tube exchangers (from Cook Critical Care, Bloomington, Ind., Sheridan Catheter Corporation, Argyle, N.Y., and Cardiomed Supplies, Gormley, Ontario, Canada) or fiberoptic bronchoscopes. These types of airway guides are commercially made, have depth markers labeled in centimeters, and are available in a wide range of outer diameters. An advantage of the tube exchanger is that it has standard adapters for either oxygen insufflation or jet ventilation. Once the single-lumen endotracheal tube is withdrawn, the new DLT can be passed by holding the tube exchanger catheter at a depth of no more than 26 cm at the teeth. Cook manufactures a 9F 83-cm-long flexible tube exchange catheter that is suitable when using a DLT. Also, a double-diameter tube exchanger can be used for DLT replacement. The tube exchanger consists of a 4.0-mm OD (outer diameter) inner part and a 7.0-mm OD outer cylindrical part, both made from polytetrafluoroethylene. The inner part can be passed through the lumen of the outer part. The advantage of this double-diameter tube exchanger is that it provides greater rigidity when exchanging a tube, thus enabling easier introduction of the DLT into the patient's trachea.[24]

In a patient with a tracheostomy who requires OLV, placement of a conventional DLT poses a problem because of the inherent shortening of the patient's upper airway as a result of the tracheostomy. To deal with this issue, manufacturers have modified the DLT. Sheridan made a 41F left-sided DLT in which the tracheal and endobronchial lumens have been shortened, and currently, Naruke Tube (Koken Medical, Shinjuku-ku, Tokyo, Japan) produces a 39F left-sided DLT made of wire-reinforced silicon.[25,26] Both of these DLTs have been used with satisfactory results in patients with permanent stomas and tracheostomies.

Complications of Double-Lumen Endotracheal Tubes

Various complications have been reported regarding the use and misuse of a DLT. Perhaps the most lethal complication arising from a DLT is an airway rupture. One of the first reports of an airway rupture with the use of a disposable DLT was done by Burton et al.[27] Two years later, Wagner et al reported the first case of a tracheal rupture with a disposable DLT.[28] The incidence of airway rupture from a DLT is certainly underreported. In a comprehensive review of the last 25 years by Fitzmaurice and Brodsky, it was found that the majority of airway injuries were associated with undersized DLTs, particularly in females who received a 35F or 37F DLT.[29] In that review, the authors did not find any report of airway trauma (i.e., bronchial rupture) with the use of a 41F DLT. A rupture of the left mainstem bronchus by the tracheal portions of a DLT has been reported by Sakuragi et al.[30] In this report, a longitudinal laceration of the left mainstem bronchus occurred that originated below the carina and extended to near the left upper-lobe bronchial orifice. The possible cause of this rupture was an undersized DLT, the endotracheal body of which had entered the left mainstem bronchus. It appears that undersized DLTs have the tendency to migrate too far distally into the bronchus, or that the endobronchial cuff requires a larger amount of air when smaller tubes are used. There are many factors that should be considered as predisposing to airway rupture. These include the following:

- Inserting a DLT too forcefully
- Placing undersized DLTs that have a tendency to migrate too far distally into the bronchus
- Overdistention of the endotracheal or endobronchial cuff by the use of nitrous oxide
- Repositioning of a DLT with the cuffs inflated
- Preexisting pathology of the airway including tumor, the use of steroids, or esophageal surgery

Airway damage during the use of a DLT can present as an unexpected air leak, as subcutaneous emphysema, or as airway bleeding and hemodynamic instability because of a tension pneumothorax. If any of the above signs are present during the case, a bronchoscopic examination should be performed to look for signs of airway disruption.

MALPOSITION OF DOUBLE-LUMEN ENDOTRACHEAL TUBES. A malpositioned DLT will fail to empty the lung, causing gas trapping during positive pressure ventilation; or it might partially collapse the ventilated (dependent) lung and eventually create severe hypoxemia as a result of bilateral shunting of blood. Further, malposition of a DLT will not protect the dependent lung against contralateral contamination of blood if hemoptysis is present. In addition, if the nondependent lung is ventilated because of a malpositioned DLT, the lung will not empty completely. In fact, the partially inflated lung will interfere with surgery. The DLT can either be located insufficiently far or too far into the appropriate bronchus. With knowledge of tracheobronchial anatomy and use of flexible fiberoptic bronchoscopy, the majority of malpositions of DLTs can be corrected if tracheobronchial anatomy is not distorted.

Some of the most common malpositions are dislodgment of the endobronchial cuff due to an overinflated cuff (which normally requires no more than 3 mL of air), surgical manipulation of the bronchus, or extension of the head and neck during lateral decubitus positioning. In a recent study, Desiderio et al found that DLTs can be moved cephalad approximately 1 cm from original placement when patients are turned to a lateral decubitus position, even when the endobronchial cuff is kept inflated while turning the patient.[31] Therefore, once the DLT is in optimal position (as demonstrated by an FOB in the supine position), only the endotracheal cuff should be kept inflated, and the endobronchial cuff should be deflated while turning the patient into the lateral decubitus position. Then, in the lateral decubitus position, the endobronchial cuff should be reinflated and the position of the tube verified by fiberoptic bronchoscopy. One way to prevent dislodgment of the DLT after the patient is in the lateral decubitus position is by placing the patient's head on folded blankets so that no flexion or extension can occur, as these movements contribute to a greater incidence of malpositions.[32] Right-sided DLTs will be more likely than left-sided DLTs to dislodge intraoperatively, and will require repositioning using fiberoptic bronchoscopy. Recent studies have demonstrated that with a better-designed right-sided DLT and greater usage of fiberoptic bronchoscopy, the incidence of malpositions is not statistically significant when right-sided DLTs are compared with left-sided DLTs (3 vs. 5 total

malpositions in 40 randomized patients) for left-sided thoracic surgery.[22] Fiberoptic bronchoscopy is recommended to correct the majority of intraoperative malpositions of DLTs. In cases in which copious secretions are present along with a malpositioned DLT, a suction tube is connected to the FOB to aid in the repositioning of the DLT. In extreme cases in which hemoptysis is present, connection of an oxygen source to the channel port of the FOB will allow oxygen insufflation and blood dispersal to aid in visual inspection of the DLT position.

Bronchial Blocking Technology for Lung Separation

Currently, there are three blocking devices available to facilitate lung separation. These include the following[3-5]:
1. Fogarty occlusion catheter
2. A single-lumen endotracheal tube with an enclosed bronchial blocker (Univent tube)
3. A wire-guided endobronchial blocker (WEB)

These bronchial blockers have a unique advantage over DLTs in that they can either be used as selective lobar blockers (single lobe) or can block the entire bronchus and produce total lung collapse. Also, these devices can be used with a conventional single-lumen endotracheal tube (from Fogarty or WEB), and, if postoperative mechanical ventilation is needed, the single-lumen endotracheal tube can be left in situ, and the blocker can be withdrawn at the conclusion of surgery without need to reintubate or replace an endotracheal tube.

Fogarty Occlusion Catheter

The Fogarty vascular embolectomy catheter can be used as a bronchial blocker device to achieve lung collapse and separation.[3] An advantage of the Fogarty catheter is that it can be passed through or alongside a single-lumen endotracheal tube in an already intubated patient without the need for a tube exchange. Another advantage of the Fogarty occlusion catheter pertains to its use in patients who cannot be intubated orally. If nasotracheal intubation is feasible, an awake nasotracheal intubation can be performed under FOB guidance, and then the Fogarty catheter is advanced through the nasotracheal tube and its position guided via fiberoptic bronchoscopy. The Fogarty catheter can also be used in a tracheostomized patient by advancing a single-lumen endotracheal tube through the stoma and then advancing the Fogarty catheter.[33]

The most commonly used Fogarty embolectomy catheter is the number 8F, although other sizes can be used. The occlusion balloons range in size from 0.5 to 3.0 mL of air. These Fogarty occlusion catheters come with a wire stylet that can be curved at the distal end to facilitate guidance to the targeted bronchus where lung collapse is desired. The Fogarty catheter is passed through the bronchoscope elbow, and guidance is facilitated by advancing the FOB next to it. After the Fogarty catheter is introduced into the target bronchus, the catheter balloon is inflated under direct vision, and the FOB is withdrawn. The optimal position of the Fogarty occlusion catheter is one that allows complete blockade of the bronchus without any detectable air leak, usually 4 mm below the tracheal carina into the targeted bronchus. A disadvantage of the Fogarty catheter as a bronchial blocker is its lack of a hollow center; therefore suction or oxygen insufflation is not possible, and lung collapse takes longer because it occurs by absorption atelectasis. Another limitation of the Fogarty catheter is that it is made of latex, so it cannot be used in patients with latex allergy.

Single-Lumen Endotracheal Tube with an Enclosed Bronchial Blocker (Univent)

Another alternative to achieve lung separation is a Univent tube.[4] This device combines the attributes of a bronchial blocker balloon and a DLT. The Univent is made of silicone and is latex free, has the general shape of a conventional single-lumen endotracheal tube, and includes a small channel housing a 2-mm diameter movable endobronchial blocker that is used to achieve selective lobar or total lung collapse. This bronchial blocker is made of flexible plastic material and has a high-volume, low-pressure cuff that requires between 2 and 8 mL of air to seal, depending on whether it is used as a selective lobar blockade or as a total bronchial blocker. The outer or proximal port of the bronchial blocker has a suction cap (Figure 8-5). The blocker also has a grip that allows rotational movement to facilitate guidance into the selected bronchus. The sizes available for Univent tubes range from 6.0- to 9.0-mm ID. (The Univent tube size designation is made by the internal diameter [ID] in millimeters). Because of the oval shape of the internal circumference, the internal radius is reduced. Also, the channel that encloses the bronchial blocker increases the anterior-posterior external diameter, which makes the tube diameter larger than the circumference of a single-lumen tube with corresponding internal diameter numbers. Table 8-4 describes the sizes available for Univent tubes compared with sizes of single-lumen endotracheal tubes and DLTs.

ADVANTAGES OF THE UNIVENT TUBE. Because of its construction with inert silicone, its reduced bulk, and its anatomic angulation, the Univent tube is thought to have less chance of causing trauma to the airway compared to DLT. There are no studies available to support this theory, however.[34]

Although the Univent tube was introduced earlier in the 1980s, the first large series of studies of its use occurred in 1987[35]. A few modifications have been made recently, including the handle grip that is incorporated as a part of the bronchial blocker and is located in the proximal portion of the blocker near the suction cap. A report by the inventor has been published, detailing his 12-year experience[36]. One of the multiple advantages of this tube is its capability for selective collapse of the entire lung (one lung) or a single lobe.[37,38] Its utility has been demonstrated in patients in whom the airway is considered difficult for direct laryngoscopy and during unanticipated difficult endotracheal intubation.[24,39-45] The Univent tube has also been found to be practical in patients who have a tracheostomy and require OLV.[46,47] Because of its relative ease of placement, the Univent tube has been used in patients with hemoptysis or in patients who have bleeding diathesis.[48,49] In addition, the Univent tube has been useful in facilitating jet ventilation during bronchial sleeve surgery or in sleeve pneumonectomy.[50,51] Among the multiple uses of the Univent tube, the capability of applying constant positive airway pressure has been reported (Table 8-5 details the indications for Univent tubes).[38,52,53]

The Univent tube has the capability of being converted to a conventional single-lumen endotracheal tube at any time during surgery by deflating the bronchial blocker and, together with the blocker shaft, withdrawing it into the main body housing. The tube is then used as a regular tube, thus making the switch from OLV to normal two-lung ventilation simple and easy. Perhaps the greatest advantage of the Univent tube is for patients who require prolonged postoperative ventilation, because there is no need of tube exchange at the conclusion of surgery if large-size Univents (i.e., 8.0- or 9.0-mm ID) are used.

CONFIRMATION OF THE PLACEMENT AND POSITIONING OF THE UNIVENT TUBE. Because the Univent tube is similar to the single-lumen tube, no study is available pertaining to selection of the proper size. Tube size selection therefore is clinically no

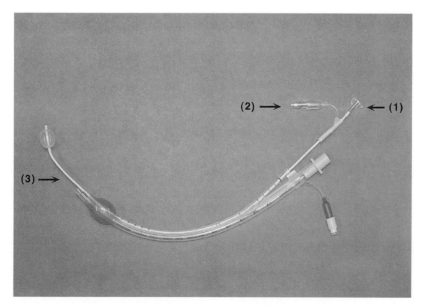

FIGURE 8-5 The Univent tube. *Arrow 1* indicates where the suction cap is located. *Arrow 2* shows the pilot balloon of the bronchial blocker cuff. *Arrow 3* shows the enclosed bronchial blocker.

TABLE 8-4

Approximate Comparative Diameters of Single-Lumen Endotracheal Tubes, Univent Tubes, and Double-Lumen Endotracheal Tubes

SINGLE-LUMEN ENDOTRACHEAL TUBES		UNIVENT TUBES		DLT (F)		BRONCHOCATH[†]	
I.D. mm	O.D. mm	I.D. mm	O.D. mm	(F)	O.D.mm*	Bronchial I.D. mm	Tracheal I.D. mm
6.5	8.9						
				26[‡]	8.7	3.5	3.5
7.0	9.5	6.0	9.7 / 11.5	28	9.3	3.2	3.1
7.5	10.2	7.0	10.7 / 12.5				
8.0	10.8	7.5	11.5 / 12.5	32	10.7	3.4	3.5
8.5	11.4	8.0	11.7 / 13.5	35	11.7	4.3	4.5
9.0	12.1			37	12.3	4.5	4.7
9.5	12.8			39	13.0	4.9	4.9
10.0	13.5	9.0	12.7 / 14.5	41	13.7	5.4	5.4

*Denotes the main body
[†]Mallinckrodt
[‡]Rüsch manufactures this DLT
I.D., internal diameter; *O.D.*, outer diameter

different from selecting a regular single-lumen endotracheal tube with a larger outer diameter. The ideal tube size is the tube that passes the glottis and vocal cords atraumatically and without any resistance while the tube is being advanced into the patient's trachea. The author believes that patients weighing more than 80 kg should receive a Univent tube of at least 7.5 or 8.0 mm ID.

Before use, the bronchial blocker is lubricated with medical-grade silicone lubricant to facilitate passage, and the bronchial and tracheal cuffs should be checked. After deflation and retraction of the bronchial cuff, standard endotracheal tube placement is performed. For placement of the right-sided Univent blocker, once the tube is in the patient's trachea, an FOB is passed. The enclosed bronchial blocker is advanced until the tip is seen and, under direct vision, it is advanced into the right mainstem bronchus. Because the right mainstem bronchus is aligned more vertically with the trachea and the anterior position of the blocker, the Univent blocker passes directly into this bronchus. Once the cuff of the blocker is placed in the right bronchus, inflation of the cuff is made with 5 to 8 mL of air until the inflated balloon blocks the bronchus. The optimal location for positioning a Univent tube in the right side is when the cuff of the blocker is inflated fully without inclusion of the origin of the right upper lobe bronchus and with no detectable leaks. In the author's clinical experience, sometimes the right upper lobe bronchus can be occluded, especially in women. To facilitate lung collapse in these cases, the bronchoscope is connected to suction and advanced to the right upper bronchus. The air that remains in the upper bronchus is evacuated, and after withdrawal of the bronchoscope, the bronchial blocker cuff is reinflated. Once the bronchial blocker blocks the targeted bronchus, applying low suction to the blocker lumen facilitates lung collapse.

Obstruction of the left mainstem bronchus can be performed in various ways. The Univent tube is positioned into the patient's trachea, and the shaft of the blocker is rotated toward the left side while advancing under direct vision; turning the patient's head also facilitates guidance of the blocker. Another method is to rotate the Univent tube 90 degrees toward the left side and then advance the blocker under direct vision. A third method is to guide the Univent tube under direct vision with fiberoptic bronchoscopy. The Univent tube is advanced near the tracheal carina where the tip of the tube sits in the entrance of the left mainstem bronchus. The blocker is advanced into the left bronchus, and the tracheal tube is withdrawn. The optimal position for the bronchial blocker in the left mainstem bronchus is one that allows visualization of the bronchial cuff 3 to 5 mm down the left main bronchus without any detectable leak when the cuff is fully inflated.[54] See Figure 8-6 for placement of a left-sided Univent tube.

Because of a shorter distance between the tracheal carina and the right upper bronchus, the Univent blocker can be used for selective lobar blockade by advancing the blocker in the bronchus intermedius, selectively collapsing the right middle and right lower lobes if needed.[37,38] The amount of air needed for the bronchial blocker to obtain a seal of the bronchus intermedius is between 3 and 5 mL.

TABLE 8-5

Specific Indications for a Single-Lumen Tube with Enclosed Bronchial Blocker (Univent Tube)

Difficult airway and one-lung ventilation
Selective lobar ventilation
Conversion to a regular endotracheal tube at any time during surgery
Small adults
During application of jet ventilation (i.e., sleeve pneumonectomy)
Absence of need to reintubate for postoperative mechanical ventilation (when Univent tubes 8.0- or 9.0-mm ID are used)

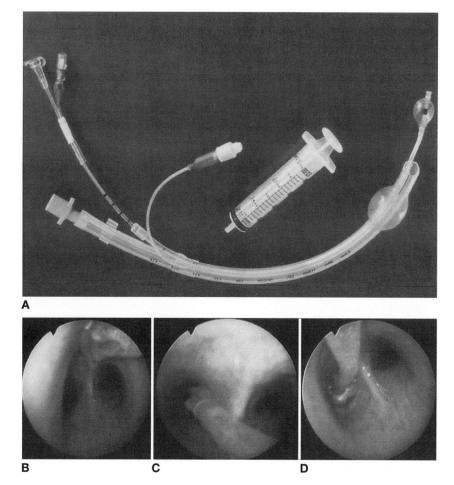

FIGURE 8-6 A, The Univent tube. **B,** A bronchoscopic view of the deflated bronchial blocker while it is being advanced near the entrance of the tracheal carina. **C,** The bronchial blocker after entering the left mainstem bronchus. **D,** A proper and optimal position of the bronchial blocker of the Univent into the left bronchus. (See also Color Plate 4.)

COMPLICATIONS OF THE UNIVENT TUBE. Various complications have been reported regarding the use of the Univent tube. Some complications have been related to problems with the tube itself. A dislodgment of the end of the tip of the bronchial blocker has been reported, as well as fragments that have been torn from the inner wall of the Univent tube.[55,56] Failure to achieve lung separation because of abnormal anatomy or difficulties in sealing the bronchus with the bronchial blocker have also been reported.[57,58]

An inclusion of the bronchial blocker into the stapling line during a right upper lobectomy has been reported.[59] This problem could be avoided by withdrawing the blocker before stapling the bronchus, if it were believed to be felt by the surgeon at the entrance of the right upper bronchus. Another serious complication reported was the obstruction of the tracheal lumen after the bronchial blocker cuff was inflated mistakenly when it was almost fully retracted, producing respiratory arrest. This complication can be prevented by cutting the pilot of the bronchial blocker balloon if mechanical postoperative ventilation is needed, through the Univent tube.[60]

A case of severe hypoxia has been reported after suctioning of the nondependent lung via the bronchial blocker lumen, creating a negative pressure pulmonary edema.[61] The presence of a pneumothorax complicating the use of the Univent tube has been reported as well.[62] Malposition and dislodgment of the bronchial blocker can occur, specifically while changing the patient's position from the supine to the lateral decubitus position or during surgery while surgical manipulation of the bronchus occurs.[63] Fiberoptic bronchoscopy is the recommended method to correct intraoperative malpositions of Univent tubes.

Comparison of Airflow Resistances Among Single-Lumen Endotracheal Tubes, Double-Lumen Endotracheal Tubes, and Univent Tubes

Airflow resistance varies among single-lumen endotracheal tubes, DLTs, and Univent tubes. Because of the relatively smaller internal diameters of the endotracheal or endobronchial lumen, the DLT might have a higher airflow resistance, thus increasing the difficulties of postoperative mechanical ventilation and weaning. It has been recommended in the past that DLTs should be replaced by a single-lumen endotracheal tube. In a recent study by Slinger et al, a comparison of airflow resistance among different sizes of disposable polyvinylchloride DLTs (35F, 37F, 39F, and 41F) was made with airflow resistance in single-lumen endotracheal tubes (sizes 6.0-, 7.5-, 8.0-, and 9.0-mm ID) and the Univent tube (6.0-, 7.5-, 8.0-, and

9.0-mm ID) in an in vitro model.[64] The DLTs were from different manufacturers (Rüsch, Sheridan, and Mallinckrodt). The study results showed that single-lumen endotracheal tubes had less airflow resistance than either a Univent or a DLT. The study also showed that Univent tubes had higher airflow resistance when compared with DLTs. Within the DLT group, Mallinckrodt DLTs had higher airflow resistance when compared with Rüsch or Sheridan models. Of particular interest in Slinger's study was that the use of smaller sizes of Univent tubes (i.e., 6.0- and 7.5-mm ID) produced a disproportionately high airflow resistance. This finding is explained by the fact that the bronchial blocker occupies a large amount of the cross-sectional area. Also, the oval shape of the Univent tube reduces the circumferential diameter.

One of the reasons for the higher airflow resistance of the Mallinckrodt DLT when compared with the Rüsch or Sheridan is the narrower lumen of the Y connector used in these other manufacturers' tubes. According to this study, DLTs from Rüsch and Sheridan should not increase the work of spontaneous ventilation. Therefore if there is a need for a short time in the postoperative period, there is no reason to replace these tubes with a single-lumen endotracheal tube. Complications such as malposition or airway trauma might arise, however, when those tubes are left in place for postoperative mechanical ventilation. Because the smaller sizes of Univent tubes (i.e., 6.0- to 7.5-mm ID) have a high flow resistance, they should be replaced with an appropriate single-lumen endotracheal tube if mechanical postoperative ventilation is needed.

Wire-Guided Endobronchial Blocker During Lung Separation

Another approach to lung separation is the use of the wire-guided endobronchial blocker (WEB), which consists of either a 7F or 9F 70-cm catheter with two (1.4-mm and 0.4-mm ID) lumens.[5] At the distal end is a high-volume, low-pressure balloon. The 1.4-mm ID lumen contains a flexible wire passing through the proximal end of the catheter and extending to the distal end, where it exits as a small flexible wire loop. This wire allows an FOB to be coupled with the WEB. This endobronchial blocker is accompanied by a three-way multiport airway adapter that is used for fiberoptic bronchoscopy, a blocker port, and a port that can be connected to the anesthesia breathing circuit. For the WEB to function properly and allow manipulation with the FOB, at least an 8.0-mm ID single-lumen endotracheal tube must be used.

The newly introduced WEB has some advantages over the DLTs and Univent tubes. For instance, it has been reported to be effective in patients who are intubated or who present with a difficult airway and require OLV during acute trauma to the chest.[65] Another advantage is that the WEB can be passed through a nasotracheal tube in patients who require nasal intubation and OLV—specifically patients with a limited mouth opening.[66,67] Also, it can be used as a selective lobar blocker in patients with a previous pneumonectomy who require selective one-lobe ventilation during thoracoscopic surgery (personal report JHC). The WEB can be used in morbidly obese patients with a history of gastroesophageal reflux who frequently require rapid-sequence induction because it uses a single-lumen endotracheal tube. Finally, because this system uses a single-lumen endotracheal tube, it maximizes the cross-sectional diameter

(internal diameter) and eliminates the need for tube exchange if mechanical postoperative ventilation is needed. (Table 8-6 depicts the indications for the wire-guided endobronchial blocker.) One of the limitations of the WEB is difficulty of use with smaller, single-lumen endotracheal tubes (less than 7.0-mm ID) because of the difficulty of navigating the WEB with the fiberoptic bronchoscope. Once the WEB is in an optimal position, movements of the patient's head can lead to easy dislodgment. Also, because the WEB's suction channel diameter is just 1.4-mm ID, suctioning of copious secretions from the nondependant lung can be limited. Once the wire loop is withdrawn, it cannot be reinserted into the WEB, so repositioning of the WEB can be troublesome. Figure 8-7 shows the wire-guided endobronchial blocker and its multiport adapter.

CONFIRMATION OF PLACEMENT AND POSITIONING OF THE WIRE-GUIDED ENDOBRONCHIAL BLOCKER. The WEB is a single unit that comes in a 7F or 9F size for use in adults, and it is passed through a standard endotracheal tube. Before placement, the endobronchial blocker cuff is inflated and tested. After testing and balloon deflation, the WEB shaft and the FOB are lubricated with medical grade silicone lubricant. This technique involves placing the endobronchial blocker through the single-lumen endotracheal tube and uses the fiberoptic bronchoscope and wire loop to guide the blocker into the appropriate mainstem bronchus (Figure 8-8). The wire loop is important if the endobronchial blocker is to be inserted into the left mainstem bronchus; otherwise, the blocker nearly always advances into the right mainstem bronchus. When passing the WEB into the left mainstem bronchus, turning the patient's head toward the right and pushing the trachea to the right at the level of the neck facilitates guidance of the WEB to the left mainstem bronchus. The bronchoscope has to be advanced far enough so that the WEB will enter the bronchus while it is being advanced. Once the deflated cuff is below the entrance of the bronchus, the bronchoscope is withdrawn; then, the cuff is fully inflated with 5 to 8 mL of air to obtain proper seal of the targeted bronchus.

After the patient is turned to the lateral decubitus position, another FOB examination is necessary to ensure that the cuff of the WEB is still positioned correctly. The wire loop can then be withdrawn to convert the 1.4-mm channel into a suction port to expedite lung collapse. It is important to remove the wire loop to avoid inclusion in the stapling line. The optimal position of the WEB in the left or in the right bronchus is when the outer surface of the blocker balloon is seen with the fiberoptic bronchoscope at least 2 to 5 mm below the tracheal carina in the targeted bronchus and proper seal is achieved (Figure 8-9).

TABLE 8-6

Specific Indications for the Wire-Guided Endobronchial Blocker

Critically ill patients
Rapid-sequence induction and one-lung ventilation
Known and unknown difficult airway
Nasotracheal intubation
Small adult patients
Selective lobar ventilation
Hemoptysis
Trauma

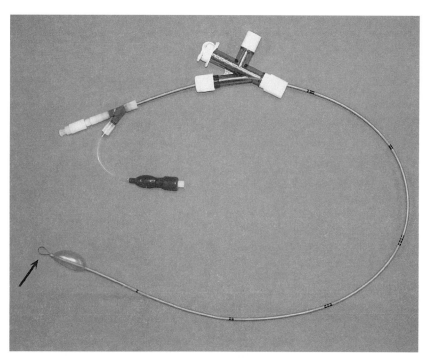

FIGURE 8-7 The wire-guided endobronchial blocker and its multiport adapter. The *arrow* indicates the distal end of the wire loop.

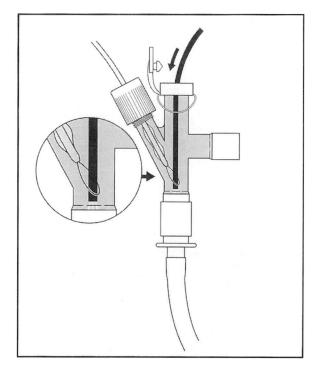

FIGURE 8-8 The multiport adapter, with coupling of the wire loop and the tip of the fiberoptic bronchoscope, navigating together within the single-lumen endotracheal tube. (Courtesy Dr. George A. Arndt.)

The small (1.4 mm) diameter of the suction channel (where the wire loop emerges) increases the time required for the lung to be collapsed. Lung collapse can be expedited, however, by attaching a barrel from a 3-mL syringe and connecting it to low suction for a few seconds. Another way to expedite lung collapse and facilitate lung separation is by deflating the WEB cuff once it is in optimal position, then passing a fiberoptic bronchoscope beyond the cuff and connecting it to a low suction, so all conducting airways are suctioned and remaining gas (air) is aspirated. Perhaps due to the relative novelty of the WEB, there are no reports of complications in the literature.

Use of Bronchial Blocking Technology During Difficult Airway and One-Lung Ventilation

A great advantage of the Fogarty occlusion catheter or the WEB is its ease of placement in patients with difficult airways.[33] This is because the safest approach to securing a difficult airway is by an awake oral or nasotracheal intubation.[67] Once intubation is achieved with a single-lumen endotracheal tube, either a Fogarty or a WEB blocker can be used by advancing any of these devices into the single-lumen endotracheal tube that has already been placed, and guiding its direction with an FOB. In cases where a small size (i.e., less than 6.5-mm ID) single-lumen endotracheal tube is employed, the tube can be exchanged for a larger size by the techniques described earlier in the chapter concerning difficult airway management.

Another alternative for providing OLV in patients with difficult airway is to use a Univent tube.[39-47] An awake intubation technique with a Univent tube over the FOB is used in cases of anticipated difficult airways. Also, the guide-wire tube

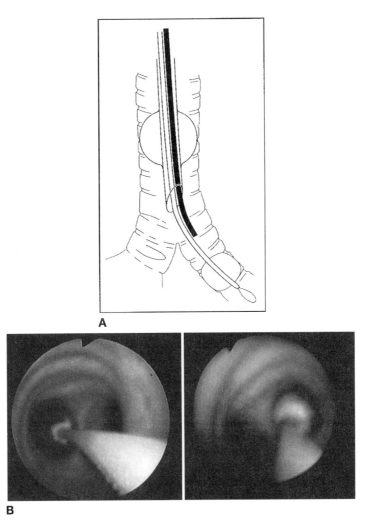

FIGURE 8-9 The fiberoptic bronchoscope for the wire-guided endobronchial blocker. **A,** Left-sided placement. **B,** Right-sided placement. (See also Color Plate 5.)

exchange technique with a Cook exchanger can be used by inserting a single-lumen endotracheal tube with an FOB during awake bronchoscopy. After the tube is in place, it is replaced with the guide-wire and is exchanged for a Univent tube of larger diameter.[24] If the Univent tube cannot be advanced beyond the epiglottis, either a 90-degrees counterclockwise rotation of the tube or the use of a laryngoscope blade to displace tissues to facilitate passage into the epiglottis is recommended. The optimal position of the Univent tube is demonstrated with fiberoptic bronchoscopy. Another use of the Univent is that it can be passed through an existing tracheostomy without any difficulties.[46,47]

Summary

Table 8-7 summarizes a practical approach to the use of these devices for lung separation, methods of size selection, and methods to confirm proper placement. Because of the greater margin of safety, the disposable left-sided DLT should be the tube of choice for the majority of cases in which lung separa-

tion is required. A disposable right-sided DLT should be an alternative when a contraindication to the placement of a left-sided DLT exists. In some cases, a right-sided DLT will be advantageous (i.e., when there is left bronchus distorted anatomy or left-sided pneumonectomy). Radiologic studies, such as a radiograph of the chest, will allow measurement of the tracheal width and predict the proper size of a left-sided DLT. In a few instances, a radiologic measurement of the left mainstem bronchial diameter from a CT scan of the chest will allow determination of the properly sized left-sided DLT. Based on clinical reports, Fogartys, Univent tubes, and/or WEB blockers might be better choices for patients with difficult airway who require lung separation or whenever a selective lobar blockade is needed. The Fogarty catheter or the WEB is suitable when nasotracheal intubation is the only choice to secure the airway and OLV is required. For all selective intubations, the method of choice for proper tube placement and bronchial blockade is fiberoptic bronchoscopy, with the patient in a supine position at first or in a lateral decubitus position later, or if a malposition occurs.[68,69]

TABLE 8-7

Summary of Lung Separation Devices and Recommendations for Placement

Device	Indication	Tube Size	Placement and confirmation
Left-sided DLT			
	• Majority of elective left or right thoracic surgical procedures	• Determined by measurements of the tracheal width from chest radiograph	FOB
Right-sided DLT			
	• Left bronchus—distorted anatomy • Left pneumonectomy		FOB with guided technique
Fogarty occlusion catheter			
	• Critically ill patient • Small bronchus • Difficult airway • Nasotracheal intubation	• Standard endotracheal tube at least 6.0-mm ID	FOB
Univent blockers			
	• Selective lobar blockade • Difficult airway requiring lung separation		FOB
WEB blockers			
	• Critically ill patient • Selective lobar blockade • Difficult airway • Nasotracheal intubation requiring lung separation	• Standard endotracheal tube at least 8.0-mm ID	FOB with guided technique

DLT, Double-lumen endotracheal tube; *FOB*, flexible fiberoptic bronchoscopy; *WEB*, wire-guided endobronchial blocker.

REFERENCES

1. Björk VO, Carlens E: The prevention of spread during pulmonary resection by the use of a double-lumen catheter, *J Thorac Surg* 20:151, 1950.
2. Robertshaw FL: Low-resistance double-lumen endobronchial tubes, *Br J Anaesth* 34:576, 1962.
3. Ginsberg RJ: New technique for one-lung anesthesia using an endobronchial blocker, *J Thorac Cardiovasc Surg* 82:542, 1981.
4. Inoue H, Shohtsu A, Ogawa J, et al: New device for one-lung anesthesia: endotracheal tube with movable blocker, *J Thorac Cardiovasc Surg* 83:940, 1982.
5. Arndt GA, Kranner PW, Rusy DA, et al: Single-lung ventilation in a critically ill patient using fiberoptically directed wire-guided endobronchial blocker, *Anesthesiology* 90:1484, 1999.
6. Lewis JW, Serwin JP, Gabriel FS, et al: The utility of a double-lumen tube for one-lung ventilation in a variety of noncardiac thoracic surgical procedures, *J Cardiothorac Vasc Surg* 6:705, 1992.
7. Brodsky JB, Macario A: Modified BronchoCath double-lumen tube, *J Cardiothorac Vasc Anesth* 9:784, 1995.
8. Sivalingam P, Tio R: Tension pneumothorax, pneumomediastinum, pneumoperitoneum, and subcutaneous emphysema in a 15-year-old Chinese girl after a double-lumen tube intubation and one-lung ventilation, *J Cardiothorac Vasc Anesth* 13:312, 1999.
9. Brodsky JD, Macario A, Mark JBD: Tracheal diameter predicts double-lumen tube size: a method for selecting left double-lumen tubes, *Anesth Analg* 82:861, 1996.
10. Chow MYH, Liam BL, Lew TWK, et al: Predicting the size of a double-lumen endobronchial tube based on tracheal diameter, *Anesth Analg* 87:158, 1998.
11. Hannallah M, Benumof JL, Silverman PM, et al: Evaluation of an approach to choosing a left double-lumen tube size based on chest computed tomographic scan measurement of left mainstem bronchial diameter, *J Cardiothorac Vasc Anesth* 11:168, 1997.
12. Brodsky JB, Benumof JL, Ehrenwerth J, et al: Depth of placement of left double-lumen endobronchial tubes, *Anesth Analg* 73:570, 1991.
13. Lieberman D, Littleford J, Horan, et al: Placement of left double-lumen endobronchial tubes with or without stylet, *Can J Anaesth* 43:238, 1996.
14. Alliaume BA, Coddens J, Deloof T: Reliability of auscultation in positioning of double-lumen endobronchial tubes, *Can J Anaesth* 39:687, 1992.
15. Klein U, Karzai W, Bloos F, et al: Role of fiberoptic bronchoscopy in conjunction with the use of double-lumen tubes for thoracic anesthesia, *Anesthesiology* 88:346, 1998
16. Benumof JL, Partridge BL, Salvatierra C, et al: Margin of safety in positioning modern double-lumen endotracheal tubes, *Anesthesiology* 67:729, 1987.
17. Slinger PD: Fiberoptic bronchoscopic positioning of double-lumen tubes, *J Cardiothorac Anesth* 3:486, 1989.
18. Stene R, Rose M, Weinger MB, et al: Bronchial trifurcation at the carina complicating use of a double-lumen tracheal tube, *Anesthesiology* 80:1162, 1994.
19. McKenna MJ, Wilson RS, Botelho RJ: Right upper lobe obstruction with right-sided double-lumen endobronchial tubes: a comparison of two tube types, *J Cardiothorac Anesth* 2:734, 1988.
20. Campos JH, Gomez MN: Pro: right-sided double-lumen endotracheal tube should be routinely used in thoracic surgery, *J Cardiothorac Vasc Anesth* 16:246, 2002.
21. Campos JH, Massa CF: Is there a better right-sided tube for one-lung ventilation? A comparison of the right-sided double-lumen tube with the single-lumen tube with right-sided enclosed bronchial blocker, *Anesth Analg* 86:696, 1998.
22. Campos JH, Massa CF, Kernstine KH: The incidence of right upper lobe collapse when comparing a right-sided double-lumen tube versus a modified left double-lumen tube for left-sided thoracic surgery, *Anesth Analg* 90:535, 2000.
23. Patane PS, Shell BA, Mahla ME: Awake fiberoptic endobronchial intubation, *J Cardiothorac Anesth* 4:229, 1990.
24. Hagihira S, Takashina M, Mori T, et al: One-lung ventilation in patients with difficult airways, *J Cardiothorac Vasc Anesth* 12:186, 1998.

25. Brodsky JB, Tobler HG, Mark JBD: A double-lumen endobronchial tube for tracheotomies, *Anesthesiology* 74:388, 1991.

26. Saito T, Naruke T, Carney E, et al: New double intrabronchial tube (Naruke tube) for tracheostomized patients, *Anesthesiology* 89:1038, 1998.

27. Burton NA, Fall SM, Lyons T, et al: Rupture of the left mainstem bronchus with a polyvinylchloride double-lumen tube, *Chest* 6:928, 1983.

28. Wagner DL, Gammage GW, Wong ML: Tracheal rupture following the insertion of a disposable double-lumen endotracheal tube, *Anesthesiology* 63:698, 1985.

29. Fitzmaurice BG, Brodsky JB: Airway rupture from double-lumen tubes, *J Cardiothorac Vasc Anesth* 13:322, 1999.

30. Sakuragi T, Kumano K, Yasumoto M, et al: Rupture of the left mainstem bronchus by the tracheal portion of a double-lumen endobronchial tube, *Acta Anaesthesiol Scan* 41:1218, 1997.

31. Desiderio DP, Burt M, Kolker AC, et al: The effects of endobronchial cuff inflation on double-lumen endobronchial tube movement after lateral decubitus positioning, *J Cardiothorac Vasc Anesth* 11:595, 1997.

32. Saito S, Dohi S, Naito H: Alteration of double lumen endobronchial tube position by flexion and extension of the neck, *Anesthesiology* 52:696, 1985.

33. Zilberstein M, Katz RI, Levy A, et al: An improved method for introducing an endobronchial blocker, *J Cardiothorac Anesth* 4:481, 1990.

34. Gayes JM: The Univent tube is the best technique for providing one-lung ventilation. pro: One-lung ventilation is best accomplished with the Univent endotracheal tube, *J Cardiothorac Vasc Anesth* 7:103, 1993.

35. Karwande SV: A new tube for single-lung ventilation, *Chest* 92:761, 1987.

36. Inoue H: Univent endotracheal tube: twelve-year experience, *J Thorac Cardiovasc Surg* 107:1171, 1994.

37. Campos JH, Ledet C, Moyers JR: Improvement of arterial oxygen saturation with selective lobar bronchial block during hemorrhage in a patient with previous contralateral lobectomy, *Anesth Analg* 81:1095, 1995.

38. Campos JH: Effects on oxygenation during selective lobar versus total lung collapse with or without continuous positive airway pressure, *Anesth Analg* 85:583, 1997.

39. Baraka A: The Univent tube can facilitate difficult intubation in a patient undergoing thoracoscopy, *J Cardiothorac Vasc Anesth* 10:693, 1996.

40. Ransom ES, Carter LS, Mund GD: Univent tube: a useful device in patients with difficult airways, *J Cardiothorac Vasc Anesth* 9:725, 1995.

41. Benumof JL: Difficult tubes and difficult airways, *J Cardiothorac Vasc Anesth* 12:131, 1998.

42. Campos JH: Difficult airway and one-lung ventilation, *Curr Rev Clin* 22:197, 2002.

43. Garcia-Aguado R, Mateo EM, Tommasi-Rosso M, et al: Thoracic surgery and difficult intubation: another application of the Univent tube for one-lung ventilation, *J Cardiothorac Vasc Anesth* 7:925, 1997.

44. Garcia-Aguado R, Mateo EM, Onrubia VJ, et al: Use of the Univent system tube for difficult intubation and for achieving one-lung anaesthesia, *Acta Anaesthesiol Scand* 40:765, 1996.

45. Takenaka I, Aoyama K, Kadoya T: Use of the Univent bronchial-blocker tube for unanticipated difficult endotracheal intubation, *Anesthesiology* 93:590, 2000.

46. Bellver J, Garcia-Aguado R, DeAndres J, et al: Selective bronchial intubation with the Univent system in patients with a tracheostomy, *Anesthesiology* 79:1453, 1993.

47. Dhamee MS: One-lung ventilation in a patient with a fresh tracheostomy using the tracheostomy tube and a Univent endobronchial blocker, *J Cardiothorac Vasc Anesth* 11:124, 1997.

48. Inoue H, Shotsu A, Ogawa J, et al: Endotracheal tube with movable blocker to prevent aspiration of intratracheal bleeding, *Ann Thorac Surg* 37:497, 1984.

49. Herenstein R, Russo JR, Moonka N, et al: Management of one-lung anesthesia in an anticoagulated patient, *Anesth Analg* 67:1120, 1988.

50. Ransom E, Detterbeck F, Klein JI, et al: Univent tube provides a new technique for jet ventilation, *Anesthesiology* 84:724, 1996.

51. Williams H, Gothard J: Jet ventilation in a Univent tube for sleeve pneumonectomy, *Eur J Anaesthesiol* 18:407, 2000.

52. Benumof JL, Gaughan S, Ozaki GT: Operative lung constant positive airway pressure with the Univent bronchial blocker tube, *Anesth Analg* 74:406, 1992.

53. Foroughi V, Krucylak PE, Wyatt J, et al: A technically simple means for administration of continuous positive airway pressure during one-lung ventilation using a Univent tube, *Anesth Analg* 81:656, 1995.

54. Hannallah MS, Benumof JL: Comparison of two techniques to inflate the bronchial cuff of the Univent tube, *Anesth Analg* 75:784, 1992.

55. Doi Y, Uda R, Akatsuka M, et al: Damaged Univent tubes, *Anesth Analg* 87:732, 1998.

56. Harioka T, Hosoi S, Nomura K: Foreign body in the trachea originated from the inner wall of the Univent tube, *Anesthesiology* 89:1596, 1998.

57. Peragallo RA, Swenson JD: Congenital tracheal bronchus: the inability to isolate the right lung with a Univent bronchial blocker tube, *Anesth Analg* 91:300, 2000.

58. Asai T: Failure of the Univent bronchial blocker in sealing the bronchus, *Anaesthesia* 54:97, 2000.

59. Thielmeier KA, Anwar M: Complications of the Univent tube, *Anesthesiology* 84:491, 1996.

60. Dougherty P, Hannallah M: A potential serious complication that resulted from improper use of the Univent tube, *Anesthesiology* 77:835, 1992.

61. Baraka A, Nawfal M, Kawkabani N: Severe hypoxemia after suction of the non-ventilated lung via the bronchial blocker lumen of the Univent tube, *J Cardiothorac Vasc Anesth* 10:694, 1996.

62. Schwartz DE, Yost CS, Larson MD: Pneumothorax complicating the use of a Univent endotracheal tube, *Anesth Analg* 76:443, 1993.

63. Campos JH, Reasoner DK, Moyers JR: Comparison of a modified double-lumen endotracheal tube with a single-lumen tube with enclosed bronchial blocker, *Anesth Analg* 83:1268, 1996.

64. Slinger PD, Lesiuk L: Flow resistances of disposable double-lumen, single-lumen, and Univent tubes, *J Cardiothorac Vasc Anesth* 12:142, 1998.

65. Grocott HP, Scales G, Schinderle D, et al: A new technique for lung isolation in acute thoracic trauma, *J Trauma* 49:940, 2000.

66. Arndt GA, DeLessio ST, Kranner PW, et al: One-lung ventilation when intubation is difficult: presentation of a new endobronchial blocker, *Acta Anaesthesiol Scan* 43:356, 1999.

67. Arndt GA, Buchika S, Kranner PW, et al: Wire-guided endobronchial blockade in a patient with a limited mouth opening, *Can J Anesth* 46:87, 1999.

68. Campos JH: Lung isolation techniques, *Anesth Clin North Am* 19:455, 2001.

69. Campos JH: Current techniques for perioperative lung isolation in adults, *Anesthesiology* 97:1295, 2002.

Anesthesia for Thoracic Diagnostic Procedures

9

Jan Ehrenwerth, MD

Sorin J. Brull, MD

ALTHOUGH thoracic diagnostic procedures have been considered to be relatively minor operations, they present a unique challenge to the anesthesiologist. Frequently, it is necessary to anesthetize a patient who is debilitated, has multisystem disease, and possesses only marginal respiratory reserve. Each of the diagnostic procedures requires special consideration for these patients. For example, during bronchoscopy the airway must be shared with the surgeon, and delivery of predictable levels of inhalation anesthetics can be difficult; mediastinoscopy might cause compression of major intrathoracic blood vessels and is occasionally associated with sudden catastrophic hemorrhage. Likewise, thoracoscopy has been known to lead to tension pneumothorax, and esophageal tears can occur during endoscopy.

Although it is theoretically possible to perform any of these diagnostic procedures under either regional or general anesthesia, there is no clear-cut advantage of one technique over the other for all patients. Rather, the choice of anesthetic technique must be individualized. The anesthesiologist should consider the patient's preoperative condition and preferences, the indications for the procedure, and its anticipated duration, as well as the anesthesiologist's familiarity with the various surgical techniques.

Preoperative Evaluation for Thoracic Diagnostic Procedures

A careful and detailed preoperative evaluation of the patient presenting for a thoracic diagnostic procedure is essential. Not only do patients who undergo these procedures often present with problems of oxygenation and ventilation, but they also can have disease processes involving several other organ systems. To minimize perioperative problems most effectively, the clinician must assess the patients' risk factors. Conditions that have been associated with increased risk of perioperative pulmonary complications include advanced age, preexisting pulmonary disease, obesity, history of smoking, cardiac dysfunction, kyphoscoliosis, neuromuscular disease, pulmonary infections, history of postoperative pulmonary complications, and poor preoperative physical condition[1] (see Chapter 18).

Warner showed that a smoking history of more than 20 pack-years is associated with an increased risk of developing postoperative pulmonary complications and that cessation of smoking for 8 weeks before surgery results in decreased postoperative respiratory compromise.[2] Even short-term smoking cessation, however, has been shown to be beneficial. Kambam demonstrated that P_{50} values return to normal and that

carboxyhemoglobin levels decrease if smoking cessation is undertaken at least 12 hours preoperatively.[3] Likewise, Smith and Landaw showed that the elevated red blood cell volume and reduced plasma volume both return toward normal in heavy smokers within a week after stopping smoking.[4] Thus, encouraging the patient to refrain from smoking preoperatively produces both long-term and short-term benefits.

The examination of the airway is of paramount importance. Assessment of neck and jaw mobility and visualization of oropharyngeal structures give important clues as to the ability to manage the airway and to instrument the trachea. Mallampati et al have described three airway classifications based on physical examination of the oropharynx.[5] Although these classifications may serve as guidelines, they are by no means absolute predictors of airway adequacy or ease of intubation. Patients' whose tracheas are difficult to intubate because of physical characteristics or previous history may be candidates for awake intubation or fiberoptic techniques.

Examination of the lungs might reveal wheezing, stridor, rales, or rhonchi. The presence of wheezing often indicates disease of the small airways and could be reversible. Wheezing can also be caused by a foreign body obstructing the large airways. Rales are associated with excess interstitial lung water from transudation of fluid. This is associated with decreased plasma oncotic pressure or increased amounts of interstitial fluid from left-sided congestive heart failure. Rhonchi are heard in patients with chronic obstructive lung disease, particularly in heavy smokers. These patients are prone to a productive cough with thick secretions, and they are at higher risk for developing perioperative atelectasis.

The presence of stridor is an extremely important clinical finding because it can indicate a significant obstruction of the airway. Furthermore, stridor can be helpful in pinpointing the area of obstruction. Inspiratory stridor is associated with extrathoracic lesions because negative pressure is generated inside the trachea during inspiration. This negative pressure allows the extrathoracic lesion to compress the airway further and worsen the obstruction. Conversely, stridor that occurs during exhalation is associated with variable intrathoracic lesions. The increase in intrathoracic pressure that occurs during exhalation further compromises the already narrowed intrathoracic segment (Figures 9-1, 9-2, and 9-3). The use of accessory muscles of respiration, substernal retractions, and tracheal tug are also indicative of an obstructive process.

Other physical signs, such as cyanosis, clubbing of the fingers, and increased anterior-to-posterior chest diameter, are usually associated with severe chronic hypoxemia and chronic

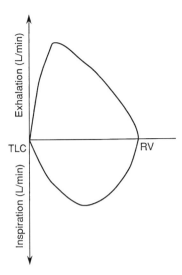

FIGURE 9-1 Schematic representation of normal flow-volume curves generated during inhalation *(bottom curve)* and exhalation *(top curve)*. *TLC,* Total lung capacity; *RV,* residual volume.

pulmonary disease. Absence of breath sounds can represent longstanding disease processes such as atelectasis, consolidation from pneumonia, or loss of parenchymal tissue. On the other hand, such an absence might indicate an acute process such as aspiration, pneumothorax, or obstruction of a main bronchus by a foreign body. Fever, leukocytosis, and sputum production should all alert the anesthesiologist to the presence of an intrapulmonary infectious process.

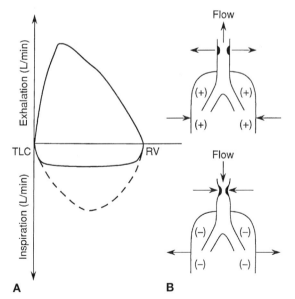

FIGURE 9-2 Schematic representation of an extrathoracic variable obstruction. The *solid lines* represent actual flow-volume curves; the *dashed line* represents a normal inspiratory pattern. Note that with the extrathoracic variable obstruction, exhalation induces a positive (+) intratracheal pressure, which in turn results in little or no resistance to flow past the narrowed segment **(A)**. Conversely, inhalation generates negative (−) intrathoracic pressure, which in turn induces negative pressure in the trachea below the point of obstruction. This negative pressure induces further obstruction and increases resistance to flow **(B)**.

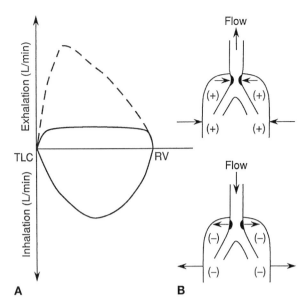

FIGURE 9-3 Schematic representation of an intrathoracic variable obstruction. Solid lines represent actual flow-volume curves, while the dashed line represents the normal expiratory pattern. During exhalation, the transthoracic positive (+) pressure is transmitted to the intrathoracic narrowed segment, which results in an increased resistance to flow **(A)**. Conversely, during inhalation, the negative (−) intrathoracic pressure distends the narrowed segment, resulting in little or no resistance to flow **(B)**.

Examination of old medical records often provides important clues as to previous problems. Frequently, patients have had multiple diagnostic procedures, and the anesthesia record can serve as a guide as to the difficulty of intubation as well as to any problems encountered during the procedure. Current diagnostic tests can be compared with previous ones to assess the progression of the disease process. Communication with the endoscopist may reveal other information about the airway obtained previously (i.e., via indirect laryngoscopy), which can help the anesthesiologist in formulating the anesthetic plan.

In addition to the history and physical assessment of the patient, laboratory data and diagnostic tests shed further light on the extent of the disease process. Analysis of room air arterial blood gases provides important information as to the status of the patient's oxygenation and ventilation. The presence of hypoxemia and hypercarbia indicates a severe disease process and, most likely, decreased pulmonary reserve. It should also warn the anesthesiologist of potential perioperative complications.

Preoperative electrocardiographic (ECG) examination can also reveal current processes usually associated with chronic pulmonary disease, such as right atrial and right ventricular hypertrophy. Comparison of a recent ECG with previous tracings can help delineate the progression of the disease and can signal development of myocardial ischemia, pulmonary hypertension, or ventricular hypertrophy.

Pulmonary function tests can be helpful in assessing the degree of impairment. Forced expiratory volume in one second (FEV_1) and forced vital capacity (FVC), performed both with and without bronchodilators, can demonstrate whether there is a reversible component of airway obstruction. If there is significant reversibility, initiation of preoperative bronchodilator therapy is indicated. Flow-volume loops can also give important clues as to the degree and location of airway obstructions (see Chapter 1).

Patients undergoing thoracic diagnostic procedures are more likely to develop postoperative pulmonary complications. Tisi recommended that preoperative spirometry be done for patients who are undergoing thoracotomy or upper abdominal operations; for those who are over 70 years of age, obese, or heavy smokers; and for those who have previous pulmonary disease.[6] Stein and Cassara found that a maximum expiratory flow rate of less than 200 L/min was predictive of patients at risk for pulmonary complications (see Chapter 18).[7]

A myriad of radiologic diagnostic procedures is currently available. These range from simple anteroposterior and lateral chest x-rays to sophisticated procedures such as tomography, computed tomography scans, magnetic resonance imaging, and arteriograms. These tests can provide invaluable information to the anesthesiologist regarding the location and degree of airway compromise (see Chapter 2). Failure to detect significant preoperative pulmonary compromise does not guarantee an uncomplicated intraoperative course. Induction of anesthesia or manipulation of the airway can unmask problems that were previously well compensated.

Bronchoscopy

Indications

Bronchoscopy evolved about 100 years ago, when Gustav Killian performed the first translaryngeal intubation of the trachea with a tube.[8,9] At first, this procedure was performed mainly to recover inhaled foreign bodies, although it was used later by Jackson for removal of excessive secretions from the pulmonary tree and for resection of endobronchial tumors.[10] New advances in technology—particularly the introduction by Ikeda of the fiberoptic bronchoscope—have permitted the broadening of the use of bronchoscopy.[11] Today, bronchoscopy is a common procedure, and both fiberoptic and rigid bronchoscopies have their own indications and involve specialized techniques. Indications for bronchoscopy can be divided into one of three categories: diagnostic, therapeutic, and preoperative evaluation of pathology.

Diagnostic Indications for Bronchoscopy

The most common indication for bronchoscopy is suspicion of bronchial neoplasm. The presenting complaints can include cough, hemoptysis, wheezing, or stridor. Cough is most often due to chronic bronchitis and is frequently associated with cigarette smoking. Sometimes a change in either the frequency or the character of the cough might be the only subtle hint of the presence of bronchogenic neoplasm. When cough is associated with other symptoms, such as stridor, it can suggest the presence of upper airway compromise from tumor. When cough is associated with wheezing, or when it leads to acute bronchospasm, it can suggest a tracheal or mediastinal tumor causing obstruction. Hemoptysis must also be regarded as an ominous sign until the presence of neoplasm is excluded. Although patients with chronic bronchitis from cigarette smok-

ing might expectorate blood-stained sputum, hemoptysis can also be the first sign of a bronchogenic neoplasm.

Other diagnostic indications for bronchoscopy include localized wheezing, atelectasis, persistent pneumonia, positive sputum cytology, and assessment of the airway. Localized wheezing or atelectasis can indicate partial endobronchial obstruction from neoplasm or from an aspirated foreign body. Bronchoscopy is useful after prolonged intubation to rule out the presence of subglottic stenosis, tracheomalacia, or, rarely, tracheoesophageal fistula. Examination of the tracheobronchial tree should also be performed after exposure to chemical fumes or smoke inhalation in order to assess the level and severity of the injury.

Bronchoscopy can also be performed when it is difficult to ascertain the correct placement of an endotracheal tube, such as in a difficult intubation or to document proper positioning of a double-lumen endotracheal tube (DLT).[12] The use of bronchoscopy with alveolar lavage has provided better diagnostic yields than both transbronchial and open-lung biopsies in patients with acquired immunodeficiency syndrome (AIDS).[13]

Therapeutic Indications for Bronchoscopy

Bronchoscopy is performed for therapeutic purposes, such as removal of aspirated foreign objects or suctioning of copious secretions that could result in atelectasis and worsening of ventilation-to-perfusion matching. When therapeutic bronchoscopy is performed after aspiration of particulate gastric contents, the removal of the particulate matter can lessen both the degree and the severity of the resulting Mendelson's syndrome. Another therapeutic indication is bronchoscopy for instillation of vasoconstrictors to decrease edema. Drainage of a lung abscess with the aid of a bronchoscope can facilitate obtaining cultures and biopsy specimens and has been used in the diagnosis and treatment of bronchial stump suture granulomas.[14]

Indications for Preoperative Assessment of Pathology with Bronchoscopy

Most patients undergoing thoracotomy for lobe resection or pneumonectomy require a preoperative bronchoscopic examination. These patients present for lung resection because of carcinoma, and preoperative bronchoscopy allows the surgeon to evaluate the extent of the tumor and to rule out malignancy of the contralateral lung.

Indications for Rigid vs. Fiberoptic Bronchoscopy

INDICATIONS FOR RIGID BRONCHOSCOPY

The rigid or open-tube endoscopic examination of the airway has been used extensively for removal of foreign bodies. It is easier to remove large foreign bodies in toto with the rigid bronchoscope, whereas the fiberoptic bronchoscope might require fragmentation of the aspirated object. Moderate or massive hemoptysis is also an indication for rigid bronchoscopy, which provides the operator with a better opportunity to suction the airway and improve the visualization of the bleeding site. In the case of a vascular tumor, the use of the rigid bronchoscope enables the endoscopist to pack the airway should massive bleeding occur during resection. In infants and small children, the rigid bronchoscope is the instrument of choice, as it allows better ventilation and control of the airway. When the patency of the airway is compromised by granulation tissue or tumor, the rigid bronchoscope could be the only instrument that can be inserted past the point of obstruction. Other advantages of the rigid technique include direct visualization of the tracheobronchial tree without the optical distortion associated with fiberoptic bronchoscopy. The rigid bronchoscope also allows the endoscopist to obtain a relatively larger biopsy specimen, thus enhancing the diagnostic yield. Finally, the rigid bronchoscope is preferred for visualization of the carina and for the assessment of its mobility and sharpness; these observations provide diagnostic clues about bronchial involvement and carcinogenic infiltration.

INDICATIONS FOR FIBEROPTIC BRONCHOSCOPY

Flexible fiberoptic bronchoscopy provides a better yield than rigid bronchoscopy in diagnosing bronchogenic carcinoma. A primary advantage of the flexible technique is improved optical resolution, which allows detailed visualization of the tracheobronchial tree. In contrast to the rigid bronchoscope, the fiberoptic bronchoscope has a flexible tip and can be maneuvered into peripheral zones of the lung (i.e., fifth division bronchi), thus improving the diagnostic and therapeutic yields of biopsy procedures and exploration. Other advantages of the fiberoptic bronchoscope include facilitation of intubation in patients who have difficult airway anatomy, facial trauma, neck injury, or an edematous airway from inhalation injury.

Fiberoptic bronchoscopy affords improved patient comfort when compared with rigid bronchoscopy. Thus the need for heavy premedication to allay fears is reduced. In patients at risk for developing hypoxia, fiberoptic bronchoscopy may be performed with the patient in a sitting or semi-sitting position, which improves the patient's ventilatory capacity. Other indications for fiberoptic bronchoscopy include patients with vertebral artery insufficiency in whom extension of the neck could induce cerebral ischemia, patients with previous cervical spine fusion, patients with atlantoaxial instability, and patients who are at risk for dental damage. Finally, video imaging (i.e., closed-circuit TV) allows closer cooperation between the endoscopist and the anesthesiologist when fiberoptic bronchoscopy is performed.

Although there are numerous reports that attest to the usefulness of fiberoptic bronchoscopy for removing aspirated foreign bodies, one disadvantage of this technique is the need to fragment the object before removal; this could lead to aspiration of small fragments distally. Another limitation of the fiberoptic bronchoscope is the relatively small size (2 mm) of the aspirating channel, limiting its usefulness for patients with hemoptysis and copious secretions.

Complications and Physiologic Changes Associated with Bronchoscopy

Many complications of bronchoscopy have been reported.[15-19] These are generally divided into two categories: complications associated with anesthesia and complications arising from the procedure itself. Hypoventilation and hypoxemia are two complications that can have potentially disastrous effects.[20-24] Both of these conditions can occur as a result of either excessive premedication or inadequate ventilation during the procedure. Because many bronchoscopies are performed under topical anesthesia, quantitative assessment of ventilation is more difficult than with general anesthesia. The use of tidal volume monitoring and capnography is difficult during regional anesthesia. Even under general anesthesia, oxygenation and ventilation can be impaired, depending on the type of bronchoscopy being performed and the method of ventilation used during the procedure. Other complications related to anesthesia include hypertension, hypotension, and tachycardia, all of which can result in myocardial ischemia.[25,26] Arhythmias are also possible and are frequently related to hypoxia and hypercarbia.[25-27]

Another potentially serious complication associated with bronchoscopy is a toxic reaction to local anesthetics. In two large retrospective studies, 73,000 bronchoscopies were reported by Credle et al and Suratt et al.[15,16] Both groups reported major complications related to local anesthetic toxicity. In both studies, tetracaine was the agent most often implicated. In Credle et al's report of more than 24,000 bronchoscopies, there were seven major complications related to topical anesthesia.[15] Excessive tetracaine was responsible for six of the seven toxic reactions, which included three cases of respiratory arrest, two seizures, one case of methemoglobinemia, and the only mortality in a patient who was not seriously ill at the time of bronchoscopy. Excessive lidocaine was responsible for a seizure and two other unspecified minor complications. Although highly effective as a topical anesthetic, tetracaine is toxic and has a low therapeutic index. The maximum recommended dose is 1.0 to 1.5 mg/kg to a total dose of 100 mg/70 kg.[28] Weisel and Tella and Adriani and Campbell have reported complications related to tetracaine administration.[29,30] One of the most difficult problems is that tetracaine toxicity can manifest itself without any warning. Indeed, the first sign of tetracaine toxicity could be a seizure or cardiovascular collapse. In contrast, lidocaine offers a much wider margin of safety than tetracaine (the maximum recommended dose of lidocaine is 5 to 7 mg/kg, depending on whether epinephrine is used). Toxicity from lidocaine is likely to include recognizable and reversible central nervous system symptoms prior to cardiovascular collapse.

The other group of complications relates to the bronchoscopic procedure itself. Severe hemorrhage following a biopsy, pneumothorax, and laceration of a bronchial wall are the most frequent problems. In addition, laryngospasm and bronchospasm can occur with manipulation of the airway or in conjunction with inadequate levels of anesthesia. Complication rates are significantly higher in asthmatics who undergo bronchoscopy, probably as a result of their increased airway reactivity.[18,31-33]

Although there are many potentially life-threatening complications related to bronchoscopy, the overall rates of morbidity and mortality are quite low. Several large-scale studies have been undertaken to assess the rate of complications with bronchoscopy.[15,16,18,19] Overall, the highest rate of complications was 8.2%, while the highest death rate was 0.1%.

The physiologic changes associated with bronchoscopy relate mainly to the cardiovascular and respiratory systems. Prys-Roberts et al noted a significant increase in sympathetic activity during laryngoscopy, which was most often manifested by tachycardia and hypertension.[25] This sympathetic response can be attenuated by a number of maneuvers. Stoelting demonstrated that intravenous lidocaine reduces the hypertensive response to laryngoscopy.[34] Similarly, other agents—including narcotics, β-blocking drugs, and sodium nitroprusside—have been used to decrease the sympathetic response.[35-38] The use of calcium channel blockers has been reported in patients at risk for developing bronchospasm related to the administration of β-blockers.[39,40] Roizen et al have demonstrated that very deep levels of inhalation anesthesia (2 to 3 minimum alveolar concentrations [MAC]) are required to block the adrenergic responses (BAR).[41] Treatment with fentanyl or alfentanil before bronchoscopy has also been shown to attenuate the hypertensive response seen in the control group, but ST-segment changes suggestive of myocardial ischemia were present in both the control and narcotic-treated groups.[42] The newer, short-acting narcotic remifentanil has been investigated recently for its ability to attenuate the ST changes in patients at risk for myocardial ischemia who were undergoing rigid bronchoscopy.[43,44] In these studies, remifentanil permitted a more rapid patient recovery than fentanyl, and the hemodynamic variables (blood pressure, heart rate) were similar in the two groups treated with fentanyl and remifentanil.[44] Although remifentanil-treated patients had a lower incidence of ST-segment depression, this did not differ significantly from that of the saline-treated patients.[43]

Bronchoscopy is frequently associated with changes in cardiac rhythm. Minor rhythm disturbances have been reported in up to 73% of the patients undergoing bronchoscopy, although major arhythmias occur in only 4% to 11% of patients.[45,46] The arrhythmias tend to be self-limited and do not cause major hemodynamic instability. Systemic absorption of topically applied anesthetics (particularly lidocaine) could have a salutary effect on cardiac dysrhythmias during bronchoscopy.

Bronchoscopy can also cause impairment of the respiratory system. Several studies have demonstrated that fiberoptic bronchoscopy induces hypoxia in awake, spontaneously breathing patients.[20,21] Salisbury et al demonstrated that fiberoptic bronchoscopy induced a decline in Po_2 in both normal volunteers and patients with chronic airway obstruction.[47] This decline in Po_2 occurred without significant changes in Pco_2 or pH. The change in Po_2 is transient and can last from 15 minutes to 4 hours.[20,47] The decline in Po_2 can be avoided by administering supplemental oxygen to the patient via a face mask or nasal cannula, or by insufflating oxygen through the suction port of the fiberoptic bronchoscope or through a nasopharyngeal airway.[48,49] Increasing the inspired oxygen concentration is accomplished more easily during general anesthesia.

Fiberoptic bronchoscopy also can affect pulmonary mechanics. Forced vital capacity and FEV_1 have been reported to decrease by 13% to 30%.[50] The proposed mechanisms for the deterioration in pulmonary mechanics during fiberoptic bronchoscopy include bronchoconstriction and airway edema. These deleterious effects of fiberoptic bronchoscopy can be eliminated by pretreating the patient with anticholinergic agents such as atropine or glycopyrrolate.[29,51,52]

Awareness during bronchoscopy is still a potentially significant problem. Moore and Seymour reported an overall 7% incidence of awareness during bronchoscopy.[53] These patients frequently receive "light" general anesthesia with a short-acting barbiturate and muscle relaxant. It is important for the anesthesiologist to remember that with this technique, patients undergoing bronchoscopy are capable of auditory awareness. Use of headphones with random noise or music might be helpful in reducing this problem. Alternatively, the use of benzodiazepines (midazolam or diazepam) has been shown to reduce the incidence of awareness in patients undergoing bronchoscopy.[54] Kestin et al reported that alfentanil with a propofol infusion provided satisfactory conditions without recall and promoted rapid emergence and recovery.[55] It remains to be seen whether the use of bispectral index (BIS) monitoring in patients undergoing bronchoscopy and sedation affects the incidence of recall.

Not infrequently, critically ill patients undergo fiberoptic bronchoscopy in the intensive care unit. They often have decreased or absent pulmonary reserve and have been ventilated mechanically for significant periods of time. Because many of these patients are awake, bronchoscopy can result in significant increases in blood pressure and heart rate with subsequent myocardial ischemia. The use of a potent narcotic such as alfentanil during tracheal suctioning in mechanically ventilated ICU patients has been reported to attenuate the marked increases in blood pressure and heart rate.[56] Lindholm et al have reviewed the potential problems of performing fiberoptic bronchoscopy in an intubated patient.[57,58] The introduction of a fiberoptic bronchoscope into an endotracheal tube may create a significant increase in airway resistance (Figure 9-4). Unless the endotracheal tube is of sufficient size, the patient's lungs will not be ventilated adequately. The increased resistance

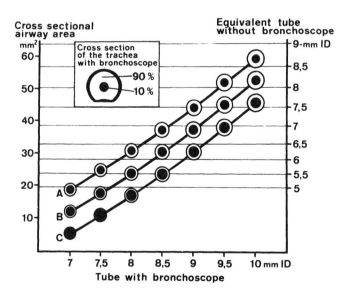

FIGURE 9-4 Schematic representation of the cross-sectional areas of endotracheal tubes of different sizes into which a fiberoptic bronchoscope has been inserted. The *outer circle* represents the internal diameter (ID) of the endotracheal tube, while the *solid circle* represents the external diameter (ED) of the bronchoscope. The different sizes of bronchoscopes represented are *(A)* 5-mm ED, *(B)* 5.7-mm ED, *(C)* 6.0-mm ED. The *white portion inside each circle* represents the area inside the endotracheal tube that remains available for air exchange. The *insert at the top-left corner* of the figure illustrates the relative relationship between a normal airway and a bronchoscope inserted in a nonintubated airway. From Lindholm CE, Ollman B, Snyder JV, et al: *Chest* 74:362, 1978.)

TABLE 9-1

Relationship of Endotracheal Tube Size and PEEP Produced by Insertion of a 5.7-mm FOB

Endotracheal tube size (mm ID)	Cross-sectional area (% occupied by the 5.7-mm FOB)	Maximum measured PEEP in patients (cmH$_2$O)
7	66	35
8	51	20
9	40	—

From Lindholm CE, Ollman B, Snyder JV, et al: Cardiorespiratory effects of flexible fiberoptic bronchoscopy in critically ill patients, *Chest* 74:362, 1978.
PEEP, Positive end-expiratory pressure; *FOB,* fiberoptic bronchoscope.

within the endotracheal tube can cause the mechanical ventilator to exceed its pressure limit and not deliver the preset tidal volume. A 5.7-mm ED adult bronchoscope inserted into a 7.0-mm ID endotracheal tube causes an increase in the peak airway pressure of up to 60 cmH$_2$O, while up to 35 cmH$_2$O of positive end-expiratory pressure (PEEP) has been reported (Table 9-1).[57] Vigorous suctioning of the airway in an intubated patient can be responsible for withdrawing as much as 300 mL of delivered tidal volume.[58] This decrease in delivered tidal volume can result in hypercarbia and hypoxemia. Therefore, when intensive care unit patients require fiberoptic bronchoscopy, the following guidelines are recommended:

1. Endoscopists should ensure that the endotracheal tube is of adequate size to accommodate the bronchoscope being used. Generally, an 8.5- to 9.0-mm endotracheal tube is necessary for most adult fiberoptic bronchoscopes.
2. Mechanically ventilated patients should be hand-ventilated with a nonrebreathing anesthesia circuit and 100% oxygen. In this manner, adequacy of ventilation and the amount of resistance generated by the bronchoscope can be assessed readily.
3. Suctioning should be performed only intermittently and for short periods.
4. The patient's mental status should be considered and appropriate sedation administered as physical condition permits.
5. Any mechanical PEEP should be removed from the circuit, as bronchoscopy itself could induce PEEP.
6. The patient's cardiovascular status should be monitored carefully, and continuous assessment of oxygen saturation with a pulse oximeter in this setting is mandatory.
7. If an indwelling arterial catheter is present, serial arterial blood gas (ABG) analyses should be performed, especially during prolonged procedures.

Methods of Ventilation during Bronchoscopy
VENTILATION DURING RIGID BRONCHOSCOPY

The original bronchoscopes were merely open tubes through which the endoscopist could operate. If general anesthesia was required, one of the following three methods of ventilation was possible:

1. Spontaneous ventilation by the patient
2. Positive pressure ventilation with oxygen delivered through the side port, while the open end of the bronchoscope was occluded
3. Apneic oxygenation

Apneic oxygenation was first described in the anesthesia literature by Frumin et al.[59] In this technique, the patient is first denitrogenated with 100% oxygen, then relaxed with neuromuscular blockers, while oxygen is delivered continuously into the trachea through a catheter or via the bronchoscope. Continuous oxygen allows the bronchoscopist to work uninterruptedly for significant periods. Because there is no ventilation, levels of carbon dioxide (CO$_2$) rise continuously. In their article, Frumin et al reported Pco$_2$ levels of up to 250 mmHg after 53 minutes of apneic oxygenation, with uneventful patient recovery.[59] Fraioli et al described a group of patients with low functional residual capacity-to-body weight ratios, in whom significant decreases in oxygenation occurred after 4 minutes and in whom apneic oxygenation could not be continued beyond 15 minutes.[60] In addition, awareness during general anesthesia with apneic oxygenation has been reported.[61]

The ventilating bronchoscope (Figure 9-5) provides a significant improvement in the care of patients undergoing bronchoscopy. This technique uses an anesthesia circuit that is attached directly to the side port of the bronchoscope. A glass window is then placed over the proximal end of the bronchoscope to occlude the bronchoscope lumen, and general anesthesia and positive pressure ventilation can be administered to the patient. This system has the advantage of allowing both inhalation and intravenous anesthesia to be administered to the patient. All anesthetic gases are easily scavenged from the circuit, and leaks around the bronchoscope can usually be managed by applying manual pressure over the larynx. Alternatively, leaks around the bronchoscope can be prevented by fitting an inflatable cuff around the bronchoscope or by packing the pharynx with moist sponges. Adequacy of ventilation can be assessed by using a respirometer or an end-tidal CO$_2$ monitor. As with any bronchoscopic procedure, continuous monitoring of arterial oxygen saturation with a pulse oximeter is mandatory. Finally, an estimation of the patient's compliance can be obtained by the anesthesiologist from the "feel" of the reservoir bag and by observing peak inspiratory pressures within the circuit. The disadvantage of this system is that the occluding window must be removed for the

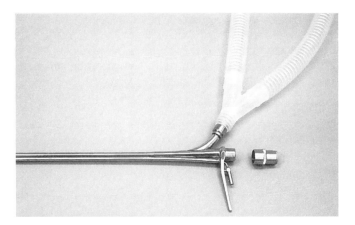

FIGURE 9-5 Rigid side-arm ventilating bronchoscope with an attached anesthesia circuit. Note that the viewing window that seals the open end of the bronchoscope has been removed for illustration purposes.

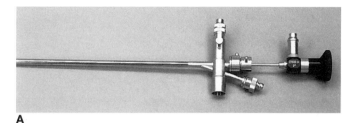

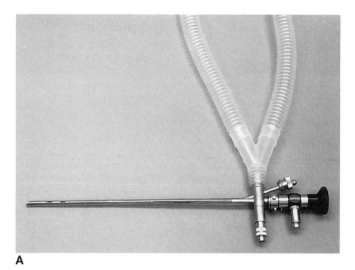

FIGURE 9-6 **A,** Rigid ventilating bronchoscope with Hopkins lens being inserted. **B,** Rigid side-arm bronchoscope containing the Hopkins lens and an attached anesthesia circuit.

endoscopist to obtain biopsy specimens or to suction the airway. The removal of the windows results in an open-ended bronchoscope through which positive pressure ventilation is not possible, while anesthetic gases are allowed to escape from the open end and pollute the operating room.

The ventilating bronchoscope system was further improved by the introduction of the Hopkins lens telescope (Figure 9-6). When inserted in a side-arm ventilating bronchoscope, the telescope gives the endoscopist an improved view of the tracheobronchial tree. In addition, this instrument has special side ports through which suction catheters and biopsy instruments can be introduced without having to open the proximal end of the bronchoscope to the atmosphere.

Another method of ventilating the patient while providing general anesthesia for bronchoscopy is to place a small endotracheal tube (5.0- to 6.0-mm ID) alongside the bronchoscope. This technique allows administration and scavaging of inhalation anesthetics as long as the proximal end of the bronchoscope remains covered. When the window of the bronchoscope is removed, anesthetic gases escape into the atmosphere. Anesthesiologists must ensure that the endotracheal tube is large enough to allow for passive exhalation. If the tube is not large enough, the end of the bronchoscope must be opened in order to allow for this. Most adults have a trachea that is able to accommodate both an endotracheal tube and a bronchoscope. In cases of tracheal narrowing or external compression, however, this technique would not be advisable.

A major enhancement to the anesthetic care of the patient undergoing bronchoscopy occurred in 1967, when Sanders introduced the ventilating attachment for the bronchoscope.[62] This consisted of a source of high-pressure oxygen (50 psi) that was intermittently jetted through a 16-gauge cannula attached to the proximal end of the bronchoscope (Figures 9-7 and 9-8). To understand how the Sanders attachment works, it is necessary to understand Bernoulli's law, which states that the velocity of a fluid flowing through a pipe is inversely proportional to the cross-sectional area.[63] Bernoulli also demonstrated that the pressure that a fluid exerts is least in the area where the speed is greatest (Figure 9-9). Thus, when the fluid is forced to flow through a constriction, the speed of the fluid increases, but the lateral wall pressure is decreased. Venturi used this information to develop his injector (Figure 9-10). By passing a high-pressure gas through a narrow orifice, there is a marked decrease in the pressure surrounding this injector. This decrease in pressure entrains surrounding gas and markedly increases the total flow. This is frequently referred to as the Sanders-Venturi technique.

The oxygen jet entrains large volumes of room air, which enables the patient to receive adequate ventilation. With this technique (to the efficacy of which a number of studies have attested), the endoscopist can work uninterruptedly through the open bronchoscope.[64-69] Giesecke et al compared the injector to the side-arm ventilating methods for bronchoscopy and found essentially similar results.[70] Both groups of patients could be ventilated and oxygenated adequately with minimal side effects.

Although the Sanders-Venturi technique had the advantage of providing adequate ventilation to the patient by entraining room air, it had the disadvantage of lowering the FIO_2 delivered to the patient to around 30%. Another disadvantage of the Sanders-Venturi is the inability to provide adequate ventilation to the patient who has decreased lung compliance; the Sanders system is capable of generating a maximum pressure of 22 cmH_2O. Cardin et al modified the Sanders technique by using the side-arm of the bronchoscope as his injector site, enabling the bronchoscopist to deliver an airway pressure of up to 55 cmH_2O with a driving pressure of only 30 psi (Figure 9-11).[64,71] Thus the investigators were able to ventilate patients with decreased pulmonary compliance more efficiently, while markedly lowering the amount of room air entrained. This significantly increased the FIO_2 delivered to the patient. Various other modifications of this technique include placing a chest tube or nasogastric tube into the trachea beside the bronchoscope, then attaching it to the jet ventilating device.[72] Nitrous oxide can also be mixed with the oxygen and jetted into the trachea for enhanced levels of anesthesia.[73,74]

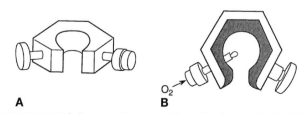

FIGURE 9-7 A diagrammatic representation of the Sanders injector. **A,** Side view. **B,** Top view. The oxygen is jetted into the side port after fitting the Sanders injector over the open end of the rigid bronchoscope.

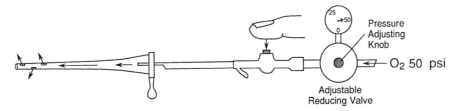

FIGURE 9-8 The Sanders attachment has been fitted to the open end of the bronchoscope and connected to a valve that allows intermittent jetting of the high-pressure oxygen via the Venturi injector. The wall oxygen at 50 psi pressure is connected to a reducing valve that allows the pressure to be adjusted from 0 to 50 psi.

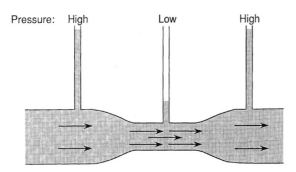

FIGURE 9-9 A schematic illustration of Bernoulli's principle. As the diameter of the pipe narrows, the speed of the fluid flowing through it increases. At the same time, the lateral wall pressure generated by the fluid flowing though the narrowed pipe segment is decreased when compared with the wall pressure of the fluid flowing through the unobstructed segment of the tube.

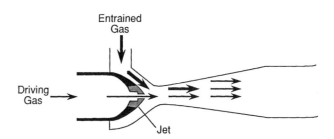

FIGURE 9-10 A diagrammatic representation of the Venturi principle. The high-pressure driving gas (oxygen) jetted through the narrow orifice creates a negative pressure around the jet orifice and entrains large amounts of surrounding gas (room air).

These systems worked well, but they required exceptional vigilance by the anesthesiologist. The best indicator of adequate ventilation is obtained by observing the patient's chest movement with inflation. Quantitative assessment of ventilation by spirometry and end-tidal CO_2 cannot be obtained. Use of pulse oximetry is required with this technique. Technology such as a transcutaneous PCO_2 monitor can also be used to assess ventilation. A hazard of using a Venturi system is that exhalation is passive and must occur either through the bronchoscope or through the open glottis. If muscle relaxation is inadequate and the vocal cords are adducted, the exhaled gas may be trapped, causing barotrauma and pneumothorax.

Several studies have demonstrated that high-frequency jet ventilation can be another useful technique for ventilation during bronchoscopy.[75-78] This technique is particularly beneficial for patients who have bronchopleural fistulae because mean airway pressure is minimal with this mode of ventilation. In addition, this technique results in no air entrainment through the proximal end of the bronchoscope, thus allowing for delivery of consistent and predictable inhalational anesthetic concentrations to the patient.[78] The high-frequency ventilation technique can also be used with the fiberoptic bronchoscope.[79]

Ventilation During Fiberoptic Bronchoscopy

The introduction of the fiberoptic bronchoscope has increased the comfort and safety of the patient undergoing bronchoscopy. The awake patient can ventilate easily around the bronchoscope, as it occupies only approximately 10% of the cross-sectional area of the trachea. If general anesthesia is used,

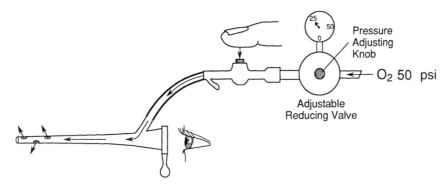

FIGURE 9-11 A schematic of the Carden modification of the Venturi injector. This modification uses the side port of the bronchoscope as the injector site, allowing reduced driving pressures and increased oxygen concentration delivery to the patient. This modification also allows the endoscopist to operate via an open-ended rigid bronchoscope.

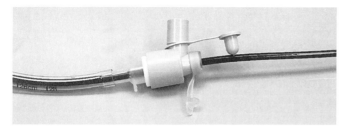

FIGURE 9-12 An endotracheal tube fitted with an elbow adapter that allows passage of the fiberoptic bronchoscope. The bronchoscope is passed through a rubber diaphragm located at the top of the elbow. The tight fit of the diaphragm around the bronchoscope allows continued ventilation during bronchoscopy.

fiberoptic bronchoscopy usually involves passing the broncho- scope through an endotracheal tube fitted with a special adap- tor (Figure 9-12). In this manner, the patient can be ventilated continuously, and end-tidal CO_2 and ventilatory volumes can be monitored easily (Figure 9-13). Because fiberoptic bron- choscopy involves the introduction of the fiberscope through the endotracheal tube, the relationship of the diameter of the bronchoscope to the diameter of the endotracheal tube becomes critical. Poiseuille's law states that flow is directly proportional to the fourth power of the radius; thus, minimal changes in the diameter of the endotracheal tube will have a great impact on the tidal volume delivered. For this reason, it has been shown that even the minimal kinking associated with a nasotracheally placed tube has a greater effect on tidal volume and airway pressure generated during ventilation than when orotracheal intubation is used.[80] Carden and Raj's modification of the endo- tracheal tube also takes advantage of the fact that flow is directly proportional to the diameter and inversely proportional to the length of the tube.[81] The Carden endotracheal tube is tapered and has a wide supraglottic portion (thus decreasing the resistance to flow), whereas the subglottic portion (where most

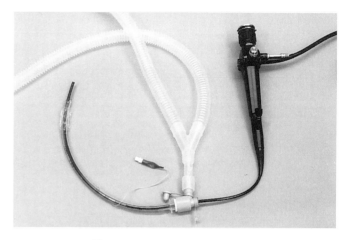

FIGURE 9-13 Fiberoptic bronchoscope inserted through an elbow (right angle) adapter into the endotracheal tube. The anesthesia circuit is attached.

of the resistance occurs) is effectively shortened to one- fourth of the normal length of 30 cm.

Lindholm et al delineated these relationships and showed that a 5.7-mm bronchoscope occupies 40% of the cross- sectional area of a 9.0-mm ID endotracheal tube, whereas the same bronchoscope occupies nearly 70% of a 7.0-mm ID endo- tracheal tube.[57,58] Fiberoptic bronchoscopes are available in several different sizes. It is important for the anesthesiologist to select an endotracheal tube of sufficient diameter to accommo- date the bronchoscope without producing a significant increase in airway pressure. A properly sized endotracheal tube also pre- vents production of PEEP and allows passive exhalation around the bronchoscope. Use of a 9.0-mm endotracheal tube for fiberoptic bronchoscopy is recommended whenever possi- ble (Figure 9-14). Although positive pressure ventilation using a standard anesthesia circle system is the most commonly employed method, other modes of ventilation have been described. Smith et al used the technique of jet ventilation

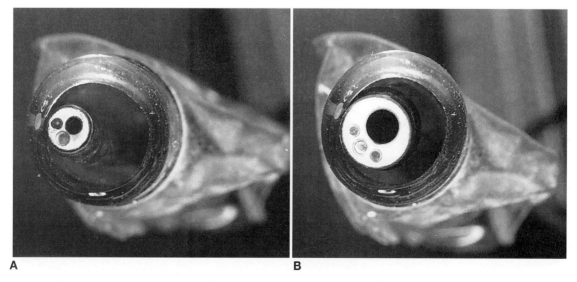

A   **B**

FIGURE 9-14 A 9.0-mm endotracheal tube containing two different-size bronchoscopes. **A,** A 4.0-mm pediatric scope. **B,** A 6.2-mm adult bronchoscope. Note that even with a 9.0-mm endotracheal tube, a significant portion of the lumen is occupied by the adult bronchoscope.

through a small chest tube that was placed in the trachea beside the fiberoptic bronchoscope.[82] A modification of this technique involves using jet ventilation through the suction channel of the fiberscope.[83]

Laser therapy for endobronchial tumors has become quite popular. The CO_2 and argon lasers have been used successfully and require a rigid bronchoscope. The Nd:YAG laser can transmit its energy along a fiberoptic cable and is therefore suitable for use with either a rigid or a fiberoptic bronchoscope. When using the Nd:YAG laser for tumor resection, severe hemorrhage can occur, because pulmonary vessels that are encased in tumor can be entered. A more detailed discussion of lasers can be found in Chapter 12.

Anesthetic Technique for Bronchoscopy

Premedication for the patient scheduled to undergo bronchoscopy depends not only on the physical status of the patient but also on the proposed surgical technique. If fiberoptic bronchoscopy under local anesthesia is planned, patients would require relatively less sedation preoperatively than if they were to undergo rigid bronchoscopy. Also, patients who are at greater risk of pulmonary complications or who have very limited pulmonary reserve should not be heavily premedicated, as this might further compromise gas exchange. For these patients, a good rapport established with the anesthesiologist during the preoperative visit might be the most valuable premedication (see Chapter 1).

Three classes of medication are given preoperatively, as follows:

1. Narcotics are administered for analgesia, to decrease the cough reflex, and to provide euphoria. Morphine has been shown to have salutary effects in mild asthmatics because of its inhibition of vagally mediated bronchoconstriction.[84] Because of its ability to induce release of histamine by the mast cells, however, morphine must be used cautiously in severe asthmatics. Alternatively, other narcotics such as meperidine, fentanyl, or hydromorphone are effective premedications.
2. Anticholinergics such as atropine (0.4 to 0.6 mg/70 kg) or glycopyrrolate (0.1 to 0.2 mg/70 kg) given intramuscularly minimize the vasovagal reflexes and diminish oral and bronchial secretions. Although not recommended in the outpatient setting, scopolamine is an excellent adjuvant to narcotic premedication because it has superior sedative, amnestic, and antisialagogue properties. Atropine and glycopyrrolate are equally effective in producing bronchodilation, whereas both atropine and scopolamine reduce the incidence of laryngospasm during induction of anesthesia.[85]
3. Benzodiazepines, such as diazepam or midazolam, can be administered as premedications because of their anxiolytic effects. Benzodiazepines are useful because of their amnestic properties and because they protect against the central nervous system toxicity of local anesthetics by increasing the seizure threshold.

The preoperative use of one other medication needs to be mentioned, if only because of its controversial role. Steroids have been suggested for the prevention of postoperative airway edema. Although several studies have attested to the usefulness of this premedication technique, most of the studies have dealt with the reduction of postoperative facial and oral edema following facial surgery.[86,87] The role of steroids in preventing airway edema postoperatively remains unclear.

Flexible Fiberoptic Bronchoscopy

The use of the fiberoptic bronchoscope allows for greater versatility on the part of the endoscopist in tailoring the anesthetic approach to the particular patient's needs and comfort. Fiberoptic bronchoscopies are frequently performed under local or topical anesthesia. The most commonly used local anesthetics for topical anesthesia include lidocaine, tetracaine, benzocaine, and cocaine. Of these, tetracaine is known to have a low therapeutic index, with a maximum safe dose of 1 to 1.5 mg/kg (100 mg/70 kg), whereas cocaine is less frequently used today because of its potential for abuse. Topicalization of the pharynx and tracheobronchial tree is therefore most easily accomplished by inhaled, nebulized lidocaine. For this purpose, 4 to 6 mL of 4% lidocaine is placed in an ultrasonic nebulizer that is attached to a facemask. This method of anesthetizing the tracheobronchial tree probably causes the least amount of discomfort to the patient, and it is also technically very easy to accomplish. Furthermore, nebulized lidocaine has been shown to be of sufficiently small size (average 6.3 μm) to be distributed over the entire mucosa of the upper and lower respiratory tracts.[88] This distribution of local anesthetic into the distal bronchioles greatly facilitates the fiberoptic examination. Neither of the two recently introduced local anesthetics (ropivacaine and levobupivacaine) has to date been investigated as a topical anesthetic during fiberoptic bronchoscopic procedures. In light of the significantly fewer central nervous system (CNS) side effects associated with the use of ropivacaine compared with lidocaine, it would be interesting to evaluate the role of these agents in this setting.[89]

The drawbacks of this method include the inability to properly anesthetize areas of the tracheobronchial tree that do not come in direct contact with the inhaled local anesthetic—for example, the area immediately below the vocal cords. The other disadvantage is that the amount of local anesthetic that is being absorbed is unknown, but for safety purposes, it must be assumed to be equal to the amount of local anesthetic that is being nebulized. Other means of anesthetizing the posterior pharynx include sprays, droppers, and anesthetic-soaked applicators such as cotton-tipped swabs, which may be placed in the posterior pharynx.

Benzocaine combined with tetracaine is available in commercially packaged aerosol sprays. The benzocaine provides rapid onset of topical anesthesia, while the tetracaine prolongs its duration. Two popular brands are Hurricaine and Cetacaine. Approximately 30 mg of benzocaine is delivered with each 0.5-second spray, and the toxic dose is 100 mg. Because benzocaine can cause methemoglobinemia, these sprays must be used very judiciously.[90]

It is important to remember that topical anesthesia only obtunds the tactile receptors of the airway, leaving intact the more deeply situated pressure receptors that are found in the posterior pharynx. Blocking of these pressure receptors is very important in order to ablate the gag reflex. In general, the abolition of the gag reflex can be accomplished by blocking the afferent pathways (including glossopharyngeal and superior laryngeal nerves) or by attenuating the hemodynamic responses by use of intravenous narcotics or local anesthetics (Figure 9-15).[91]

Glossopharyngeal nerve blockade can be accomplished by injection of local anesthetic into the lateral pharyngeal wall at the root of the tongue, as the lingual branch of the glossopharyngeal nerve is relatively superficial as it traverses the posterior aspect of the palatoglossal arch (Figure 9-16). A 26- or 27-gauge, short (½- to ⅝-inch) needle is used, and a negative aspiration test must be performed to ensure that injection is not made into the carotid artery. A total dose of 40 mg of lidocaine (2 mL of 1% lidocaine on each side) provides 10 to 15 minutes of anesthesia. If a longer duration is desired, the block is performed with an epinephrine-containing solution (1:200,000). The superior laryngeal nerve block may be accomplished by injecting local anesthetic (2 to 3 mL of 2% lidocaine) at the tip of the superior thyroid cornu (Figure 9-17). The superior laryngeal nerve can also be blocked topically by applying local anesthetic-soaked pledgets to the pyriform sinuses bilaterally.

Finally, anesthetizing areas immediately underneath the vocal cords can be accomplished by injecting local anesthetic directly into the trachea through the cricothyroid membrane (i.e., transtracheal injection of 2 to 3 mL of 4% lidocaine). Injection of the local anesthetic should be performed rapidly while the patient is taking a vital capacity breath because this is usually followed by a forceful cough. To prevent the needle from puncturing and injuring the structures posterior to the trachea as the patient coughs and lunges forward, a surgical clamp can be snapped on the needle at the level of its skin entry before injecting the local anesthetic. Alternatively, a 22-gauge Teflon intravenous catheter may be introduced percutaneously into the trachea, and the needle withdrawn before injecting the local anesthetic.[92] This Teflon catheter is malleable enough so that the tissues are not injured when the patient coughs.

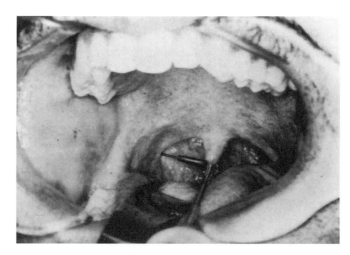

FIGURE 9-16 Glossopharyngeal nerve block using with an angled peroral tonsillar needle. (From Cooper M, Watson RL: *Anesthesiology* 43:372, 1975.)

Before performing any topical anesthesia, it must be remembered that anesthesia of the larynx and trachea is relatively contraindicated in patients with a full stomach because obtundation of protective airway reflexes might place them at increased risk for aspiration of gastric contents. Furthermore, local anesthetic toxicity is enhanced in the face of hypercarbia and acidosis. Therefore the anesthesiologist must be very vigilant to ensure proper ventilation and oxygenation of the patient during the entire perioperative period.

A safe and technically easy fiberoptic bronchoscopic examination can be performed during general anesthesia. For this technique, maintenance may be provided by intermittent boluses or by continuous infusion of intravenous agents, such as narcotics (fentanyl, sufentanil, remifentanil or alfentanil), ketamine, etomidate, sodium thiopental, or propofol.

Fiberoptic bronchoscopy can also be performed with general anesthesia using potent inhalation agents. For this technique, several options are possible. The first involves passing of the fiberoptic bronchoscope through the patient's endotracheal tube, which has been fitted with an adaptor (Figure 9-12). This method allows continuous ventilation of the patient while the bronchoscopic examination is being performed and also has the benefit of scavenging of exhaled gases.

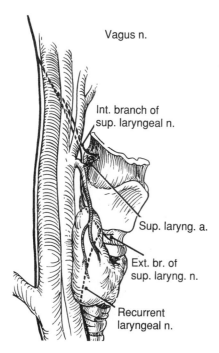

Vagus n.

Int. branch of
sup. laryngeal n.

Sup. laryng. a.

Ext. br. of
sup. laryng. n.

Recurrent
laryngeal n.

FIGURE 9-15 Diagram of the nerve supply of the larynx. (From Gaskill JR, Gillies DR: *Arch Otolaryngol* 84:654, 1966.)

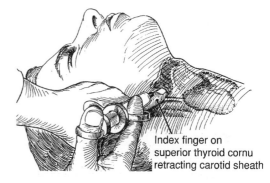

Index finger on
superior thyroid cornu
retracting carotid sheath

FIGURE 9-17 Percutaneous block of the internal branch of the superior laryngeal nerve. (From Gaskill JR, Gillies DR: *Arch Otolaryngol* 84:654, 1966.)

The second option involves passing the fiberscope into the trachea beside an existing, smaller sized endotracheal tube. This technique has the disadvantage of not scavenging the anesthetic gases, as inflating the endotracheal tube cuff allows no further maneuvering of the fiberoptic bronchoscope. A third method involves jet ventilation with oxygen via a catheter placed perorally into the trachea. Anesthesia and muscle relaxation are then accomplished with intravenous agents.[82] Alternatively, oxygen can be delivered via the suction channel of the fiberscope.[82,83] Topicalization of the airway is beneficial in patients undergoing general anesthesia for bronchoscopy because it reduces the anesthetic requirements, attenuates the cough reflex, and allows faster emergence from anesthesia.

Rigid Bronchoscopy

Although the literature describes the use of local anesthesia for performance of rigid bronchoscopy, most of the techniques involving topical or local anesthesia since the introduction of flexible bronchoscopy have been performed with the fiberoptic bronchoscope.[93-95] Thus, rigid bronchoscopy is most often performed with a general anesthetic technique.

Depending on the preoperative evaluation of the patient, the airway might first need to be secured by an awake fiberoptic intubation. Alternatively, an adequate airway might allow induction of anesthesia with a barbiturate/relaxant technique, followed by intubation with either an endotracheal tube or directly with the rigid bronchoscope.

After induction of anesthesia, the specific anesthetic technique depends on the type of rigid bronchoscope used. When using an open-ended bronchoscope with mass apneic oxygenation, jet ventilation, or a Sanders-Venturi technique, anesthesia must consist of intravenous agents plus muscle relaxation. Although it is technically possible to deliver a nitrous oxide/oxygen mixture via the Sanders attachment, this is not recommended because of operating room pollution.[72]

Modification of the open end of a closed-ended bronchoscope by the addition of a window or a Hopkins telescope to the proximal end allows the use of a semiclosed anesthesia circle system. This circle system facilitates an inhalation anesthetic technique while allowing waste anesthetic gases to be properly scavenged. If the closed system is opened by frequent removal of the window, the primary anesthetic technique should be converted to an intravenous general anesthetic to prevent operating room pollution.

Whether performed with a rigid or a fiberoptic instrument, bronchoscopy is a highly stimulating procedure that requires an adequate depth of anesthesia. This level of anesthesia must be maintained until the end of the procedure. Rapid emergence and recovery of protective airway reflexes are desirable. The use of short-acting agents such as propofol, cisatracurium, rocuronium, remifentanil, sevoflurane, and desflurane can facilitate these goals.[96]

Mediastinoscopy

In 1954, Harken et al reported a new procedure for the tissue diagnosis of mediastinal disease employing a modified laryngoscope (Figures 9-18 and 9-19).[97] This approach (cervical mediastinal exploration) was later refined in 1959 by Carlens,

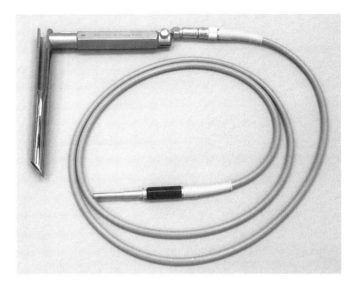

FIGURE 9-18 A mediastinoscope with attached fiberoptic light cable.

who reported the technique of anterior cervical mediastinoscopy.[98] The anatomic basis for development of this procedure for tissue diagnosis of mediastinal tumors rests on the lymphatic drainage of the lungs that proceeds from the hilar nodes to the subcarinal, paratracheal, and, finally, to the supraclavicular lymph nodes. The major indications for performance of mediastinoscopy are evaluation of lymph node involvement in patients with carcinoma of the lung, and obtaining a tissue biopsy of suspected tumors. Patients with bilateral lymph node involvement are an absolute contraindication for thoracotomy, whereas unilateral involvement does not constitute a contraindication to definitive surgery.[99]

Contraindications to mediastinoscopy can be classified as either absolute or relative. The absolute contraindications include the following[100,101]:

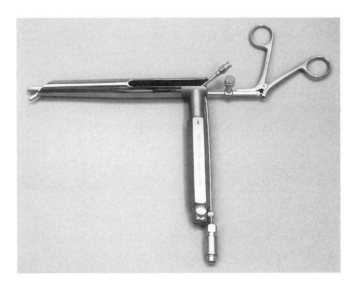

FIGURE 9-19 A mediastinoscope through which a biopsy forceps has been inserted.

1. Anterior mediastinal tumors
2. Inoperable tumor
3. Previous recurrent laryngeal nerve injury
4. Extremely debilitated patients
5. Ascending aortic aneurysm and
6. Previous mediastinoscopy

The relative contraindications to mediastinoscopy include thoracic inlet obstruction and the presence of a superior vena cava syndrome.

The tumors that can be identified during mediastinoscopy include primary malignant tumors such as lymphoma as well as bone, vascular, or connective tissue tumors. Secondary malignant mediastinal tumors might originate from lung and pericardium. Mediastinoscopy has also proved to be a valuable tool in the diagnosis of benign tumors such as thymic, tracheal, and bronchial cysts, thymic lymphomas or hyperplasia, nervous system tumors, thyroid masses, (i.e., goiter), or aneurysms of the ascending aorta, as well as enlarged nodes associated with sarcoidosis. Less common mass lesions present in the mediastinum include pheochromocytoma, teratoma, myxoma, thymoma, lipoma, and hiatal hernia.[102]

Four approaches to mediastinoscopy have been described. In the early 1900s, von Hacker described the method of reaching the retroesophageal space by introducing the mediastinoscope along the anterior border of the sternocleidomastoid muscle and passing medial to the vessels within the carotid sheath.[103] In 1954, Harken et al described a technique of entering the mediastinum by introducing a laryngoscope through a lateral supraclavicular incision.[97] The anterior mediastinotomy, first described by McNeill and Chamberlain in 1966,[104] involves a vertical incision on either the right or the left side of the chest, over the lateral sternal border, through which the mediastinum can be entered.[105] The disadvantage of all these techniques is that they allow only for unilateral exploration and biopsy. If bilateral exploration were necessary, the same procedure would have to be repeated on the contralateral side. Such bilateral thoracic incision would expose the patient to the risk of flail chest. In 1959, Carlens introduced a midline approach for mediastinoscopy via a suprasternal incision.[98] This approach allows for safe bilateral exploration and biopsy of tissue from both the paratracheal and the subcarinal areas.

Preoperative Evaluation for Mediastinoscopy

Preoperative evaluation of the patient scheduled to undergo mediastinoscopy is extremely important in decreasing or preventing the incidence of perioperative morbidity and mortality. As with all preoperative patients, a complete history and physical examination should be performed. Particular attention should be paid to respiratory symptoms such as wheezing, dyspnea, and orthopnea. It is also important to ascertain whether the respiratory symptoms are exacerbated by exercise or by assuming the supine position. Presence of these respiratory changes should raise the suspicion of major airway obstruction secondary to a mediastinal mass. Dyspnea has been reported to be an important indicator of airway obstruction. In one study, 9% of patients with a mediastinal mass compressing the trachea had dyspnea as their presenting complaint.[106] Dysphagia as a preoperative finding could indicate the presence of a large mediastinal mass impinging on both the trachea and the esophagus.

If the preoperative evaluation reveals a potentially serious airway obstruction because of a mediastinal mass, a preoperative course of chemotherapy or radiation has been suggested to shrink the size of the tumor and decrease the likelihood of respiratory compromise during induction and maintenance of anesthesia.[107] Although this course of therapy can be effective in patients with mediastinal tumors, it is of no value in patients with airway obstruction secondary to a substernal goiter.[108]

Preoperative workup should include chest x-rays with posteroanterior and lateral views, tomograms, computed tomography scan of the chest and neck, and pulmonary function tests such as flow-volume loops. If tracheal deviation is suspected, then specific studies (neck films and/or tomograms) should be obtained to evaluate the location and extension of the mass as well as the degree of airway compromise. Flow-volume loops in both the upright and supine positions are particularly useful in determining whether the obstruction is fixed and whether it is intrathoracic or extrathoracic (see Figures 9-1, 9-2, and 9-3). Patients with oat-cell carcinoma of the lung might have the Eaton-Lambert syndrome, which is associated with prolonged recovery from nondepolarizing muscle relaxants.

Mediastinal tumors have been associated with development of superior vena cava obstruction.[109] Mediastinoscopy in these patients is particularly hazardous because of the increased risk of major venous bleeding. Presenting symptoms in patients with caval obstruction (superior vena cava syndrome) include shortness of breath (83% of cases), cough (70%), and orthopnea (64%).[110,111]

Anesthetic Technique for Mediastinoscopy

Patients undergoing mediastinoscopy could already be at increased risk of pulmonary complications because of airway obstruction, so premedication is probably best avoided. Thorough preoperative discussion of plans and proposed techniques, however, will allow the anesthesiologist to form a good rapport with the patient. In the majority of cases, this will be sufficient to allay most patients' fears. If anxiolysis is necessary, the combination of benzodiazepines and opioids should be avoided for their synergistic respiratory depressant effect, and benzodiazepines alone (0.25 to 0.5 mg intravenously) should be administered.

Anesthetic management of patients for mediastinoscopy can involve either local or general anesthesia. Advocates of mediastinoscopy under local anesthesia consider this a safer technique in the very debilitated patient.[112-114] They report superior results and numerous advantages such a shortened operating time, decreased patient discomfort after the procedure, and early detection and correction of pneumothorax or bilateral recurrent laryngeal nerve paralysis.[112]

Today, however, general anesthesia is the technique of choice at most institutions if the patient scheduled for mediastinoscopy has no preoperative signs or symptoms of airway obstruction.[101,103,115-119] In many cases, mediastinoscopy can be performed as an outpatient procedure. These patients usually have minimal postoperative pain, and if problems occur they are usually detected intraoperatively. Because of the potential for sudden and severe hemorrhage, however, these procedures should not be done at a freestanding outpatient facility.[120] In these patients, the general anesthetic technique can involve inhalation or intravenous agents, or, most commonly, a combination of the two. The occurrence of a pneumothorax during mediastinoscopy must be anticipated. It is therefore prudent to avoid the use of nitrous oxide, which can increase the size of the pneumothorax and lead to tension pneumothorax.

Other intraoperative considerations include the possibility of innominate artery compression by the mediastinoscope. To detect this complication, several measures have been advocated. They include constant palpation of the right radial or carotid pulse, placement of a right indwelling radial artery catheter, or monitoring of the continuous plethysmographic tracing of a pulse oximeter.[119,121] The danger of innominate artery compression is that falsely low blood pressure readings will be obtained. Simultaneous measurement of blood pressure in the left arm ensures that therapeutic decisions will not be based on erroneous readings.[122]

The possibility of sudden and massive hemorrhage as a complication of mediastinoscopy exists. The innominate artery and vein, the azygos vein, and the aorta are all possible sources of hemorrhage (Figure 9-20).[120] For this reason, typed and cross-matched blood must be available. Preoperative placement of at least two large-bore intravenous catheters is advised. In the particular case of superior vena caval obstruction, placement of an intravenous catheter in the lower extremity ensures venous access below the level of obstruction.

Following intubation, the use of muscle relaxants provides the endoscopist with an operative field that is safe from sudden

movements, which might lead to injury of the adjacent organs by the mediastinoscope. Nondepolarizing muscle relaxants must be used judiciously for patients undergoing mediastinoscopy, because airway collapse from loss of muscle tone has been reported.[107,123-126] In addition, the existence of the myasthenic syndrome must be kept in mind when using nondepolarizing muscle relaxants.

If the preoperative work-up is indicative of airway compromise secondary to compression, the anesthetic management is more controversial and depends on whether a tissue diagnosis exists. If it does, the most prudent course of action would be to proceed with preoperative chemotherapy or radiotherapy in order to shrink the tumor size and decrease the degree of obstruction. In a series of 98 cases, Piro et al reported a 7% (5/74) incidence of airway complications in patients not receiving preoperative radiation therapy.[127] In contrast, there were no reported cases of airway complications in the 24 patients who underwent preoperative radiotherapy.

If tissue diagnosis of the mediastinal mass does not exist and the patient has signs and symptoms of airway compromise, the most prudent management would be to obtain percutaneous needle biopsy under local anesthesia, followed by radiation and then general anesthesia for mediastinoscopy.[107]

When airway obstruction is present preoperatively, general anesthesia is fraught with problems. Acute tracheal collapse, inability to ventilate the patient, and subsequent death have been reported in patients with mediastinal masses.[107,125,128-130]

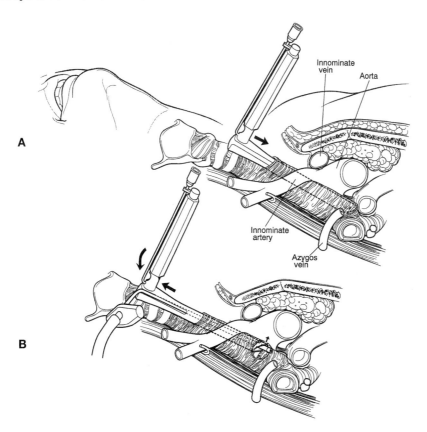

FIGURE 9-20 A, The proximity of the mediastinoscope to major blood vessels is illustrated. **B,** A suction device is introduced beside the scope. This can cause compression of the innominate artery. (From Ponn RB, Federico JA: Mediastinoscopy and staging. In Kaiser LR, Kron IL, Spray TI [eds]: *Mastery of cardiothoracic surgery,* Philadelphia, 1998, Lippincott-Raven.)

In the event that circumstances do not permit preoperative shrinkage of the obstructive tumor by radiotherapy, special precautions must be taken when inducing general anesthesia.[131] First, the location of the obstruction should be defined, if possible. Second, a variety of different-sized rigid bronchoscopes, endotracheal tubes (including wire reinforced), and a fiberoptic bronchoscope should be available. Third, in patients with large mediastinal masses that compress the distal trachea and the mainstem bronchi, the ability to institute cardiopulmonary bypass quickly is preferable.

In the case of extrathoracic variable obstruction, fiberoptic intubation under topical anesthesia should be performed in the awake patient. This allows the anesthesiologist to inspect the tracheobronchial tree and to ensure placement of the endotracheal tube below the level of obstruction. If fiberoptic intubation cannot be accomplished, an endotracheal tube can be inserted through a tracheotomy or crycothyrotomy performed under local anesthesia. General anesthesia, muscle relaxation, and positive pressure ventilation can then be safely undertaken in most circumstances.

Intrathoracic obstructing masses create the most challenging management dilemmas, the following three in particular:
1. The extent of airway compromise might be difficult to ascertain preoperatively.
2. The tumor might compress the distal trachea and both mainstem bronchi, so that introduction of an endotracheal tube distal to the compromised area is not feasible.
3. Positive pressure ventilation and muscle relaxation will worsen the intrathoracic obstruction because the distending, negative intrathoracic pressure generated by spontaneous inspiration is lost.

Endotracheal intubation should therefore be performed in the spontaneously ventilating patient. Anesthesia maintenance should likewise consist of a technique that permits spontaneous ventilation by the patient. If muscle relaxation and/or positive pressure ventilation become unavoidable, collapse of the airway can ensue. In this situation, the only recourse would be rapid institution of partial cardiopulmonary bypass.[132,133] In the case of an intrathoracic obstructing mass involving the trachea and only one of the mainstem bronchi, the use of a DLT might provide a patent airway.

Complications of Mediastinoscopy

When performed by an experienced endoscopist, mediastinoscopy has a lower morbidity and mortality than exploratory thoracotomy.[116] The incidence of major respiratory complications is directly related to the size of the preoperative mediastinal mass and to the extent of the disease within the mediastinum and the thoracic cage.[115,116]

In a collective series of 9543 cases, nine deaths were directly attributable to mediastinoscopy or the anesthetic technique.[118] Mortality was 0.09%, and morbidity was 1.5%. In this literature review, the most common complication was hemorrhage, followed by pneumothorax, recurrent nerve injury, infection, tumor spread, phrenic nerve injury, esophageal injury, chylothorax, air embolism, and hemiparesis. Failure to achieve hemostasis from the inferior thyroid venous plexus makes mediastinoscopy technically more complicated, and it can produce a significant wound hematoma. In up to 10% of

patients, the right bronchial artery could pass anteriorly across the trachea and down the anterior aspect of the right bronchus. This anatomy may render the bronchial artery particularly susceptible to injury by the mediastinoscope. Esophageal perforation might also occur during paratracheal lymph node dissection and biopsy, particularly if tracheal deviation is present preoperatively.[103] Other reports of complications during mediastinoscopy include laceration of the left pulmonary artery, compression of the innominate artery simulating cardiac arrest, acute tracheal collapse following mediastinoscopy, right bronchial artery hemorrhage, and transient hemiparesis.[118,122,128,134,135]

Mediastinoscopy is a procedure that has very well-defined indications and contraindications. It has proven to be a procedure that can be performed safely under either local or general anesthesia. Preoperative evaluation of the patient with particular emphasis on the degree of airway compromise because of obstruction is crucial. If the safety caveats are followed, mediastinoscopy is a relatively safe procedure with a mortality rate of less than 1:1000 and a morbidity rate of less than 2%. Depending on the indications, the diagnostic yield with mediastinoscopy varies between 38% in patients with carcinoma to nearly 100% in patients with sarcoidosis.[118]

There are several unique postoperative concerns for patients who have had a mediastinoscopy. Vocal cord paralysis as a result of injury to the recurrent laryngeal nerve can lead to stridor and airway compromise. Furthermore, diaphragmatic weakness or paralysis can be the result of intraoperative injury to the phrenic nerves. Finally, hemorrhage into the mediastinum can lead to cardiovascular collapse from cardiac tamponade.

Thoracoscopy

Thoracoscopy is a procedure that was first introduced in 1910 by Jacobaeus for the diagnosis and treatment of effusions secondary to tuberculosis. Today, thoracoscopy is used for the diagnosis of pleural effusions and for biopsy and preoperative evaluation of primary malignant lesions of the lung and pleura.[136-143] Other diagnostic indications for thoracoscopy include the diagnosis of cardiac herniation after a pneumonectomy and the identification of the origin of a bronchopleural fistula.[136,144,145] Recently, thoracoscopy has been used for therapeutic maneuvers. Retrieval of intrathoracic foreign bodies, such as a sheared catheter or a surgical sponge, has been reported.[146] Other therapeutic uses of thoracoscopy include chemical pleurodesis for recurrent pneumothorax and drainage of pleural effusions or empyemas. In the early 1990s, a thoracoscopic approach to esophageal myotomy for the treatment of achalasia was used with excellent results.[147] Recently, thoracoscopy was used to visualize direct injections of fibrin sealant to obliterate air leaks.[148] Thoracoscopy has also been used in trauma patients to assess the degree of injury and sometimes to coagulate bleeding vessels.[149] Jones et al reported that emergency thoracoscopy prevented an unnecessary thoracotomy in 16 out of 36 (44%) patients who had sustained thoracic trauma.[150] Thoracoscopic pericardiectomy was reported in elderly patients with massive pericardial effusions from uremic pericarditis.[151] Thoracic sympathectomy (for the treatment of

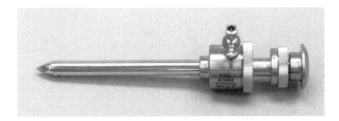

FIGURE 9-21 A thoracoscope with the trocar in place.

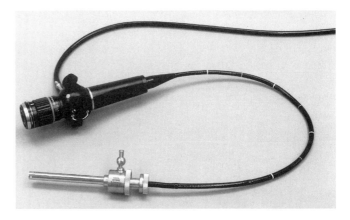

FIGURE 9-23 The thoracoscope sheath through which a fiberoptic bronchoscope has been inserted.

hyperhidrosis) also has been reported via a thoracoscopic technique.[152,153] Other reported uses of thoracoscopy include diagnosis and treatment of mediastinal tumors, including thymectomy for myasthenia gravis patients.[143,154] Contraindications to the performance of thoracoscopy include presence of dense ipsilateral adhesions or previous obliteration of the pleural space, critically ill patients, or patients in shock.[155,156]

Thoracoscopy is generally regarded as a safe procedure. Reported complications include postoperative bleeding, intrapleural hemorrhage, subcutaneous emphysema, and postoperative pneumothorax. Overall, the procedure is extremely well tolerated, even by debilitated patients.[146,157]

Thoracoscopy is usually performed by introducing a sheath with a trocar into the pleural space (Figure 9-21). The trocar is then removed, and any number of viewing instruments can be placed into the pleural space via the sheath (Figure 9-22). Commonly, a rigid telescope with various viewing angles is used. In addition, a fiberoptic bronchoscope (Figure 9-23) has been reported to be extremely useful for examination of the lung and pleural space; the same is true of rigid bronchoscopes, laparoscopes and mediastinoscopes.[158-161] An additional sheath sometimes can be introduced, thus allowing the endoscopist to have an unobstructed view to suction or take biopsy specimens of the operative site. Some surgeons prefer the rigid thoracoscope, while others prefer the fiberoptic scope. The rigid thoracoscope is reported to provide a better field of vision and better overall lighting, while the fiberoptic version is more maneuverable.[136]

Most surgeons currently use the video-assisted thoracoscopic surgery (VATS) technique. VATS involves a high-resolution camera connected to a rigid thoracoscope, which has an integrated fiberoptic light source that transmits a magnified image to a video monitor. The thoracoscope and camera are inserted into the chest via a disposable port. Other instruments, such as miniature staplers, can then be introduced through additional ports. The use of the video monitor allows the anesthesiologist to observe the progress of the surgical procedure and facilitates teaching. In addition, a video recorder can be used to record the entire procedure for later review (Figures 9-24, 9-25, 9-26, 9-27, and 9-28).

Once the thoracoscope is introduced, the operative lung is deflated selectively to allow a complete inspection of the pleura and adjacent organs. During VATS procedures, it is especially critical that the operative lung be completely collapsed. This can be accomplished with a DLT or a bronchial blocker (BB).[162]

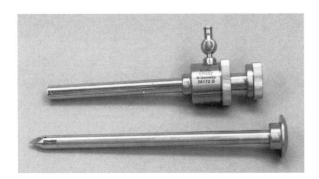

FIGURE 9-22 A thoracoscope with the trocar removed and ready to accept viewing or surgical biopsy instruments.

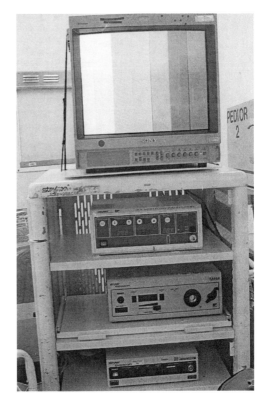

FIGURE 9-24 A video tower used for VATS.

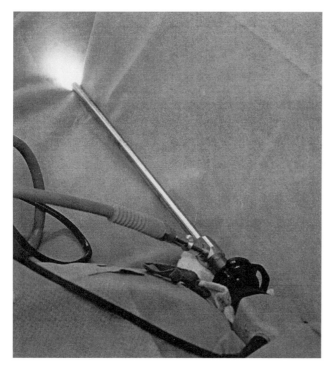

FIGURE 9-25 The VATS telescope with the camera and light source attached.

Bauer et al compared a left-sided DLT with the Wiruthan bronchial blocker (Willy Rusch AG, Kernan, Germany) for one-lung ventilation during thoracoscopy.[163] The investigators discussed unsuccessful placement attempts, malpositions, time to place the DLT or BB, and the quality of lung deflation. The group in which a left-sided BB was used had a higher incidence of unsuccessful attempts at placement and malpositions; the left-sided BB took longer to place than the DLT or right-sided BB. The quality of lung deflation was judged as poor in 44% of the right-sided BB group and as fair to excellent in the DLT and left-sided BB groups. Overall, the authors concluded that the DLT was superior to the BB.

In some cases, the surgeon might want to insufflate CO_2 into the pleural space to augment the collapse of the operative lung. This is safe as long as the pressure is less than 10 mmHg and the flow is limited to 1 to 2 L/min.[164] High pressures or flow can cause sudden contralateral mediastinal shift that results in cardiovascular collapse. Other complications of carbon dioxide insufflation include decreased venous return, increased left ventricular afterload, and the potential for carbon dioxide embolism.[165]

Although adequate oxygenation is usually maintained during one-lung ventilation, occasionally patients become hypoxic. The traditional treatment for this was CPAP to the nonventilated lung, with or without PEEP to the ventilated lung. During VATS procedures, however, the use of CPAP to the nonventilated lung is not possible, as it obscures the surgeon's view.

Nitric oxide (NO) is a potent vascular smooth muscle vasodilator. It was once hoped that administration of inhaled NO to the ventilated lung would decrease shunt and improve oxygenation during one-lung ventilation.[166] The results of several studies have been disappointing, however.[162] A study by Moutafis compared two-lung ventilation to one-lung ventilation in three groups of patients.[167] One group received 100% oxygen; a second group received O_2 and NO; and a third group received O_2, NO, and intravenous almitrine. Almitrine increases hypoxic pulmonary vasoconstriction, whereas NO vasodilates the ventilated lung. The results showed significant decreases in PO_2 in the groups receiving oxygen and oxygen plus NO; however, oxygenation was maintained at near-control levels in the group receiving O_2, NO, and almitrine.[167] This latter combination of the three agents could prove to be a useful technique in VATS when oxygenation is a problem.

Preoperative assessment of patients undergoing thoracoscopy should include the same considerations as for the patients undergoing bronchoscopy. Thoracoscopy can be done under either general or regional anesthesia without difficulty.[137,145,168] For

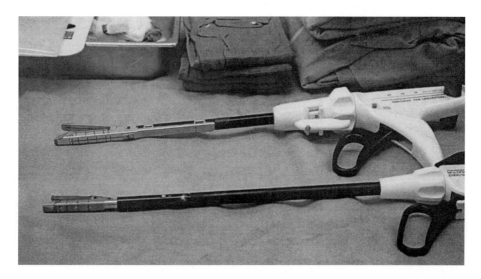

FIGURE 9-26 Miniature staplers used in VATS.

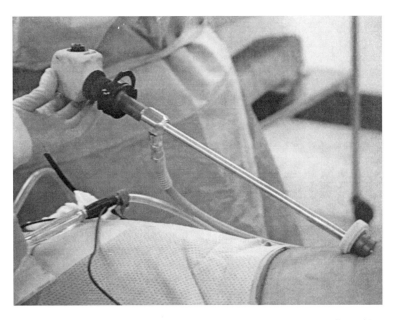

FIGURE 9-27 The VATS telescope with attached camera inserted through a disposable port.

relatively minor surgical procedures (e.g., ablation of persistent air leaks by selective injection of fibrin sealant or talc pleurodesis), local anesthesia with moderate ("conscious") sedation has been used successfully.[148,169] Regional anesthesia for thoracoscopy consists of performing intercostal nerve blocks at least two segments above and below the anticipated operative site. Intercostal nerve blocking, however, does not anesthetize the visceral pleura, which requires the application of topical local anesthetics. It is also advisable to perform a stellate ganglion block in order to obtund the cough reflex and prevent injury to adjacent viscera. Alternatively, intravenous narcotics can be used to depress the cough reflex.

Compared with general anesthesia, regional anesthesia has the advantage of improving the patient's ability to cough post-operatively and provides postoperative analgesia secondary to intercostal nerve blockade. Regional anesthesia might also be better tolerated by debilitated patients. The major disadvantage of regional anesthesia is that the patient must breathe spontaneously while the operative lung is collapsed. Although this can be tolerated for short periods of time, it probably is not advisable for longer procedures. Finally, the placement of talc or other sclerosing agents into the pleura is frequently uncomfortable for the awake patient.

When general anesthesia is selected for thoracoscopy, a DLT is recommended so that ventilation and oxygenation can be controlled and monitored carefully. A DLT also allows selective deflation of the operative lung during the procedure. In some instances, bilateral thoracoscopy is performed, and

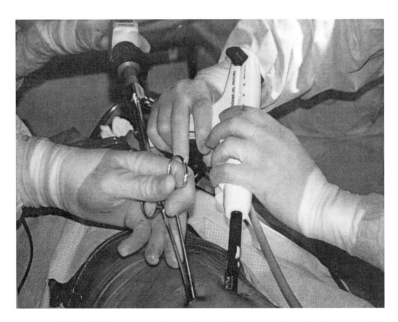

FIGURE 9-28 VATS with the surgeon using a clamp and the camera to guide placement of the stapler.

each lung can be collapsed and ventilated successively as needed by the surgeon. Furthermore, the double-lumen tube allows the lung to be reexpanded under the direct vision of the surgeon, which is helpful in the case of a lung trapped by adhesions or in the case of a bronchopleural fistula. The patient's oxygenation and ventilation are more easily monitored and controlled with capnography and pulse oximetry during general anesthesia. For longer surgical procedures, placement of an indwelling arterial catheter for blood gas monitoring is indicated.

General anesthesia for thoracoscopy can be accomplished with either intravenous or potent inhalation agents. As with bronchoscopy, the use of short-acting intravenous agents is important to allow rapid emergence and prompt recovery of airway reflexes. The same goal can be achieved by using potent inhalation anesthetics, which have the additional advantage of delivering high concentrations of inspired oxygen during one-lung anesthesia.

At the end of the surgical procedure, the patient should be monitored in a postoperative recovery room setting regardless of the type of anesthetic used. Because of the surgically induced pneumothorax, these patients should be transported from the operating room to the recovery room while supplemental oxygen is being administered. Postoperative thoracoscopy patients are at higher risk of sudden pulmonary decompensation and postoperative bleeding. Therefore recovery room personnel must maintain a high index of suspicion when caring for these patients. Continuous pulse oximetry, along with all of the other routine monitoring techniques, must be used.

Overall, VATS is well tolerated and is associated with decreased postoperative pain, faster return to preoperative status, and shorter hospital stays. VATS is superior to traditional thoracotomy for many thoracic diagnostic procedures.

Esophagoscopy

In 1853, the French physician Desormeaux was first to introduce the endoscope to visualize the interior of the bladder; a decade later (1865), he used this instrument to visualize the esophagus.[9] One hundred fifty years later, indications for esophagoscopy include removal of a foreign body, dilatation of strictures, evaluation and biopsy of esophageal lesions, and sclerotherapy for bleeding esophageal varices.[170-172] Because many of the patients undergoing esophagoscopy cannot eat, preoperative assessment should include evaluations of fluid balance and nutritional status, serum albumin, and serum electrolytes. Patients with esophageal cancer need careful preoperative screening because they might have had prior chemotherapy with adriamycin, doxorubicin, or bleomycin. Adriamycin and doxorubicin can cause severe cardiomyopathy and congestive heart failure, which are dose related and can be fatal.[173] Life-threatening pulmonary toxicity can occur in up to 25% of patients receiving bleomycin. Symptoms include cough and dyspnea and can progress to hypoxia and pulmonary fibrosis. The anesthesiologist should be cognizant of the predisposition to pulmonary toxicity in bleomycin-treated patients who receive high oxygen concentrations during anesthesia.[173]

Patients undergoing esophagoscopy present a unique challenge to the anesthesiologist. Routine measures taken to prevent aspiration of gastric contents on induction of anesthesia could be inadequate or even contraindicated. For instance, oral antacids and H_2-receptor blockers could be ineffective in the patient with achalasia. Patients with esophageal diverticula or strictures might not be able to empty the esophagus completely. Therefore food retained above the level of the lesion can be aspirated during induction. The use of intravenous agents that decrease gastric secretions and facilitate gastric emptying might be useful for these patients.[174]

Furthermore, when performing Sellick's maneuver, the application of cricoid pressure might actually dislodge retained food from the esophagus, with tracheal aspiration as the result. Foreign bodies in the esophagus can also constitute a contraindication to rapid-sequence induction. A large foreign body (e.g., a chicken bone) could cause esophageal perforation during application of cricoid pressure. Similarly, a sharp foreign body such as an open safety pin could likewise lead to an esophageal perforation.

Esophageal perforation during endoscopy is of particular concern, as it is associated with a high incidence of morbidity and mortality.[175,176] Esophagoscopy can be performed either with a rigid or a flexible fiberoptic esophagoscope. Both of these procedures can be performed with topical anesthesia plus sedation or with general anesthesia. General anesthesia is usually preferred for rigid esophagoscopy, particularly when a foreign body is present, as coughing and bucking during the procedure can lead to esophageal perforation (Figure 9-29). The use of a wire-reinforced endotracheal (ET) tube can prevent compression of the tube by the rigid esophagoscope. Obstruction of the ET tube can be detected by observing increases in the airway pressure or the development of an obstructive pattern on the capnogram.[174]

Awake intubation should be performed in any situation in which cricoid pressure is contraindicated. A small-sized or a wire-reinforced endotracheal tube might be necessary when a large rigid foreign body impinges on or obstructs the trachea. An awake fiberoptic intubation allows identification of any tracheal narrowing and enables the anesthesiologist to place the endotracheal tube precisely below the level of obstruction. Correct placement is particularly important in the case of a tracheoesophageal fistula, to ensure that the endotracheal tube is located below the level of the communication. It is important to remember that during emergence from anesthesia following esophagoscopy, patients are still at significant risk for aspiration of gastric contents. Thus the anesthesiologist must be certain that the patients are fully awake and able to protect their airways prior to extubation.

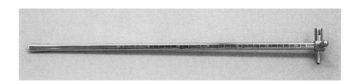

FIGURE 9-29 A rigid esophagoscope.

REFERENCES

1. Vaughn GC, Downs JB: Perioperative pulmonary function. Assessment and intervention, *Anesthesiol Rev* 17:19, 1990.
2. Warner MA, Divertie MB, Tinker JH: Preoperative cessation of smoking and pulmonary complications in coronary artery bypass patients, *Anesthesiology* 60:380, 1984.
3. Kambam JR, Chen LH, Hyman SA: Effect of short-term smoking halt on carboxyhemoglobin levels and P_{50} values, *Anesth Analg* 65:1186, 1986.
4. Smith RJ, Landaw SA: Smokers polycythemia, *N Engl J Med* 298:6, 1978.
5. Mallampati SR, Gatt SP, Gugino, LD, et al: A clinical sign to predict difficult tracheal intubation: a prospective study, *Can Anaesth Soc J* 32:429, 1985.
6. Tisi GM: Preoperative evaluation of pulmonary function: validity, indications and benefits, *Am Rev Respir Dis* 119:293, 1979.
7. Stein M, Cassara EL: Preoperative pulmonary evaluation and therapy for surgery patients, *JAMA* 211:787, 1970.
8. Sackner MA: Bronchofiberoscopy: state of the art, *Am Rev Respir Dis* 111:62, 1975.
9. Hagopian EJ, Mann C, Galibert L-A, Steichen FM: The history of thoracic surgical instruments and instrumentation, *Chest Surg Clin North Am* 10:9, 2000.
10. Jackson C: Bronchoscopy; past, present and future, *N Engl J Med* 199:759, 1928.
11. Ikeda S, Yanai N, Tshikawa S: Flexible bronchofiberscope, *Keio J Med* 17:1, 1968.
12. Smith G, Hirsch N, Ehrenwerth J. Placement of double-lumen endobronchial tubes: correlation between clinical impressions and bronchoscopic findings, *Br J Anaesth* 58:1317, 1986.
13. McKenna RJ, Campbell A, McMurtrey MJ, et al: Diagnosis for interstitial lung disease in patients with acquired immunodeficiency syndrome (AIDS): a prospective comparison of bronchial washing, alveolar lavage, transbronchial lung biopsy, and open-lung biopsy, *Ann Thorac Surg* 41:318, 1986.
14. Baumgartner WA, Mark JBD: Bronchoscopic diagnosis and treatment of bronchial stump suture granulomas, *J Thorac Cardiovasc Surg* 81:553, 1981.
15. Credle WF, Jr, Smiddy JF, Elliott RC: Complications of fiberoptic bronchoscopy, *Am Rev Respir Dis* 109:67, 1974.
16. Suratt PM, Smiddy JF, Gruber B: Deaths and complications associated with fiberoptic bronchoscopy, *Chest* 69:747, 1976.
17. Zavala DC: Complications following fiberoptic bronchoscopy: the "good news" and the "bad news," *Chest* 73:783, 1978.
18. Lukomsky GI, Ovchinnikov AA, Bilal A: Complications of bronchoscopy: comparison of rigid bronchoscopy under general anesthesia and flexible fiberoptic bronchoscopy under topical anesthesia, *Chest* 79:316, 1981.
19. Pereira W, Kounat DM, Snider GL: A prospective cooperative study of complications following flexible fiberoptic bronchoscopy, *Chest* 73:813, 1978.
20. Albertini RE, Harrell JH, Kurihara N, Moser KM: Arterial hypoxemia induced by fiberoptic bronchoscopy, *JAMA* 230:1666, 1974.
21. Dubrawsky C, Awe RJ, Jenkins DE: The effect of bronchofiberscopic examination on oxygenation status, *Chest* 67:137, 1975.
22. Kleinholtz EJ, Fussel J: Arterial blood gas studies during fiberoptic bronchoscopy, *Am Rev Respir Dis* 108:1014, 1973.
23. Hoffman S, Bruderman I: Blood-pressure and blood-gas changes during anesthesia for bronchoscopy using a modified method of ventilation, *Anesthesiology* 37:95, 1972.
24. Miller EJ: Hypoxemia during fiberoptic bronchoscopy, *Chest* 75:103, 1979 (letter).
25. Prys-Roberts C, Greene LT, Meloche R, et al: Studies of anaesthesia in relation to hypertension II: haemodynamic consequences of induction and endotracheal intubation, *Br J Anaesth* 43:531, 1971.
26. Prys-Roberts C, Foex P, Biro GP, et al: Studies of anaesthesia in relation to hypertension V: adrenergic beta-receptor blockade, *Br J Anaesth* 45:671, 1973.
27. Luck JC, Messeder OH, Rubenstein MJ, et al.: Arrhythmias from fiberoptic bronchoscopy, *Chest* 74:139, 1978.
28. Wood M: Local anesthetic agents. In Wood M, Wood AJJ (eds): *Drugs and anesthesia,* ed 2, Baltimore, 1990, Williams & Wilkins.
29. Weisel W, Tella RA: Reaction to tetracaine (Pontocaine) used as topical anesthetic in bronchoscopy, *JAMA* 147:218, 1951.
30. Adriani J, Campbell D: Fatalities following topical application of local anesthesia to mucous membranes, *JAMA* 162:1527, 1956.
31. Poe RH, Dass T, Celebic A: Small airway testing and smoking in predicting risk in surgical patients, *Amer J Med Sci* 283:57, 1982.
32. Olsson GL: Bronchospasm during anaesthesia: a computer-aided incidence study of 136,929 patients, *Acta Anaesthesiol Scand* 31:244, 1987.
33. Gass GD, Olsen GN: Preoperative pulmonary function testing to predict postoperative morbidity and mortality, *Chest* 89:127, 1986.
34. Stoelting RK: Circulatory changes during direct laryngoscopy and tracheal intubation: influence of duration of laryngoscopy with or without prior lidocaine, *Anesthesiology* 47:381, 1977.
35. Martin DE, Rosenberg H, Aukburg SJ, et al: Low-dose fentanyl blunts circulatory responses to tracheal intubation, *Anesth Analg* 61:680, 1982.
36. Inada E, Cullen DJ, Nemeskal R, et al: Effect of labetalol on the hemodynamic response to intubation: a controlled randomized double-blind study, *Anesthesiology* 67:A31, 1987.
37. Maharaj RJ, Thompson M, Brock-Utne JG, et al: Treatment of hypertension following endotracheal intubation: a study comparing the efficacy of labetalol, practolol and placebo, *S Afr Med J* 63:691, 1983.
38. Stoelting RK: Attenuation of blood pressure response to laryngoscopy and tracheal intubation with sodium nitroprusside, *Anesth Analg* 58:116, 1979.
39. Townley RG: Calcium channel antagonists in coronary artery spasm and bronchial spasm, *Chest* 82:401, 1982.
40. Russi EW, Marchette B, Yerger L, et al: Modification of allergic bronchoconstriction by a calcium antagonist: mode of action, *Am Rev Respir Dis* 127:675, 1983.
41. Roizen MR, Horrigan RW, Frazer BM: Anesthetic doses blocking adrenergic (stress) and cardiovascular responses to incision: MAC BAR, *Anesthesiology* 54:390, 1981.
42. Wark KJ, Lyons J, Feneck RO: The haemodynamic effects of bronchoscopy, *Anaesthesia* 41:162, 1986.
43. Prakash N, McLeod T, Gao Smith F: The effects of remifentanil on haemodynamic stability during rigid bronchoscopy, *Anaesthesia* 56:576, 2001.
44. Natalini G, Fassini P, Seramondi V, et al: Remifentanil vs. fentanyl during interventional rigid bronchoscopy under general anaesthesia and spontaneous assisted ventilation, *Eur J Anaesthesiol* 16:605, 1999.
45. Elguindi AS, Harrison GN, Abdulla AM, et al: Cardiac rhythm disturbances during fiberoptic bronchoscopy: a prospective study, *J Thorac Cardiovasc Surg* 77:557, 1979.
46. Shrader DL, Lakshminarayan S: The effect of fiberoptic bronchoscopy on cardiac rhythm, *Chest* 73:821, 1978.
47. Salisbury BG, Metzger LF, Altose MD, et al: Effect of fiberoptic bronchoscopy on respiratory performance in patients with chronic airways obstruction, *Thorax* 30:441, 1975.
48. Harless KW, Scheinhorn DJ, Tannen RC, et. al: Administration of oxygen with mouth-held nasal prongs during fiberoptic bronchoscopy, *Chest* 74:237, 1978 (letter).
49. Britton RM, Nelson KG: Improper oxygenation during bronchofiberoscopy, *Anesthesiology* 40:87, 1974.
50. Neuhaus A, Markowitz D, Rotman HH, et al: The effects of fiberoptic bronchoscopy with and without atropine premedication on pulmonary function in humans, *Ann Thorac Surg* 25:393, 1978.
51. Belen J, Neuhaus A, Markowitz D, et al: Modification of the effect of fiberoptic bronchoscopy on pulmonary mechanics, *Chest* 79:516, 1981.
52. Thorburn JR, James MFM, Feldman C, et al: Comparison of the effects of atropine and glycopyrrolate on pulmonary mechanics in patients undergoing fiberoptic bronchoscopy, *Anesth Analg* 65:1285, 1986.
53. Moore JK, Seymour AH: Awareness during bronchoscopy, *Ann R Coll Surg Engl* 69:45, 1987.
54. Toft P, Romer U: Comparison of midazolam and diazepam to supplement total intravenous anaesthesia with ketamine for endoscopy, *Can J Anaesth* 34:466, 1987.
55. Kestin IG, Chapman JM, Coates MB: Alfentanil used to supplement propofol infusions for oesophagoscopy and bronchoscopy, *Anaesthesia* 44:994, 1989.
56. Brocas E, Dupont H, Paugam-Burtz C, et al: Bispectral index variations during tracheal suction in mechanically ventilated critically ill patients: effect of an alfentanil bolus, *Intensive Care Med* 28:211, 2002.
57. Lindholm CE, Ollman B, Snyder JV, et al: Cardiorespiratory effects of flexible fiberoptic bronchoscopy in critically ill patients, *Chest* 74:362, 1978.
58. Lindholm CE: Flexible fiberoptic bronchoscopy in the critically ill patient, *Ann Otol* 83:786, 1974.
59. Frumin MJ, Epstein RM, Cohen G: Apneic oxygenation in man, *Anesthesiology* 20:789, 1959.
60. Fraioli RL, Sheffer LA, Steffenson JL: Pulmonary and cardiovascular effects of apneic oxygenation in man, *Anesthesiology* 39:588, 1973.

61. Barr AM, Wong RM: Awareness during general anaesthesia for bronchoscopy and laryngoscopy using the apnoeic oxygenation technique, *Br J Anaesth* 45:894, 1973.

62. Sanders RD: Two ventilating attachments for bronchoscopes, *Delaware Med J* 39:170, 1967.

63. MacIntosh R, Mushin WW, Epstein HG: *Physics for the anaesthetist*, Philadelphia, 1963, FA Davis.

64. Carden E: Positive pressure ventilation during anesthesia for bronchoscopy: a laboratory evaluation of two recent advances, *Anesth Analg* 52:402, 1973.

65. Sullivan MT, Neff WB: A modified Sanders ventilating system for rigid-wall bronchoscopy, *Anesthesiology* 50:473, 1979.

66. Morales GA, Epstein BS, Cinco B, et al: Ventilation during general anesthesia for bronchoscopy, *J Thorac Cardiovasc Surg* 57:873, 1969.

67. Spoerel WE: Ventilation through an open bronchoscope (preliminary report), *Can Anaesth Soc J* 16:61, 1969.

68. Duvall AJ, Johnsen AF, Buckley J: Bronchoscopy under general anesthesia using the Sanders ventilating attachment, *Ann Otol Rhinol Laryngol* 78:490, 1969.

69. Carden E: Recent improvements in techniques for general anesthesia for bronchoscopy, *Chest* 73:697, 1978.

70. Giesecke AH, Gerbershagen HU, Dortman C, et al: Comparison of the ventilating and injection bronchoscopes, *Anesthesiology* 38:298, 1973.

71. Carden E, Trapp WG, Oulton J: A new and simple method for ventilating patients undergoing bronchoscopy, *Anesthesiology* 33:454, 1970.

72. Gillick JS: The inflation-catheter technique for ventilation during bronchoscopy, *Anesthesiology* 40:503, 1974.

73. El-Naggar M: The use of a small endotracheal tube in bronchoscopy, *Br J Anaesth* 47:390, 1975.

74. Carden E, Schwesinger WB: The use of nitrous oxide during ventilation with the open bronchoscope, *Anesthesiology* 39:551, 1973.

75. Vourc'h G, Fischler M, Michon F, et al: High-frequency jet ventilation v. manual jet ventilation during bronchoscopy in patients with tracheobronchial stenosis, *Br J Anaesth* 55:969, 1983.

76. Rouby JJ, Viars P: Clinical use of high-frequency ventilation, *Acta Anaesthesiol Scand* 33:134, 1989.

77. Eriksson I, Sjostrand U: Effects of high-frequency positive pressure ventilation (HFPPV) and general anesthesia on intrapulmonary gas distribution in patients undergoing diagnostic bronchoscopy, *Anesth Analg* 59:585, 1980.

78. Borg U, Eriksson I, Sjostrand U: High-frequency positive pressure ventilation (HFPPV): a review based upon its use during bronchoscopy and for laryngoscopy and microlaryngeal surgery under general anesthesia, *Anesth Analg* 59:594, 1980.

79. Schlenkhoff D, Droste H, Scieszka S, et al: The use of high-frequency jet ventilation in operative bronchoscopy, *Endoscopy* 18:192, 1986.

80. Wright PE, Marini JJ, Bernard GR: In vitro versus in vivo comparison of endotracheal tube airflow resistance, *Am Rev Respir Dis* 140:10, 1989.

81. Carden E, Raj PP: Special new low resistance to flow tube and endotracheal tube adapter for use during fiberoptic bronchoscopy, *Ann Otol* 84:631, 1975.

82. Smith RB, Lindholm CE, Klain M: Jet ventilation for fiberoptic bronchoscopy under general anesthesia, *Acta Anaesth Scand* 20:111, 1976.

83. Satyanarayana T, Capan L, Ramanathan S, et al: Bronchofiberscopic jet ventilation, *Anesth Analg* 59:350, 1980.

84. Eschenbacher WL, Bethel RA, Baushay HA, et al: Morphine sulfate inhibits bronchoconstriction in subjects with mild asthma whose responses are inhibited by atropine, *Am Rev Respir Dis* 130:363, 1984.

85. Gal TJ, Suratt PM, Lu JY: Glycopyrrolate and atropine inhalation: comparative effects on normal airway function, *Am Rev Respir Dis* 129(5):871-873, 1984.

86. Schaberg SJ, Stuller CB, Edwards SM: Effect of methylprednisolone on swelling after orthognathic surgery, *J Oral Maxillofac Surg* 42:356, 1984.

87. Shieh HL, Hutton CE, Kafrawy AH, et al: Comparison of meclofenamate sodium and hydrocortisone for controlling the postsurgical inflammatory response in rats, *J Oral Maxillofac Surg* 46:777, 1988.

88. Christoforidis AJ, Tomashefski JF, Mitchell RI: Use of an ultrasonic nebulizer for the application of oropharyngeal, laryngeal and tracheobronchial anesthesia, *Chest* 59:629, 1971.

89. Hartmannsgruber MW, Silverman DG, Halaszynski TM, et al: Comparison of ropivacaine 0.2% and lidocaine 0.5% for intravenous regional anesthesia in volunteers, *Anesth Analg* 89:727, 1999.

90. Rosenblatt WH: Airway management. In Barash PB, Cullen BF, Stoelting RK (eds): *Clinical anesthesia*, Philadelphia, 2001, Lippincott Williams & Wilkins.

91. Steinhaus JE, Gaskin L: A study of intravenous lidocaine as a suppressant of cough reflex, *Anesthesiology* 24:285, 1963.

92. Stiffel P, Hameroff SR: A modified technique for transtracheal anesthesia, *Anesthesiology* 51:274, 1979.

93. Cooper M, Watson RL: An improved regional anesthetic technique for peroral endoscopy, *Anesthesiology* 43:372, 1975.

94. Gaskill JR, Gillies DR: Local anesthesia for peroral endoscopy using superior laryngeal nerve block with topical application, *Arch Otolaryng* 84:654, 1966.

95. Kandt D, Schlegel M: Bronchologic examinations under topical ultrasonic aerosol inhalation anesthesia, *Scand J Resp Dis* 54:65, 1973.

96. Steegers PA, Foster PA: The use of propofol in a group of older patients undergoing oesophagoscopy, *SAMJ* 73:279, 1988.

97. Harken DE, Black H, Clauss R, et al: A simple cervicomediastinal exploration for tissue diagnosis of intrathoracic disease, *N Engl J Med* 251:1041, 1954.

98. Carlens E: A method for inspection and tissue biopsy in the superior mediastinum, *Dis Chest* 36:343, 1959.

99. Pearson FG: Lung cancer: the past 25 years, *Chest* 89:200S, 1986.

100. Weissberg D, Herczeg E: Perforation of thoracic aortic aneurysm: a complication of mediastinoscopy, *Chest* 78:119, 1980 (letter).

101. Vaughan RS: Anaesthesia for mediastinoscopy, *Anaesthesia* 33:195, 1978.

102. Burkell CC, Cross JM, Kent HP, et al: Mass lesions of the mediastinum, *Curr Probl Surg* 100:1, 1969.

103. Foster ED, Munro DD, Dobell ARC: Mediastinoscopy: a review of anatomical relationships and complications, *Ann Thorac Surg* 13:273, 1972.

104. McNeill TM, Chamberlain JM: Diagnostic anterior mediastinotomy, *Ann Thorac Surg* 2:532, 1966.

105. Stemmer EA, Calvin JW, Steedman RA, et al: Parasternal mediastinal exploration to evaluate resectability of thoracic neoplasms, *Ann Thorac Surg* 12:375, 1971.

106. Oldham HN Jr: Mediastinal tumors and cysts, *Ann Thorac Surg* 11:246, 1971.

107. Neuman GG, Weingarten AE, Abramowitz RM, et al: The anesthetic management of the patient with an anterior mediastinal mass, *Anesthesiology* 60:144, 1984.

108. Shambaugh GE, Seed R, Korn A: Airway obstruction in substernal goiter: clinical and therapeutic implications, *J Chron Dis* 26:737, 1973.

109. Tonnesen AS, Davis FG: Superior vena caval and bronchial obstruction during anesthesia, *Anesthesiology* 45:91, 1976.

110. Mackie AM, Watson CB: Anaesthesia and mediastinal masses: a case report and review of the literature, *Anaesthesia* 39:899, 1984.

111. Lochridge SK, Knibble WP, Doty DB: Obstruction of the superior vena cava, *Surgery* 85:14, 1979.

112. Ward PH, Stephenson SE Jr, Harris PF: Exploration of the mediastinum under local anesthesia, *Ann Otol Rhinol Laryngol* 75:368, 1966.

113. Selby JH Jr, Leach CL, Heath BJ, et al: Local anesthesia for mediastinoscopy: experience with 450 consecutive cases, *Am Surg* 44:679, 1978.

114. Morton JR, Guinn GA: Mediastinoscopy using local anesthesia, *Amer J Surg* 122:696, 1971.

115. Prakash UBS, Abel MD, Hubmayr RD: Mediastinal mass and tracheal obstruction during general anesthesia, *Mayo Clin Proc* 63:1004, 1988.

116. Philips PA, Van De Water JM: Mediastinoscopy vs. exploratory thoracotomy, *Arch Surg* 105:48, 1972.

117. Flynn JR, Rossi NP, Lawton RL: Significance of mediastinoscopy in carcinoma of the lung, *Arch Surg* 94:243, 1967.

118. Ashbaugh DG: Mediastinoscopy, *Arch Surg* 100:568, 1970.

119. Petty C: Right radial artery pressure during mediastinoscopy, *Anesth Analg* 58:428, 1979.

120. Ponn RB, Federico JA: Mediastinoscopy and staging. In Kaiser LR, Kron IL, Spray TI (eds): *Mastery of cardiothoracic surgery*, Philadelphia, 1998, Lippincott-Raven.

121. Trinkle JK, Bryant LR, Hiller AJ, et al: Mediastinoscopy: experience with 300 consecutive cases, *J Thorac Cardiovasc Surg* 60:297, 1970.

122. Lee JH, Salvatore A: Innominate artery compression simulating cardiac arrest during mediastinoscopy: a case report, *Anesth Analg* 55:748, 1976.

123. Sibert KS, Biondi JW, Hirsch NP: Spontaneous respiration during thoracotomy in a patient with a mediastinal mass, *Anesth Analg* 66:904, 1987.

124. Bittar D: Respiratory obstruction associated with induction of general anesthesia in a patient with mediastinal Hodgkin's disease, *Anesth Analg* 54:399, 1975.

125. Bray RJ, Fernandes FJ: Mediastinal tumour causing airway obstruction in anaesthetized children, *Anaesthesia* 37:571, 1982.
126. Levin MB, Bursztein S, Heifetz M: Cardiac arrest in a child with an anterior mediastinal mass, *Anesth Analg* 64:1129, 1985.
127. Piro AJ, Weiss DR, Hellman S: Mediastinal Hodgkin's disease: a possible danger for intubation anesthesia, *Int J Radiat Oncol Biol Phys* 1:415, 1976.
128. Barash PG, Tsai B, Kitahata LM: Acute tracheal collapse following mediastinoscopy, *Anesthesiology* 44:67, 1976.
129. Keon TP: Death on induction of anesthesia for cervical node biopsy, *Anesthesiology* 55:471, 1981.
130. Todres ID, Reppert SM, Walker PF, et al: Management of critical airway obstruction in a child with a mediastinal tumor, *Anesthesiology* 45:100, 1976.
131. Younker D, Clark R, Coveler L: Fiberoptic endobronchial intubation for resection of an anterior mediastinal mass, *Anesthesiology* 70:144, 1989.
132. Wilson RF, Steiger Z, Jacobs J, et al: Temporary partial cardiopulmonary bypass during emergency operative management of near total tracheal occlusion, *Anesthesiology* 61:103, 1984.
133. Hall KD, Friedman M: Extracorporeal oxygenation for induction of anesthesia in a patient with an intrathoracic tumor, *Anesthesiology* 42:493, 1975.
134. Lee CM, Grossman LB: Laceration of left pulmonary artery during mediastinoscopy, *Anesth Analg* 56:226, 1977.
135. Dalton ML, Gerken MV, Neely WA: Right bronchial artery hemorrhage complicating mediastinoscopy, *Contemp Surg* 24:75, 1984.
136. Bloomberg AE: Thoracoscopy in perspective, *Surg Gyn Obstet* 147:433, 1978.
137. Baumgartner WA, Mark JBD: The use of thoracoscopy in the diagnosis of pleural disease, *Arch Surg* 115:420, 1980.
138. Rodgers BM, Ryckman FC, Moazam F, et al: Thoracoscopy for intrathoracic tumors, *Ann Thorac Surg* 31:414, 1981.
139. Miller JI, Hatcher CR Jr: Thoracoscopy: a useful tool in the diagnosis of thoracic disease, *Ann Thorac Surg* 26:68, 1978.
140. Boutin C, Viallat JR, Cargnino P, et al: Thoracoscopic lung biopsy: experimental and clinical preliminary study, *Chest* 82:44, 1982.
141. Poulos C, Ponn R, Tranquilli M, et al: Thoracoscopy for diagnosis of chest disease, *Conn Med* 52:201, 1988.
142. Canto A, Blasco E, Casillas M, et al: Thoracoscopy in the diagnosis of pleural effusion, *Thorax* 32:550, 1977.
143. Cirino LMI, Milanez de Campos JR, Fernandez A, et al: Diagnosis and treatment of mediastinal tumors by thoracoscopy, *Chest* 117:1787, 2000.
144. Rodgers BM, Moulder PV, DeLaney A: Thoracoscopy: new method of early diagnosis of cardiac herniation, *J Thorac Cardiovasc Surg* 78:623, 1979.
145. Williams A, Kay J: Thoracic epidural anesthesia for thoracoscopy, rib resection, and thoracotomy in a patient with a bronchopleural fistula postpneumonectomy, *Anesthesiology* 92:1482, 2000.
146. Oakes DD, Sherck JP, Brodsky JB, et al: Therapeutic thoracoscopy, *J Thorac Cardiovasc Surg* 87:269, 1984.
147. Ali A, Pellegrini CA: Laparoscopic myotomy: technique and efficacy in treating achalasia, *Gastrointest Endosc Clin North Am* 11:347, 2001.
148. Thistlethwaite PA, Luketich JD, Ferson PF, et al: Ablation of persistent air leaks after thoracic procedures with fibrin sealant, *Ann Thorac Surg* 67:575, 1999.
149. Lowdermilk GA, Naunheim KS: Thoracoscopic evaluation and treatment of thoracic trauma, *Surg Clin North Am* 80:1535, 2000.
150. Jones JW, Kitahama A, Webb WR, et al: Emergency thoracoscopy: a logical approach to chest trauma management, *J Trauma* 21:280, 1981.
151. Nakamoto H, Suzuki T, Sugahara S, et al: Successful use of thoracoscopic pericardiectomy in elderly patients with massive pericardial effusion caused by uremic pericarditis, *Am J Kidney Dis* 37:1294, 2001.
152. Reardon PR, Preciado A, Scarborough T, et al: Outpatient endoscopic thoracic sympathectomy using 2-mm instruments, *Surg Endosc* 13:1139, 1999.
153. Lin TS: Endoscopic clipping in video-assisted thoracoscopic sympathetic blockade for axillary hyperhidrosis. An analysis of 26 cases, *Surg Endosc* 15:126, 2001.
154. Yim APC, Kay RLC, Izzat MB, et al. Video-assisted thoracoscopic thymectomy for myasthenia gravis, *Semin Thorac Cardiovasc Surg* 11:65, 1999.
155. McFadden PM, Robbins RJ: Cardiothoracic and vascular surgery. Thoracoscopic surgery, *Surg Clin North Am* 78:763, 1998.
156. Dieter RA, Jr, Kuzycz GB: Complications and contraindications of thoracoscopy, *Int Surg* 82:232, 1997.
157. Weissberg D, Kaufman M, Zurkowski Z: Pleuroscopy in patients with pleural effusion and pleural masses, *Ann Thorac Surg* 29:205, 1980.
158. Ben-Isaac FE, Simmons DH: Flexible fiberoptic pleuroscopy: pleural and lung biopsy, *Chest* 67:573, 1975.
159. Senno A, Moallem S, Quijano ER, et al: Thoracoscopy with the fiberoptic bronchoscope, *J Thorac Cardiovasc Surg* 67:606, 1974.
160. Gwin E, Pierce G, Boggan M, et al: Pleuroscopy and pleural biopsy with the flexible fiberoptic bronchoscope, *Chest* 67:527, 1975.
161. Kaiser LR: Diagnostic and therapeutic uses of pleuroscopy (thoracoscopy) in lung cancer, *Surg Clin North Am* 67:1081, 1987.
162. Brodsky JB, Fitzmaurice B: Modern anesthetic techniques for thoracic operations, *World J Surg* 25:162, 2001.
163. Bauer C, Winter C, Hentz X, et al: Bronchial blocker compared to double-lumen tube for one-lung ventilation during thoracoscopy, *Acta Anaesthesiol Scand* 45:250, 2001.
164. Shah JS, Bready LL: Anesthesia for minimally invasive surgery: laparoscopy, thoracoscopy, hysteroscopy, *Anesthesiol Clin North Am* 19:153, 2001.
165. Tobias JD-Anaesthetic implications of thoracoscopic surgery in children, *Paediatr Anaesth* 9:103, 1999.
166. Cohen E: One-lung ventilation: prospective from an interested observer, *Minerva Anestesiol* 65:275, 1999.
167. Moutafis M, Liu N, Dalibon N, et al: The effects of inhaled nitric oxide and its combination with intravenous almitrine on PaO₂ during one-lung ventilation in patients undergoing thoracoscopic procedures, *Anesth Analg* 85:1130, 1997.
168. Rusch VW, Mountain C: Thoracoscopy under regional anesthesia for the diagnosis and management of pleural disease, *Amer J Surg* 154:274, 1987.
169. Mares DC, Mathur PN: Medical thoracoscopic talc pleurodesis for chylothorax due to lymphoma, *Chest* 114:731, 1998.
170. Wilson RH, Campbell WJ, Spencer A, et al: Rigid endoscopy under general anaesthesia is safe for chronic injection sclerotherapy, *Br J Surg* 76:719, 1989.
171. Bornman PC, Kahn D, Terblanche J, et al: Rigid versus fiberoptic endoscopic injection sclerotherapy, *Ann Surg* 208:175, 1988.
172. Bendig DW: Removal of blunt esophageal foreign bodies by flexible endoscopy without general anesthesia, *Am J Dis Child* 140:789, 1986.
173. Mohindra P, Yacoub JM: Anesthetic management of the cancer patient undergoing noncardiac thoracic surgery, *Int Anesthesiol Clin* 36:45, 1998.
174. Plummer S, Hartley M, Vaughan RS: Anaesthesia for telescopic procedures in the thorax, *Br J Anaesth* 80:223, 1998.
175. Wolloch Y, Zer M, Dintsman M, et al: Iatrogenic perforations of the esophagus, *Arch Surg* 108:357, 1974.
176. Steyn JH, Brunnen PL: Perforation of cervical oesophagus at oesophagoscopy, *Scot Med J* 7:494, 1962.

Tracheostomy and Tracheal Resection and Reconstruction 10

Roger S. Wilson, MD

Tracheostomy

General Considerations

Tracheostomy, a common surgical procedure, is performed using a variety of techniques. Indications for tracheostomy include the following:

1. Upper airway obstruction
2. Access for tracheal toilet
3. Routing for administration of positive pressure ventilation
4. Airway protection from aspiration of gastric and/or pharyngeal contents

The incidence of complications—including hypoxia, cardiac arrest, injury to structures immediately adjacent to the trachea, pneumothoraces, and hemorrhage—should be minimal when performed electively. Elective tracheostomy is most frequently performed as an open surgical procedure and should be done in the operating room under "ideal" operating conditions. In general, the best operating conditions are provided with prior endotracheal intubation and with the patient adequately anesthetized or sedated with use of additional local anesthesia.

Anesthetic requirements are variable and are dictated by the state of patient awareness and the nature and extent of other systemic disease. If necessary, the procedure can be done safely with local infiltration supplemented with intravenous sedative and/or narcotic drugs. The advantage of this approach, especially when used for a critically ill patient, is that it allows for the administration of high concentrations of inspired oxygen. In patients whose cardiovascular stability is not a problem, general anesthesia with intravenous and/or inhalation agents may be used, with or without supplemental local infiltration. Use of nitrous oxide is dictated by the level of inspired oxygen concentration. Monitoring techniques are determined by the extent of comorbidity, with emphasis on cardiopulmonary function.

Surgical Procedure

The patient is placed in the supine position, the neck extended with the help of either a rolled towel or an inflatable thyroid bag placed beneath the shoulders. The head can be positioned in a "doughnut" or a head-dish for additional stability. These maneuvers provide for maximal surface exposure and, in most patients, bring the trachea from the intrathoracic to the cervical position. After appropriate preparation of the skin and surgical draping, the procedure is accomplished through a short horizontal incision placed at the level of the second tracheal ring (Figure 10-1). The strap muscles are separated in the midline, and the thyroid isthmus is divided and sutured appropri-

ately to obtain hemostasis. Specific identification of the location of the tracheal rings is made by counting down from the easily palpable cricoid cartilage. The second and third rings are opened vertically in the midline for access to the trachea. The tracheostomy tube should be placed so that it does not erode the first ring and press against the cricoid cartilage. In addition, the opening should not be placed too low, or the tip of the tube and its cuff will be too close to the carina. Low placement of the tracheostomy tube is also hazardous because the innominate artery crosses anteriorly to the trachea low in the neck and the possibility of erosion into the vessel by either the cuff or tip of the tracheostomy tube exists. Segments of the trachea should not be removed because this might lead to a greater loss of tracheal wall stability and predispose the remaining segments to stenosis once healing is accomplished after removal of the tube. The lateral tracheal walls are retracted with the help of thyroid pole retractors, and the appropriately sized tracheostomy tube is inserted into the airway, after slow withdrawal of the previously placed oral or nasal endotracheal tube to a more proximal position in the trachea. Once the tracheostomy tube is positioned and an adequate airway is demonstrated through positive pressure ventilation and visual inspection of chest wall expansion, the previously placed endotracheal tube is removed from the trachea. The wound is closed appropriately, skin sutures are placed through the flange ends, and "trach-tape" or a tie is secured around the neck.

Complications

Complications can occur during the intraoperative and postoperative periods. Intraoperative complications generally occur as a result of anesthesia, underlying disease, or surgical procedure. Surgical complications generally fall into three major categories, including hemorrhage, injury to structures adjacent to the trachea, and no airway cannula. Bleeding from the surgical incision is usually controlled easily but can be complicated by the difficulty of exposure. Vascular structures (such as the thyroid isthmus) might bleed easily when divided for exposure. Injuries to adjacent structures include damage to recurrent laryngeal nerves, entrance into major vessels, and rare (but possible) laceration of the esophagus. The inability to cannulate the trachea is possible because of inadequate surgical exposure, an inability to bring the trachea to a superficial location, or selection of a tracheostomy tube too large to fit into the tracheal stoma. Careful planning and appropriate selection of tubes can avoid such complications. In the presence of prior endotracheal intubation, the danger of loss of the airway is minimized.

196

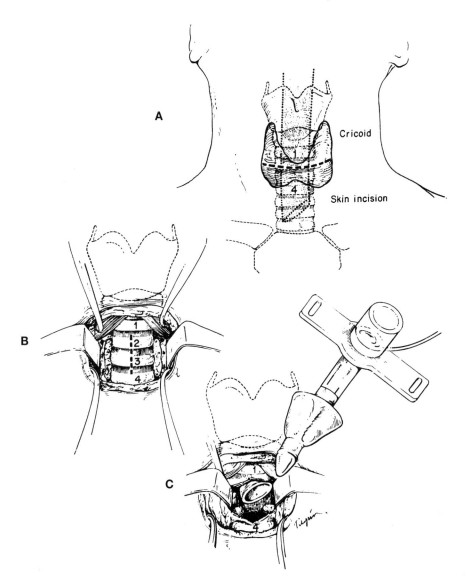

FIGURE 10-1 Technique of tracheostomy. **A,** With an endotracheal tube in place, a horizontal skin incision is made 1 to 2 cm below the cricoid cartilage. **B,** Strap muscles are spread in the midline and the thyroid isthmus is divided. A vertical incision is made in the second and third cartilaginous rings. **C,** With thyroid pole retractors holding back the cut edge of the trachea, the endotracheal tube is withdrawn and the tracheostomy tube is inserted. (From Grillo HC: *Surg Gynecol Obstet* 129: 347, 1969.)

Long-term complications resulting from the use of endotracheal and tracheostomy tubes is considered in the discussion of types of tracheostomy tubes and cuffs.

Emergency Tracheostomy

Occasionally, an "emergency" tracheostomy is necessary, dictated by the urgency of providing an airway when rapidly progressing airway obstruction exists.[1,2] Such obstruction can occur after head and neck trauma, upper-airway compromise because of allergic reactions, angioneurotic edema, epiglottitis, or local infection after neck surgery (e.g., thyroidectomy or anterior approach for cervical fusion). Postoperative problems of this type result from hemorrhage with external compression and potential for total airway obstruction. The ability to accomplish airway control with an endotracheal tube might not be possible. Appropriate emergency procedures include needle tracheostomy, cricothyroidotomy, and standard tracheostomy. Needle tracheostomy is often of limited success because flow through the catheter or needle requires a high-pressure gas source and the immediate availability of appropriate connecting devices between the gas source and the needle or catheter. With this technique, ventilation—and hence, CO_2 elimination—is difficult. This maneuver is potentially life-saving for only a limited time. Formal emergency tracheostomy in general is not technically feasible, owing to the lack of adequate instruments and lighting and the time required to accomplish it before major circulatory and/or cerebral complications occur.

The technique of cricothyroidotomy has become increasingly popular and has been described in numerous publications.[3,4] One advantage is that it can be done quickly with a minimum amount of equipment. A rolled towel is placed under the shoulders to put the neck in a hyperextended position.

A small transverse incision is made through the skin into the cricothyroid membrane with a #11 scalpel blade; the incision is spread with a surgical clamp or a knife handle or with a digital technique. A small (5.0 or 6.0 mm) pediatric endotracheal tube or tracheostomy tube is placed through the cricothyroid membrane into the trachea. This technique has the advantages of simplicity, speed, and minimal bleeding. It also provides an airway sufficient for adequate gas exchange. Potential complications of this technique include the following:

- Injury to the cricoid or thyroid cartilages, with the potential for laryngeal stenosis
- Injury to the esophagus
- Hemorrhage from the anterior jugular vein
- Injury to the carotid artery or internal jugular vein
- Infection at the cricothyroid incision

These complications are generally avoidable if the incision is correctly placed, if a small tube is used, and if the duration of use of the cricothyroidotomy is limited to a short time period (i.e., hours or days). Although it might be advisable to convert the cricothyroidotomy to a standard tracheostomy as soon as the patient's overall condition permits, opinion regarding this decision is not uniform.

Tracheostomy Tube Design

Tracheostomy tubes come in a wide variety of types. They differ in several respects, including the following[5]:
1. Rigidity
2. Flange shape
3. Length
4. Internal/external diameter
5. Angle or curvature of the tube body
6. Cuff shape and characteristics

Tube characteristics for several manufacturers are detailed in Table 10-1.

Recognition that tracheal intubation with cuffed endotracheal and tracheostomy tubes can produce injury has stimulated improvement in the design of both tubes and cuffs. The pathogenesis of tracheal injuries produced by "cuff pressure" has been well documented.[6-9] Complications include tracheal stenosis or disruption of the tracheal wall, with the potential for development of a tracheoesophageal fistula or a fistula into a major vessel such as the innominate artery. A number of cuff designs and techniques have been developed in the hope of minimizing tracheal injury.[10,11] Approaches have included intermittent cuff inflation and deflation; inflation of cuffs during inspiration only; underinflation with a minimal leak technique; use of double-cuff tubes; and design of high-volume, low-pressure cuffs. This last design has proved to be the most effective way of reducing tracheal injury.[12]

The large-residual-volume, low-pressure cuff has been designed in several configurations by a variety of manufacturers. The general design of this cuff is such that it occludes the lumen of the trachea by conforming to the existing configuration of the cross-sectional area without deforming it. This is depicted in Figure 10-2. Improved design of the cuff per se does not totally eliminate tracheal injury. Several precautions must be undertaken regardless of the type of cuff used. The cuff must not be inflated beyond the minimum volume and pressure required to provide a minimal leak.

TABLE 10-1

Size and Length of Tracheostomy Tubes

BIVONA FOME-CUF

Size	I.D.	O.D.	Length
5	5.0 mm	7.3 mm	60 mm
6	6.0 mm	8.7 mm	70 mm
7	7.0 mm	10.0 mm	80 mm
8	8.0 mm	11.0 mm	88 mm
9	9.0 mm	12.3 mm	98 mm
9.5	9.5 mm	13.3 mm	98 mm

PORTEX—D.I.C.

Size	I.D.	O.D.	Length
6	6.0 mm	8.5 mm	64 mm
7	7.0 mm	9.9 mm	70 mm
8	8.0 mm	11.3 mm	74 mm
9	9.0 mm	12.6 mm	80 mm
10	10.0 mm	14.0 mm	80 mm

SHILEY—LPC

Size	I.D.	O.D.	Length
4	5.0 mm	9.4 mm	65 mm
6	6.4 mm	10.8 mm	76 mm
8	7.6 mm	12.2 mm	81 mm
10	8.9 mm	13.8 mm	81 mm

TRACOE FLEX

Size	I.D.	O.D.	Length
4	4.0 mm	7.2 mm	65 mm
6	6.0 mm	9.2 mm	73 mm
8	8.0 mm	11.5 mm	76 mm
10	10.0 mm	13.5 mm	80 mm
12	12.0 mm	15.9 mm	83 mm

Excessive pressure within the inflated cuff (generally assumed to be greater than 25 mmHg) potentially increases the risk of tracheal injury. Although lateral wall pressure (pressure at the point of surface contact between cuff and tracheal wall) is more important than intracuff pressure, the latter is monitored because of ease of measurement. Excessive cuff pressure is frequently encountered when the tracheostomy tube that has been selected is too small, requiring overinflation of the cuff to completely fill the void between the tube and the trachea. When this occurs, alternative measures—for example, an increase in tracheostomy tube size, selection of a tracheostomy tube with a larger cuff, or acceptance of a larger leak—must be undertaken.

Care and Maintenance of the Tracheostomy

Adequate care must be provided to the tracheal stoma to prevent injury and to limit local infection. The care should focus on removal of secretions from the region of the stoma and the surrounding skin. Tracheostomy dressings should be changed regularly (i.e., every 8 hours). The technique should include use of sterile gloves and cotton-tip applicators with hydrogen peroxide to cleanse the stoma site. Tracheostomy tapes, which often become soiled, should be changed on a regular basis.

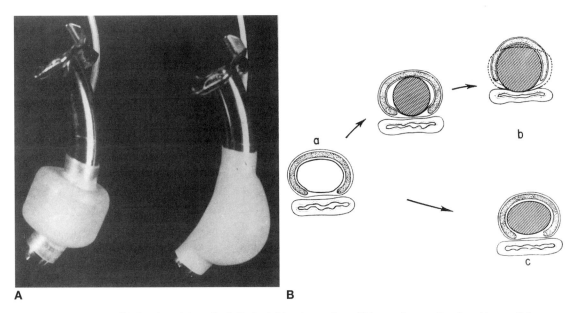

FIGURE 10-2 Tracheostomy tube cuffs. **A,** On the left is a large-volume, high-compliance cuff, adjacent to a partially inflated standard high-pressure cuff. **B,** When the high-pressure cuff is inflated, the eccentrically shaped trachea *(a)* is not sealed until the airway is deformed with use of high cuff pressures *(b)*. This is in contrast to the low-pressure cuff *(c)*, which fills the eccentrically shaped trachea and provides occlusion without exerting significant pressure. (From Cooper JD, Grillo HC: *Ann Surg* 169: 334, 1969.)

Tracheostomy tubes with an inner cannula are beneficial in cases in which secretions (which generate increased risk) are abundant. The advantage of this tube design is that it allows removal of the inner cannula for cleaning without having to remove the tracheostomy tube from the airway.

It is advisable to change the tracheostomy tube on a regular schedule to ensure that the tube can be removed easily. Difficulty with removal occurs as the stoma heals down around the shaft of the tube, the stoma size being reduced so that when the tube is partially withdrawn, the bulk of the cuff precludes removal from the airway.[13] Elective removal and reinsertion of a new tracheostomy tube on a weekly basis obviate this problem. Elective tube changes should be postponed until 72 to 96 hours after original surgical placement; inadequate development of the stomal tract during the first few days makes such changes dangerous.

Elective tube change should be accomplished with a well-structured flow of action. The nature of the changing procedure should be explained to the patient. If mechanical ventilation is being used, 100% inspired oxygen should be administered for several minutes before the procedure is performed. A laryngoscope, an endotracheal tube, and a self-inflating manual resuscitation bag should be readily available. The patient is positioned flat in bed and a rolled towel placed under the shoulders to provide better visualization of the neck area. After suctioning of the airway, the cuff is deflated and the tube withdrawn. A similar-size tracheostomy tube should be repositioned in the stoma, the cuff inflated, and adequacy of tube placement ascertained by auscultation of breath sounds, with spontaneous or positive pressure ventilation delivered through the tracheostomy tube. If the patient needs to be returned to mechanical ventilation, the adequacy of breath sounds must again be reconfirmed by use of chest auscultation after the tube is secured in place.

Percutaneous Tracheostomy

Percutaneous tracheostomy, which has been used to some extent for the past 50 years, is an alternative to the open surgical approach. The most popular technique, known as *percutaneous dilatational tracheostomy* (PDT), was originally described by Ciaglia in 1985.[14] Multiple modifications of the approach have been described in subsequent years. In principle, the technique employs the use of serial dilators introduced into the trachea over a guide wire and is generally done with bronchoscopic visualization. Modifications to improve this technique have included design of special dilating forceps and use of a single-tapered dilator rather than multiple-sized ones. Several commercial PDT kits are currently available, providing all of the necessary equipment for efficient and expedient application.

It is likely that the general trend toward minimally invasive surgery and the increase in procedures done by nonsurgical, interventional specialists will continue to promote use of this bedside procedure. Advocates of this technique frequently focus on use in critically ill patients in an intensive care unit (ICU) setting. Obvious advantages in this setting include avoidance of inherent risks associated with transport to and from the operating room, availability of existing monitoring, and cost savings with respect to operating room charges and anesthesia fees. Although multiple published studies have attempted to compare the risk and benefits of the percutaneous procedure with the open procedure, problems with study design and the multiple variables that exist in patient populations, techniques, and operator experience create problems in analysis of outcomes.[15,16] Two recently published meta-analyses summarize the potential difference in complications with both approaches. Stomal infection, bleeding, and trauma to structures adjacent to the trachea are some of the most commonly cited complications.

Tracheal Resection and Reconstruction

Etiology of Injuries

Although tracheostomy is one of the most ancient of surgical procedures, techniques of tracheal resection have been advanced only during the last several decades.[17] Currently, all but the most extensive benign and malignant lesions are potentially surgically resectable. Techniques of tracheal surgery and anesthesia have been developed and refined to a considerable degree. In addition, there have been heightened awareness and understanding of tracheal disease including neoplastic, inflammatory, and traumatic disease. The etiologies of tracheal injury are numerous and are outlined in Table 10-2.

CONGENITAL LESIONS

As outlined by H.C. Grillo, there are a variety of congenital lesions involving the trachea.[18] The extent ranges from those incompatible with life (e.g., tracheal agenesis or atresia) to regional segmental stenoses. Congenital tracheal stenosis can be associated with a number of other anomalies, such as an aberrant left pulmonary artery or a pulmonary artcry sling, which produces compression of the posterior tracheal wall. This occurs when the left pulmonary artery originates from the proximal portion of the right pulmonary artery and passes behind the trachea to the left lung. Complete tracheal rings are common in this anomaly, and surgical correction of the vascular anomaly does not necessarily improve airway obstruction. In contrast, vascular ring malformations, when they compress the trachea without associated primary tracheal anomalies, are generally improved by surgical correction. Tracheal compromise of this type occurs with a double aortic arch, a right aortic arch or a ligamentum arteriosum.

In general, surgical repair of pediatric tracheal abnormalities must be approached with caution. The small cross-sectional area of the airway, with its potential for obstruction from edema and secretions, increases the surgical risk in infancy or childhood. In addition, other increased risks of surgery and anesthesia might preclude operation at this time. If possible, it is preferable to use alternative measures (such as tracheostomy) to temporize until some later stage of life.

NEOPLASTIC LESIONS

Primary neoplastic lesions, although uncommon, can develop in the trachea (Table 10-3).[19] In several published series, squamous cell carcinoma and adenoid cystic carcinoma are the most common lesions, with a variety of other rare tumors having been cited in all series.[19-21]

Although extensive knowledge concerning the natural history of these lesions is not clear, it is evident that both squamous cell carcinoma and adenoid cystic carcinoma are amenable to early, aggressive therapy and are potentially curable. Squamous cell carcinoma can present as a well-localized lesion of the exophytic type or as an ulcerating lesion. Experience suggests that spread takes place first to regional lymph nodes adjacent to the trachea and then extends directly into mediastinal structures. Adenoid cystic carcinoma infiltrates the airway in a submucosal fashion, often for longer distances than is evident on gross endoscopic examination. Some lesions of high malignancy have spread by direct invasion into the pleura and lungs by the time the diagnosis is made. The opportunity for complete removal of this type of tumor occurs at the time of the initial surgery, with wide resections of the margins. Currently, experience with the many other types of tumors that can invade the trachea is limited, and for this

◗ TABLE 10-2

Etiology of Tracheal Lesions

Congenital lesions	Tracheal agenesis/atresia	
	Congenital stenosis	
	Congenital chondromalacia	
Neoplastic lesions	Primary neoplasms	Squamous cell carcinoma
		Adenoid cystic carcinoma (cylindroma)
		Carcinoid adenoma
		Carcinosarcoma-chondrosarcoma
	Secondary neoplasms	Bronchogenic carcinoma
		Esophageal carcinoma
		Tracheal carcinoma
		Breast carcinoma
		Head/neck carcinoma
Postintubation injuries	Laryngeal stenosis	
	Cuff injury	
	Ulceration/fistula	
	Granuloma formation	
Posttracheostomy injuries	Cuff lesions	
	Stoma lesions	
Trauma	Penetrating	
	Blunt injuries	Cervical
		Intrathoracic
Infection		

TABLE 10-3

Primary Tracheal Tumors

Benign	Squamous papillomata	Multiple
		Solitary
	Pleomorphic adenoma	
	Granular cell tumor	
	Fibrous histiocytoma	
	Leiomyoma	
	Chondroma	
	Chondroblastoma	
	Schwannoma	
	Paraganglioma	
	Hemangioendothelioma	
	Vascular malformation	
Intermediate	Carcinoid	
	Mucoepidermoid	
	Plexiform neurofibroma	
	Pseudosarcoma	
Malignant	Adenocarcinoma	
	Adenosquamous carcinoma	
	Small cell carcinoma	
	Atypical carcinoid	
	Melanoma	
	Chondrosarcoma	
	Spindle cell sarcoma	
	Rhabdomyosarcoma	

reason, generalizations concerning their natural histories are difficult.

Primary tumors of the trachea present in several ways. Shortness of breath, especially on exertion, is often the primary symptom. As the tumor grows, this symptom begins to worsen, producing limitations with even minimal levels of exercise. Wheezing, which is often confused and misdiagnosed as bronchial asthma, is a common feature. Stridor, with repeated attacks of respiratory obstruction due to a combination of tumor and secretions, can occur as well. A history of position-dependent airway obstruction—especially in the case of exophytic lesions—is possible. Obstruction can occur in a specific position (such as a lateral position) and be relieved in other positions. This finding is important when the patient's history is taken during the preanesthesia visit because induction of anesthesia in such patients must occasionally be undertaken in a specific position to ensure initial patency of the airway. Patients can also present with episodes of unilateral and bilateral pneumonia that are often unresponsive to antibiotics and physiotherapy. Hemoptysis might accompany several of the aforementioned findings or present as the sole symptom.

Secondary neoplasms can occur throughout the tracheobronchial tree. It is not uncommon for structures adjacent to the airway to involve the trachea by metastases or by direct extension. Bronchogenic, laryngeal, and esophageal carcinoma can invade the trachea and main bronchi. In general, metastases of this nature are associated with far-advanced disease and obviate tracheal surgery except for purposes of palliation.

Secondary neoplasms occurring from thyroid malignancies represent perhaps one area in which combined primary resection of the tumor and tracheal reconstruction are warranted. Not uncommonly, late recurrences of carcinoma originating in the thyroid have appeared in the trachea and larynx. Resection

of these slow-growing, late lesions has produced excellent palliation for several years.

A variety of other tumors can involve the trachea, including metastases from head and neck carcinoma, carcinoma of the breast with mediastinal involvement, and lymphoma. In general, tracheal reconstruction is not indicated in such cases. A recently published review of a 26-year experience with surgical management of primary tracheal tumors at the Massachusetts General Hospital supported an aggressive surgical approach.[19] Of the tumors in 198 patients who were evaluated, 147 (74%) were surgically excised. Overall 10-year survival for squamous cell carcinoma was approximately 33%, whereas survival for adenoid cystic neoplasms was 45%. Surgical mortality for resection was 5%; among 7 deaths in 132 patients, 6 occurred after carinal resection and reconstruction.

INJURIES
Direct laryngeal and tracheal trauma can occur from both penetrating and blunt injuries to the cervical portion of the airway.[22] The presentation of penetrating injuries (including knife wounds or gunshot wounds) is dependent on the severity of the injuries and coexisting trauma to other vital structures such as nerves and vessels.

Blunt injuries can damage the cervical trachea severely and are often complicated in their presentation.[23] Direct blows to the cervical area can be sufficient to lacerate or even completely sever the trachea. Supporting tissues might hold the damaged area together, providing an airway that is adequate enough to allow enough time for the patient to reach an emergency facility. Total disruption of this airway is often produced at the time of intubation or attempts at emergency tracheostomy. If the airway is adequate, all maneuvers (e.g., tracheostomy and/or intubation) should be held in abeyance until clinical evaluation and diagnostic tests are performed to delineate the severity of the injury. Adequate facilities—ideally, a well-equipped operating room—should be available for optimum management. Laryngeal fracture can occur as a primary or concomitant injury in such cases. The surgical management of such lesions, as described by Montgomery in 1968, is best undertaken after healing of the acute injury.[24]

The intrathoracic trachea and bronchi, like other intrathoracic organs, might also be disrupted during indirect closed-chest trauma.[25,26] One area particularly susceptible to injury is the membranous wall of the trachea, which can be lacerated in a vertical direction with extension at the level of the carina into the right or left mainstem bronchus. Such injuries often present as a pneumothorax that commonly fails to respond completely to tube thoracostomy and suction. The inability to reexpand a collapsed lung or the persistence of an excessive air leak should always raise the question of tracheal or major disruption. Incomplete separation of the bronchi might occur and present only as a late stenosis after discharge from the hospital.

INFECTION
Although rare, stricture of the trachea can result from pulmonary tuberculosis or other infectious etiologies, including diphtheria, syphilis, and typhoid, all of which have been described previously. Rarely are chronic inflammatory conditions of the trachea involved with stenosis. Fibrosing mediastinitis and systemic diseases such as Wegener's granulomatosis or amyloidosis can produce benign strictures.

POSTINTUBATION AND TRACHEOSTOMY INJURIES

The use of endotracheal or tracheostomy tubes has been shown to produce a variety of tracheal lesions. These have been described in detail in several articles.[6,7] As shown in Figure 10-3, lesions can be produced by the cuff in any of the areas where it contacts the tracheal wall. Laryngeal injury occurs with use of either oral or nasal endotracheal tubes and at the stoma site with tracheostomy tubes.

Endotracheal intubation can produce a variety of injuries involving the nares, larynx, and trachea, with most injuries resulting from pressure necrosis.[6] At the laryngeal level, the vocal cords are a common site of injury. The extent of injury varies from edema and local irritation to more serious ulceration and erosion (often at the posterior commissure), with subsequent scar formation and/or granulomata. Although the majority of laryngeal lesions reverse themselves naturally over time, a number require surgical correction. Initial symptoms include hoarseness, sore throat, and stridor. Progression of edema with resulting airway obstruction might require reintubation and, in a limited number of cases, tracheostomy.

Subglottic stenosis can occur as a result of mucosal erosion at the level of the cricoid cartilage. The true incidence of this lesion is unknown. Subglottic stenosis poses a difficult problem owing to limitations in surgical repair when the lesion is severe.

Cuff-related lesions from either tracheostomy or endotracheal tubes are similar. The presumed mechanism involves a force applied against the tracheal wall, producing necrosis. Although many etiologic factors have been considered (including local infection and toxicity of cuff materials), it is apparent that the single most important factor is the direct pressure exerted by the inflated cuff against the tracheal mucosa.[8,9] The degree of injury produced depends on a number of factors, including the length of time the pressure is applied, the healing abilities of the patient, and the total amount of tissue injury produced. The extent of injury might vary from superficial ulceration with minimal sequelae, to extensive erosion involving destruction of cartilage with the potential for fistula formation. The pathophysiology and visual confirmation of such lesions both in the experimental model and in patients have been described extensively.[12] The natural evolution of this injury relates to cicatrization during the healing process, which produces a circumferential stenosis (Figure 10-3).

Tracheomalacia likewise can be the consequence of a cuff-related injury. This occurs at the level of the cuff, where progressive lateral force weakens a tracheal segment and local inflammation destroys the cartilage. Tracheomalacia also occurs between the level of the tracheostomy stoma and the cuff, where inflammatory changes—perhaps due to pooling of secretions and local bacterial infection—lead to thinning of cartilaginous structures without significant injury to the mucosa itself. Such segmental injuries produce a functional obstruction, particularly when a maximal respiratory effort during inspiration or expiration is produced. The tracheal stoma is a frequent site of stenosis. The mechanism is most likely related to a significant loss of anteriolateral tracheal wall and subsequent cicatricial healing, producing an anteriolateral stricture, as shown in Figure 10-3. Factors leading to the development of such an injury include extensive surgical resection of anterior tracheal wall, local infection of the tissue in the stomal area, and pressure necrosis created by leverage between ventilator tubing and the tracheostomy tube.

Granulation tissue can develop at several sites in the airway, including the stoma and the tip of the tracheostomy or endotracheal tube (where it impinges on the anterior tracheal wall). Such lesions produce airway obstruction, which can be position-related and ball-valve in nature.

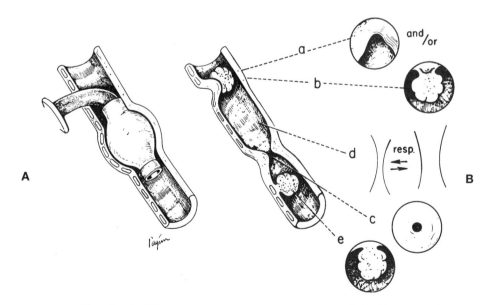

FIGURE 10-3 Sites of tracheal injury. **A,** A cuffed tracheostomy tube is shown in situ with dilation of the trachea at the level of the high-pressure cuff. **B,** Sites of possible tracheal injuries are shown as follows: *(a)* erosion of the stoma and subsequent healing produce an anterolateral stricture; *(b)* granuloma also may form at this level; *(c)* at the level of pressure exerted by the cuff, circumferential erosion will result in a circumferential stenosis; *(d)* between the stoma and the level of the cuff, thinning of the tracheal wall with potential loss of cartilage may occur; and *(e)* the tube tip may produce erosion and/or granulomata. (From Cooper JD, Grillo HC: *Ann Surg* 169: 334, 1969.)

Life-threatening complications of tracheal injuries include tracheoesophageal fistula and fistula formation between the airway and major vessels. Tracheoesophageal fistulas are usually manifest by unexplained recurrent episodes of aspiration pneumonia, often associated with an increase or a change in the character of tracheal secretions. Presenting features during mechanical ventilation might include the presence of air in the gastrointestinal tract and/or the inability to maintain adequate tidal volume and minute ventilation. Tracheo-innominate artery fistulas manifest themselves by sudden, massive, life-threatening hemorrhage from the tracheobronchial tree or through the stoma. Such lesions are often heralded by minor episodes of bleeding from the stoma as erosion first begins to develop.

Diagnostic Evaluation

Diagnostic evaluation for patients with obstructive lesions of the airway consists of detailed history and physical examination, pulmonary function studies, roentgenographic studies, and bronchoscopy. The indications for each study and the potential benefit derived from the information vary from patient to patient. In addition, the severity and urgency of airway compromise often dictate the diagnostic regimen that is followed. In life-threatening situations in which there is a high index of suspicion as to the nature of the tracheal pathology, diagnosis might consist only of bronchoscopy. In the patient presenting for elective surgery with symptoms indicative of airway obstruction, however, a detailed evaluation is generally warranted.[28]

HISTORY AND PHYSICAL EXAMINATION

The signs and symptoms produced by airway obstruction are affected by the anatomic location, the degree of airway obstruction, and the presence of preexisting cardiopulmonary disease. The clinical symptoms generally consist of dyspnea (especially with effort), wheezing (which may present as frank stridor), difficulty in clearing secretions, and eventually, airway obstruction and associated inability to clear mucus. These non-specific symptoms are frequently misdiagnosed. It is not uncommon, especially in cases of tracheal tumors, to find that patients have been diagnosed with asthma. In many cases, suspicion as to some other diagnosis is aroused only when the "asthma" fails to respond to usual treatment modalities, which often include the use of corticosteroids. It is essential to remember that in any patient with a history of recent intubation and/or tracheostomy, the development of any of the above symptoms should be considered secondary to a tracheal lesion until proved otherwise. Preexisting cardiopulmonary disease often limits exercise. In such cases, tracheal stenosis can progress to a severe stage before symptoms become apparent.

Physical examination is essential but often of limited value. Audible stridor, either occurring at rest or provoked by a maximal expiratory effort with an open mouth, is a common finding. Chest auscultation frequently reveals diffuse inspiratory and expiratory wheezing, which often if difficult to differentiate from that typical of asthma. Auscultation of the upper cervical airway might reveal high-pitched inspiratory and expiratory sounds characteristic of obstruction to air flow.

PULMONARY FUNCTION STUDIES

Although standard spirometry is of limited value in diagnosing obstructive lesions, the use of flow-volume loops has been shown to be highly reliable.[29] With standard spirometry, measured air flow during inspiration and expiration could be reduced. Maximal expiratory and/or inspiratory flow is affected to a far greater degree than is the one-second forced expiratory volume. The ratio of peak expiratory flow to FEV_1 has been used as an index of obstruction. When this ratio is 10:1 or greater, it is suggestive of airway obstruction. The flow-volume loop is the most specific test for the diagnosis of upper airway obstruction. During a forced expiration from total lung capacity, the maximal flow achieved during the first 25% of the vital capacity is dependent on effort alone. In the case of fixed airway obstruction, the peak expiratory flow is markedly reduced, producing a characteristic plateau. With fixed intrathoracic or extrathoracic lesions, the inspiratory flow has the same characteristic plateau. In the case of a variable obstruction (such as is seen with tracheomalacia), the maximal cutoff of inspiratory or expiratory flow depends on the location of the lesion. Extrathoracic or cervical lesions produce a plateau during inspiration with minimal effect on expiratory flow, whereas intrathoracic lesions (which are variable) tend to demonstrate alterations in the expiratory flow curve with minimal or no effect on inspiration. In general, stenoses that are circumferential—such as those produced by cuff lesions—are fixed in origin. Tumors and tracheomalacia frequently produce a variety of intermittent obstructions. It is theoretically possible to estimate the functional impairment of the tracheal lesion by using a restricted orifice in the patient's mouthpiece as he or she undergoes the flow-volume study. When the limited orifice begins to show additional effect on the flow-volume loop, it can be assumed that the intrinsic lesion has reduced the trachea to that cross-sectional area. In general, airway obstruction must reach 5 to 6 mm in cross-sectional diameter before signs and symptoms become clinically evident. The peak expiratory flow rate decreases to approximately 80% of normal when the airway diameter is reduced to 10 mm (see Chapters 1 and 3).

RADIOLOGIC STUDIES

Routine and special radiologic studies often precisely demonstrate the location and extent of the tracheal pathology (Figures 10-4 and 10-5).[30,31] In addition to the standard posteroanterior and lateral chest radiographs, the oblique views are of additional benefit. The latter often shows the full extent of the trachea when mediastinal structures are rotated to the side. Lateral cervical views are of value in demonstrating detailed laryngotracheal relationships and deformities impinging on the anterior or posterior tracheal walls. When necessary, fluoroscopy is done to determine the functional nature of the lesion, to demonstrate the presence of airway malacia, and to evaluate glottic function. Once areas of disease are identified, linear tomograms of the trachea (in both anteroposterior and lateral projections) and computed tomography (CT) of the chest are used to obtain definition and the exact position of the lesions. In general, contrast material should not be used because of the risk of producing airway obstruction. Magnetic resonance imaging (MRI) is useful to detail soft tissue and to characterize the lesion using sagittal and coronal views. Patients presenting with significant symptoms might not tolerate the positioning required for MRI scans.

Evaluation of patients with endotracheal tubes in place must be undertaken with caution because optimal examination with radiologic techniques can only be done when the endotracheal

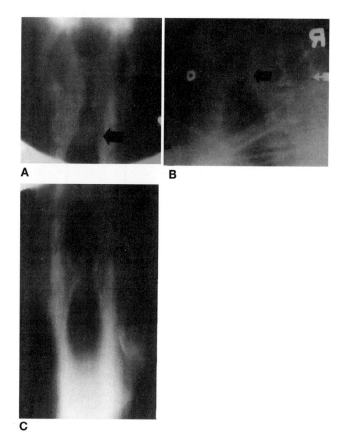

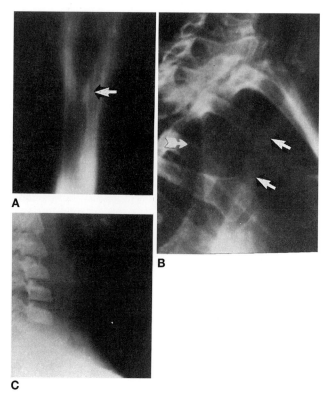

FIGURE 10-4 Radiographs of benign tracheal lesions. **A,** Details of the larynx and upper trachea are shown, with a large granuloma indicated by the arrow. **B,** The same lesion shown in detail on a soft tissue lateral view of the neck. The arrow indicate the granuloma within the air column. **C,** Laminagraph showing stomal stenosis. Above may be seen the normal upper surface of the vocal cords and the bell-shaped subglottic larynx, which terminates at the bottom of the cricoid. (From Grillo HC, Donahue DM: *J Thorac Cardiovasc Surg* 109: 486, 1995.)

FIGURE 10-5 Other tracheal lesions are shown. **A,** Detail of a cuff stenosis on a tracheal laminagraph is shown. The bell shape of the lower larynx may be seen above with a segment of normal trachea, which tapers abruptly to a narrow stenotic segment. The trachea opens up to a normal diameter below this segment. **B,** Detail from an oblique view shows the trachea air column reaching a point of maximum narrowing between the two white arrows. **C,** Ball-like anterior granuloma is shown on a lateral neck view in the lower part of a long cervical trachea. The granuloma formed at the site of anterior erosion where the tip of the tube had pressed against the tracheal wall. (From Grillo HC, Donahue DM: *J Thorac Cardiovasc Surg* 109: 486, 1995.)

or tracheostomy tube has been removed. Although the airway might be adequate immediately after decannulation, it is not uncommon for compromise to occur in a matter of minutes afterward. Hence, any decannulation, especially when done in the x-ray department, must be performed under close supervision of someone trained and properly equipped to reinstitute tracheal intubation.

BRONCHOSCOPY

Bronchoscopy, with both rigid and flexible techniques, is generally the most definitive diagnostic procedure. In general, bronchoscopy is deferred until the time of the proposed corrective operation in order not to precipitate airway obstruction secondary to edema or hemorrhage. The anesthetic approach for bronchoscopy in this population is discussed next.

Anesthetic Management

Various approaches to the induction and the maintenance of anesthesia during surgery for tracheal reconstruction have been described.[32-35] The surgical and anesthetic techniques described in this chapter have been used by Dr. H.C. Grillo, his colleagues, and the thoracic anesthesia group for several hundred patients who have undergone tracheal resection and reconstruction at the Massachusetts General Hospital since 1962.[36-46]

PREOPERATIVE ASSESSMENT

Based on the diagnostic studies just discussed, preoperative workup should localize the nature, location, and extent of the trachea requiring reconstruction. The preoperative assessment from the anesthesiologist's vantage point should consider, among other things, the degree of airway limitation, the presence of preexisting disease (especially of the lungs or heart), and the potential problems in the postoperative period. The patient should be evaluated with the understanding that intraoperative difficulties associated with the airway, as well as potential problems during induction, could cause the individual undue stresses from hypoxia, hypercarbia, and/or cardiovascular instability. The general approach to the anesthetic technique used and possible alternatives during the procedure must be based on these factors as well as on the anticipated surgical approach.

In most cases, bronchoscopy is done at the time of the contemplated surgical correction. Advantages of this approach are the following:

1. Only one anesthetic is required for total correction.
2. Appropriate invasive monitoring need only be undertaken once.

3. Airway compromise after bronchoscopy, in the presence of existing disease, should not become a life-threatening postoperative problem.

Careful detail must be undertaken to evaluate the anatomic configuration and function of the upper airway. Inspection of jaw motion, adequacy of the oral pharynx, and problems relating to mask fit must be viewed with great concern in the preoperative period because prolonged induction with inhalation agents relies heavily on the ability to maintain an adequate natural airway in lieu of the distal airway problems. Arterial blood gases, although possibly affected by preexisting chronic and acute parenchymal lung disease, are seldom deranged in the presence of pure upper airway stenosis. Occasionally, if obstruction is severe enough, a compensatory hypocarbia can result. Hypercarbia occurs, as with asthma, only as an extremely late event. When severe airway compromise exists in the preoperative period, prophylactic measures may be used. These include use of increased inspired oxygen concentrations, increased humidity, and topical steroids or racemic epinephrine. During the course of the workup, a patient is generally admitted to an ICU if his airway is thought to be extremely marginal. This measure permits close and continuous observation, available monitors, and required equipment and personnel if emergency intubation should become necessary.

The use of preoperative medication is governed by the extent of airway obstruction. In patients with minimal airway obstruction, the need for tranquilizers, sedatives, and/or drying agents is dictated by the usual criteria. The obvious concern when faced with airway obstruction is to avoid oversedation and central respiratory depression. In cases in which anxiety and emotional instability make patient management difficult, appropriate sedation with small doses of tranquilizers and/or barbiturates is relatively safe. In patients in whom airway obstruction is severe—especially when there is obvious stridor and use of accessory respiratory muscles—the administration of atropine and other drying agents should be avoided. Atropine has been reported to produce drying of secretions, creating a situation in which inspissated plugs form and become impacted in the narrow portion of the airway, creating a close to total obstruction of the airway. When in doubt, all premedication should be withheld until the patient arrives in the operating room and is under the close supervision of the anesthesiologist and surgeon.

In those patients in whom airway obstruction exists but has been bypassed by an endotracheal tube, a tracheostomy tube, or a T-tube, the use of premedication is governed by the patient's needs and the conditions compatible with safe induction of anesthesia.

MONITORING

The standard approach for monitoring the otherwise uncomplicated patient is to use an electrocardiogram, blood pressure cuff, pulse oximeter, esophageal stethoscope, and radial arterial catheter. The arterial catheter not only is useful for instantaneous monitoring of blood pressure during the intraoperative and postoperative periods but is of even greater benefit in facilitating sampling of arterial blood to follow the efficiency of gas exchange. The selection of the site of cannulation is governed not only by the availability of such vessels but also by the fact that the right radial artery is often lost owing to compression or

deliberate sacrifice of the innominate artery, which crosses the trachea (and, hence, the operative field) anteriorly from left to right. For this reason, the left radial artery is preferred. In addition, when the approach is via a right thoracotomy and surgical exposure dictates that the right arm be prepared into the surgical field, the left radial, left brachial, dorsalis pedis, or femoral arteries generally are used.

A central venous catheter is appropriate when it is anticipated that vasopressor support or other intravenous medications requiring such a route will be utilized during the intraoperative period. In general, the use of central venous pressure and pulmonary artery catheters are dictated by the severity of preexisting cardiopulmonary disease. After intubation, placement of an esophageal stethoscope not only provides useful information pertaining to breath sounds, heart tones, and rhythm, but it also provides a foreign body that guides the surgeon in helping to identify the esophagus within the surgical field. Measurement of end-tidal gases should also be performed during this operative procedure.

AIRWAY EQUIPMENT

In addition to a conventional anesthesia machine and appropriate monitoring, it is necessary to provide several other important pieces of equipment. It is beneficial to have an anesthesia machine with the capabilities of delivering high-flow oxygen, in excess of 20 L/min. This is particularly useful during the induction phase (when air leaks can pose problems) and during rigid bronchoscopy. In addition, appropriate equipment should be provided to facilitate laryngoscopy and topical anesthesia. The choice of a laryngoscope blade is not as important as the individual's ability to use any given one with facility. A long bronchial sprayer with lidocaine 4% is useful for topicalization of the pharynx and tracheal mucous membranes. The most important equipment to be kept readily available is a variety of tubes for endotracheal intubation, ranging in size from 20F to 30F. The optimal size to provide an adequate airway, suction secretions, and permit enough room for surgical manipulation and suturing of the airway is 28F. In general, the tube size is selected when visualization of the airway is accomplished during rigid bronchoscopy, and the decision is made as to whether it is feasible to intubate through the stenosis or rely on a tube placed above it. Recently, several published reports have described the use of the laryngeal mask airway (LMA) in patients with tracheal stenosis.[47-49] Given the limited experience to date, it would seem prudent not to use the LMA approach in situations in which critical stenosis exists.

ANESTHESIA MANAGEMENT

Once the patient is positioned comfortably on the operating room table in the supine position with an appropriate intravenous catheter and monitoring in place, the induction of anesthesia commences. In patients in whom airway obstruction is of minor significance, owing to either a good natural airway or the presence of an intratracheal appliance, anesthesia can be induced with thiopental or a similar agent. When airway conditions are consistent with a high degree of obstruction, it is desirable to undertake a gentle, controlled inhalation induction with a volatile anesthetic. Relaxants should be avoided if at all possible, placing reliance on spontaneous ventilation and assisted breaths because the ability to intubate the larynx and provide an airway is not always guaranteed. In many cases in which airway obstruction is severe, it is impossible with mask and positive pressure ventilation to provide adequate gas flow through a limited orifice. During spontaneous ventilation, however, the patient is able to breathe adequately, even in the anesthetized state.

Anesthesia is administered until there is assurance that the patient can tolerate direct laryngoscopy. Laryngoscopy is then performed, and at this time topical anesthesia, generally with lidocaine 4%, is applied to the oral pharynx and glottis. The mask is reapplied, volatile agent-oxygen is administered, and a judgment is made as to whether the patient has responded unfavorably to this procedure. If conventional signs—including tachycardia, hypertension, tearing, or any other manifestations of light anesthesia—are evident, continued induction is carried out for an adequate period of time. When conditions again are favorable, a second laryngoscopy is undertaken, and an attempt is made to topicalize the trachea by inserting the tracheal spray immediately below the vocal cords. When an adequate depth of anesthesia is present, bronchoscopy can be undertaken.

During bronchoscopy, it is critical for the anesthesiologist to make a visual inspection of the status of the airway with regard to the nature and extent of the lesion. This measure is important in terms of appreciating the difficulty of endotracheal tube placement and selection of the appropriate size of tube. There are several potential problems that must be considered at this time. Lesions involving the upper third of the trachea—especially those in the subglottic area—pose special problems with placement owing to cuff position. A lesion that is located high in the airway, where the tube cannot be passed through the lesion because of the limited orifice, does not allow the cuff to pass below the vocal cords and results in inability to attain a complete seal of the airway. Selection of a tube that is small enough to pass through the lesion with the cuff below it produces additional problems because of decreased internal diameter (especially when size 20F to 24F tubes are used) and creates problems of potential airway obstruction with secretions and blood during the operative procedure. Lesions located in the middle and lower thirds of the trachea are less problematic with respect to position. The tube must be passed through the lesion itself to maintain adequacy of ventilation until the trachea is transected, and the lesion must be dilated at the time of bronchoscopy to provide adequacy of the airway. Dilatation must be considered with great caution owing to the risk of significant airway damage, which might be complicated by bleeding or perforation into other structures such as the esophagus or great vessels. Dr. H.C. Grillo's approach has been to dilate strictures if the airway measures less than 5 mm in diameter. Dilatation is done under direct vision with several rigid pediatric ventilating bronchoscopes. A dilator passed through a large bronchoscope can perforate the tracheobronchial wall easily, especially if the stricture is in the distal trachea. If the airway measures more than 5 mm, an endotracheal tube is generally passed to a point above the stricture in lesions of the mid- to lower trachea; in lesions of the upper trachea, the tube is passed through it. Caution must be exercised when tumors are present in the airway because of the potential for direct trauma if passage of the endotracheal tube results in obstruction from a dislodged piece of tumor, with or without serious hemorrhage

in the airway. Strictures of the anterior tracheal wall or stoma strictures are generally easily dealt with, as the mobile posterior membranous tracheal wall usually allows passage of an endotracheal tube or gas flow if the tube is positioned above the lesion.

Once bronchoscopy is completed, endotracheal intubation with the appropriate size of endotracheal tube is performed. This procedure is done in the usual manner with the sniffing position and direct laryngoscopy. As the tube is advanced down the airway, passage of the tube through the area of stricture can often be felt. Once the tube is thought to be in the appropriate position, the chest is auscultated in standard fashion to ensure bilateral lung ventilation. The tube is then secured, the eyes are taped, and an esophageal stethoscope is passed. Anesthesia is maintained with an inhalation agent and oxygen or—in cases in which normal pulmonary function exists and an adequate airway is present—with a combination of nitrous oxide and oxygen to supplement the anesthetic. Relaxants are avoided, and ventilation is generally accomplished by hand.

Surgical Positioning

As shown in Figure 10-6, several approaches to surgical positioning are used depending on the extent and location of the tracheal lesion. For most lesions located in the upper half of the trachea, an anterior collar incision is used with or without a vertical partial sternal split. For this incision, the patient is positioned supine, with a thyroid bag or bolster placed under the shoulders and the head on a supporting doughnut. The back of the table is elevated approximately 10 to 15 degrees to position the cervical and sternal area parallel to the floor when the head is in the fully extended position. The arms are either left at the side or extended on arm boards at 90 degrees angles. Exploration of the lesion is done through the anterior collar incision, and the sternum is divided later on if this is deemed necessary for surgical exposure.

Lesions of the lower half of the trachea are approached through a right posterolateral thoracotomy incision in the fourth interspace or in the bed of the fourth rib. The position for this incision is a standard left lateral decubitus position, with the right arm draped and prepared so that it can be moved into the surgical field for easier access to the neck. In this position, it is necessary to have intravenous and monitoring catheters in the left upper or lower extremities. A thoracotomy can be done and a collar incision added to free the trachea if there is need to perform a laryngeal release. In special cases of extensive or unusual lesions involving a greater area of the trachea, a vertical incision can be extended into the right and left fourth intercostal spaces from the sternal incision, as shown in Figure 10-6.

Reconstruction of the Upper Trachea

For lesions of the upper half of the trachea, the surgical approach is shown in Figure 10-7. A low, short collar incision is made across the neck, and a T-incision is extended vertically over the sternum. Anterior dissection of the trachea is carried from the cricoid cartilage to the carina, with care taken not to injure the innominate artery or other structures adjacent to the trachea. Dissection around the back of the trachea is done at a point inferior to the lesion. If the patient has not been intubated

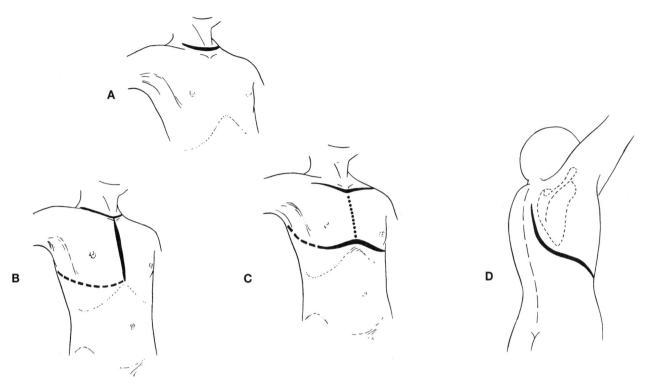

FIGURE 10-6 Incisions for tracheal resection. **A,** Standard collar incision for the majority of benign strictures and neoplastic lesions of the upper trachea. **B,** Sternotomy extension: the dotted line shows an extension that may be carried through the fourth interspace to provide total exposure of the trachea from cricoid to carina. **C,** Technique for raising a large bipedicle flap for total exposure and use in cases in which mediastinal tracheostomy is required. **D,** Posterolateral thoractomy, carried through the bed of the fourth rib or the fourth interspace for exposure of the lower half of the trachea. (From Grillo HC: *Surg Gynecol Obstet* 129: 347, 1969.)

through the stricture, caution must be undertaken during this dissection because it is possible through release of the external supporting structure of the trachea to produce progressive (and eventually, complete) airway obstruction.

During this portion of the cervical procedure, anesthesia is maintained through a previously placed oral endotracheal tube. At the point at which it is anticipated that the trachea will be divided, nitrous oxide is eliminated from the anesthetic gas

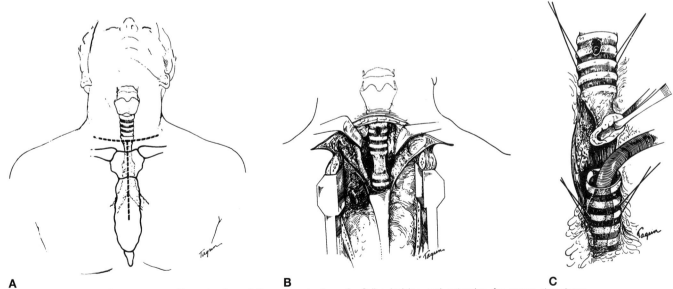

FIGURE 10-7 Reconstruction of the upper trachea. **A,** Collar incision and extension for upper sternotomy. **B,** Dissection is carried down to isolate the damaged segment. **C,** Circumferential dissection is carried out immediately beneath the level of pathology. Traction sutures are in place and the distal airway intubated via the operating field. (From Grillo HC: *Ann Surg* 162: 734, 1965.)

mixture, and anesthesia is maintained with a volatile agent and oxygen alone. At this point, a tape is placed around the trachea below the lesion, and lateral traction sutures are placed through the full thickness of the tracheal wall in the midline on either side at a point no more than 2 cm below the point of division of the trachea. It is important to anticipate the placement of these sutures so that the cuff on the endotracheal tube can be deflated to prevent it from being injured by the suture needle. The trachea is then transsected below the lesion, as demonstrated in Figure 10-7, *C*, and the distal trachea is intubated across the operative field with a flexible armored tube. The necessary sterile connecting equipment—consisting of corrugated tubings and a Y-piece—are then passed to the anesthesiologist for connection to the anesthesia machine. The ability to ventilate the lungs is then assessed by use of positive pressure. The surgical dissection continues to free and excise the injured portion of the trachea.

Once adequacy of the tracheal lumen and the extent of the tracheal resection have been determined, an attempt is made to approximate the two free ends of the trachea. This is accomplished by use of traction sutures, with the anesthesiologist flexing the neck by grasping the head from above. When it is deemed possible to reanastomose the tracheal ends directly,

intermittent sutures are placed into the trachea in a through-and-through manner, with anesthesia continuing through the tube positioned in the distal airway. In cases in which it is not possible to bring the ends together owing to undue tension, a laryngeal release is performed. Once all sutures have been placed, the distal armored tube is removed, and the oral endotracheal tube, which has remained in the proximal portion of the trachea, is advanced through the anastomosis into the distal trachea under direct vision (Figure 10-8). Care must be taken at this point not to pass the tube too far distally in the trachea because subsequent flexion of the neck for surgical foreshortening of the trachea can potentiate right mainstem bronchial intubation. Before this exchange, the airway is suctioned to remove aspirated blood. Anesthesia is then administered through the oral endotracheal tube into the distal trachea as the sutures are tied down to produce an airtight anastomosis. After all sutures have been placed, the patient's neck is flexed, and the head is supported in the position shown in Figure 10-8, *B*.

On completion of the operation, the patient should be breathing spontaneously; extubation should be anticipated either under "awake" conditions or under moderately deep anesthesia. The selection of the "awake" technique, which is designed to afford a good airway, must be balanced against the

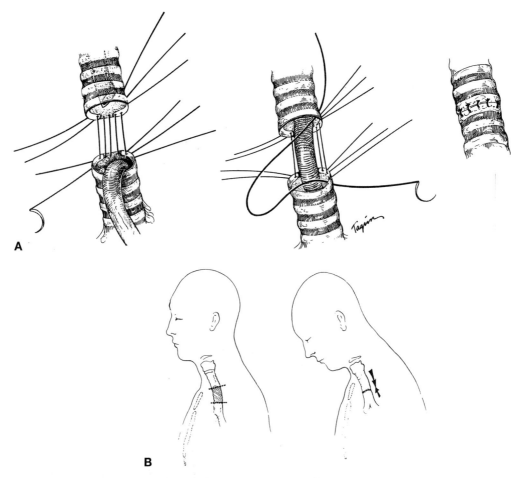

FIGURE 10-8 Details of anastomotic technique. **A,** Original endotracheal tube positioned in the upper trachea with the distal trachea intubated. Once all sutures are in place, the endotracheal tube is advanced and the sutures are tied in serial fashion. **B,** With cervical flexion, the maximum amount of approximation is obtained. (From Grillo HC: *Ann Surg* 162: 734, 1965.)

occasional need to reintubate the patient if laryngeal difficulty and/or other aspects of unresected tracheal disease promote airway obstruction. In most cases, it is prudent to extubate patients at a deeper level of anesthesia and maintain the airway, thus avoiding the potential for struggling, bucking, and excessive motion that could injure the suture line. In patients in whom intubation was difficult because of upper airway pathologic condition, it is prudent to allow the patient to awaken, supporting the head and neck during the excitement phase to avoid excessive motion. It is generally preferable to attempt extubation in the operating room, where the quality of air patency can be evaluated quickly. Under such controlled circumstances, reintubation or diagnostic bronchoscopy can be done more easily and safely than in the recovery room or ICU. Once the airway and ventilation are judged to be adequate, the patient can be transported safely, with supplemental oxygen, to the recovery room or intensive care unit.

Reconstruction of the Lower Trachea

The basic incision and surgical approach for the lower trachea have been described in the foregoing sections. The general principles concerning intubation and early maintenance of anesthesia are similar to those described for the upper trachea, with the exception of tube selection. In dealing with lower tracheal (and especially, carinal) lesions, it is advantageous to have a tube that is adequate in length to enter either mainstem bronchus. For this purpose, an armored tube with an added extension of some 4 to 5 inches on the proximal portion is used to provide both flexibility at the distal end and adequate length for bronchial intubation (Figure 10-9). This tube is generally passed with the aid of a stylet and positioned according to the anatomic location and extent of the lesion.

During the thoracotomy and surgical resection of the trachea, positive pressure ventilation is used while maintaining the ability of the patient to ventilate spontaneously; often, spontaneous breathing is needed during periods of discontinuity of the airway, when positive pressure ventilation is not possible. Although ventilation is impaired because of the open thorax, adequate gas exchange has been maintained with high-flow insufflation of oxygen and anesthetic agent while relying on the dependent lung for the bulk of ventilation.

In general, resection involving the distal trachea and carina is carried out with the endotracheal tube in a position that is proximal to the lesion. Surgical exposure and resection are much the same as previously described for upper tracheal lesions. Once the trachea is divided, it is common to find that the distal tracheal stump is too short to hold the endotracheal tube and cuff. Under these circumstances, it frequently is impossible to ventilate both lungs adequately. Generally, the left mainstem bronchus is intubated through the operative field, and ventilation and anesthesia are carried out entirely via the left lung while the diseased segment is excised. Although it is theoretically possible to eliminate perfusion to the right lung temporarily with pulmonary artery clamping, this is technically very difficult and entails the potential hazard of injury to the right pulmonary artery. In cases in which adequate oxygenation and ventilation are not attainable with one lung, an easy approach is to advance a second tube into the right mainstem bronchus, preferably in the bronchus intermedius. A second anesthesia machine and sterile tubings are used to maintain continuous positive airway pressure (5 cmH$_2$O) with oxygen to the nondependent lung, whereas ventilation is carried out in the dependent left lung (see Chapter 8). With lesions of the distal trachea not involving the carina, anastomosis and tube positioning are carried out in much the same way as for the upper tracheal lesions. This process is depicted in Figure 10-10. Once the anastomosis is complete, it is prudent to withdraw the endotracheal tube back into the proximal trachea so that ventilation goes through the area of anastomosis.

In resections involving the carina in which end-to-end and end-to-side anastomosis between trachea and right and left mainstem bronchi must be carried out, a variety of tube manipulations and combinations of the previously considered maneuvers must be undertaken (Figure 10-11). Generally, the right mainstem bronchus is anastomosed to the distal trachea, and the left bronchus is reimplanted in end-to-side fashion into the bronchus intermedius or the distal trachea. It is not uncommon during such procedures to have significant periods of one-lung

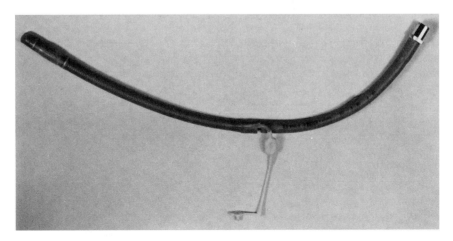

FIGURE 10-9 Armored endotracheal tube with extension for bronchial intubation.

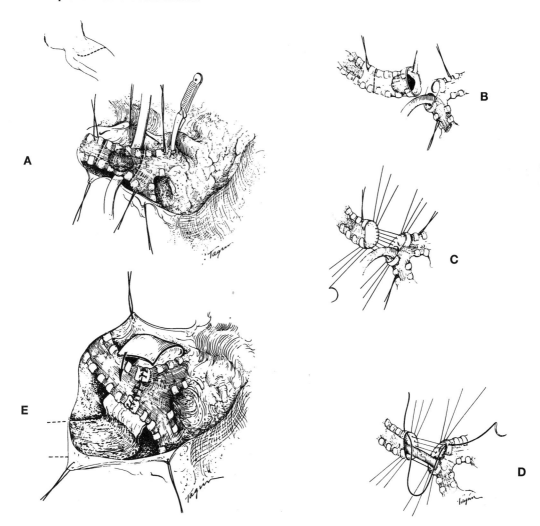

FIGURE 10-10 Transthoracic approach. **A,** The lesion in the distal trachea has been isolated and the right pulmonary artery is shown to be clamped, although this is not done routinely. **B,** The trachea has been divided above the carina and the left main bronchus intubated. **C,** Anastomotic sutures are placed by a procedure similar to that used in the upper trachea. **D,** The endotracheal tube has been advanced through the anastomosis and the remaining sutures appropriately placed. **E,** Anastomosis completed with a pedicle pleural flap secured for additional support. (From Grillo HC: *Surg Gynecol Obstet* 129: 347, 1969.)

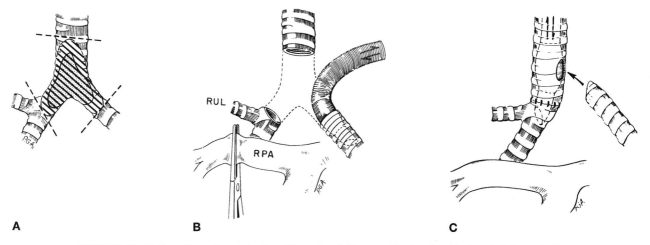

FIGURE 10-11 Resection and reconstruction of the carina. **A,** Tumor position is outlined by the stippled area. **B,** With the tube positioned in the left main bronchus, the right lung is mobilized and the stump of the right mainstem bronchus sutured into the trachea. **C,** The left main bronchus is anastomosed in end-to-side fashion into the trachea. (From Grillo HC: *Thorax* 28: 667, 1973.)

anesthesia, with the need to insufflate the second lung dictated by the level of arterial oxygenation.[46]

Once all the anastomoses have been completed and adequacy of ventilation is assured by quality of breath sounds and visual inspection of chest wall expansion, closure of the surgical wound is undertaken in standard fashion.

When a right thoracotomy has been used for surgical dissection, the decision as to whether to extubate the airway is of major importance. The potential for inadequacy of ventilation and pulmonary toilet must be balanced against the problems of continued intubation, potential infection, and direct trauma to the suture line. Provided no significant parenchymal lung disease was present preoperatively, it is generally possible to extubate patients after thoracotomy and major carinal reconstruction without undue consequences. Exceptions are generally those patients in whom bilateral thoracotomy has been undertaken and in whom significant postoperative pain is expected to limit cough and ventilation. These patients require tracheal intubation and some amount of mechanical ventilatory support. After thoracotomy, the procedures for extubation are similar to those described for the upper airway approach. An exception is that the patient is generally taken out of the lateral position and placed supine before extubation. This positioning facilitates adequate exposure if reintubation is deemed necessary. The patient is transported to the recovery area once stability of circulation and adequacy of ventilation are achieved.

Postoperative Care

Postoperative patients are admitted to the ICU for a minimum period of 24 hours. Patients are monitored with electrocardiogram, arterial pressure, and serial arterial blood gases. A radiograph of the chest is obtained shortly after admission to ensure that no pneumothorax is present. Sufficient oxygen is administered with a high-flow humidified system through a facemask to provide adequate arterial oxygenation and thinning of secretions. The head is maintained in the flexed position by a number of firm pillows placed behind the occiput and sutures located from the chin to the anterior chest. Chest physical therapy and routine nursing procedures are dictated by the nature of other underlying diseases and the ability to effectively maintain gas exchange and pulmonary toilet. Blind nasotracheal suctioning is undertaken with caution in those patients whose ability to cough is inadequate to raise secretions. This is best done by physicians, chest physical therapists, or nurses trained specifically in this procedure. Potential complications include perforation of the anastomotic site and tracheal irritation with subsequent edema and airway obstruction, which can induce vomiting and aspiration. In cases in which abundant secretions are a problem, frequent transoral flexible fiberoptic bronchoscopy can be used to provide pulmonary toilet. This is especially true in cases in which the carina has been resected and secretions tend to pool in major bronchi without being propelled by normal mechanisms into the trachea. The need for emergency intubation because of hemorrhage, airway obstruction, or dehiscence of the anastomosis arises with extreme rarity.

In case of inadequate ventilation, with increasing levels of carbon dioxide and/or deterioration of oxygenation, endotracheal intubation is undertaken. This procedure must be done with caution, generally with the aid of sedation and topical

anesthesia; the tube is placed either nasally or orally, with direct visualization of the larynx. This measure can be accomplished with the patient maintained in the flexed position without producing undue stress on the suture line. After intubation, the need for ventilation is reassessed after pulmonary toilet has been achieved, and therapy is directed at minimizing both positive pressure on the airway and the time during which the intubation is maintained. Minimizing intubation time is especially important in cases in which the endotracheal tube passes through the anastomosis (high tracheal reconstructions) because of the potential for dehiscence in an early stage of recovery. When prolonged intubation (generally considered more than 2 to 3 days) is anticipated, elective tracheostomy should be seriously considered. The hazards of the tracheostomy are dictated by body habitus, the location of the anastomosis, and the ability to safely dissect and position the tracheostomy tube following the reconstructive surgery.

Upper-airway obstruction resulting from laryngeal edema is an infrequent complication. It has occurred most commonly when there has been a high anastomosis or previous history of laryngeal disease. When there is a history of cord paralysis and/or recurrent episodes of laryngeal edema, or when the trachea is anastomosed directly to the larynx at the cricoid cartilage, prophylactic measures are taken to avoid laryngeal edema. This therapy includes use of high humidity and inhalation of topical steroids and racemic epinephrine. Dexamethasone and racemic epinephrine, 0.5 mL of a 1:200 dilution in 2.5 mL water, are administered with a nebulizer every 4 hours. Schedules are arranged so that inhalation of one or the other drug is achieved every 2 hours. This regimen is continued for a minimum of 24 hours, or longer if laryngeal edema (as evidenced by stridor and hoarseness) persists.

Patients should be kept in the ICU for a period of 1 or more days until it is deemed safe to return them to a general surgical floor. This decision is dictated by the ability to discontinue cardiovascular monitoring, the need for repeated measurement of arterial blood gases, and the quality of nursing care. In most cases in which the procedure has been uncomplicated, patients are able to sit out of bed in a chair on the day after surgery and are often able to begin taking clear liquids and/or soft solids by the first postoperative day.

REFERENCES

1. Heffner JE, Miller KS, Sahn SA: Tracheostomy in the intensive care unit. Part 1: indications, technique, management, *Chest* 90:269, 1986.
2. Heffner JE, Miller KS, Sahn SA: Tracheostomy in the intensive care unit. Part 2: complications, *Chest* 90:432, 1986.
3. Sise MJ, Shackford SR, Cruickshank JO, et al: Cricothyroidotomy for long-term tracheal access. A prospective analysis of morbidity and mortality in 76 patients, *Ann Surg* 200:13, 1984.
4. Cole RR, Aguilar EA: Cricothyroidotomy versus tracheotomy: an otolaryngologist's perspective, *Laryngoscope* 98:131, 1988.
5. Wilson DJ: Airway appliances and management. In Kacmarek R, Stoller J (eds): *Current respiratory care,* Toronto, 1988, BC Decker.
6. Lindholm CE: Prolonged endotracheal intubation, *Acta Anesthesiol Scand* 33(Suppl):1969.
7. Stauffer JL, Olson DE, Petty TL: Complications and consequences of endotracheal intubation and tracheostomy. A prospective study of 150 critically ill adult patients, *Am J Med* 70:65, 1981.
8. Ching NPH, Ayres SM, Spina RC, et al: Endotracheal damage during continuous ventilatory support, *Ann Surg* 179:123, 1974.

9. Cooper JD, Grillo HC: The evolution of tracheal injury due to ventilatory assistance through cuffed tubes. A pathologic study, *Ann Surg* 169:334, 1969.

10. Carroll RG, McGinnis GF, Grenvik A: Performance characteristics of tracheal cuffs, *Int Anesthesiol Clin* 12:111, 1974.

11. Crawley BE, Cross DE: Tracheal cuffs. A review in dynamic pressure study, *Anesthesia* 30:4, 1975.

12. Cooper JD, Grillo HC: Experimental production and prevention of injury due to cuffed tracheal tubes, *Surg Gynecol Obstet* 129:1235, 1969.

13. Pavlin EG, Nelson E, Pulliam J: Difficulty in removal of tracheostomy tubes, *Anesthesiology* 44:69, 1976.

14. Ciaglia P, Firshing R, Syniec C: Elective percutaneous dilatational tracheostomy: a new simple bedside procedure, *Chest* 87:715, 1985.

15. Dulguerov P, Gysin C, Perneger TV, et al: Percutaneous or surgical tracheostomy: a meta-analysis, *Crit Care Med* 27:1617, 1999.

16. Freeman BD, Isabella K, Lin N, et al: A meta-analysis of prospective trials comparing percutaneous and surgical tracheostomy in critically ill patients, *Chest* 118:1412, 2000.

17. Grillo HC: Notes on the windpipe, *Ann Thorac Surg* 47:9, 1989.

18. Grillo HC: Congenital lesions, neoplasms and injuries of the trachea. In Sabiston DC, Spencer FC (eds): *Gibbon's surgery of the chest,* Philadelphia, 1982, WB Saunders.

19. Grillo HC, Mathisen DJ: Primary tracheal tumors: treatment and results, *Ann Thorac Surg* 49:69, 1990.

20. Pearson FG, Todd TRJ, Cooper JD: Experience with primary neoplasms of the trachea, *J Thorac Cardiovasc Surg* 88:511, 1984.

21. Perelman MI, Koroleva N, Birjukov J, et al: Primary tracheal tumors, *Semin Thorac Cardiovasc Surg* 8:400, 1996.

22. Mathisen DJ, Grillo HC: Laryngotracheal trauma, *Ann Thorac Surg* 43:254, 1987.

23. Jones WS, Mavroudis C, Richardson JD, et al: Management of tracheobronchial disruption resulting from blunt trauma, *Surgery* 95:319, 1984.

24. Montgomery WW: The surgical management of supraglottic and subglottic stenosis, *Ann Otol Rhinol Laryngol* 77:534, 1968.

25. Chesterman JT, Satsangi PN: Rupture of the trachea and bronchi by closed injury, *Thorax* 21:21, 1966.

26. Deslauriers J, Beaulieu M, Archambault G, et al: Diagnosis and long-term follow-up of major bronchial disruptions due to nonpenetrating trauma, *Ann Thorac Surg* 33:33, 1982.

27. Hood RM, Sloan HE: Injuries of the trachea and major bronchi, *J Thorac Cardiovasc Surg* 38:458, 1959.

28. Kryger M, Bode F, Antic R, et al: Diagnosis of obstruction of the upper and central airways, *Am J Med* 61:85, 1976.

29. Hyatt RE, Black LF: The flow-volume curve. A current perspective, *Am Rev Respir Dis* 107:191, 1973.

30. MacMillan AS, James AE Jr, Stitik FP, et al: Radiologic evaluation of post-tracheostomy lesions, *Thorax* 26:696, 1971.

31. Pearson FG, Andrews MJ: Detection and management of tracheal stenosis following cuffed tube tracheostomy, *Ann Thorac Surg* 12:359, 1971.

32. Geffin B, Bland J, Grillo HC: Anesthetic management of tracheal resection and reconstruction, *Anesth Analg* 48:884, 1969.

33. Clarkson WB, Davies JR: Anesthesia for carinal resection, *Anesthesia* 33:815, 1978.

34. Ellis RH, Hinds CJ, Gadd LT: Management of anesthesia during tracheal resection, *Anesthesia* 31:1076, 1976.

35. Pisonneault C, Fortier J, Donati F: Tracheal resection and reconstruction, *Can J Anaesth* 46:439, 1999.

36. Grillo HC: Circumferential resection and reconstruction of mediastinal and cervical trachea, *Ann Surg* 162:734, 1965.

37. Grillo HC: Terminal or mural tracheostomy in the anterior mediastinum, *J Thorac Cardiovasc Surg* 51:422, 1966.

38. Grillo HC: The management of tracheal stenosis following assisted respiration, *J Thorac Cardiovasc Surg* 57:521, 1969.

39. Grillo HC: Surgical approaches to the trachea, *Surg Gynecol Obstet* 129:347, 1969.

40. Grillo HC: Reconstruction of the trachea. Experience in 100 consecutive cases, *Thorax* 28:667, 1973.

41. Grillo HC, Donahue DM, Mathisen DJ, et al: Postintubation tracheal stenosis: treatment and results, *J Thorac Cardiovasc Surg* 109:486, 1995.

42. Grillo HC, Donahue DM: Postintubation tracheal stenosis, *Semin Thorac Cardiovasc Surg* 8:370, 1996.

43. Muehrcke D, Grillo HC, Mathisen DJ, Reconstructive airway operation after irradiation, *Ann Thorac Surg* 59:14, 1995.

44. Mitchell JD, Mathisen DJ, Wright CD, et al: Clinical experience with carinal resection, *J Thorac Cardiovasc Surg* 117:39, 1999.

45. Donahue DM, Grillo HC, Wain JC, et al: Reoperative tracheal resection and reconstruction for unsuccessful repair of postintubation stenosis, *J Thorac Cardiovasc Surg* 114:934, 1997.

46. Mathisen DJ: Carinal reconstruction: techniques and problems, *Semin Thorac Cardiovasc Surg* 8:403, 1996.

47. Catala JC, Garcia Pedrajas F, Carrera J, et al: Placement of an endotracheal device via the laryngeal mask airway in a patient with tracheal stenosis, *Anesthesiology* 84:239, 1996 (letter).

48. Asai T, Fujise K, Uchida M: Use of the laryngeal mask in a child with tracheal stenosis, *Anesthesiology* 75:903, 1991.

49. Asai T, Fujise K, Uchida M: Laryngeal mask and tracheal stenosis, *Anaesthesia* 48:81, 1993 (letter).

Pulmonary Resection

Pulmonary Resection

11

Pulmonary Resection

Pulmonary Resection   11

Philip M. Hartigan, MD
Simon C. Body, MB, ChB
David John Sugarbaker, MD, FCCP

AT the beginning of the 20th century, infections of the chest (primarily tuberculosis and empyema) were the primary indication for pulmonary resection surgery. The advent of antibiotics and the epidemic rise in the incidence of smoking-related lung cancer have shifted the focus of thoracic surgery. Treatment of lung cancer is now overwhelmingly the principal indication for pulmonary resection. Additional indications include the treatment of a bronchopleural fistula, empyema, or fibrothorax, as well as the resection of lung bullae, blebs, cysts, abscesses, and pulmonary arteriovenous malformations. Lung volume reduction surgery as a treatment for emphysema is covered in Chapter 12.

This chapter reviews surgical and anesthetic issues for pulmonary resection, beginning with some general considerations regarding surgical approaches. The premise throughout is that an appreciation of both surgical issues and anesthetic considerations is important for optimal collaboration with the surgeon in the anesthetic care of patients undergoing thoracic surgery.

Thoracic Incisions for Pulmonary Resection

Commonly used thoracic incisions for pulmonary resection are listed in Table 11-1. Understanding and anticipating the steps of opening and closing thoracic incisions are of value. Appropriate depth of anesthesia to minimize the sympathetic response and provide for a prompt emergence requires timing and anticipation. Attention to surgical entry into the pleural space allows for timing and evaluation of one-lung ventilation (OLV). Observing the absence of free movement of the lung when viewed through the pleura can alert the surgical team of the potential for adhesions and increased blood loss, or of difficulty in achieving exposure. A motionless surgical field is particularly crucial when work is performed on major vessels or bronchial structures. Knowledge of when to be particularly vigilant for blood loss aids in the estimate of intravascular volume. The need for inspiratory positive pressure hold maneuvers can be anticipated to test the integrity of bronchial stumps, or to recruit lung units when reexpanding the atelectatic lung. A well-timed sigh maneuver during chest closure helps expel air and fluid from the pleural space and ensure a well-reexpanded lung. If ribs are fractured or reapproximated with difficulty, greater postoperative pain can be anticipated. In general, awareness and anticipation of events aid in the early recognition of trouble and more elegant coordination with the surgical team.

Posterolateral Thoracotomy Incision

The standard posterolateral incision historically has been the most widely used because of the generous exposure provided to all portions of the ipsilateral lung and hilum. Compared with more limited incisions, disadvantages of this approach include the time required to open and close the chest and the attendant pain, healing, and postoperative respiratory dysfunction attributable to the extensive amount of soft tissue and/or muscle transected. The adoption of endoscopic stapling devices in the past decade has made more limited variations of the posterolateral incision practical for most lung surgery. Nevertheless, full posterolateral incisions still have a place for select extensive or difficult pulmonary resections.

The posterolateral skin incision extends from the anterior axillary line, at the level of the inframammary crease, in a posterior direction along the inferior border of the scapula, before swinging cephalad to run parallel to the spine, midway between the spine and the scapular border (Figure 11-1). The serratus anterior, latissimus dorsi, and the lower portion of the trapezius muscles are divided to expose the rib cage. Rhomboid and pectoralis major muscles might need to be partially divided as well, depending on the need for exposure. The pleura is usually entered at the level of the fifth interspace, which is identified by elevating the scapular wing and counting down from the first rib. The pleural space may be entered either by going in through the periosteal bed or by dividing the intercostals and parietal pleura along the inferior border of the intercostal space (to avoid the neurovascular bundle) (Figure 11-2). The transperiosteal route is advocated by some in the belief that periosteal borders provide stronger tissue for closure than intercostal muscle. If the need for an intercostal muscle flap is anticipated, the transperiosteal option for pleural entry is preferable. Most surgeons resect a small portion of rib to achieve mobility and prevent rib fracture by retraction. Dividing a rib is more painful than resecting a portion of rib. Resection of a long segment of rib provides little exposure advantage over resection of a small portion, but it might be indicated for repeat thoracotomies.[1] Positive inflation pressure to the operative lung should be avoided during incision of the pleura. Exposure of the pleural space to atmospheric pressure should result in rapid deflation of the lung, barring severe obstructive disease, adhesions, or technical problems with lung isolation.

Minor variations on the posterolateral incision might be dictated by the position and size of the lesion targeted, as well as by surgical preference and experience. The exposure

TABLE 11-1
Thoracic Incisions for Pulmonary Resection

Posterolateral
Limited variants of posterolateral
Muscle-sparing, limited thoracotomies
   Anterolateral muscle-sparing
   Vertical axillary muscle-sparing
   Posterolateral muscle-sparing
Anterior (anterolateral)
Bilateral transsternal
Median sternotomy
Thoracoabdominal
Video-assisted thoracoscopic surgery (VATS)

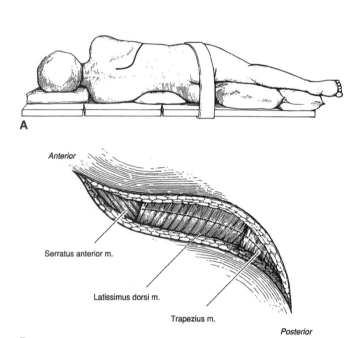

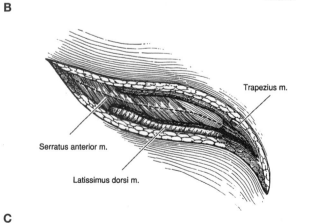

FIGURE 11-1 Posterolateral thoracotomy skin incision **A,** followed by division of the latissimus dorsi and trapezius muscles **B,** and subsequently by division of the serratus anterior muscle layer **C,** (From Moores DWO, Foster ED, McKneally MF: Incisions. In Pearson FG [ed]: *Thoracic surgery,* New York, 1995, Churchill Livingstone.)

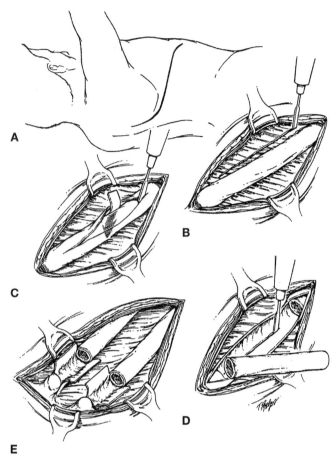

FIGURE 11-2 The options for entering the pleural space after posterolateral thoracotomy **A,** include dividing the intercostal muscle from the superior rib edge with electrocautery **B,** reflecting the periosteum off the superior rib edge, and entering through the periosteal bed without rib resection **C,** subperiosteal rib resection **D,** and an intercostal approach with short-segment rib resection posteriorly **E,** (From Heitmiller RF: Thoracic incision. In Bave AE, Geha AS, Hammond GL, et al [eds]: *Glenn's thoracic and cardiovascular surgery,* ed 6, Stanford, Conn, 1995, Appleton & Lange.)

advantages must be balanced against the morbidity, which is attributable chiefly to the pain and the functional impairment imposed by muscle transection. Injury or entrapment of the intercostal neurovascular bundle, transection of the long thoracic nerve, frozen shoulder, brachial plexopathy, rib fracture by retraction, bleeding, and infection are among the potential complications of this incision.

Limited Lateral Thoracotomy and Other Variants of the Posterolateral Incision

The limited lateral thoracotomy is illustrative of the various limited versions of the posterolateral incision, which are increasingly being used in an effort to minimize the trauma, pulmonary dysfunction, and recovery time of pulmonary resections. The limited lateral incision is essentially just the lateral aspect of a posterolateral incision, with or without sparing of the muscles. A transverse skin incision is made from the anterior axillary line at the level of the submammary fold to a point several centimeters below the scapular tip (Figure 11-3). In the nonmuscle-sparing technique, the chest wall is exposed by

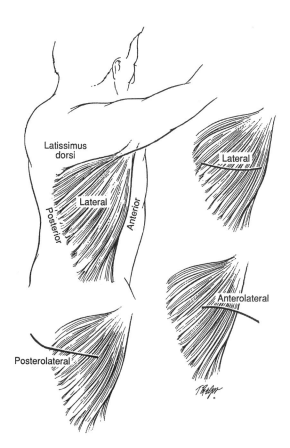

FIGURE 11-3 Limited lateral, posterolateral and anterolateral thoracotomy incisions. (From Heitmiller RF: Thoracic incision. In Bave AE, Geha AS, Hammond GL, et al [eds]: *Glenn's thoracic and cardiovascular surgery,* ed 6, Stanford, Conn, 1995, Appleton & Lange.)

dividing the latissimus dorsi. The pleural space may be entered as described previously. Rib resection is usually not required, but partial rib resection can be elected to improve exposure and prevent fracture. Extension of the incision to a wider or even full posterolateral incision remains an option. Exposure with the lateral incision is more limited but is adequate for most uncomplicated pulmonary resections, including pneumonectomy, lobectomy, lesser resections, bleb or bullae resection, and decortication. The premium on excellent lung isolation is high, and improvements in the provision of single-lung anesthesia were necessary precursors to the development of more limited thoracotomy incisions. More posterior, anterior, or axillary variations on this theme might be dictated by the lesion targeted or by surgical experience and preference. The assumption that such limited thoracotomy incisions result in improved postoperative pain, cough, mobility, and recovery is generally accepted but has not been proven rigorously.

Muscle-Sparing Thoracotomy

There is confusion surrounding the terminology for the various muscle-sparing thoracotomy incisions. Heitmiller organizes them into three groups, depending on the relationship of the skin incision to the latissimus dorsi muscle.[2] The "anterolateral" muscle-sparing approach is essentially a limited anterior/lateral thoracotomy with posterior retraction rather

than division of the latissimus dorsi. The serratus anterior is either partially divided or retracted as well. Considerable blunt subcutaneous dissection to create large skin flaps is required to mobilize the muscle groups. The pleura is entered as described previously, usually at the fourth or fifth interspace, and two rib retractors are usually used at right angles to create a square or rectangular chest wall opening. "Vertical axillary" incisions use a midaxillary, longitudinal incision, anterior and posterior skin flaps, and posterior retraction of the latissimus dorsi (Figure 11-4). The only muscles transected are the intercostals (to enter the chest). "Posterolateral" muscle-sparing thoracotomies use modified posterolateral skin incisions, with various degrees of division or detachment and anterior retraction of the latissimus dorsi and serratus anterior muscles.

Functionally, the muscle-sparing approaches share the advantages of smaller, less painful incisions and minimal tran-

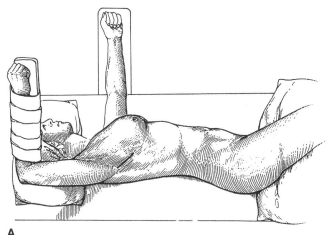

A

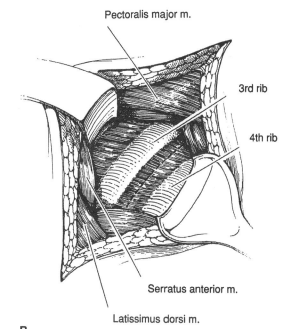

B

FIGURE 11-4 Vertical axillary muscle-sparing thoracotomy skin incision **A,** with retraction of the latissimus dorsi, serratus anterior, and pectoralis muscles **B,** (From Moores DWO, Foster ED, McKneally MF: Incisions. In Pearson FG [ed]: *Thoracic surgery,* New York, 1995, Churchill Livingstone.)

section of muscle. In most cases, the only muscles transected in muscle-sparing incisions are the intercostals. Both early (pain and decreased pulmonary function) and late (frozen shoulder, persistent incisional pain, reduced arm strength) complications of posterolateral incisions are believed to be alleviated by limited muscle-sparing techniques.[3] Compared with posterolateral incisions, muscle-sparing lateral thoracotomies are associated with improved early postoperative forced expiratory volume (FEV_1), early shoulder girdle muscle strength, and reduced perceived pain and narcotic use.[4,5] Late differences in pulmonary function, however, become clinically insignificant between the two techniques.[6] Disadvantages of muscle-sparing limited thoracotomies include an increased incidence of seroma formation and more limited exposure.

The vertical axillary thoracotomy incision differs from the others in that it provides a longitudinal, cosmetically appealing incision with a more apical exposure of the chest. The pleura is often entered at the fourth interspace. This type of incision is well suited for apical bleb disease, first rib resection, sympathectomy, and most pulmonary resections, though it is not recommended when difficult hilar dissections are anticipated.[7] Upper-lobe lesions are best handled through the fourth interspace. Middle- and lower-lobe lesions are better reached via the fifth interspace when using an axillary approach. Brachial plexus injury is possible with the more severe abduction of the arm required to expose the axilla.

Anterior (Anterolateral) Thoracotomy

Anterior thoracotomy incisions provide good exposure to the anterior portions of the upper lobes and to the pericardium and anterior mediastinum. They are less suitable for resections involving lower lobes—particularly on the left side of the body—because of the need to retract the heart. A curvilinear skin incision is made from the sternum to the midaxillary line (Figure 11-5). In men, the level of the incision is determined by the site of the lesion. In women, an inframammary incision is created, and a flap is developed for more apical access to the chest. Pectoralis major and minor muscles are divided, and for major resections, one or two costal cartilages might be divided parasternally. The pleural space may be entered as described

for posterolateral incisions and extended posteriorly, with division of the serratus anterior muscle and posterior retraction of the latissimus dorsi. Most of the limited pulmonary resections previously performed via anterior thoracotomies to avoid the morbidity of full posterolateral incisions are now better carried out through video-assisted thoracic surgery (VATS) or limited muscle-sparing thoracotomy incisions. Despite the limited access they offer to the posterior thorax, anterior thoracotomies are useful in trauma situations because the patient is nearly supine, allowing access to the abdomen and to mediastinal (or even contralateral) structures for exploration or resuscitation. Anesthesiologists and surgeons performing anterior thoracotomies must be cognizant of the vulnerability of internal mammary artery coronary grafts.

Bilateral Trans-sternal Thoracotomy

Although their primary use is for bilateral lung transplantation, bilateral trans-sternal thoracotomy incisions are also advocated as potential alternatives to median sternotomy for bilateral pulmonary resections or simultaneous treatment of bilateral spontaneous pneumothorax.[8] Alternative nomenclature includes the "clam-shell," "crossbow," or "transverse thoracosternotomy" incision. The patient is positioned supine with both arms padded and extended up over the face, with elbows bent and forearms secured to a rigid ether screen or stand. Some surgeons prefer to use a towel roll placed longitudinally under the back. The incision essentially consists of bilateral anterior thoracotomies as previously described, joined by a transverse sternotomy (Figure 11-6). The pleural space is entered at the fourth or fifth interspace as previously described. The pleural spaces may be opened one at a time to optimize single-lung ventilation. The advantages of this approach are superb exposure of both pleural cavities and mediastinum without the need

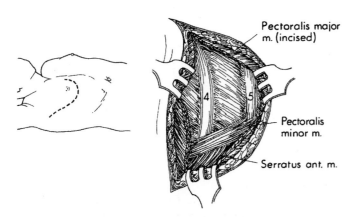

FIGURE 11-5 Anterior (anterolateral) thoracotomy incision. (From Fry WA: Thoracic incision. In Shields TW, LoCicero J, Ponn RB [eds]: *General thoracic surgery,* ed 5, Philadelphia, 200, Lippincott, Williams, & Wilkins.)

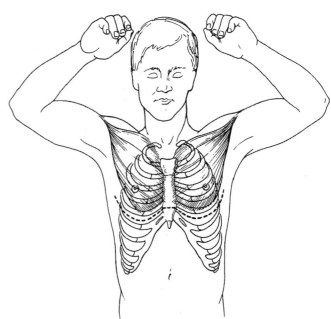

FIGURE 11-6 Bilateral trans-sternal thoracotomy incision. (From Boyd AD, Glassman LR: Thoracic incisions. In Kaiser LR [ed]: *Mastery of cardiothoracic surgery,* Philadelphia, 1998, Lippincott-Raven.)

to reposition the patient from one lateral decubitus position to another. Incisional pain is severe and often necessitates postoperative ventilation. Other potential complications include early sternal instability and wound infections.

Median Sternotomy

Median sternotomy, most commonly performed for surgery of the heart and mediastinum, has been employed for pneumonectomies, lobectomies, and lesser resections, as well as for bilateral pulmonary metastasectomies, bilateral bullectomies, and lung volume reduction surgery. This is also a useful approach for transpericardial repair of a postpneumonectomy bronchopleural fistula. Hilar structures to the left lower lobe (particularly the left inferior pulmonary vein) are difficult to reach from this incision. For this reason, median sternotomy is not recommended for left-sided pneumonectomies or left-sided lower lobectomies.[9]

Advantages of a median sternotomy approach include excellent exposure to proximal great vessels, the heart, anterior mediastinum, and anterior hilar structures, with less pain and early pulmonary dysfunction than alternatives such as bilateral trans-sternal incisions or full posterolateral thoracotomies. No muscles are divided with this approach. Compared with posterolateral thoracotomies for pulmonary resection, median sternotomy has improved vital capacity and peak flow spirometry measurements as well as faster recovery of pulmonary function.[10] In patients with prior thoracotomy incisions and recurrent disease, median sternotomy offers more adhesion-free access to the hilum. Disadvantages include limited exposure to the posterior mediastinum (especially left lower lobe hilar structures) and the potential for cardiac lacerations. Ceasing ventilation during sternotomy is widely thought to reduce the probability of pulmonary or cardiac laceration. Other complications include sternal wound infections (1% to 5%), mediastinitis, sternal instability, subxiphoid hernia, and brachial plexus injury, which has been attributed to undetected first rib fractures.[11] Sternal retractors are generally placed low in the sternum in an attempt to minimize fractures of the upper ribs. Cosmetic objections by female patients can sometimes be alleviated by performing the sternotomy via lower, more limited skin incisions.

Oxygenation during OLV in the supine position for median sternotomy approaches can be more problematic than for a thoracotomy approach in the lateral decubitus position. The reason is that gravity aids the reduction in pulmonary blood flow to the nondependent, operative lung in the lateral decubitus position, whereas hypoxic pulmonary vasoconstriction (HPV) must act alone to reduce operative lung shunt in the supine position. Bardoczky et al demonstrated significantly lower PaO_2 levels when OLV was initiated in the supine position compared with the lateral decubitus position in 24 thoracic surgical patients (Figure 11-7).[12] At an FIO_2 of 1.0, PaO_2 was 61% higher in the lateral decubitus position compared with the supine position. Arterial oxygen levels normally decline to a lower plateau after initiation of OLV. Watanabe et al found that the rate of decline tended to be steeper and that the plateau PaO_2 was lower following initiation of OLV in the supine position compared with the lateral decubitus position.[13] The maximal response of HPV in the supine position occurs within 15 minutes after initiation

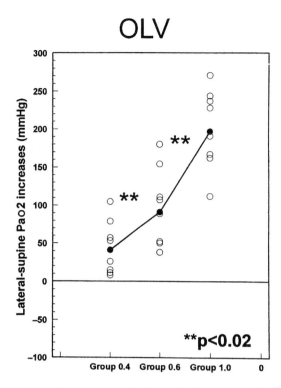

FIGURE 11-7 Values represent the changes in the mean (●) and individual (○) PaO_2 values (mmHg) when OLV was initiated in the lateral decubitus position compared with the supine position (baseline), at different FIO_2 values (0.4, 0.6, and 1.0), for 24 patients with chronic obstructive pulmonary disease. (From Bardoczky GI, Szegedi LL, d'Hollander AA, et al: *Anesth Analg* 90:35, 2001.)

of OLV.[14] If oxygenation remains marginal after 15 minutes of OLV for supine, median sternotomy procedures, maneuvers to augment oxygenation (PEEP, CPAP, intermittent reexpansion of the operative lung, etc.) should be employed. If it does not interfere with the progress of surgery, tilting the table to a semilateral position (nonoperative side down) might improve oxygenation marginally.[13]

Thoracoabdominal Incisions

The thoracoabdominal incision is indicated primarily for surgery of the upper abdomen or retroperitoneal region, or for simultaneous exposure of the lower chest and upper abdomen (thoracoabdominal aneurysms, tumors of the gastroesophageal junction, etc.). Rarely would this approach be used for pulmonary resection.

The patient is positioned with the shoulders in the lateral decubitus position and the hips rotated toward supine. The incision runs from the posterior axillary line along the eighth interspace, across the costal margin anteriorly, to the abdominal midline halfway between the umbilicus and the xiphoid. The pleural space is accessed via the seventh or eighth intercostal space after division of the external oblique and serratus anterior muscles. The peritoneal cavity is accessed by dividing the anterior rectus sheath, rectus muscle, and posterior rectus sheath. The diaphragm may be opened as needed with care to avoid injury to the phrenic nerve and its branches. Lung isolation is generally helpful to surgical exposure. Acute postoperative incisional pain is severe, and depending on the extent of the incision, it could be difficult to achieve adequate spread of local anesthetic through a thoracic epidural catheter to cover the entire incision completely. For this reason, patients with thoracoabdominal incisions often require postoperative ventilation.

Closure of Thoracotomy Incisions

Chest tubes (usually two) are inserted through separate stab wounds prior to closure. Generally, one chest tube is placed anteriorly and superiorly for evacuation of air, and a second tube is placed posteriorly and inferiorly for drainage of fluid and blood. The tubes exit the chest at an angle and are tunnelled for several centimeters to prevent fistula formation and to direct the tubes without creating an acute angle, which might cause kinking. Chest tubes generally exit through anterior and midaxillary positions inferior to the incision, to optimize drainage and patient comfort. Complete reinflation of the lungs should be confirmed visually by the surgeon and anesthesiologist prior to closure of the chest. Recruitment of atelectatic lung units is best accomplished by prolonged (5 to 15 seconds) inspiratory positive pressure hold maneuvers by the anesthesiologist. The peak pressure employed to reexpand the lungs generally needs to be in the range of 20 to 40 cmH$_2$O, measured at the inspiratory circuit. The minimal effective pressure should be employed. If excessive pressures are required, fiberoptic bronchoscopy should be employed to rule out obstruction of the operative lumen or airway by blood, secretions, or tube malposition. Ribs are reapproximated with heavy absorbable sutures. If a rib has been resected, heavy paracostal sutures are passed around the remaining superior and inferior ribs to approximate the opposing intercostal muscles. As the chest is closed, care is taken to avoid entrapment of intercostal neurovascular structures. Divided muscles are then reapproximated, followed by closure of the skin incision. The chest tubes should be placed on continuous suction when the chest is closed to prevent tension pneumothorax and to maintain lung expansion.

Video-Assisted Thoracic Surgery

In the past decade, the concept of video-assisted thoracic surgery (VATS) has developed and become widely embraced in the United States.[15-17] Recent developments in fiberoptic light sources, video endoscopic technology, endoscopic stapling devices, and endoscopic surgical instruments were essential prerequisites to this development. For pulmonary resection, VATS has largely supplanted open thoracotomy techniques for uncomplicated wedge resections and segmentectomies. Anesthesia for VATS is discussed in Chapter 12.

Common Thoracic Surgical Procedures: Surgical and Anesthetic Considerations

General Anesthetic Considerations

The most commonly performed pulmonary resections include wedge resections, segmentectomies, lobectomies, and pneumonectomies. The basic surgical considerations and events of these procedures, as well as of sleeve resections and extrapleural pneumonectomies, deserve to be understood by the enlightened anesthesiologist. Specific anesthetic implications for these procedures tend to be dictated more by the incision and the patient's coexisting pathophysiology than by the amount of

pulmonary parenchyma resected. In general, for thoracotomy approaches, the issues reviewed in detail in Chapters 7 and 8 would apply with respect to lung isolation, OLV, monitoring, the conduct of anesthesia, and postoperative pain control. Only anesthetic considerations that are not generally applicable to all thoracotomies are discussed in these pages for the different procedures. For most lesser resections (wedge and segmental), the anesthetic implications discussed for VATS approaches apply. In general, anesthetics should be tailored to provide for rapid postoperative extubation for all pulmonary resections, if possible. Invasive monitoring and the amount of intravenous access should be dictated by the incision, the patient's comorbidities, and the proximity of the lesion to other vital structures. Conservative intravenous fluid management is recommended for lobectomies and pneumonectomies out of respect for the potential for (and serious consequences of) postpneumonectomy pulmonary edema (see the discussion that follows).

Wedge Resections

Small, nonanatomic, parenchymal-sparing pulmonary resections are commonly referred to as "wedge" resections. Wedge resections are indicated for diagnosis of an indeterminate pulmonary nodule, metastasectomies that are expected to prolong life, and for resection of stage I or II lung cancer in patients who would not tolerate more definitive resection (lobectomy/pneumonectomy). Currently, VATS is overwhelmingly the surgical approach of choice. Open approaches, usually with a limited, muscle-sparing thoracotomy, are indicated for patients in whom VATS is contraindicated, where the capability for VATS is lacking, or for certain combined procedures. The location of VATS ports is determined by the location of the lesion.

Localization of the nodule can be problematic with the VATS approach. For this reason, many surgeons restrict the VATS approach to lesions located in the peripheral third of the lung.[16] Peripheral nodules can appear through the thoracoscope as a convexity of the pleural surface, a dimpling of the pleura, or an irregularity of color or texture of the pleural surface. Often the surgeon must stroke the surface or "palpate" the lung with ring forceps to localize the nodule. Occasionally, it is necessary to enlarge an accessory port to admit a finger for digital palpation. Preoperative wire localization, dye marking, or coil injection, as well as intraoperative fluoroscopic or ultrasound guidance, have been described but are not commonly used.[17] Wires can become dislodged with collapse of the lung.

Once located, the nodule is grasped with a clamp from one accessory port while a stapling device is applied in several bites from opposing angles and ports. Margins on the order of 2 cm are generally sought.[15] Electrocautery or neodymium:yttrium aluminum garnet (Nd:YAG) lasers are alternative techniques for excision and have their advocates.[18]

Segmentectomy

Segmentectomy refers to the excision of a discrete bronchopulmonary segment, including the lymph node groupings associated with the bronchus and its pulmonary artery. It is primarily indicated for patients with suppurative pulmonary lesions (tuberculosis, bronchiectasis, etc.) who fail medical management, and for the treatment of early (T$_1$N$_0$) lung cancer in select patients.[18] It is controversial whether segmentectomy provides comparable results to lobectomy for primary lung cancer. In a randomized trial, Ginsberg et al compared outcomes following lobectomy vs. lesser resections for non–small cell lung cancer and found improved outcomes in the lobectomy group.[19] Because segmentectomies were grouped with nonanatomic wedge resections in that study, the question remains unanswered for true segmentectomies. Current standards, therefore, call for lobectomy for the surgical treatment of isolated lung cancer, reserving segmental resections for patients who cannot tolerate lobectomy.

Segmentectomies are usually performed via limited thoracotomy or VATS incisions, which are positioned according to the segment sought. After entry into the chest, the hilar structures are exposed by incising the pleura as it reflects upon the hilum, and the major fissure is opened. The pulmonary arterial branches and segmental bronchus are identified, ligated, and divided. In suppurative lung disease, the bronchus is divided first to limit contamination. Otherwise, the order of division is variable, dictated by the segment and the anatomy. Stapling devices or interrupted fine absorbable sutures are used to divide the bronchus. Additional coverage of the stump is usually not necessary. Retraction and blunt dissection are then employed to separate the remainder of the diseased segment, clamping, ligating, and dividing small airways and vessels as needed. When anatomic planes are followed, significant airleaks are unlikely. Two chest tubes are generally employed as described for thoracotomy incisions. Alveolar leaks will seal with reexpansion, but stump leaks should be recognized prior to closure by applying an inspiratory hold maneuver with saline in the chest. Persistent air leaks can lead to a persistent pleural space, to empyema, and a bronchopleural fistula (see below).

The priority for excellent lung isolation is high, particularly if a VATS approach is employed. Blood loss is rarely significant. In order to delineate anatomic segments, the anesthesiologist could be asked to inflate the lung temporarily prior to clamping the bronchus. As the remaining lung is then redeflated, the segment subserved by the clamped bronchus will deflate more slowly. Intersegmental collaterals often exist, allowing air to escape even when the bronchus is clamped. Despite this, temporary reinflation of segments is often helpful.

Lobectomy

Currently, lobectomy is the accepted standard surgical treatment for localized non–small cell lung cancer and is the most commonly performed oncologic thoracic resection.[20] Standard lobectomy for cancer involves anatomic resection of the lobar parenchyma as well as the N_1 hilar, interlobar, and segmental lymph nodes draining the area. Although posterolateral thoracotomy is the classic and most convenient incision for lobectomies, anterolateral, median sternotomy (except for left lower lobe), and, increasingly, muscle-sparing lateral thoracotomy incisions have been used. VATS lobectomies are currently investigational and not yet recommended as an accepted alternative.[21] The expectation that the VATS approach for lobectomies would result in reduced morbidity, mortality, recovery time, and hospital stay compared with open resection has not been conclusively proven to date.[21]

In the open technique, the pleural space is entered through the fifth intercostal space or through the periosteal bed of the fifth rib. Often, a segment of rib is excised to facilitate atraumatic rib retraction. After mobilization of the lung, the mediastinal pleura is incised to access the hilum. Node sampling is performed as indicated, and the appropriate fissure is opened by sharp and blunt dissection. Crucial steps include the identification of the lobar branch of the pulmonary artery, and dissection of the artery from its fibrous sheath. The pulmonary artery is a delicate, thin-walled structure that can have anomalous anatomy. Proximal control is mandatory prior to difficult dissections. Division of the artery, veins, and bronchus is usually accomplished with stapling devices. The integrity of the bronchial stump is tested by the application of positive pressure with a saline-filled hemithorax. Additional reinforcement of the bronchial stump is not routinely performed, as the remaining lung usually provides coverage following reinflation. Two chest tubes are placed as described previously, and the remaining lung is reinflated as the chest is closed.

VATS lobectomies begin with an eighth intercostal thoracoscopic port, which provides a panoramic view of the hemithorax. A utility thoracotomy incision (4 to 6 cm) is generally created from the anterior edge of the latissimus dorsi to the anterior axillary line. This incision provides instrument or digital access to hilar structures without resection or undue retraction of ribs. One or two additional access ports are usually needed. With long-handled or endoscopic instruments and stapling devices, the hilum is dissected, the lobar vessels and bronchus are divided, and the fissure is completed. The specimen is removed through the utility incision, with a retrieval bag if malignant seeding is a possibility.

Sleeve Resections

"Sleeve resection" is a general term referring to the excision of a discrete segment of the airway followed by the anastomosis of the remaining distal segment. In a "sleeve lobectomy," a lobe is removed together with a segment of the mainstem bronchus, followed by reattachment of the remaining lobe(s) (Figure 11-8). Sleeve resections involving the carina are called "carinal resections," while those above the carina are called "tracheal resections" (see Chapter 10). Sleeve lobectomies are most commonly performed for broncial carinoma as an alternative to pneumonectomy, in order to preserve lung function.

Sleeve lobectomies are technically similar to lobectomies except for the bronchoplasty. Preoperative bronchoscopy is essential. Posterolateral incisions are usually employed. Care is taken to preserve the bronchial arterial supply to the bronchial margins. The bronchus should not be "skeletalized" of its surrounding vascular tissue prior to its division. Bronchial divisions should be made squarely, as wedge resections or angled anastomoses tend to kink. The anastomosis is performed end-to-end or telescoped if a size discrepancy exists. Reinforcement with a vascular flap (pericardial, pleural, omental, or intercostal muscle) is generally performed.

Despite the greater degree of technical complexity, sleeve lobectomies carry no higher perioperative mortality than pneumonectomies.[22] The advantage of preserved pulmonary function can make surgery feasible in elderly or frail patients who would not tolerate a pneumonectomy. Long-term success is comparable to pneumonectomy in some series.[23] Complications include bronchial stricture or kinking, fistula

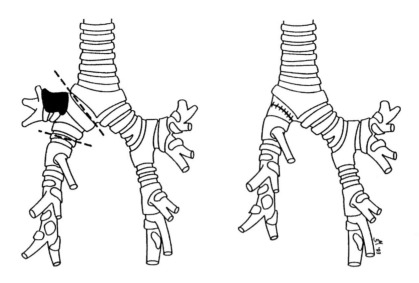

FIGURE 11-8 Right upper lobe sleeve resection. (From Shields TW: *Clin Chest Med* 14:121, 1993.)

formation, or dehiscence of the bronchial anastomosis. Stricture may be treated with a stent. Dehiscence may require completion pneumonectomy, which carries a mortality rate of 15% to 20%.[24,25]

ANESTHETIC CONSIDERATIONS SPECIFIC TO SLEEVE RESECTIONS

A double-lumen endotracheal tube (DLT) seated in the contralateral bronchus is the best means of achieving lung isolation for sleeve resections. Ipsilaterally situated DLTs or bronchial blockers can interfere with surgery or disrupt the anastomosis. While the bronchus is open to atmosphere, continuous positive airway pressure (CPAP) to the operative lung cannot be provided by the traditional tracheal lumen route. If, during OLV, hypoxemia develops that fails to respond to other maneuvers (e.g., positive end-expiratory pressure [PEEP] to the nonoperative lung), a catheter may be passed into the distal operative bronchus, either via the tracheal lumen of the DLT or over the field, to provide supplemental oxygen by insufflation or jet ventilation. Alternatively, the distal operative bronchus can be intubated over the field temporarily with a small endotracheal tube to deliver supplemental oxygen (as is done with tracheal resections).

Pneumonectomy

Pneumonectomy consists of excision of one entire lung together with its visceral pleura. It is most commonly indicated for lung cancer that is centrally located, adherent to hilar structures, or crossing the fissure. Although more common in developing coutries, advanced bronchiectasis or chronic suppurative diseases can occasionally be indications for pneumonectomy. Reported operative mortality ranges from 4% to 8%, and morbidity for survivors is significant.[26]

A central surgical point is that the final decision to proceed with pneumonectomy is an intraoperative decision based on intraoperative staging. Preoperative staging underestimates the extent of disease in nearly 50% of patients.[27] Bronchoscopy immediately before surgery must assure at least 2 cm of mainstem bronchus grossly free of tumor. Evaluation of mediastinal lymph nodes, exclusion of pleural metastases, and chest wall, diaphragmatic, spinal or mediastinal tumor invasion must be established intraoperatively prior to division of any major vessel or airway. In addition, the major hilar structures must be evaluated circumferentially to rule out mediastinal extension prior to resection. In addition, the patient must have an adequate pulmonary reserve to tolerate a pneumonectomy. This is an imprecise process, usually based on the calculated postoperative FEV_1 and modified by differential V/Q scans and objective and subjective estimates of exercise tolerance. This topic is covered in detail in Chapter 1.

Thoracotomy for pneumonectomy is usually performed through a standard posterolateral incision or a limited variation thereof. The pleura is entered as previously described, and the chest is evaluated systematically to establish that the cancer is localized. The mediastinal pleura is incised and the pulmonary artery, the superior and inferior pulmonary veins, and the mainstem bronchus are circumferentially evaluated for resectability. For right pneumonectomies, the azygous vein and inferior pulmonary ligament are often divided to improve access to the hilum, though some surgeons spare the azygous vein (Figures 11-9 and 11-10). Appropriate lymph nodes are harvested and evaluated as indicated. The hilar structures can be divided in any order. The claim that ligating the artery before the veins leads to the loss of less blood trapped within the lung has not been substantiated. Occasionally, the pulmonary veins must be ligated intrapericardially. Advocates exist for both stapler and manual closure of the bronchus, though most favor the former. A leak test is generally performed at this point, and the bronchial stump is then covered with a pericardial fat pad, parietal pleura, an intercostal muscle flap, pericardium, or some other vascularized tissue. The bronchial stump should be as short as possible to present a minimal pocket for the collection of secretions. Bronchial vessels are potential sources of bleeding, which should be recognized prior to closure. The thoracotomy is closed without the usual thoracostomy tubes because there is no lung to reexpand, and because suction applied to the empty hemithorax could cause mediastinal shift or cardiac herniation with hemodynamic collapse. Some surgeons advocate a drainage catheter, which can be useful to assess bleeding or for

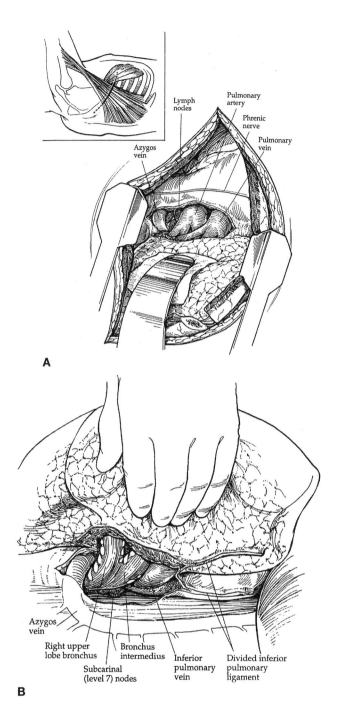

A

B

FIGURE 11-9 Exposure for pulmonary resection. **A,** View of anterior right hilar structures. **B,** Posterior right hilar view after division of the mediastinal pleura and inferior pulmonary ligament. (From DeCamp MM Jr, Liptay MJ, Sugarbaker DJ: Pulmonary resections. In Nyhus LM, Baker RJ, Fischer JE [eds]: *Mastery of surgery,* ed 3, Boston, 1997, Little Brown.)

adding or removing air.[28] Most advocate removing 0.75 to 1.5 L of air from the empty chest to medialize the mediastinum and trachea. A postoperative chest x-ray is the best means of evaluating the position of the mediastinum.

ANESTHETIC CONSIDERATIONS SPECIFIC TO PNEUMONECTOMIES

The anesthetic issues that apply generally to thoracotomies are reviewed in Chapter 7. Continuous intraarterial blood pressure monitoring is justified by the potential need for arterial

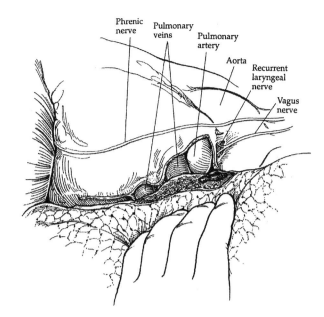

FIGURE 11-10 Anterior view of the left hilar and mediastinal structures. (From DeCamp MM Jr, Liptay MJ, Sugarbaker DJ: Pulmonary resections. In Nyhus LM, Baker RJ, Fischer JE [eds]: *Mastery of surgery,* ed 3, Boston, 1997, Little Brown.)

blood gas measurements. Many practitioners employ central venous pressure monitoring to help guide intravascular fluid management. A significant increase in central venous pressure with test-clamping of the pulmonary artery (PA) would suggest a compromised capacity of the right ventricle to accommodate the afterload imposed by a pneumonectomy. If a pulmonary artery catheter (PAC) is employed, care must be exercised to prevent its entrapment by the stapling of the operative pulmonary artery. Although PACs usually float to the right lung, abnormalities of pulmonary blood flow distribution associated with pulmonary pathology make this rule of thumb less reliable in thoracic surgical cases. Many advocate withdrawal of the PAC to the pulmonic valve before PAC crossclamping to prevent entrapment. If the catheter is withdrawn and refloated after PA crossclamping there is potential for disruption of the PA staple line.

Practitioners must be aware of potential pitfalls in the interpretation of PAC data during pneumonectomy cases. Pulmonary artery occlusion pressure (PAOP) is considered an accurate reflection of left atrial pressure only if there is an uninterrupted column of blood between the catheter tip and the left atrium (West's zone III of the lung), a premise that may be violated during OLV in the lateral decubitus position with an open hemithorax. It is well known that positive-end-expiratory pressure (PEEP) may falsely elevate PAOP measurements. Intrinsic PEEP is frequently present in unmeasured amounts during OLV of thoracic surgical patients and may further confound PAC measurement.

PA occlusion pressure measured by inflating the balloon in the nonoperative PA after contralateral PA crossclamp may yield spuriously low values.[29] The reason is that balloon inflation may occlude a sufficient amount of the remaining pulmonary arterial tree and reduce left atrial filling as a function of the measurement process. PA catheters are infrequently utilized for pulmonary resection surgery. If right- or left-side ventricular filling or function needs to be assessed intraoperatively, transesophageal echocardiography is an alternative and probably a safer and superior technology.

Following induction and bronchoscopy, lung isolation is generally best accomplished by intubating the nonoperative bronchus with an appropriately sided DLT. A left-sided DLT can be used for left pneumonectomies, but it must be pulled back at the time of bronchial crossclamping. In such a case, there is risk that the DLT might inadvertently advance and disrupt the stump. Bronchial blockers work well for left pneumonectomies, but because the right mainstem is shorter than the left, they are more likely to become dislodged when used for right pneumonectomies. When bronchial blockers are used for pneumonectomies, they must be withdrawn at the time of bronchial crossclamping, with the ventilator paused so that it does not reinflate the operative lung when the balloon is deflated. Although right-sided DLTs might provide poor lung isolation when the right mainstem bronchus is anomalously short, placement of a bronchial blocker through the tracheal lumen has been shown to be effective in rescuing an ill-fitting right DLT.[30]

The choice of agents and conduct of the anesthetic should be tailored to the goal of rapid postoperative extubation. Prior to closure, the bronchial stump is tested with 20 to 40 cmH$_2$O of positive pressure as described previously. Following closure, the patient is turned supine, the DLT is exchanged for a single-lumen ETT, and a fiberoptic bronchoscopic evaluation of the stump and clean-out of the remaining lung are performed. The return to the supine position can result occasionally in hypotension or even cardiovascular collapse, owing to embarrassment of venous return from mediastinal shift, or herniation of the heart into the empty thoracic cavity. Immediate return to the preexisting lateral decubitus position is the life-saving maneuver to correct a case of cardiac herniation. Cardiac herniation is more common in right pneumonectomies. Less threatening drops in blood pressure upon resumption of the supine position might be attributable to shift of the mediastinum in either direction. A shift of the trachea could suggest which direction, and whether to add or remove air from the chest drain. A portable chest radiograph is the best way to guide the medialization of the mediastinum. It is obviously undesirable to administer an added dose of drug through the thoracic epidural in the 15 minutes before this position change, as this process can result in diagnostic confusion.

Postpneumonectomy pulmonary edema (PPE) is an incompletely understood phenomenon, occurring in 2% to 4% of pneumonectomy patients and carrying a mortality in excess of 50%.[31] The risk is higher for right pneumonectomies than for left, possibly because of the more compromised lymphatic drainage of the residual lung that occurs following right-sided resections. Earlier reports suggested that excess intravascular fluid administration was causally related to the development of PPE.[32-33] Subsequent studies failed to support that association; however, more restrictive fluid management strategies were employed in those later studies.[34,35] There is some evidence of increased pulmonary capillary permeability in the remaining lung following pneumonectomy.[35] Shear stress from abruptly increased capillary flow and ventilator-associated lung injury have a been postulated as potential mechanisms for this increased permeability.[36] Whether fluid administration is causally related to PPE, it is apparent that in the presence of increased pulmonary capillary permeability, unnecessary crystalloid administration exacerbates the degree of pulmonary edema. Because blood loss during pneumonectomy is usually modest, restricting fluids to less than 20 mL/kg for the first 24 hours is generally possible without hemodynamic instability. No series has found an increased incidence of PPE when this strategy is employed.[37]

Extrapleural Pneumonectomy

Initially described for the treatment of tuberculous empyema, extrapleural pneumonectomy (EPP) is now chiefly performed for the local control of malignant pleural mesothelioma (MPM). Untreated, diffuse MPM has a median survival of 4 to 12 months. Significant survival improvement has been achieved in selected patients by EPP followed by radiation and chemotherapy when performed at centers experienced in this procedure, despite the inherent morbidity and mortality risks associated with the surgery.[38]

MPM has been causally linked to asbestos exposure. The geometry of the amphibole type allows it to reach the subpleural space, where it becomes a continuous carcinogenic stimulus.[38] Contributing etiologic factors include cigarette smoking and, possibly, exposure to the simian virus (SV40) through polio vaccines used in the 1950s. New cases of MPM appear annually at a rate of 2000 to 3000 cases/year, and this trend is expected to continue well into the twenty-first century because of the long latency period between asbestos exposure and diagnosis. Of the three major subtypes of MPM (epithelial, sarcomatous, and mixed), the epithelial type is associated with the most favorable prognosis.[39]

The technique of EPP includes the following five basic steps[38]:
1. Incision and exposure of the parietal pleura
2. Dissection of the parietal pleura from the chest wall, diaphragm, and mediastinum
3. Control of the pulmonary vessels and bronchus, followed by subcarinal node dissection
4. En bloc resection of lung, pleura, pericardium, and diaphragm
5. Reconstruction of the diaphragm and pericardium (on the right side)

A generous posterolateral incision with resection of the sixth rib is required. Blunt and sharp dissection are employed to separate the parietal pleura from the chest wall and subsequent structures while attempting to maintain an intact pleural envelope to prevent seeding of extrapleural structures (Figure 11-11). This process of blunt and sharp pleural dissection continues apically, laterally, medially, and inferiorly, with packing along the way to stem blood loss. Notable vulnerable vascular structures encountered in this process include superior and inferior vena cavae, the pulmonary artery, the azygous vein, and the internal mammary artery and vein. The ipsilateral hemi-diaphragm is dissected bluntly from the peritoneum, following a radial incision of the diaphragm. The specimen is removed, and a pericardial fat pad is used to bolster the bronchial stump. Right-sided pericardial defects are reconstructed with a fenestrated prosthetic patch such as Gor-Tex (WL Gore & Associates, Inc., Flagstaff, Arizona).

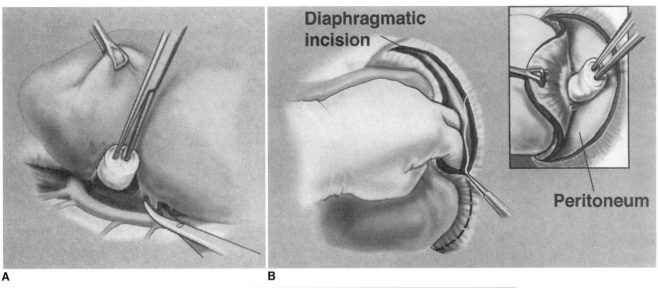

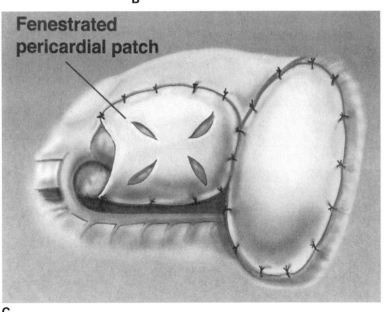

FIGURE 11-11 Right extrapleural pneumonectomy. **A,** The right lung is dissected medially, away from the azygous vein along an extrapleural plane. **B,** Dissection of the pleural envelope off of the diaphragm and *(inset)* blunt dissection of the diaphragm from the peritoneum. **C,** Diaphragmatic and fenestrated pericardial patches to prevent herniation. (From Garcia JP, Richards WG, Sugarbaker DJ: Surgical treatment of malignant mesothelioma. In Kaiser LR [ed]: *Mastery of cardiothoracic surgery,* Philadelphia, 1998, Lippincott-Raven.)

A similar but impermeable patch is used to reconstruct the diaphragm. Hemostasis of the legion minor chest wall vessels is sought with electrocautery and/or an argon beam coagulator. The chest is closed as described for pneumonectomies, usually with a red rubber catheter left in place.

ANESTHETIC CONSIDERATIONS SPECIFIC TO EXTRAPLEURAL PNEUMONECTOMIES

In addition to the previously described issues that apply to thoracotomies and pneumonectomies, EPP surgery is characterized by significantly greater blood loss due to the innumerable small chest wall vessels avulsed in the process of blunt dissection of the pleura. Correspondingly more generous intravenous access, fluid administration, warming maneuvers, and invasive hemodynamic monitoring are appropriate. There is potential for disruption of major blood vessels causing rapid, acute bleeding in addition to the more gradual, continuous losses from chest wall vessels. Disruption of internal mammary arteries is possible, and patients with ipsilateral internal mammary artery coronary bypass grafts are at high risk of coronary ischemia and myocardial infarction.

The weight of the tumor together with the traction required to achieve blunt dissection can inhibit venous return and reduce compliance in the dependent lung. The temptation to correct venous return with enthusiastic volume expansion with crystalloid is to be avoided. As soon as the heavy specimen is removed, both compliance and venous return will improve. Use of blood products and vasoconstrictors and judicious administration of crystalloid will usually temporize until the specimen is removed. The issue of PPE has been discussed previously and applies to EPP surgery as well.

The risks of cardiac herniation and hemodynamic collapse upon resumption of the supine position are particularly important to be aware of for EPP because of the generous pericardial window created in right-sided resections. The pericardial patch should prevent these problems, but dehiscence of the patch is possible. In addition, a tamponade-like effect can result if the patch is too tight. Despite these limitations, extubation at the completion of surgery remains an achievable priority in nearly all cases. When blood losses and fluid shifts result in significant airway edema, the switch from a DLT to a single-lumen tube for the terminal bronchoscopic evaluation can be treacherous. Strategies for handling this eventuality include using a stylette ("tube changer") or using a bronchial blocker instead of a right-sided DLT (for a left EPP) to obviate the need to change tubes.

Miscellaneous Pulmonary Resections

Bronchopleural Fistula

Bronchopleural fistula (BPF) refers to a persistent abnormal communication between the tracheobronchial tree and the pleural cavity, which can occur from a variety of causes (Table 11-2). Two thirds are related to surgery and could be "central" (because of breakdown of pneumonectomy/lobectomy stumps) or "peripheral" (because of breakdown of distal staple lines).[40] The vast majority of small, peripheral BPFs, whether medical or surgical, heal with appropriate drainage and conservative management.

The incidence of BPF varies from 4.5% to 20% following pneumonectomy or 0.5% following lobectomy, and it carries a high mortality risk (18% to 50%).[41-44] BPFs are more common following right pneumonectomies and manual vs. stapled bronchial closures. Predisposing factors include the following:

- Technical difficulties with bronchial closure
- Residual tumor at the bronchial stump
- Preoperative irradiation of the hilum
- Diabetes
- Infection
- Long bronchial stumps
- Completion pneumonectomy for persistent or recurrent inflammatory disease

At least 50% of pneumonectomy/lobectomy suture or staple closures separate and subsequently heal by secondary intent.[45] The integrity of the peribronchial tissue, therefore, tends to be as important as the technique of closure.[46] The importance of respecting the peribronchial tissue, protecting the bronchial arterial supply, and reinforcing pneumonectomy stumps with vascular tissue (e.g., omental pedicle flap) is emphasized as a surgical issue.[41]

The presentation and treatment of postsurgical BPFs depend on the size of the air leak, the type of resection (pneumonectomy vs. lesser resection), and the time of presentation. The surgical management of postsurgical air leaks is not standardized, but certain principles are generally agreed upon (Table 11-3).

Postpneumonectomy BPFs tend to be the most problematic and carry the highest mortality risk. A distinction is appropriate between BPFs that present early (during the first several days after surgery), and delayed (weeks to years later). Whereas the former results from stump dehiscence and calls for early reclosure, the latter is usually accompanied by an empyema, requiring clearance of the infection prior to definitive closure. Acute dehiscences present as sudden, large increases in air leak evident in the thoracostomy tube drainage system (if present), with various degrees of respiratory distress.[47] Because the mediastinum has not yet become fibrosed and stabilized, there can be contralateral mediastinal shift with compromise of remaining lung function.[40] Chest radiographs exhibit a sudden drop in the air-fluid level, and patients are in peril of flooding the remaining lung with potentially infected fluid from the pneumonectomy cavity.

Immediate management for such a stump dehiscence calls for positioning the patient so as to decrease the probability of further soiling the contralateral lung, supporting respiration, and establishing effective drainage if such is not already in place. Thoracentesis of the pneumonectomy space is rarely helpful and risks infecting the pleural space.[48] Depending on

TABLE 11-2
Causes of Bronchopleural Fistula

Breakdown of suture/staple line following lung resection	
Rupture of cavity	Cyst
	Abscess
	Bulla
	Bleb
Erosion of bronchial wall by infection	Empyema
	Pneumonia
	Tuberculosis
Erosion of bronchial wall by neoplasm	
Penetrating trauma	
Pulmonary infarction	
Iatrogenic	Medical/surgical procedures	Barotrauma from mechanical ventilation
		Thoracentesis
		Transbronchial biopsy
	Anesthetic procedures	Traumatic intubation
		Traumatic use of endotracheal tube changer

TABLE 11-3
General Principles for Surgical Management of Bronchopleural Fistulae

Prompt drainage of pleural space
Protect against soilage of remaining lung tissue
Appropriate antibiotics
Respiratory support
Early diagnostic bronchoscopy
Early reoperation and reclosure for large central stump dehiscences that occur in the early postoperative period
Address infections before attempting reclosure
Reinforce stumps with vascularized tissue
Obliteration of residual pleural space
Minimize tension on and airflow through the fistula

the size of the leak, respiratory support could require just supplemental oxygen, or intubation of the contralateral bronchus with a DLT (or endobronchial tube) followed by single-lung positive pressure ventilation. Bronchoscopy confirms the diagnosis and helps evaluate the size of the fistula and the amount of stump available to effect a repair. Barring infection or residual tumor at the stump, early reoperation and reclosure of the stump are indicated. Reinforcement of the new stump with a vascularized flap of some sort is mandatory. Most surgeons would approach reoperation for stump dehiscence through the original thoracotomy incision. Small (<3 mm), early air leaks following pulmonary resection are approached more conservatively by some, with a trial of drainage, antibiotics, serial bronchoscopic evaluations, and possibly the bronchoscopic application of a sealant material (e.g., fibrin glue).[47] Sealant material serves to close the opening physically and to initiate an inflammatory fibrotic response.[40]

Delayed postpneumonectomy BPFs are almost invariably associated with an infected pleural space (empyema) and can be difficult to diagnose. Patients often present with insidious deterioration marked by fever, cough, expectoration of purulent or serosanguinous fluid, and (possibly) aspiration of fluid or pus to the remaining lung. An auscultatory squeak can be heard when the Valsalva maneuver is performed. Because the chest tube drain is generally not in place at this point, the physiology is that of a true pneumothorax and potential tension pneumothorax. Early establishment of effective thoracostomy drainage, antibiotic therapy, and respiratory support are called for. Computed tomography can be helpful in delineating the empyema cavity and identifying loculations to guide chest tube placement.

Unlike acute dehiscences, the presence of an established infection precludes immediate stump reclosure. The empyema must be addressed as will shortly be discussed (see "Anesthetic Considerations for Empyemas and Decortication") with closed and/or open drainage procedures, systemic and cavitary antibiotics, nutritional support, débridements, and repeated dressing changes and packing of the cavity with antibiotic-soaked packing material. With open drainage procedures, the packing also serves to decrease the airleak across the fistula. With successful treatment of the empyema, many postpneumonectomy

BPFs heal with 4 to 6 weeks of packing and open drainage, barring residual tumor or excessive airflow across the fistula.[49] In other cases, surgical reclosure could be required or favored. Surgical approaches for reclosure include repeat ipsilateral thoracotomy, contralateral right thoracotomy (or VATS) for left pneumonectomy BPFs (left thoracotomies do not provide sufficient exposure for right-sided BPFs), or a trans-sternal, transpericardial approach. As discussed previously, buttressing of the new stump with vascularized tissue (usually omental flap) is imperative. Obliteration of the pleural cavity can be accomplished by transposition of extrathoracic muscle flaps (latissimus dorsi, serratus anterior, pectoralis major), or limited thoracoplasty (rare). Reclosure and obliteration of the space may be performed as single or multistaged procedures. Carinal resection might be required if the affected stump is too short (Figure 11-12). Advocates of the trans-sternal, transpericardial approach argue that it avoids the inflammation and dense adhesions of the previous thoracotomy and provides excellent exposure if a carinal resection becomes necessary.[49]

Bronchopleural fistulae associated with lobectomies or lesser resections usually resolve with conservative management, as long as chest tube suction accomplishes effective reexpansion of the remaining lung. Acute postlobectomy BPFs present with sudden increases in air leaks. Delayed BPFs, occurring after the chest tube has been removed, produce the reappearance of an air-fluid level and the symptoms of empyema described above. Respiratory distress can result from the soilage of remaining lung, from collapse of remaining ipsilateral lung (pneumothorax), and/or from mediastinal shift and tension pneumothorax if air trapping occurs. Identification of occult bronchopleural fistulae can occasionally be aided by radionuclide inhalation or dye techniques. Detachable balloons, deployed via a bronchoscope, have been used to both localize and treat small, distal fistulae.[50] A Heimlich valve (a one-way valve on a drain) sometimes is employed with good effect for persistent small air leaks. Fibrin glue applied through a bronchoscope can be used to treat some small, distal fistula.[51] Rarely do nonpneumonectomy BPFs require operative repair. When they do, the principles outlined in Table 11-3 would apply.[50] Recalcitrant BPFs following lobectomies or sleeve resections might require completion pneumonectomy, which

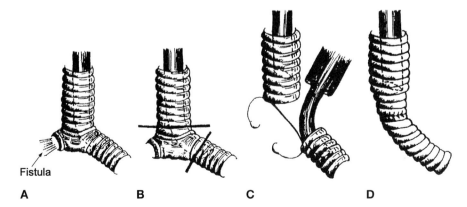

FIGURE 11-12 **A,** Right bronchopleural fistula. **B,** Carinal resection. **C,** Intubation of the left mainstem bronchus. **D,** Completed anastomosis of the left main bronchus to the trachea. (From Topcuoglu MS, Kayhan C, Ulus T: *Ann Thorac Surg* 69:394, 2000.)

carries a high risk of refistulization. Large air leaks following lung volume reduction surgery or bullectomy—in which a large-area parenchymal staple line has been disrupted—can also prove difficult to close by conservative measures. A VATS approach to restapling is generally employed for such situations. Pleurodesis is also employed for persistent, distal, small airleaks or for recurrent (first contralateral or second ipsilateral) spontaneous pneumothoraces.

Chest tube management is important in patients with BPF. The goals of chest tubes are to drain the pleural space and promote the reexpansion of remaining ipsilateral lung (if any). Toward this end, large-diameter, low-resistance tubes placed on strong suction would be advantageous. Excessive chest tube suction in mechanically ventilated patients, however, could increase fistula airflow, "steal" tidal volume from remaining lung units, or trigger an inspiration-cycled ventilator. In patients undergoing pneumonectomy, excessive suction can cause mediastinal shift, hemodynamic compromise, or even cardiac herniation. Carbon dioxide excretion is enhanced by high fistula and chest tube airflows and can lead to acid-base imbalances. Insufficient suction, or a chest tube that is too small for the fistula flow, leads to collapse of remaining lung and risks tension pneumothorax. In efforts to reduce fistula airflow and loss of tidal volume, synchronized inspiratory occlusion of the chest tube has been reported.[52] In efforts to promote recruitment of residual lung and prevent loss of PEEP through the fistula, synchronized expiratory positive pressure to the pleural space via the chest tube (equal to applied PEEP) has been attempted.[53,54] Chest tubes have also been used as conduits to apply sclerosing agents with the goal of promoting pleural symphysis.[40]

Bronchopleural fistulae are dreaded complications of pulmonary resection and carry a high mortality risk. Death usually results from sepsis, respiratory failure, malnutrition, or, dramatically, from erosion into the pulmonary arterial stump. The impetus for early extubation of patients following pulmonary resection lies in part in the belief that positive pressure ventilation increases the probability of stump dehiscence. This widely held and intuitive hypothesis has not been, and is unlikely to ever be, tested rigorously. Postoperative mechanical ventilation following pulmonary resection has been associated with bronchopleural fistulae, but a causative relationship has not been established.[41,55] Modern options for ventilator modes (including pressure-support ventilation) might well offer minimal risk to a technically adequate stump closure. Nevertheless, the earliest possible extubation remains the standard goal for pulmonary resection.

ANESTHETIC CONSIDERATIONS FOR BRONCHOPLEURAL FISTULA

Anesthesiologists may encounter patients with a BPF in several settings, including diagnostic bronchoscopy, repair of acute stump dehiscence, debridement or decortication of an empyema, establishment of a closed or open drainage system, or definitive fistula closure with muscle-flap obliteration of a cavity. Anesthesiologists also can serve as consultants regarding optimal ventilation or lung isolation in a mechanically ventilated patient with a BPF in an intensive care unit. Unifying goals of BPF management include minimization of airflow across the fistula, adequate gas exchange in the unaffected lung, avoidance of tension pneumothorax, and protection

against contamination of the remaining lung. For patients with a BPF following a lobectomy or lesser resection, expansion of the remaining ipsilateral lung postoperatively and in the ICU are also beneficial for ultimate closure of the fistula.

Regardless of the procedure planned, most surgeons will want to begin with a fiberoptic evaluation as a first step. If a chest tube is not already in place, one should be established and placed on underwater seal prior to initiating positive pressure ventilation. Often, the size of the BPF will be evident from the extent of the chest tube air leak or from a preceding bronchoscopic evaluation. Patients with a pinhole fistula with minimal air leak can tolerate traditional intravenous inductions and conventional two-lung positive pressure ventilation through a single-lumen endotracheal tube for the duration of the bronchoscopy, with minimal risk of cross-contamination or ventilatory insufficiency. The resistance of such small fistulae guarantees that most of the tidal volume will distribute to functional lung. A patent drainage system guards against a tension pneumothorax. Care should obviously be paid to the depth of insertion of the endotracheal tube, to avoid further disrupting a vulnerable pneumonectomy stump, if applicable.

Intermediate (several millimeters) or large BPFs deserve more respect for their capacity to "steal" tidal volume and cross-contaminate unaffected lung. Such patients might achieve adequate expansion of remaining lung during negative-pressure breathing, but during positive pressure mechanical ventilation, the majority of the tidal volume will pass preferentially through the low-resistance fistula. Several anesthetic options exist for the initial bronchoscopy. The most conservative option is an awake bronchoscopy, with topical anesthesia, sedation, and the head of the bed raised. With excellent topical anesthesia, many patients accept a laryngeal mask airway (LMA) or bite block to facilitate bronchoscopy. Judicious use of ultrashort-acting narcotics and distal airway topical anesthesia via the bronchoscope help prevent coughing. Alternatively, an intravenous induction with short-acting agents, intubation with a single-lumen endotracheal tube, and immediate bronchoscopy during a period of apnea can work very well. With thorough preoxygenation, the bronchoscopic examination can usually be completed before significant desaturation occurs. If the patient becomes hypoxic, the endotracheal tube can be advanced temporarily over the bronchoscope into the unaffected bronchus. With the cuff inflated, the oxygen saturation can be restored, and the tube can then easily be pulled back to complete the examination. Another alternative is to establish lung isolation with a DLT immediately and perform the evaluative bronchoscopy through the tracheal lumen of the DLT using a pediatric bronchoscope. The positioning of the DLT should be performed under direct fiberoptic observation to ensure that it does not inadvertently further disrupt a proximal bronchial stump. The other option is an inhalation induction while maintaining spontaneous ventilation. Disadvantages to this approach are that it takes time, thus enlarging the window for potential coughing and cross-contamination. In addition, the kinetics of an inhalation induction might be disrupted, depending on the extent of the air leak. Maintenance of a reliable anesthetic depth can be awkward when frequent suctioning from the bronchoscope combine with coughing and loss of agent through the fistula. Careful titration of total intravenous anesthesia (TIVA) can also accomplish induction while maintaining spontaneous respiration, but the margin between inadequate and excessive depth (apnea) could be narrow. Supplemental topical anesthesia to the airway can pave the way for bronchoscopy at a lighter plane of anesthesia.

Following bronchoscopy, the most convenient means of managing patients with large air leaks is to establish lung isolation rapidly by intubating the unaffected bronchus with a DLT (or endobronchial tube). Here again, it is important that the DLT be guided into place under direct fiberoptic guidance, to ensure rapid, accurate placement, and to prevent further disruption of an already compromised bronchial stump. Once in place with the bronchial cuff inflated, conventional OLV via the bronchial lumen can be employed without air leak through the fistula or risk of soiling the unaffected lung. If the patient's oxygen saturation declines during the intubation process, small tidal volume breaths of 100% oxygen through the bronchial lumen (or facemask) will generally temporize sufficiently to complete the intubation. Meticulous preoxygenation should precede the intubation, and short-acting induction agents should be used to allow return to spontaneous ventilation if undue difficulty is encountered. Raising the head of the bed and tilting the patient "fistula-side down" reduce the chances of cross-contamination. Alternatively, the placement of a protective DLT can be performed in an awake patient with sedation and topical anesthesia, or in an anesthetized, spontaneously breathing patient, as described previously for bronchoscopy.

Nonpneumonectomy patients with a large BPF and inadequate single-lung oxygenation might require alternative support in the operating room (or in the ICU for a period of time until the fistula closes). The options include conventional two-lung ventilation, unconventional two-lung ventilation (high-frequency or independent-lung ventilation), or, rarely, extracorporeal membrane oxygenation (ECMO). Conventional two-lung ventilatory techniques can adopt several strategies to minimize fistula airflow. In general, airleak flows are closely tied to mean airway pressures.[56] Ventilator settings aimed at reducing mean airway pressure and fistula airflow include small tidal volumes and rapid respiratory rates. When the BPF is in a distal airway, it might be possible to place a bronchial blocker in the appropriate lobar bronchus.[57] As mentioned previously, one-way valves in the chest tube apparatus, synchronized to the ventilator, can be timed to occlude (increase fistula airflow resistance) during inspiration. Conventional extrinsic PEEP is not practical with a BPF because the fistula releases the pressure, though some have attempted to infuse air into the chest during expiration to create a backpressure equal to the set PEEP.[53] In general, such in-line chest tube valve systems require close supervision and are prone to malfunction from the blood and pus passing through them.

Independent lung ventilation (ILV) is an alternative technique. The patient must be intubated with a double-lumen endotracheal tube, and the unaffected lung is ventilated conventionally. The remaining lung on the side of the fistula may be ventilated at different settings, synchronously or asynchronously, usually with a separate ventilator.[58,59] ILV seeks to optimize lung recruitment and gas exchange in two lungs of markedly different compliance, while minimizing airflow

across the fistula. Management of two ventilators is complex, labor intensive, and requires close monitoring. Others have described the use of a variable-resistance valve placed in the lumen that serves the lung with the fistula.[59] Titration of the resistance of the valve decreases tidal volume, airway pressure, and fistula leak in the diseased lung, diverts tidal volume to the unaffected lung, and allows a measure of ILV with a single ventilator. Rather than independently ventilating the BPF side, the use of continous positive airway pressure (CPAP), adjusted to a level just below the opening pressure of the fistula, has also been suggested.[58] ILV with high-frequency ventilation to the fistula side, and conventional positive pressure ventilation to the unaffected lung, have been described also.[61]

The term "high-frequency ventilation" (HFV) encompasses a spectrum of alternative ventilation techniques, collectively characterized by respiratory rates in excess of 60 per minute. High-frequency positive pressure ventilation (HFPPV), high-frequency jet ventilation (HFJV), and high-frequency oscillation ventilation (HFOV) are subsets of HFV, roughly defined as indicated in Table 11-4.

Among those subtypes, HFJV is the most commonly employed alternative technique for patients with a BPF. Potential advantages of HFJV with relevant applications are listed in Table 11-5. The potential to achieve comparable (or improved) gas exchange at lower peak and mean airway pressures is the key advantage of HFJV in patients with a BPF. High peak airway pressures could increase the caliber of a fistula opening or extend a proximal dehiscence. Transfistula airflow is proportional to the difference between the mean pressures proximal and distal to the opening. In addition to theoretically reducing fistula stress and airflow, HFJV might improve recruitment and expansion of residual lung. With conventional ventilation—because the fistula possesses low resistance and infinite compliance—a significant portion of the tidal volume is "stolen" from functional lung, and extrinsic PEEP is decompressed by the fistula. With HFJV, the short expiratory time (0.1 to 0.2 seconds) leads to entrapment of air within functional lung to improve inflation and recruitment. Adjusting the HFJV parameters to optimize lung expansion results in increased airway peak and mean airway pressures, and, consequently, increased fistula airflow. The mechanism of gas delivery in HFJV is complex and incompletely understood. In

---

TABLE 11-4

Types of High-Frequency Ventilation

Type of HFV	Rate/Min	Type of Ventilator	Gas Entrainment	Process	
				Inspiration	Exhalation
HFPPV	60 to 100	Volume	No	Active*	Passive†
HFJV	100 to 400	Jet Pulsation	Yes	Active	Passive
HFOV	400 to 2400	Piston pump	Yes	Active	Passive

From Benumof J: High-frequency and high-flow apneic ventilation during thoracic surgery. In Benumof J: *Anesthesia for thoracic surgery,* ed 2, Philadelphia, 1995, WB Saunders.
HFV, High-frequency ventilation; *HFPPV,* high-frequency positive pressure ventilation; *HFJV,* high-frequency jet ventilation; *HFOV,* high-frequency oscillation ventilation.
*Caused by the ventilator.
†Caused by elastic recoil of lung.

TABLE 11-5

Potential Advantages of HFJV

Advantage	Application
Adequate gas exchange at lower peak and mean airway pressures	BPF in OR or ICU
Less hemodynamic compromise due to lower airway and intrathoracic pressures	ICU, OR procedures with closed chest
Motionless surgical field	Pulmonary resection, tracheal surgery
Small-bore catheter delivery apparatus	Patients with stenotic airways; tracheal reconstruction
Improved surgical access and view	Laryngeal surgery
Eliminates need for flammable endotracheal tube	Laser airway surgery

addition to mass movement of air, it could involve various degrees of enhanced molecular diffusion (Taylor dispersion), high-velocity gas flow, coaxial gas flow, and Pendelluft movement.[62]

Disadvantages of HFJV include the lack of standardization and unfamiliarity of the equipment, an inability to monitor distal airway pressures or end-tidal CO_2, and an inability to use potent inhalation agents without polluting the operating room. Potential complications include barotrauma from hyperinflation or direct pressure effect, airway dissection, mucosal damage due to shear stress, gastric distention, and tracheobronchitis from excessive drying and cooling due to expansion of gases at the jet orifice.[63] Important to the safe application of HFJV are training and familiarity with the equipment, adequate warming and humidification systems, close monitoring of blood pressures and arterial blood gasses, and a means of monitoring airway pressures—preferably with an automatic shutdown device to discontinue gas flow at high airway pressures. Airway pressure must be measured at least 10 cm distal to the jet orifice to prevent being confounded by the subatmospheric pressures in the entrainment zone close to the jet.[63] In addition, a means of monitoring fistula airflow is recommended to allow appropriate titration of HFJV parameters.[64]

Despite the theoretical advantages and multiple reports of the successful application of HFJV in patients with BPF, it has not proved universally advantageous in terms of gas exchange, fistula flow, and airway pressures.[56,65-69] The question of whether HFJV is superior to conventional ventilation for such patients is complicated by the broad diversity of HFJV techniques and settings, the lack of adequately controlled prospective trials, and the variability of the mechanical properties of BPFs (and lungs) between patients and within a given patient over time. A recent review described at least 27 different modifications of HFJV equipment and delivery techniques.[63] Despite these technical and methodologic impediments to generalized acceptance, the compelling theoretical advantages suggest that HFJV should be considered for patients with bilateral or large BPF airleaks who are difficult to manage by conventional ventilatory techniques, provided that adequate technical expertise with the equipment is available. Patients with relatively normal lung compliance and a large proximal fistula are most likely to benefit.[68]

Empyema and Decortication

Empyema is defined as purulent or infected material within the pleural space. Thus, an empyema can result from the pleural accumulation of infected fluid or the infection of accumulated pleural fluid. Causes of empyema are listed in Table 11-6.

The most common sequence of events usually involves inflammation of the pleura resulting in an expanding pleural effusion. If initially sterile, the effusion might become infected by the primary source (e.g., pneumonia), or by a secondary source (e.g., hematogenously or following thoracentesis). Persistent inflammation leads to fibrin deposition, pleural thickening, and the formation of a coagulum of viscous, suppurative effusion, usually with the formation of loculations. The lung becomes restricted by the fluid and eventually by the thickened visceral pleura (fibrothorax). Symptoms include fever, cough (often productive of purulent sputum), pleuritic chest pain, and various degrees of dyspnea. Diagnosis is usually made by aspiration of frank pus or infected fluid from a radiographically apparent pleural effusion.

The general treatment strategy for nonsurgical empyema is to establish effective drainage, administer appropriate antibiotics, and correct the underlying cause. Drainage techniques vary in accordance with the maturity of the empyema.[70] Early postpneumonic pleural effusions in which the fluid is of low viscosity and without pus or loculations can be drained by a trial of simple aspiration or percutaneous placement of a drainage catheter. When pleural aspirates are frankly purulent or viscous and productive of positive cultures, tube thoracostomy continuous drainage with saline and antibiotic irrigation is indicated. Effusions that appear uniloculate at this stage often have fibrinous strands criss-crossing the pleural space and impairing drainage. Irrigation with fibrinolytics has been useful in some trials, but not in others.[71,72] Thoracoscopic drainage and breakdown of septae are often necessary. Advanced and complicated empyemas with loculations, viscous pus, grossly thickened pleura, and trapped lung require a VATS or thoracotomy incision to decorticate, break down loculations, and establish definitive drainage (Figure 11-13).[70]

Postsurgical empyemas following pneumonectomy are usually associated with a BPF (see the foregoing discussion). Even in the absence of an air leak, a BPF should be suspected and actively sought by bronchoscopy. Following initial stabilization with a thoracostomy drainage tube and antibiotics, surgical

TABLE 11-6

Causes of Empyema

Pulmonary infections (postpneumonic)
Postsurgical (lung, mediastinal, subdiaphragmatic surgery)
Bronchopleural fistula
Septicemia
Iatrogenic (e.g., following thoracentesis)
Trauma
Subdiaphragmatic infections/peritonitis
Esophageal perforation
Rupture of infected pleural bleb
Lung abscess
Spontaneous pneumothorax

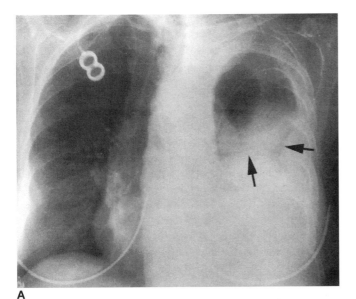

A

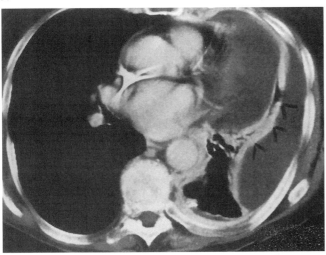

B

FIGURE 11-13 Empyema and loculated pleural effusion. **A,** Lobulated contours *(arrows)* of peripheral opacity on posteroanterior chest x-ray suggests loculation. **B,** Computed tomographic scan demonstrates two locules of fluid separated by contrast-enhanced lung (arrowheads). (From Curtis A, Miller WT: Radiographic evaluation of the lungs and chest. In Shields TW, LoCicero J, Ponn RE [eds]: *General thoracic surgery,* ed 5, Philadelphia, 2000, Lippincott Williams & Wilkins.)

debridement of necrotic tissue and loculations by a thoracotomy or VATS approach is usually indicated. If a BPF is present, open drainage procedures are generally employed in the form of a Clagett procedure, Eloesser flap, or modifications thereof. The original Clagett procedure involved opening the anterior portion of the preexisting thoracotomy incision, removing a 3-inch segment of the seventh rib at the anterior or midaxillary line, and suturing the superficial fascia down to the periosteum of the resected rib.[73] The resulting open drain was packed with antibiotic-soaked dressings. After 2 to 3 days, systemic symptoms of the empyema abated, and patients were sent home for 6 to 8 weeks of frequent dressing changes, after which the wound was closed in layers and the hemithorax was filled with antibiotic solution.[73] If a BPF is present, a well-vascularized muscle flap

is mobilized to cover the stump and fistula (modified Clagett procedure).[48] An Eloesser flap is a similar open drainage system, involving a limited thoracotomy and rib resection with suturing of a flap of skin to the pleura, to create an epithelium-lined sinus. Most surgeons advocate obliteration of postpneumonectomy empyema cavities with extrathoracic muscle flaps (Figure 11-14).

When empyema complicates lobectomy or lesser resections, the acute treatment consists of the same closed chest tube drainage with antibiotics. Simple drainage is often sufficient for empyemas following lower lobectomies, because the remaining lung tends to fill the space. Apical resections or upper lobectomies are more likely to require open drainage or a muscle-flap closure to obliterate the empyema space.[74]

If a fibrothorax has developed, decortication is essential to allow full reexpansion of the remaining lung. Decortication refers to the process of stripping or peeling off the restricting fibrous layer. A fibrothorax usually results from an empyema, but it can also be seen in association with a hemothorax or any long-standing extensive pleural inflammatory process. Decortication is usually indicated when closed drainage or thoracoscopic efforts have failed to clear the pleural space and symptomatic pulmonary restrictive physiology has developed as a result of a fibrothorax.[75] A VATS approach might suffice when the process is early or limited, but most established fibrothoraces require a thoracotomy incision for effective decortication.[76] By blunt and sharp dissection, the parietal pleura is stripped from the chest wall, along with the fibrinous peel in the area of interest. To various degrees, the visceral pleura might also require removal. Bleeding results from the avulsion of numerous small blood vessels in the chest wall. Air leaks result from the disruption of numerous alveoli on the surface of the lung during visceral pleurectomy. Both bleeding and air leaks generally resolve with full reexpansion of the lung. Failure to obliterate the space by full reexpansion or transposition

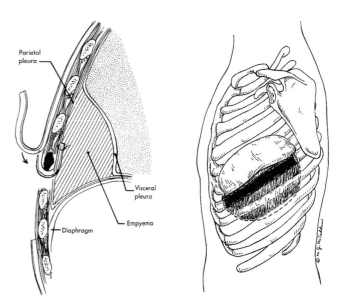

FIGURE 11-14 Schematic of Eloesser flap for open drainage of an empyema. (From Cohen RG, DeMeester TR, LaFontaine E: The pleura. In Sabiston DC, Spencer FC [eds]: *Surgery of the chest,* ed 6, Philadelphia, 1995, WB Saunders.)

of muscle flaps invites the reaccumulation of fluid and the recurrence of empyema (as well as significant postoperative bleeding and air leak).

ANESTHETIC CONSIDERATIONS FOR EMPYEMAS AND DECORTICATION

The principal anesthetic issue for patients with empyemas is to prevent the contamination of uninfected lung. If a BPF coexists, the ventilatory considerations previously described would apply also. Preoperatively, effective drainage, antibiotic therapy, intravenous hydration, and nutritional and metabolic support are ideal. Often, loculations prevent optimal drainage of the empyema. The patient should be assessed for the degree to which he or she is debilitated by chronic infection. CT scans should be viewed to assess residual loculated fluid or pus and the effect of the empyema or fibrothorax on remaining lung.

An initial bronchoscopic evaluation is usually performed to clean out and assess the affected bronchus or stump. This can be done with either sedation or general anesthesia. Lung isolation is then best accomplished with a DLT positioned under fiberoptic observation to prevent disruption of a bronchial stump, if applicable. Confirmation of correct placement and adequate bronchial balloon inflation should be unambiguously confirmed by fiberoptic bronchoscopy prior to turning the patient to the lateral decubitus position. Frequent suctioning of infected material from the tracheal lumen is often necessary during the case and should be performed assiduously prior to deflating the bronchial cuff at the end of the case. Reexpansion of functional lung that had been restricted by empyema or fibrothorax is an important step as the chest is closed. A final bronchoscopic cleaning and evaluation for the presence of a BPF usually are performed by the surgeon prior to emergence.

Thoracic epidural analgesia is usually not necessary for empyema cases, and there is a theoretic risk of hematogenous seeding of the catheter from bacteremia. With appropriate preoperative antibiotics, the risk of an epidural abscess from a thoracic epidural is likely remote, but worth considering.

If a fibrothorax is present, there could be significant restrictive physiology requiring frequent, low tidal-volume ventilations. Decortication might actually be easier if the affected lung is inflated rather than deflated, and some surgeons will request this. Decortication often results in significant blood loss and air leaks, which will be alleviated by reexpansion of remaining ipsilateral lung at the end of the case (or by obliteration of the space in the case of postpneumonectomy empyemas).

Lung Abscess

A lung abscess is a suppurative, cavitary lesion within the lung parenchyma, often with an air-fluid level. Historically, lung abscesses were important causes of pneumonia-associated deaths. Currently, antibiotics control most lung abscesses, occasionally with the aid of surgery, though debilitated, malnourished, or immunosuppressed individuals remain particularly vulnerable.

Aspiration (often related to alcoholism or a seizure disorder) by an individual with poor dental hygiene is the most common scenario leading to a lung abscess. The resulting pyogenic pneumonitis leads to bacterial proliferation, leukocyte accumulation, liquefaction necrosis, and formation of a fibrinous cavitary wall. Periodic partial drainage into a bronchocavitary fistula produces the classic air-fluid level. The most common anaerobic agent is *Bacteroides*, though other pyogenic bacteria, mycobacteria, fungi, and parasites can be causative agents. Among other potential etiologies of lung abscesses are pneumonia, foreign-body aspiration, BPF, obstructive bronchial carcinoma, pulmonary infarction, and infectious emboli from right-sided endocarditis.

Symptoms are similar to those for empyema. Intermittent fever, night sweats, weight loss, a cough productive of putrid, purulent sputum, and a history suggestive of aspiration and/or poor dental hygiene are suggestive. Serial chest radiography reveals a pulmonary infiltrate that gradually organizes into a cavitary lesion with a central lucency, with or without an air-fluid level. CT scans help distinguish a peripheral abscess from an empyema. Ninty-five percent of lung abscesses occur in the superior segments of the lower lobes and the axillary subsegment of the right upper lobe.[74]

Treatment consists of 6 to 8 weeks of antibiotics, with adequate drainage facilitated by chest physiotherapy. Fiberoptic bronchoscopy is indicated to obtain pus for culture and sensitivity testing, to rule out a malignancy or foreign body, or to aid drainage. CT-guided percutaneous drainage is indicated when the abscess does not drain adequately internally. Occasionally, closed-chest tube thoracostomy or open pneumonostomy is required to achieve drainage. Indications for surgical intervention include failure to respond to medical management, suspicion of carcinoma, significant hemoptysis, and complications of lung abscess, such as bronchopleural fistula or empyema. If symptoms precede antibiotic treatment by more than 12 weeks, or if the abscess is greater than 4 cm in diameter, the likelihood that antibiotics alone will be sufficient is low.[77] Surgical resection is also usually recommended for persistent cavities that are large (more than 6 cm) or thick walled. An algorithm for the management of lung abscesses is provided in Figure 11-15.

ANESTHETIC CONSIDERATIONS

Protection of uninfected lung from contamination, as described for the management of patients with empyema, is the central anesthetic consideration for patients with lung abscesses. Patients with abscesses are more likely to have a history of alcoholism and poor dentition, and are less likely to have had recent lung resection surgery. In other respects, patients with lung abscesses should be treated as described for patients with an empyema.

Pulmonary Arteriovenous Malformations

Pulmonary arteriovenous malformations (AVMs) are congenital, abnormal communications between pulmonary arteries and veins. Dysgenesis of the microvasculature during development results in the coalescence of capillaries and venules to form a vascular sac joining dilated feeding arteries to pulmonary veins.[78] Functionally, they represent right-to-left intrapulmonary shunts, which fail to perform gas exchange or filtering functions. Other abnormal pulmonary arteriovenous communications can exist. Systemic AVMs between the bronchial arteries and pulmonary veins representing left-to-right shunts might exist but are exceedingly rare and functionally more benign. Acquired intrapulmonary vascular shunts can occur from traumatic or surgically associated arteriovenous fistulas or

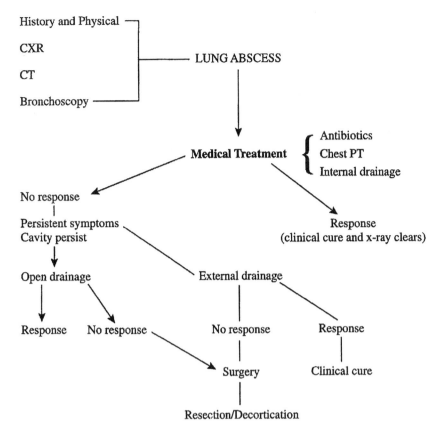

FIGURE 11-15 Algorithm for the management of lung abscess. *CT,* Computed tomography; *CXR,* chest x-ray; *PT,* pneumothorax. (From Miller JI: Bacterial infections of the lungs and bronchial compressive disorders. In Shields TW, LoCicero J, Ponn RE [eds]: *General thoracic surgery,* ed 5, Philadelphia, 2000, Lippincott Williams & Wilkins.)

from remodeling of the microvasculature in association with the hepatopulmonary syndrome, portal hypertension, or schistosomiasis.[78] Only the macroscopic congenital pulmonary AVMs for which intervention is indicated are germane to this discussion.

The consequences and natural history of macroscopic pulmonary AVMs are not benign. Hypoxemia occurs in proportion to the amount of cardiac output passing through the AVM. Paradoxic embolization can result in transient ischemic attacks, embolic strokes, and brain abscesses. Rupture or bleeding can result in hemoptysis or hemothorax. Most brain abscesses contain anaerobes suggestive of an oral origin, emphasizing the importance of antibiotic prophylaxis prior to dental procedures. Pulmonary AVMs are more common in females, and their size appears to be influenced by estrogen and progesterone. Pregnancy enhances the growth of pulmonary AVMs and increases the risk of hemorrhage and stroke.[79,80] Arterial oxygenation tends to improve during pregnancy, and the fetus tends to fare well, but maternal hypoxemia markedly deteriorates after delivery to levels below prepregnancy values.[78]

Eighty percent of angiographically demonstrable pulmonary AVMs are associated with the congenital syndrome of hereditary hemorrhagic telangiectasias (HHT) (formerly called Rendu-Osler-Weber disease).[78] The remainder are idiopathic or developmental. The distinction is relevant because HHT has associated disease and a more dire prognosis. Extrapulmonary lesions associated with HHT include systemic AVMs and facial, mucocutaneous, and gastrointestinal telangiectasias. Patients with HHT exhibit frequent spontaneous epistaxis, characteristic telangiectasia, polycythemia, hypoxemia, exertional dyspnea, and migraine headaches. Bleeding from gastrointestinal telangiectasia or epistaxis can convert polycythemia to anemia in some. Most important, pulmonary AVMs in patients with HHT are more likely to be multiple and to produce a more predictable progression of neurologic and hypoxemic complications.[81] The prevalence of neurologic events in patients with pulmonary AVMs is as high as 40%, and the probability increases with age, the size and number of AVMs, and the total shunt flow over time.[82] This ongoing threat of neurologic complications justifies intervention when possible. The pattern of inheritance in HHT is autosomal dominant. If a diagnosis of HHT is established, relatives should be screened for pulmonary AVMs.

The characteristic radiographic appearance of pulmonary AVMs is one of a lobulated, well-defined opacity connected to the hilum by broad linear shadows representing dilated feeding vessels (Figure 11-16). Lesions are multiple and bilateral and occur in caudal lung zones in the vast majority of cases.[82] Occasionally, a solitary lesion might be misinterpreted as a nodule. Auscultation can reveal a rough, humming, continuous bruit, which is accentuated in systole and with deep inspiration. On fluoroscopy, lesions are pulsatile and become

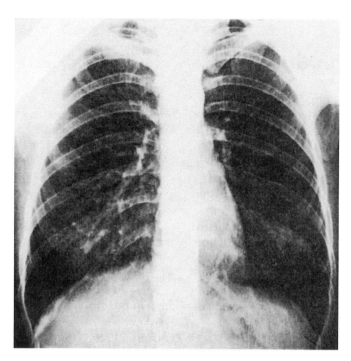

FIGURE 11-16 Chest x-ray of a patient with multiple pulmonary arteriovenous fistulas in the lower lobes. (From Dines DE et al: *Mayo Clin Proc* 58:176, 1995.)

smaller with the Valsalva maneuver. Computed tomography (CT) is noninvasive and more sensitive than chest x-ray as a screening tool. Contrast angiography is the accepted study to define the feeding vessels prior to intervention, although three-dimensional magnetic resonance angiography (MRA) was shown to be a promising potential alternative in recent reports.[83,84] Contrast echocardiography is a sensitive, noninvasive technique for detection of pulmonary arteriovenous shunts, but its place as a screening test remains undefined.[85] A test with a positive result consists of the echocardiographic detection of microcavitations in the left atrium three to six cardiac cycles following the intravenous injection of agitated saline (the earlier appearance of contrast would suggest an intracardiac shunt). Perfusion lung scintigraphy can estimate the magnitude of shunt. Blood gas abnormalities are relatively insensitive screening tests.

Treatment (resection or obliteration) is justified for essentially all radiographically detectable or symptomatic pulmonary AVMs to prevent neurologic sequelae.[81] Even asymptomatic pulmonary AVMs should be addressed for patients with HHT. Surgical excision is recommended for most single or selected multiple lesions. AVMs with a systemic blood supply should be excised surgically.[86] Coexisting pulmonary hypertension is considered a contraindication to surgical excision by some.[81] The choice of surgical approach (thoracotomy vs. VATS) is dictated by the size and location of the lesion and its feeding vessels. Radiographically guided embolization techniques using balloons or coils are evolving and are increasingly preferred for many multiple or bilateral pulmonary AVMs.[81] The technique involves the percutaneous positioning of stainless steel coils or detachable balloons into the feeding vessels to occlude flow and create a thrombosis of

the AVM. Advantages of embolotherapy are that it can be performed under local anesthesia, it is less invasive, and it more precisely targets the AVM with less destruction of functional lung parenchyma. Potential complications include failures of embolization, vascular damage, partial recanalization, ectopic deposition of a coil, delayed bacterial contamination of a thrombus, and pulmonary infarction. The rates of these complications are low, and increasingly effective embolotherapy is sparing many patients from surgery. Successful closure of a large pulmonary AVM using a transcatheter double umbrella device (Cardioseal) normally designed for closure of intracardiac communications has been reported.[87]

ANESTHETIC CONSIDERATIONS FOR PULMONARY AVMS

Patients with pulmonary AVMs might come to surgery for primary resection of one or more lesions or because of the failure of embolotherapeutic efforts. The central anesthetic considerations include provision of adequate oxygenation in the presence of the right-to-left shunt, effective lung isolation, and avoidance of embolic complications.

The magnitude of the shunt can be quite variable. In one series, shunt magnitude varied from 4% to 60% of the cardiac output.[82] It is unusual to have insurmountable difficulties with oxygenation. Because most pulmonary AVMs occur in basal regions of the lung, shunt flow is usually reduced (and oxygenation improved) when patients move from the upright to the supine position. Lateral decubitus positioning (with the lesion nondependent) further engages gravity's aid in reducing shunt blood flow. Patients with bilateral, large AVMs are more complex and should have the larger lesion resected first. Conditions that might redirect blood flow from the dependent to the nondependent lung (hypoxemia, hypercarbia, acidosis, excessive airway pressures including intrinsic or extrinsic PEEP) should be minimized. Increases in pulmonary vascular resistance result in relative increases in flow through low-resistance AVMs. CPAP to the nondependent lung would be expected to have a reduced effectiveness as a rescue maneuver because of the nondependent lung AVM. The usual expected obligatory shunt in the nondependent lung during OLV is likely to be larger as a result of the AVM and the absence of HPV within the AVM. An F_{IO_2} of 100% should be employed during the OLV phase. High inspired concentrations of oxygen do not improve oxygenation directly from a pure shunt such as an AVM, but they might do so indirectly by reducing pulmonary vascular resistance and thereby the fraction of cardiac output through the shunt. Management is simplified as soon as the feeding arteries to the AVM are crossclamped. Nevertheless, it must be remembered that coexisting residual microscopic or macroscopic pulmonary AVMs are likely to be present, particularly in patients with HHT.

Separation of the lungs can be accomplished by any of the usual techniques. Effective lung separation not only aids surgical access to the hilum but also protects against blood contamination of the contralateral lung. Assiduous attention to de-airing maneuvers and use of air filters are important, even after excision of the target AVM, because of the frequent existence of multiple lesions. Nitrous oxide should be avoided in deference to the threats of both air emboli and hypoxemia.

Blood loss for a pulmonary AVM procedure is likely to be greater than for a comparable pulmonary resection for cancer.

An arterial catheter might be useful for hemodynamic monitoring as well as for comparison of arterial blood gasses before and after excision of the AVM. Further invasive hemodynamic monitoring should be dictated by the patient's perceived cardiovascular reserve. Pulmonary AVMs are usually associated with normal pulmonary arterial and right-sided heart pressures. Many patients, however, present in their fourth or fifth decade and might have significant coexisting disease. In a recent case report, contrast transesophageal echocardiography together with a pulmonary artery catheter proved useful to diagnose and partially localize a traumatic pulmonary arteriovenous fistula.[88] If a pulmonary artery catheter is used, care must be taken to ensure that it is not in the field of resection at the time of crossclamping.

Most patients with pulmonary AVMs have HHT. Their propensity for epistaxis argues against the nasal route for intubations, gastric tubes, or temperature probes. Oral telangiectasia might be noted during intubation, but these rarely are a source of bleeding. A history of neurologic complications should be sought. Either polycythemia or anemia could be present, depending on the patient's history of bleeding from gastrointestinal telangiectasias. A prior history of blood transfusions is not uncommon.

Lung Cysts and Bullae

Lung cysts and bullae can be considered together as thin-walled air- or fluid-filled cavities within the pulmonary parenchyma. There are many potential causes in adults, which can be classified broadly as acquired or residual congenital pulmonary cysts or bullae (Table 11-7). They might be sources of infection, pneumothorax, or air trapping, leading to space-occupying lesions that impair adjacent lung function. Anesthetic issues are comparable and are considered collectively. Cysts resulting from trauma are omitted from surgical and anesthetic discussion because they tend to resolve spontaneously. Mediastinal cysts are also excluded, although they can impinge on pulmonary parenchyma.

CONGENITAL PULMONARY CYSTS AND BULLAE

Bronchogenic Cysts. Congenital bronchogenic cysts are products of abnormalities in the tracheobronchial budding process of lung organogenesis. They can occur peripherally within the lung parenchyma (70%) or centrally attached to the mediastinum or hilum. Peripheral bronchogenic cysts result when the distal tip of a developing bronchial arborization becomes separated from the parent branch. The small groups of sequestered cells develop into thin-walled cysts lined with ciliated columnar or cuboidal epithelium with a fibromuscular

TABLE 11-7

Lung Cysts and Bullae

Congenital pulmonary cysts and bullae	Bronchogenic cysts Congenital cystic adenomatoid malformation Pulmonary sequestration Congenital lobar emphysema
Acquired pulmonary cysts and bullae	Bullous emphysema Pulmonary hydatid cyst Traumatic lung cyst Pneumatocele

base and occasionally with cartilage or bronchial glands.[89] Central bronchogenic cysts develop similarly from earlier budding errors. Widespread congenital cysts producing a so-called honeycomb lung are incompatible with life.

Bronchogenic cysts become problematic if they become enlarged and exert a mass effect on functional lung or mediastinal structures ("tension cyst"), if they rupture and create a pneumothorax, or if they become infected. Small cysts without communications to a bronchus are asymptomatic and can be noted incidentally as round, clearly demarcated lesions on chest radiographs. Communicating cysts often produce air-fluid levels, are prone to recurrent infection, and can trap air by a ball-valve mechanism, thus risking rapid expansion or rupture. Infected cysts can be obscured by surrounding pneumonia or might be difficult to differentiate from an empyema. CT scans help differentiate cystic lesions from solid ones. The symptoms of an infected cyst include the familiar syndrome of fever, cough, expectoration of purulent sputum, and occasional hemoptysis. Should a tension cyst cause acute cardiopulmonary instability, emergent needle aspiration of the cyst might serve as a temporizing solution. Conservative surgical excision of bronchogenic cysts is generally recommended, whether a bronchial communication is evident.

Congenital cystic adenomatoid malformation. Congenital cystic adenomatoid malformations (CCAMs) are rare pulmonary lesions derived from the abnormal proliferation of terminal bronchioles, with failure of normal alveolar maturation. CCAM lesions usually arise from a single lobe, have variable numbers and sizes of cysts, and usually do not communicate directly with the tracheobronchial tree (Figure 11-17). Various classifications have been imposed on CCAM subtypes, but the most important prognostic feature is the size of the mass.[90] In utero, the mass effect of large lung tumors can cause maternal polyhydramnios (from fetal esophageal compression) and fetal hydrops (from mediastinal shift and cardiac/superior vena caval compression). Ultrasonographic studies prompted by maternal polyhydramnios usually make the diagnosis. Without prenatal intervention, fetal hydrops usually results in fetal or neonatal demise. Although it is available in only a few centers, in utero fetal surgery (resection or thoracoamniotic shunt placement) performed at 24 to 32 weeks have yielded excellent outcomes.[90] Intermediate-sized CCAMs can cause various degrees of neonatal respiratory compromise by their mass effects. Emergency neonatal surgery could be required to decompress functional lung tissue, which might be hypoplastic. Approximately 15% of CCAMs will shrink or disappear during gestation.[90] Small, primarily cystic lesions might be well tolerated and escape detection until later in life. In adults, CCAM could be an incidental finding or a source of recurrent infections. Abnormal communications with the tracheobronchial tree can develop and provide a source of fluid and infection in the cysts. Carcinomas, apparently arising within CCAM lesions, have been reported.[91] Surgical excision (usually lobectomy) is recommended for symptomatic or asymptomatic CCAM lesions.

Pulmonary sequestration. Pulmonary sequestrations are masses of nonfunctioning lung tissue without a connection to the tracheobronchial tree. They have an anomalous systemic arterial supply that usually arises from the aorta above or

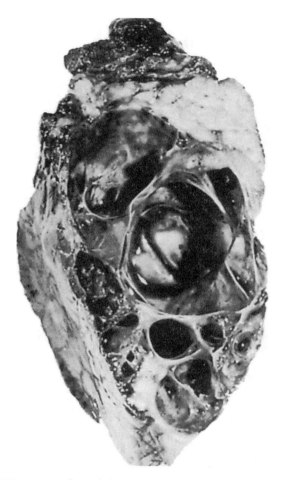

FIGURE 11-17 Congenital cystic adenomatous malformation. (From Reynolds M: Congenital lesions of the lung. In Shields TW, LoCicero J, Ponn RE [eds]: *General thoracic surgery*, ed 5, Philadelphia, 2000, Lippincott Williams & Wilkins.)

below the diaphragm. There are two categories: intralobar and extralobar. Early accessory lung buds (fifth or sixth week of gestation) give rise to intralobar pulmonary sequestrations, which are completely enclosed within a lobe. Extralobar pulmonary sequestrations are thought to arise from accessory lung buds that appear later in development. The extralobar form is a completely separate mass with its own visceral pleura. On ultrasound examination, extralobar sequestrations might be indistinguishable from microcystic CCAMs. Like CCAMs, the mass effect of pulmonary sequestrations can cause fetal hydrops, fetal demise, or neonatal respiratory compromise. Unlike CCAMs, the majority (68%) of pulmonary sequestrations spontaneously shrink or involute during gestation.[90] The development of fetal hydrops is ominous and justifies antenatal intervention if available. This usually consists of drainage of polyhydramnios or thoracoamniotic shunting.

Intralobar pulmonary sequestrations are more likely to escape early detection and often present with recurrent infections in the second or third decade of life. The source of infections could be via the pores of Kohn. Infection might lead to abscess formation, which can cloud the diagnosis. Associated anomalies are uncommon, and venous drainage is more predictably through the inferior pulmonary vein. The systemic

arterial supply usually arises from the abdominal aorta and penetrates the diaphragm. The treatment for intralobar sequestration is usually lobectomy, as inflammatory changes often preclude an anatomic segmentectomy.

Small extralobar sequestrations might also escape early detection until revealed by recurrent infections or an incidental x-ray. Extralobar sequestrations usually occur in the left chest, but can also be found in the mediastinum or beneath the diaphragm. They are more commonly associated with other congenital anomalies, including congenital diaphragmatic hernias. The arterial supply and venous drainage might be more variable, and infections can result from communications with the foregut.[89] Surgical excision of extralobar sequestrations is usually straightforward because of its separate visceral pleura. The principal surgical consideration for both types of sequestration is to correctly identify and control the anomalous feeding and draining vessels.

Congenital lobar emphysema. Congenital lobar emphysema is a rare condition of newborns and infants characterized by the isolated hyperinflation of a lobe in the absence of extrinsic bronchial compression.[89] Causes of this include hypoplasia, dysplasia, or absence of bronchial cartilage, leading to dynamic obstruction and air trapping within the affected lung. In many cases, the cause is unknown. This is most commonly a disorder of an upper lobe or of the right middle lobe presenting in the first six months of life. Tachypnea, cyanosis, and wheezing, with hyperresonance and decreased breath sounds on the affected side, characteristically prompt an x-ray and the expectation of a tension pneumothorax. Careful inspection for vascular markings is necessary to make this distinction. Physiologically, the effect is identical. A chest CT can be useful in excluding extrinsic causes of bronchial compression from enlarged lymph nodes, bronchogenic cysts, or anomalous blood vessels. The surgical treatment of choice is lobectomy.[92] Bronchoscopy should immediately precede surgery to rule out reversible endobronchial lesions or a foreign body and to assess the extent of bronchial collapse. The hazards of general anesthesia are such that surgeons must be prepared to open and decompress the emphysematous hemithorax upon induction if necessary (see the discussion that follows).

ACQUIRED PULMONARY CYSTS AND BULLAE

Bullous emphysema. Emphysematous bullae are thin-walled subpleural air sacs formed as a result of the destructive process of emphysema. Blebs are intrapleural collections of air bounded by thin layers of the visceral pleura. Blebs tend to be more unstable than bullae and more prone to spontaneous rupture. Both can expand to impressive dimensions and impair the respiratory function of the remainder of the lung, rupture (pneumothorax), or, rarely, become infected or cause hemoptysis. Giant bullae, by definition, occupy more than 50% of the affected hemithorax (Figure 11-18). Bullae freely communicate with the bronchial tree through multiple small openings. They could appear to be a single sac with a narrow neck, a coalescence of many parent bullae with a broad neck, or a widespread diffuse pattern involving multiple lobes.

Classically, the origin and progressive enlargement of bullae have been attributed to the trapping of air by a presumed ball-valve mechanism in the bronchial communications. This concept was challenged in the 1980s by dynamic CT scan

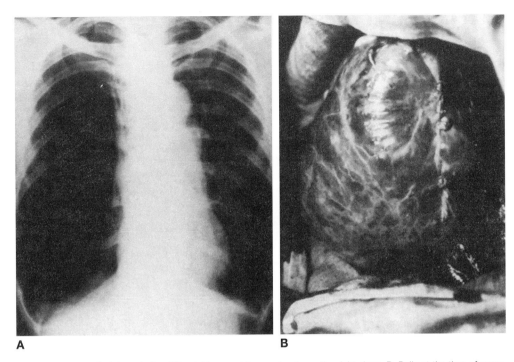

A   **B**

FIGURE 11-18 **A,** A large bulla of the right upper lob occupies the entire right chest. **B,** Bulla at the time of operation. (From Ferguson TB Jr, Ferguson TB: Congenital lesions of the lung and emphysema. In Sabiston DC, Spencer FC [ed]: *Surgery of the chest,* ed 6, Philadelphia, 1995, WB Saunders.)

observations and intrabullous pressure measurements that were found to be incompatible with that hypothesis. Currently, it is thought that bullae enlarge because of compliance differences between the surrounding lung and the enlarged airspaces that form from emphysematous destruction of alveolar walls. During inspiration, air preferentially enters the more compliant airspace (bulla) at the expense of inflation of less compliant surrounding parenchyma. Air can be "trapped" within bullae more because of the preferential inflation and reduced elastic recoil (relative to surrounding lung tissue) than from any physical ball-valve mechanism in the bronchial communications. Nevertheless, expiratory airflow obstruction that is characteristic of emphysema contributes to the expansion of bullae over time. Superimposed ball-valve mechanisms have been postulated for cases of sudden, rapid expansion of a preexisting bulla.

Large bullae or blebs impair respiration and exercise tolerance in several ways. As space-occupying lesions, they impair expansion of adjacent lung parenchyma. The reduction in the volume of adjacent, functional lung results in decreased elastic recoil. Small airways are in part held open by a "traction effect" of surrounding parenchyma. Emphysema leads to increased airways resistance, in part because of a decrease in this traction effect. Large bullae exacerbate this tendency by further reducing the volume of functional lung. Distortion of bronchial anatomy can further increase airway obstruction. In severe cases, bullae or blebs can exert a compressive effect on airways or on intrathoracic vascular structures. The mechanics of respiration are disadvantaged by the flattened diaphragm and hyperexpanded rib cage of bullous emphysema. Bullae can be sources of increased deadspace and work of breathing. Most bullae, however, have such limited ventilation that they contribute little to deadspace.[93]

Rupture of a bulla or bleb results in a pneumothorax, which is pathophysiologically similar to a bronchopleural fistula. An initial spontaneous pneumothorax in a young person generally resolves with simple tube thoracostomy treatment (or conservative treatment if smaller than 20% of the lung). Older patients with rupture of a large emphysematous bulla often have large air leaks, loculated air spaces, and a poorer response to chest-tube therapy. Symphysis between the parietal pleura and lung can take much longer or can require pleurodesis.

Surgical bullectomy (or blebectomy) is indicated when an unruptured bulla grows to affect respiratory function significantly and leads to dyspnea. Most authors agree that prophylactic bullectomy is justified in the nondyspneic patient if the bulla occupies more than half the hemithorax, compresses normal lung, or has enlarged significantly following a period of radiographic observation. A compressive effect is deduced from evidence of vascular displacement or crowding in adjacent parenchyma, hilar or mediastinal displacement, displacement of fissures, or anterior mediastinal herniation of the lung. The improvement in volume, elastic recoil, airway traction, and respiratory mechanisms for the remaining lung must be weighed against the significant operative risks imposed by the advanced COPD and coexisting diseases that invariably accompany emphysematous bullae.

The goal of bullectomy surgery is to reduce or eliminate the space-occupying effect of the bulla while preserving all functional lung. This goal can be achieved by bullectomy, plication, or intracavitary tube suction and drainage of the bulla.[94] Plication involves folding the visceral pleura upon itself to create a more robust, multilayered tissue for the purchase of staples or sutures. Operative bullectomy should involve lobectomy only if the entire lobe is destroyed. Bullectomy can be performed via various thoracotomy incisions, but a VATS approach is increasingly common. Bilateral apical bullectomies can be performed by separate staged procedures or by a single median sternotomy approach. Surgical considerations include proper identification of the base of the bulla and elimination of air leaks and residual space. Air leaks tend to be the most problematic phenomena. Plication techniques, stapling devices, pleurodesis, and the buttressing of staple lines with Teflon, bovine pericardium,or other reinforcing material have been employed toward this end (see the section on lung volume reduction surgery in Chapter 12). Pleural tenting procedures, in which a region of overlying parietal pleura is freed from the chest wall, is sometimes employed to provide a cover to obliterate the pleural space following bullectomy. Rapid postoperative extubation is sought to minimize positive airway pressures against the staple line.

Pulmonary hydatid cysts. Hydatid cysts of the lung are watery, parasitic cysts, containing larvae of the dog tapeworm, *Echinococcus granulosus*. Echinococcosis is a relatively common cause of pulmonary cysts in endemic regions—and increasingly, among travelers. Endemic areas are typically sheep- and cattle-raising regions (Australia, New Zealand, South America, and some Mediterranean regions). Cysts can be several millimeters in diameter or grow to nearly fill the hemithorax in which they are contained. The serumlike, crystal-clear, watery hydatid fluid suspends larvae within and is surrounded by a thin transparent membrane (endocyst) and an outer laminated membrane.

Hydatid cysts can grow in diameter by as much as 5 cm/yr and become medically problematic in several ways. By mass effect, they can exert pressure on adjacent structures (bronchus, great vessels, esophagus, etc.). Spontaneous or traumatic rupture may occur, sending fluid, parasites, or laminated debris into adjacent tissue, bronchus, pleura, or the circulation (systemic emboli).

Hypersensitivity reactions, bronchospasm, and anaphylaxis can result. Surrounding tissues can develop secondary echinococcosis, and the residual cavity can become infected and develop into an abscess. Drainage into the bronchi might cause only minor coughing and expectoration of fluid and laminated debris, or it might cause dramatic expulsion of fluid with respiratory distress or asphyxiation, depending on the amount of fluid involved. Similarly, rupture into the pleural space might cause only minor symptoms (mild dyspnea, fever, cough or chest pain), or it could result in a large hydropneumothorax, severe dyspnea, shock, suffocation, or anaphylaxis. Rupture becomes more dangerous and more likely as cysts become larger. It is recommended that any cyst larger than 7 cm be removed.[95]

Radiographically, hydatid cysts appear as smoothly outlined, dense spherical opacities. Medical treatment (benzimidazole compounds) has limited efficacy and significant side effects and are recommended only for patients considered inoperable (due to disseminated disease, difficult location, etc.). Surgical goals are complete removal of the intact unruptured cyst and maximal preservation of functional lung. Small, intact, peripheral cysts are often easily enucleated without loss of lung parenchyma. Segmentectomy or lobectomy is indicated when single or multiple cysts occupy most of the segment or lobe. Patients with suppurative cysts should be prepared for surgery

with postural drainage and antibiotics. Bronchiectasis, pulmonary fibrosis, or surrounding suppurative infection unresponsive to preoperative treatments are indications for larger resections. If bilateral cysts occur, the larger one should be excised first.

Enucleation involves blunt separation of the laminated layer from the surrounding pericystic zone (fibrous reactive host layer), with care to prevent rupture. Lung isolation, or reduced airway pressure during dissection, can be helpful in preventing early herniation of the cyst. Increased airway pressure at the time of delivery might aid delivery of the cyst.[95] The multiple bronchial openings in the residual cavity must then be identified and closed. Multiple "leak tests" with saline in the residual opening could be required to locate all bronchial openings. An alternative surgical strategy is to inject hypertonic saline into the cyst to sterilize it, followed by aspiration of the contents and removal of the evacuated cyst.

Pneumatocele. Pneumatoceles are thin-walled, air-filled spaces generated by pulmonary infections. They usually appear in the first week of a pneumonia and resolve spontaneously within 6 weeks. *Staphylococcus aureus* is the most common etiologic agent.[96] Pneumatoceles can appear as radiolucent zones, often initially obscured by the underlying pneumonia, which become more clearly visible on chest radiographs as the pneumonia resolves. As with other lung cysts, potential complications of pneumatoceles include secondary infection and enlargement as a result of air entrapment, with possible rupture or displacement and compression of normal lung. Adverse hemodynamic consequences can result from either a tension pneumothorax or a tension pneumatocele. The latter is unusual and is presumed to result from a one-way valve mechanism, usually in the setting of positive pressure mechanical ventilation.[97] Occasionally, surgical decompression is required and has been performed by percutaneous needle aspiration, catheter drainage, or chest tube drainage under CT or fluoroscopic guidance. Rarely is thoracoscopic or open surgical drainage or excision required.

Anesthetic considerations for resection of lung cysts and bullae. The hazards and pathophysiology of lung cysts and bullae are similar and may be considered jointly. In general, small, asymptomatic, uninfected cysts without bronchial communications (e.g., hydatid cysts, small residual CCAMs, or pulmonary sequestrations) may be treated like any limited resection. Loculi that are infected, which are large enough to exert compressive effects on adjacent vital structures, or which communicate with bronchi sufficiently to pose a risk of air trapping, rapid enlargement, or rupture, pose additional risk.

Infected cysts should be assumed to communicate with the tracheobronchial tree and to pose a potential risk of contaminating the contralateral lung with suppurative material. A roll under the shoulder of the uninfected side, with the head of the bed slightly raised during induction, might be helpful. The best protection is to secure effective lung isolation rapidly. DLTs have the advantage (over bronchial blockers or endobronchial intubations) of a channel for suctioning pus from the operative lung. In general, patients should not come to the operating room in a septic state. Whenever possible, percutaneous or chest tube drainage with antibiotic treatment of cysts in septic patients should precede surgical excision. The risk of "seeding" a thoracic epidural catheter is low if such decompression and antibiotic treatment have occurred. Nevertheless, the possibility of an epidural abscess should be considered when estimating the risks and benefits of postoperative pain options. In general, anesthetic management issues for infected cysts are similar to those for pulmonary abscesses.

The "compressive" effects of large, symptomatic, parenchymal lung cysts or bullae are usually limited to compression of adjacent lung tissue. Such patients generally tolerate single-lung anesthesia well from a gas exchange standpoint because they are already "auto-pneumonectomized" to an extent by their lesion. Exceptions are patients with bilateral lesions, in which case the most compromised lung should be operated on first. Nitrous oxide will cause expansion of air-filled cysts or bullae, whether or not they communicate directly with the bronchial tree. Following excision of the compressive lesion, attention should be paid to effective reexpansion of functional lung by recruitment maneuvers previously described. Patients tend to benefit from the recruitment of functional lung, as well as from the restoration of favorable respiratory mechanics following removal of large, compressive lesions. Adults with bullous emphysema and severe obstructive airways disease undergoing bullectomy should be treated similarly to patients undergoing lung volume reduction surgery (see Chapter 12). Most bullectomies (or plications) are performed through VATS incisions, though some centers prefer the median sternotomy approach. Hypoxemia during OLV is more likely with the supine position compared with the lateral decubitus position, due to increased blood flow through the operative (unventilated) lung as a function of gravity.[98]

Most air-filled, enlarging cystic lesions and all bullae should be assumed to communicate with the bronchial tree; therefore, they have the potential to trap air during positive pressure ventilation. Rapid expansion of lesions could lead to a compressive effect with both hemodynamic and respiratory consequences. Rupture of a cyst or bulla with a closed chest causes a pneumothorax, which could become a tension pneumothorax. Hyperexpansion of intact giant cysts and bullae have cardiovascular effects identical to those of tension pneumothorax. Potential mechanisms of hypotension include the following:

1. Decreased venous return due to increased intrathoracic pressure
2. Extrinsic restriction of diastolic ventricular filling (tamponade effect)
3. Mediastinal shift
4. Ventricular interdependence

The essence of therapy is to restore venous return and reduce the volume of the tension cyst or bulla. Vasopressors, volume-expanding fluids, generous venous access, and a surgeon prepared to decompress the chest should all be available prior to induction of patients with giant cysts or bullae. Prevention is best accomplished by rapidly establishing lung isolation by any means and by limiting positive pressure ventilation volumes and pressures prior to lung isolation. High-risk patients can be intubated with a DLT while awake (or while asleep and breathing spontaneously), though this is rarely necessary.

Patients with bilateral lesions can develop an expanding pneumothorax or hyperexpansion of cysts/bullae in the nonoperative lung. This development can present as hypoxemia and hypotension during OLV and be difficult to diagnose. Decreased dependent-lung breath sounds, diminished compliance, and a rising mediastinum provide clues. HFJV has been advocated for patients with bilateral bullae and indeed could be useful in the hands of anesthesiologists skilled in the technical aspects of its use.[99,100] If those skills are lacking, the advantages of HFJV probably do not outweigh the risks.

Postoperative air leaks are a major source of morbidity, particularly for bullectomies. Exposing the staple line to the minimal necessary ventilatory pressures and volumes and tailoring the anesthetic to provide for rapid return of spontaneous ventilation are worthy goals. Although it is acknowledged that peak inspiratory pressures (and even plateau pressures) are imperfect reflections of the distal airway pressures at the staple line, no direct means of monitoring staple line stress exists. If significant air leaks are present after resection, or if the surgeon communicates concern about the integrity of the tissue at the staple line, the ventilator should be adjusted to minimize the volume stress to that lung, even if achieving that aim requires permissive hypercapnia. Air leaks often improve when the patient is returned to the supine position. If the air leak is still extensive, the patient should either be reexplored immediately or given a trial of postoperative ventilation with a pressure-controlled ventilator and the chest tube placed to water seal.

Carcinoid Tumors

Carcinoid tumors are rare, predominantly gastrointestinal tumors, well known to anesthesiologists for their potential to secrete vasoactive mediators and illicit the "carcinoid syndrome." They account for 1% of bronchial tumors, where they typically grow slowly and prove responsive to primary surgical resection. Problems from pulmonary carcinoid tumors relate to their potential to cause bronchial obstruction, metastasize, elaborate mediators, and to cause valvular heart disease.

The identification and classification of carcinoid tumors are evolving. Carcinoid tumors arise from neuroendocrine cells, exhibit positive reactions to silver stains and neuroendocrine markers, and typically contain numerous membrane-bound neurosecretory granules.[101] Previously classified as adenomas because of their typically indolent behavior, carcinoid tumors are now recognized to represent a spectrum with varying degrees of malignancy in their histology and behavior. The distinction between "typical" and "atypical" pulmonary carcinoids has prognostic and therapeutic significance.[101]

The typical form is more common and usually presents as an isolated, slow-growing, histologically more benign mass in lobar, segmental, or (occasionally) mainstem bronchi. Although they can produce obstructive symptoms, their slow progression could lead to a long-standing misdiagnosis of bronchial asthma. On bronchoscopy, they appear as purplish or pink vascular soft tumors covered by intact epithelium. They may grow predominantly intraluminally or (more commonly) extraluminally, with just the "tip of the iceberg" visible. Primary, parenchymal-sparing surgical excision (often by sleeve resection) is the accepted treatment, typically yielding a 90% 5-year survival rate.[102] Endoscopic resections via a rigid bronchoscope run a significant risk of excessive bleeding and incomplete resection. Such techniques are indicated only for select subsets of patients, for palliation or treatment of nonoperative candidates, or for temporary relief of obstruction prior to later, definitive surgical resection.[102] The neodymium:yttrium-aluminum-garnet (Nd:YAG) laser has been useful for establishing hemostasis when endoscopic techniques are used, but it is not recommended for excision.

Ten percent of pulmonary carcinoids are histologically more malignant and can resemble small cell carcinoma. These "atypical" carcinoids tend to present more peripherally, at a later age (fifth decade), and with lymphatic or distant metastasis already established. Their behavior is less aggressive than that of small cell tumors, but more aggressive than typical carcinoids. Treatment by surgical excision usually requires lymph node dissection as well and yields a 5-year disease-free survival rate of less than 60%.[102] Pulmonary carcinoids are relatively unresponsive to chemotherapy. The role of adjuvant chemotherapy and radiation for atypical pulmonary carcinoid tumors is not yet established.

The symptoms of pulmonary carcinoid tumors usually relate to bronchial obstruction. Wheezing, a persistent cough, recurrent infection, or hemoptysis may be seen. Hemoptysis results from inflammation or ulceration of the overlying mucosa and could be accentuated in females during menses. Rarely, obstruction might create a ball-valve mechanism that leads to air trapping distal to the tumor.

The carcinoid syndrome is a collection of signs and symptoms related to the release of vasoactive amines and peptides from the tumor to the systemic circulation. The symptoms occur episodically and can be quite variable. It is important to note that such symptoms are neither common nor pathognomonic. True carcinoid syndrome occurs in fewer than 5% of cases, and other tumors can release vasoactive substances. The most common symptom is flushing. Other signs and symptoms are listed in Table 11-8.

Serotonin and histamine are the most commonly identified mediators. Other mediators include dopamine, substance P, neurotensin, prostaglandins, and kallikrein.[101,103] Serotonin is produced from the amino acid tryptophan, released in response to adrenergic stimulation, and broken down to 5-hydroxy indole acetic acid (5-HIAA), which appears in the urine. Serotonin can cause hypertension, hypotension, increased GI motility, hypoproteinemia (due to tryptophan depletion), and hyperglycemia. The amphibaric effect of serotonin is not completely understood.[104] Profound diarrhea occasionally has sig-

TABLE 11-8

Signs and Symptoms of Carcinoid Syndrome

Cutaneous flushing
Bronchospasm
Hypotension/hypertension
Abdominal pain
Nausea/vomiting
Valvular heart disease
Diarrhea
Hepatomegaly
Hyperglycemia
Hypoalbuminemia
Pellagra

nificant effects on intravascular volume and electrolytes. Elevated serotonin levels can cause drowsiness and delayed emergence from anesthesia.[105] Serotonin has also been implicated in carcinoid heart disease (see the discussion that follows). Although urine 5-HIAA levels are commonly measured, up to 20% of patients with carcinoid syndrome have normal levels.[105,106] Histamine release has been implicated in flushing and bronchospasm.[105] Kallikreins are protease enzymes that generate bradykinins and tachykinins. Bradykinin causes vasomotor relaxation (hypotension and flushing), and tachykinins (neuropeptide K, neurokinin A, vasoactive intestinal peptide, substance P) can contribute to flushing, hypotension, and cardiac disease.

Carcinoid heart disease occurs in one half to two thirds of patients with carcinoid syndrome and consists of regurgitant or stenotic valvular dysfunction related to the collagenous plaques on the surfaces of valves and cordae tendonae.[101,107] Grossly, the plaques appear as a pearly white coating causing thickening of leaflets, fusion of commissures, and foreshortening of leaflets and cordae.[107] Right-sided lesions are more common, with tricuspid regurgitation a nearly universal finding. The pulmonic valve often exhibits both stenosis and regurgitation. Untreated symptomatic right-sided carcinoid heart disease leads to death by right-side heart failure in less than 1 year on average. Valve replacement surgery is associated with high morbidity and mortality in this population.[108] Left-sided carcinoid heart disease is much less common. This could be related to the fact that most carcinoid tumors arise in the intestines and drain into systemic veins. Whether pulmonary carcinoid tumors are more likely to give rise to left-sided cardiac disease than intestinal carcinoid tumors is not known. Patients who develop carcinoid heart disease have higher serum serotonin and urine 5-HIAA levels than those who do not, but treatment that reduces these levels does not result in regression of cardiac lesions.[109]

ANESTHETIC CONSIDERATIONS FOR CARCINOID TUMORS

Avoiding a "carcinoid crisis" (severe hypotension or hypertension due to tumor mediator release) and issues related to bronchial obstruction are usually the principal anesthetic concerns for patients undergoing resection of the rarely secreting pulmonary carcinoid tumors. VATS or at least limited thoracotomy incisions are usually employed for resection. Continuous intraarterial blood pressure monitoring is indicated to detect carcinoid crisis promptly. Central venous pressure monitoring might be helpful as a central route for drug delivery and for assessing intravascular volume, which can be complicated by coexisting valvular disease.

The somatostatin analog, octreotide, is the principal weapon against carcinoid crisis and should at least be available in the OR for all carcinoid cases. Release of mediators can be triggered by adrenergic surges or surgical manipulation of carcinoid tumors. Octreotide is thought to inhibit the release of mediators and to block the receptor sites of many of the vasoactive substances. Eighty percent of carcinoid tumors have large numbers of high-affinity somatostatin binding sites.[101,110] In patients with histories suggestive of carcinoid syndrome, a convenient approach is to run an infusion of octreotide at approximately 50 μg/hr beginning prior to induction, with titration to blood pressure changes intraoperatively and gradual weaning during the postoperative period. Alternatively—

TABLE 11-9

Agents Used to Prevent or Treat Symptoms of Carcinoid Syndrome

Octreotide (somatostatin analog)
H_1 & H_2 receptor antagonists
Aprotinin (inhibits kallikrein)
Corticosteroids
α-Methyl-dopa
Glucagon
5-hydroxy tryptamine receptor antagonists
Ketanserin
Cyproheptadine
Methysergide
α- and β-Adrenergic receptor antagonists
Para-chlorophenylalanine
Methotrimeprazine

because of its rapid and reliable absorption—octreotide can be administered as a subcutaneous bolus (50 to 100 μg) followed by additional intravenous boluses (25 to 50 μg) as needed or prior to tumor manipulation.[103] Hypertensive as well as hypotensive carcinoid crises should respond to octreotide.[104] The effectiveness of octreotide is such that the many alternative treatments (Table 11-9) have become relegated to the status of second-tier agents.

Avoidance of adrenergic stimulation is as important as octreotide prophylaxis. Preoperative sedation, a smooth induction and emergence, avoidance of hypoxemia and hypercarbia, and adequate anesthetic depth for the levels of stimulation therefore assume a high priority. Thoracic epidural anesthesia would be expected to be beneficial toward this end. Close attention to the conduct of surgery allows for anticipation of tumor manipulation. Many drugs commonly used in anesthesia can have undesirable effects on carcinoid mediator release. Indirect sympathomimetic agents, paradoxically, can exacerbate hypotension by stimulating mediator secretion. β_2-Adrenergic agonists commonly used to treat bronchospasm can stimulate mediator release also and exacerbate hypotension and bronchospasm. Corticosteroids, inhaled ipratropium bromide, antihistamines, and octreotide have been recommended to treat or prevent bronchospasm in patients with carcinoid syndrome.[103] Adequate anesthetic depth might be the best defense against stimulus-induced intraoperative bronchospasm. The oft-published claim that succinylcholine could trigger mediator release from fasciculation-induced squeeze of tumors has not been documented and should not prevent its use when indicated. Drugs with significant histamine-releasing effects are probably best avoided. The antiemetic ondansetron might have secondary benefit in this population as a serotonin antagonist.[103] Emergence and postoperative pain management should be guided by an appreciation of the potential for residual functional tumor or metastases.

Strategies for airway management and lung isolation should be guided by the assessed risk of major airway obstruction. Fortunately, obstructive tracheal or carinal carcinoid tumors are exceedingly rare. One such case report exists, and the anesthetic management has been described.[111] The general principles of airway management for patients undergoing tracheal resection apply and have been discussed in detail elsewhere in this text (see Chapter 10). The potential for tracheal or major bronchial obstruction is usually evident from positional symptomatology, radiographic studies (CT or MRI scans), or flow-volume loops, if available. Most patients will have been examined bronchoscopically prior to surgery, so that the topography and risk are known. Rarely, the degree of obstruction will necessitate maintenance of spontaneous respiration to maintain patency. In such cases, the options include an awake intubation with upper- and lower-airway topical anesthesia, or a spontaneous breathing inhalation induction followed by intubation while asleep. The need to avoid adrenergic stimulation in patients with carcinoid syndrome makes such intubation techniques delicate.

Anesthesiologists might also encounter patients with carcinoid tumors undergoing flexible fiberoptic bronchoscopy for assessment and diagnostic biopsy. As discussed previously, the index of concern for airway obstruction should determine the induction technique. Biopsy can produce impressive bleeding from these vascular tumors. Intravenous access should be accordingly generous. Mediator release could be triggered by biopsy or from airway stimulation with light anesthesia. Patients with a history of carcinoid syndrome might benefit from invasive intraarterial monitoring, even though the procedure is minimally invasive. Total intravenous anesthesia (with an octreotide infusion) provides more reliable anesthetic depth and suppression of mediator release than inhalation techniques because of the unpredictable effects of intermittent suction and obstruction on gas delivery.

Additional anesthetic considerations for resection of carcinoid tumors center on associated pathology. The potential for carcinoid cardiac disease should be assessed carefully. An echocardiogram to assess valve function preoperatively is indicated for all patients with carcinoid syndrome. In cases of severe valvular disease, consideration should be given to pre-resection valve surgery or combined valve replacement and pulmonary resection.[112] The presence of carcinoid heart disease and high preoperative urinary 5-HIAA levels have been associated with severe perioperative complications, including death.[113] Preoperative correction of intravascular volume depletion, electrolyte imbalances, and hyperglycemia should take place when possible. Hypoproteinemia may affect drug bioavailability. Bronchial carcinoids have been associated with other endocrinopathies, secondary to excessive release of ACTH (Cushing's syndrome), melanocyte-stimulating hormone (MSH), and antidiuretic hormone (ADH). Multiple endocrine adenomatosis syndrome (MEA) has also been associated with carcinoid tumors.[102] Evidence of such coexisting disorders should be sought preoperatively, and a multidisciplinary approach could be appropriate for complex cases.

REFERENCES

1. Fry WA: Thoracic incisions. In Shields TW, LoCicero J, Ponn RB (eds): *General thoracic surgery,* ed 5, Philadelphia, 2000, Lippincott Williams & Wilkins.
2. Heitmiller RF: Thoracic incisions. In Bave Ae, Geha AS, Hammond GL, et al (eds): *Glenn's thoracic and cardiovascular surgery,* ed 6, Stamford CT, 1996, Appleton and Lange.

3. Crawford FA, Kratz JM: Thoracic incisions. In Sabiston DC, Spencer FC (eds): *Surgery of the chest,* ed 6, Philadelphia, 1995, WB Saunders.

4. Lemmer JL, Gomez M, Symreng T, et al: Limited lateral thoracotomy, improved postoperative pulmonary function, *Arch Surg* 125:873, 1990.

5. Hazelrigg SR, Landreneau JL, Boley TM, et al: The effects of muscle sparing versus standard posterolateral thoracotomy on pulmonary function, muscle strength, and postoperative pain, *J Thorac Cardiovasc Surg* 101:394, 1991.

6. Ponn RB, Ferreini A, D'Agostino RS, et al: Comparison of late pulmonary function after posterolateral and muscle sparing thoracotomy, *Ann Thorac Surg* 53:673, 1992.

7. Heitmiller RF: Thoracic incisions. In Bave AE, Geha AS, Hammond GL, et al (eds): *Glenn's thoracic and cardiovascular surgery,* ed 6, p 73, Stamford, Conn, 1996, Appleton and Lange.

8. Fry WA: Thoracic incisions. In Shields TW, LoCicero J, Ponn RB (eds): *General thoracic surgery,* ed 5, Philadelphia, 2000, Lippincott Williams & Wilkins.

9. Shields TW: General features of pulmonary resections. In Shields TW, LoCicero J, Ponn RB (eds): *General thoracic surgery,* ed 5, Philadelphia, 2000, Lippincott Williams & Wilkins.

10. Cooper JD, Nelems JM, Pearson FG: Extended indications for median sternotomy in patients requiring pulmonary resections, *Ann Thorac Surg* 26:413, 1978.

11. Van der Salm TJ, Cereda JM, Cutler BS: Brachial plexus injury following median sternotomy, *J Thorac Cardiovasc Surg* 80:447, 1980.

12. Bardoczky GI, Szegedi LL, d'Hollander AA, et al: Two-lung and one-lung ventilation in patients with chronic obstructive pulmonary disease. The effects of position and FIO_2, *Anesth Analg* 90:35, 2001.

13. Watanabe S, Noguchi E, Yamada S, et al: Sequential changes of arterial oxygen tension in the supine position during one-lung ventilation, *Anesth Analg* 90:28, 2001.

14. Bindslev L, Jolin A, Hedenstierna G, et al: Hypoxic pulmonary vasoconstriction in the human lung. Effect of repeated hypoxic challenges during anesthesia, *Anesthesiology* 62:621, 1985.

15. Jaklitsch MT, Harpole DH, Roberts JR, et al: Video-assisted techniques in thoracic surgery. In Loughlin KR, Brooks DC (eds.): *Principles of endosurgery,* Cambridge, Mass, 1996, Blackwell Science.

16. Mentzer SJ, Sugarbaker DJ: Thoracoscopy and video-assisted thoracic surgery. In Brooks DC (ed): *Current techniques in laparoscopy, Curr Med* 20:1, 1994.

17. Manncke K, Rosin RD (eds): *Minimal access thoracic surgery,* London, 1998, Chapman and Hall.

18. LoCicero J: Segmentectomy and lesser pulmonary resections. In Shields TW, LoCicero J, Ponn RB (eds): *General thoracic surgery,* ed 5, Philadelphia, 2000, Lippincott Williams & Wilkins.

19. Ginsberg RJ, Rubinstein LV: Randomized trial of lobectomy versus limited resection for T_1N_0 non-small cell lung cancer, *Ann Thorac Surg* 60:615, 1995.

20. Fell SC, Kirby TJ: Technical aspects of lobectomy. In Shields TW, LoCicero J, Ponn RB (eds): *General thoracic surgery,* ed 5, Philadelphia, 2000, Lippincott Williams & Wilkins.

21. McKenna RJ: Video-assisted thoracic surgery for wedge resection, lobectomy, and pneumonectomy. In Shields TW, LoCicero J, Ponn RB (eds): *General thoracic surgery,* ed 5, p 455, Philadelphia, 2000, Lippincott Williams & Wilkins.

22. Schirren J, Muley T, Vogt-Moykopf I: Sleeve lobectomy. In Shields TW, LoCicero J, Ponn RB (eds): *General thoracic surgery,* ed 5, Philadelphia, 2000, Lippincott Williams & Wilkins.

23. Mehran RJ, Deslauriers J, Peraux M, et al: Survival related to nodal status after sleeve resection for lung cancer, *J Thorac Cardiovasc Surg* 107:576, 1994.

24. Van Schil PE, Brutel de la Riviere A, Knaepen PJ, et al: Completion pneumonectomy after bronchial sleeve resection, incidence, indications, and results, *Ann Thorac Surg* 53:1042, 1992.

25. Kawahara K, Akamine S, Takahashi T, et al: Management of anastomotic complications after sleeve lobectomy for lung cancer, *Ann Thor Surg* 57:1529, 1994.

26. Goldstraw P: Pneumonectomy and its modifications. In Shields TW, LoCicero J, Ponn RB (eds): *General thoracic surgery,* ed 5, Philadelphia, 2000, Lippincott Williams & Wilkins.

27. Gernando HC, Goldstraw P: The accuracy of clinical evaluative intrathoracic staging in lung cancer as assessed by postsurgical pathologic staging, *Cancer* 65:2503, 1990.

28. Sugarbaker DJ, DeCamp MM, Liptay MJ: Pulmonary resection. In Nyhus LM, Baker RJ, Fischer JE (eds): *Master of surgery,* ed 3, Boston, 1997, Little Brown.

29. Wittnich C, Trudel I, Zidulka A, et al: Misleading "pulmonary wedge pressure" after pneumonectomy. Its importance in postoperative fluid therapy, *Ann Thorac Surg* 42:192, 1986.

30. Nino M, Body SC, Hartigan PM: The use of a bronchial blocker to rescue an ill-fitting double-lumen endotracheal tube, *Anesth Analg* 91:1370, 2000.

31. Slinger PD: Perioperative fluid management for thoracic surgery. The puzzle of post pneumonectomy pulmonary edema, *J Cardiothorac Vasc Anesth* 91:1370, 1995.

32. Zeldin RA, Normandin D, Landtwing D, et al: Postpneumonectomy pulmonary edema. *J Thorac Cardiovasc Surg* 87:259, 1984.

33. Verheijan-Breemhar L, Bogaard JM, van den Berg B, et al: Post-pneumonectomy pulmonary oedema, *Thorax* 43:323, 1988.

34. Turnage S, Lunn I: Postpneumonectomy pulmonary edema. A retrospective analysis of associated variables, *Chest* 103:1646, 1993.

35. Waller DA, Gebitekin C, Saunders NR, et al: Noncardiogenic pulmonary edema complicating lung resection, *Ann Thorac Surg* 55:140, 1993.

36. Van der Weff YD, van der Houwen HK, Heijamans PIM, et al: Postpneumonectomy pulmonary edema. A retrospective analysis of incidence and possible risk factors, *Chest* 111:1278, 1997.

37. Slinger PD: Anesthesia for lung resection surgery. In Thys DM, Hillel Z, Schwartz AJ (eds): *Textbook of cardiothoracic anesthesiology,* p 772, New York, 2001, McGraw-Hill.

38. Sugarbaker DJ, Norberto JJ, Swanson SJ: Extrapleural pneumonectomy in the setting of multimodality therapy for diffuse malignant pleural mesothelioma, *Semin Thorac Cardiovasc Surg* 9:373, 1997.

39. Swanson SJ, Grondin SC, Sugarbaker DJ: Technique of pleural pneumonectomy in diffuse mesothelioma. In Shields TW, LoCicero J, Ponn RB (eds): *General thoracic surgery,* ed 5, Philadelphia, 2000, Lippincott Williams & Wilkins.

40. Baumann MH, Sahn SA: Medical management and therapy of bronchopleural fistulas in the mechanically ventilated patient, *Chest* 97:721, 1990.

41. Cerfolio RJ: The incidence, etiology, and prevention of postresectional bronchopleural fistula, *Semin Thorac Cardiovasc Surg* 13:3, 2001.

42. Steiger Z, Wilson RF: Management of bronchopleural fistulas, *Surgery* 158:267, 1984.

43. Ellis JH, Sequeira FW, Weber TR, et al: Balloon catheter occlusion of bronchopleural fistulae, *AJR* 138:157, 1982.

44. Hankins JR, Miller JE, Attar S, et al: Bronchopleural fistula. Thirteen-year experience with 77 cases, *J Thorac Cardiovasc Surg* 76:755, 1978.

45. Smith DE, Karish AF, Chapman JP, et al: Healing of the bronchial stump after pulmonary resection, *J Thorac Cardiovasc Surg* 46:548, 1963.

46. Cohen RG, DeMeester TR, Lafontaine E: The pleura. In Sabiston DC, Spencer FC (eds): *Surgery of the chest,* ed 6, Philadelphia, 1995, WB Saunders.

47. Shields TW, Ponn RB: Complications of pulmonary resection. In Shields TW, LoCicero J, Ponn RB (eds): *General thoracic surgery,* ed 5, Philadelphia, 2000, Lippincott Williams & Wilkins.

48. Deschamps C, Allen MS, Miller DL, et al: Management of postpneumonectomy empyema and bronchopleural fistula, *Semin Thorac Cardiovasc Surg* 13:13, 2001.

49. Ginsberg RJ, Saborio DV: Management of the recalcitrant postpneumonectomy bronchopleural fistula. The trans-sternal transpericardial approach, *Semin Thorac Cardiovasc Surg* 13:20, 2001.

50. Cooper WA, Miller JI: Management of bronchopleural fistula after lobectomy, *Semin Thorac Cardiovasc Surg* 13:89, 2001.

51. Glover W, Chavis T, Daniel TM, et al: Fibrin glue applications through the fiberoptic bronchoscope: closure of bronchopleural fistulas, *J Thorac Cardiovasc Surg* 93:470, 1987.

52. Gallagher TJ, Smith RA, Kirby RR, et al: Intermittent inspiratory chest tube occlusion to limit bronchopleural cutaneous airleaks, *Crit Care Med* 4:328, 1976.

53. Downs JB, Chapman RL: Treatment of bronchopleural fistula during continuous positive pressure ventilation, *Chest* 69:363, 1976.

54. Phillips YY, Lonigan RM, Joyner LR: A simple technique for managing a bronchopleural fistula while maintaining positive pressure ventilation, *Crit Care Med* 7:351, 1979.

55. Alger FJ, Alvarez A, Aranda JL, et al: Prediction of early bronchopleural fistula after pneumonectomy. a multivariate analysis, *Ann Thorac Surg* 72:1662, 2001.

56. Albeda SM, Hansen-Flaschen JH, Taylor E, et al: Evaluation of high-frequency jet ventilation in patients with bronchopleural fistulas by quantitation of the airleak, *Anesthesiology* 63:551, 1985.

57. Otruba Z, Oxorn DL Lobar bronchial blockade in bronchopleural fistula, *Can J Anaesth* 39:176, 1992.

58. Rafferty TD, Palma J, Motoyama EK, et al: Management of a bronchopleural fistula with differential lung ventilation and positive end-expiratory pressure, *Respir Care* 25:654, 1980.

59. Hillman KM, Barber JD: Asynchronous independent lung ventilation, *Crit Care Med* 8:390, 1980.

60. Carvalho P, Thompson WH, Riggs R, et al: Management of a bronchopleural fistula with a variable resistance valve and a single ventilator, *Chest* 111:1452, 1997.

61. Feeley TW, Keating D, Nashimura T: Independent lung ventilation using high-frequency ventilation in the management of a bronchopleural fistula, *Anesthesiology* 69:420, 1988.

62. Benumof J: High-frequency and high-flow apneic ventilation during thoracic surgery. In Benumof J (ed): *Anesthesia for thoracic surgery*, ed 2, p 432, Philadelphia, 1995, WB Saunders.

63. Ihra G, Gockner G, Kashanipour A, et al: High-frequency jet ventilation in European and North American institutions, developments and clinical practice, *Eur J Anaesthesiol* 17:418, 2000.

64. Power DJ, Cline CD, Rodman GH: Effect of chest tube suction on gas flow through a bronchopleural fistula, *Crit Care Med* 13:99, 1985.

65. Derdarian SS, Rajagopal KR, Abbrecht PH, et al: High-frequency positive pressure jet ventilation in bilateral bronchopleural fistulae, *Crit Care Med* 10:119, 1982.

66. Ritz R, Benson M, Bishop MJ: Measuring gas leakage from bronchopleural fistulas during high-frequency jet ventilation, *Crit Care Med* 12:836, 1984.

67. Orlando R, Gluck EH, Cohen M, et al: Ultra-high-frequency jet ventilation in a bronchopleural fistula model, *Arch Surg* 123:591, 1988.

68. Bishop MJ, Benson MS, Sato P, et al: Comparison of high-frequency jet ventilation with conventional mechanical for ventilation for bronchopleural fistula, *Anesth Analg* 66:833, 1987.

69. Spinale FG, Linker RW, Crawford FA, et al: Conventional versus high-frequency jet ventilation with a bronchopleural fistula, *J Surg Res* 46:147, 1989.

70. Wells FC: Empyema thoracis. What is the role of surgery? *Resp Med* 84:97, 1990.

71. Tuncozgur B, Ustunsoy H, Sivrikoz MC, et al: Intrapleural urokinase in the management of parapneumonic empyema, a randomized controlled trial, *Int J Clin Pract* 55:658, 2001.

72. Cameron R: Intrapleural fibrinolytic therapy vs. conservative management in the treatment of parapneumonic effusions and empyema, *Cochran Database Syst Rev* 3:CD002312, 2000.

73. Clagett OT, Geraci JE: A procedure for the management of postpneumonectomy empyema, *J Thorac Cardiovasc Surg* 45:141, 1963.

74. Miller JI: Postsurgical empyemas. In Shields TW, LoCicero J, Ponn RB (eds): *General thoracic surgery,* ed 5, Philadelphia, 2000, Lippincott Williams & Wilkins.

75. Rice TW: Fibrothorax and decortication of the lung. In Shields TW, LoCicero J, Ponn RB (eds): *General thoracic surgery,* ed 5, Philadelphia, 2000, Lippincott Williams & Wilkins.

76. Swanson SJ, Sugarbaker DJ: Surgery and pleural space. Fibrothorax, thoracoscopy, and pleurectomy. In Baum GL, Crapo JD, Celli BR, et al (eds): *Textbook of pulmonary diseases,* ed 5, Philadelphia, 1998, Lippincott-Raven.

77. Barnett TB, Herring CL: Lung abscess. initial and late results or medical therapy, *Arch Int Med* 127:217, 1971.

78. Hughes JMB, Luce JM: Pulmonary arteriovenous malformations and other pulmonary vascular abnormalities. In Murray JF, Nadel JA (eds): *Textbook of respiratory medicine*, ed 3, Philadelphia, 2000, WB Saunders.

79. Shovlin CL, Winstock AR, Peters AM, et al: Medical complications of pregnancy in hereditary haemorrhagic telangiectasia, *Q J Med* 88:879, 1995.

80. Ference BA, Shannon TM, White RJ, et al: Life-threatening pulmonary hemorrhage with pulmonary arteriovenous malformations and hereditary hemorrhagic telangiectasia, *Chest* 106:1387, 1994.

81. Shields TW: Congenital vascular lesions of the lungs. In Shields TW, LoCicero J, Ponn RB (eds): *General thoracic surgery,* ed 5, Philadelphia, 2000, Lippincott Williams & Wilkins.

82. Dutton JA, Jackson JE, Hughes JM, et al: Pulmonary arteriovenous malformations. results of treatment with coil embolization in 53 patients, *Am J Roentgenol* 165:1119, 1995.

83. Maki DD, Siegelman ES, Roberts DA, et al: Pulmonary arteriovenous malformations, three-dimensional gadolinium-enhanced MR angiography—initial experience, *Radiology* 19:243, 2001.

84. Goyen M, Ruehm SG, Jagenburg A, et al: Pulmonary arteriovenous malformation. Characterization with time-resolved ultrafast 3D MR angiography, *J Magn Reson Imaging* 13:458, 2001.

85. Feinstein JA, Moore P, Rosenthal DN, et al: Comparison of contrast echocardiography versus cardiac catheterization for detection of pulmonary arteriovenous malformations, *Am J Cardiol* 90:281, 2002.

86. Lyerly HK, Sabiston DC: Pulmonary arteriovenous fistulas. In Sabiston DC, Spencer FC (eds): *Surgery of the chest,* ed 6, Philadelphia, 1995, WB Saunders.

87. Apostolopoulou SC, Kelekis NL, Papagiannis J, et al: Transcatheter occlusion of a large pulmonary arteriovenous malformation with use of a Cardioseal device, *J Vasc Interv Radiol* 12:767, 2001.

88. Margreiter J, Dessi A, Mair P, et al: Pulmonary arteriovenous fistula detected with transesophageal contrast echocardiography, *J Cardiothorac Vasc Anesth* 15:755, 2001.

89. Reynolds M: Congential lesions of the lung. In Shields TW, LoCicero J, Ponn RB (eds): *General thoracic surgery*, ed 5, p 937, Philadelphia, 2000, Lippincott Williams & Wilkins.

90. Adzick NS: The fetus with a lung mass. In Harrison MR, Evans MI, Adzick NS, et al (eds): *The unborn patient; the art and science of fetal therapy,* Philadelphia, 2001, WB Saunders.

91. Granata C, Gambini C, Balducci T, et al: Bronchioalveolar carcinoma arising in congenital cystic adenomatoid malformation in a child. A case report and review on malignancies originating in congenital cystic adenomatoid malformation, *Pediatr Pulmonol* 25:62, 1998.

92. Raynor AC, Capp MP, Sealy WC, et al: Lobar emphysema of infancy, *Ann Thorac Surg* 4:374, 1967.

93. Pride NB, Barter CE, Hugh-Jones P: The ventilation of bullae and the effect of their removal on thoracic gas volume and test of pulmonary function, *Am Rev Respir Dis* 107:83, 1973.

94. Deslauriers J, Le Blanc P: Bullous and bleb diseases, emphysema of the lung, and lung volume reduction surgery. In Shields TW, LoCicero J, Ponn RB (eds): *General thoracic surgery,* ed 5, Philadelphia, 2000, Lippincott Williams & Wilkins.

95. Aletras H, Symbas PN: Hydatid disease of the lung. In Shields TW, LoCicero J, Ponn RB (eds): *General thoracic surgery,* ed 5, 2000, Lippincott Williams & Wilkins.

96. Dines DE: Diagnostic significant of pneumatocele of the lung, *JAMA* 204:79, 1968.

97. Shen H, Lu FL, Wu H, et al: Management of tension pneumatocele with high-frequency oscillatory ventilation, *Chest* 121:284, 2002.

98. Bardoczky GI, Szegedi LL, d'Hollander AA, et al: Two-lung and one-lung ventilation in patients with chronic obstructive pulmonary disease. The effects of position and F_iO_2, *Anesth Analg* 90:35, 2001.

99. McCarthy G, Coppel DL, Gibbons JR, et al: High-frequency jet ventilation for bilateral bullectomy, *Anaesthesia* 42:411, 1987.

100. Normandale JP, Feneck RO: Bullous cystic lung disease, *Anaesthesia* 40:1192, 1985.

101. Kulke MH, Mayer RJ: Carcinoid tumors, *N Engl J Med* 340:858, 1999.

102. Ginsberg RJ: Carcinoid tumors. In Shields TW, LoCicero J, Ponn RB (eds): *General thoracic surgery,* ed 5, Philadelphia, 2000, Lippincott Williams & Wilkins.

103. Graham GW, Unger BP, Coursin DB: Perioperative management of selected endocrine disorders, *Anesthesiol Clin* 38:31, 2000.

104. Warner RRP, Mani S, Profeta J, et al: Octreotide treatment of carcinoid hypertensive crisis, *Mt Sinai J Med* 61:349, 1994.

105. Vaughan DJA, Brunner MD: Anesthesia for patients with carcinoid syndrome, *Int Anesthesiol Clin* 35:129, 1997.

106. Lawrence JP, Ishizuka J, Haber B, et al: The effect of somatostatin on 5-hydroxytryptamine release from a carcinoid tumour, *Surgery* 108:1131, 1990.

107. Simula DV, Edwards WD, Tazelaar D, et al: Surgical pathology of carcinoid heart disease. A study of 139 valves from 75 patients spanning 20 years, *Mayo Clin Proc* 77:139, 2002.

108. Robiolio PA, Rigolin VH, Harrison JK, et al: Predictors of outcome of tricuspid valve replacement in carcinoid heart disease, *Am J Cardiol* 75:485, 1995.

109. Pellikka PA, Tajik AJ, Khandheria BK, et al: Carcinoid heart disease, clinical and echocardiographic spectrum in 74 patients, *Circulation* 87:1188, 1993.

110. Reubi JC, Lang JW, Maurer R, et al: Distribution and biochemical characterization of somatostatin receptors in tumors of the human central nervous system, *Cancer Res* 47:5758, 1987.

111. Kannan S, Puri GD, Chari P: Anesthetic management of a patient with an obstructing carcinal carcinoid for tumor excision and pneumonectomy, *J Cardiothorac Vasc Anesth* 12:192, 1998.

112. Lennon PF, Hartigan PM, Friedberg JS: Clinical management of patients undergoing concurrent cardiac surgery and of pulmonary resection, *J Cardiothorac Vasc Anesth* 12:587, 1998.

113. Kinney MA, Warner ME, Nagorney DM: Perianesthetic risks and outcomes of abdominal surgery for metastatic carcinoid tumors, *Br J Anaesth* 87:447, 2001.

Anesthesia for Specific Thoracic Procedures

Erin A. Sullivan, MD

Jean S. Bussières, MD, FRCPC

Edda M. Tschernko, MD

12

THIS chapter reviews the anesthetic considerations and perioperative management for specific thoracic surgical procedures. These procedures include video-assisted thoracoscopic surgery, endobronchial surgery, whole-lung lavage, lung volume reduction surgery, surgery for hemoptysis, thoracic outlet syndrome, transthoracic vertebral surgery, adult diaphragmatic surgery, superior vena cava syndrome, and pectus excavatum.

Video-Assisted Thoracoscopic Surgery

In 1921, the Swedish physician Jacobaeus reported the first series of thoracoscopic procedures as a technique to diagnose and treat pulmonary tuberculosis and pleural effusions.[1] The advent of modern thoracic anesthesia and thoracic surgical techniques has been paramount to the development of video-assisted thoracoscopic surgery (VATS). This minimally invasive surgical technique, initially performed solely for diagnostic purposes, has been advocated for a variety of both diagnostic and therapeutic procedures (Table 12-1). Compared with conventional thoracotomy, VATS decreases the impairment of early postoperative pulmonary function, decreases postoperative pain, and could promote a more rapid recovery, in this way reducing total length of hospital stay and total cost of care.[2-4] Although VATS offers many advantages for patients who would otherwise be considered as too high-risk for conventional thoracotomy, it does present some potential complications. Complications associated with VATS include infection, hemorrhage, hemodynamic instability, prolonged air leak, "down lung" syndrome, tumor seeding, reexpansion pulmonary edema, cardiac arrhythmias, chronic pain, and nerve injury.[5,6] The potential for conversion of a VATS procedure to an open thoracotomy always exists and should be considered carefully when formulating the anesthetic plan. The incidence of conversion from VATS to a thoracotomy has been reported to range from 1% to as high as 20%.[7,8] Indications for conversion to thoracotomy can be found in Table 12-2.

Anesthetic Considerations for VATS

PREOPERATIVE EVALUATION

The preoperative assessment and management of patients scheduled for thoracic surgery have been described thoroughly in Chapter 1. Because patients scheduled for VATS often present with similar comorbidities and indications for surgery as those scheduled for open thoracotomy, and because there is no reliable means to predict whether a VATS will be converted to an open procedure, the preoperative evaluation of these groups of patients should be similar.[9] The anesthesiologist should do the following:

1. Review the patient's history and perform a physical examination.
2. Review pertinent laboratory studies, including hematology, serum chemistry, and coagulation studies.
3. Review the patient's chest radiograph and any other special radiologic imaging studies.
4. Review the electrocardiogram and results of other applicable cardiac studies such as echocardiography, stress tests, and cardiac catheterization.
5. Review the patient's pulmonary function studies and use this information to assess the impact of the surgical procedure on the patient's postoperative pulmonary function.

Options for pain management—including intercostal nerve block, intravenous patient-controlled analgesia, thoracic paravertebral block, and thoracic epidural anesthesia—should be discussed with the patient. Although many anesthesiologists do not use thoracic epidural anesthesia for most VATS procedures, this mode of pain management should be offered to the patient preoperatively in the event that the VATS is converted to an open thoracotomy. Under this circumstance, the thoracic epidural catheter can be placed after the patient is awake in the postanesthesia care unit.

INTRAOPERATIVE MANAGEMENT

Many of the same principles that apply to the patient undergoing open thoracotomy also apply to VATS (see Chapters 4 and 7). Historically, VATS was performed with patients under local anesthesia with intravenous sedation. Today, VATS is most commonly performed with a general anesthetic technique with controlled ventilation and a bronchial blocking device in order to provide effective lung isolation. Standard monitors—including an electrocardiogram, pulse oximetry, noninvasive blood pressure cuff, and capnography—are employed. Some studies have reported the use of only noninvasive monitoring during VATS; however, these studies involved relatively healthy patients undergoing simple procedures.[10] Depending on the patient's preexisting comorbidities as well as the complexity of the procedure, it could be appropriate to use invasive monitors such as an arterial catheter, central venous pressure catheter, or pulmonary artery catheter. It is important to realize that the data

TABLE 12-1

Indications for Diagnostic and Therapeutic Thoracoscopy

Pulmonary parenchymal and pleural disease	Biopsy, staging (malignancies)
	Tuberculosis
	Mesothelioma
	Interstitial fibrosis
	Solitary nodules
	Evaluation of traumatic thoracic injury
	Pleurodesis
	Drainage of pleural effusions
	Lung volume reduction surgery
	Pulmonary wedge resection, lobectomy
	Resection of bullae, blebs, and granulomas
	Decortication
	Empyemectomy
	Diaphragmatic disease
Esophageal disease	Biopsy, staging (malignancies)
	Vagotomy
	Heller myotomy
	Zenker's diverticulum
	Antireflux procedures
	Minimally invasive esophagectomy
Mediastinal masses	Lymphoma, metastatic disease
	Thymectomy
	Chylothorax
Cardiovascular procedures	Patent ductus arteriosus ligation
	Internal mammary artery dissection
	Pericardial window, stripping
	Thoracoscopic mid-CAB
Miscellaneous	Sympathectomy (hyperhydrosis, chronic reflex pain syndrome)
	Transthoracic anterior vertebral surgery
	Removal of intrathoracic foreign bodies (sheared catheters, surgical sponge)

From Shah JS, Bready LL: Anesthesia for thoracoscopy. In Benumof JL, Joshi GP (eds): *Anesthesia for minimally invasive surgery: laparoscopy, thoracoscopy, hysteroscopy,* Philadelphia, 2001, WB Saunders.
CAB, Coronary artery bypass.

obtained from pulmonary artery catheter monitoring during thoracoscopy might be negatively impacted by hypoxic pulmonary vasoconstriction, single-lung ventilation, surgical manipulation, and catheter position.[11,12] Transesophageal echocardiography (TEE) might also be an extremely useful and accurate intraoperative monitor for assessment of cardiac fill-

TABLE 12-2

Indications for Conversion from Thoracoscopy to Thoracotomy

Unsatisfactory operative lung deflation/isolation
Extensive pulmonary resection or pneumonectomy required
Extensive pleural adhesions
Centrally located pulmonary lesion
Lesion too large for thoracoscopic resection
Excessive bleeding
Surgical complications resulting from attempted thoracoscopy

ing and function during those VATS procedures that do not involve esophageal resection.

VATS can be performed with local, regional, or general anesthesia; as stated previously, however, the choice is highly dependent on the severity of the patient's cardiopulmonary status as well as on the complexity of the surgical procedure itself.[13,14] Various regional anesthetic techniques have been successfully used either alone or in combination: thoracic paravertebral blocks, intercostal nerve blocks plus ipsilateral stellate ganglion block, thoracic epidural anesthesia, and field blocks.[15] Regional anesthetic techniques require careful patient selection for VATS of brief duration. Patients who are uncooperative or who have a potentially difficult airway should not be considered for VATS with the use of regional anesthesia alone. Potential complications resulting from this anesthetic approach include the following:

- Failure of the regional technique to produce satisfactory surgical conditions
- Hypoxemia and hypercapnia as a result of paradoxic respirations
- Hemodynamic compromise secondary to the creation of an open pneumothorax and mediastinal shift

All of these complications require conversion to general anesthesia, sometimes on an emergency basis.

Most anesthesiologists use a general anesthetic technique with controlled ventilation and a bronchial blocking device for their patients undergoing VATS. Effective lung isolation and deflation of the operative lung are essential for the success of the VATS procedure because the surgeon must work within the confines of a closed thoracic cavity. To facilitate satisfactory operative lung deflation, it might be helpful to ventilate the lungs with oxygen (rather than with an air/oxygen mixture) before lung isolation, particularly if the patient has poor pulmonary elastic recoil or chronic obstructive pulmonary disease (COPD). Tidal volumes should be adjusted to 5 to 7 mL/kg in order to minimize mediastinal shifting, which could further inhibit the surgeon's ability to perform VATS successfully. Because the application of continuous positive airway pressure (CPAP) to the operative lung might be detrimental to the success of VATS, it is recommended that small increments of positive end-expiratory pressure (PEEP) be applied to the nonoperative lung if the patient's oxygenation is compromised during single-lung ventilation (details of lung separation are discussed in Chapter 8). Depending on the surgical procedure and the likelihood of conversion to an open thoracotomy, a regional anesthetic technique such as thoracic epidural anesthesia may be combined with the general anesthetic. Selection of specific anesthetic agents should be individualized and based on the preexisting condition of the patient as well as on the anticipated length of the procedure. The goal for a general anesthetic approach is to provide satisfactory intraoperative anesthesia and analgesia using agents that facilitate tracheal extubation at the conclusion of surgery and minimize the occurrence of postoperative respiratory depression.[16]

POSTOPERATIVE MANAGEMENT

Postoperative management of the patient undergoing VATS is similar to that of the patient undergoing thoracotomy. Although thoracoscopy is reported to be less painful and cause less respiratory dysfunction when compared with open thoracotomy, a vigilant approach must be maintained with regard to postoperative pain management and pulmonary therapy.

The degree of postoperative pain experienced by patients undergoing VATS is highly variable and dependent on the surgical procedure performed. Procedures involving uncomplicated thoracoscopic pulmonary resection tend to produce pain limited to the intercostal port insertion sites and to the chest tubes. In many instances, this pain can be managed effectively with intravenous patient-controlled analgesia (e.g., morphine or hydromorphone), intravenous nonsteroidal medications (unless otherwise contraindicated) or oral analgesic medications. At the other end of the pain spectrum are those procedures involving the pleura, such as pleural stripping or instillation of pleural sclerosing agents to minimize the reoccurrence of spontaneous pneumothorax or pleural effusions. These procedures are extremely painful and require more aggressive modalities of pain management, such as thoracic epidural analgesia. Inadequate pain management for these patients ultimately leads to postoperative respiratory failure, particularly for those with limited pulmonary reserve (see Chapter 20).

It is just as important to provide satisfactory postoperative pulmonary therapy for patients who have had a thoracoscopic procedure as a thoracotomy. Judicious and appropriate use of bronchodilators, chest physiotherapy, and incentive spirometry as well as early patient ambulation help minimizes the risk of operative morbidity and promote a timely functional recovery.

Endobronchial Surgery

Endobronchial tumors produce a gradual obstruction of the mainstem bronchi that leads to severe dyspnea and collapse of the affected lung. Several therapies are currently available for the palliative treatment of these life-threatening lesions: laser therapy, insertion of bronchial stents, and a new experimental technique, photodynamic therapy.

Laser Therapy

The term *laser* is an acronym for "light amplification by stimulated emission of radiation." When a gaseous medium such as argon (Ar) or carbon dioxide (CO_2) is stimulated by an energy source, it emits energy in the form of light. Through a series of repeated reflections, the emitted light begins to exhibit the characteristics of a laser: coherence (light waves in phase with respect to time and space), collimation (same direction), and monochromaticity (same wavelength).

The effect that a laser exerts on tissue is dependent on its wavelength (measured in nanometers) and its power density (W/cm^2). The excited medium (e.g., Ar, CO_2) from which the laser derives its name determines the emitted wavelength. Longer wavelengths tend to be highly absorbed by tissues and are converted to heat energy at a more shallow tissue penetration depth. Lasers with shorter wavelength tend to scatter. The CO_2 laser emits a long wavelength (10,600 nm) and is useful for precise cutting of tissues due to its high tissue absorption and shallow tissue penetration depth. In contrast to the CO_2 laser, the neodymium-yttrium-aluminum-garnet (Nd-YAG) laser emits a shorter wavelength (1.064 nm) and is an effective tool for tumor debulking.[17]

The extinction length (EL) of a laser is defined as that distance or depth of tissue within which 90% of the laser beam energy is absorbed. The EL for the CO_2 laser in most tissues and water is 0.03 mm.[17] The EL for the Nd-YAG laser is 60 mm in water and 1-3 mm in soft tissue.[17] Complications of Nd-YAG laser therapy can occur as late as 48 hours after initial treatment due to edema formation, hemorrhage, and luminal obstruction.[17]

The power density of a laser is defined as the amount of energy per unit area. It is usually expressed as watts per square centimeter (W/cm^2). The absorption of most medical lasers by tissue leads to production of heat rather than ionization. The heat resulting from lasers with a low flux (rate of energy delivery) coagulates proteins and vaporizes intracellular water, leading to cell lysis. Therefore the low flux of the Nd-YAG laser primarily coagulates proteins and causes carbonization to occur over a large tissue area. On the other hand, the high flux of the CO_2 laser yields almost immediate cellular vaporization, and carbonization occurs only at the tissue edge.

An inhomogeneous tissue substance and low tissue absorption tend to increase scattering, thus increasing the cross-sectional area of the laser beam. The end result is that the critical volume—defined as the volume in which 90% of the interaction with the material occurs—is increased. The critical volume for the Nd-YAG laser is 300 to 900 times greater than that for the CO_2 laser, which accounts for a wider range of heating and more edema formation than occurs with the CO_2 laser. Van der Spek et al have likened the effects of the Nd-YAG laser on tissue to an iceberg in the sense that only the tip of the affected tissue is visible.[17] They furthermore stated that "when a high flux is used, the center of the 'iceberg' may undergo vaporization, with rapid expansion of the tissues, resulting in a limited explosion of the overlying tissue—the popcorn effect."[17]

PRACTICAL APPLICATIONS OF LASERS FOR AIRWAY PROCEDURES

In 1974, the CO_2 laser was first reported as a useful surgical technique during bronchoscopy.[18] Today, the laser is commonly used for the resection of airway tumors and other lesions, such as laryngeal papillomata, subglottic stenosis, and vascular malformations. Cancer tissue is reported to be more vulnerable to laser destruction than is normal tissue, thus making laser therapy a viable option for palliation of endobronchial tumors. The criteria established for laser resection of endobronchial tumors includes extension of the lesion into the bronchial wall (but not beyond the cartilage) and an axial length of less than 4 cm.[19]

Lasers are useful for the palliative treatment of obstructive malignancies of the esophagus, trachea, and mainstem bronchi. In contrast to external radiation and chemotherapy, laser therapy produces no systemic toxicity, nor is it dose limited. Symptomatic relief occurs almost immediately with laser therapy but could take several weeks with chemotherapy and external radiation.[20,21]

HAZARDS OF LASER THERAPY

The hazards associated with laser therapy include atmospheric contamination, perforation of a vessel or structure, embolism, and energy transfer to an inappropriate location. During the period of January 1989 through June 1990, 21 laser injuries were reported to the Food and Drug Administration: 2 minor, 12 serious, and 7 fatal.[22] Of these reported the following injuries[22]:

- 24% resulted from gas embolism.
- In 24%, there was perforation of an organ or vessel.

- 19% involved eye exposure or injury.
- Airway fire occurred in 14% of the reported cases.
- 9% of injuries resulted in other burns.
- There was a 9% incidence of miscellaneous injury.

Smoke and plume (fine particulate matter that is small enough to penetrate to the level of the alveoli) are released as a byproduct of laser tissue vaporization and might be teratogenic, mutagenic, and/or a vector for viral infection.[23] The mutagenicity of laser condensate has been reported in vitro to be one-half that of electrocautery.[24] Although some studies have reported that smoke plume serves as a vector for viral infection via transmission of viral DNA particles (mostly condylomas and skin warts), this topic remains controversial, particularly with regard to transmission of the human immunodeficiency virus (HIV).[25] One study described the detection of noninfectious DNA fragments found in a CO_2 laser plume from HIV-infected tissue pellets, while yet another study concluded that HIV was not detected in electrosurgical smoke plume at all.[26] Other studies have indicated that although laser plume does not appear to contain viable tumor cells, it might contain viable bacterial spores.[27,28]

The most effective means of preventing dissemination of the laser plume is to use an efficient smoke evacuator at the surgical site.[29] In addition, smoke evacuators might help to eliminate laser plume that would otherwise cause visual obstruction of the surgeon and reduce the potential for ignition. High-efficiency surgical masks that filter small particles of plume (0.3 μm or more) are also effective in minimizing the dissemination of potentially harmful laser plume.

Another hazard associated with laser therapy for endobronchial lesions is the inadvertent perforation of a large blood vessel or bronchus. Airway hemorrhage occurs most often during laser of an endobronchial lesion that completely occludes a mainstem bronchus. In this instance, the direction of the mainstem bronchus is distorted, and the possibility of bronchial and vascular perforation exists. Because blood vessels measuring greater than 5 mm in diameter are not coagulable by laser, life-threatening hemorrhage can occur, resulting in hypoxemia, hypoventilation, and hemodynamic compromise. Other complications resulting from inadvertent perforation of the trachea or bronchi include pneumothorax, pneumomediastinum, and tracheoesophageal fistula.

Venous gas embolization has been reported during Nd-YAG resection of endobronchial lesions.[30-32] Two of these reviews reported several deaths resulting from cardiovascular collapse, described as severe bradycardia, shock, myocardial infarction, and cardiac arrest.[31,32] Possible etiologies of venous gas embolism during Nd-YAG surgery could include entrainment of helium (used as a coolant gas) or air/oxygen (from a jet ventilation device or vigorous bag mask ventilation) into a pulmonary vein during airway hemorrhage.

The wavelengths of all currently available medical lasers are transmitted through air and reflected by smooth metal surfaces. Inadvertent triggering of the laser at the wrong time can result in damage to the eyes, tissue burns, ignition of surgical drapes, and—of particular concern to anesthesiologists—airway burns.

It is imperative that all operating room personnel and the patient be provided with proper eye protection during the conduct of laser surgery. Eye injury from CO_2 lasers may result in serious corneal injury, while the Nd-YAG laser can cause retinal damage. The patient's eyes should be protected first by taping the eyelids closed and then by covering the eyes with saline-soaked pads. Operating room personnel should be provided with special eyewear designed for the wavelength of the laser in use. For CO_2 lasers, any clear glass or plastic lenses will suffice because the glass and plastic lenses are opaque to far infrared. Contact lenses do not offer sufficient protection. Nd-YAG lasers require specially coated lenses that are opaque to near infrared. All windows into the operating room should be covered during laser procedures, as lasers other than the far-infrared CO_2 types produce beams that pass through glass. Specific warning signs should be posted on the outside door of the operating room to prevent other personnel from entering while the laser is in use.

Perhaps the most feared complication of laser use during airway surgery is an airway fire. The estimated incidence of endotracheal tube fires is 0.5% to 1.5%.[33] Many of these fires, when handled appropriately, result in minimal or no harm to the patient; however, catastrophic consequences are possible.

An oxygen-rich atmosphere can potentiate the ignition of any hydrocarbon material, including tissue, plastic, and rubber. Fires can result from direct laser illumination, reflected laser light, or smoke plume. Most endotracheal fires are initially confined to the external surface of the endotracheal tube, which causes local thermal destruction. Should a fire remain unrecognized and progress to the oxygen-rich environment on the interior of the endotracheal tube, combustion will occur, blowing heat and toxic byproducts of combustion distal into the pulmonary parenchyma. A similar circumstance occurs during inadvertent puncture and deflation of the tracheal cuff of the endotracheal tube. Specific management of airway fires is discussed later in this section.

ANESTHETIC CONSIDERATIONS FOR LASER THERAPY

Deep intravenous sedation combined with topical airway anesthesia and general anesthesia has been used for laser therapy of the airway. Likewise, laser therapy has been delivered with the assistance of both flexible fiberoptic bronchoscopy and rigid bronchoscopy. General anesthesia is preferred for rigid bronchoscopy and has been recommended for flexible fiberoptic bronchoscopy.[34] For some patients, awake fiberoptic intubation or a general anesthetic induction technique that initially preserves spontaneous ventilation might be necessary, as the use of neuromuscular blocking agents could potentially convert a partial airway obstruction into a complete airway obstruction. Standard monitoring is used for laser therapy; invasive monitors could be appropriate for some patients.

The mixture of airway gases becomes an important issue during laser therapy. Combustion of excess oxidizers can lead to the serious events described previously. Most clinicians recognize the need to reduce the FIO_2 to less than 0.4 or to the minimum oxygen concentration consistent with adequate patient oxygenation. Nitrous oxide is also an oxidizer capable of combustion. In fact, adding nitrous oxide to oxygen could be just as dangerous as administering a high concentration of oxygen alone.[35] The use of an oxygen/air mixture appears to be acceptable.

The use of a helium/oxygen mixture has been reported to prevent the ignition and fires of nonwrapped, unmarked PVC endotracheal tubes.[36] Some anesthesiologists prefer helium as a diluent to nitrogen because it has a higher thermal conductivity than nitrogen. Helium also has a lower density, permitting the use of a smaller endotracheal tube without turbulence and high flow resistance. It should be noted that the use of helium prevents an accurate measurement of anesthesia gases by most mass spectrometry units because they have no collector plates for helium. In such instances, erroneously high values for other gases such as oxygen, carbon dioxide, nitrogen, nitrous oxide, and the volatile anesthetic gases will be observed.

Although the volatile anesthetic agents that are currently used are nonflammable and nonexplosive in clinically relevant concentrations, they can undergo pyrolysis during an airway fire, thus producing potentially toxic compounds. It is for this reason that some do not recommend the use of volatile anesthetics during airway laser therapy.

External ignition of an endotracheal tube during laser therapy is due to the transfer of heat between the laser itself and the tube; internal ignition, on the other hand, is due to laser perforation of the tube with support of combustion by the gases entrained inside the tube. When endotracheal intubation for laser therapy is indicated, the endotracheal tube may be protected by wrapping metallic tape in an overlapping fashion along its entire length, exclusive of the tracheal cuff and the tip distal to the cuff. An overlap of half the tape width has been recommended to provide both good protection and a smooth surface.[37] There are many tapes available that appear to be metallic but are not; these tapes will not reflect the laser. Tapes should be tested prior to use by firing the laser at the tape. The reflected beam from reflective tape can cause an airway burn; therefore a tape with a matte finish, which results in a more diffuse reflected beam, is preferred. Wet muslin can also be used as an effective protective endotracheal tube wrapping; however, it is bulky and can ignite if it dries out. Alternatively, a number of endotracheal tube types are designed specifically for use during airway laser surgery. Although these special endotracheal tubes might offer some advantage over endotracheal tubes wrapped with metal tape, reports of airway fires resulting in serious airway injury have been documented with them as well.[38,39] The use of an oil-based ointment for lubrication of all endotracheal tubes used during laser therapy should be avoided, as this lubricant might be combustible.

The tracheal cuff of the endotracheal tube should be inflated with saline. In the event that the tracheal cuff should rupture, the saline will help to extinguish a fire. Some anesthesiologists advocate the use of saline-soaked pledgets to pack the tracheal cuff to further reduce the possibility of tracheal damage should the cuff rupture. Care must be taken to retrieve the pledgets in order to avert potential airway obstruction at the conclusion of the procedure.

Rigid bronchoscopy has been used widely as an alternative technique to endotracheal intubation for laser therapy of endobronchial lesions. Rigid bronchoscopy provides good visibility and permits easier retrieval of debris that might accumulate in the airway. The rigid bronchoscope maintains a patent airway and substantially decreases the risk of fire because it is constructed of metal that is nonignitable and nonflammable. The metal is capable of reflecting the laser beam and thereby producing indirect tissue damage. The same precautions for administration of gases used during general endotracheal anesthesia for laser therapy also apply to administration of general anesthesia with rigid bronchoscopy. Although the steel bronchoscope is not combustible, use of high oxygen concentrations might cause carbonized tissue to ignite.

Rigid bronchoscopy requires the administration of intravenous general anesthesia (e.g., propofol) as well as neuromuscular blockade. Ventilation and oxygenation of the patient are achieved using a number of techniques that could include intermittent positive pressure ventilation, the Sanders injection system, and high-frequency positive pressure (jet) ventilation.

MANAGEMENT OF AIRWAY FIRES

If an airway fire should occur during laser therapy, the surgeon and anesthesiologist must act quickly, decisively, and in a controlled fashion, with clear communication being of the utmost importance. The laser should be discontinued immediately followed by termination of ventilation, removal of the oxygen source, and, finally, extubation of the trachea. This sequence of procedures serves to decrease inhalation of the toxic products of combustion and decrease the amount of oxidizing agents and fuel present to perpetuate the fire. The flaming material should be extinguished in a bucket of water. Subsequently, the patient should be ventilated with 100% oxygen via bag mask with maintenance of general anesthesia. Rigid bronchoscopy should follow in order to evaluate the airway for damage as well as to remove any debris. If there is any evidence of airway damage detected during rigid bronchoscopy, the patient's trachea should be reintubated. If damage to the airway is severe, a low tracheotomy may be indicated. Postoperatively, the patient could require prolonged endotracheal intubation and mechanical ventilation. Steroids might help to decrease airway edema.

Tracheal and Bronchial Stents

Tracheal and bronchial stents are used to prevent airway obstruction due to internal or external compression of the trachea and bronchi. These stents can provide either temporary or definitive therapy for a number of obstructive conditions including endobronchial tumors, mediastinal masses, and tracheal or bronchial strictures. Previously, the only options available for treatment of these lesions were laser excision, dilation, or conventional surgical excision.

There are two types of stents: metallic and Silastic (Dumon). Rigid bronchoscopy is the conventional approach for stent placement; however, the self-expanding metallic stents can be placed using flexible fiberoptic bronchoscopy. Although the metallic stents are more stable and not as prone to dislodgement as the Silastic stents, they are much more difficult to remove.

Optimal anesthetic management for tracheal and bronchial stents is achieved with general anesthesia and neuromuscular blockade, although some practitioners use flexible fiberoptic bronchoscopy and deep intravenous sedation. Care must be exercised when anesthetizing patients with severe symptoms of airway obstruction.

Photodynamic Therapy

Photodynamic therapy (PDT) is a new treatment available for palliation of obstructive esophageal and tracheobronchial malignancies as well as several other forms of cancer. PDT requires the use of a photoactive drug (photosensitizer) and light (visible or infrared).[40] The photosensitizer tends to accumulate preferentially in the tumor. Upon exposure to a light source (visible or infrared), the photosensitizer absorbs the light, and a series of chemical reactions occur, leading to the direct or indirect production of cytotoxic species (free radicals and singlet oxygen).[41] This cytotoxic reaction with the subcellular organelles and macromolecules leads to selective necrosis and apoptosis of the cancer cells that host the photosensitizer. One advantage of PDT is that it does not involve the generalized destruction of noncancerous cells. PDT also acts on the vascular supply to the tumor by reducing blood flow and subsequently causing tumor necrosis.

Only tumors that are located superficially and that can be reached by direct light or light delivered through an optical fiber are susceptible to this therapy. At the present time, the application of PDT for palliative therapy of cancerous lesions in humans is still considered to be relatively experimental.

Whole-Lung Lavage

This section reviews the historical considerations of whole-lung lavage, its indications, the details of the technique, the possible complications, and finally, the benefits of this unusual treatment modality. It is important to differentiate whole-lung lavage from bronchoalveolar lavage. Bronchoalveolar lavage is a diagnostic tool performed with patients under local anesthesia, which uses only 300 mL of liquid in one segment of the lung with the aid of the fiberoptic bronchoscope. Whole-lung lavage is a treatment modality that requires more than 10 L of normal saline instilled through a double-lumen tube in one whole lung while the patient is under general anesthesia.

Historical Considerations

In 1928, Vicente described a technique resembling modern whole-lung lavage: he placed a catheter by way of the mouth in the dependent lung of an awake human patient who was breathing room air in the lateral decubitus position. He then flushed saline solution to aid in the removal of secretions (Figure 12-1, *A*). This technique was used to treat such conditions as bronchiectasis, chronic bronchitis, and lung abscess.[42,43]

In 1963, Ramirez-Rivera described pulmonary segmental flooding through an endobronchial, semipermanent catheter positioned transtracheally in an awake, spontaneously breathing patient (Figure 12-1, *B*).[44-46] In 1965, Ramirez-Rivera described the whole-lung lavage technique performed on a patient under local anesthesia and 1 year later with the patient under general anesthesia (Figure 12-1, *C*).[47,48] In 1982, Spragg introduced the modern technique of whole-lung lavage (Figure 12-2).[49]

Indications for Whole-Lung Lavage

Whole-lung lavage is the most effective treatment modality for symptomatic pulmonary alveolar proteinosis. This lung disease is caused by an alveolar accumulation of a lipoprotein material

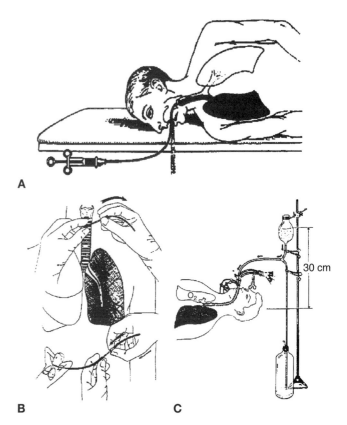

FIGURE 12-1 Evolution of whole-lung lavage. **A,** Patient is awake in the lateral decubitus position and an oral catheter is placed into the dependent lung. (From Vicente G: *Presse Méd* 1267, 1929.) **B,** Patient is awake in semisupine position, then a transtracheal catheter is positioned with its tip 5 cm beyond the carina. A slow infusion of 100 mL of warm isotonic saline is then performed. (From Ramirez-Rivera J et al: *Arch Intern Med* 112:422, 1963.) **C,** The improved technique for lavaging the lung with DLT was first described with the patient under local anesthesia and a year later, under general anesthesia. (From Ramirez-Rivera J: *Dis Chest* 50:582, 1966.)

that has the characteristic of surfactant.[50] Primary pulmonary alveolar proteinosis, first reported by Rosen in 1958, is a rare disorder of unknown cause and variable natural history.[51,52] Thought to be a nonspecific pulmonary reaction to several insults, it creates a true alveolar-capillary blockade. The patient presents with dyspnea and hypoxemia made worse by exercise. Spontaneous remission can occur, but the therapeutic decision in pulmonary alveolar proteinosis depends on the progression of the illness and the extent of the physiologic impairment. The usual goal of whole-lung lavage is improvement in the clinical, physiologic, and radiologic aspects of the patient. The prognosis for pulmonary alveolar proteinosis has improved greatly since the introduction of whole-lung lavage by Ramirez in 1965.

Recent data suggest that an abnormality in the granulocyte-macrophage colony stimulating factor (GM-CSF) receptor or ligand might be involved in the pathogenesis of pulmonary alveolar proteinosis. GM-CSF is required for normal surfactant homeostasis. Some studies conducted with GM-CSF administered subcutaneously obtained an overall response rate of 43%. It was concluded that GM-CSF appears to benefit a subset of

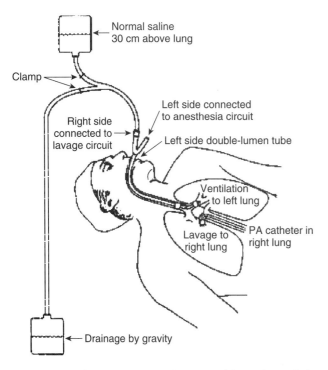

FIGURE 12-2 Modern perspective: description of the modern technique. (From Benumof JL: Anesthesia for special elective therapeutic procedures. In Benumof JL [ed]: *Anesthesia for thoracic surgery,* ed 2, Philadelphia, 1995, WB Saunders.)

patients with adult pulmonary alveolar proteinosis and could represent a novel alternative to repeated whole-lung lavage in treating the disease.[54]

Other pathologic states were also treated by whole-lung lavage but with variable success: cystic fibrosis, asthma, chronic obstructive lung disease, radioactive dust inhalation, alveolar microlithiasis, lipoid pneumonitis or exogenous lipoid pneumonia, and silicosis.[55-66]

Preoperative Evaluation

Typically, in pulmonary alveolar proteinosis, the pulmonary function test indicates a restrictive pattern. Carbon monoxide diffusing capacity is usually reduced by an order of magnitude similar to the severity of the hypoxemia. Radiologic imaging, CT scans, and ventilation-perfusion scans help to determine the most impaired lung so that one can be lavaged first.[67] The other lung is treated a few days or a few weeks later. If there is any doubt about the diagnosis, a lung biopsy should be performed.

Technique for Whole-Lung Lavage

In this author's institution, the team is composed of trained and experienced staff consisting of an anesthesia technician, a nurse, a physiotherapist, and an anesthesiologist.

MONITORING

In addition to the standard monitors, an arterial catheter is used for beat-to-beat measurement of blood pressure and blood gases analysis. Some clinicians also suggest the use of continuous intra-arterial blood gas monitoring, a pulmonary artery catheter, continuous monitoring of mixed venous oxygen saturation, and transesophageal echocardiography.[68-73] The

pulmonary artery catheter may be used as a therapeutic aid to divert blood flow away from the lavaged lung by inflating the balloon.

A ventilator monitor (Ventilator module, System Sirecust 400, Siemens AG UB med, Erlangen, Germany) can be used in conjunction with the Servoventilator 900C (Siemens-Elema AB, Ventilator Division, S-171 95 Solna, Sweden) to transfer the flow and pressure values from the ventilator and to compute the compliance on a breath-to-breath basis. Side-stream spirometry (Datex Division of Instrumentarium Corp., Finland) used to measure the patient airway pressures, volumes, flow, compliance, and resistance coupled to the Capnomac Ultima (Datex Division of Instrumentarium Corporation, Finland) can yield the same result[68].

ANESTHETIC TECHNIQUE FOR WHOLE-LUNG LAVAGE

Only a light premedication is used. Preoxygenation is mandatory. General anesthesia is induced and maintained with intravenous agents such as sufentanil, propofol, and a neuromuscular blocking agent. Volatile anesthetics are rarely used. The procedure for unilateral lavage lasts from 3 to 4 hours.

LUNG SEPARATION

A disposable left double-lumen endotracheal tube with a carinal hook is used. The carinal hook offers greater stability of the tube with respect to the numerous manipulations that occur during the lung lavage. Accurate placement of the tube is confirmed with fiberoptic bronchoscopy, and adequacy of the airway seal is confirmed by a pressure-volume loop obtained from side-stream spirometry.[67,68]

In order to measure the effectiveness of the whole-lung lavage objectively, gas exchange and pulmonary mechanics are obtained from both lungs simultaneously and then from each lung separately both before and after the procedure.

LUNG LAVAGE

The patient is placed in the supine position. In order to improve the effectiveness of the lavage, ventilation of the patient's lungs with an F_{IO_2}, of 1.0 is initiated for a few minutes to facilitate denitrogenation.[67] One-lung ventilation is established in the nonlavaged lung. A disposable irrigation and drainage system (Figure 12-3) is used to instill approximately 1 L of warm normal saline solution (37° C). The irrigating liquid is suspended 30 cm above the patient's midthoracic level; then, with the assistance of a small amount of suction (less than 20 cmH_2O), the saline is drained rapidly into a container positioned 60 cm below the patient's midthoracic level. This process is repeated 10 times or more if necessary to obtain a clear effluent lavage fluid.

Supplemental mechanical maneuvers are used to increase the efficacy of the whole-lung lavage. These techniques consist of manual chest physiotherapy, percussion, vibration, and pressure applied during the filling and drainage phases.[74] A flannel cloth is used to protect the patient's skin from irritation that the repetitive percussion might provoke. Positional manipulations are very useful for irrigating and draining all the different segments of the lung.[67] The full lateral position is used at least once during the procedure. When the lavaged lung is in the nondependent position, care must be taken to avoid the risk of leakage into the dependent, ventilated lung.

After three cycles of lavage and drainage, manual ventilation of the lavaged lung is frequently used midway to facilitate

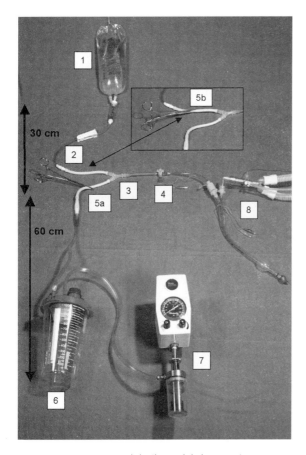

FIGURE 12-3 Irrigation and drainage system.
1. Normal saline bag
2. Large-bore tubular set for bladder irrigation
3. Y-adaptor
4. Three-way stopcock for enteral feeding
5a. Clamp on the drainage-side tubing during instillation phase
5b. Clamp on the instillation-side tubing during drainage phase
6. Vacuum bottle
7. Suction unit
8. #5 endotracheal tube, swivel adaptor, and double-lumen tube

the evacuation of the alveolar material.[75] Near the conclusion of the procedure, high-frequency jet ventilation is used between lavage cycles to increase the elimination of the material. Strict in-and-out balance of lavage liquid must be recorded.

Complications
DESATURATION
An increase in the blood flow to the nonventilated lung occurs during the drainage phase. This causes a decrease in arterial oxygen saturation (Figure 12-4).[67] During that time, if necessary, temporary partial unilateral pulmonary artery balloon occlusion may be employed with a pulmonary artery catheter positioned under fluoroscopy in the artery of the lavaged lung. Blood flow is diverted from the lavaged, nonventilated lung to the nonlavaged, ventilated lung to improve oxygenation.[49,76] The use of nitric oxide with or without

almitrine infusion has been described.[77] Others have performed whole-lung lavage under hyperbaric conditions.[78] Recently, the use of extracorporeal membrane oxygenation (ECMO) has been described to perform bilateral, simultaneous whole-lung lavage.[79] The use of PEEP on the ventilated lung helps improve oxygenation during the filling phase but might worsen the Pao_2 during the drainage phase.[80]

LEAKAGE
Pulmonary compliance of the nonlavaged lung must be monitored continuously to diagnose any liquid spillage from the lavaged lung. The mechanisms of liquid spillage are different depending on which lung is being treated. When whole-lung lavage is performed in the right lung, excessive pressure originates in the trachea; when leaking occurs, there is flooding of the left lung (Figure 12-5, *A*). When leaking originates from the left side during left lung lavage, it is caused by excessive pressure in the left lung or by displacement of the double-lumen tube. Thus leakage from the lung to the trachea and finally to the right lung occurs (Figure 12-5, *B*).

If a decrease in the compliance of the ventilated lung occurs, it is important to suspect flooding of the ventilated lung. At that time, confirmation by fiberoptic bronchoscopy and treatment with vigorous suctioning and inflation of the involved lung should be performed. It is essential to assess the function of the nonlavaged lung before continuing the lavage in order to ensure that the flooded lung can maintain adequate oxygenation during subsequent one-lung ventilation. When flooding of the nonlavaged lung occurs, maintenance of postoperative ventilation is required in order to allow recovery.[66] The best treatment for this complication is prevention, which can be accomplished by secure fixation of the double-lumen tube, by using a double-lumen tube with a carinal hook, and by being careful not to dislodge the double-lumen tube during patient and head manipulations. Other complications, such as pneumothorax and hydrothorax, are rare.

Conclusion of the Whole-Lung Lavage Procedure
When the effluent lavage fluid is clear, the procedure is complete. Usually, 10 to 15 L are instilled (up to 50 L) and more than 90% is recovered, leaving a recuperation deficit of less than 10%. At the end of the procedure, the lavaged lung is thoroughly suctioned.

The effluent liquid of the whole-lung lavage appears different depending on the patient's underlying disease. The sediment might seem milky following whole-lung lavage for pulmonary alveolar proteinosis, and it can appear sandy if lung lavage is performed for silicosis (Figure 12-6). After reintubation with a single-lumen endotracheal tube, fiberoptic bronchoscopy is performed to visualize the occurrence of undetected leakage that might have occurred during the procedure. During the fiberoptic bronchoscopy inspection, this author regularly observed local irritation of the distal tracheal mucosa secondary to the movement of the double-lumen tube during whole-lung lavage. The use of a double-lumen tube with a carinal hook has decreased the incidence of irritation noticeably.

Mechanical ventilation with PEEP is continued, usually for less than 2 hours, to restore lung function until the patient awakens in the recovery room. Alveolar infiltrates seen on the

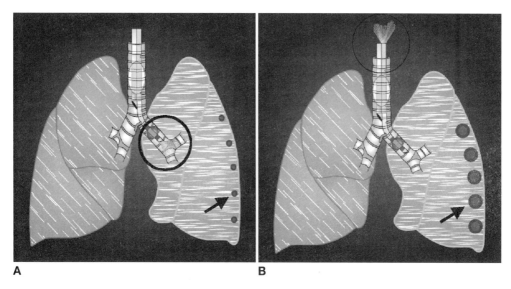

FIGURE 12-4 Desaturation. **A,** During the filling phase *(circle),* there is reduction of blood flow to the nonventilated lung by compression of the pulmonary blood vessels *(arrow).* **B,** During the drainage phase *(circle),* there is reperfusion of the nonventilated lung *(arrow),* creating a shunt, leading to desaturation.

chest x-ray immediately after whole-lung lavage usually clear within 24 hours. Observation of the patient in the intensive care unit for 24 hours is a routine part of the procedure.

Postoperative Management of Whole-Lung Lavage

Following whole-lung lavage, pulmonary compliance and oxygenation decrease significantly in the lavaged lung compared with its baseline value and with the non-lavaged lung. In pulmonary alveolar proteinosis, lavage is performed on one lung. A few days later, whole-lung lavage of the contralateral lung is completed. Before the next contralateral lavage, compliance and oxygenation should recover to their baseline values as measured prior to the first lavage.[66] At the time of subsequent lavage, oxygenation is usually not a problem because the treated (and now near-normal) lung is used to support gas exchange during the procedure.[67]

Following whole-lung lavage, patients usually exhibit a marked subjective improvement that correlates with increases in Pao$_2$ (at rest and exercise), vital capacity, diffusing capacity, and clearing of the chest roentgenogram. Some patients require lavage every few months, whereas others remain in remission for several years. The disease can eventually show a late recurrence.[67] In the authors' experience, less than 50% of patients need more than the initial bilateral whole-lung lavage. Whole-lung lavage proves to be successful for patients with pulmonary alveolar proteinosis, not only because the lavage removes an enormous accumulation of alveolar lipoproteinaceous material,

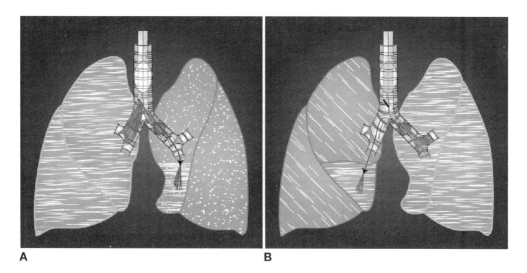

FIGURE 12-5 Leakage from the lavage lung to the nonlavage lung. **A,** During right-lung lavage, excessive pressure in the trachea promotes flooding in the left (ventilated) lung. **B,** During left-lung lavage, excessive pressure in the left lung or displacement of the DLT promotes flooding of the right (ventilated) lung.

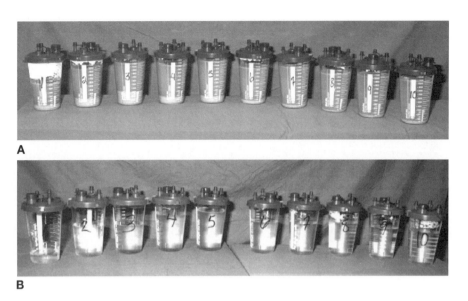

FIGURE 12-6 Product from whole-lung lavage. **A,** Product from pulmonary alveolar proteinosis appears milky. **B,** Product from silicosis appears sandy.

but also because it interrupts the pathogenic loop and temporarily restores the activity and function of the macrophages.

Pediatric Whole-Lung Lavage

Whole-lung lavage has been used in the pediatric and neonatal population with some success. Whole-lung lavage is technically difficult in infants and small children because it is difficult to isolate the lungs safely and adequately during lavage. Small double-lumen tubes (Bronchopart, size 26F, 28F, and 32F, Willy Rusch AG, 71394 Kernen, Germany or Broncho-Cath size 28F and 32F, Mallinckrodt Medical, Athlone, Ireland) are now available for use in children greater than 8 to 10 years

old or weighing more than 30 kg. Small fiberoptic bronchoscopes are also available to verify and adjust the final position of this double-lumen tube. If the placement of a double-lumen tube is possible, the whole-lung lavage technique for the child is similar to that of an adult.

If the airway is too small for insertion of a double-lumen tube, whole-lung lavage is technically more challenging. Different methods to isolate both lungs have been described and are summarized in Figures 12-7, 12-8, and 12-9. Airway isolation has been obtained for infants as small as 2 kg.[81,82] Ideally, whole-lung lavage is performed as with a double-lumen tube in place, but with much more attention to the stability of the airway devices.

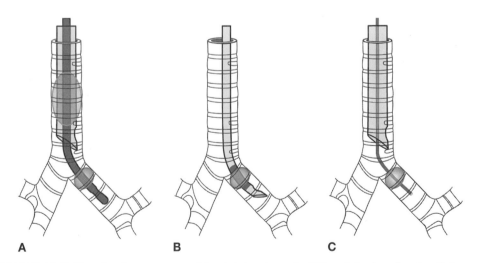

FIGURE 12-7 Alternative airway management for whole-lung lavage in children. **A,** A urinary Fogarty catheter, positioned with fiberoptic bronchoscopy guidance in a mainstem bronchus, is used to isolate and lavage one lung. **B,** A long, cuffed endobronchial tube is used to isolate and lavage one lung. Final positioning is confirmed by fiberoptic bronchoscopy. **C,** A 5F double-lumen Swan-Ganz catheter is introduced through the sidearm of a rigid 3.5-mm bronchoscope into a mainstem bronchus. It is used to isolate and to lavage one lung of a 2-kg infant. The bronchoscope served to ventilate the contralateral lung. The procedure is monitored under direct vision with a video monitor, ensuring correct position of the bronchoscope and the catheter at all times. (From Moazam F, Schmidt JH, Chesrown SE, et al: *J Red Surg* 20(4): 398, 1985.)

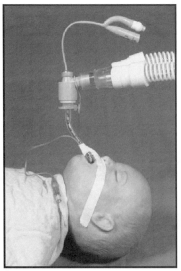 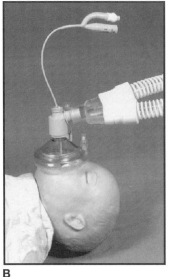 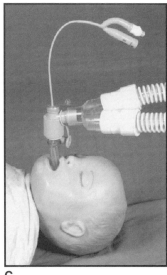

A   B   C

FIGURE 12-8 Endotracheal tube, anesthesia mask, or laryngeal mask. **A,** The Fogarty catheter is introduced through a bronchoscope adapter attached to a 6-mm diameter endotracheal tube that ventilates the contralateral lung. (From Ciravegna B, Sacco O, Moroni C, et al: *Pediatr Pulmonol* 23(3):233, 1997.) **B,** Alternatively, the proximal part of the tube can be passed through a bronchoscope adapter attached to a tight-fitting anesthesia mask that ventilates the contralateral lung. (From McKenzie B, Wood RE, Bailey A: *Anesthesiology* 70(3): 550, 1989.) **C,** Alternatively, a laryngeal mask can be used instead of the anesthesia mask. It could be easier to manage the ventilation with a ventilator rather than with manual ventilation.

When the techniques just described cannot be applied, particularly in patients weighing <10 kg, ECMO can be used to oxygenate the patient while bilateral simultaneous whole-lung lavage is performed. Different approaches for vascular cannulation have been described.[83,84] Finally, one case report describes the use of partial liquid ventilation with perflubron (LiquidVent; Alliance Pharmaceuticals Corporation and Hoechst Marion Roussel) and ECMO for 4 days following whole-lung lavage in a 3.4- kg infant at 6 weeks of age.[85]

Conclusion

After more than 35 years of evolution, whole-lung lavage is an efficient and safe technique. This procedure can be adapted to a large variety of patients and diseases.

Lung Volume Reduction Surgery

Chronic obstructive pulmonary disease (COPD) is the major cause of pulmonary disability in the United States and Europe.[86] Specific guidelines for the diagnosis and care of patients with COPD are given by the American Thoracic Society.[87] The cardinal physiologic defect in emphysema is a decrease in elastic recoil of the lung tissue. This results in the principal physiologic abnormalities of emphysema: decreased maximum expiratory airflow, leading to air trapping and hyperinflation and severely limited exercise capacity.[88,89] The destruction of the alveolar-capillary membrane surface leads to a reduction in diffusing capacity. Emphysema is usually the result of cigarette smoking but can also be caused by α-1-antitrypsin deficiency.[90,91] It is a chronic progressive disorder that ultimately leads to disability and early death. Emphysema is estimated to be present in 2 million adults in the United States,

and, along with other forms of COPD, it accounts for about 90,000 deaths annually.

Current Therapy for Emphysema

Guidelines for the diagnosis and management of emphysema are established by the American Thoracic Society.[87] The goals of therapy for emphysema are to halt the progressive decline in lung function, prevent exacerbations of the disease, improve exercise capacity and quality of life, and prolong survival. The only treatment that has been shown to alter the rate of progression of COPD is cessation of smoking.[92] Influenza immunization and pneumococcal vaccination are recommended for the prevention of life-threatening infection.[87] Exacerbations of bronchospasm and infection are treated with steroids and antibiotics, respectively.[93,94] Furthermore, β-adrenergic agonists and anticholinergics are recommended for treatment of COPD and asthma.[87] Although these interventions are believed to shorten the duration of individual episodes and to minimize symptoms, there is little evidence that they either alter the natural history of the disease or reduce mortality. Bronchodilators improve lung function, exercise capacity, and quality of life in patients with COPD but are of limited benefit to patients without reversible airway disease.[87] Pulmonary rehabilitation—including aerobic exercise conditioning, education, and psychologic support—improves exercise capacity in patients with COPD and might reduce the rate of hospitalization.[95,96]

Long-term home oxygen therapy in chronically hypoxemic patients is the only treatment for COPD that has been documented to decrease mortality rates.[97,98] Adjunctive forms of therapy, such as the use of mucolytics to control respiratory

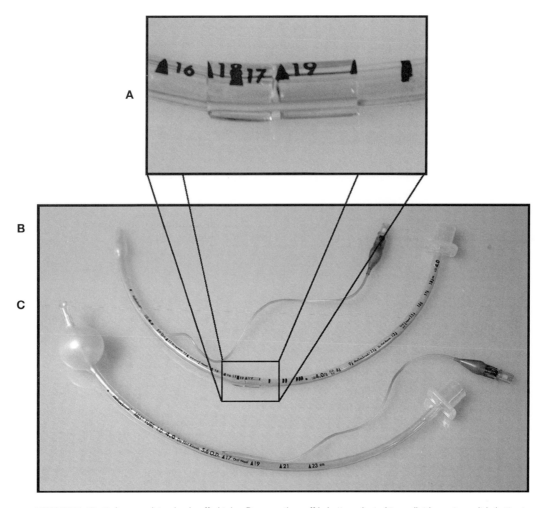

FIGURE 12-9 Long endotracheal cuffed tube. Because the cuff is better adapted to pediatric anatomy, it is better to use a long, handmade small endotracheal tube **(A),** rather than the MLT version (Mallinckrodt Inc., St. Louis, MO 63134), which features a larger cuff for adult use **(B).** It is easier to produce a long version of a small endotracheal tube with an exterior sleeve 3 cm long and obtained from a tube 1 mm larger than the interior tubes, to join the two parts of the new tube together **(C).**

secretions or narcotics to reduce the sensation of dyspnea, have been used in selected COPD patients.[87] In end-stage COPD patients, single- or double-lung transplantation has been used as a last resort, but this option is limited by financial resources and the number of donor organs.

Lung Volume Reduction Surgery for Emphysema

The failure of medical treatment alone to produce long-term improvement of symptoms has promoted the introduction of various surgical procedures over the last 90 years. Surgical procedures such as phrenic nerve paralysis, thoracoplasty, denervation of the lung, and stabilization and fixation of the trachea provided minimal or no benefit.[99]

In 1957, Brantigan and Mueller first introduced the technique for surgical excision of lung tissue to reduce the volume of hyperinflated lung parenchyma; they named this procedure "lung volume reduction surgery" (LVRS).[100] Although 75% of patients reported clinical improvement, the lack of objective documentation for benefit from the procedure in conjunction

with an operative mortality of 18% prevented widespread acceptance of the procedure.

In 1995, Cooper et al reported a modified Brantigan procedure in which emphysematous lung tissue was resected from both lungs via a median sternotomy approach. In the initial series of 20 selected patients undergoing LVRS with this method, there was no operative mortality, and the operation produced an 82% increase in forced expiratory volume in one second (FEV_1). Thus, with improvements in both surgical and anesthetic techniques that occurred in the interim, Cooper et al reintroduced a very promising surgical procedure for treatment of end-stage emphysema decades after the procedure was first attempted.[101]

Lung volume reduction surgery (i.e., bilateral resection of 20% to 30% of the total lung volume) was found to be associated with significant improvement of lung function, significant alleviation of dyspnea, and improvement of exercise tolerance in selected patients with severe emphysema.[101] To date, it seems that some patients undoubtedly exhibit marked improvement after LVRS, and numerous studies have tried to elucidate the mechanisms of improvement. About 20% of patients, however, show no objective or subjective improvement.[102,103] Furthermore, some centers report early operative mortality rates ranging from 2.5% to 13.3%.[104,105] Currently, it is generally accepted that careful patient selection for LVRS is crucial for a successful outcome; however, there are no established criteria for patient selection available, and predictors for outcome after LVRS remain under investigation. In their workshop summary from the National Heart Lung and Blood Institute, Weinmann and Hyatt stated that a precondition for successful conduct of LVRS is "the obvious need for highly experienced surgical, anesthetic, and critical care teams."[104] LVRS is an especially challenging procedure for the anesthesiologist, as it requires a profound knowledge of anesthesia for thoracic surgery, pain therapy, and respiratory mechanics in both the anesthetized and awake patient suffering from end-stage emphysema.

Mechanisms of Functional Improvement After LVRS

The anesthesiologist must possess a thorough knowledge of the physiologic mechanisms of improvement after LVRS in order to provide optimal patient care. It is essential to have a thorough understanding of the pathophysiology of COPD.[87,104,106-113] Maximal air flow in normal and diseased lungs is determined by the pulmonary elastic recoil and the characteristics of the airway. The defining characteristic of COPD is a reduction of maximal expiratory flow. As the disease progresses, patients must breathe at a higher lung volume in order to achieve the flows necessary to meet their ventilatory requirements. Total lung capacity (TLC), the maximum lung volume that patients can achieve, increases due to diminished elastic recoil of the lung and remodeling of the rib cage and diaphragm. This adaptive response is limited, however. In end-stage COPD, the end-inspiratory volume approaches TLC. Patients are dyspneic at rest and are unable to increase ventilation enough during exercise to maintain a normal Pao_2 and $Paco_2$ because they are already breathing near or at maximal flows when at rest. In addition, there can be marked abnormalities in ventilation-perfusion matching.

Shortly after the reintroduction of LVRS, investigators started to examine the mechanism of functional improvement following LVRS during rest and during exercise. The main focus of these studies was postoperative alterations in ventilatory mechanics and diaphragmatic function.

Postoperative Alterations in Pulmonary Function Testing

LVRS is known to produce marked changes in several parameters of pulmonary function testing. Most notably, there is a significant increase in FEV_1. Table 12-3 depicts the average changes that can be expected 3 to 6 months following surgery; it must be noted, however, that a significant number of subjects (approximately 20%) exhibit no significant improvement in pulmonary function testing after LVRS.[104]

Postoperative Alterations in Pulmonary Mechanics

Several investigators showed an improvement in elastic recoil, a reduction in expiratory flow limitation, a decrease in DPH (dynamic pulmonary hyperinflation), and a decrease in work of breathing (WOB) during resting conditions after LVRS.[108] Expiratory flow limitation becomes most apparent in the pressure-volume curve obtained from a subject, in which the x-axis depicts transpulmonary pressure and the y-axis depicts volume. In patients with COPD, inspiration is not markedly altered, whereas expiration is characterized by a very flat slope of the pressure-volume curve (Figure 12-10). O'Donnell et al and Gelb et al demonstrated that the slope of expiration becomes markedly steeper in the pressure-volume curve of patients after LVRS (Figure 12-10), indicating a significant reduction in expiratory airflow limitation.[109,113] Thus it seems accepted to date that improvement in expiratory airflow leads to a favorable functional improvement in selected emphysema patients after LVRS.

Another issue was the time course of improvement in pulmonary mechanics after surgery. Cooper et al reported that patients were successfully extubated in the operating room at the conclusion of surgery following bilateral resection of 20% to 30% of lung volume.[101] This was surprising, as an FEV_1 of 800 mL was considered previously as a criterion for inoperability in patients scheduled for lung resection.[114] Therefore, it had to be suspected that pulmonary mechanics improved almost immediately after LVRS. To test this hypothesis, pulmonary mechanics were assessed before and within 24 hours after surgery and additionally at later time intervals. Improvements in WOB (Figure 12-11), intrinsic positive end-expiratory pressure ($PEEP_i$ = a measure for DPH), and pulmonary resistance (R_L) were present as early as 24 hours after LVRS.[115,116] These findings indicate that early extubation after bilateral lung resection in patients with FEV_1 less than 800 mL is possible and can be explained by early improvement in pulmonary mechanics following the procedure.

TABLE 12-3

Average Baseline and Postoperative Values for Lung Volume Reduction Surgery

Test	Baseline Values	Postoperative Values
Total lung capacity (TLC)	130%–140% of predicted	20% decrease
Residual volume (RV)	>200% of predicted	30% decrease
Forced vital capacity (FVC)	50%–70% of predicted	30%–40% increase
Forced expiratory volume in 1 second (FEV_1)	25%–30% of predicted	50%–60% increase
Carbon monoxide diffusing capacity (DL_{CO})	30%–40% of predicted	No change
6-minute walk test	700–1200 ft	20%–30% increase

From Weinmann GG, Hyatt R: *Am J Respir Crit Care Med* 154:1913-1918, 1996.

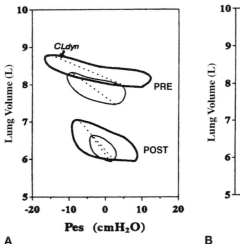
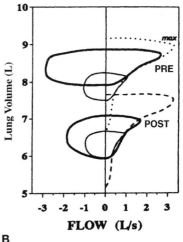

A   **B**

FIGURE 12-10 In one representative subject, pressure-volume **(A)** and flow-volume **(B)** relations are shown during a typical tidal breath at rest *(thin lines)* and during an equivalent level of exercise *(thick lines)* before and after volume reduction surgery. Comparisons were made at similar levels of ventilation before surgery (rest = 19.7 L/min; exercise = 37.4 L/min) and after surgery (rest = 20.4 L/min; exercise = 34 L/min). *Dotted* (presurgery) and *dashed* (postsurgery) *lines* **(B)** indicate the maximal expiratory flow-volume envelopes performed at rest. *Cldyn,* Dynamic compliance. (From O'Donnell DE, Webb KA, Bertley JC, et al: *Chest* 110:23, 1996.)

Several investigators demonstrated that improvement in exercise capacity was due to improved pulmonary mechanics,[113,117,118] In exercise tests with continuous monitoring of pulmonary mechanics, significant decreases in $PEEP_i$, WOB, and R_L were found after LVRS.[118]

Postoperative Alterations in Diaphragmatic Function

Benditt et al found improved diaphragmatic pressure generation in patients undergoing exercise tests 3 months after LVRS.[119] Investigations at other institutions produced similar results.[120,121] Improved diaphragmatic pressure generation, however, was found not to be demonstrated earlier than three months after surgery (Table 12-4).[115] Diaphragmatic force generation was not significantly different from preoperative values after one month following LVRS.[115] Thus, it seems likely that the improvement in diaphragmatic function is a late benefit of LVRS.

To date, it appears that there is a group of highly selected end-stage emphysema patients who benefit from LVRS by means of early improvement of pulmonary mechanics and by somewhat later improvement in diaphragmatic function. The duration of these improvements remains unclear.

Optimal Criteria for LVRS

PATIENT SELECTION

General Criteria for Patient Selection. General criteria for patient selection and recommendations for screening procedures are described by Weinmann and Hyatt.[104] These selection criteria may vary between institutions. Distinct selection criteria for LVRS candidates were published by Daniel et al and are shown in Table 12-5.[122]

Whether patients with significant hypercapnia should undergo LVRS is controversial.[104,123] Furthermore, some institutions report significant coronary artery disease (coronary

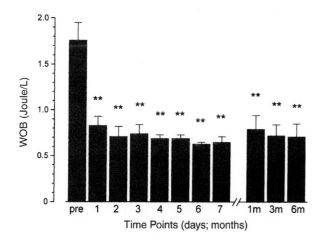

FIGURE 12-11 Changes in work of breathing (WOB) at various time points after lung volume reduction surgery (LVRS).
*$P < 0.001$.

TABLE 12-4		
Mean Transdiaphragmatic (P_{di}) and Esophageal (P_{es}) Pressures: Lung Volume Reduction Surgery		
Time of Testing	**P_{di} (mmHg)**	**P_{es} (mmHg)**
Preoperative	64.4 ± 4.5	53.2 ± 3.6
1 month postoperative	76.6 ± 7.6	55.3 ± 6.0
3 months postoperative	$90.2 \pm 13.2^*$	$68.1 \pm 5.4^*$
6 months postoperative	$87.0 \pm 7.6^*$	$70.8 \pm 3.8^*$

From Tschernko EM, Wisser W, Wanket, et al: *Thorax* 52:545-550, 1997.
*$P < 0.05$
Mean transdiaphragmatic (P_{di}) and esophageal (P_{es}) pressure of patients with emphysema before LVRS as well as 1, 3, and 6 months after LVRS.

From Daniel TM, Barry BK, Chan MD, et al: *Ann Surg* 223(5):526, 1996.

TABLE 12-5

General Inclusion Criteria for LVRS

Diagnosis of COPD
Patient history, physical examination, lung function test, chest x-ray, etc.
Smoking cessation for >1 month
Age <75 years
FEV_1 15%–35% of predicted
$Paco_2$ <55 mmHg
Prednisone requirement <20 mg/day
PAP_{sys} <50 mmHg
No previous thoracotomy or pleurodesis
Absence of symptomatic coronary artery disease
Absence of chronic asthma or bronchitis
Commitment to preoperative and postoperative supervised pulmonary rehabilitation for 6 weeks

COPD, Chronic obstructive pulmonary disease; *FEV₁,* forced expiratory volume in one second; *Paco₂,* arterial carbon dioxide pressure in mmHg; *PAP_sys,* systolic pulmonary arterial pressure in mmHg.

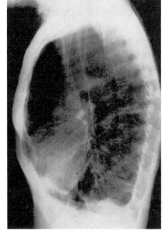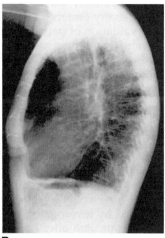

FIGURE 12-12 A lateral chest x-ray is shown. **A,** The patient is shown before lung volume reduction surgery (LVRS): The thorax is barrel-shaped with high transparency of the lungs, a large retrosternal air-filled space, and a flattened-to-concave diaphragm. **B,** The chest x-ray of the same subject shown 3 months after LVRS. The lung fields are less transparent, the air-filled retrosternal space has decreased significantly, and the diaphragm exhibits an almost normal, convex shape.

artery stenosis >70%) diagnosed in 15% of their asymptomatic LVRS candidates and thus, they recommend left and right heart cardiac catheterization preoperatively.[124] This invasive cardiac screening seems justified by several case reports of myocardial infarction during and after LVRS. Other institutions recommend limiting cardiac screening to transthoracic echocardiography.[104] In general. it is reasonable for centers with less experience to employ strict criteria for patient selection to minimize patient morbidity and mortality.

Morphologic Criteria for Patient Selection. The chest x-ray should provide evidence of hyperinflated lungs, large intercostal spaces, retrosternal airspace, flattened diaphragm, and high transparency of the lungs as shown in the left panel of Figure 12-12. For a precise morphologic evaluation, a high-resolution computer tomograph (HR-CT) of the chest is essential for identification of nonhomogenous areas within the lungs.[125] HR-CT locates the target areas for resection. An ideal

anatomic precondition for LVRS is marked inhomogeneity of the lung structure, where normal lung tissue and severely destroyed, overdistended tissue are present in the same lung (Figure 12-13, *A*). Homogenous distribution of the disease proves to be an unfavorable precondition (Figure 12-13, *B*). Several authors have demonstrated that patients presenting with severe inhomogeneity are very likely to benefit from LVRS.[126-128] Two reasons might account for this:

- Compressed, normal lung tissue is released after removing adjoining hyperinflated, nonfunctional, destroyed tissue, and in this way the pulmonary mechanics of the remaining tissue are improved.

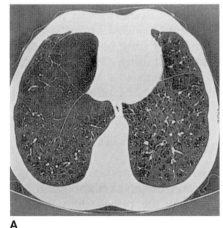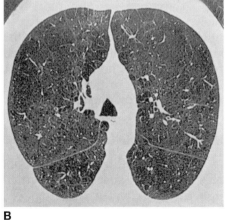

FIGURE 12-13 A, A high-resolution computed tomography (HR-CT) scan of a patient presenting with inhomogeneous distribution of emphysema. Parenchymal destruction is greater in the ventral portions of the lung; thus the functional portions are easily distinguished from nonfunctional segments. **B,** An HR-CT of a patient with homogenous distribution of emphysema. It is much more difficult to determine which segments need to be resected.

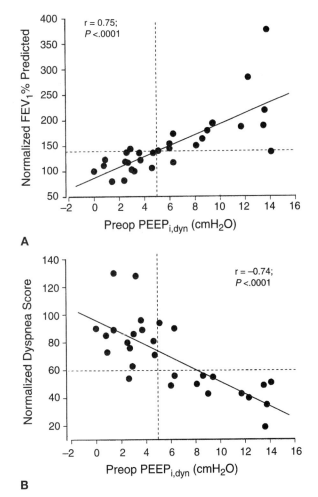

FIGURE 12-14 A, Circles represent single data pairs of patients. The x-value is preoperative dynamic end-expiratory pressure (PEEP$_{i,dyn}$), and the y-value is normalized forced expiratory volume in one second (FEV$_1$%) 3 months after lung volume reduction surgery (LVRS). The horizontal dotted line represents an increase in predicted FEV$_1$% of 40% after LVRS. Circles above this line represent patients with an increase in FEV$_1$% >40%, and circles below this horizontal dotted line represent patients with an increase in FEV$_1$% <40%. The vertical dotted line separates patients with preoperative PEEP$_{i,dyn}$ <5 cmH$_2$O from patients with preoperative PEEP$_{i,dyn}$ >5 cmH$_2$O. Thus the plot is divided into four parts containing the false-negative cases (upper-left part), the true positive cases (upper-right part), the true negative cases (lower-left part), and the false positive cases (lower-right part) for a threshold value of PEEP$_{i,dyn}$ ≥5 cmH$_2$O. The straight, solid line represents the line of linear regression, r is the correlation coefficient, and p is the level of significance. **B,** Circles represent single data pairs of patients. The x-value is preoperative dynamic end-expiratory pressure (PEEP$_{i,dyn}$), and the y-value is the normalized dyspnea score 3 months after lung volume reduction surgery (LVRS). The horizontal dotted line represents a decrease of dyspnea score of 40% after LVRS. Circles above this line represent patients with a decrease <40%, and circles below this horizontal dotted line represent patients with a decrease >40%. The vertical dotted line separates patients with preoperative PEEP$_{i,dyn}$ <5 cmH$_2$O from patients with preoperative PEEP$_{i,dyn}$ >5 cmH$_2$O. Thus, the plot is divided into four parts containing the true negative cases (upper-left part), the false positive cases (upper-right part), the false negative cases (lower-left part), and the true positive cases (lower-right part) for a threshold value of PEEP$_{i,dyn}$ ≥ 5 cmH$_2$O. The straight, solid line represents the line of linear regression, r is the correlation coefficient, and p is the level of significance.

- Surgery is easier to perform if the target areas are clearly visible. In many centers, lung perfusion scintigraphy is still routinely performed for screening LVRS candidates primarily to rule out ventilation-perfusion mismatch. However, chest computed tomography has been shown to be superior compared to lung perfusion scintigraphy for the evaluation of patients.[129]

The evaluation of lung morphology is semiquantitative and difficult to standardize. Only about 25% of patients present with inhomogeneous distribution of the disease. Therefore, the evaluation of preoperative functional criteria as predictors seems important.

Functional Criteria for Patient Selection. Currently, a preoperative FEV$_1$ less than 20% of the predicted value in combination with homogenous morphology or a carbon monoxide diffusion capacity less than 20% of the predicted value is regarded as contraindication for surgery. These patients were found to have significantly increased mortality after LVRS compared with conventional medical treatment alone.[130]

Pulmonary mechanics are severely impaired in patients with emphysema, and LVRS leads to a significant improvement.[108-111,118] Several parameters characterizing pulmonary mechanics show specific changes after LVRS. These parameters were tested by investigators as preoperative predictors for outcome after LVRS. FEV$_1$ is frequently chosen to represent outcome because it correlates well with mortality in emphysema patients. Furthermore, outcome is frequently characterized by changes seen in pressure-volume loops and by changes in dyspnea score because severe dyspnea leads to an impaired quality of life.

Ingenito et al hypothesized that patients with markedly elevated inspiratory resistance are likely to have airway disease predominating and are thus unlikely to show improvement of expiratory flow after LVRS, which would limit any benefit from the procedure.[131] The investigators proved their hypothesis by demonstrating that preoperative inspiratory lung resistance correlated negatively with changes in FEV$_1$ ($r = -0.63$; $P < 0.001$). In contrast, patients with elevated expiratory lung resistance showed good improvement (Figure 12-14).

Preoperative PEEP$_i$, a correlate of dynamic pulmonary hyperinflation, and postoperative gain in normalized FEV$_1$% were found to be well correlated ($r = 0.69$, $P < 0.0002$), as shown in Figure 12-15.[132] A cutoff point of preoperative PEEP$_1$ of 5 cmH$_2$O had a positive predictive value of 86% and a negative predictive value of 92% in predicting a change in FEV$_1$% of more than 40% after LVRS.[132] Similar results were found for changes in dyspnea score.

Despite these and other promising methods to predict outcome following LVRS, most require time-consuming, sophisticated measuring techniques and are difficult to incorporate into standard clinical practice. As a result, none of the evaluated parameters has gained widespread acceptance to date.

Preoperative Patient Preparation
PHARMACOLOGIC PREPARATION

Most of the patients presenting for LVRS require long-term bronchodilator therapy (β-adrenergic agonists), steroid therapy (inhalation or systemic), and mucolytic therapy. Additionally, these patients frequently require antibiotics. Most centers

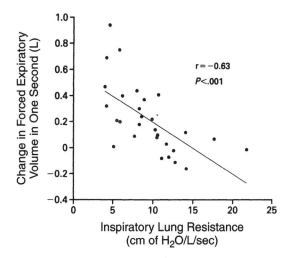

FIGURE 12-15 Data pairs of preoperative inspiratory lung resistance ($cmH_2O/L/sec$) and change in forced expiratory volume in one second (FEV_1) 3 months after lung volume reduction surgery (LVRS) are shown. The straight, solid line represents the line of linear regression, r is the correlation coefficient, and P is the level of significance. An inverse relationship between preoperative inspiratory lung resistance and improvement in FEV_1 is depicted. (From Ingenito EP, Evans RB, Loring SH, et al: *N Engl J Med* 338:1181-1185, 1998.)

recommend continuation of bronchodilator and mucolytic therapy before LVRS, including the day of surgery. The patient must be free from respiratory infections for at least three weeks prior to LVRS and require no antibiotic therapy preoperatively. In terms of steroid therapy the goal is to gradually reduce the dose of systemic steroids prior to LVRS.

Many patients have received long-term theophylline therapy before LVRS, and some patients experience toxic symptoms while theophylline blood levels are in the therapeutic range.[133] The main side effects are nervousness, tremor, and tachycardia. Theophylline therapy should be discontinued before LVRS if the patient shows significant side effects or if the serum levels reach more than 20 ng/mL.

PREOPERATIVE EXERCISE PROGRAM

Almost all centers advocate a preoperative exercise program for their patients. The optimal training program is supervised by a specialized nurse and physician and lasts for at least 6 weeks before surgery. Training consists of walking for a distance on a flat surface, bicycle ergometer training, and weight lifting. These exercises are combined with a special diet. Leg exercise is usually better tolerated than arm exercise. The following are advantages of an exercise program before surgery:

- The patient's willingness to cooperate can be assessed.
- Endurance and exercise tolerance are increased, which will be helpful for early mobilization after surgery.[101]
- Maximum oxygen consumption can be increased in many subjects.[96]

PSYCHOLOGIC PREPARATION

Patients presenting for LVRS are frequently very anxious secondary to the dyspnea and asthmatic crises they experienced in the past. Psychologic factors can induce an asthma attack that is a dangerous complication during the perioperative period. Anxiety is associated with an increase in respiratory

frequency leading to an increase in dynamic pulmonary hyperinflation and dyspnea.[134] Therefore it is important that the anesthesiologist be able to establish a good relationship with the patient before surgery. The optimal psychologic preconditions are likely to be achieved when the preoperative preparation, preoperative visit, insertion of the thoracic epidural catheter, administration of general anesthesia, and early postoperative therapy are conducted by the same physician or by a team well known to the patient. Anxiolytic therapy might be necessary during the preoperative and perioperative periods.

Anesthesia for LVRS

THORACIC EPIDURAL ANALGESIA

It is now generally accepted that thoracic epidural analgesia (TEA) is mandatory for optimal postoperative pain management following LVRS. A thoracic epidural catheter is inserted at the T_3 to T_4 or T_4 to T_5 vertebral level in the awake patient immediately before surgery[4]. The spread of anesthesia and analgesia should be assessed carefully before induction of general anesthesia in order to avoid inadequate pain management that could cause ventilatory depression during the immediate postoperative period. A local anesthetic such as bupivacaine or ropivacaine can be used for TEA, preferably in combination with an opioid. Because patients with emphysema tend to be volume depleted, it is important that they be adequately volume loaded (1 to 2 mL/kg) before TEA is fully activated so that severe hypotension can be avoided. A potent vasopressor such as norepinephrine or phenylephrine should be available before TEA is activated. Ropivacaine is frequently preferred over bupivacaine as the local anesthetic because it causes less circulatory depression and helps to reduce the incidence of hypotension.

Most anesthesiologists providing care to patients for LVRS are convinced that TEA is crucial to reduce perioperative patient morbidity and mortality. Unfortunately, there are no controlled studies available to validate this theory. Some anesthesiologists might consider such a study unethical, as patients would potentially be denied optimal pain management. In patients with normal lung function undergoing lung resection, there is evidence that sufficient postoperative analgesia with TEA can reduce morbidity and mortality; however, other authors emphasize that the influence of TEA on outcome after lung resection has not been proven.[135,136] Nevertheless, the use of TEA has been established worldwide as the means for intraoperative and postoperative analgesia for patients undergoing LVRS. In order to guarantee optimal analgesia, TEA should be maintained until all chest drains are removed.

GENERAL ANESTHESIA FOR LVRS

Monitoring. Monitoring for LVRS should include a six-lead ECG, pulse oximetry, invasive blood pressure monitoring, a temperature probe for continuous core temperature measurement, and a central venous catheter to assess central venous pressure. The routine use of a pulmonary artery catheter is controversial; however, continuous monitoring of pulmonary artery pressure (PAP) might be helpful because PAP can increase substantially during single-lung ventilation, potentially causing acute right ventricular failure. Transesophageal echocardiography might also be useful for intraoperative cardiac monitoring.

ANESTHETIC DRUGS FOR LVRS

During endotracheal intubation with a double-lumen tube, the intravenous analgesic requirement can be reduced substantially if the pharynx and larynx are carefully anesthetized with a topical anesthetic spray (e.g., 2% lidocaine).[137] Following intubation, analgesia should be maintained with TEA. It is important to mention that intubation of a poorly anesthetized emphysema patient can precipitate life-threatening bronchospasm.[138]

To facilitate tracheal extubation as early as possible after LVRS and avoid prolonged air leakage associated with prolonged positive pressure ventilation, only short-acting drugs should be used for sedation and neuromuscular blockade during general anesthesia. Propofol is thus a suitable choice for sedation. If the patient is susceptible to bronchospasm, a volatile inhalation anesthetic such as sevoflurane or isoflurane might be preferred over an intravenous agent. Frequently, neuromuscular blocking agents with short duration and absence of histamine liberation (e.g., vecuronium or cisatracurium) are chosen.

Mechanical Ventilation During LVRS

Optimal mechanical ventilation for LVRS must provide sufficient arterial oxygenation while strictly avoiding air trapping, which can potentiate the threat of pneumothorax.[134] Air trapping can be minimized by using moderate tidal volumes (9 mL/kg or less during ventilation of both lungs and 5 mL/kg or less during single-lung ventilation), low respiratory frequencies (12 breaths/minute or less during ventilation of both lungs and 16 breaths/minute or less during single-lung ventilation), and a prolonged expiratory time (I:E = 1:3 during double- and single-lung ventilation). If the preoperative HR-CT exhibits a substantial difference in the quality of lung tissue between the right and left lung, it could be more desirable to resect the less functional lung first.

It is important to limit airway pressure (35 cmH$_2$O or less) generated by the ventilator in order to avoid barotraumas that could result in a pneumothorax or tension pneumothorax. The anesthesiologist should pay constant attention to the inspired and expired volumes during mechanical ventilation. For this purpose, it is necessary to monitor the configuration of the end-tidal CO$_2$ waves closely. In most patients undergoing LVRS, the anesthesiologist will have to accept elevated values of end-tidal and Pa$_{CO_2}$ (arterial carbon dioxide tension) during single-lung ventilation. This permissive hypercapnia is the price for the prevention of barotrauma during mechanical ventilation for LVRS. P$_a$CO$_2$ values will return to the normal range soon after the procedure, when both lungs can be ventilated again.

Patient Warming During LVRS

Sufficient patient warming can be achieved with warming blankets, heating mats, and warm intravenous fluid infusions. Core body temperature and the peripheral temperature of the patient should be maintained within the normal range. A decrease in the body heat content of the patient will lead, ultimately, to shivering after extubation, along with increased carbon dioxide production and oxygen consumption. It is frequently impossible for the patient with end-stage emphysema to meet the increased ventilatory demands caused by shivering.

Shivering is an undesirable complication that could lead to reintubation in the postoperative period.

Early Extubation After LVRS

It is difficult to avoid air leakage entirely, despite the use of new surgical techniques that use staplers buttressed with bovine pericardium. Air leakage can be exacerbated by positive pressure ventilation, whereas the negative intrapleural pressure generated during spontaneous breathing minimizes air leakage. Therefore early extubation after LVRS is of prime importance. Several criteria must be satisfied before the patient can be extubated (Table 12-6). Should the patient fail to meet all of these criteria, it is reasonable to stabilize the patient in a quiet environment such as an intensive care unit or the post-anesthesia care unit before extubation. Successful extubation will usually be possible within 1 to 2 hours and is not harmful to the patient. This is preferable to premature extubation in the operating room followed by prolonged episodes of arterial hypoxemia.

Summary

Patient selection is of crucial importance for a successful outcome after LVRS. The anesthesiologist must be actively involved in patient selection because he or she will be responsible for the patient's immediate perioperative management. Patient history and preoperative status, as well as the results obtained from the evaluation of chest x-rays, HR-CT scans, and catheterization of the right heart, should be weighed carefully during the patient selection process. The careful selection and preoperative preparation of patients are essential to minimize perioperative complications and obtain a successful outcome. Furthermore, it must be emphasized that the role of the anesthesiologist is of crucial importance for the successful conduct of LVRS.

To date, it is unclear whether LVRS is superior to conventional medical therapy alone for the long-term treatment of patients with end-stage emphysema, as there appears to be a progressive decline in pulmonary function following the procedure. The National Emphysema Treatment Trial (NETT), a multicenter, randomized, prospective study, compares patients with end-stage emphysema undergoing LVRS plus conventional medical therapy with those receiving medical therapy alone. It is the intent of the study to clarify this important question in the near future.

TABLE 12-6

Extubation Criteria After LVRS

1. Patient awake and cooperative
2. Patient breathing sufficiently, such as rapid shallow breathing index (respiratory frequency per min/tidal volume in L) <70
3. Sufficient arterial oxygenation: Sao$_2$ ≥92 while patient is breathing spontaneously (Fio$_2$ ≤0.35)
4. Adequate pain management achieved
5. Patient core temperature >35.5° C
6. No shivering
7. Stable hemodynamic conditions

Hemoptysis

Massive hemoptysis occurs in less than 0.5% of all patients who are admitted to the hospital for pulmonary dysfunction.[140] More than 90% of patients presenting with massive hemoptysis also have a history of chronic pulmonary infection. Some common infectious etiologies include tuberculosis and bronchiectasis. Neoplasms account for the majority of the noninfectious causes of bronchial hemorrhage. Chronic inflammation of the airways promotes vascularization of the high-pressure bronchial arteries that might subsequently erode or perforate, thus causing massive hemoptysis.[141]

Cardiovascular etiologies include mitral stenosis, arteriovenous malformations, pulmonary embolism, and pulmonary artery perforation/rupture secondary to the placement of a pulmonary artery catheter.[142] Pulmonary artery catheter-related rupture of a pulmonary artery has a reported incidence of 0.1% to 0.2%.[143,144] This event can present as either hemoptysis or hemothorax. Rao et al reported a series of 4684 patients who underwent pulmonary artery catheterization; four of these patients experienced pulmonary artery rupture.[143] Of these four incidents, three occurred during cardiac surgery and full anticoagulation, and one resulted from excessive inflation of the pulmonary catheter balloon. Mortality from massive hemoptysis usually results from hypoxia rather than exanguination and is more likely if the patient is anticoagulated. The differential diagnosis for massive hemoptysis is shown in Table 12-7.

Anesthetic Management of Massive Hemoptysis

Surgery is indicated in the patient who has required multiple blood transfusions, persistent hemoptysis, or deterioration of

TABLE 12-7
Causes of Massive Hemoptysis

Infection
Tuberculosis
Bronchiectasis
Bronchitis
Lung abscess
Necrotizing pneumonia

Neoplasm
Bronchogenic carcinoma
Metastatic carcinoma
Mediastinal tumor
Endobronchial polyp

Cardiovascular disease
Mitral stenosis
Pulmonary arteriovenous malformation
Pulmonary embolism
Pulmonary vasculitis

Miscellaneous causes
Pulmonary artery catheterization
Cystic fibrosis
Pulmonary contusion/laceration
Reperfusion of pulmonary vasculature after pulmonary embolectomy

From Benumof JL: Anesthesia for emergency thoracic surgery. In Benumof JL (ed): *Anesthesia for thoracic surgery*, Philadelphia, 1987, WB Saunders.

pulmonary function.[145] Contraindications to surgery include inoperable pulmonary carcinoma, failure to localize the site of hemorrhage, and the presence of severe bilateral pulmonary disease. For those patients with either a contraindication for surgery or those who refuse surgery, selective bronchial artery embolization may be attempted.

Although a chest x-ray might help to localize the site of bleeding, the x-ray might not necessarily be precise. Bronchoscopy is a much more precise technique for determining both the cause and the source of bleeding. Insertion of a rigid bronchoscope facilitates ventilation and suctioning of the airway. Flexible fiberoptic bronchoscopy may be used in those situations when the patient is not actively bleeding or when bleeding is confined to the upper lobes. Bronchoscopy can serve as both a diagnostic and a therapeutic intervention. Topical iced saline and vasoconstrictors may be administered via the bronchoscope. In some instances, this can be sufficient to stop the bleeding. More recently, selective intrabronchial spraying of fibrin precursors has been administered through the suction port of a flexible fiberoptic bronchoscope.[146,147]

The goals for successful anesthetic management of the patient with massive hemoptysis include proper airway management with successful isolation of the bleeding lung, volume resuscitation, and maintenance of satisfactory arterial blood gases. Standard monitors are applied, and large-bore intravenous catheters should be placed to facilitate volume resuscitation. Invasive monitors, such as arterial and central venous catheters, might be indicated. Supplemental oxygen should be administered, and the patient should initially be positioned with the bleeding lung in the dependent position to minimize spillage and contamination of the other lung. Although coughing can exacerbate bleeding, this reflex should not be obliterated in the awake patient with an unsecured airway. After the patient's airway is secured, coughing may be suppressed in an attempt to decrease bleeding; suctioning of the airway in an intubated patient diminishes the need for an intact cough reflex.

If the patient presents at the time of surgery with a single-lumen endotracheal tube already in place, options include either using a bronchial blocking device placed with the assistance of a fiberoptic bronchoscope or changing the tube to a double-lumen endotracheal tube. It could be necessary, however, to perform an awake fiberoptic intubation in order to secure the patient's airway safely. This can be accomplished using a single-lumen endotracheal tube followed by placement of a bronchial blocker to facilitate lung isolation. Alternatively, a mainstem bronchial intubation of the unaffected lung can be performed with the assistance of the fiberoptic bronchoscope. Ideally, a double-lumen endotracheal tube should be used to facilitate surgical exposure and provide for selective suctioning of the affected lung as well as differential pulmonary ventilation if necessary. Following resection of the bleeding pulmonary segment, the patient should remain intubated and mechanically ventilated.

Thoracic Outlet Syndrome

Thoracic outlet syndrome (TOS) involves compression of the subclavian vessels and nerves of the brachial plexus in the region of the thoracic outlet. The thoracic outlet is bounded by the first rib inferiorly, the scalenus anterior muscle anteriorly, the scalenus muscle posteriorly, and the clavicle.[148] Compression of the neurovascular structures of the upper extremity can occur secondary to the following:

- Bone—cervical rib, long transverse process of C_7, abnormal first rib, osteoarthritis
- Muscles—scalenes
- Trauma—neck hematoma, clavicular fracture
- Fibrous bands—congenital and acquired
- Neoplasm

TOS is most common in women between the ages of 18 and 35 years. Symptoms most commonly develop as a result of neural compromise; however, vascular or neurovascular symptoms have also been reported.[148] In lower brachial plexus compression, the symptoms can manifest as shoulder pain and parasthesias along the distribution of the ulnar nerve. Upper brachial plexus compression can produce facial, jaw, or ear pain associated with parasthesias radiating down the lateral aspect of the arm. Compression of the subclavian artery produces fatigue, weakness, ischemic pain, parasthesias, and a cold upper extremity. Thrombosis with distal embolization occurs rarely but can produce ischemic changes or Raynaud's phenomenon. Atypical angina (pseudoangina) has also been reported. Venous compression or occlusion usually manifests as edema, venous distention, formation of collaterals, and cyanosis of the upper extremity. Several maneuvers that may be performed to evaluate a patient suspected of having TOS have been described.[149] A loss or decrease of the radial pulse or the reproduction of neurologic symptoms suggest a positive test.

Treatment of TOS is initially nonsurgical and is successful in 50% to 90% of patients.[150] Surgical intervention is indicated for those who fail conservative therapy or who have progression of sensory or motor symptoms, excessively prolonged ulnar or median nerve conduction velocities, narrowing or occlusion of the subclavian artery, and thrombosis of the axillary/subclavian vein. The initial surgical approach for TOS is resection of the first rib via a transaxillary, supraclavicular, infraclavicular, transthoracic, or posterior technique.[151] Complications that can result from resection of the first rib include brachial plexus injuries, vascular injuries, pleural effusion, winged scapula, and infection. The rate of recurrence of symptoms following surgery has been reported as approximately 1%.[152]

Anesthetic Management of TOS Surgery

Patients presenting for TOS surgery are generally young and healthy. Preoperative workup includes standard chest x-ray and cervical spine films, which may reveal bony abnormalities such as a cervical rib or degenerative changes. CT scans, MRI scans, and cervical myelograms may be obtained to rule out cervical disc disease or narrowing of the intervertebral foramina. If the degree of vascular impairment cannot be determined clinically or if an aneurysm or venous thrombosis is suspected, then Doppler studies, angiograms, or venograms could be warranted. Other preoperative testing should be performed as indicated by the patient's medical history and physical examination.

Standard monitoring inclusive of a noninvasive blood pressure cuff, electrocardiogram, pulse oximetry, and capnography should be used. The noninvasive blood pressure cuff and the intravenous catheter should be placed on the unaffected limb.

An arterial cannula could be indicated for some patients. Thoracic epidural analgesia is beneficial for intraoperative and postoperative pain management and is used frequently in conjunction with general endotracheal anesthesia. A double-lumen endotracheal tube could facilitate the surgical exposure, particularly if surgery is performed via the transthoracic approach. It is usually feasible to extubate the patient at the conclusion of surgery unless otherwise indicated.

Transthoracic Vertebral Surgery

Surgeons recorded the first thoracic spine surgery in the 1600s. The results of early thoracic spine surgery were riddled with failure and complications. Modern advances in surgical technique and anesthesiology have greatly improved surgical outcomes; however, the risk of postoperative complications remains significant. Unique characteristics of the thoracic spine and thoracic spinal cord help account for these complications following surgical manipulation. For example, the ratio of the size of the spinal cord to the spinal canal is larger in the thorax than in other areas of the spine. Furthermore, the blood supply of the thoracic spinal cord can be tenuous and variable, especially between T_4 and T_9. The direct blood supply from the radicular and intramedullary vessels is limited, and collateral circulation at the microcirculatory level is sparse, thus making this "watershed zone" particularly vulnerable.

The majority of spinal procedures have been performed with a posterior approach. During the 1960s, the anterior approach to spinal surgery was developed as a treatment for spinal deformities of polio victims and for vertebral tuberculosis.[153] Today, transthoracic vertebral surgery via the anterior approach is used for the treatment of traumatic, neoplastic, and degenerative conditions of the spine. The main advantage of the anterior approach is that it minimizes manipulation of the spinal cord and permits optimal exposure of the spine for multilevel discectomies and placement of intervertebral body grafts.[154] The disadvantages of this technique are the risk of injury to the major vessels in the mediastinum as well as the risk of developing an often debilitating postthoracotomy syndrome.

Thoracoscopic anterior spinal surgery was developed in 1992, with the first published report appearing in 1993.[155] Thoracoscopy provides superior visualization and access to the ventral spinal cord and allows for a more complete decompression of midline lesions. When compared with the conventional thoracotomy approach to anterior thoracic spine surgery, thoracoscopy is associated with less blood loss, less chest tube drainage, fewer postoperative complications, a decreased need for analgesics, and a shorter hospital stay.[156] Intercostal pain and postthoracotomy syndrome are less common and less severe following transthoracic vertebral surgery with thoracoscopy.

Anesthetic Management and Considerations for Transthoracic Vertebral Surgery

It is essential for the anesthesiologist to be familiar with the surgical procedure in order to optimize the anesthetic management. Transthoracic vertebral surgery typically involves the levels of T_5 to T_{10} approached anteriorly with either a conventional thoracotomy incision plus rib resection or VATS. Either of these techniques poses a risk to the lung parenchyma, thoracic duct, or the great vessels. The risk of spinal cord injury and the amount of intraoperative blood loss depends on the extent and difficulty of the vertebral disease and the reconstruction. Intraoperative somatosensory evoked potentials (SSEPs) are commonly used to detect potential spinal cord compromise. Optimal surgical exposure is obtained by collapsing the ispilateral lung.

Taking the above requirements for optimal surgical exposure and potential complications into account, the goals for anesthetic management of these patients is clear. Standard monitors, including a noninvasive blood pressure cuff, electrocardiogram, pulse oximetry, and capnography, are used. Adequate intravenous access should be obtained in anticipation of significant blood loss. If the patient's peripheral venous access is poor or the patient has a significant cardiac history, consideration should be given to securing central venous access. Pulmonary artery catheterization could be a consideration for some patients if their comorbid history so dictates. An arterial cannula can be considered, particularly because single-lung ventilation will be required for surgical exposure. A double-lumen endotracheal tube or other bronchial blocking device should be used for the reason previously stated. Details regarding the management of single-lung ventilation are found in Chapter 4. The patient is placed in the lateral decubitus position for the procedure.

The choice of agents for maintenance of general anesthesia must be tailored toward optimizing the signals obtained during SSEP monitoring. Compromise or injury of a neurologic pathway is manifested as an increase in the latency and/or a decrease in the amplitude of evoked potential waveforms. Anesthetic factors capable of producing this pattern of alteration must be controlled carefully. Studies regarding the effects of intravenous agents demonstrate that induction doses of thiopental, etomidate, and fentanyl preserve SSEP recordings.[157] It is recommended that constant anesthetic drug levels should be maintained in order to obtain satisfactory SSEP recordings. The intermittent bolus administration of intravenous agents and stepwise changes in the volatile anesthetics during maintenance anesthesia should be avoided, especially during those times when neurologic injury might occur. A continuous intravenous anesthetic technique offers one method for achieving these goals. Volatile anesthetic agents may be used as long as the end-tidal concentrations do not exceed 0.5 MAC.

Physiologic factors such as temperature, systemic blood pressure, PaO_2, and $PaCO_2$ can alter SSEPs as well; therefore, it is important to maintain normothermia and an adequate systemic blood pressure to ensure optimal perfusion of the spinal cord and other vital organs. Studies report that during scoliosis surgery, SSEP changes have been observed that resolved with increases in systemic blood pressure. This suggests that spinal cord manipulation during "acceptable" limits for systemic blood pressure could cause significant ischemia and potential neurologic damage.[158]

The goals at the conclusion of surgery are to have the patient fully awake and extubated in the operating room as long as satisfactory extubation criteria are met. Early extubation allows for a full neurologic assessment of the patient as well as the early detection and treatment of any deficits that might have resulted from surgical manipulation.

Adult Diaphragmatic Surgery

Injuries to the diaphragm occur in 0.8% to 1.6% of all patients with multiple traumatic insults.[159] Frequently, patients with diaphragmatic rupture are relatively free of symptoms, with the result that the diagnosis is often delayed. The classification of traumatic ruptures of the diaphragm was described by Carter, who designated all patients diagnosed immediately following injury as type I ruptures and those with a delayed diagnosis as types II and III.[160] In type II patients, the diagnosis is established on the basis of the patient's symptoms or as an incidental finding during recovery from the primary injury. Type III ruptures typically encompass those patients sustaining acute ischemia or perforation of the herniated organs after recovery from the primary traumatic injury. The majority of diaphragmatic ruptures involve the left hemidiaphragm.

The acuity of the injury can play a role regarding the surgical approach for repair of the diaphragm. In the situation of an emergency operation following acute injury (Carter type I rupture), it is more likely that the exploratory laparotomy will be performed in the conventional manner with an open incision. Alternatively, if the injury is either Carter type II or type III, a laparoscopic approach may be used. There have been reports, however, of laparoscopic treatment of type I diaphragm rupture.[161,162]

Anesthetic Considerations and Management for Adult Diaphragmatic Surgery

The anesthetic management of adult patients with diaphragmatic rupture is dictated by the acuity of the injury and whether the surgical approach will be open or laparoscopic. Those patients who present at the time of traumatic injury with a Carter type I rupture tend to require aggressive treatment. Patients with Carter type II rupture are usually scheduled for elective surgery. Carter type III rupture can present for urgent surgical intervention and might also require aggressive resuscitation due to the severe metabolic and hemodynamic disturbances that result from ischemia or perforation of a viscus.

In addition to standard monitoring, the choice for using invasive monitors such as an arterial, central venous pressure, or pulmonary artery catheters should be based on the patient's medical history and condition at the time of surgery. A diaphragmatic injury, whether acute or chronic, might permit migration of abdominal contents into the thorax, thus compressing the lung and producing abnormalities in gas exchange. The heart might also be compressed, resulting in arrhythmias.

These patients should all be treated as having a full stomach because the competence of the esophagogastric junction is impaired. For those patients with other associated acute traumatic injuries at the time of surgery, special attention must be directed toward potential cervical spine injury when selecting the method to secure the patient's airway. Patients should be adequately preoxygenated, and either a rapid-sequence induction with maintenance of cricoid pressure and direct laryngoscopy or an awake fiberoptic intubation should be performed. A single-lumen endotracheal tube is used to secure the airway in either case.

The choice of anesthetic agents is also dependent on the status of the patient at the time of surgery. Patients presenting with severe hypovolemia might require agents that only minimally depress the cardiovascular system and hemodynamic compensatory mechanisms (e.g., central catecholamine output and baroreceptor reflexes). Whenever possible, intravascular volume should be restored prior to the induction of general anesthesia. Etomidate has been shown to demonstrate the least cardiovascular depressant activity.[163] Alternatively, ketamine may be considered because of its sympathomimetic effects. A rapid-acting neuromuscular blocking agent should be used initially if a rapid-sequence induction is used. Maintenance of anesthesia may occur with the volatile anesthetic agents (if the patient's condition allows), with neuromuscular blocking agents, and with an appropriate dose of opioids.

Metabolic disturbances, if present, should be corrected. Laparoscopy can exacerbate preexisting metabolic disturbances because of the insufflation of CO_2. Other resuscitative measures—such as administration of crystalloids and colloids and transfusion of blood and blood products—should be performed as needed. The surgical approach itself could affect fluid management. Creation of a pneumoperitoneum during laparoscopy could result in acute hemodynamic instability in the hypovolemic patient secondary to a decrease in venous return. In the absence of intraabdominal bleeding, a conventional exploratory laparotomy promotes less acute fluid shifting.

Patients scheduled for elective repair of a diaphragmatic rupture usually meet the criteria for extubation at the conclusion of surgery. Those who present for urgent or emergency surgical intervention could require postoperative mechanical ventilation and intensive care, particularly if they require aggressive intraoperative resuscitation.

Patients undergoing laparoscopic procedures to repair a diaphragm rupture might require less narcotic analgesia and have shorter hospital stays than those who have an open abdominal procedure. This outcome is also highly dependent on the acuity of the injury and on the presence or absence of associated trauma.

Superior Vena Cava Syndrome

A number of benign and malignant processes can cause obstruction of the superior vena cava and lead to superior vena cava syndrome. Malignant etiologies include bronchial carcinoma and malignant lymphoma. Benign etiologies include thrombosis of the superior vena cava secondary to central venous hyperalimentation and pacemaker catheters, idiopathic mediastinal fibrosis, mediastinal granuloma, and multinodular goiter. The pathophysiology of the syndrome is secondary to increased venous pressure of the vessels draining into the superior vena cava that cause symptoms, such as the following:

- Edema of the head, neck, and upper extremities
- Increased jugular venous distention
- Dilated collateral veins over the upper extremities and chest wall
- Cyanosis
- Headache
- Mental confusion

A majority of patients exhibit dyspnea, cough, and orthopnea due to obstruction of the airways by engorged veins and mucosal edema. Contrast medium-enhanced computerized tomography or magnetic resonance imaging is usually adequate to establish the diagnosis of superior vena cava obstruction and to assist with the differential diagnosis of the etiology. Venography confirms the diagnosis. Percutaneous needle biopsy is the most common initial method used to establish a histologic diagnosis prior to initiation of empirical therapy. Should percutaneous needle biopsy fail to establish the histologic diagnosis, thoracotomy, sternotomy, bronchoscopy, or lymph node biopsy could be necessary.

Following histologic diagnosis, most patients are able to receive optimal therapy with percutaneous stenting, irradiation, corticosteroid therapy, multiagent chemotherapy, and anticoagulant or fibrinolytic therapy. Percutaneous stenting is promising for the treatment of superior vena cava syndrome, especially for patients who have malignancies.[164,165] A major advantage of this therapy is that the self-expanding stents may be placed with the use of local anesthesia during radiologic manipulation. Complications from the procedure are rare, and recurrence of symptoms is uncommon.

For patients who have failed initial therapy or those with near-to-complete obstruction of the superior vena cava, surgical bypass or resection of the obstructing lesion via median sternotomy is indicated.[166]

Anesthetic Considerations and Management for Superior Vena Cava Syndrome

A careful assessment of the patient's airway should be performed because edema might be present in the mouth, oropharynx, and hypopharynx. Additionally, external compression of the airway, fibrosis limiting range of neck flexion and extension, and compression of the recurrent laryngeal nerve and trachea could be present. Many patients with significant respiratory compromise must maintain the sitting position to achieve adequate ventilation. Preparation of the patient for an awake fiberoptic intubation is warranted.

In addition to standard monitors, a radial arterial pressure catheter is suggested. Depending on the patient's other comorbid conditions, the use of a central venous catheter or pulmonary artery catheter inserted via the femoral vein may be necessary. Peripheral venous access should include a large-bore venous catheter inserted into the lower extremity prior to induction of general anesthesia. Consideration should be given to the placement of additional intravenous catheters after the induction of general anesthesia, as blood loss during surgery can be significant due to a high central venous pressure or to unexpected arterial bleeding.

Postoperatively, patients with persistent superior vena cava obstruction are at increased risk for respiratory failure secondary to acute laryngospasm, acute bronchospasm, impairment of the muscles of respiration, and increased airway obstruction due to tumor. It is therefore prudent to maintain endotracheal intubation and mechanical ventilation during the immediate postoperative period unless the obstruction has been relieved and the patient's airway is not compromised.

Pectus Excavatum

Pectus excavatum is the most common anterior chest wall deformity and is characterized by posterior depression of the sternum and lower costal cartilages. The incidence is 1 in 1000 live births with a 3:1 male-female predominance.[167] A family history of pectus excavatum has been identified in 37% of cases, thus supporting a genetic predisposition.[168] Approximately 20% of cases are associated with other musculoskeletal abnormalities, such as scoliosis and Marfan's syndrome. Congenital heart disease is present in 1.5% of patients with pectus excavatum.[169]

Most patients with pectus excavatum are asymptomatic at the time of presentation. Some patients do report dyspnea or pain during exercise that radiates along the costal cartilages. Cardiac murmurs and arrhythmias may be noted in those with mitral valve prolapse. Pulmonary assessment is obtained with pulmonary function studies, exercise studies, and ventilation-perfusion scans. Cardiovascular assessment is performed using echocardiography or angiography. Patients with pectus excavatum who manifest severe cardiopulmonary symptoms demonstrate a restrictive pattern on their pulmonary function studies and evidence of right ventricular outlet obstruction on echocardiography and angiography.

Indications for surgical intervention include cosmesis, psychosocial factors, and the presence of cardiovascular or pulmonary insufficiency. The repair consists of excision of all abnormal cartilage with preservation of the perichondrial sheaths of the cartilage, sternal osteotomy with anterior fixation of the sternum, and the use of a retrosternal strut to secure the sternum firmly in an anterior position for approximately 6 months to 1 year. The retrosternal struts are removed through a small incision on the lateral chest over an end of the strut. Complications of the surgical procedure are rare but include pneumothorax and wound infection. Satisfactory repair is achieved when the procedure is performed during childhood. Results are much less favorable when full growth is attained.

Anesthetic Considerations and Management for Pectus Excavatum

Because the majority of patients presenting for repair of pectus excavatum are asymptomatic, anesthetic management is usually straightforward. Standard monitoring and a general anesthetic technique combined with thoracic epidural analgesia is optimal. For those patients exhibiting symptoms of restrictive pulmonary disease and/or right ventricular outlet obstruction, the use of invasive monitoring (e.g., arterial catheter, central venous monitoring, pulmonary artery catheter) and intraoperative transesophageal echocardiography may be warranted. Patients can usually be extubated in the operating room at the conclusion of surgery. Effective postoperative pain management can be achieved with thoracic epidural analgesia.

REFERENCES

1. Jacobeus H: Cauterization of adhesions in pneumothorax: treatment of tuberculosis. *Surg Gynecol Obstet* 32:49, 1921.
2. Hazelrigg SR, Nunchuck SK, Landreneau RJ: Cost analysis for thoracoscopy: thoracoscopic wedge resection, *Ann Thorac Surg* 56:633, 1993.
3. Ferson PF, Landreneau RJ, Dowling RD, et al: Comparison of open versus thoracoscopic lung biopsy for diffuse infiltrative pulmonary disease, *J Thorac Cardiovasc Surg* 106:194, 1993.
4. Rubin JW, Finney NR, Borders BM, et al: Intrathoracic biopsies, pulmonary wedge excision and management of pleural disease: is video-assisted closed chest surgery the approach of choice? *Ann Surg* 60:860, 1994.
5. Inderbitzi RG, Grillet MP: Risk and hazards of video-thoracoscopic surgery: a collective review, *Eur J Cardiothorac Surg* 10:483, 1996.
6. Krasna MJ, Deshmukh S, McGlaughlin JS: Complications of thoracoscopy, *Ann Thorac Surg* 61(4):1066, 1996.
7. Jancovici R, Lang-Lazdunski L, Pons F, et al: Complications of video-assisted thoracic surgery: a five-year experience, *Ann Thorac Surg* 61:533, 1996.
8. Walker WS, Pugh GC, Craig SR, et al: Continued experience with thoracoscopic major pulmonary resection, *Int Surg* 81:255, 1996.
9. Horswell JL: Anesthetic techniques for thoracoscopy, *Ann Thorac Surg* 56:624, 1993.
10. Lewis RJ, Caccavale RJ, Sisler GE, et al: One hundred consecutive patients undergoing video-assisted thoracic operations, *Ann Thorac Surg* 54:421, 1992.
11. Nadeau S, Noble W: Misinterpretation of pressure measurements from the pulmonary artery catheter, *Can Anaesth Soc J* 33:352, 1986.
12. Tuman K, Carroll G, Ivankovich A: Pitfalls in interpretation of the pulmonary artery catheter data, *J Cardiothorac Anesth* 3:625, 1989.
13. Plummer S, Hartley M, Vaughan R: Anaesthesia for telescopic procedures in the thorax, *Br J Anaesth* 80:223, 1998.
14. Nezu K, Kushibe K, Tojo T, et al: Thoracoscopic wedge resection of blebs under local anesthesia with sedation for treatment of a spontaneous pneumothorax, *Chest* 111:230, 1997.
15. Mulder D: Pain management principles and anesthesia techniques for thoracoscopy, *Ann Thorac Surg* 56:630, 1993.
16. Weiss S, Aukburg S: Thoracic anesthesia. In Longnecker D, Tinker J, Morgan G (eds): *Principles and practice of anesthesiology,* ed 2, St. Louis, 1998, Mosby.
17. van der Spek AFL, Sparge PM, Norton ML: The physics of lasers and implications for their use during airway surgery, *Br J Anaesth* 60:709, 1988.
18. Strong MS, Vaughan CW, Polany J, et al: Bronchoscopic carbon dioxide laser surgery, *Ann Otol* 83:769, 1974.
19. Boyce JR: Laser therapy for bronchoscopy, *Anesth Clin North Am* 7:597, 1989.
20. Gelb AF, Epstein JB: Laser in treatment of lung cancer, *Chest* 86:662, 1984.
21. Unger M: Bronchoscopic utilization of the Nd-YAG laser for obstructing lesions of the trachea and bronchi, *Surg Clin North Am* 64:931, 1984.
22. U.S. Food and Drug Administration: Special report: laser safety. *Laser Nurs* 4:3, 1990.
23. Kokosa J, Eugene J: Chemical composition of laser-tissue interaction smoke plume, *J Laser Appl* 2:59, 1989.
24. Tomita Y, Mihashi S, Nagata K, et al: Mutagenicity of smoke condensates induced by CO_2-laser and electrocauterization, *Mutat Res* 89:145, 1981.
25. Baggish MS, Poiesz BJ, Joret D, et al: Presence of human immunodeficiency virus DNA in laser smoke, *Lasers Surg Med* 11:197, 1991.
26. Johnson GK, Robinson WS: Human immunodeficiency virus-i (HIV-I) in the vapors of surgical power instruments, *J Med Virol* 33:47, 1991.
27. Voohries RM, Lavyne MH, Strait TA, et al: Does the CO_2 laser spread viable brain tumor cells outside the surgical field? *J Neurosurg* 60:819, 1984.
28. Byrne PO, Sisson PR, Oliver PD, et al: Carbon dioxide laser irradiation of bacterial targets *in vitro, J Hosp Infect* 9:265, 1987.
29. Smith JP, Moss CE, Bryant CJ, et al: Evaluation of a smoke evacuator used for laser surgery, *Lasers Surg Med* 9:276, 1989.
30. Dullye KK, Kaspar MD, Ramsay MAE, et al: Laser treatment of endobronchial lesions, *Anesthesiology* 86:1387, 1997.
31. Dumon F, Shapshay S, Bourcereau J, et al: Principles for safety in application of neodymium-YAG laser in bronchology, *Chest* 86:163, 1984.
32. Vourc'h G, Fischler M, Personne C, et al: Anesthetic management during Nd:YAG laser resection for major tracheobronchial obstructing tumors, *Anesthesiology* 61:636, 1984.
33. Hermens JM, Bennett MJ, Hirschman CA: Anesthesia for laser surgery, *Anesth Analg* 62:218, 1983.
34. George PJM, Garrett CPO, Nixon C, et al: Treatment for tracheobronchial tumors: local or general anesthesia, *Thorax* 42:656, 1987.
35. Wolf GL, Simpson JI: Flammability of endotracheal tubes in oxygen and nitrous oxide enriched atmosphere, *Anesthesiology* 67:236, 1987.
36. Pashayan AG, Gravenstein JS, Cassis NJ, et al: The helium protocol for laryngotracheal operations with CO_2 laser: a retrospective review of 523 cases, *Anesthesiology* 68:801, 1988.
37. Williamson R: Why 70 watts to evaluate metal tapes for CO_2 laser surgery? *Anesth Analg* 72:414, 1991.
38. Ossoff RH: Laser safety in otolaryngology-head and neck surgery: Anesthetic and educational considerations for laryngeal surgery, *Laryngoscope* 99:1, 1989.

39. Emergency Care Research Institute: Laser-resistant endotracheal tubes and wraps, *Health Devices* 19:112, 1990.

40. Dougherty TJ: Photodynamic therapy, *J Photochem Photobiol* 58:895, 1993.

41. Girotti AW: Photosensitized oxidation of cholesterol in biological systems: reaction pathways, cytotoxic effects and defense mechanisms, *J Photochem Photobiol B: Biol* 22:171, 1994.

42. Vicente G: Le lavage des poumons, *Presse Med*: 1266, 1929.

43. Rogers RM, Braunstein MS, Shuman JF. Role of bronchopulmonary lavage in the treatment of respiratory failure: a review, *Chest* 62(5):95S, 1972.

44. Ramirez-Rivera J, Schultz RE, Betton RE: Pulmonary alveolar proteinosis. A new technique and rationale for treatment, *Arch Intern Med* 112:419, 1963.

45. Ramirez-Rivera J: The strange beginnings of diagnostic and therapeutic bronchoalveolar lavage, *PRHS* 11(1):27, 1992.

46. Rodi G., Lotti G, Galbusera C, et al: Whole-lung lavage. *Monaldi Arch Chest Dis* 50(1):64, 1995.

47. Ramirez-Rivera J, Kieffer RF, Ball WC: Bronchopulmonary lavage in man, *Ann Intern Med* 63(5):819, 1965.

48. Ramirez-Rivera J: Bronchopulmonary lavage, *Dis Chest* 50(6):581, 1966.

49. Spragg RG, Benumof JL, Alfery, DD: New method for the performance of unilateral lung lavage, *Anesthesiology* 57(6):535, 1982.

50. Persson A: Pulmonary alveolar proteinosis. In Fishman AP (ed), et al: *Fishman's pulmonary diseases and disorders,* ed 3, New York. 1998, McGraw-Hill.

51. Rosen SH, et al: Pulmonary alveolar proteinosis, *New Engl J Med* 258:1123, 1958.

52. Goldstein LS, Kavuru Mani S, Curtis-McCarthy P, et al: Pulmonary alveolar proteinosis, *Chest* 114(5):1357, 1998.

53. Wasserman K, Mason GR: Pulmonary alveolar proteinosis. In Murray JF. Nadel JA (eds): *Textbook of respiratory medicine,* ed 2, Philadelphia, 1994, WB Saunders.

54. Seymour JF, Presneill J, Otto D, et al: Therapeutic efficacy of granulocyte macrophage colony-stimulating factor in patient with idiopathic acquired alveolar proteinosis, *Am J Respir Crit Care Med* 163:524, 2001.

55. Braunstein MS, Fleegler B: Failure of bronchopulmonary lavage in cystic fibrosis, *Chest* 66(1):96, 1974.

56. Lober CW, Saltzman HA, Kylstra JA: Volume-controlled lung lavage in a woman with cystic fibrosis, *Chest* 68(3):382,1975.

57. Dahm LS, Ewing CW, Harrison GM, et al: Comparison of three techniques of lung lavage in patients with cystic fibrosis, *Chest* 72(5):493, 1977.

58. Spock A: State of the art of lung lavage in patients with cystic fibrosis. In: *Intl Conf Cystic Fibrosis* 113, 1977.

59. Adkins MO, Chan JC, Brodsky JB: Unsuccessful unilateral bronchopulmonary lavage for a patient with severe cystic fibrosis, *J Card Anesth* 3(4):481, 1989.

60. Chang HY, Chen CW, Chen CY, et al: Successful treatment of diffuse lipoid pneumonitis with whole-lung lavage, *Thorax* 48(9):947, 1993.

61. Wong CA, Wilsher ML: Treatment of exogenous lipoid pneumonia by whole-lung lavage, *Aust NZ J Med* 24(6):734, 1994.

62. Ciravegna B, Sacco O, Moroni C, et al: Mineral oil lipoid pneumonia in a child with anoxic encephalopathy: treatment by whole-lung lavage, *Pediatr Pulmonol* 23(3):233, 1997.

63. Danel C, Israël-Biet D, Costabel U, et al: Therapeutic applications of bronchoalveolar lavage, *Eur Respira J* 5:1173, 1992.

64. Mason GR, Abraham JL, Hoffman L, et al: Treatment of mixed-dust pneumoconiosis with whole-lung lavage, *Am Rev Respir Dis* 126(6):1102, 1982.

65. Wilt JL, Banks DE, Weissman DN, et al: Reduction of lung dust burden in pneumoconiosis by whole-lung lavage, *JOEM* 38(6):619, 1996.

66. Bussières JS, St-Onge S, Saey D, et al: Feasibility, safety and efficacy of whole-lung lavage in silicosis, *Can J Anesth* 46(5):A43, 1999.

67. Benumof JL: Anesthesia for special elective therapeutic procedures. In Benumof JL (ed): Anesthesia for thoracic surgery, ed 2, p 548, Philadelphia, 1994, WB Saunders.

68. Bardoczky GI, Engelman E, D'Hollander A: Continuous spirometry: an aid to monitoring ventilation during operation, *Br J Anesth* 71:747, 1993.

69. Takahashi S, Saito S, Mizutani T, et al.: Continuous intra-arterial blood gas monitoring during bronchopulmonary lavage for pulmonary alveolar proteinosis, *Masui* 47(5):626-631, 1998.

70. Cohen E, Eisenkraft JB: Bronchopulmonary lavage: effects of oxygenation and hemodynamic, *J Cardiothorac Anesth* 4(5):609, 1990.

71. McMahon CC, Irvine T, Conacher ID: Transoesophageal echocardiography in the management of whole-lung lavage, *Brit J Anaesth* 81:262, 1998.

72. Loubser PG: Validity of pulmonary artery catheter-derived hemodynamic information during bronchopulmonary lavage, *J Cardiothorac Vasc Anesth* 11(7):885, 1997.

73. Swenson JD, Astler KL, Bailey FL: Reduction in left ventricular filling during bronchopulmonary lavage demonstrated by transesophageal echocardiography, *Anesth Analg* 81(3):634-637, 1995.

74. Hammon WE, McCaffree DR, Cucchiara AJ: A comparison of manual to mechanical chest percussion for clearance of alveolar material in patients with pulmonary alveolar proteinosis, *Chest* 103(5):1409, 1993.

75. Bingisser R, Kaplan V, Zollinger A, et al.: Whole-lung lavage in alveolar proteinosis by a modified lavage technique, Chest 113(6):1718, 1998.

76. Eisenkraft JB, Neustein SM: Anesthetic management of therapeutic procedures of the lungs and airways. In Kaplan JA: *Thoracic anesthesia*, ed 2, p 425, New York, 1991, Churchill Livingstone.

77. Moutafis M, Dalibon N, Colchen A, et al.: Improving oxygenation during bronchopulmonary lavage using nitric oxide inhalation and almitrine infusion, *Anesth Analg* 89:302, 1999.

78. Biervliet JD, Peper JA, Roos CM, et al: Whole-lung lavage under hyperbaric conditions. In Erdmann W (ed): *Oxygen transport to tissue XIV,* p 115, New York, 1992, Bruley, Plenum Press.

79. Cohen ES, Elpern E, Silver MR: Pulmonary alveolar proteinosis causing severe hypoxic respiratory failure treated with sequential whole-lung lavage utilizing venovenous extracorporeal membrane oxygenation, *Chest* 120:1024, 2001.

80. Julien T, Caudine M, Barlet H, et al: PEEP effect on PaO_2 during bronchopulmonary lavage for alveolar proteinosis, *Ann Fr Anesth Reanim* 5:173, 1986.

81. Mckenzie B, Wood RE, Bailey A: Airway management for unilateral lung lavage in children, *Anesthesiology* 70(3):550, 1989.

82. Moazam F, Schmidt JH, Chesrown SE, et al: Total lung lavage for pulmonary alveolar proteinosis in an infant without the use of cardiopulmonary bypass, *J Red Surg* 20(4):398, 1985.

83. Hiratzka LF, Swan DM, Rose EF, et al.: Bilateral simultaneous lung lavage utilizing membrane oxygenator for pulmonary alveolar proteinosis in an 8-month-old infant. *Ann Thorac Surg* 35(3):313, 1983.

84. Lippmann M, Mok MS, Wasserman K: Anaesthetic management for children with alveolar proteinosis using extracorporeal circulation, *Br J Anaesth* 49:173, 1977.

85. Tsai WC, Lewis D, Nasr SZ, et al: Liquid ventilation in an Infant with pulmonary alveolar proteinosis, *Pediatr Pulmonol* 26:283, 1998.

86. National Heart, Lung, and Blood Institute: Division of lung disease workshop report, the definition of emphysema, *Am Rev Respir Dis* 132:182, 1985.

87. American Thoracic Society: Standards for the diagnosis and care of patients with chronic obstructive pulmonary disease (COPD) and asthma, *Am Rev Respir Dis* 136(1):225, 1986.

88. Potter, WA, Olafsson S, Hyatt RE: Ventilatory mechanics and expiratory flow limitation during exercise in patients with obstructive lung disease, *J Clin Invest* 50:910, 1971.

89. Stubbing DC, Rengelly LD, Morse JLC, et al: Pulmonary mechanics during exercise in subjects with chronic airflow obstruction, *J Appl Physiol* 49:511, 1980.

90. Carrell RW, Jeppsson JO, Laurell CB, et al: Structure and variation of the human alpha-1-antitrypsin, *Nature* 298:329, 1982.

91. Janus ED, Phillips NT, Carrell RW: Smoking, lung function and alpha-1-antitrypsin deficiency, *Lancet* 1:152, 1985.

92. Buist AS, Sexton GJ, Nagy JM, et al: The effect of smoking cessation and modification on lung function, *Am Rev Respir Dis* 114:115, 1976.

93. Sahn SA: Corticosteroid therapy in chronic obstructive pulmonary disease, *Pract Cardiol* 11(8):150, 1985.

94. Tager I, Speizer FE: Role of infection in chronic bronchitis, *N Engl J Med* 292:563, 1975.

95. Belman MJ, Mittman C, Weir R: Ventilatory muscle training improves exercise capacity in chronic obstructive pulmonary disease patients, *Am Rev Respir Dis* 121:273, 1980.

96. Hughes RL, Davison R: Limitations of exercise reconditioning in COLD, *Chest* 83:241, 1983.

97. Anthonisen NR: Long-term oxygen therapy, *Ann Intern Med* 99:519, 1983.

98. Nocturnal Oxygen Therapy Trail Group: Continuous or nocturnal oxygen therapy in hypoxemia chronic obstructive lung disease: a clinical trail, *Ann Intern Med* 91:391, 1980.

99. Carter MG, Gaensler EA, Kyllonen A: Pneumoperitoneum in the treatment of pulmonary emphysema, *N Engl J Med* 243:549, 1950.

100. Brantigan OC, Mueller E: A surgical approach to pulmonary emphysema, *Am Rev Respir Dis* 80:194, 1959.

101. Cooper JD, Trulock EP, Triantafillou AN, et al: Bilateral lung volume reduction) for chronic obstructive pulmonary disease, *J Thorac Cardiovasc Surg* 109:106, 1995.

102. Miller JI, Lee RE, Mansour KA: Lung volume reduction surgery: lessons learned, *Ann Thorac Surg* 61:1464, 1996.

103. Naunheim KS, Ferguson MK: The current status of lung volume reduction operations for emphysema, *Ann Thorac Surg* 62:601, 1996.

104. Weinmann GG, Hyatt R: Evaluation and research in lung volume reduction surgery, *Am J Respir Crit Care Med* 154:1913, 1996.

105. Wisser W, Tschernko E, Senbaklavaci O, et al: Functional improvement after volume reduction: sternotomy versus videoendoscopic approach, *Ann Thorac Surg* 63:822, 1997.

106. Babb TG, Viggiano R, Hurley B, et al: Effect of mild-to-moderate airflow limitation on exercise capacity, *J Appl Physiol* 70:223, 1991.

107. Tobin MJ: Respiratory muscles in disease, *Clin Chest Med* 9:263, 1988.

108. Dueck R, Cooper S, Kapelanski D, et al: A pilot study of expiratory flow limitation and lung volume reduction surgery, *Chest* 116:1762, 1999.

109. Gelb AF, Zamel N, McKenna RJ, et al: Mechanism of short-term improvement in lung function after emphysema resection, *Am J Respir Crit Care Med* 154:945, 1996.

110. Marchand E, Gayan-Ramirez G, De Leyn P, et al: Physiological basis of improvement after lung volume reduction surgery for severe emphysema: where are we? *Eur Respir J* 13(3):686, 1999.

111. Sciurba FC, Rogers RM, Keenan RJ, et al: Improvement in pulmonary function and elastic recoil after lung-reduction surgery for diffuse emphysema, *N Engl J Med* 334:1095, 1996.

112. Tschernko EM, Wisser W, Hofer S, et al: Influence of lung volume reduction on ventilatory mechanics in patients suffering from severe COPD, *Anesth Analg* 83:996, 1996.

113. O'Donnell DE, Webb KA, Bertley JC, et al: Mechanisms of relief of exertional breathlessness following unilateral bullectomy and lung volume reduction surgery emphysema, *Chest* 110:18, 1996.

114. American College of Physicians: Preoperative pulmonary function testing, *Ann Intern Med* 112:793, 1990.

115. Tschernko EM, Wisser W, Wanke T, et al: Changes in ventilatory mechanics and diaphragmatic function after lung volume reduction surgery in patients with COPD, *Thorax* 52:545, 1997.

116. Tschernko EM, Wisser W, Hofer S, et al: Influence of lung volume reduction on ventilatory mechanics in patients suffering from severe COPD, *Anesth Analg* 83:996, 1996.

117. Hoppin FG: Theoretical basis for improvement following reduction-pneumoplasty in emphysema, *Am J Respir Crit Care Med* 155:520, 1997.

118. Tschernko EM, Gruber EM, Jaksch P, et al: Ventilatory mechanics and gas exchange during exercise before and after lung volume reduction surgery, *Am J Respir Crit Care Med* 158:1424, 1998.

119. Benditt JO, Wood DE, McCool D, et al: Changes in breathing and ventilatory muscle recruitment patterns induced by lung volume reduction surgery, *Am J Respir Crit Care Med* 155:279, 1997.

120. Baydur A: Improvements in lung and respiratory muscle function following lung volume reduction surgery, *Chest* 116:1507, 1999.

121. Lahrmann H, Wild M, Wanke T, et al: Neural drive to the diaphragm after lung volume reduction surgery, *Chest* 116:1593, 1999.

122. Daniel TM, Barry BK, Chan MD, et al: Lung volume reduction surgery: case selection, operative technique, and clinical results, *Ann Surg* 223(5):526, 1996.

123. Wisser W, Klepetko W, Senbaklavaci O, et al: Chronic hypercapnia should not exclude patients from lung volume reduction surgery, *Eur J Cardiothorac Surg* 14:107, 1998.

124. Thurnheer R, Muntwyler J, Stammberger U, et al: Coronary artery disease in patients undergoing lung volume reduction surgery for emphysema, *Chest* 112(1):122, 1997.

125. Weder W, Thurnheer R, Stammberger U, et al: Radiologic emphysema morphology is associated with outcome after surgical lung volume reduction, *Ann Thorac Surg* 64:313, 1997.

126. Hamacher J, Block KE, Stammberger U, et al: Two years' outcome of lung volume reduction surgery in different morphologic emphysema types, *Ann Thorac Surg* 68:1792, 1999.

127. Rogers RM, Coxson HO, Sciurba FC, et al: Preoperative severity of emphysema predictive of improvement after lung volume reduction surgery: use of CT morphometry, *Chest* 118:1240, 2000.

128. Saltman SH: Can CT measurement of emphysema severity aid patient selection for lung volume reduction surgery? *Chest* 118:1231, 2000.

129. Thurnheer R, Engel H, Weder W, et al: Role of lung perfusion scintigraphy in relation to chest computed tomography and pulmonary function in the evaluation of candidates for lung volume reduction surgery, *Am J Respir Crit Care Med* 159(1):301, 1999.

130. National Emphysema Treatment Trial Research Group: Patients at high risk of death after lung-volume-reduction surgery, *N Engl J Med* 345(15):1075, 2001.

131. Ingenito EP, Evans RE, Loring SH, et al: Relation between preoperative inspiratory lung resistance and the outcome of lung-volume-reduction surgery for emphysema, *N Engl J Med* 338:1181, 1998.

132. Tschernko EM, Kritzinger M, Gruber EM, et al: Lung volume reduction surgery: preoperative functional predictors for postoperative outcome, *Anesth Analg* 88:28, 1999.

133. Weinberg M, Hendeles L: Methylxanthines. In Weiss EB, Segal MS, Stein M (eds): *Bronchial asthma. Mechanisms and therapeutics*, ed 2, Boston, 1985, Little, Brown.

134. Tuxen DV, Lane S: The effects of ventilatory pattern on hyperinflation, airway pressures, and circulation in mechanical ventilation of patients with severe air-flow obstruction, *Am Rev Respir Dis* 136:872, 1987.

135. Ballantyne JC, Carr DB, deFerranti S, et al: The comparative effects of postoperative analgesic therapies on pulmonary outcome: cumulative meta-analyses of randomized, controlled trials, *Anesth Analg* 86(3):598, 1998.

136. Warner DO: Preventing postoperative pulmonary complications, *Anesthesiology* 92:1467, 2000.

137. Loehning RW, Waltemath CL, Bergman NA: Lidocaine and increased respiratory resistance produced by ultrasonic aerosols, *Anesthesiology* 44:306, 1976.

138. Brandus V, Joffe S, Benoit CV, et al: Bronchial spasm during general anesthesia, *Canad Anesth Soc J* 17:269, 1970.

139. The National Emphysema Treatment Trial Research Group: Rationale and design of The National Emphysema Treatment Trial: a prospective randomized trial of lung volume reduction surgery, *Chest* 116:1750, 1999.

140. Benumof JL: Anesthesia for emergency thoracic surgery. In Benumof JL (ed): *Anesthesia for thoracic surgery*, p 375, Philadelphia, 1987, WB Saunders.

141. Wedel M: Massive hemoptysis. In Moser KM, Spragg RG (eds): *Respiratory emergencies*, ed 2, p 194, St Louis, 1982, Mosby.

142. Reich DL, Thys DM: Mitral valve replacement complicated by endobronchial hemorrhage: spontaneous, traumatic, or iatrogenic? *J Cardiothorac Anesth* 2:359, 1988.

143. Rao TLK, Gorski DW, Laughlin S, et al: Safety of pulmonary artery catheterization, *Anesthesiology* 57:A116, 1982.

144. McDaniel DD, Stone JG, Faltas AN, et al: Catheter-induced pulmonary artery hemorrhage, *J Thorac Cardiovasc Surg* 82:1, 1981.

145. Benumof JL: Anesthesia for emergency thoracic surgery. In Benumof JL (ed): *Anesthesia for thoracic surgery*, p 376, Philadelphia, 1987, WB Saunders.

146. Bense L: Intrabronchial selective coagulation treatment of hemoptysis: report of three cases, *Chest* 97:990, 1990.

147. Tsukamoto T, Sasaki H, Nakamura II: Treatment of hemoptysis patients by thrombin and fibrinogen-thrombin infusion therapy using a fiberoptic bronchoscope, *Chest* 96:473, 1989.

148. Atasoy E: Thoracic outlet compression syndrome, *Orthop Clin North Am* 27:265, 1996.

149. Sunderland S: *Nerves and nerve injuries*, ed 2, p 69, Edinburgh; New York, 1978, Churchill Livingstone.

150. Pang D, Wessel HB: Thoracic outlet syndrome, *Neurosurgery* 22:105, 1988.

151. Mackinnon SE, Patterson AT: Supraclavicular first rib resection, *Semin Thorac Cardiovasc Surg* 8:208, 1996.

152. Urschel HC, Razzuk M: Upper plexus thoracic outlet syndrome: Optimal therapy, *Ann Thorac Surg* 63:935, 1997.

153. Hodgson AR, Stock FE, Fang HSY, et al: Anterior spinal fusion: the operative approach and pathological finding in 412 patients with Potts disease of the spine, *Br J Surg* 48:172, 1980.

154. Stillerman CB, Weiss MH: Surgical management of thoracic disc herniation and spondylosis. In Menezes AH, Sonntag VKH (eds): *Principles of spinal surgery*, p 581, New York, 1996, McGraw-Hill.

155. Mack MJ, Regan JJ, Bobechko WP, et al: Application of thoracoscopy for diseases of the spine, *Ann Thorac Surg* 56:736, 1993.

156. Dickman CA, Karahalios DG: Thoracoscopic spinal surgery, *Clin Neurosurg* 43:392, 1996.

157. McPherson RW, Sell B, Traytsman RJ: Effects of thiopental, fentanyl and etomidate on upper extremity somatosensory evoked potentials in humans, *Anesthesiology* 65:584, 1986.

158. Grundy BL, Nash CL, Brown RH: Arterial pressure manipulation alters spinal cord function during correction of scoliosis, *Anesthesiology* 54:249, 1981.

159. Kearney PA, Roahana SW, Burney RE: Blunt rupture of the diaphragm: mechanism, diagnosis and treatment, *Ann Emerg Med* 18:1326, 1989.

160. Carter BN, Guiseffi J, Felson B: Traumatic diaphragmatic hernia, *Am J Roentgol* 65:56, 1951.

161. Power M, McCoy D, Cunningham AJ: Laparoscopic-assisted repair of a traumatic ruptured diaphragm, *Anesth Analg* 78:1187, 1994.

162. Livingston DH, Bartholomew BJ, Blackwood J: The role of laparoscopy in abdominal trauma, *J Trauma* 33:471, 1992.

163. Wauquier A, Hermans C, Van den Broeck W, et al: Resuscitative drug effects in hypovolemic hyptensive animals. I: Comparative cardiovascular effects of an infusion of saline, etomidate, thiopental, or pentobarbital in hypovolemic dogs, Janssen Research Products, 1981.

164. Gross CM, Kramer J, Waigand J, et al: Stent implantation in patients with superior vena cava syndrome, *Am J Roentgenol* 169:429, 1997.

165. Tanigawa N, Sawada S, Mishima K, et al: Clinical outcome of stenting in superior vena cava syndrome associated with malignant tumors: Comparison with conventional treatment, *Acta Radiol* 39:669, 1998.

166. Stanford W, Doty DB: The role of venography and surgery in the management of patients with superior vena cava obstruction, *Ann Thorac Surg* 41:158, 1986.

167. Clausner A, Hoffmann-v Kapp-herr S: Gegenwartiger stand der trichterbrust, *Dtsch Med Wochenschr* 120:881, 1995.

168. Shamberger RC, Welch KJ: Surgical repair of pectus excavatum, *J Pediatr Surg* 23:319, 1988.

169. Schamberger RC, Welch KJ, Castameda AR, et al: Anterior chest wall deformities and congenital heart disease, *J Thorac Cardiovasc Surg* 96:427, 1988.

Anesthesia for Esophageal and Mediastinal Surgery
13

James B. Eisenkraft, MD
Steven M. Neustein, MD

Esophageal Surgery

The advent of anesthetic techniques to manage patients during thoracic surgery has permitted the development of a variety of surgical treatments for esophageal disease. These anesthetic techniques include the use of double-lumen endobronchial tubes to provide one-lung anesthesia and collapse of the lung on the side ipsilateral to the thoracotomy incision. The surgical diseases discussed in this section include tumors, hiatus hernia, rupture and perforation, achalasia, stricture, and esophagorespiratory tract fistula. It is essential to understand the pathophysiology of these lesions to safely anesthetize those patients who present for surgical treatment.

The esophagus is a muscular tube that extends from the pharynx, through the neck and thorax, to the abdomen. In adults, it averages 23 cm to 25 cm in length. The esophagus enters the superior mediastinum posterior to the trachea and the left recurrent laryngeal nerve and anterior to the vertebral bodies. It traverses to the posterior mediastinum and slightly to the left, passing posterior to the left mainstem bronchus (Figure 13-1). It continues posterior to the pericardium and left atrium and anterior to the descending aorta. Throughout the entire thoracic cavity, the right side of the esophagus is adjacent to the right mediastinal pleura and lung. On the left side at the level of T_5 to T_7, interposed between the left mediastinal pleura and the esophagus, are the aortic arch, common carotid artery, subclavian artery, and descending aorta. The esophagus continues a short distance in the abdomen until it joins the stomach at the cardia.

The blood supply to the esophagus is from the inferior thyroid arteries in the neck, the bronchial and intercostal arteries and the aorta in the thorax, and the left gastric artery in the abdomen. Venous drainage from the upper esophagus is to the inferior thyroid veins, from the middle esophagus to the azygos veins, and from the lower esophagus to the gastric veins. These venous systems anastomose with one another, and the azygos and gastric veins form connections between the systemic and portal venous systems.

The esophagus receives both vagal and sympathetic innervation. The vagus nerves lie on either side of the esophagus and form a plexus around it. The esophageal wall consists of two muscular layers: an inner circular layer and an outer longitudinal layer. The outer layer in the proximal esophagus is primarily striated muscle; distally, it is mainly smooth muscle.

The peristaltic wave, which normally takes 5 to 10 seconds to pass from the pharynx to the stomach, is predominantly under vagal control.[1] An increase in intraabdominal pressure results in an increase in the lower esophageal pressure such that the barrier pressure (the difference in pressures between the stomach and esophagus) remains unchanged.[2] Drugs that decrease lower esophageal sphincter pressure include anticholinergics, sodium nitroprusside, dopamine, β-adrenergic agonists, tricyclic antidepressants, and opioids.[3] Drugs that increase lower esophageal sphincter pressure include anticholinesterases, metoclopramide, prochlorperazine, and metoprolol (Table 13-1).[2]

The following sections discuss the anesthetic management of patients with hiatus hernia, esophageal cancer, intrathoracic esophageal rupture and perforation, achalasia, and esophagorespiratory tract fistula.

Surgical Diseases and Treatment
HIATUS HERNIA

Although most patients with gastroesophageal reflux have a sliding hiatus hernia, most patients with a hiatus hernia do not have significant reflux.[3] Patients with heartburn have a lowered barrier pressure and may be at increased risk for regurgitation of gastric contents. Two types of hiatus hernia have been described. Type I hernias, also called *sliding hernias*, make up

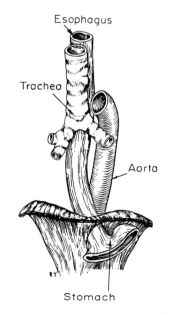

FIGURE 13-1 The esophagus and its anatomic relations. (From Orringer MB, Marshall B, Iannettoni MD: *Ann Surg* 230:392, 1999.)

269

TABLE 13-1

Effects of Drugs on Lower Esophageal Sphincter Pressure

Increase	Decrease	No Change
Metoclopramide	Atropine	Propranolol
Domperidone	Glycopyrrolate	
Prochlorperazine	Dopamine	Cimetidine
Cyclizine	Sodium nitroprusside	Ranitidine
Edrophonium	Ganglion blockers	Atracurium
Neostigmine	Thiopental	Nitrous oxide
Histamine	Tricyclic antidepressants	
Succinylcholine	β-Adrenergic agonists	
Pancuronium	Halothane	
Metoprolol	Enflurane	
α-Adrenergic stimulants	Opioids	
Antacids	Nitrous oxide	

From Aitkenhead AR: Anesthesia for esophageal surgery. In Gothard JW (ed): *Thoracic anesthesia*, London, 1987, Bailliere-Tindall.

approximately 90% of esophageal hiatal hernias. In this type, the esophagogastric junction and fundus of the stomach have herniated axially through the esophageal hiatus into the thorax.[3] Although the hernia may move cephalad and caudad in response to pressure changes in the chest and abdomen, the term *sliding* refers not to this movement, but to the presence of a partial sac of parietal peritoneum. The lower esophageal sphincter is cephalad to the diaphragm and might not respond appropriately to increased abdominal pressure. Thus, a reduced barrier pressure during coughing or breathing leads to regurgitation. The type II or *paraesophageal hiatus hernia* is characterized by portions of the stomach herniating into the thorax next to the esophagus. In the presence of a type II hernia, the esophagogastric junction is still located in the abdomen. The most common complications from type II hernias are blood loss, anemia, and gastric volvulus.

Obese patients with a hiatus hernia usually have impaired respiratory function due to both the obesity (when present) and the presence of the stomach in the thorax.[4] The total lung volume and the maximum breathing capacity are reduced, and the residual volume is increased.[4,5]

Patients presenting for esophageal surgery should have a preoperative chest x-ray, which might reveal evidence of aspiration or reduced lung volume. Patients with aspiration pneumonia should be treated with chest physiotherapy and antibiotics, and bronchospasm should be treated if present. Coexisting lung disease and obesity are indications for pulmonary function testing in any patient scheduled to undergo thoracotomy.

Patients with an incompetent lower esophageal sphincter are at risk for reflux and aspiration and should receive preoperative treatment to increase the pH of the gastric juice. One choice is the administration of an H_2-blocker, such as ranitidine or cimetidine. The oral or intravenous dose of cimetidine is 300 mg, four times daily. Alternative oral dosing regimens are 400 mg, twice daily, or 800 mg, once daily. When given intravenously, cimetidine should be given slowly, as rapid intravenous administration over two minutes might cause hypotension.[6] Bradycardia and heart block can also occur.[7,8] With continued

administration, there can be central nervous system effects that can include confusion, agitation, seizures, and coma.[9] Cimetidine can also lead to delayed awakening from anesthesia.[10] Metabolism of drugs with a high hepatic extraction (e.g., lidocaine, propranolol, and diazepam) might be delayed. This could be due to reduced liver blood flow and inhibition of the mixed function oxidase system.[11]

Ranitidine is a more potent inhibitor of gastric parietal cell hydrogen ion secretion than cimetidine. There are fewer side effects from ranitidine.[12] Central nervous system effects are less likely, probably because of the decreased ability of ranitidine to cross the blood-brain barrier. Although cardiac effects are unusual, bradycardia has been reported in association with intravenous administration.[13] Both ranitidine and cimetidine decrease liver blood flow. The oral dose of ranitidine is 150 mg, twice daily, but the intravenous dose is 50 mg every 6 to 8 hours. The intravenous route is preferred over the oral route because esophageal emptying is likely to be delayed in the presence of esophageal dysfunction. The medication should be administered both the night before and on the morning of surgery.

Omeprazole, 20 mg, administered orally the night before surgery, has been shown to reduce both the acidity and the volume of gastric contents.[14] The patients in this study were undergoing esophageal resection for cancer. No patient had more than 25 mL of gastric material with a pH below 2.5. Another alternative is sodium citrate (Bicitra), a nonparticulate antacid. Particulate antacids are harmful if aspirated and should, therefore, be avoided. Also, the whitish color of most antacids will obscure the surgeon's view if esophagoscopy is planned.

Metoclopramide, 10 to 20 mg intravenously over a period of 3 to 5 minutes, can be administered to increase lower esophageal sphincter tone. Anticholinergics can be administered if necessary but will decrease the tone of the lower esophageal sphincter (Table 13-1).

The goal of surgical repair of a sliding hernia is to obtain competence of the gastroesophageal junction. Because restoration of the normal anatomy is not always successful in preventing subsequent reflux, several antireflux operations have been developed, the so-called *wrap-around procedures*. An example of such a procedure is the Nissen fundoplication. This can be performed via an abdominal or thoracic incision and entails wrapping the distal esophagus with the fundus of the stomach.[3]

Nissen fundoplication can now also be performed laparoscopically, which allows for a faster recovery with less postoperative pain. During these cases, there is a risk of esophageal or gastric perforation during passage of the esophageal bougie.[15] Such a perforation, if it occurs, could require conversion from the minimally invasive laparoscopic to the open surgical procedure, and a thoracotomy may become necessary. Pyriform sinus perforation has also been reported with the use of an esophageal bougie.[16]

Paraesophageal hiatal hernia can also be repaired laparoscopically. An anterior hemifundoplication can be added; this procedure has been reported to cure preexisting gastroesophageal reflux and can prevent the development of reflux postoperatively.[17] In one series, only one of 38 patients required a conversion to an open procedure.[15] A left-sided hydrothorax has been reported to occur during laparoscopic Nissen fundoplication.[18] This complication was probably due to transudation of intraabdominal irrigation fluid through a diaphragmatic perforation.

Laparoscopic fundoplication is well tolerated in children, and postoperative analgesic requirements have been reported to be minimal.[19] In another series of children, there was transient hypoxia postoperatively in 25% of cases.[20] Difficulties during thoracoscopy in children include poor visualization and suturing.[21]

ESOPHAGEAL CANCER

Because of its distensibility, the esophagus proximal to an obstruction can become dilated and filled with food (Figure 13-2). This material is not exposed to the acid milieu of the stomach and so becomes infected with bacterial growth. Regurgitated liquid can lead to aspiration pneumonitis and atelectasis in patients with poor laryngeal reflexes. Even with prolonged fasting, the esophagus might not be empty above the obstruction, and the patient is thus at risk for aspiration of infected material on induction of general anesthesia. In the presence of esophageal obstruction, suctioning of the esophagus proximal to the obstruction with a large-bore nasogastric tube might decrease, but not totally eliminate, the risk of aspiration.

Although chemotherapy alone is ineffective for either squamous cell carcinoma or adenocarcinoma, combined therapy with radiation and surgery is often undertaken because the disease is likely to be systemic by the time of diagnosis. The chemotherapeutic agents used most often are antibiotic derivatives, such as doxorubicin and bleomycin.[22] In addition to myelosuppression, doxorubicin may lead to a dose-related cardiomyopathy in either an acute or slowly progressive manner. Ten percent of patients might develop the acute form, in which the ECG shows nonspecific ST-T wave changes and decreased QRS voltage, and there might also be premature ventricular

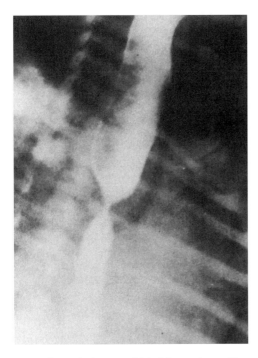

FIGURE 13-2 Cancer in the upper third of the esophagus. The esophageal lumen is almost occluded by the tumor, and the proximal esophagus is distended, forming a pouch. (From Rao TLK and El-Etr. AA: Esophageal and mediastinal surgery. In Kaplan JA [ed]: *Thoracic anesthesia,* New York, 1983, Churchill Livingstone.)

contractions, supraventricular tachyarrhythmias, cardiac conduction abnormalities, and left-axis deviation.[23] With the exception of decreased QRS voltage, these changes resolve within 1 to 2 months of discontinuing treatment. The slowly progressive form of cardiomyopathy is characterized by the slow onset of symptoms and then is followed by rapidly progressive heart failure. Cardiomyopathy is unlikely if the total dose of doxorubicin has been less than 500 mg/m^2 of body surface area.[23]

Bleomycin is used to treat esophageal squamous cell carcinoma. This agent causes only minimal myelosuppression, but pulmonary toxicity occurs in 5–10% of patients, with death resulting in 2% of patients taking bleomycin. The presence of pulmonary toxicity is initially manifested by cough, dyspnea, and basilar rales that then can develop into a mild or severe form.[24] Although there can be exertional dyspnea and a normal resting PaO$_2$ with the mild form, in the severe form there is resting hypoxemia, with interstitial pneumonia and fibrosis appearing on the chest x-ray.[25] There can be an increased alveolar-arterial difference for oxygen and reduced diffusion capacity.[24] These patients are at increased risk for developing acute respiratory distress syndrome postoperatively.[26] It has been hypothesized that exposure to an increased FIO$_2$ (leading to superoxide and other free radicals) might be responsible; however, there are data that contradict this.[27] The development of interstitial fluid in the lungs may be due to impaired lymphatic drainage secondary to the fibrotic changes. Patients over the age of 70 years who have received radiation treatment and more than 400 U of bleomycin were found to be at increased risk for toxicity.[24] The use of bleomycin has fallen out of favor in recent years due to its pulmonary toxicity. Other drugs that can be used include cis-platinum, vinblastine, or 5-fluorouracil.[28]

Radiation is another treatment used for esophageal cancer. It is much more effective for squamous cell carcinoma than for adenocarcinoma. Complications of this form of treatment include pneumonitis, pericarditis, bleeding, myelitis, and tracheoesophageal fistula.[1]

The three types of surgical treatment of esophageal carcinoma are esophagectomy with gastric replacement, esophagogastrectomy, and replacement of the esophagus with the colon. Esophagectomy and esophagogastrectomy are done by several different surgical approaches, depending on the location of the tumor and the preference of the surgeon (Table 13-2). For esophagectomy with gastric replacement (Ivor Lewis procedure), the stomach is first mobilized via an abdominal incision. Following a right thoracotomy, tumor resection is performed, which can lead to surgical compression of the vena cava and heart, causing hypotension. The stomach is pulled up into the chest and anastomosed to the proximal esophagus. For esophageal tumors involving the stomach, an esophagogastrectomy is performed via a left thoracoabdominal incision. Following the resection, the jejunum is anastomosed to the proximal esophagus. Recently, esophagectomy has been described with totally endoscopic surgery.[29]

Replacement of the esophagus with colon, which can be used to treat lesions throughout the esophagus, keeps the stomach intact. It is usually performed for tumors within 20 cm of the cricopharyngeus muscle.[2] The approach can vary depending on the level of the lesion—a left thoracoabdominal

TABLE 13-2

Surgical Approaches for Esophagectomy and Esophagogastrectomy

Surgery	Incisions	Anesthetic Considerations
Laparotomy and right thoracotomy "Ivor Lewis" (Lower and some middle-third esophageal lesions)	2 incisions: Upper Abdominal midline, then right thoracotomy approximately fifth, sixth intercostal spaces	One-lung ventilation Repositioning supine to right-lateral intraoperatively
Trans-hiatal "Orringer"	2 incisions: Upper	Hemodynamic instability from cardiac compression during blunt intrathoracic dissection
(Lower third lesions. May be used for mid-third in some centers)	Abdominal midline then left neck	Possibility of occult perforation of tracheobronchial tree during blunt dissection (leave tracheal tube uncut in case of need to advance into bronchus) No vascular access in left neck
Left-side thoracoabdominal Lower esophageal lesions only	1 incision: Left lateral thoracotomy extended to left upper lateral abdominal	One-lung ventiltion desirable
Combined chest, abdominal and neck ("three hole") (upper/midesophageal lesions)	3 incisions: Right thoracotomy, then laparotomy, then left neck	One-lung ventilation necessary Repositioning lateral to supine intraoperatively No vascular access in left neck
Thoracoscopy plus laparotomy or combined with laparoscopy (Upper/midesophageal lesions)	1 or 2 incisions, plus video port access Thoracoscopy to avoid blunt dissection in chest Neck incision at end	One-lung ventilation necessary Potentially prolonged surgery

approach being used for low thoracic lesions, and separate upper abdominal and right thoracic incisions for higher thoracic lesions.[2]

In the presence of an unresectable tumor, the placement of a wide-bore tube, such as a Celestin tube, can provide palliation of dysphagia. For insertion of such a tube, a gastrostomy is first performed. A catheter is passed from the stomach retrograde past the lesion and into the pharynx. The wide-bore tube to be used for palliation is sutured to the catheter and pulled past the lesion into the stomach. One risk involved in this procedure is esophageal perforation.

Surgery is always necessary if the plan is to cure the patient of esophageal cancer, rather than to palliate.[30] In one recent series, transhiatal esophagostomy was feasible in 99% of cases. In this report, the stomach was used as a replacement for the esophagus in 96% of cases. There was a 4% mortality rate. The most common complications were anastomotic leak (13%) and atelectasis or pneumonia (2%). Intrathoracic hemorrhage, recurrent laryngeal nerve injury, chylothorax, and tracheal laceration also occurred, but each occurred in less than 1% of patients.[31]

A mediastinal abscess can occur following esophagectomy.[32] Thoracoscopy may be used for esophageal mobilization, pharyngoscopy, and esophagectomy. In one series, morbidity and mortality were not reduced with esophagectomy, compared with patients who underwent transhiatal mobilization.[33] In general, advances in thoracic anesthesia have led to a decrease in mortality in cancer patients undergoing noncardiac thoracic surgery.[34]

BENIGN ESOPHAGEAL STRICTURE

Chronic reflux of acidic gastric contents can lead to ulceration, inflammation, and eventually stricture of the esophagus. Reflux is the most common cause of benign stricture formation in the lower esophagus. The pathologic changes are reversible if the acidic gastric contents cease their contact with the esophageal mucosa. Surgery might be necessary if medical treatment and dilatations are inadequate (Figure 13-3). There

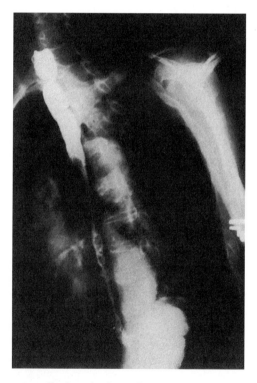

FIGURE 13-3 Esophageal stricture. Twenty-four hours following a barium swallow, contrast material can still be seen in the esophagus. (From Rao TLK and El-Etr AA: Esophageal and mediastinal surgery. In Kaplan JA [ed]: *Thoracic Anesthesia*, New York, 1983, Churchill Livingstone.)

are two types of surgical repair, both of which are usually approached via a left thoracoabdominal incision. Gastroplasty after esophageal dilatation interposes the fundus of the stomach between esophageal mucosa and the acidic milieu of the stomach. The remaining fundus can be sewn to the lower esophagus to create a valvelike effect.[2] The second type of repair is resection of the stricture and the creation of a thoracic end-to-side esophagogastrostomy. Vagotomy and antrectomy are performed to eliminate stomach acidity, and a Roux-en-Y gastric drainage procedure is performed to prevent alkaline intestinal reflux.

INTRATHORACIC ESOPHAGEAL RUPTURE AND PERFORATION

A rupture is a burst injury often due to uncoordinated vomiting, straining associated with weightlifting, childbirth, defecation, or crush injuries to the chest and abdomen. The rupture is usually located within 2 cm of the gastroesophageal junction, and is usually on the left side.[2] The rupture is due to a sudden increase in abdominal pressure with a relaxed lower esophageal sphincter and an obstructed esophageal inlet. In contrast to a perforation, in the presence of a rupture, the stomach contents enter the mediastinum under high pressure and the patient becomes symptomatic much more abruptly.

There are multiple causes of esophageal perforation, including foreign bodies, endoscopy, bougienage, traumatic tracheal intubation, and oropharyngeal suctioning at birth.[1,35-38] Iatrogenic causes are most common, with upper gastrointestinal endoscopy being the most frequent.[37] Other etiologies of iatrogenic esophageal perforation include endoesophageal intubation, esophageal obturator airways, esophageal balloon tamponade, and nasogastric tubes.[38] An endoscope will most likely cause a perforation at the upper esophageal sphincter, which is the narrowest point in the esophagus.[2] Perforations resulting from bougienage are most often at the level of the lesion. A perforation from traumatic attempts at tracheal intubation usually occurs near the cricopharyngeus muscle.[2] At this level, the cricopharyngeus muscle and the cervical vertebrae can compress the esophageal lumen.[35] Hyperextension of the neck might increase the likelihood of perforation during instrumentation.

In addition to pain, patients with intrathoracic esophageal perforation or rupture can develop hypotension, diaphoresis, tachypnea, cyanosis, emphysema, and hydrothorax or hydropneumothorax.[2,35] Radiologic studies might reveal subcutaneous emphysema, pneumomediastinum, widening of the mediastinum, pleural effusion, and pneumoperitoneum.[39] An esophagogram with either barium or iodinated water-soluble contrast material can localize the injury. Air might be seen in the mediastinum on a computed tomography (CT) scan of the chest.[37] These patients should receive antibiotics, and they require intravascular volume repletion as determined by central venous pressure monitoring. The patients could also require supplementary oxygen and even inotropic support of the circulation if arterial pressure remains low despite the administration of fluids. A large hydrothorax or hydropneumothorax, if present, should be drained preoperatively to improve circulatory and respiratory function.[2]

Important principles of treatment for a perforation of the thoracic portion of the esophagus include drainage and prevention of further contamination.[39] Esophagoscopy might first be needed to localize the rupture or perforation.[2] A right-sided thoracotomy is used when the injury is in the lower third of the esophagus.[1] In the presence of a healthy esophageal wall and an unobstructed esophagus, a primary closure can be performed. When the injury is at the lower end of the esophagus, it can be repaired with a portion of the stomach.

Esophagectomy is performed if an operable esophageal carcinoma is present. If the patient's medical condition is very poor, it might be more prudent to avoid a thoracotomy by iso-

lating the esophagus. The esophagus is divided in the neck, and a cervical esophagostomy is created. The distal esophagus is divided from an abdominal incision, and a feeding gastrostomy is placed.[2]

ACHALASIA

Achalasia is a disorder in which there is a lack of peristalsis of the esophagus and a failure of the lower esophageal sphincter to relax in response to swallowing. It is thought to have a neurogenic etiology, and many patients either are missing or have degeneration of the ganglion cells of Auerbach's plexus. This plexus, the plexus myentericus, is a nerve plexus consisting of unmyelinated fibers and postganglionic autonomic cell bodies in the esophageal wall. Clinically, the patients have esophageal distention that may lead to chronic regurgitation and aspiration.

As it is not currently possible to correct the motility disorder, the goal of treatment is to alleviate the distal obstruction. This can be done by either esophageal dilatation or by surgery. Dilatation, which carries with it the risk of perforation, can be achieved by mechanical, hydrostatic, or pneumatic means. The surgical repair consists of a Heller myotomy, which is an incision through the circular muscle of the esophagogastric junction. The myotomy is often combined with a hiatus hernia repair to prevent subsequent reflux.[40-42] This treatment is controversial, however, and some investigators have reported that myotomy without a fundoplication relieves dysphagia without causing reflux.[43-45] The procedure is usually performed via a thoracic incision, but an abdominal approach is also possible. A thoracic approach is required for extension of the myotomy more proximally, which can be continued by some surgeons to the level of the aortic arch.[40] The esophagomyotomy provides the best results and is the preferred treatment unless the patient is a poor surgical risk or refuses surgery, in which case an esophageal dilation can be performed.[3] Failure to provide initial relief of dysphagia reflects an inadequate myotomy, whereas later recurrence might be due to either reapposition of severed muscle or stricture from postmyotomy gastroesophageal reflux and esophagitis.[46]

The Dor operation is a modification of the procedure in which a stent is inserted into the muscular defect created by the myotomy in order to prevent muscular reapposition and, thus, recurrent dysphagia.[46,47] Good results following the Dor operation have been reported in 17 patients, with only one patient experiencing mild persistent dysphagia.[46]

The Heller myotomy can now be performed laparoscopically. This approach is associated with less postoperative pain, shorter hospital stay, and better treatment of dysphagia, when compared with the open abdominal approach.[48] Complications may include pneumothorax and atelectasis.[49] Intraoperative endoscopy is performed to evaluate the effectiveness of the myotomy. Manometry may also be performed to determine whether there is residual high pressure.[50]

ESOPHAGORESPIRATORY TRACT FISTULA

Esophagorespiratory tract fistula in an adult is most often due to malignancy.[51,52] Occasionally, the fistula is benign and could be due to injury by a tracheal tube or from trauma or inflammation.[51] Rarely, an adult might present with congenital benign tracheoesophageal fistula without esophageal atresia. Of the malignant fistulae, approximately 85% are secondary to esophageal cancer.[53] The incidence of fistula formation in the presence of esophageal cancer ranges from 5% to 18%.[54,55] Palliation is the usual treatment, as there is often local tumor extension, the patients have received radiation, and long-term survival is poor.[53-55] It is controversial as to whether the palliation should take the form of endoesophageal intubation or esophageal bypass and exclusion.[51] There is a higher perioperative morbidity and mortality (25% to 40%)[56,57] from esophageal bypass than from esophageal intubation (20% to 30%),[58] but the palliation afforded by esophageal bypass surgery is better and survival could be slightly longer.[53,56-60] The goal of palliation is to eliminate the passage of esophageal contents into the respiratory tract and to restore continuity to the alimentary tract. Regardless of the technique used for esophageal bypass or exclusion, the fistula still exists at the end of the operation but has effectively been removed from the alimentary tract. In this procedure, the esophagus is divided in two places—at the cardia of the stomach and proximally in the neck. The fundus of the stomach is connected to the proximal portion of the divided esophagus. The stomach, jejunum, or colon may be used as the connection, which can be placed in either a presternal or a retrosternal position. The isolated portion of esophagus can be drained either internally or externally.

Drainage of the isolated esophagus has been recommended in patients with poor pulmonary function, as these patients might not be able to tolerate the additional secretions that would accumulate without such drainage.[51] Preoperatively, these patients are likely to experience dysphagia, abdominal or substernal pain, and severe coughing associated with eating or drinking. Chronic aspiration will lead to hypoxemia, pneumonia, fever, sepsis, dyspnea, and sputum production.

In addition to the fistula, aspiration might also be due to recurrent laryngeal nerve dysfunction secondary to tumor extension. Because of the juxtaposition of the esophagus and aorta, there could be a connection between these two structures. If present, such a communication could be disrupted by any manipulation of the fistula, leading to severe hemorrhage.[61] Aortography might not identify the fistula because it is clotted, but the aortic lumen might be altered in appearance because of invasion by tumor.[62] Esophageal bypass and exclusion are very hazardous in the presence of an esophagoaortic fistula and are more likely to result in death than in palliation.[51]

Localization of the fistula preoperatively is part of the preoperative evaluation. In contrast to the pediatric patient with esophagorespiratory tract fistulae, which usually connect the distal esophagus to the posterior tracheal wall, these fistulae might connect to any part of the respiratory tract.[51] In most cases, the fistula can be seen on esophagography, but aspiration of barium is a complication of this study.[63-65] Bronchoscopy has been recommended as the best method for fistula identification, but success rates of only 50% to 75% have been reported.[63,65]

ZENKER'S DIVERTICULUM

Zenker's diverticulum is actually a diverticulum of the lower pharynx . Because it arises from a weakness at the junction of the thyropharyngeus and cricopharyngeus muscles just proximal to the esophagus, it can be managed by general surgeons; by ear, nose, and throat surgeons; or by thoracic surgeons. It is commonly considered as an esophageal lesion for the following two reasons:

- Its location is proximal to the upper esophagus.
- The underlying cause might be a failure of the upper esophageal sphincter to relax during swallowing, with an increase in pressure in the lower pharynx, leading to localized dilation and eventually to the formation of a diverticulum.

Early symptoms can be nonspecific, with dysphagia and complaints of food sticking in the throat. As the diverticulum enlarges, patients describe noisy swallowing, regurgitation of undigested food, and supine coughing spells. Recurrent aspiration and pneumonia can develop in the later stages.[66]

The major concern for anesthesia is the possibility of aspiration on induction of general anesthesia for excision of the diverticulum.[67] The possibility of aspiration intraoperatively and postoperatively should also be considered in a patient with a Zenker's diverticulum having anesthesia for any other type of surgery. Because the diverticulum fills with relatively alkaline oral secretions, aspiration is less likely to be fatal than aspiration of stomach contents. Even prolonged fasting does not ensure that the diverticulum will be empty. The best method to empty the diverticulum is to have the patient express and regurgitate the contents immediately prior to induction. Many of these patients are accustomed to doing this on a regular basis at home. As the diverticulum orifice is almost always above the level of the cricoid cartilage, cricoid pressure during a rapid-sequence induction does not prevent aspiration; it has been reported to contribute to aspiration by causing the sac to empty into the pharynx.[2] Surgical excision is usually done through an incision in the lower left neck.

The safest method of managing the airway for these patients might be awake fiberoptic intubation. The majority of such patients, however, have been managed without incident using a modified rapid-sequence induction without cricoid pressure, with the patient supine and in a head-up position (20 to 30 degrees). Other considerations for these patients include the possibility of perforation of the diverticulum when passing an oro- or nasogastic tube, or an esophageal bougie. In addition, placing a pack in the pharynx above the glottis around the tracheal tube may decrease the risk of aspiration during surgery.

Anesthetic Considerations for Esophageal Surgery

PREOPERATIVE EVALUATION AND PREPARATION

A thorough preoperative evaluation is essential. Patients with esophageal obstruction have dysphagia when ingesting solids, progressing to dysphagia when ingesting liquids, and they frequently develop poor nutritional status. Improving the nutritional status prior to surgery can lead to decreased morbidity and mortality.[68,69] In addition to a poor nutritional status, patients with esophageal disease can suffer from chronic aspiration, leading to a poor preoperative respiratory status.

During and following thoracotomy for esophageal surgery, there is a high incidence of supraventricular tachyarrhythmias because of manipulation of the heart and lungs. Although digitalis given preoperatively might decrease the incidence of arrhythmias, there is some risk of digitalis toxicity.[70] When digitalis is given preoperatively, it is not possible to titrate the dose to clinical effect, making the possibility of toxicity more likely.[71,72] Preoperative digitalization is controversial. Many of the patients with esophageal cancer are elderly, a circumstance that further increases the chances of coexisting cardiopulmonary dysfunction. Other preoperative considerations include chemotherapeutic treatment for cancer and the use of antacids, H_2-blockers, and metoclopramide in patients with hiatus hernia. These treatments have been discussed in the preceding sections.

MONITORING

In addition to the routine monitors, an arterial catheter is needed for continuous blood pressure monitoring and intermittent arterial blood sampling. Continuous blood pressure monitoring is indicated, as there could be arrhythmias with resulting hypotension due to surgical intrathoracic manipulation and blood loss. Central venous access is indicated to allow central delivery of medications that might be needed to treat arrhythmias and hypotension, and for measurement of central venous pressure to guide fluid administration. If indicated by the patient's preoperative cardiac status, a pulmonary arterial catheter might be needed. Continuous pulse oximetry is particularly important because there can be periods of hypoxemia and hemoglobin desaturation during one-lung anesthesia.

INDUCTION OF ANESTHESIA

Because patients presenting for esophageal surgery might be at risk for aspiration, either an awake tracheal intubation or a rapid-sequence induction with cricoid pressure is indicated. Additionally, a patient with mediastinal lymphadenopathy might have tracheal compression and collapse of the airway with the onset of muscle relaxation. Ventilation might be possible only by passage of a tracheal tube beyond the obstruction (see the Mediastinal Mass section later in this chapter).

A range of 30 to 44 Newtons has been recommended as the force to be used for applying cricoid pressure. One study found that a wide range of force was used, and technique was frequently poor among anesthesia assistants.[73] The use of a simulator for training led to an improvement in cricoid pressure application technique. In a right-handed person, use of the left hand to apply cricoid pressure could be more likely to be associated with either inadequate or excessive force.[74]

It could be necessary to release the cricoid pressure in order to place an intubating laryngeal mask airway. In this study, the use of cricoid pressure reduced the success rate of intubation through a laryngeal mask airway from 84% to 52% ($P = 0.03$).[75]

Application of cricoid pressure has been reported to decrease lower esophageal sphincter tone, but this effect does not cause reflux clinically.[76,77] An excellent discussion regarding the application of cricoid pressure is to be found in a recent review.[78]

CHOICE OF TRACHEAL TUBE

For lower esophageal resections via a left thoracoabdominal incision, it is not absolutely necessary to collapse the left lung with a double-lumen endotracheal tube, although this might be the practice in some centers. A single-lumen tracheal tube can be placed, and surgical exposure can be obtained by retraction of the left lung. For esophageal surgery via a thoracotomy, it is usually necessary to place a double-lumen endotracheal tube to collapse the ipsilateral lung. Although some authors have advocated placing a left-sided double-lumen tube irrespective of the side of the thoracotomy, a right-sided double-lumen tube offers some advantages for a right-sided thoracotomy for esophageal surgery.[2] The major risk in using a right-sided double-lumen

tube is collapse of the right upper lobe. This risk is unlikely to be significant during a right thoracotomy, however, as the right lung will be collapsed in any case. On the other hand, obstruction of the left upper lobe, which can occur during use of a left-sided double-lumen tube, is likely to cause hypoxemia during a right thoracotomy with collapse of the right lung. Additionally, a right-sided double-lumen tube is technically easier to place in the correct bronchus, an important consideration in a patient who is at risk for aspiration.

Many anesthesiologists prefer not to use a double-lumen tube when a rapid-sequence induction with cricoid pressure is planned. Another option would be to use a Univent tube (Univent, Fuji Systems Corp., Tokyo, Japan). This consists of a single-lumen tube that houses a channel along its concave side, inside of which is located a bronchial blocker. The tube is rotated in such a way that the concave side of the tube faces the side to be blocked, and the blocker is advanced while the bronchus to be blocked is visualized utilizing fiberoptic bronchoscopy. It could be difficult to advance the blocker to the left mainstem bronchus, due to a more angulated takeoff. The fiberoptic bronchoscope can be used to guide the Univent tube into the left mainstem bronchus, and then the blocker can be advanced as the tube is withdrawn. Disadvantages of the Univent tube are that it is bulky and might not be able to be advanced into the mainstem bronchus. The Univent tube could also be difficult to pass between the vocal cords because of its large external diameter (see Chapter 8).

At the end of the case, if the patient is to remain tracheally intubated, the Univent tube does not have to be changed. The blocker is withdrawn completely into its channel. Postoperative caregivers must receive careful instruction about the Univent tube if it is left in place. If the blocker should be inflated while it is in the trachea, complete respiratory obstruction can occur.

In the case of a difficult intubation, it might only be possible to place a standard single-lumen tube (which has a smaller external diameter than the Univent tube) for the same size internal diameter. A Fogarty (embolectomy) catheter can be placed, during visualization with a bronchoscope, into the mainstem bronchus of the lung to be blocked. Before inflation of the blocker, suction must be applied to deflate the lung. Once the balloon on the Fogarty catheter or other blocker is inflated, gas will not exit the lung via the tracheal tube, but there will be a slow absorption of oxygen.

It might be preferable to use smaller tidal volumes when a blocker is used, so as to lessen the airway pressure. Some gas could pass beyond the blocker in the face of higher airway pressure but not be exhaled (exhalation is passive). Progressive inflation of the deflated lung would result in such a case.

INTRAOPERATIVE CONSIDERATIONS AND MANAGEMENT

Hypotension can occur because of hypovolemia from blood loss, inferior vena cava compression, or surgical manipulation of the heart. If hypotension occurs, the surgeon should be notified to determine whether it is due to surgical compression. Another potential complication is surgical trauma to the trachea. This can be managed by ventilating only via the bronchial lumen of the double-lumen endobronchial tube (if one is present in the bronchus of the lung being ventilated) or by advancing a single-lumen endotracheal tube beyond the tracheal rupture into the bronchus.[79] For this reason, when managing an esophagectomy with a single-lumen tube, it is extremely important not to routinely cut the single-lumen tube to a shorter length.

High concentrations of nitrous oxide are contraindicated when bowel is present in the chest because bowel distention can occur, resulting in respiratory impairment and, possibly, interference with surgical exposure. In addition, one-lung anesthesia should be conducted with a high inspired concentration of oxygen. A patient with relatively normal lungs undergoing esophageal surgery could be more likely to experience hypoxemia during one-lung ventilation than a patient presenting for lung resection. This is because the patient presenting for lung surgery could already have limitation of blood flow to the diseased lung and, thus, less ventilation/perfusion mismatching during one-lung anesthesia. Also, during lung resection, the surgeon ligates the pulmonary artery or a branch thereof, which decreases the shunt.

The surgeon might request the anesthesiologist to pass an oropharyngeal bougie to facilitate the surgical repair. The bougie is then removed. To test the integrity of the anastomosis or repair, methylene blue is injected via a nasoesophageal or oroesophageal tube, the lower end of which has been carefully positioned by the surgeon in relation to the anastomosis. If the patient is to remain tracheally intubated at the end of a procedure in which a double-lumen endobronchial tube has been used, reintubation with a single-lumen endobronchial tube must be done very carefully and checked immediately, as unrecognized esophageal intubation and ventilation could result in acute disruption of the suture line.

ANESTHETIC MANAGEMENT FOR ESOPHAGEAL DILATATION

Indications for esophageal dilatation include achalasia, stricture, and collagen diseases involving the esophagus (e.g., scleroderma, myopathies, and spasm).[80] If an esophageal dilatation is to be performed, the patient will require a general anesthetic. Before induction, the esophagus should be suctioned with wide-bore tubing. A rapid-sequence induction with cricoid pressure applied, or an awake intubation if a difficult airway is suspected, should be performed. Retching and bucking can increase the possibility of esophageal perforation and subsequent mediastinitis and should, therefore, be avoided. Agents such as atropine, which decrease the tone of the esophageal body, should be avoided, as good tone is necessary for successful rupture of muscle fibers produced by the dilatation. One older technique that has been described uses neuroleptanesthesia (droperidol and fentanyl) and a succinylcholine infusion.[80] A more modern approach would be to use propofol and a short-acting muscle relaxant, such as mivacurium. The trachea should not be extubated until the patient is fully awake and able to protect his or her airway because aspiration remains a risk postoperatively.

ANESTHETIC MANAGEMENT FOR ESOPHAGORESPIRATORY TRACT FISTULA SURGERY

Anesthetizing the patient with an esophagorespiratory tract fistula carries with it unique considerations that distinguish this from other types of esophageal surgery. Because positive pressure ventilation can result in loss of inspired gas through the fistula and inadequate ventilation, spontaneous ventilation should be maintained during induction until gentle ventilation by mask has been shown to provide effective gas exchange. The lung on the same side as the fistula is likely to be less com-

pliant because of chronic aspiration, allowing the contralateral lung to receive most of the ventilation. Some authors have recommended avoidance of positive pressure ventilation before tracheal intubation because of the possibility of gas flow through the fistula, which can cause abdominal distention, secondary respiratory insufficiency, and even hypotension and cardiac arrest.[81-83] This can be accomplished either as an awake intubation or following an inhalation induction, which is likely to be slow and stormy as a result of poor respiratory function and the presence of secretions. Routine gastrostomy under local anesthesia has been recommended prior to induction to serve as a vent if positive pressure ventilation by mask should become necessary.[83,84] Because of the risk of leakage and mediastinitis, however, gastrostomy is not available as an option if the stomach is to be moved into the thorax. High-frequency jet ventilation is another alternative that can be used to reduce gas loss through the fistula (see Chapter 12).[85]

Unless the fistula is located high enough in the trachea that the cuff of a single-lumen tube can make a seal distal to the fistula (which is rare), a double-lumen endobronchial tube will be needed. Such a tube protects the contralateral lung from contamination and provides the ability to ventilate it without applying positive pressure to the fistula.[86] Because a double-lumen tube might not always pass to the intended side when placed blindly, it could be useful to use a flexible fiberoptic bronchoscope to position the tube under direct vision so as to minimize the possibility of disrupting the fistula. A right-sided double-lumen tube should be used for a fistula in the distal trachea, left mainstem bronchus, or left lung, and a left-sided double-lumen tube should be used for a fistula in the right mainstem bronchus or right lung. If the site of the fistula cannot be determined preoperatively, a right-sided double-lumen tube should be placed because in terms of statistical probability, the fistula is most likely to communicate with the trachea or the left mainstem bronchus. Right-sided ventilation should be attempted first. Either gastric distention or loss of delivered tidal volume indicates presence of a right-sided fistula, and left-lung ventilation should then be used instead. If two-lung ventilation becomes necessary, a nasogastric tube can be passed to vent the stomach, but there could be loss of tidal volume through the vent. If two-lung ventilation is used, the excluded esophageal portion must be drained to protect against disruption of the suture line.[51] A method of airway management for a pericarinal fistula in an adult has been described using bilateral endobronchial tubes placed with fiberoptic bronchoscopy.[87]

At the conclusion of the procedure, resumption of spontaneous ventilation is preferred. Postoperatively, positive-pressure ventilation can be harmful in a number of different ways. It can disrupt the esophageal suture lines if the excluded esophageal segment has not been drained. It can also lead to loss of tidal volume (if the fistula is drained externally) and to abdominal distention (if the fistula is drained internally).[51] Another potential complication of continued positive pressure ventilation is disruption of the fistula. It is, therefore, important to optimize the patient's respiratory function intraoperatively by suctioning secretions, avoiding excessive intravenous sedation, and providing good postoperative analgesia with either intrathecal or epidural opioids. In one series, 9 of 18 patients had postoperative ventilation, which was required for periods ranging from three days to three weeks.[57] High-frequency jet ventilation is an attractive alternative if postoperative ventilation is required, as this technique applies only minimal pressure to the airway.

Postoperative Considerations

Postoperative complications include hypotension, which is most likely because of hypovolemia or hemorrhage. Patients who have been receiving total parenteral nutrition might be at risk for delayed awakening due to hypoglycemia or hyperosmolar coma. The rate of administration of parenteral nutrition should be either reduced, stopped, or substituted with 10% dextrose.

Respiratory complications are common following thoracic esophageal surgery, especially in the presence of obesity and coexisting lung disease (e.g., aspiration pneumonia). Incisional pain can lead to hypoventilation, hypoxemia, and atelectasis. Administration of intrathecal or epidural opioids provides analgesia with minimal sedation and might improve respiratory function. The patient might have received subcutaneous heparin to prevent deep venous thrombosis; the use of intrathecal or epidural opioids is controversial in such cases due to the possibility of epidural hematoma.

There is a high incidence of postoperative complications following thoracotomy for esophageal perforation or rupture. If present, mediastinitis often leads to severe septicemia with anaerobic or gram-negative organisms. The chance of primary repair dehiscence is more than 50%.[2] Patients should remain tracheally intubated at the conclusion of a thoracic repair of an esophageal perforation or trauma due to the likelihood of infection, respiratory impairment, hypotension from blood loss, hypothermia, arrhythmias, or fluid transudation.

Additional complications following esophageal bypass and exclusion for esophageal respiratory tract fistula include pneumothorax if either pleural cavity is accidentally entered from a retrosternal approach. Aspiration can occur due to recurrent laryngeal nerve injury from cervical dissection.

Mediastinal Mass

Patients with a mediastinal mass pose special problems for the anesthesiologist. While some mediastinal masses can produce obvious superior vena cava obstruction, they also can cause compression of the major airways and/or heart, which could be less obvious and become apparent only following induction of (or emergence from) general anesthesia.

Thoracoscopy has been utilized for mediastinal surgery. A 2 × 2 cm pericardial cyst, located between the superior vena cava and right atrium, was removed by video-assisted thoracoscopic surgery.[88] The same author had previously reported excision of a mediastinal thymic cyst via thoracoscopy.[89] Thoracoscopy has been used for resection of paraesophageal tumors and for neurogenic tumor located in the posterior mediastinum.[90] It has also been used for resection of esophageal cyst.[91]

The most common anesthesia complication related to such a mass is tracheobronchial obstruction, although the mechanical (compression) complications produced by such tumors depend on the part of the mediastinum in which they are located.

Patients presenting with mediastinal masses often need anesthesia for diagnostic procedures (e.g., node biopsy or bronchoscopy) as well as for therapeutic surgery (e.g., thoracotomy or laparotomy). Numerous case reports attest to serious potential problems that can develop during these cases. These complications will be considered briefly.

Tracheal and Bronchial Compression

Complete airway obstruction has been reported and can develop acutely during induction of anesthesia, intubation, patient positioning, maintenance, or recovery. In a review of 22 case reports, this complication was found in 20 cases.[92] Five of these 20 had respiratory symptoms or signs preoperatively and, in three cases, the symptomatology varied with patient position.

In three cases, inhalation induction of anesthesia precipitated airway obstruction, which was not completely alleviated by intubation. Indeed, in some cases, intubation made an incomplete obstruction complete until a longer tube with a smaller diameter was passed beyond the obstruction. It has been suggested that loss of chest wall muscle tone and loss of the expansile forces of spontaneous inspiration following the administration of neuromuscular blocking drugs might abolish the extrinsic support of a bronchus (or trachea) that has been critically narrowed. This mechanism also explains tracheobronchial obstruction that occurs in a patient in the supine position, which is relieved by a change in position or by return of spontaneous respiration.[93]

If tracheobronchial compression or distortion is present, tracheal intubation can cause complete airway obstruction if the distal orifice of the tube abuts the tracheal wall or is occluded by a narrowed section or acute angle in the airway. Such obstruction has been relieved by passing either a long tube of small internal diameter or a bronchoscope beyond the stenotic region.[92-94] In some cases, respiratory obstruction due to edema develops during recovery, requiring reintubation.[96] Large negative airway pressures developed by vigorously attempted spontaneous inspirations can cause distal airway collapse and/or pulmonary edema.[97]

ANESTHETIC MANAGEMENT

The anesthetic management of the patient with tracheobronchial obstruction due to mediastinal tumor is based on an appreciation of the potential for total airway obstruction and the chemosensitivity and/or radiosensitivity of most mediastinal tumors. An algorithm for the anesthetic management of these patients has been proposed (Figure 13-4).[98] If, during the preoperative evaluation, the patient evidences dyspnea or positional dyspnea and is scheduled for biopsy, the procedure should be performed under local anesthesia. If the tumor is believed to be radiosensitive or chemosensitive, these treatments should be instituted and their benefits assessed by x-ray, computed tomography (CT), or magnetic resonance imaging (MRI) before any surgical procedure is undertaken. If the patient is not dyspneic, a flow-volume loop test of pulmonary function should be performed in both the sitting and supine positions. This test is helpful in assessing potentially obstructing lesions of the airway and will distinguish between intra- and extrathoracic obstructions. Figures 13-5 and 13-6 show how radiation therapy to an anterior mediastinal mass can improve vital capacity and expiratory flow rate. The effects of a large mediastinal tumor on gas

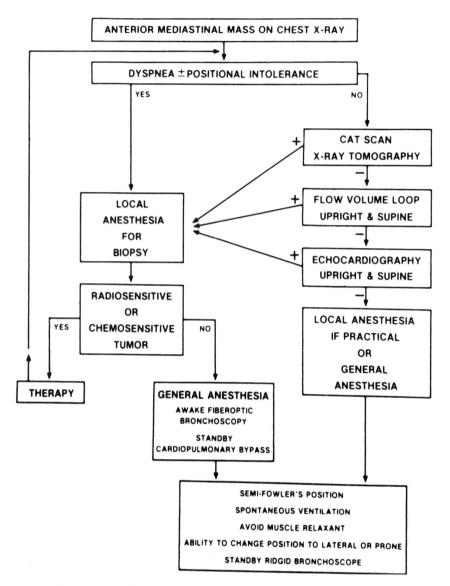

FIGURE 13-4 Flow chart depicting the preoperative evaluation of the patient with an anterior mediastinal mass. A plus sign (+) indicates a positive finding; a minus sign (–) indicates a negative workup. (From Neuman GG, Weingarten AE, Abramowitz RM, et al: *Anesthisiology* 60:144, 1984.)

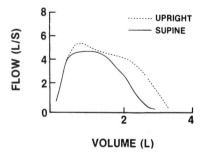

FIGURE 13-5 Flow-volume loop before radiation therapy in the upright and supine positions. Note marked reduction in vital capacity and expiratory flow rates. The expiratory flow rate plateaus, which is indicative of an intrathoracic airway obstruction. (From Neuman GG, Weingarten AE, Abramowitz RM, et al: *Anesthisiology* 60:144, 1984.)

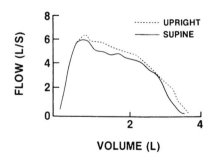

FIGURE 13-6 Flow-volume loop after radiation therapy in the upright and supine positions. There is improvement in expiratory flow rates and vital capacity, with minimal change when supine. (From Neuman GG, Weingarten AE, Abramowitz RM, et al: *Anesthisiology* 60:144, 1984.)

exchange have been described in detail by Fletcher and Nordstrom.[99] Other useful studies include a chest CT scan—which can reveal anatomic airway obstruction—and echocardiography in the upright and supine positions, which will show the effect of the tumor on the heart. If the results of the flow-volume, CT, and echocardiography studies are negative, the patient can receive general anesthesia if indicated. Local anesthesia would still be considered the ideal method of management in case the normal studies represented false-negative results. In one case, flow-volume loops demonstrated marked decreases in forced expiratory volume at 1 second and peak expiratory flow rate in the supine position, suggesting the potential for airway obstruction. Following radiotherapy, repeat studies showed improved function, and the planned procedure was then performed under local anesthesia.[99]

Preoperative radiation therapy can distort tissue histology and prevent an accurate histologic diagnosis. Furthermore, in pediatric patients, it could be difficult to obtain tissue with patients under local anesthesia. Ferrari and Bedford reported a series of 44 patients, 18 years of age or younger, with anterior mediastinal mass who underwent general anesthesia prior to treatment with radiation or chemotherapy even in the presence of cardiovascular and respiratory symptoms.[100] Although none of their patients died as a result of the anesthetic or operative experience, seven did develop airway compromise. The authors concluded that "in the absence of life-threatening preoperative airway obstruction and severe clinical symptoms, general anesthesia may be safely induced prior to radiation therapy," and that "the benefit of obtaining an accurate tissue diagnosis and initiating an appropriate therapeutic regimen outweigh the possible risks inherent in anesthetizing children with anterior mediastinal masses."[101] Others have disagreed with the conclusion that general anesthesia is "safe" when the reported rate of life-threatening complications is 16% to 20%.[101,102]

When the patient is to receive general anesthesia, a careful evaluation of the airway using a fiberoptic bronchoscope should be performed first.[101] Indeed, the fiberoptic bronchoscope can be used as a means to intubate the trachea. Some have recommended that general anesthesia then be induced with the patient in the lateral decubitus position so that the tumor falls away from the airway. One advantage of spontaneous ventilation is that during spontaneous inspiration, the normal transpulmonary pressure gradient tends to distend the airways and maintains their patency, even in the presence of extrinsic compression.[103] Neuromuscular blocking drugs should be avoided. If airway obstruction occurs during general anesthesia, it can be relieved by passage of a rigid ventilating bronchoscope or anode (reinforced/armored) tube beyond the obstruction. In some cases, obstruction can be relieved by direct laryngoscopy, allowing the laryngoscopist to lift up the laryngeal structures, thus replacing the lost muscle tone caused by a neuromuscular blocking drug.[104] Relief of obstruction can also be achieved by changing the position of the patient from supine to lateral or prone.[105] If the surgical procedure undertaken is via a median sternotomy, the extramural pressure on the airway is relieved when the chest is opened, thus decreasing the degree of obstruction. In one reported case, following opening of the chest, the inspiratory and expiratory flows were normalized, although the inspiratory pressure pattern remained abnormal.[99] When the chest was closed following a biopsy, the flows again became abnormal.

Airway obstruction and pulmonary edema are potential complications in the postoperative period. Obstruction can be due to expansion of the tumor caused by edema secondary to surgical manipulation and can necessitate reintubation of the airway.[97] Vigorous attempts at inspiration against an obstructed airway can lead to negative-pressure pulmonary edema once the obstruction has been relieved.

The use of femorofemoral cardiopulmonary bypass before the induction of anesthesia has been reported.[106] There might be airway obstruction, even following an awake intubation.[107] In this report, an awake intubation was performed in a patient who had a large anterior mediastinal mass; the patient had minimal respiratory symptoms but did have a narrowing of the trachea and both mainstem bronchi on CT scan. Ventilation became difficult during the anesthetic. The authors recommended that patients with >50% compression of the trachea or mainstem bronchi have the femoral vessels cannulated in case cardiopulmonary bypass should become necessary.[108] Other risk factors include preoperative respiratory symptoms and mediastinal mass >50% of thoracic diameter. In a series of children with anterior mediastinal masses, general anesthesia was considered safe if the CT scan indicated a tracheal area that was at least 50% of predicted and peak expiratory flow rates of 50% of predicted.[108]

Bilateral pneumothorax occurring during neck surgery has been reported.[109] This patient underwent resection of a parathyroid tumor that extended into the mediastinum. The anesthetic was uneventful until tracheal extubation, at which time the patient developed cyanosis. Bilateral pneumothoraces were detected by chest x-ray. These were treated successfully using bilateral chest tubes. Pneumothorax could have been due to injury to the parietal pleura.[99]

The laryngeal mask airway has been used to manage a patient with a large anterior mediastinal mass. The patient was maintained with a light general anesthetic and was breathing spontaneously.[110]

Superior Vena Cava, Pulmonary Arterial, and Cardiac Involvement

Obstruction of the superior vena cava (SVC) is most often due to a malignant tumor, usually on the right side. Etiologies include bronchial carcinoma, malignant lymphoma, and benign causes, such as SVC thrombosis induced by a pulmonary artery catheter. The syndrome is most severe if the tumor is growing rapidly, because a collateral circulation does not have adequate time to develop (Figure 13-7) (see Chapter 12).[111]

The SVC syndrome is characterized by engorged veins in the upper part of the body caused by an increased peripheral venous pressure; edema of the head, neck, and arms; dilated veins over the chest wall, which represent anastomotic pathways; and cyanosis. Respiratory symptoms include dyspnea, cough, and orthopnea, possibly due to venous engorgement in the airway. Changes in mental status can occur due to an increase in cerebral venous pressure. The SVC syndrome can be exacerbated or first noted during anesthesia, and the combination of decreased venous return from the upper part of the

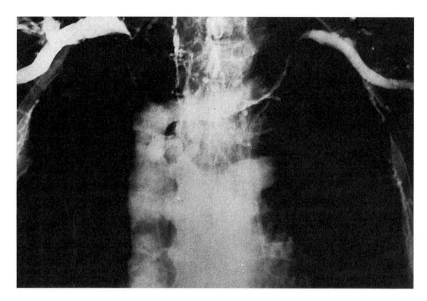

FIGURE 13-7 Venogram showing superior vena cava obstruction. Note bilateral obstruction to venous return from innominate veins due, in this case, to a large anterior mediastinal tumor.

body coupled with pharmacologic vasodilatation can result in severe hypotension.[112]

Mediastinal tumors can compress the pulmonary artery, causing a flow murmur, decrease in cardiac output, and decrease in pulmonary perfusion. This situation has been known to be fatal.[113] In another case in which tumor enveloped the pulmonary artery, the patient became severely cyanosed after induction of anesthesia but subsequently was safely anesthetized after establishment of extracorporeal oxygenation by femorofemoral bypass under local anesthesia.[114]

Large mediastinal lymphomas have been associated with arrhythmias under anesthesia because of pericardial or myocardial involvement.[115] In addition, a large thymoma was reported to have compressed the heart, simulating cardiac tamponade.[116]

A 14-year-old child was reported to have developed hypoxemia and hypotension following induction of anesthesia. She had been diagnosed erroneously with a pericardial effusion and had presented to the operating room for drainage. Intraoperative transesophageal echocardiography (TEE) was used and revealed the presence of an anterior mediastinal mass. The tumor was then debulked and the patient recovered well.[117]

A change in neck position can lead to airway compression in an anesthetized patient with a mediastinal mass.[118] Death can occur even from an asymptomatic mediastinal mass.[119] Patients who are at highest risk could require radiation or chemotherapeutic treatment of the tumor before receiving the anesthetic, but these procedures could interfere with subsequent attempts at tissue diagnosis.[120]

ANESTHESIA CONSIDERATIONS

In general, anesthesia considerations are similar to those for patients with tracheobronchial compression. All diagnostic procedures ideally should be performed with patients under local anesthesia. If general anesthesia is required, the same positional considerations should be taken into account. When severe and potentially untreatable airway obstruction seems likely, an extracorporeal oxygenator and support team should be immediately available.

If SVC obstruction is present, a preoperative course of mediastinal irradiation is a priority unless the syndrome is mild.[103,111] Such patients should be brought to the operating room in an upright position so as to reduce airway edema. It has been recommended that a radial arterial catheter be inserted in all patients and that, depending on the patient's medical condition, a central venous catheter be placed via the femoral vein.[121] A wide-bore intravenous cannula should be inserted in a lower extremity vein. The veins of the SVC drainage region (arms and neck) should be avoided because of the obstruction and unpredictable effects of drugs administered via these routes. No attempts at central venous cannulation via the SVC should be made because the risk of perforation and major hemorrhage is high, and any pressure readings obtained would likely be erroneous. If an awake fiberoptic intubation with the patient in the sitting position is planned, the patient should first receive a drying agent. Extreme care should be taken to avoid airway trauma during intubation, as the increased venous pressure and congestion make hemorrhage more likely. Topical anesthesia of the airway in these patients can best be achieved by inhalation of nebulized local anesthetic (lidocaine, 4 mL of 4%, with or without 10 mg of phenylephrine). The local anesthetic provides anesthesia for the trachea and avoids the necessity of a transtracheal injection of local anesthetic. The latter is usually associated with coughing, which can exacerbate any hemorrhage.

During surgery, massive hemorrhage, respiratory obstruction, or fatal exacerbation of the SVC obstruction might occur. Compatible blood should be kept available in the operating room in the event of severe hemorrhage. If SVC obstruction develops during anesthesia, diuretics and steroids might be of benefit.[112] No information is available as to whether spontaneous or controlled ventilation is preferable, although it should be remembered that coughing, straining, and the supine or Trendelenburg positions exacerbate the syndrome.[122]

Following diagnostic procedures in patients with SVC obstruction in whom the obstruction has not been relieved, acute respiratory failure can develop, necessitating reintubation and ventilatory support.[123] These patients, therefore, require intense observation during the recovery period.

Myasthenia Gravis and Thymic Surgery

Myasthenia gravis (MG) is an uncommon condition, but one of particular interest to the thoracic anesthesiologist because of the relationship between the thymus gland and the disease mechanism. Thymectomy is now considered to be the treatment of choice for most patients with MG.[124,125]

Clinical Aspects

The worldwide prevalence of MG is 1 per 20,000 to 30,000 population, and the incidence is two to five new cases per million per year. The disorder affects females more than males (3:2 ratio), and there appear to be two peak ages for incidence: the third decade for females and the fifth for males.[126,127] Although several different types of MG (congenital, neonatal, D-penicillamine-induced, and acquired autoimmune MG) have been described, only acquired autoimmune MG will be discussed here, as it is the variety most likely encountered by the thoracic anesthesiologist. The reader is referred to a number of excellent reviews for more information on the other types of MG.[128,129]

Acquired autoimmune MG is a chronic neuromuscular disorder characterized by weakness and fatigability of voluntary muscles, with improvement following inactivity. The onset of MG is often slow, insidious, and difficult to pinpoint. Any muscle or muscle group can be affected, and the condition is characteristically associated with periods of relapse and remission. Most commonly, the onset is ocular (diplopia, ptosis) and, if the disease remains localized to the eyes for two to three years, progression to generalized MG becomes less likely.[126]

In some patients, the condition might be generalized and may even involve the bulbar musculature, resulting in difficulties in breathing, chewing, swallowing, and speech. Peripheral neuromuscular involvement can result in difficulty walking or using the arms and hands. Vague complaints are not uncommon, and emotional overlay has resulted in substantial delays in diagnosis. The disease can also present an unexpected response to certain drugs.[130-132]

A classification of the severity of MG is difficult because the clinical spectrum is so broad; therefore, a number of systems have been described. The classification most commonly used is shown in Table 13-3.

PATHOPHYSIOLOGY

There have been great advances in the understanding of the pathophysiology of MG.[133,134] The fundamental abnormality in MG is a decrease by 70% to 90% in the number of postsynaptic acetylcholine receptors (AchRs) at the endplates of affected neuromuscular junctions, which causes a decrease in the margin of safety of neuromuscular transmission.[135,136] When the number of AchRs is normal, 75% of receptors must be occupied or occluded (by an antagonist, e.g., curare) to produce a threshold clinical decrease in neuromuscular function; for an almost complete block, 92% of receptors must be occupied by an antagonist.[137] Patients with MG, who might be lacking 70% to 90% of their receptors, are therefore on or close to the steep part of the receptor occlusion-transmission decrement relationship curve and are especially sensitive to anything that might adversely affect neuromuscular transmission.

It has long been known that burn patients develop resistance to nondepolarizing neuromuscular blocking drugs, perhaps because of upregulation of nicotinic receptors.[138] Recently, it has been reported that MG is improved in the postburn period.[139]

AUTOIMMUNE ASPECTS

Anti-AchR antibodies have been detected in some 90% of patients with MG. The actual titer of antibodies is not always directly related to disease severity and, in some patients with MG, no antibodies are detectable.[140] The antibodies produce their effects by causing a complement-mediated lysis of the postsynaptic membrane, by directly blocking the AchRs, and by modulating the turnover rate of AchRs in such a way that the degradation rate exceeds the rate of synthesis and incorporation into the postsynaptic membrane. Electron-micrographic studies of the motor-endplate area in affected muscles show a loss of synaptic folds (thus decreasing the area), a widening of the synaptic cleft, and decreased numbers of AchRs, as assessed by binding of α-bungarotoxin.[141]

DIAGNOSIS OF MYASTHENIA GRAVIS

The diagnosis should be suspected from the patient's history, and confirmation should be sought with pharmacologic, electrophysiologic, and immunologic testing. Because fatigue is the most characteristic feature, the patient cannot sustain or repeat muscular contraction. The electrical counterpart of this phenomenon is the progressive decline or decrement (fade) of

---

TABLE 13-3		
Clinical Classification of Myasthenia Gravis		
I.	*Ocular*—involvement of ocular muscles only. Mild with ptosis and diplopia. Electrophysiologic (EMG) testing of other musculature is negative for MG.	
IA.	*Ocular*—peripheral muscles showing no clinical symptoms, but showing a positive EMG for MG.	
II.	*Generalized*	
A.	*Mild*—slow onset, usually ocular, spreading to skeletal and bulbar muscles. No respiratory involvement. Good response to drug therapy. Low mortality rate.	
B.	*Moderate*—same as group IIA, but progressing to more severe involvement of skeletal and bulbar muscles. Dysarthria, dysphagia, difficulty chewing. No respiratory involvement. Patient's activities limited. Fair response to drug therapy.	
III.	*Acute fulminating*—rapid onset of severe bulbar and skeletal weakness with involvement of muscle respiration. Progression usually within 6 months. Poor response to therapy. Patient's activities limited. Low mortality rate.	
IV.	*Late severe*—severe MG developing at least 2 years after onset of group I or group II symptoms. Progression of disease may be gradual or rapid. Poor response to therapy and poor prognosis.	

Adapted from Osserman KE and Genkins G: *Mt Sinai J Med* 38:862, 1971.
EMG, Electromyogram; *MG*, myasthenia gravis.

the muscle action potentials evoked by repetitive stimulation of a motor nerve. Both the mechanical and electrical fades are characteristically improved with intravenous edrophonium, 2 to 10 mg (the Tensilon test).

Electromyography (EMG) is commonly used to confirm the diagnosis. The median, ulnar, or deltoid nerve is stimulated at 3 Hz for 3 seconds while muscle action potentials are recorded via surface electrodes. A positive test result for MG is characterized by a decrement of more than 10% when comparing the amplitude of the fifth with that of the first response (T_5/T_1). This fade is found in more than 95% of patients with MG if three or more muscle groups are tested.[142]

Myasthenic patients are characteristically sensitive to curare and, when the EMG is equivocal, a regional curare test can be performed in a limb that has been isolated by a tourniquet.[143,144] If the symptoms are limited to the bulbar musculature, a generalized curare test might be needed, which requires the presence of an anesthesiologist in the event that severe respiratory distress ensues.[145] In equivocal cases, a positive result of a test for anti-AchR antibodies is diagnostic. A negative result of this test in a patient with generalized weakness virtually excludes MG as the diagnosis.

MEDICAL TREATMENT

Anticholinesterases represent the most common initial therapy in the medical management of MG. These drugs (Table 13-4) prolong the action of acetylcholine at the neuromuscular junction and might also exert a nicotinic agonist effect of their own on the AchRs. Pyridostigmine (Mestinon) is used most commonly and is administered orally (60 mg tablets; 12 mg/mL solution) every 3 to 4 hours. Being quaternary amines, anticholinesterases are highly ionized in (and, therefore, poorly absorbed from) the gastrointestinal tract. If the patient is unable to accept oral preparations, pyridostigmine may be given parenterally in 1/30 of the usual oral dose. Serum concentration of pyridostigmine is related to the clinical response, which peaks at 1.5 to 2.0 hours following an oral dose and wanes by 4 hours after administration.[146] For those patients who are extremely weak on awakening in the morning, pyridostigmine is available in slow-release capsules (180 mg) for a prolonged overnight effect. Neostigmine (Prostigmin) has a shorter onset and duration of action and may be given orally, subcutaneously, or intravenously.

Patients with MG learn to regulate their anticholinesterase medications and to titrate dosage against optimum effect in those muscles most severely affected by the condition. This can result in certain nonessential muscle groups being either overdosed or underdosed, while the most important muscles (e.g., respiratory,

bulbar) are adequately controlled. Some patients can develop a psychological dependence on their anticholinesterase therapy and be reluctant to decrease or stop it preoperatively.[129]

Overdose of anticholinesterase can lead to the muscarinic effects of acetylcholine, manifested by colic, diarrhea, miosis, lacrimation, and salivation. Atropine (an antimuscarinic) is not routinely administered to patients receiving pyridostigmine, as it would mask the foregoing signs of overdosage. Atropine is used, however, in cases of severe muscarinic side effects.

MYASTHENIC EMERGENCIES (CRISES)

Myasthenic Crisis. In untreated cases, a myasthenic crisis can represent the onset of the condition. In treated cases, it is manifested as gradually increasing weakness and, perhaps, the involvement of previously unaffected muscles. Myasthenic crisis can be due to omission or underdosage with anticholinesterase.

Cholinergic Crisis. Cholinergic crisis is rare and due to overdosage with anticholinesterase, which causes a depolarization block of neuromuscular transmission. Symptoms can include salivation, sweating, abdominal cramps, urinary frequency and urgency, fasciculations, and weakness. It is treated by ventilatory support, antimuscarinic agents (atropine), and cessation of all anticholinesterase therapy until the crisis is resolved.

Distinction between a myasthenic and cholinergic crisis may be made with an edrophonium (Tensilon) test. Edrophonium, 2 to 10 mg intravenously, is administered and causes transient improvement in the case of a myasthenic crisis, but exacerbation or no improvement in a cholinergic crisis. Crises may also be distinguished by examining the pupils, which are dilated (mydriatic) in a myasthenic crisis but constricted (miotic) in a cholinergic crisis.

Desensitization Crisis. The third and rarest type of crisis, desensitization crisis, is associated with inefficacy of anticholinesterase medication and has been attributed to endplate desensitization.[147] Supportive measures and immunotherapy are the required treatments.

IMMUNOSUPPRESSIVE THERAPY

Because MG has an immunologic basis, glucocorticoids and azathioprine have been used to suppress the immune response. Indications for steroid therapy vary widely among different centers and include patients with ocular MG as well as patients with severe disease who are unsuitable for, or respond poorly to, thymectomy.[129] Steroids may exert a direct therapeutic effect at the neuromuscular junction in addition to having a thymolytic and/or lympholytic effect. Patients commonly show a clinical deterioration when steroid therapy (usually prednisone, 1 mg/kg on alternate days) is begun, and improvement usually takes several weeks. High-dose methylprednisolone has been suggested for the perioperative management of patients undergoing thymectomy and in the medical management of MG.[148,149]

Azathioprine (1 to 2 mg/kg/day) has been effective in producing clinical improvement and reducing antibody titers.[150] Cyclophosphamide (1 to 2 mg/day) has also been used effectively. A trial of cyclosporine therapy in MG suggests that this drug might similarly have a place in the medical management of these patients.[151] New antibodies have been found in patients with seronegative MG, possibly defining an immunologically distinct form of MG. A new immunosuppressant, mycopheno-

---

TABLE 13-4

Anticholinesterase Drugs Used to Treat Myasthemia Gravis

| Drug | Dosage (mg) | | | Efficacy |
	Oral	IV	IM	
Pyridostigmine (Mestinon)	60	2.0	2.0-4.0	1
Neostigmine (Prostigmin)	15	0.5	0.7-1.0	1
Ambenonium (Mytelase)	6	NA	NA	2.5

NA, Not available.

late mofetil, could be another option in the therapy of MG. Other work suggests the possibility of developing a vaccine against MG.[152]

PLASMAPHERESIS

Plasma exchange can produce transient improvement in muscle strength and decreases in anti-AchR antibody titers. It is used in severe cases of MG and, prior to thymectomy, has been reported to improve postoperative respiratory function.[153-155] Anesthetic implications of preoperative plasmapheresis include decreases in plasma pseudocholinesterase levels and prolonged paralysis following succinylcholine.[156]

ROLE OF THE THYMUS GLAND

Blalock pioneered thymectomy as a treatment for MG, when, following removal of a cyst from the thymic region of a patient with severe MG, dramatic improvement ensued.[157] Abnormalities are found in 75% of thymus glands removed from patients with MG. Of these, 85% show hyperplasia of germinal centers and proliferation of B cells, while 15% show thymoma, a frequently invasive tumor of the thymus. Only 30% of patients with thymoma, however, have symptomatic MG.

Following thymectomy, 80% of patients with MG will be improved or go into remission, and it is believed that cells of the thymus gland are related in some way to the production of the antibodies responsible for the condition.[127,158] Recent evidence suggests that the thymus produces a chemotactic factor that attracts appropriate white blood cells that form the anti-AchR antibodies. The myasthenic patients who improved after thymectomy had greater chemotactic activity than those who showed no improvement. It was postulated that stromal cells within the thymus gland of MG patients selectively attract peripheral helper T-cells and potentially facilitate activation of these T-cells. Activated T-cells, in turn, activate B-cells to produce anti-AchR antibody.[159]

MEDICAL VS. SURGICAL MANAGEMENT

A retrospective study of 80 patients with MG treated medically matched with 80 patients treated surgically (groups similar in terms of age, sex, severity, and duration of MG) showed that the surgically treated patients lived longer and had more clinical improvement than the group treated medically.[160] The difference was most marked among the female patients. Early thymectomy is now considered the treatment of choice for most patients with MG, exceptions being those in Osserman group I (Table 13-3).[126,161]

THYMECTOMY

The thymus gland lies behind the sternum in the anterior mediastinum. The traditional surgical approach is via a sternum-splitting incision (median sternotomy), which permits total exposure but could be associated with some morbidity in terms of postoperative ventilatory need. An alternative surgical approach is via the transcervical route, an approach similar to that used for suprasternal mediastinoscopy.[161] Controversy surrounds the question of which is the best surgical approach. Although a more radical procedure can be achieved via the transsternal route, the morbidity is greater, and equally good outcome results have been claimed following transcervical thymectomy.[162-164] Performance of a transcervical thymectomy does not preclude subsequent exploration by a median sternotomy or anterior thoracotomy (Chamberlain approach) in the

event that the MG is not improved by transcervical thymectomy. The converse also holds true. In the presence of a large mediastinal mass or suspected thymoma, however, a transsternal approach is usually preferred.[165] Success has also been reported with minimally invasive video-assisted thymectomy.[166,167]

Anesthetic Management for Thymectomy

PREOPERATIVE EVALUATION

Ideally, patients with MG should undergo elective surgery while in remission.[168] Given that early thymectomy is now the treatment of choice for MG, however, most patients have active disease when admitted for thymectomy. Patients should have their physical and emotional states optimized as much as possible. Those with severe disease are often admitted several days prior to surgery; milder cases are admitted on the day of surgery. A physical examination should include assessment of the airway and evaluation of muscle power and the ability to chew and swallow. Ideally, lung function studies and arterial blood gas analysis should be obtained preoperatively, especially if postoperative respiratory difficulties are anticipated. The chest x-ray, CT scan, or MRI should be examined to determine the presence of a tumor. In those patients with bulbar symptoms, nutritional status can be evaluated by measuring serum protein, electrolyte, and hemoglobin concentrations.

OPTIMIZING THE PHYSICAL CONDITION

If found, nutritional, fluid balance, or other deficiencies should be corrected. Patients with dysphagia could require nasogastric feeding via a tube. Any infections should be treated, bearing in mind that certain antibiotics (e.g., aminoglycosides) can exacerbate the muscle weakness. Other (autoimmune) diseases sometimes associated with MG (e.g., thyroid, rheumatoid) should be sought, ruled out, or treated adequately. In cases with severe bulbar involvement, the tracheobronchial tree might need to be cleared of secretions. This may require bronchoscopy.

MANAGEMENT OF DRUG THERAPY

The perioperative management of anticholinesterase therapy varies among institutions. One effective practice is that on admission, the daily dosage of pyridostigmine is decreased by 20% by reducing the size of each dose and/or increasing the interval between successive doses. The rationale for this is to prevent possible overdosing because, following thymectomy, the anticholinesterase requirement is usually decreased.

The surgical, anesthetic, and perioperative procedures—including the possible need for postoperative ventilation—should be explained fully to the patient. Education in breathing exercises and use of an incentive spirometer are also helpful.

Thymectomy is usually scheduled to be the first case of the day, particularly if the usual morning dose of pyridostigmine is to be withheld. Premedication should be with agents that do not cause respiratory depression, and opioids should, therefore, generally be avoided. Oral diazepam to reduce anxiety and intramuscular atropine or glycopyrrolate to decrease secretions are usually satisfactory. Unless the patient is physically or psychologically dependent on it, pyridostigmine is not administered on the morning of surgery. The patient, therefore, will tend to be weak on arrival to the operating room and requires less drug—whether potent inhaled agents or neuromuscular blockers—to produce relaxation. If, however, it should be indicated, $\frac{1}{30}$ of the usual oral dose is given intramuscularly. Those patients receiving chronic steroid therapy require additional parenteral coverage during the perioperative period.

MONITORING

Standard monitoring for thymectomy should be used in all patients with MG. Invasive hemodynamic monitoring is used if indicated by other existing cardiovascular conditions. Neuromuscular transmission should be monitored using a peripheral nerve stimulator (blockade monitor) and (ideally) a recording device to quantify the response to supramaximal peripheral nerve stimulation. Mechanical (mechanomyographic [MMG]) responses may be recorded and displayed using a force transducer and recording system. More recently introduced modalities for clinical monitoring of neuromuscular function in the operating room include an integrated EMG monitoring system (Datex-Ohmeda Neuromuscular Transmission Monitor) in the AS3 or S5 monitoring systems or the Accelograph acceleration monitor (Biometer, Inc., Copenhagen, Denmark).[169,170] Both systems have been used to assess neuromuscular function quantitatively in patients with MG, and both devices provide digital readouts of the T_1/control and T_4/T_1 ratios (as well as an optional hard copy printout).[170,171]

INDUCTION AND MAINTENANCE OF GENERAL ANESTHESIA

Induction of anesthesia is achieved easily with propofol or thiopental sodium. With the patient breathing N_2O and O_2, baseline MMG, EMG, or accelerographic recordings should be obtained to establish baseline neuromuscular responses in the nerve-muscle group monitored (usually the ulnar nerve and the adductor pollicis if using MMG or accelerography, or the ulnar nerve and first dorsal interosseous, adductor pollicis brevis, or hypothenar muscles if using the EMG monitor). Anesthesia can be deepened with a potent inhaled volatile agent (now usually isoflurane, desflurane, or sevoflurane) until direct laryngoscopy is possible, when the larynx is sprayed with lidocaine (4 mL of 4% in adults) and the trachea is intubated without the use of muscle relaxants. The lungs are then mechanically ventilated according to end-tidal or arterial blood gas CO_2 tensions. Temperature and breath sounds are monitored using an esophageal stethoscope and temperature probe.

Transcervical thymectomy is performed via a suprasternal incision (similar to that used for mediastinoscopy); therefore, the patient is positioned with the neck extended as much as possible with a folded sheet(s) under the shoulders and a "donut" to support the occiput. The transcervical approach to the thymus is anterior to the innominate vessels, whereas for mediastinoscopy an instrument is passed behind the vessels. Because retraction is only anteriorly (upward) on the sternum, innominate vessel compression and pseudocardiac arrest are not usually problems. Dissection in the anterior mediastinum via a small ("keyhole" or "minimally invasive") incision is not without risk or complications, which include hemorrhage and pneumothorax. Hemorrhage is uncommon, but it is important to preoperatively identify suitable venous access sites in the lower limbs so that if hemorrhage does occur in structures draining to the SVC, blood and fluids administered can reach the right atrium via the inferior vena cava. This has been lifesaving in patients who have suffered major hemorrhage during mediastinoscopic procedures. Pneumothorax, if it occurs, is

usually right-sided and due to adherence of the thymus to the pleura. It is usually identifiable at the time of surgery and can be drained. The transcervical thymectomy procedure usually lasts approximately 80 minutes but can vary according to surgeon and surgical difficulty.

During the surgical procedure, the potent inhaled anesthetic agent is titrated according to hemodynamic response and depth of anesthesia required. It is discontinued when closure begins. Nitrous oxide is discontinued on skin closure, and tracheal extubation is performed when the patient is awake, responsive, and able to generate negative inspiratory pressures of more than -20 cmH$_2$O.

Following tracheal extubation, all patients are carefully monitored in the post-anesthesia care unit. Once able to swallow soft food (custard, Jello), they are given their usual oral dose of pyridostigmine. In cases of mild respiratory distress, nausea, or difficulty swallowing, pyridostigmine in $\frac{1}{30}$ of the oral dose is administered intravenously or intramuscularly.

A chest x-ray is obtained routinely in the post-anesthesia care unit to rule out the presence of significant pneumothorax. Once the patient has been stable for 2 to 3 hours following oral pyridostigmine, he or she is discharged to the floor. Following transcervical thymectomy, most patients can be discharged to home by the second postoperative day. Those patients with more severe myasthenia who require postoperative ventilation and admission to the intensive care unit have a more prolonged hospital stay.

The transcervical approach to thymectomy has several advantages over the transsternal approach. The thoracic cage is not disrupted, so vital capacity is not decreased.[165] Thus, the need for postoperative mechanical ventilation is less likely following transcervical rather than transsternal thymectomy.

The management of anesthesia for transsternal thymectomy is essentially similar to that for transcervical thymectomy, except that the requirement for postoperative ventilation is perhaps more likely. The transsternal approach is used most commonly for patients with large thymic tumors and thymomas and for reexploration following transcervical thymectomy. Because these represent more extensive surgical procedures, arterial and central venous cannulae are generally indicated for hemodynamic monitoring purposes.

Choice of Anesthetic Technique
POTENT INHALED VOLATILE ANESTHETICS

Inhalation anesthesia, avoiding the use of neuromuscular blocking drugs, probably represents the most popular anesthetic technique because the effects of the inhaled agents are considered to be readily controllable and reversible. Myasthenic patients, however, appear to be more sensitive than normal individuals to the neuromuscular depressant effects of these agents.[172,173] In normal (i.e., not myasthenic) patients, low concentrations of inhaled agents are known to potentiate the effects of nondepolarizing neuromuscular blocking drugs, but, when given alone, produce neuromuscular depression only at high concentrations (e.g., more than 3% enflurane).[174] In myasthenic patients, 1% enflurane caused a 37% decrease in the T_4/T_1 ratio, and higher concentrations further decreased the T_1/control and T_4 ratios.[172] In a group of eight Chinese myasthenic patients, 1.5% isoflurane in 60% N_2O caused a 40% decrement in the train-of-four ratio, demonstrating that myasthenics are also more sensitive to the relaxant effects of isoflurane.[173] The sensitivity to potent inhaled agents varies widely among myasthenics; the responses to enflurane and isoflurane in two such patients are shown in Figures 13-8 and 13-9.

Of the potent inhaled anesthetics, the ethers seem to have greater neuromuscular depressant effects compared with the alkane, halothane. Indeed, one myasthenic patient who was receiving 3% halothane was reported to show little or no relaxation.[175] Another study found that isoflurane possesses approximately twice as strong a neuromuscular blocking effect as halothane in myasthenic patients. The newer inhaled anesthetics, desflurane and sevoflurane, are much less soluble than the older agents and therefore should offer greater control of muscle relaxation (i.e., more rapid onset and offset of action on muscle). Successful uses of both desflurane and sevoflurane in patients with MG have been reported.[176-180]

NEUROMUSCULAR BLOCKING DRUGS

Certain myasthenic patients can show inadequate relaxation with, or be unable hemodynamically to tolerate potent, inhaled agents, in which case a balanced technique involving neuromuscular blocking drugs may be selected.

DEPOLARIZING AGENTS (SUCCINYLCHOLINE)

Based on several clinical case reports and studies, myasthenic patients demonstrate resistance to succinylcholine.[181-186] Clinically, the use of succinylcholine has been generally without incident, despite the occasional earlier onset of phase 2 block.[181-188] The ED_{50} and ED_{95} (the effective dose producing 50% and 95% decreases in twitch response) for succinylcholine in normal patients are 0.17 and 0.31 mg/kg, respectively. In myasthenic patients, these values are 0.33 and 0.82 mg/kg, that is, 2.0 and 2.6 times the normal values. Because the doses of succinylcholine in common clinical use (1.0 to 1.5 mg/kg) represent three to five times the ED_{95} in normal individuals, adequate intubating conditions should be achievable in MG patients when these doses are used. If a rapid-sequence tracheal intubation is required, however, the data suggest that a dose of at least 1.5 to 2.0 mg/kg could be needed to produce rapid onset of excellent intubating conditions.[184-186] The mechanism whereby myasthenic patients are resistant to succinylcholine is unknown but is probably related to the decreased number of AchRs at the motor endplate.[134]

It should also be recognized that if the patient has received anticholinesterase therapy prior to succinylcholine, the dura-

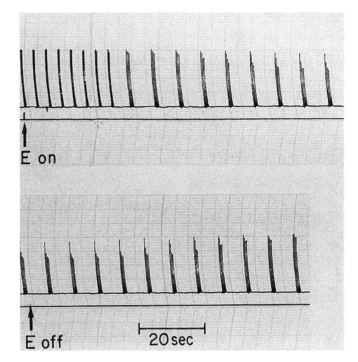

FIGURE 13-8 Continuous mechanomyogram (force-transducer) of responses to train-of-four stimulation (2 Hz) in a sensitive myasthenic patient. At *E on*, enflurane, 1% inspired concentration, was begun. Note the rapid onset of the decrease in first twitch height compared with control (T_1/C) and the decrease in fade ratio (T_4/T_1). At *E off*, enflurane was discontinued, and the recovery of T_1/C and T_4/T_1 ratio is observed after this brief (1¼ minute) exposure to enflurane. (From Eisenkraft. JB: Myasthenia gravis and thymic surgery: anesthetic considerations. In Gothard JW [ed]: *Thoracic anesthesia,* London, 1987, Baillierc-Tindall.)

tion of action will be prolonged, even though the potency in terms of relaxation produced might not be affected.[189]

NONDEPOLARIZING NEUROMUSCULAR BLOCKING DRUGS

Patients with MG are characteristically sensitive to the effects of the nondepolarizing neuromuscular blocking drugs. Pancuronium and *d*-tubocurarine have been used without complications, but careful titration of small doses against quantified effect is essential if uncontrolled, prolonged paralysis is to be avoided.[181-186]

In myasthenic patients, the regional curare test shows both an increased response and a prolonged effect, suggesting an increased affinity between AchR and relaxant.[143] Because

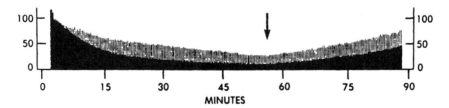

FIGURE 13-9 Integrated electromyographic (EMG) recording (Datex 221 Neuromuscular Tranmission Monitor) demonstrating the effect of isoflurance on the T_4/T_1 (fade) ratio. The EMG monitor tracing shows the responses to T_1 and T_4. At time 0, isoflurane adminstration was commenced; at the arrow, it was discontinued. Note the slow recovery of both T_1/controls and T_4/T_1 ratios after a prolonged (approximately 55 minutes) expossrue as compared with Figure 13-8. (From Eisenkraft. JB: Myasthenia gravis and thymic surgery: anesthetic considerations. In Gothard JW [ed]: *Thoracic anesthesia,* London, 1987, Baillierc-Tindall.)

d-tubocurarine and pancuronium have long elimination half-lives, most anesthesiologists avoid using these agents in patients with MG. The intermediate-duration relaxants (e.g., cisatracurium, rocuronium, atracurium, mivacurium, and vecuronium) offer significant advantages over their long-acting predecessors and have been used safely in patients with MG.

Atracurium has been used in at least 18 patients with MG.[190,191] The potency data reported are very much a function of methodology used, but they suggest that the ED_{95} in MG patients is approximately one fifth that of normal patients.[192] The time course of the blockade is normal.

An advantage of atracurium is that with an elimination half-life of only 20 minutes, even if an overdose were given, the prolongation of relaxation would be relatively short. Rapid breakdown could also make reversal of residual blockade unnecessary, which might be advantageous in a patient who is sensitive to anticholinesterases.[192] Cisatracurium could have similar advantages.[193]

Vecuronium has also been used successfully in patients with MG. It has a slightly longer elimination half-life than atracurium (55 minutes vs. 20 minutes), but it possesses other potential advantages. The ED_{95} for vecuronium in patients with MG has been reported to be 40% to 50% of that in controls, and duration of action might also be prolonged.[194-198] Itoh et al found a difference in sensitivity to vecuronium between patients with ocular and those with generalized MG, the latter being more sensitive.[199-201]

Mivacurium has also been used in patients with MG. In one report of four cases, the authors concluded that provided anticholinesterase therapy is withheld in the immediate postoperative period, mivacurium appears to be a safe and appropriate neuromuscular blocker in this group of patients. The cumulative dose required to establish full neuromuscular block was 60 to 90 μg/kg, and a maintenance infusion commencing at 3 μg/kg/min was recommended, guiding by monitoring of response.

Another report of the use of mivacurium in one MG patient taking pyridostigmine, 120 mg qid, also discusses the relationship between plasma cholinesterase, acetylcholinesterase, and anticholinesterase drugs.

Whichever nondepolarizing relaxant is chosen for use in a myasthenic patient, it is strongly recommended that all patients be considered sensitive and that small ($^1/_{10}$ normal) incremental doses be titrated against quantified effect using MMG, EMG, or accelographic monitoring. In this way, excessive doses can be avoided while providing adequate relaxation and the potential for reversal of residual blockade. Preanesthetic train-of-four fade was found to predict the atracurium requirement in MG patients.[202] The site of monitoring might also be important; monitoring of the orbicularis oculi could overestimate the blockade.[203]

A prospective study of the effect of preoperative administration of pyridostigmine on the sensitivity of subsequently administered nondepolarizing relaxant has not been reported. In one pharmacodynamic study of vecuronium in patients with MG, however, there did not appear to be a significant difference between the ED_{50} and ED_{95} values in four patients who did receive preoperative pyridostigmine compared with six who did not.[204]

REVERSAL OF RESIDUAL NEUROMUSCULAR BLOCKADE

There are numerous reports of the uneventful reversal of residual neuromuscular blockade produced by nondepolarizing relaxants in patients with MG. Use of pyridostigmine in 1.0 to 2.0 mg increments intravenously with atropine, 0.4 mg, added to the first dose and additional 0.2 mg increments being given as needed to prevent muscarinic side effects, has been advocated, although small incremental doses of neostigmine can be used too.[181-186] Because atracurium and vecuronium are associated with a rapid spontaneous recovery of neuromuscular function, reversal might not always be necessary following these agents.[190] Although the potential for cholinergic crisis exists when anticholinesterases are used for reversal, crisis seems to be rare. One group reversed residual relaxation because of atracurium using two doses of neostigmine, 2.5 mg intravenously, given 5 minutes apart; the group used a similar technique following vecuronium in patients with MG.[123,190] Reference to Table 15-3 indicates that neostigmine, 5 mg intravenously, is equivalent to pyridostigmine, 600 mg given orally, much greater than the 320 mg average total oral daily pyridostigmine doses in these patients, yet no instance of cholinergic crisis was reported.[190,194]

Edrophonium might be the drug of choice for reversing residual relaxation because the time from administration to peak onset of effect is the least of all the anticholinesterase agents, making titration of dose against monitored effect that much easier.

OTHER TECHNIQUES

Because muscle relaxation (due to potent inhaled anesthetic agents or neuromuscular blocking drugs) is not absolutely necessary for most cases of thymectomy (transsternal or transcervical), anesthetic techniques have been used that avoid muscle relaxant agents. Anesthesia for transcervical thymectomy has been provided satisfactorily using fentanyl/etomidate or fentanyl/Althesin (alphadolone/alphadolone) infusions together with N_2O (50%) in oxygen. Bradycardia occurred during induction of anesthesia, and most of the patients required naloxone postoperatively. All patient were tracheally extubated in the operating room, and none required tracheal reintubation.[205]

Combined regional and general anesthesia techniques have also been used to provide good surgical conditions and improved postoperative analgesia in patients undergoing transsternal thymectomy. The use of thoracic or lumbar epidural anesthesia in combination with light general anesthesia has been reported to provide excellent intra- and postoperative conditions for both surgeon and patient.[206-209]

In an alternative technique, subarachnoid morphine (Duramorph, 5.0 to 7.5 μg/kg) has been administered immediately following induction of general anesthesia. The opioid resulted in a decreased requirement for inhaled anesthetic, early tracheal extubation, excellent postoperative analgesia, and improved respiratory function in the early postoperative period. Data from this study remain unpublished.

RESPONSES OF PATIENTS IN REMISSION

Some MG patients become asymptomatic when receiving steroid therapy. Such patients have been reported both as sensitive to, and as showing normal response to, curare.[210,211] In one patient who was studied both during relapse and remission using the regional curare test, little difference in sensitivity was noted between both occasions.[143]

Patients in true remission (i.e., asymptomatic when not undergoing any therapy) are reported to demonstrate increased sensitivity to vecuronium and atracurium.[192,212] A report of responses to succinylcholine during true remission suggests that the patient showed a normal response to this drug (i.e., no resistance).[213]

SENSITIVITIES TO OTHER MEDICATIONS

Medications that possess neuromuscular blocking properties should be avoided or used with caution in myasthenic patients.[214] Such drugs include antiarrhythmics (quinidine, procainamide, and calcium channel blockers), diuretics, or other drugs causing hypokalemia, such as nitrogen mustards (thiotepa), quinine, and aminoglycoside antibiotics (gentamicin, neomycin, and colistin). Dantrolene sodium has been reported as not increasing the neuromuscular deficit in one patient with MG who had a strongly positive family history for malignant hyperthermia and was scheduled for thymectomy.[215]

Postoperative Ventilatory Requirement

Patients with MG are more likely to develop postoperative respiratory failure; indeed, it has been reported that surgery is the leading cause of respiratory failure among these patients, the most common type of procedure undergone being thymectomy.[216]

When thymectomy was originally introduced as a treatment for myasthenia, a tracheostomy was routine because all patients were ventilated electively in the postoperative period. Until 1967, at The Mount Sinai Hospital, New York City, New York, elective tracheostomy was performed in all patients scheduled for thymectomy. Since that time, the earlier diagnosis and performance of surgery, together with improved medical, surgical, and anesthesia management, have resulted in tracheostomy being the exception rather than the rule for myasthenic patients.

A number of studies have attempted to identify preoperatively those myasthenic patients who are most likely to develop postoperative ventilatory failure and who, therefore, need prolonged ventilatory support. Most of these studies have addressed transsternal thymectomy, given that as many as 50% of patients undergoing this procedure might require a prolonged period of ventilation afterward.

In 1974, Mulder et al suggested that a tracheotomy was indicated if bulbar muscle weakness, a past history of respiratory or myasthenic crisis, or a vital capacity of less than 2 L was present.[217] In 1975, Loach et al reported that ventilation was required if vital capacity was less than 2 L and that further risk factors were the presence of thymoma, bulbar symptoms (particularly dysphagia), and an age over 50 years.[218] In the latter study of 28 patients, 14 needed postoperative ventilation, usually for 12 days or longer.

Leventhal et al reported a retrospective analysis of experience with 24 myasthenic patients who had undergone transsternal thymectomy at the Hospital of the University of Pennsylvania.[219] Of these 24 patients, eight required prolonged ventilation (defined as more than 3 hours, but in general more than 18 hours) and were compared with 16 patients who did not. Four risk factors were identified, and a predictive scoring system was developed to identify those patients who would

need ventilation postoperatively. The risk factors and points assigned to each were as follows:
1. A duration of MG more than 6 years (12 points)
2. A history of chronic respiratory disease other than respiratory disease or failure directly due to MG (10 points)
3. A daily pyridostigmine dose requirement less than 750 mg 48 hours before surgery (8 points)
4. A preoperative vital capacity less than 2.9 L (4 points)

It was found that those patients with a score 10 points or more were more likely to need prolonged ventilation.[219] When applied to the 24 patients on whom it was based, this predictive model was correct in 22 of the 24 cases (91%), with no false-negative (i.e., no patients incorrectly predicted to be ready for extubation) and two false-positives (2 of 16 patients were incorrectly predicted to need ventilation when they did not). When tested in an additional 18 patients at the same institution, the predictions were 78% correct, with no false-negatives.[220]

The predictive scoring system was tested in 27 patients who had undergone thymectomy (4 transcervical, 23 transsternal) in a hospital in Vancouver, Canada, and was found to be of limited value, with a sensitivity of only 43%. These investigators reported the scoring system to be of even less value in myasthenic patients undergoing other forms of surgery.[221]

Others likewise have failed to validate the scoring system.[222-224] Gracey et al stated that, "the most important preoperative observation signifying need for postoperative mechanical ventilation was the severity of bulbar involvement (Osserman groups III and IV), usually indicated by significant dysarthria and dysphagia along with borderline respiratory function."[222]

Expiratory weakness, by reducing cough efficacy and the ability to remove secretions, has been suggested as the main predictive determinant. Younger et al studied expiratory function in 32 patients with MG who underwent transsternal thymectomy.[225] Preoperative clinical lung function and expiratory muscle pressure data were analyzed in an attempt to identify preoperative factors that correlated with duration of postoperative ventilatory support. Ten of the 32 patients (31%) needed support for more than 3 days, and duration of ventilation correlated best with maximal static expiratory pressure. This observation is significant, as anesthesiologists usually use peak negative inspiratory pressure (–25 mmHg or –20 cmH$_2$O) as one of the criteria for evaluating the adequacy of spontaneous ventilation and determining when mechanical ventilation may be discontinued. Furthermore, Pavlin et al studied the recovery of airway protection in normal, conscious volunteers who received intravenous d-tubocurarine.[226] They reported that although ventilation might be adequate at a maximum inspiratory pressure of –25 mm Hg, the muscles of airway protection are still nonfunctional, although all patients who could accomplish a head-lift for 5 seconds could perform airway-protective maneuvers. Thus, both adequacy of ventilation as well as ability to protect the airway and clear secretions are essential prerequisites before considering withdrawal of ventilatory support and tracheal extubation.

Ringqvist and Ringqvist measured respiratory mechanics in a group of nine patients with untreated myasthenia and found that maximum inspiratory force was decreased less than the maximum expiratory pressure.[227] It therefore seems desirable to assess both inspiratory and expiratory forces, especially in those patients thought to be at greatest risk for postoperative respiratory failure.

Postoperative respiratory failure appears to be less common following transcervical rather than transsternal thymectomy. The reason this is most likely is because there is no disruption of the thoracic cage with its associated decrease in vital capacity. It can also be argued that the transsternal thymectomy series has included patients with more severe myasthenia than the transcervical series, hence the apparently lower morbidity with the transcervical approach. In one study of 22 patients who underwent transcervical thymectomy, none required postoperative ventilation.[165] A review of transcervical thymectomy patients at The Mount Sinai Medical Center, New York, indicated that only 8 of 92 (8.7%) needed postoperative ventilation for more than 3 hours.[228] The predictive scoring system of Leventhal et al was also tested in these 92 patients and found to be of no value, having a sensitivity of only 37.5%.[219,223] Analysis of The Mount Sinai Medical Center MG patient data indicates that the risk factors associated with the need for postoperative ventilation following transcervical thymectomy are severity of disease (Osserman groups III and IV), a previous history of respiratory failure due to myasthenia, and concurrent corticosteroid therapy for myasthenia.[228]

Redfern et al reported their experience of anesthesia for 30 myasthenic patients who underwent transsternal thymectomy in the United Kingdom.[229] Of these, only 3 (10%) developed postoperative respiratory failure in relation to myasthenia. A fourth patient required reintubation for severe stridor due to prolapse of an arytenoid cartilage. The requirement for postoperative ventilation in the other three patients could have been related to cholinergic crisis caused by a relative overdose of neostigmine.[229,230]

It is evident that the accurate preoperative prediction of postoperative respiratory failure in MG is not completely elaborated.[231] Such a project is made difficult by the small numbers of patients available for study, the analysis of data obtained retrospectively, the wide variety of patient disease states, and the management techniques used. Meanwhile, each patient should be treated on his or her individual merits and controlled ventilation discontinued only when clinically indicated. Those patients with the most severe myasthenia are at greatest risk for ventilatory failure and should be monitored carefully. Short-term ventilation via a soft cuff (low-pressure, high-volume) oro- or nasotracheal tube is suitable for most patients requiring ventilatory assistance. Tracheostomy is now usually performed only in those patients likely to need long-term (more than 10 days) ventilation.

Techniques to Decrease the Need for Postoperative Ventilation
PREOPERATIVE PLASMAPHERESIS
Patients with severe myasthenia have been treated successfully with plasmapheresis, and it has been suggested that plasmapheresis be performed preoperatively in high-risk groups (Osserman groups III and IV).[153-155] In one study of 37 myasthenic patients undergoing thymectomy, it was found that those patients with respiratory weakness who had received preoperative plasmapheresis required significantly less time on mechanical ventilation and in the intensive care unit than a similarly weak group who did not receive this treatment preoperatively.[154] Others have also found plasmapheresis to be a worthwhile adjuvant in the preparation of myasthenics (Osserman group IV) for thymectomy.[155] The anesthetic implications of plasmapheresis have been mentioned previously.[156]

HIGH-DOSE STEROIDS
It has been reported that the preoperative administration of methylprednisolone, 1 g, significantly reduced the morbidity (in terms of neuromuscular function and respiratory complications) of transsternal thymectomy.[148] Of 32 patients who underwent transsternal thymectomy, all were tracheally extubated within 2 hours of surgery, and none required postoperative ventilatory support.

PREOPERATIVE ADMINISTRATION OF ANTICHOLINESTERASE
Anticholinesterase therapy is generally withheld on the day of surgery. If neuromuscular blocking drugs are to be avoided altogether, however, and if profound relaxation is not essential, a case can be made for giving the usual morning dose of anticholinesterase. One study has compared two groups of myasthenic patients undergoing transsternal thymectomy.[232] In one group, the usual dose of pyridostigmine was administered preoperatively; in the other, it was withheld. The requirement for postoperative ventilatory support was found to be higher in the group that had not received pyridostigmine preoperatively. By administering oral pyridostigmine preoperatively, the peak effect occurred approximately 3 hours later, when it would be expected that the operation would be complete and the patient prepared for tracheal extubation.

Postoperative Considerations
During the postoperative period, pain relief is commonly provided by opioid analgesics (traditionally meperidine), but in reduced dosages. The analgesic effects of morphine have been reported to be increased by anticholinesterases, which prompted the recommendation that the dose of opioid analgesics be reduced by one-third in patients receiving anticholinesterase agents.[185,233] The mechanism for any potentiation, if it exists, is not elaborated.

As mentioned previously, spinal opioids have been used successfully to provide intra- and postoperative analgesia. In one report, a thoracic (T_6 to T_7) epidural catheter was placed in each of two patients undergoing transsternal thymectomy.[206] Postoperative analgesia was achieved in one patient with 100 μg of fentanyl in 10 mL of 0.9% sodium chloride, followed by a continuous epidural infusion of fentanyl, 4 μg/mL in 0.9% sodium chloride. Following extubation, the patient remained pain-free overnight in the intensive care unit, receiving epidural fentanyl, 48 μg/hr (12 mL/hr). In a second patient, postoperative analgesia was achieved with epidural fentanyl, 75 μg in 10 mL of 0.9% sodium chloride. In the intensive care unit, the patient received epidural fentanyl by infusion at 10 mL/hr (4 μg/mL). Satisfactory analgesia and no complications were reported with this technique. In another report, anesthesia for transsternal thymectomy was provided by a combination of 2% epidural lidocaine (15 mL injected at L_1 to L_2) and light general anesthesia (N_2O/O_2, 3 L/2 L; isoflurane, 0.4% to 1.2%).[209] The patient received 0.8 mg of epidural hydromorphone in the operating room and again in the postanesthesia care unit. After extubation on the following day, patient-controlled analgesia with morphine was instituted. When the latter proved unsatisfactory, a further dose of 1 mg of hydromorphone was administered epidurally; this was effective in improving respiratory parameters. The following day, the patient was discharged to the floor with a reduced patient-controlled maintenance dose of analgesia.[209]

An alternative technique is the use of subarachnoid morphine. As mentioned previously, this has been used in doses of 5.0 to 7.5 μg/kg prior to the start of transsternal thymectomy; it provided satisfactory analgesia for 24 to 30 hours postoperatively (unpublished data).

Following tracheal extubation, myasthenic patients should be observed carefully for signs of respiratory distress or choking on secretions. Avoidance of infections and attention to clearing secretions are essential.

Effects of Thymectomy

Often, in the immediate postoperative period, patients show a dramatic improvement in their clinical conditions.[231,234] For this reason, the dosage of anticholinesterase is routinely reduced preoperatively. However, the immediate improvement is usually short-lived, and lasting improvement or a remission might take months or years to occur. In general, it is reported that within one year following thymectomy, 30% of patients go into remission and 80% are clinically improved.[234,235] Although the natural history of all patients with MG is to eventually go into remission, the prevention of disease progression and the earlier onset of remission are both enhanced by thymectomy. It has also been reported that there is an increased incidence of extrathymic neoplasia among patients with MG, but that the incidence reverts to normal following thymectomy.[235,236]

Myasthenic Syndrome

Myasthenic syndrome could represent a nonmetastatic effect of bronchial carcinoma and might be humorally mediated. In a review of 50 cases of Lambert-Eaton myasthenic syndrome (LEMS), however, carcinoma was detected in only 25 patients (50%), of whom 21 had small cell lung cancer.[237] The latter carcinoma was evident within 2 years of onset of LEMS for more than 5 years. The main neurologic features of the syndrome are proximal lower limb weakness (100%), depressed tendon reflexes (92%) with posttetanic potentiation (78%), and autonomic features, particularly dry mouth (74%), and ptosis (54%).[237] Analysis indicated that a patient who presented with LEMS had a 62% chance of having an underlying small cell carcinoma of the lung and that this risk declined sharply after two years, becoming very low by 5 years. It was suggested that in cases associated with small cell carcinoma of the lung, antigenic determinants on tumor cells initiated the autoimmune response.[237]

LEMS occurs more commonly among males than females. The main symptoms are weakness and easy fatigability of the proximal muscles of the extremities (especially the thighs). Involvement of muscle innervated by cranial nerves occurs in 70% of cases. In contrast to MG, in which there is fatigue on exertion, in LEMS there is a transient increase in strength on activity that precedes weakness, and muscle pain is common.

There is increased sensitivity to all neuromuscular blocking drugs, both depolarizing and nondepolarizing.[238,239] The neuromuscular transmission defect in LEMS is presynaptic and similar to that produced by an excess of magnesium ions, botulinum toxin, or neomycin, all of which decrease the number of quanta of acetylcholine released by a nerve impulse from the motor nerve terminal.[134,240] This is secondary to destruction of the active release zones in the nerve terminal and is believed to be of autoimmune etiology.[241,242]

The electrophysiologic characteristics of LEMS are as follows[243]:

1. An abnormally low amplitude of muscle action potential in response to a single supramaximal stimulus,
2. A decremental response at low rates (1 to 3 Hz) of nerve stimulation
3. Marked facilitation of the response at high rates of stimulation (50 Hz) and after 10 seconds of maximum contraction of the muscle
4. Posttetanic facilitation

Differences between MG and myasthenic syndrome are shown in Table 13-5.

Treatment of LEMS differs from that of classic MG. Although both conditions improve with local cooling, patients with LEMS respond poorly to anticholinesterase drugs.[239,243] The most successful treatment has been with so-called facilitatory agents, which act to increase the release of acetylcholine from the motor nerve terminal by selectively blocking potassium channels.[244,245] These agents include guanidine in doses of 10 to 35 mg/kg/day. This drug could cause renal failure, hypotension, and bone marrow depression.[246] Other agents that have been used are caffeine, calcium, germine, and 4-aminopyridine.[247-249] Treatment is not uniformly successful and is often limited by drug side effects, particularly central nervous system stimulation. In this rare condition, 3,4-diaminopyridine causes less central nervous system depression and might be the drug of choice.[250] The maximum daily dose is 100 mg, given in divided doses.

The possible coexistence of LEMS should always be considered when evaluating a patient with bronchial carcinoma for anesthesia because affected patients are reported to be extremely sensitive to all muscle relaxants.[143,251] One patient with a 6-month history of LEMS who was being treated with 3,4-diaminopyridine, 30 mg orally every 6 hours, demonstrated normal response to succinylcholine, but a marked sensitivity to vecuronium as well as a slow recovery time.[252] Reversal of residual neuromuscular blockade with neostigmine was largely ineffective, but was improved by oral 3,4-diaminopyridine. This patient received nitrous oxide (70%) and isoflurane (0.5%) in oxygen for anesthesia maintenance. The authors concluded that if such a patient requires anesthesia, the 3,4-diaminopyridine should be continued up to the time of surgery and that, if possible, neuromuscular blocking drugs should be avoided or used sparingly with close monitoring.[252]

In patients with LEMS, use of a potent inhaled anesthetic might represent the most conservative course of management.[253] If a neuromuscular blocking drug is needed, cisatracurium might represent the most appropriate choice. Should the condition be suspected by clinical observation preoperatively, the diagnosis could be confirmed by EMG.

TABLE 13-5

Differences Between Myasthenia Gravis and the Myasthenic (Lambert-Eaton) Syndrome

	Myasthenia Gravis	Myasthenic Syndrome
Sex	Female > Male	Male > Female
Presenting symptoms	External ocular muscle bulbar and facial weakness	Proximal limb weakness (legs > arms)
Other symptoms	Fatigue on activity	Increased strength on activity precedes fatigue
	Muscle pains uncommon	Muscle pain common
	Reflexes normal	Reflexes reduced or absent
EMG	Initial muscle action potential relatively normal	Initial muscle action potential abnormally small
	Decremental response on high-frequency stimulation ("fade")	Decremental response at low rates of stimulation, incremental response on high-frequency stimulation
Response to blocking drugs	Sensitivity to nondepolarizing blockers	Sensitivity to both nondepolarizing and depolarizing blockers
	Resistance to depolarizing blockers	
	Good response to anticholinesterases	Poor response to anticholinesterases
Pathologic state	Thymoma present in 20% to 25% of patients	Small-cell bronchogenic carcinoma usually present

Adapted from Telford RJ and Holloway TE: *Br J Anesth* 64:363, 1990.

Pancoast's Syndrome

A Pancoast tumor is an apical carcinoma of the bronchus that invades the brachial plexus, resulting in pain in the arm by invasion and compression of the lower roots of the plexus. It is recognized that muscles that are partially or totally denervated demonstrate increased sensitivity to cholinergic nicotinic agonists. These muscles respond to succinylcholine by developing a contracture instead of the paralysis observed in normally innervated striated muscle. Reports of the development of contracture in such a denervated muscle during anesthesia are rare. It is reported, however, that a patient with a right-sided Pancoast tumor, in response to succinylcholine, developed fasciculations over most of the body except for the right arm, which became rigid as the rest of the body relaxed.[254] The rigidity gradually wore off within 3 to 4 minutes, at which time muscle power returned to the rest of the body. If such a tumor is present or suspected, use of a nondepolarizing neuromuscular blocking drug could be preferable, as it should produce relaxation without contractures.

REFERENCES

1. Greenhow DE: Esophageal surgery. In Marshall BE, Longnecker DE, Fairley HB (eds): *Anesthesia for thoracic procedures*, p451, Boston, 1988, Blackwell Scientific Publications.
2. Aitkenhead AR: Anesthesia for esophageal surgery. In Gothard JW (ed): *Thoracic anesthesia*, p181, London, 1987, Bailliere-Tindall.
3. Pairolero PC, Trastek VF, Payne WS: Esophagus and diaphragmatic hernias. In Schwartz SI, Shires GI, Spencer FL (eds): *Principles of surgery*, p1103, New York, 1989, McGraw-Hill.
4. Semyk J, Arborelius M Jr, Lilja B: Respiratory function in esophageal hiatus hernia I. Spirometry, gas distribution and arterial blood gases, *Respiration* 32:93, 1975.
5. Semyk J, Arborelius M, Jr, Lilja B: Respiratory function in esophageal hiatus hernia II. Regional lung function, *Respiration* 32:103, 1975.
6. Iberti TJ, Paluch TA, Helmer L, et al: The hemodynamic effects of intravenous cimetidine in intensive care patients; a double-blind, prospective study, *Anesthesiology* 64:87, 1986.
7. Cohen J, Weetman AP, Dargie HJ, et al: Life-threatening arrhythmias and intravenous injection of cimetidine, *Br Med J* 2:768, 1979.
8. Shaw RG, Mashford ML, Desmond PV: Cardiac arrest after intravenous injection of cimetidine, *Med J Aust* 2:629, 1980.
9. Schentag JJ, Cerra FB, Calleri G, et al: Pharmacokinetic and clinical studies in patients with cimetidine-associated mental confusion, *Lancet* 1:177, 1979.
10. Viegas OJ, Stoops CA, Ravindran RS: Reversal of cimetidine-induced postoperative somnolence, *Anesthesiol Rev* 9:30, 1982.
11. Feely J, Wilkinson GR, Wood AJ: Reduction of liver blood flow and propranolol metabolism by cimetidine, *N Engl J Med* 304:692, 1981.
12. Zeldis JB, Friedman LS, Isselbacher KJ: Ranitidine: a new H2-receptor antagonist, *N Engl J Med* 309:1368, 1983.
13. Camarri E, Chirone E, Fanteria G, et al: Ranitidine-induced bradycardia, *Lancet* 2:100, 1982.
14. Yamanaka Y, Mammoto T, Kita T, et al: A study of 13 patients with gastric tube in place after esophageal resection: use of omeprazole to decrease gastric acidity and volume, *J Clin Anesth* 13:370, 2001.
15. Lowham AS, Filipi CJ, Hinder RA, et al. Mechanisms and avoidance of esophageal perforation by anesthesia personnel during laparoscopic foregut surgery, *Surg Endosc* 10:979, 1996.
16. Nagata C, Yano T, Hara S, et al: Accidental pyriform sinus perforation with Savary-Gilliard esophageal bougie during general anesthesia, *Masui* 49:639, 2000.
17. Athanasakis H, Tzortzinis A, Tsiaoussis J, et al: Laparoscopic repair of paraesophageal hernia, *Endoscopy* 33:590, 2001.
18. Sudoh Y, Kawamoto M, Ohsawa Y, et al: Hemilateral hydrothorax and atelectasis during laparoscopic Nissen fundoplication, *Masui* 45:4761, 1996.
19. Rowney DA, Aldridge LM: Laparoscopic fundoplication in children: anaesthetic experience in 51 cases, *Paediatr Anaesth* 10:291, 2000.
20. Sfez M, Guerard A, Desruelle P: Cardiorespiratory changes during laparoscopic fundoplication in children, *Paediatr Anaesth* 5:89, 1995.
21. Schier F, Waldschmidt J: Thoracoscopy in children, *J Pediatr Surg* 31:1640, 1996.
22. Rao TLK, El-Etr AA: Esophageal and mediastinal surgery. In Kaplan JA (ed): *Thoracic anesthesia*, New York, 1983, Churchill Livingstone.
23. Stoelting RK: *Pharmacology and physiology in anesthetic practice*, Philadelphia, 1987, JB Lippincott.
24. Crooke ST, Bradner WT: Bleomycin: a review, *J Med* 7:333, 1976.
25. Luna MA, Bedrossian CW, Lichtiger B, et al: Interstitial pneumonitis associated with bleomycin therapy, *Am J Clin Pathol* 58:501, 1972.
26. Goldiner PL, Carlon G, Cuitkovic E, et al: Factors influencing postoperative morbidity and mortality in patients treated with bleomycin, *Br Med J* 1:1664, 1978.
27. Lamantia KR, Glick JH, Marshall BE: Supplemental oxygen does not cause respiratory failure in bleomycin, *Anesthesiology* 60:65, 1984.
28. DeVita VT: Principles of cancer therapy. In Braunwald E, Isselbacher KJ, Petersdorf RG, et al (eds): *Harrison's principle of internal medicine*, p431, New York, 1987, McGraw-Hill.
29. Luketich JD, Schauer PR, Christie NA, et al: Minimally invasive esophagectomy, *Ann Thorac Surg* 70:906, 2000.
30. Pompili MF, Mark JB: The history of surgery for carcinoma of the esophagus, *Chest Surg Clin N Am* 10:145, 2000.
31. Orringer MB, Marshall B, Iannettoni MD: Transhiatal esophagectomy: clinical experience and refinements, *Ann Surg* 230:392, 1999.

32. Hashimoto T, Ishizawa Y, Yamamoto T, et al: Mediastinal abscess diagnosed after its rupture into the trachea in a patient after esophagectomy, *Masui* 44:434, 1995.

33. Law SY, Fok M, Wei WI, et al: Thoracoscopic esophageal mobilization for pharyngolaryngoesophagectomy, *Ann Thorac Surg* 70:418, 2000.

34. Mohindra P, Yacoub JM: Anesthetic management of the cancer patient undergoing noncardiac thoracic surgery, *Int Anesthesiol Clin* 36:45, 1998.

35. Topsis J, Kinas H, Kandall S: Esophageal perforation—a complication of neonatal resuscitation, *Anesth Anal* 69:532, 1989.

36. Krasna I, Rosenfeld D, Benjamin B, et al: Esophageal perforation in the neonate: an emerging problem in the newborn nursery, *J Pediatr Surg* 22:784, 1987.

37. Sakurai H, McElhinney J: Perforation of the esophagus: experience at Bronx VA Hospital 1969, *Mt Sinai J Med* (NY) 54:487, 1987.

38. O'Neill JE, Giffin JP, Cottrell JE: Pharyngeal and esophageal perforation following endotracheal intubation, *Anesthesiology* 60:487, 1984.

39. Sarr MG, Pemberton JH, Payne WS: Management of instrumental perforations of the esophagus, *J Thorac Cardiovasc Surg* 84:211, 1982.

40. Little AG, Soriano A, Ferguson MK, et al: Surgical treatment of achalasia: results with esophagomyotomy and Belsey repair, *Ann Thorac Surg* 45:489, 1988.

41. Murray GF, Battaglini JW, Keagy BA, et al: Selective application of fundoplication in achalasia, *Ann Thorac Surg* 37:285, 1966.

42. Belsey R: Functional disease of the esophagus, *J Thorac Cardiovasc Surg* 52:164, 1966.

43. Ellis FH Jr, Gibb SP, Crozier RE: Esophagomyotomy for achalasia of the esophagus, *Ann Surg* 192:157, 1980.

44. Thompson D, Shoenut JP, Thenholm BG, et al: Reflux patterns following limited myotomy without fundoplication for achalasia, *Ann Thorac Surg* 43:550, 1987.

45. Pai GP, Ellison RG, Rubin JW, et al: Two decades of experience with modified Heller's myotomy for achalasia, *Ann Thorac Surg* 38:201, 1984.

46. Desa LA, Spencer J, McPherson S: Surgery for achalasia cardiae: the Dor operation, *Ann R Coll Surg Engl* 72:128, 1990.

47. Dor J, Humbert P, Paoli JM, et al: Traitment du reflux par la technique dite de Heller-Nissen modifie, *Presse Med* 50:2563, 1967.

48. Ali A, Pellegrini CA: Laparoscopic myotomy: technique and efficacy in treating achalasia, *Gastrointest Endosc Clin N Am* 11:347, 2001.

49. Finley RJ, Clifton JC, Stewart KC, et al. Laparoscopic Heller myotomy improves esophageal emptying and the symptoms of achalasia, *Arch Surg* 13:892, 2001.

50. Tatum RP, Kahrilas PJ, Manka M, et al: Operative manometry and endoscopy during laparoscopic Heller myotomy. An initial experience, *Surg Endosc* 13:1015, 1999.

51. Hindman B, Bert A: Malignant esophagorespiratory tract fistulas: anesthetic considerations for exclusion procedures using esophageal bypass, *J Cardiothorac Anesth* 1:438, 1987.

52. Wesselhoeft C, Keshishian J: Acquired nonmalignant esophagotracheal and esophagobronchial fistulas, *Ann Thorac Surg* 6:187, 1968.

53. Duranceau A, Jamieson C: Malignant tracheoesophageal fistula, *Ann Thorac Surg* 37:346, 1984.

54. Little AG, Fergisson M, Demeester TR, et al: Esophageal carcinoma with respiratory tract fistula, *Cancer* 15:1522, 1984.

55. Schuchmann GF, Heydorn WH, Hall RV, et al: Treatment of esophageal carcinoma: a retrospective review, *J Thorac Cardiovasc Surg* 79:67, 1980.

56. Angorn I: Intubation in the treatment of carcinoma of the esophagus, *World J Surg* 18:417, 1974.

57. Colan A, Nicolaou N, Delikaris P, et al: Pessimism concerning palliative bypass procedures for established malignant esophagorespiratory fistulas: a report of 18 patients, *Ann Thorac Surg* 37:108, 1984.

58. Girardet R, Rensdell H Jr, Wheat M Jr: Palliative intubation in the management of esophageal carcinoma, *Ann Thorac Surg* 18:417, 1974.

59. Symbas P, McKeown P, Hatcher C Jr, et al: Tracheoesophageal fistula from carcinoma of the esophagus, *Ann Thorac Surg* 38:382, 1984.

60. Weaver R, Matthews H: Palliation and survival in malignant esophagorespiratory fistula, *Br J Surg* 67:539, 1980.

61. Bryant LR, Bowlin J, Malette W, et al: Thoracic aneurysms with aorticobronchial fistula, *Ann Surg* 168:79, 1968.

62. Graeber G, Farrell B, Neville J Jr, et al: Successful diagnosis and management of fistulas between the aorta and the tracheobronchial tree, *Ann Thorac Surg* 29:555, 1980.

63. One G, Kwong K: Management of malignant esophagobronchial fistula, *Surgery* 67:293, 1970.

64. Steiger Z, Wilson R, Leichman L, et al: Management of malignant bronchoesophageal fistulas, *Surg Gynecol Obstet* 157:201, 1983.

65. Campion J, Bourdelat D, Launois B: Surgical treatment of malignant bronchoesophageal fistulas, *Am J Surg* 146:641, 1983.

66. Thiagarajah S, Lear E, Keh M: Anesthetic implications of Zenker's diverticulum. *Anesth Analg* 70:109, 1990.

67. Aouad MT, Berzina CE, Baraka AS: Aspiration after anesthesia in a patient with a Zenker diverticulum, *Anesthesiology* 92:1873, 2000.

68. Moghissi K, Hornshaw J, Teasdale PR: Parenteral nutrition in carcinoma of the esophagus treated by surgery: nitrogen balance and clinical studies, *Br J Surg* 64:125, 1977.

69. Heatley RV, Williams RHP, Lewis MH: Preoperative intravenous feeding—a controlled trial, *Postgrad Med J* 55:541, 1979.

70. Juler GL, Stemmer EA, Connolly JE: Complications of prophylactic digitalization in thoracic surgical patients, *J Thorac Cardiovasc Surg* 68:352, 1969.

71. Shields TW, Unik GT: Digitalization for prevention of arrhythmias following pulmonary surgery, *Surg Gynecol Obstet* 126:743, 1968.

72. Burman SO: The prophylactic use of digitalis before thoracotomy, *Ann Thorac Surg* 14:359, 1972.

73. Meek T, Gittins N, Duggan JE. Cricoid pressure: knowledge and performance amongst anaesthesia assistants, *Anaesthesia* 54:59, 1999.

74. Cook TM, Godfrey I, Rockett M, et al. Cricoid pressure: which hand? *Anaesthesia* 55:648, 2000.

75. Harry RM, Nolan JP: The use of cricoid pressure with the intubating laryngeal mask, *Anaesthesia* 54:656, 1999.

76. Tournadre JP, Chassard D, Berrada KR, et al: Cricoid cartilage pressure decreases lower esophageal tone, *Anesthesiology* 86:7, 1997.

77. Skinner HJ, Bedford NM, Girling KJ, et al. Effect of cricoid pressure on gastroesophageal reflux in awake patients, *Anaesthesia* 54:798, 1999.

78. Ng A, Smith G: Gastroesophageal reflux and aspiration of gastric contents in anesthetic practice, *Anesth Analg* 93:494, 2001.

79. Sung HM, Nelems B: Tracheal tear during laryngopharyngectomy and transhiatal oesophagectomy: a case report, *Can J Anaesth* 36:333, 1989.

80. Owitz S, Pratilas V, Pratilas M, et al: Anesthetic and pharmacologic considerations in esophageal dilatation, *Anesthesiol Rev* 8:21, 1981.

81. Calverley RK, Johnson AE: The anesthetic management of tracheoesophageal fistula: a review of ten years' experience, *Can Anaesth Soc J* 19:270, 1972.

82. Grant D, Thompson G: Diagnosis of congenital tracheoesophageal fistula in the adolescent and adult, *Anesthesiology* 49:139, 1978.

83. Baraka A, Slim M: Cardiac arrest during IPPV in a newborn with tracheoesophageal fistula, *Anesthesiology* 32:564, 1970.

84. Myers CR, Love JW: Gastrostomy as a gas vent in repair of tracheoesophageal fistula, *Anesth Analg* 47:119, 1968.

85. Turnball AD, Carlon G, Howland WS, et al: High-frequency jet ventilation in major airway or pulmonary disruption, *Ann Thorac Surg* 32:468, 1981.

86. Grebenik C: Anaesthetic management of malignant tracheoesophageal fistula, *Br J Anaesth* 63:492, 1989.

87. Au CL, White SA, Grant RP: A novel intubation technique for tracheoesophageal fistula in adults, *Can J Anaesth* 46: 688, 1999.

88. Koshino T, Inoue N, Abe T: A case report of video-assisted thoracoscopic resection for a pericardial cyst, *Kyobu Geka* 51:599, 1998.

89. Asakura S, Mori A, Katoh H, et al: Thoracoscopic treatment of mediastinal thymic cyst, *Kyobu Geka* 47:861, 1994.

90. Watanabe M, Takagi K, Aoki T, et al: Thoracoscopic resection of mediastinal tumors, *Nippon Kyobu Geka Gakkai Zasshi* 42:1016, 1994.

91. Kawamura M, Takahashi Y, Kusanagi Y, et al: A case of esophageal cyst resected by thoracoscopic surgery, *Nippon Kyobu Shikkan Gakkai Zasshi* 32:1022, 1994.

92. Mackie AM, Watson CB: Anaesthesia and mediastinal masses, *Anaesthesia* 39:899, 1984.

93. Bray RJ, Fernandes FJ: Mediastinal tumour causing airway obstruction in anaesthetized children, *Anaesthesia* 37:571, 1982.

94. Amaha K, Okutsu Y, Nakamura Y: Major airway obstruction by mediastinal tumour. A case report, *Br J Anaesth* 45:1082, 1973.

95. Shambaugh BE, Seed R, Korn A: Airway obstruction in a substernal goiter. Clinical and therapeutic implications, *J Chronic Dis* 26:737, 1973.

96. Piro AJ, Weiss DR, Hellman S: Mediastinal Hodgkin's disease: a possible danger for intubation anesthesia, *Int J Radiat Oncol Biol Phys* 1:415, 1976.

97. Price SL, Hecker BR: Pulmonary oedema following airway obstruction in Hodgkin's disease, *Br J Anaesth* 59:518, 1987.

98. Neuman GG, Weingarten AE, Abramowitz RM, et al: The anesthetic management of the patient with an anterior mediastinal mass, *Anesthesiology* 60:144, 1984.
99. Fletcher R, Nordstrom L: The effects on gas exchange of a large mediastinal tumor, *Anaesthesia* 41:1135, 1986.
100. Ferrari LR, Bedford RF: General anesthesia prior to treatment of anterior mediastinal masses in pediatric cancer patients, *Anesthesiology* 72:991, 1990.
101. Tinker TD, Crane DL: Safety of anesthesia for patients with anterior mediastinal masses: I (correspondence), *Anesthesiology* 73:1060, 1990.
102. Zornow MH, Benumof JL: Safety of anesthesia for patients with anterior mediastinal masses: II (correspondence), *Anesthesiology* 73:1061, 1990.
103. Silbert KS, Biondi JW, Hirsch NP: Spontaneous respiration during thoracotomy in a patient with mediastinal mass, *Anesth Analg* 66:904, 1987.
104. DeSoto H: Direct laryngoscopy as an aid to relieve airway obstruction in a patient with a mediastinal mass, *Anesthesiology* 67:116, 1987.
105. Prakash UBS, Abel MD, Hubmay RD: Mediastinal mass and tracheal obstruction during general anesthesia, *Mayo Clin Proc* 63:1004, 1988.
106. Tempe DK, Arya R, Dubey S, et al: Mediastinal mass resection: Femorofemoral cardiopulmonary bypass before induction of anesthesia in the management of airway obstruction, *J Cardiothorac Vasc Anesth* 15:233, 2001.
107. Goh MH, Liu XY, Goh YS: Anterior mediastinal masses: an anaesthetic challenge, *Anaesthesia* 54:670, 1999.
108. Shamberger RC: Preanesthetic evaluation of children with anterior mediastinal masses, *Semin Pediatr Surg* 8:61,1999.
109. Masui K, Ishiyama T, Kumazawa T: Bilateral pneumothorax following lower neck and upper mediastinal surgery, *Masui* 48:652, 1999.
110. Hattamer SJ, Dodds TM: Use of the laryngeal mask airway in managing a patient with a large anterior mediastinal mass: a case report, *AANA J,* 64:497, 1996.
111. Lokich JJ, Goodman R: Superior vena cava syndrome. Clinical management, *JAMA* 231:58, 1975.
112. Tonnesen AS, Davis FG: Superior vena caval obstruction during anesthesia, *Anesthesiology* 45:912, 1976.
113. Gutman JA, Haft JI: Mediastinal tumor presenting as a heart murmur: diagnosis and treatment, *J Med Soc NJ* 76:364, 1979.
114. Hall DK, Friedman M: Extracorporeal oxygenation for induction of anesthesia in a patient with an intrathoracic tumor, *Anesthesiology* 42:493, 1975.
115. Keon TP: Death on induction of anesthesia for cervical node biopsy, *Anesthesiology* 55:471, 1981.
116. Canedo MI, Otken L, Stefadouros MA: Echocardiographic features of cardiac compression by a thymoma simulating cardiac tamponade and obstruction of the superior vena cava, *Br Heart J* 39:1038, 1977.
117. Lin CM, Hsu JC: Anterior mediastinal tumour identified by intraoperative transesophageal echocardiography, *Can J Anaesth* 48:78, 2001.
118. Stamme C, Lubbe N, Mahr KH, et al: Mediastinal tumor and airway obstruction in general anesthesia. Case report and review of the literature, *Anasthesiol Intensivmed Notfallmed Schmerzther* 29:512, 1994.
119. Viswanathan S, Campbell CE, Cork RC: Asymptomatic undetected mediastinal mass: a death during ambulatory anesthesia, *J Clin Anesth* 7:151, 1995.
120. Robie DK, Gursoy MH, Pokorny WJ: Mediastinal tumors—airway obstruction and management, *Semin Pediatr Surg* 3:259, 1994.
121. Benumof JL: Anesthesia for special elective therapeutic procedures.In: *Anesthesia for thoracic surgery,* p366, Philadelphia, 1987, WB Saunders.
122. Steen SN: Superior vena cava obstruction during anesthesia, *NY State J Med* 69:2906, 1969.
123. Quong GG, Brigham BA: Anaesthetic complications of mediastinal masses and superior vena caval obstruction, *Med J Aust* 2:487, 1980.
124. Vincent A, Drachman DB: Myasthenia gravis, *Adv Neurol* 88:159, 2002.
125. Abel M, Eisenkraft JB: Anesthetic implications of myasthenia gravis, *Mt Sinai J Med* (NY) 69:31, 2002.
126. Osserman KE, Genkins G: Studies in myasthenia gravis—review of a 20-year experience in over 1200 patients, *Mt Sinai J Med* (NY) 38:862, 1971.
127. Herrmann C, Lindstrom JM, Kessey JC, et al: Myasthenia gravis—current concepts, *West J Med* 142:797, 1985.
128. Engel AG: Myasthenia gravis and myasthenic syndromes, *Ann Neurol* 16:516, 1984.
129. Havard CWH, Scadding GK: Myasthenia gravis: pathogenesis and current concepts in management, *Drugs* 26:174, 1983.
130. Kornfeld P, Horowitz SH, Genkins G, et al: Myasthenia gravis unmasked by antiarrhythmic agents, *Mt Sinai J Med* (NY) 43:10, 1976.
131. Elder BF, Beal H, DeWald W, et al: exacerbation of subclinical myasthenia by occupational exposure to an anesthetic, *Anesth Analg* 50:363, 1971.
132. Wojciechowski APJ, Hanning CD, Pohl JEF: Postoperative apnoea and latent myasthenia gravis, *Anaesthesia* 39:51, 1985.
133. Lindstrom JM: Acetylcholine receptors and myasthenia, *Muscle Nerve* 23:453, 2000.
134. Naguib M, Flood P, McArdle JJ, et al: Advances in neurobiology of the neuromuscular junction. Implications for the anesthesiologist, *Anesthesiology* 96:202, 2002.
135. Fambrough DM, Drachman DB, Satyamurti S: Neuromuscular junction in myasthenia gravis: decreased acetylcholine receptors, *Science* 182:293, 1973.
136. Albuquerque EX, Rash JE, Meyer RF, et al: An electrophysiological and morphological study of the neuromuscular junction in patients with myasthenia gravis, *Exp Neurol* 51:536, 1976.
137. Paton WDM, Waud DR: The margin of safety of neuromuscular transmission, *J Physiol* 191:59, 1967.
138. Martyn JA, White DA, Gronert GA, et al: Up- and down-regulation of skeletal muscle acetylcholine receptors. Effects on neuromuscular blockers, *Anesthesiology,* 76:822, 1992.
139. Uchara K, Kobayashi M, Hirasaki A, et al: Myasthenia gravis is improved temporarily at postburn period, *Masui* 50:521, 2001.
140. Lindstrom JM, Seybold ME, Lennon VA, et al: Antibody to acetylcholine receptor in myasthenia gravis: prevalence, clinical correlates and diagnostic value, *Neurology* 26: 1054, 1976.
141. Tsujihata M, Hazama R, Ishii N, et al: Ultrastructural localization of acetylcholine receptor at the motor endplate: myasthenia gravis and other neuromuscular diseases, *Neurology* 30:1203, 1980.
142. Ozdemir C, Young RR: The results to be expected from electrical testing in the diagnosis of myasthenia gravis, *Ann NY Acad Sci* 274:203, 1976.
143. Brown JC, Charlton JE: A study of sensitivity to curare in myasthenic disorders using a regional technique, *J Neurol Neurosurg Psychiatry* 38:27, 1975.
144. Balestrieri FJ, Prough DS: Diagnostic value of systemic curare testing, *Anesthesiology* 57:226, 1982.
145. Cohan SL, Pohlmann JLW, Mikszewski J, et al: The pharmacokinetics of pyridostigmine, *Neurology* 26:536, 1976.
146. Glaser G: Crisis, precrisis and drug resistance in myasthenia gravis, *Ann NY Acad Sci* 135:335, 1966.
147. Bolooki H, Schwartzman RJ: High-dose steroids for the perioperative management of patients with myasthenia gravis undergoing thymectomy. A preliminary report, *J Thorac Cardiovasc Surg* 75:754, 1978.
148. Arsura E, Brunner NG, Namba T, et al: High-dose intravenous methylprednisolone in myasthenia gravis, *Arch Neurol* 42:1149, 1985.
149. Niakan E, Harati Y, Rolak LA: Immunosuppressive drug therapy in myasthenia gravis, *Arch Neurol* 43:155, 1986.
150. Tindall RSA, Rollins JA, Phillips JT, et al: Preliminary results of a double-blind, randomized placebo-controlled trial of cyclosporine in myasthenia gravis, *N Engl J Med* 316:719, 1987.
151. Ciafaloni E, Sanders DB: Advances in myasthenia gravis, *Curr Neurol Neurosci Rep* 2:89, 2002.
152. d'Empaire G, Hoaglin DC, Perlo VP, et al: Effect of prethymectomy plasma exchange on postoperative respiratory function in myasthenia gravis, *J Thor Cardiovasc Surg* 89:592, 1985.
153. Gracey Dr, Howard FM, Divertie MB: Plasmapheresis in the treatment of ventilator-dependent myasthenia gravis patients. Report of four cases, *Chest* 85:739, 1984.
154. Spence PA, Morin JE, Katz M: Role of plasmapheresis in preparing myasthenic patients for thymectomy: initial results, *Can J Surg* 27:303-305, 1984.
155. Lumley J: Prolongation of suxamethonium following plasma exchange, *Br J Anaesth* 52:1149, 1980.
156. Blalock A, Mason MG, Morgan HJ, et al: Myasthenia gravis and tumors of the thymic region, *Ann Surg* 110:544, 1939.
157. Mulder DG, Graves M, Herrmann C: Thymectomy for myasthenia gravis: recent observations and comparisons with past experience, *Ann Thorac Surg* 48:551, 1989.
158. Annoh T, Torisu M: Immunologic studies of myasthenia gravis II: a new chemotactic factor for lymphocytes found in patients with myasthenia gravis, *Surgery* 105:615, 1989.
159. Buckingham JM, Howard FM, Bernatz PE, et al: The value of thymectomy in myasthenia gravis. A computer-assisted matched study, *Ann Surg* 184:453, 1976.

160. Heiser JC, Rutherford RB, Fingel SP: Thymectomy for myasthenia gravis. A changing perspective, *Arch Surg* 117:533, 1982.

161. Jaretski A, Bethea M, Wolff M, et al: A rational approach to total thymectomy in the treatment of myasthenia gravis, *Ann Thorac Surg* 24:120, 1977.

162. Papatestas AE, Genkins G, Kornfeld P: Comparison of the results of transcervical and transsternal thymectomy in myasthenia gravis, *Ann NY Acad Sci* 377:766, 1981.

163. Schrager JB, Deeb ME, Brinster MR, et al: Transcervical thymectomy for mysthenia gravis achieves results comparable to thymectomy by sternotomy, *Ann Thorac Surg* 24:320-327, 2002.

164. Donnelly RJ, LaQuaglia MP, Fabir B, et al: Cervical thymectomy in the treatment of myasthenia gravis, *Ann R Coll Surg Engl* 66:305, 1984.

165. Yim AP: Paradigm shift in surgical approaches to thymectomy, *ANZ J Surg* 72:40, 2002.

166. Yim AP, Kay RL, Izzat MB, et al: Video-assisted thoracoscopic thymectomy for myasthenia gravis, *Semin Thorac Cardiovasc Surg* 11:65, 1999.

167. Krucylak PE, Naunhcim KS: Preoperative preparation and anesthetic management of patients with myasthenia gravis, *Semin Thorac Cardiovasc Surg* 11:47, 1999.

168. Nilsson E, Meretoja DA: Force and EMG responses of vecuronium in myasthenia gravis, *Anesthesiology* 71:A812, 1989.

169. Viby-Mogensen J, Jensen E, Werner M, et al: Measurement of acceleration: a new method of monitoring neuromuscular function, *Acta Anaesth Scand* 32:45, 1987.

170. Weber S: integrated electromyography: is it the new standard for clinical monitoring of neuromuscular blockade? *Int J Clin Monit Comput* 4:53, 1987.

171. Eisenkraft JB, Papatestas AE, Sivak M: Neuromuscular effects of halogenated agents in patients with myasthenia gravis, *Anesthesiology*, 61(S):A307, 1984.

172. Rowbottom SJ: Isoflurane for thymectomy in myasthenia gravis, *Anaesth Intensive Care* 17:444, 1989.

173. Lebowitz MH, Blitt CD, Walts LF: Depression of twitch response to stimulation of the ulnar nerve during Ethrane anesthesia in man, *Anesthesiology* 33:52, 1970.

174. Ward S, Wright DJ: Neuromuscular blockade in myasthenia gravis with atracurium besylate, *Anaesthesia* 62:692, 1984.

175. Nilsson E, Muller K: Neuromuscular effects of isoflurane in patients with myasthenia gravis, *Acta Anaesthesiol Scand* 34:126, 1990.

176. Hubler M, Litz RJ, Albrecht DM: Combination of balanced and regional anaesthesia for minimally invasive surgery in a patient with myasthenia gravis, *Eur J Anaesthesiol* 17:325, 2000.

177. Baraka AS, Taha SK, Kawkabam N: Neuromuscular interaction of sevoflurane—cisatracurium in a myasthenic patient, *Can J Anaesth* 47:562, 2000.

178. Kiran U, Choudhury M, Saxena N, et al: Sevoflurane as a sole anaesthetic for thymectomy in myasthenia gravis, *Acta Anaesthesiol Scand* 44:351, 2000.

179. Baraka A, Siddik S, el Rassi T, et al: Sevoflurane anesthesia in a myasthenic patient undergoing transsternal thymectomy, *Middle East J Anesthesiol* 15:603, 2000.

180. Baraka A, Afifi A, Muallem M, et al: Neuromuscular effects of halothane, suxamethonium and tubocurarine in a myasthenic undergoing thymectomy, *Br J Anaesth* 43:91, 1971.

181. Stanski DR, Lee RF, MacCannell KL, et al: Atypical cholinesterase in a patient with myasthenia gravis, *Anesthesiology* 46:298, 1977.

182. Wainwright AP, Brodrick PM: Suxamethonium in myasthenia gravis, *Anaesthesia* 42:950, 1987.

183. Eisenkraft JB, Book WJ, Mann SM, et al: Resistance to succinylcholine in myasthenia gravis. A dose-response study, *Anesthesiology* 69:760, 1988.

184. Foldes FF, Nagashima H: Myasthenia gravis and anesthesia.In Oyama T (ed): *Endocrinology and the anaesthetist. Monographs in anaesthesiology*, vol 2, p171, New York, 1984, Elsevier.

185. Ginsberg H, Varejes L: The use of a relaxant in myasthenia gravis, *Anaesthesia* 10:177, 1955.

186. Miller JD, Lee C: Muscle diseases. In Katz J, Benumof JL, Kadis LB (eds): *Anesthesia and uncommon diseases*, p619, Philadelphia, 1990, WB Saunders.

187. Azar I: The response of patients with neuromuscular disorders to muscle relaxants: a review, *Anesthesiology* 61:173, 1984.

188. Foldes FF, McNall PG: Myasthenia gravis: a guide for anesthesiologists, *Anesthesiology* 23:837, 1962.

189. Bell CF, Florence AM, Hunter JM, et al: Atracurium in the myasthenic patient, *Anaesthesia*, 39:961, 1984.

190. Smith CE, Donati F, Bevan DR: Cumulative dose-response curves for atracurium in patients with myasthenia gravis, *Can J Anaesth* 36:402, 1989.

191. Eisenkraft JB: Myasthenia gravis and thymic surgery—anaesthetic considerations, In Gothard JW (ed): *Thoracic anaesthesia*, London, 1987, Bailliere-Tindall.

192. Baraka A, Siddik S, Kawkabani N: Cisatracurium in a myasthenic patient undergoing thymectomy, *Can J Anaesth* 46:779, 1999.

193. Hunter JM, Bell CF, Florence AM, et al: Vecuronium in the myasthenic patients, *Anaesthesia* 40:848, 1985.

194. Eisenkraft JB, Book WJ, Papatestas AE: Sensitivity to vecuronium in myasthenia gravis—a dose-response study, *Can J Anaesth* 37:301, 1990.

195. Buzello W, Noeldge G, Krieg N, et al: Vecuronium for muscle relaxation in patients with myasthenia gravis, *Anesthesiology* 64:507, 1986.

196. Nilsson E, Meretoja AO: Vecuronium dose-response and maintenance requirements in patients with myasthenia gravis, *Anesthesiology* 73:28, 1990.

197. Itoh H, Shibata K, Nitta S: Comparison between sevoflurane and propofol neuromuscular effects in a patient with myasthenia gravis: effective doses of vecuronium, *Anesthesiology* 95:803, 2001.

198. Itoh H, Shibata K, Nitta S: Difference in sensitivity to vecuronium between patients with ocular and generalized myasthenia gravis, *Br J Anaesth* 87:885, 2001.

199. Paterson IG, Hood JR, Russell SH, Weston MD, Hirsch NP: Mivacurium in the myasthenic patient, *Br J Anaesth* 73:474-478, 1994.

200. Seigne RD, Scott RP: Mivacurium chloride and myasthenia gravis, *Br J Anaesth* 72:468-469, 1974.

201. Mann R, Blobner M, Jelen-Esselborn S, et al: Preanesthetic train-of-four fade predicts the atracurium requirement of myasthenia gravis patients, *Anesthesiology* 93:346, 2000.

202. Itoh H, Shibata K, Yoshida M, et al: Neuromuscular monitoring at the orbicularis oculi may overestimate the blockade in myasthenic patients, *Anesthesiology* 93:1194, 2000.

203. Eisenkraft JB, Book WJ, Papatestas AE: Sensitivity to vecuronium in myasthenia gravis—a dose-response study, *Can J Anaesth* 37:301, 1990.

204. Florence AM: Anesthesia for transcervical thymectomy in myasthenia gravis, *Ann R Coll Surg Engl* 66:309, 1984.

205. Burgess FW, Wilcosky B: Thoracic epidural anesthesia for transsternal thymectomy in myasthenia gravis, *Anesth Analg* 69:529, 1989.

206. Akpolat N, Tilgen H, Gursoy F, et al: Thoracic epidural anaesthesia and analgesia with bupivacaine for transsternal thymectomy for myasthenia gravis, *Eur J Anaesthesiol* 14:220, 1997.

207. Abe S, Takeuchi C, Kaneko T, et al: Propofol anesthesia combined with thoracic epidural anesthesia for thymectomy for myasthenia gravis—a report of eleven cases, *Masui* 50:1217, 2001.

208. Gorback MS: Analgesic management after thymectomy, *Anesthesiol Rep* 2:262, 1990.

209. Lake CL: Curare sensitivity in steroid-treated myasthenia gravis, *Anesth Analg* 57:132, 1978.

210. Fillmore RB, Herren AL, Perlo AF: Curare sensitivity in myasthenia gravis, *Anesth Analg* 57:515, 1978.

211. Lumb AR, Calder I: 'Cured' myasthenia gravis and neuromuscular blockade, *Anaesthesia* 44:828, 1989.

212. Abel M, Eisenkraft JB, Patel N: Sensitivity to succinylcholine in myasthenia gravis during true remission: a dose-effect study, *Anaesthesia* 43:30, 1991.

213. Barrons RW: Drug-induced neuromuscular blockade and myasthenia gravis, *Pharmacotherapy* 17:1220, 1997.

214. Mora CT, Eisenkraft JB, Papatestas AE: Intravenous dantrolene in a patient with myasthenia gravis, *Anesthesiology* 64:371, 1986.

215. Gracey DR, Divertie MB, Howard FM: Mechanical ventilation for respiratory failure in myasthenia gravis. Two years' experience with 22 patients, *Mayo Clin Proc* 85:739, 1983.

216. Mulder DG, Hermann C, Buckberg GB: Effect of thymectomy in patients with myasthenia gravis, *Am J Surg* 128:202, 1974.

217. Loach AB, Young AC, Spalding JMK, et al: Postoperative management after thymectomy, *Br Med J* 1:309, 1975.

218. Leventhal R, Orkin FK, Hirsch RA: Prediction of the need for postoperative mechanical ventilation in myasthenia gravis, *Anesthesiology* 53:26, 1980.

219. Orkin FK, Leventhal SR, Hirsch RA: Predicting respiratory failure following thymectomy, *Ann NY Acad Sci* 377:862, 1981.

220. Grant RP, Jenkins JC: Prediction of the need for postoperative mechanical ventilation in myasthenia gravis, *Can Anaesth Soc J* 29:112, 1982.

221. Gracey DR, Divertie MB, Howard FM, et al: Postoperative respiratory care after transsternal thymectomy in myasthenia gravis. A three-year experience in 53 patients, *Chest* 86:67, 1984.

222. Eisenkraft JB, Papatestas AE, Kahn CH, et al: Predicting the need for postoperative mechanical ventilation in myasthenia gravis, *Anesthesiology* 65: 79, 1986.

223. Naguib M, el Dawlatly AA, Ashour M, et al: Multivariate determinants of the need for postoperative ventilation in myasthenia gravis, *Can J Anaesth* 43:1006, 1996.

224. Younger DS, Braun NMT, Jaretzki A, et al: Myasthenia gravis: determinants for independent ventilation after transsternal thymectomy, *Neurology* 34:336, 1984.

225. Pavlin EG, Holle RH, Schoene RB: Recovery of airway protection compared with ventilation in humans after paralysis with curare, *Anesthesiology* 70:381, 1989.

226. Ringqvist I, Ringqvist T: Respiratory mechanics in untreated myasthenia gravis with special reference to the respiratory forces, *Acta Med Scand* 190:499, 1971.

227. Eisenkraft JB, Papatestas AE, Pozner JN, et al: Prediction of ventilatory failure following transcervical thymectomy in myasthenia gravis, *Ann NY Acad Sci* 505:888, 1987.

228. Redfern N, McQuillan PJ, Conacher I, et al: Anaesthesia for transsternal thymectomy in myasthenia gravis, *Ann R Coll Surg Engl* 68:289, 1987.

229. Eisenkraft JB, Papatestas AE: Anaesthesia for transsternal thymectomy in myasthenia gravis, *Ann R Coll Surg Engl* 70:257, 1988.

230. Chevalley C, Spiliopoulos A, de Perrot M, et al: Perioperative medical management and outcome following thymectomy for myasthenia gravis, *Can J Anaesth* 48:446, 2001.

231. Pandit SK, Kothary S, Orringer M: Preoperative anticholinesterase therapy in myasthenic patients for thymectomy, abstracted, *Anaesthesia*, suppl 1982.

232. Slaughter D: Neostigmine and opiate analgesia, *Arch Int Pharmacodyn Ther* 83:143, 1950.

233. Oosterhuis HJ: Observations of the natural history of myasthenia gravis and the effect of thymectomy, *Ann NY Acad Sci* 377:679, 1981.

234. Papatestas AE, Genkins G, Kornfeld P: The relationship between the thymus and oncogenesis. A study of the incidence of non-thymic malignancy in myasthenia gravis, *Br J Cancer* 24:635, 1971.

235. Vessey MP, Doll R: Thymectomy and cancer, *Br J Cancer* 26:53, 1972.

236. O'Neill JH, Murray NMF, Newsom-Davis J: The Lambert-Eaton myasthenic syndrome. A review of 50 cases, *Brain* 111:577, 1988.

237. Anderson HJ, Churchill-Davidson HC, et al: Bronchial neoplasm with myasthenia; prolonged apnoea after administration of succinylcholine, *Lancet* 2:1291, 1953.

238. Pascuzzi RM: Myasthenia gravis and Lambert-Eaton syndrome, *Ther Apher* 6:57, 2002.

239. Lambert EH, Eaton LM, Rooke ED: Defect of neuromuscular transmission associated with malignant neoplasm, *Am J Physiol* 178:612, 1956.

240. Fukunaga H, Engel AG, Osame M, et al: Paucity and disorganization of presynaptic membrane active zones in the Lambert-Eaton myasthenic syndrome, *Muscle Nerve* 5:686, 1982.

241. Lang B, Newson-Davis J, Wray D, et al: Autoimmune aetiology for myasthenic syndrome. *Lancet* 2:224, 1981.

242. Elmquist D, Lambert EH: Detailed analysis of neuromuscular transmission in a patient with the myasthenic syndrome sometimes associated with bronchogenic carcinoma, *Mayo Clin Proc* 43:689, 1968.

243. Vizi ES, van Dijk, Foldes FF: The effect of 4-aminopyridine on acetylcholine release, *J Neural Transm* 41:265, 1975.

244. Lundh H: Effects of 4-aminopyridines on neuromuscular transmissions, *Brain Res* 153:307, 1978.

245. Norris FH, Eaton JM, Nielke CH: Depression of bone marrow by guanidine, *Arch Neurol* 30:184, 1974.

246. Takamori M: Calcium, caffeine and Eaton-Lambert syndrome, *Arch Neurol* 27:285, 1972.

247. Cherington M: Guanidine and germine in Eaton-Lambert syndrome, *Neurology* 26:944, 1976.

248. Agoston S, VanWeeden T, Westra P, et al: Effects of 4-aminopyridine in Eaton-Lambert syndrome, *Br J Anaesth* 50:383, 1978.

249. Lundh H, Nilsson D, Rosen I: Novel drug of choice in Eaton-Lambert syndrome, *J Neurol Neurosurg Psychiatry* 46:684, 1983.

250. Wise RP: A myasthenic syndrome complicating bronchial carcinoma, *Anaesthesia* 17:488, 1962.

251. Telford RJ, Hollway TE: The myasthenic syndrome: anaesthesia in a patient treated with 3,4 diaminopyridine, *Br J Anaesth* 64:363, 1990.

252. Itoh H, Shibata K, Nitta S: Neuromuscular monitoring in myasthenic sydrome, *Anaesthesia* 56:562-567, 2001.

253. Brim JD: Denervation supersensitivity. The response to depolarizing muscle relaxants, *Br J Anaesth* 45:222, 1973.

Pulmonary Transplantation

14

Paul S. Myles, MB, BS, MD, MPH, FCARCSI, FANZCA*

Pulmonary transplant recipients have end-stage disease that in other circumstances would contraindicate surgery; if surgery proceeds, it usually mandates postoperative care in an intensive care unit (ICU), often with prolonged mechanical ventilation and difficulty with ventilator weaning. The introduction of pulmonary transplantation has given patients with end-stage pulmonary disease a means to improve their overall health status and survival.[1] This has resulted in many anesthesiologists being confronted with such patients—both those awaiting transplantation and those who have undergone transplantation and require other types of surgery.[2-5] Many of the important issues associated with their management are common to both groups, and so an understanding of those issues is essential for all anesthesiologists.

Issues that arise for pulmonary transplantation patients include the following[6-12]:

- Optimization of mechanical ventilation and one-lung ventilation (OLV)
- Management of intraoperative hypoxia and hypercapnia
- Pulmonary hypertension and right ventricular (RV) failure
- Use of inhaled nitric oxide (NO) and transesophageal echocardiography (TEE)
- Understanding of the pathophysiology of cardiopulmonary bypass (CPB)
- Maintenance of other vital organ functions
- Postoperative pain management

Critical incidents during pulmonary transplantation are common and often life-threatening and can challenge even the most experienced and adept anesthesiologist.[11,13-20]

Several anesthetic interventions can result in marked and immediate improvement of the patient during and after transplantation. Some of these allow the procedure to be completed without cardiopulmonary bypass, thus avoiding its known adverse effects.[21-24] Other interventions can improve oxygenation and right-side ventricular function and provide a rapid recovery, allowing tracheal extubation in the operating room or soon afterwards. The anesthesiologist, therefore, has a crucial role to play in patient outcome after pulmonary transplantation. Knowledge of these issues can also be helpful in the nontransplant setting.[2,4,25]

Recent advances in anesthesia and critical care—the introduction of short-acting anesthetic drugs, multi-modal analgesic techniques, inhaled NO and other selective pulmonary vasodilators, acceptance of hypercapnia and avoidance of pulmonary hyperinflation, and TEE assessment of right ventricular function—have all provided the anesthesiologist with effective interventions for managing patients with end-stage pulmonary disease. These, along with other advances in immunology, immunosuppressant therapy, and infection surveillance, have led to gradual improvement in long-term survival after pulmonary transplantation.[1]

As with other types of specialized surgery, outcome after pulmonary transplantation can be improved with increasing experience and case load, with larger institutions having more favorable results.[26,27] Accumulating experience within an institution is also associated with improved outcome—at the author's institution, a 50% reduction in early (less than 90 days) postoperative mortality was observed over the first 7 years of the lung transplantation program, and recent data suggest ongoing improvements in survival (Figure 14-1).[28] Survival after pulmonary transplantation has continued to improve worldwide in the last decade.[1] Approximately 75% of recipients are alive at 1 year and 55% at 5 years after transplantation. There is better survival in recipients with emphysema and poorer survival in those with congenital heart disease and pulmonary hypertension.[1]

The major causes of late mortality are opportunistic infection and bronchiolitis obliterans. Common opportunistic infections can be bacterial *(Staphylococcus, Streptococcus, Pseudomonas, Mycoplasma, Pneumocystis)*, viral *(Cytomegalovirus, Influenza)*, and fungal *(Candida, Aspergillus)* in origin.[29]

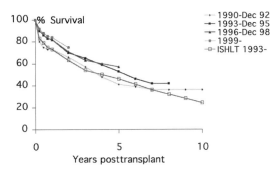

FIGURE 14.1 Survival after pulmonary transplantation at the Alfred Hospital, Melbourne, Australia. There has been an apparent improvement in survival with increasing experience.

*The author would like to thank David Bain and Greg Snell, Alfred Hospital, Melbourne, for assistance with the provision of TEE images, and provision of some data used in this chapter, respectively.

Bronchiolitis obliterans is a fibrosing process thought to be caused by chronic low-grade rejection (and possibly infection) and is the eventual cause of death in about 50% of pulmonary transplant recipients.

Pulmonary Allograft Procurement and Preservation

The establishment of criteria for the diagnosis of brain death, although neither universally adopted nor consistent, has led to a increase in organ donation.[30] Potential pulmonary allograft donors are screened for absence of infection, previous surgery, marked contusion or aspiration, and a history of heavy smoking.[31] Acceptable donor lung function is confirmed by absence of x-ray infiltrates and near-normal gas exchange, suggested by an PaO_2 of more than 300 mmHg while receiving 100% oxygen.

Physiologic derangements can occur in the brain-dead donor, and they require special care.[32,33] These include loss of temperature regulation, hypovolemia, hypokalemia, and an acute hormonal deficiency state that commonly includes a reduction in circulating thyroid hormone. Up to 40% of donors have systolic dysfunction and ventricular arrhythmias.[32] Ongoing medical care after the diagnosis of brain death must be optimal in order to preserve donor organ function.

Intraoperative management of the donor is determined by the organs that are being harvested. In the operating room, the multiorgan donor is placed supine and undergoes an extensive midline sternotomy-laparotomy incision from neck to pubis. Commonly administered drugs include a broad-spectrum antibiotic, a nondepolarizing muscle relaxant (to suppress movements associated with spinal reflex activity), and methylprednisolone, 1 g. During dissection and pulmonary allograft procurement, the donor might require large volumes of fluid resuscitation and is at risk of hypothermia. It is usual for the pulmonary donor to receive an epoprostenol infusion at 1 to 10 ng/kg/min for 10 to 20 minutes during dissection in order to optimize pulmonary blood flow and subsequent pneumoplegia distribution. It is recommended that 5 cmH_2O positive end-expiratory pressure (PEEP) be applied during allograft excision in order to minimize atelectasis. Following excision, the allograft can have 5 cmH_2O continuous positive airway pressure (CPAP) applied to maintain partial inflation; it is then stored in ice at 0 to 4° C for transfer to its eventual destination.

Administration of inhaled NO during excision can improve early allograft function, possibly by attenuating ischemic and oxidant injury during storage and reperfusion. In a small study, dogs that received inhaled NO at 60 ppm at the time of harvest had an 80% reduction in pulmonary vascular resistance (PVR), with concomitant reductions in neutrophil sequestration and markers of oxidant injury, both of which are associated with improved oxygenation.[34]

Allograft ischemic time is considered to be a limiting factor in pulmonary transplantation, but the shortage of donor organs has led to an extension of the timing criteria. Some institutions have experience of long pulmonary ischemic times.[27,35,36] Ueno et al compared early allograft function and outcomes (incidence of rejection, duration of mechanical ventilation, ICU and hospital length of stay) among those who had short (less than 5 hours, n = 20), intermediate (5 to 8 hours, n = 39), and long (more than 8 hours, n = 15) ischemic times. Early allograft function was impaired in those with long ischemic times, but there were no significant differences in other outcomes.[36] This suggests that the acceptable ischemic time in pulmonary transplantation could be longer than previously thought. Also, there is an association between donor age and pulmonary ischemic times with subsequent recipient mortality.[1] Ischemic times of up to 8 hours of pulmonary allografts from donors less than 40 years of age have a negligible effect on recipient mortality, whereas for organs from older donors there is a twofold increase in recipient mortality for ischemic times longer than 6 hours.[1]

A shortage of donor organs (and in some patients, the existence of a contraindication to transplantation) has furthered the expansion of lung volume reduction surgery.[4,37] This could be an alternative or deferring procedure in patients with emphysema. Optimism for this approach is tempered by lack of long-term outcome data (see Chapter 12).[38]

Evaluation of the Pulmonary Transplant Recipient

Initial clinical evaluation of a patient with end-stage pulmonary disease and assessment of the patient's suitability for transplantation include characterization of the underlying pulmonary disease, exclusion of other organ dysfunction, and assessment of the patient's suitability to tolerate and continue lifelong immunosuppressant medication.[7,39,40] A thorough respiratory system evaluation, including details of previous respiratory events (e.g., pneumothorax, pleurisy) and thoracic surgical procedures, is important. Previous thoracic surgery can be associated with technical difficulties at the time of transplantation, such as prolonged dissection, difficulty with surgical exposure, and excessive bleeding.

The principal investigations are those that characterize the disease and its severity. Thus, whether the disease pattern is predominantly obstructive or restrictive, knowledge of the patient's exercise capacity and need for home oxygen therapy are fundamental. Essential investigations include the following[6,7,39,41-46]:

- Chest x-ray
- Arterial blood gases (ABGs)
- Spirometry
- Ventilation:perfusion scan
- Echocardiography (and sometimes catheterization and coronary angiography)
- Measures of renal function (electrolytes, creatinine clearance)
- Hematology
- Blood group measurements
- Viral serology

ABO blood group and HLA compatibility are used to match the donor allograft, and the chest x-ray can help estimate the size of the recipient's thoracic cavity to assist donor allograft size-matching.

Many potential recipients have risk factors for coronary artery disease, which, if found to be present, might contraindicate pulmonary transplantation. Traditional assessment includes coronary angiography, but many institutions have

TABLE 14-1

The Number of Pulmonary Transplant Procedures Reported to the Registry of the International Study of Heart and Lung Transplantation

Transplant Procedures	Up to 1984	1995–1999
Heart-lung	1957	741
Single lung	3014	3500
Bilateral sequential lung	1819	2815

From Hosenpud JD, Bennett LE, Keck BM, et al: *J Heart Lung Transplant* 19:909, 2000.

adopted a selective approach to this invasive investigation.[40] Snell et al analyzed 243 referrals for pulmonary transplantation, for which 85 of 101 patients underwent coronary angiography on the basis of predetermined risk factors that included age over 50 years, male gender, hypertension, hypercholesterolemia, diabetes, angina, or a history of smoking. Almost a third (32%) of the selected patients had proven coronary artery disease, and in some of these, revascularization was performed before their definitive transplant procedure. Subsequent outcome appeared to be acceptable.[43]

Potential pulmonary transplant recipients can be divided conveniently into the following four groups[1,39,46,47]:

1. Chronic obstructive pulmonary disease (COPD, e.g., emphysema)
2. Suppurative pulmonary disease (e.g., cystic fibrosis)
3. Restrictive pulmonary disease (e.g., pulmonary fibrosis)
4. Pulmonary hypertension (with or without congenital heart disease)

The most common types of pulmonary transplantation are single-lung transplantation (SLTx) and bilateral sequential lung transplantation (BSLTx), with heart-lung transplantation (HLTx) becoming a very uncommon procedure (see Tables 14.1 and 14.2).[1-7,15-17,21,29-31] There has been a change in the pattern of transplantation, whereby HLTx has been replaced in favor of BSLTx, with the aim being to preserve the native heart and avoid cardiac allograft atherosclerosis.[1]

Patient Preparation and Monitoring

The pulmonary transplant recipient is usually informed of the impending operation two to four hours before operating room scheduling.[47] This can be a time of conflicting emotions for the patient and his or her family. Often, there is a sense of relief and excitement, and yet heightened anxiety. The patient's emotional state might also adversely affect cardiopulmonary status, with increased dyspnea, tachycardia, and hypertension. As in other circumstances, reassurance and a clear explanation of the procedures can be worthwhile.

Many end-stage pulmonary disease patients receive inhaled bronchodilator and steroid therapy. Missed doses can aggravate the extent of airway obstruction, so it is important that these medications be continued up until the time of surgery. The routine use of high-dose methylprednisolone during pulmonary transplantation should provide additional protection against reversible airflow obstruction, and it is recommended that the initial loading dose be administered before induction of anesthesia.

Routine premedication includes immunosuppressant drugs (azathioprine and cyclosporine) and might include an anxiolytic (e.g., IM midazolam, 5 mg) and bronchodilator therapy (e.g., albuterol, 500 mg, and ipratropium, 250 µg, via nebulizer). Sedative agents, such as benzodiazepines or opioids, should be used with caution in these patients because they can result in further carbon dioxide (CO_2) retention and/or hypoxia, both of which can exacerbate pulmonary hypertension or result in agitation or CO_2 narcosis. Supplemental oxygen is usually required during transfer to the operating room.

Routine monitoring for pulmonary transplantation includes pulse oximetry, electrocardiography (ECG) and, following intravascular catheterizations, invasive systemic arterial, central venous, and pulmonary arterial pressures. Following tracheal intubation, capnography, inhalation agent monitoring, and temperature monitoring are employed. The role of TEE is discussed in the following sections.

There have been recent descriptions of other monitoring devices that could be beneficial during pulmonary transplantation.[6,8,47-49] Modifications of the pulmonary artery catheter that

TABLE 14-2

Pattern of Preexisting Disease and Type of Pulmonary Transplant Recipients at Alfred Hospital, Melbourne, Australia. Fewer HLTx Procedures are Currently Performed in Favor of Increasing Popularity of BSLTx

Preexisting Disease	HLTx (n = 51)	BSLTx (n = 179)	SLTx (n = 171)
Suppurative pulmonary disease (n = 126) Cystic fibrosis, bronchiectasis, agammaglobulimemia	8	117	1
Obstructive pulmonary disease (n = 171) α₁ antitrypsin deficiency, emphysema, sarcoidosis	10	31	130
Interstitial pulmonary disease (n = 51) Idiopathic pulmonary fibrosis, scleroderma, bronchiolitis obliterans	3	11	37
Pulmonary hypertension (n = 54) Primary pulmonary hypertension, congenital heart disease	30	20	4

HLTx, Heart-lung transplantation; *BSLTx*, bilateral sequential lung transplantation; *SLTx*, single-lung transplantation.

measure continuous cardiac output, mixed venous oximetry, and RV ejection fraction have been evaluated in the transplant setting but do not yet appear to have an established role. Another fairly recent innovation is continuous ABG monitoring, whereby intravascular sensors measure arterial blood pH, Pa_{CO_2}, and Pa_{O_2} continuously via a peripheral arterial cannula.[50] Because of the potential for significant and sometimes rapid acid-base disturbances during both the intraoperative and postoperative periods, these devices could be of some use during pulmonary transplantation. This is costly technology and so might be indicated only for selected high-risk patients undergoing BSLTx and HLTx procedures.[47] Such patients often have profound disturbances of cardiopulmonary function during surgery; hypercapnia is usual and can be severe (Figure 14-2).

Intraoperative hypothermia is common after pulmonary transplantation because the thoracic organs are exposed to room temperature, the surgical procedure can be prolonged, and the patients often have reduced body mass and lose heat readily. Intraoperative hypothermia can be avoided using forced-air warming, which has the added benefit of reducing postoperative shivering.[51] Prevention of hypothermia is an important component of care if tracheal extubation is planned at the end of the procedure. Avoidance of hypothermia has also been shown to reduce infection rates, at least after colorectal surgery, and this consideration is likely to be important in pulmonary transplantation as well.[52]

Anesthesia

Specific anesthetic management for pulmonary transplantation depends on the type of procedure performed (HLTx, SLTx, or BSLTx) and in many cases can be adapted from routine cardiothoracic practice. At several critical stages, the anesthesiologist must be particularly vigilant and remain responsive to life-threatening critical incidents. These include the following[6,9,11,13-16,18-20]:

- Induction of anesthesia
- Commencement of mechanical ventilation
- Institution of OLV
- Pulmonary artery (PA) clamping
- PA unclamping and reperfusion of the pulmonary allograft

Single-Lung Transplantation

The most common indications for SLTx are COPD (43%) and pulmonary fibrosis (20%).[1] If the patient's evaluation indicates that a single donor lung allograft will result in adequate long-term function, SLTx is indicated. This procedure has the benefits of increasing the number of recipients who can be served by a single donor, facilitating a shorter operative and allograft ischemic time, preserving one native lung (which can provide some security in the event of allograft failure), and promoting good long-term survival.

Anesthetic management for single-lung transplanation is similar to that for many other thoracic surgical procedures requiring OLV; in most cases, tracheal extubation can occur at the end of the procedure. Key features of anesthetic management include use of short-acting anesthetic drugs, maintenance of normothermia, and optimal postoperative analgesia. A double-lumen tube (DLT) is required, and mechanical ventilation should be modified according to the patient's underlying condition. Nearly all SLTx procedures can be performed without cardiopulmonary bypass.

Bilateral Sequential Lung Transplantation

The most common indications for BSLTx are cystic fibrosis (32%) and COPD (18%). BSLTx has largely replaced HLTx because of the advantages of avoiding concomitant cardiac transplantation and (in most cases) being able to avoid cardiopulmonary bypass.[1,7,27] Optimal anesthetic and surgical management can lead to avoidance of cardiopulmonary bypass in about 75% of cases; however, some institutions routinely

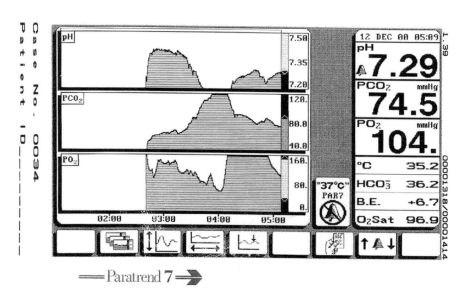

FIGURE 14-2 Continuous arterial blood gas monitoring (Paratrend 7, Agilent Technologies, USA) in a patient with severe cystic fibrosis undergoing bilateral sequential lung transplantation. Intravenous sedation was administered for insertion of pulmonary artery and epidural catheters at 03:10; anesthesia and mechanical ventilation commenced at 04:05; one-lung ventilation commenced at 04:40.

perform all their BSLTx procedures with cardiopulmonary bypass.[12]

Anesthetic management for BSLTx can be demanding.[6,8,9,47] There are many stages throughout the procedure when the anesthesiologist is called upon to stabilize the patient. A DLT is required unless the procedure is to be done with cardiopulmonary bypass, and mechanical ventilation should be modified according to the patient's underlying condition. Some patients can recover from anesthesia immediately, with tracheal extubation occuring in the operating room or soon afterward.

Heart-Lung Transplantation

There are still occasional patients who require HLTx, most commonly those with congenital heart disease or primary pulmonary hypertension.[1,6,8,47] The care of these patients is particularly demanding for the anesthesiologist, with most having significant pulmonary hypertension and right ventricular dysfunction, and some having had previous cardiac surgery.

Induction of anesthesia can seriously impair myocardial contractility and the balance between pulmonary and systemic circulations. Anesthetic management should include maintenance of myocardial contractility and avoidance of pulmonary vasoconstriction. A standard single-lumen tracheal tube is used, and routine mechanical ventilation can be employed in most circumstances. Antifibrinolytics to reduce perioperative bleeding and blood transfusion are often indicated.

Patients with congenital heart disease and pulmonary hypertension usually electively undergo mechanical ventilation beyond 12 to 24 hours.[22]

Choice of Anesthetic Drugs

The anesthetic plan is determined by the type of procedure and whether early recovery and tracheal extubation in the operating room are planned. Most patients undergoing SLTx (and some undergoing BSLTx) can be recovered immediately after surgery.[6,47,53] Early recovery after surgery and anesthesia is facilitated by use of new, short-acting anesthetic drugs, such as propofol and sevoflurane, and the new opioid, remifentanil. Remifentanil can support a substantial hypnotic dose reduction, which can attenuate adverse effects and speed recovery time.

There is now good evidence that anesthetic drug titration can be guided by bispectral index (BIS) monitoring.[54,55] Gan et al found that BIS monitoring led to a 25% reduction in propofol use and a concomitant 35% enhancement in speed of recovery ($P < 0.001$) in general surgical patients.[54] Similarly, Song et al found a 30% to 55% reduction in times to verbal responsiveness ($P < 0.05$) with sevoflurane and desflurane in BIS-titrated groups.[55] Thus it is likely that BIS-guided anesthesia might achieve a faster and more reliable recovery after pulmonary transplantation, which in turn could reduce the need for postoperative mechanical ventilation in selected cases.

Patients undergoing pulmonary transplantation may be at an increased risk of awareness because of the reduced uptake of volatile agents at the commencement of surgery, a reduction in hypnotic drug administration in response to acute hemodynamic disturbances, and when planning for early awakening and tracheal extubation in the operating room.[56] BIS monitoring could have a role to play in this regard, in that anesthetic drug administration can be more reliably titrated and hypotension less likely to occur.[57]

Propofol and the inhalation agents, particularly isoflurane and sevoflurane, have bronchodilator properties.[58,59] These could be beneficial for patients with airflow obstruction. In other circumstances, choice of intravenous or inhalation anesthesia is determined largely by preference. Because most recipients are not particularly at risk of myocardial depression, standard concentrations of volatile agent or intravenous propofol anesthesia, 3 to 5 mg/kg/hr, can be used. A larger opioid component of anesthesia can be useful in reducing the myocardial depressant and vasodilating properties of the standard induction agents in patients undergoing HLTx (or BSLTx with cardiopulmonary bypass), particularly if their underlying disease suggests a complicated postoperative course and early tracheal extubation is not anticipated. Remifentanil is particularly effective, as it allows both maximal stress ablation and (because of its rapid elimination) early tracheal extubation, whereas sufentanil or fentanyl is suitable if a period of postoperative mechanical ventilation is planned.

Induction of Anesthesia

Preoxygenation should precede induction of anesthesia.[60] Induction of anesthesia and commencement of mechanical ventilation can result in significant hypotension.[6,13,17,18] This is due to the vasodilating and myocardial depressant properties of the anesthetic agents, as well as to increases in intrathoracic pressure and PVR. Although most pulmonary transplant recipients have normal myocardial function and usually have only slightly elevated pulmonary arterial pressure, they can have hyperresponsive pulmonary vasculature because of medial wall hypertrophy.[24,39,42,44,45,61] This condition makes them susceptible to pulmonary hypertension and right ventricular dysfunction. A careful titrated induction of anesthesia using any of the induction agents is suitable for most patients, provided there is meticulous observation and maintenance of systemic and pulmonary arterial pressures. These are usually supported by preemptive intravascular volume loading to maintain ventricular preload.

In patients with impaired ventricular function or greater degrees of pulmonary hypertension—most notably, those with primary pulmonary hypertension or cyanotic congenital heart disease—induction of anesthesia needs to be modified further. These patients are at increased risk of profound systemic hypotension and circulatory arrest.[9,17,18,42] Such patients should be optimized before induction of anesthesia, which could require commencement of an inotrope infusion, usually in conjunction with a selective pulmonary vasodilator such as inhaled NO.[62-65] Induction of anesthesia should not commence in this higher risk group of patients without a surgeon being present in the operating room. If severe hypotension or cardiac arrest ensues, attending surgeons could be required to institute emergency cardiopulmonary bypass, usually via femoral cannulation. In those at highest risk, insertion of femoral cannulae before induction of anesthesia should be considered.

The airway should be secured rapidly following induction of anesthesia. This process is facilitated by a rapid-onset neuromuscular blocking drug such as succinylcholine, 1.5 mg/kg, or rocuronium, 0.9 to 1.2 mg/kg. For patients undergoing SLTx and most of those undergoing BSLTx, a method of pulmonary isolation is required. The most common device is a disposable polyvinylchloride DLT, although the Univent tube (Fuji Systems, Japan) or a bronchial blocker is employed occasionally.[6-9,16] Endobronchial tube position should then be checked with fiberoptic bronchoscopy to ensure optimal positioning. Most patients can be managed with a left-sided DLT, with the bronchial cuff positioned just distal to the carina so that it does not impinge on the bronchial anastomosis. In patients with suppurative pulmonary disease, it is prudent to aspirate both lumens with 8–12F suction catheters; this cannot be achieved through the narrow suction port of the fiberoptic bronchoscope. Bronchial suction might need to be repeated regularly. There are occasions when pulmonary ventilation might be impaired or pulmonary isolation compromised; this requires vigilance and manipulation of the endobronchial device.[16]

Initially, an FIO_2 of 1.0 is chosen, and this can be reduced after pulmonary allograft implantation.[42,66,67] Although used on some occasions in some institutions, nitrous oxide is best avoided during pulmonary transplantation, as it can increase PVR, and the recipient is then at risk of air embolism following reperfusion of the allograft.[68]

Mechanical Ventilation

Mechanical ventilation is associated with many potential complications during pulmonary transplantation.[11,13,15,47,69,71] Barotrauma (pneumothorax, air leak via a tracheal/bronchial anastomosis, increased PVR and right ventricular dysfunction) can result from the direct effects of high airway pressure, and "volotrauma" (leading to circulatory collapse) can result from dynamic hyperinflation (DHI).[72]

Mechanical ventilation of patients with end-stage pulmonary disease should be adapted according to the patient's underlying disease process. The risk of the complications just discussed is in part dependent on the ventilator settings chosen, and these should be determined by the patient's status and the desired PaO_2 and $PaCO_2$ values.[11,42,72-76] The standard normal values of PaO_2 (100 mmHg) and $PaCO_2$ (40 mmHg) are often inappropriate in this population, as the patient might have adapted to levels outside the normal range. Thus, the patient's preoperative ABG results can be used to guide ventilator man-

agement, with the result that many patients can tolerate a reduced minute ventilation. This will lead to an increase in $PaCO_2$ (a situation known as permissive hypercapnia), which is usually well-tolerated.[74] Levels of $PaCO_2$ as high as 60 mmHg are commonly accepted during pulmonary transplantation, and values as high as 120 mmHg have been reported without adverse sequelae.[4,11,15,25,47,74] Permissive hypercapnia could reduce the risk of pulmonary barotrauma and DHI.

Patients with severe airflow obstruction (asthma, cystic fibrosis, emphysema) are at greatest risk of DHI, or "gas-trapping," during mechanical ventilation (Figure 14-3).[11,13,15,47,71,73,77] DHI results in residual PEEP and so is also known as "auto-PEEP" or "intrinsic PEEP."[70,73,76,78-80] Auto-PEEP results in overinflation of the lungs, reduction in venous return, and direct cardiac compression. Lesser degrees of auto-PEEP are common during pulmonary transplantation, particularly early after induction when there is a tendency to hyperventilate the lungs at the same time that anesthetic drug-induced myocardial depression and vasodilation occur. The resultant tamponade effect can lead to severe hypotension and cardiac arrest.[11,13,15,71,73]

The most important directives are to remain aware of the possibility of DHI and maximize expiratory time so that the lungs have time to empty before the next inspiratory cycle begins (Figure 14-4). If hypotension remains troublesome or of uncertain etiology, then a period of circuit disconnection—the apnea test—should resolve the situation and both diagnose and treat DHI.[11,13,47] DHI can also be detected by noting systolic pressure variation during the respiratory cycle.[81,82] This reflects the relative underfilling of the heart during inspiration, when the hyperinflated lungs impede venous return. Minor degrees of DHI-induced hypotension can also be treated with intravascular volume replacement and/or use of vasoconstrictor agents.

DHI can occur during OLV, particularly in patients with airflow obstruction.[12] Ducros et al measured the amount of auto-PEEP and trapped gas volume (ΔFRC) during two-lung and one-lung ventilation. They found a negative correlation between these measures of DHI and the FEV_1/FVC ratio (Figure 14-5).[77] The adverse hemodynamic effects of DHI are generally attenuated following surgical exposure and pleural opening because intrathoracic pressure is reduced; this permits an increase in minute ventilation and CO_2 clearance.

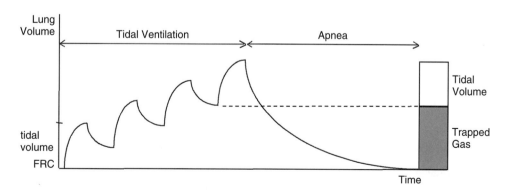

FIGURE 14-3 Development of dynamic hyperinflation during mechanical ventilation and schematic representation of lung deflation during apnea. *FRC,* Functional residual capacity. (From Tuxen DV: Acute severe asthma. In Oh TE [ed]: *Intensive care manual,* ed 3, Sydney, 1990, Butterworth.)

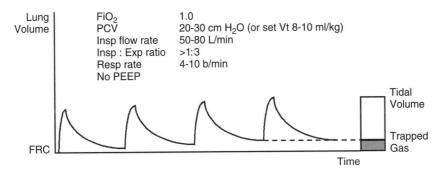

FIGURE 14-4 Reduction in dynamic hyperinflation (volume of trapped gas) with maximized expiratory time. *FRC*, Functional residual capacity; *PCV*, pressure control ventilation; *Vt*, tidal volume; *PEEP*, positive end-expiratory pressure. (Adapted from Myles PS, Ryder IG, Weeks AM: *J Cardiothorac Vasc Anesth* 111:100, 1997.)

The key to optimal ventilator management in patients with airflow obstruction is to maximize expiratory time (Figure 14-4). This is achieved by increasing inspiratory flow rate so that the same tidal volume can be delivered with a shorter inspiratory time, and accepting a smaller minute volume (i.e., a lower respiratory rate). These settings increase peak inspiratory pressure, but it must be understood that this does not equate to increased alveolar pressure—peak airway pressure primarily reflects resistance in the breathing circuit and major airways and is not transmitted to the pulmonary tissues. In fact, these ventilator settings are less likely than standard settings to cause pulmonary stretch injury, known as *volotrauma*.[72,73]

In general, PEEP is not recommended in patients with severe airflow obstruction, though there is some evidence that if extrinsically-applied PEEP is less than intrinsic PEEP, DHI will not be aggravated.[76]

An alternative mode of ventilation is high frequency jet ventilation (HFJV), which, theoretically at least, can reduce the risk of barotrauma because it operates at lower airway pressure.[83-85] HFJV has been found useful in patients with bronchopleural fistula and giant bullae.[83-84] Conacher has reported success with a modified form of HFJV in patients at risk of DHI, including many pulmonary transplant recipients using prolonged expiratory pauses to assist lung emptying.[85] A recent clinical trial, however, failed to demonstrate the superiority of HFJV in pulmonary transplantation when compared with conventional mechanical ventilation that included the ventilator settings just recommended.[86]

Patients with restrictive pulmonary diseases can usually be ventilated with a normal respiratory pattern and could gain additional benefit from PEEP.[42,87-89] Because positive pressure ventilation also increases PVR, patients with primary or secondary pulmonary hypertension could initially be adversely affected early after induction.[87] Correction of hypoxia and hypercapnia, however, might ultimately result in better hemodynamic control. The extent to which PEEP is transmitted to the circulation is dictated by the underlying pulmonary disease. Patients with interstitial pulmonary disease (low pulmonary compliance) are less likely to transmit intrapulmonary pressure compared with those who have emphysema (high pulmonary compliance).

The recent ARDSNet trial could have some relevance for intraoperative ventilatory management in patients with restrictive pulmonary disease. This trial enrolled 861 critically ill patients with acute lung injury or acute respiratory distress syndrome (ARDS) and randomly allocated them to "traditional tidal volume" (12 mL/kg) or "lower tidal volume" (6 mL/kg) groups. Ventilator management was directed toward reducing plateau pressure and pulmonary stretch-injury—patients receiving low tidal volumes had a mean plateau pressure of 25 cmH_2O, while the traditional tidal volume group had a mean plateau pressure of 33 cmH_2O. The investigators found a 22% survival advantage in the low tidal volume group (31% vs. 40%, $P = 0.007$).[88] This is consistent with a previous study demonstrating that, by reducing alveolar overdistention, PEEP and low tidal volumes were superior to traditional ventilation in ARDS.[89] Thus, it seems reasonable to reduce tidal volumes and mean airway pressure to less than 30 cmH_2O in patients with restrictive pulmonary disease undergoing pulmonary transplantation.

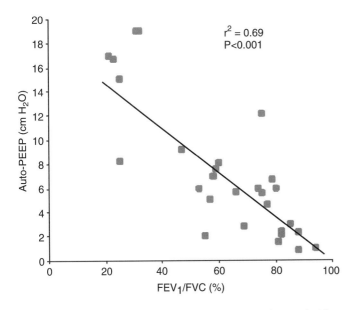

FIGURE 14-5 Relationship during OLV between the degree of airflow obstruction (FEV_1/FVC) and dynamic hyperinflation (auto-PEEP). (From Ducros L, Moutafis M, Castelain MH, et al: *J Cardiothorac Vasc Anesth* 13:35, 1999.)

One-Lung Ventilation

Patients with end-stage pulmonary disease might not tolerate OLV. For most patients, the sooner the hilum of the lung can be dissected and the pulmonary artery ligated, the better; to this end, most surgeons ligate each branch of the pulmonary artery as they proceed.[27] This procedure enhances pulmonary blood flow to the ventilated lung and also blunts the acute changes in PVR. Cardiopulmonary bypass is required in those patients who cannot tolerate OLV.[16,9,24,42] Maneuvers to improve oxygenation during OLV include all of those used during nontransplant thoracic surgery, such as intermittent lung inflation, providing CPAP to the nonventilated lung, or providing PEEP to the ventilated lung.[90] Hypoxia during OLV appears to be less of a problem in patients with emphysema; this can be explained by DHI-induced intrinsic PEEP (Figure 14-5).[2,77,91,92]

Pressure-controlled ventilation may be a superior mode of ventilation during OLV. Tugrul et al, in a crossover trial of 48 thoracic surgical patients, found that pressure-controlled ventilation, when compared with volume-controlled ventilation, resulted in lower airway pressures, decreased shunt, and improved oxygenation during OLV.[93]

Volatile agents are known to impair hypoxic pulmonary vasoconstriction in a dose-related fashion, but this effect is considered to be of minimal consequence in clinical practice.[94,95] Nevertheless, Abe et al found that propofol-based anesthesia was associated with reduced shunt fraction and improved oxygenation when compared with a period of volatile-based anesthesia during OLV.[96] For this reason, it is worth considering conversion to, or preference for, a total intravenous anesthetic technique for pulmonary transplantation.

Other steps that are frequently overlooked when attempting to improve oxygenation during OLV are to recheck DLT position with fiberoptic bronchoscopy, and to suction excess secretions that can cause regional atelectasis. Inhaled NO is not effective in improving oxygenation in most cases, but when combined with a pulmonary vasoconstrictor such as almitrine, pulmonary blood flow to areas of well-ventilated lung can be maximized; this combination can improve oxygenation during OLV.[97,98]

The foregoing information supports the following steps to improve gas exchange and cardiovascular function during mechanical ventilation and OLV[25]:

1. If restrictive pulmonary disease exists, use PEEP and reduced tidal volume (6 mL/kg).
2. Increase inspiratory flow rate (I:E ratio >1:3), and reduce respiratory rate (6 to 10 breaths/min).
3. Permissive hypercapnia with its higher $PaCO_2$ is clinically acceptable.
4. Use pressure-controlled ventilation.
5. Use total intravenous anesthesia.
6. Use inhaled NO and a pulmonary vasoconstrictor in combination.

Role of Nitric Oxide

NO is formed from L-arginine by the enzyme NO synthase, of which there are two distinct forms of the enzyme: constitutive and inducible.[99] NO is a highly lipophilic molecule that readily diffuses across endothelial and epithelial cell membranes into adjacent smooth muscle cells. There, it causes vasodilation via soluble guanylate cyclase and cyclic guanosine 3′,5′-monophosphate production. Endogenous NO regulates vascular tone and inhibits platelet activation and adhesion.[99] Local production is controlled by the constitutive isoform of NO synthase. An inducible form also exists; this form plays a role in inflammatory processes that include leukocyte activation and migration and smooth cell proliferation. Some factors have been shown to induce NO synthase; these include endotoxin, interleukins, tumor necrosis factor, bradykinin, and glutamate.[99-102] NO is thought to have antimicrobial activity.[99,103] The effects of NO are localized because it is rapidly metabolized by hemoglobin to form methemoglobin; NO has a plasma half-life of less than 12 seconds.

NO is available as a gas mixture in nitrogen. When inhaled, NO uptake occurs in well-ventilated regions of the lung, diverting pulmonary blood flow to well-ventilated alveoli.[104] Clinical studies have clearly established that inhaled NO is a selective pulmonary vasodilator and can lead to a marked improvement in right ventricular function, shunt fraction, and oxygenation.[62-65,98-99,104-106] Because of its short half-life, NO has no direct effect on the systemic circulation.

Randomized trials have demonstrated improved gas exchange using inhaled NO in critical-care patients with acute lung injury.[106,107] Similar benefits have been reported in pulmonary transplantation.[14,108-115] Maximal pulmonary vasodilation is achieved at a dose of 5–40 ppm, whereas improvement in pulmonary blood flow distribution in acute lung injury occurs at a dose of 1 to 10 ppm.[106] Inhaled NO, at a dose of 20 to 40 ppm, has been shown to reduce PVR and reverse RV failure, leading to improved cardiac output.[14,62,64,65,104,105] This is achieved without causing systemic hypotension.

Inhaled NO might ablate the reperfusion injury and protect the donor lung allograft.[34,108-110,112,113] Anecdotally, inhaled NO appears to offer beneficial effects not only during but also after pulmonary transplantation.[34,110-112] Kemming et al studied eight patients in the ICU with poor gas exchange and pulmonary hypertension after transplantation. There was a dose-dependent decrease in pulmonary arterial pressure of 3.0 mmHg, 4.5 mmHg, and 6.0 mmHg at 1, 5, and 8 ppm, respectively. There also was an improvement in oxygenation.[115]

Not all patients benefit from inhaled NO. Patients with COPD rely on hypoxic regulation of perfusion according to segmental pulmonary ventilation; NO interferes with this regulatory mechanism and can worsen gas exchange in these patients.[116] Thus, it appears that patients with increased shunt (e.g., ARDS), rather than those with poor ventilation-perfusion matching (eg. COPD), are most likely to benefit from NO.

Other vasodilator drugs have been used by the inhaled route in order to optimize selective pulmonary vasodilation. Like NO, inhaled epoprostenol and milrinone appear to have selective effects similar to those of NO and could likewise improve right ventricular function in patients with pulmonary hypertension.[64,117]

Pulmonary Hypertension and Right Ventricular Function

Pulmonary transplant recipients commonly have a degree of pulmonary hypertension. There is usually a fixed component, but because of the intimal and smooth muscle hypertrophy within the vessel wall, many recipients have a reactive component that can cause sudden, dramatic increases in PVR leading to acute right ventricular failure. The reversible component has sometimes been quantified during the preoperative evaluation, using either echocardiography or cardiac catheterization to determine pulmonary arterial and right-sided pressures, as well as the effect of pulmonary vasodilator administration. Right ventricular afterload is usually summarized by the transpulmonary gradient, calculated as mean pulmonary arterial pressure minus pulmonary capillary wedge pressure; values greater than 15 mmHg indicate markedly elevated PVR.

Patients with severe pulmonary hypertension are usually stabilized on medical therapy that includes a calcium antagonist and warfarin anticoagulation, with severe cases receiving domiciliary oxygen and, in some cases, intravenous epoprostenol.[118,119] Long-term inhalation of NO has also been used in severe cases.[65]

The right ventricle has special characteristics that must be appreciated. The pulmonary circulation is dynamic and is highly responsive to vasoconstrictive stimuli such as vasoactive drugs, hypercarbia, acidosis, agitation, or pain. An acute increase in PVR can lead to an immediate deterioration in right ventricular function. Note that the ability of the right ventricle to cope with such events is inversely proportional to the general status of the patient. Those with long-standing pulmonary hypertension have a "trained" right ventricle because of compensatory right ventricular hypertrophy and can generally cope with such changes, but other patients develop acute right ventricular failure even after moderate increases in PVR. Such changes occur quickly but can often be corrected before dramatic irreversible processes begin.

The most dangerous period of anesthesia is at induction, when anesthetic drugs induce myocardial depression and vasodilation, and when mechanical ventilation increases PVR. This can result in profound hypotension, which can threaten coronary perfusion, especially to the right ventricle. The right coronary artery supplies the sinoatrial node in 65% of patients and the atrioventricular node in 85% of patients. Although right coronary artery flow is biphasic (including systole and diastole) in healthy subjects, in patients with pulmonary hypertension and right ventricular hypertrophy blood flow assumes the characteristics of left coronary flow, being dependent on the diastolic phase of the cardiac cycle. This is why hypotension associated with acute right ventricular failure commonly manifests as severe bradycardia or asystole and can lead to an irretrievable situation if not corrected. Cardiac arrest at induction of anesthesia for pulmonary transplantation has been reported.[17,18]

The interrelationship between the right and left ventricles is a crucial determinant in pulmonary transplantation.[47,120-123] If the right ventricle is impaired, it will not pump sufficient blood flow to fill the left ventricle, which in turn will fail and not provide the sufficient systemic perfusion pressure needed for right coronary artery flow and right ventricular perfusion (Figure 14-6). Right ventricular failure is associated with flattening of the interventricular septum towards the left ventricular (LV) cavity, and because of underfilling and impaired contractility, there is further impairment of left ventricular

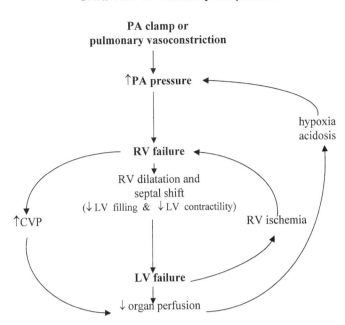

FIGURE 14-6 The effect of ventricular interaction. An acute rise in pulmonary arterial (PA) pressure can result in acute right ventricular (RV) failure, leading to right ventricle dilatation, septal shift towards the left ventricle, and left ventricular failure. *CVP,* Central venous pressure; *LV,* left ventricular. (From Myles PS: *Semin Cardiothorac Vasc Anesth* 2:140, 1998.)

function—which, in turn, aggravates right ventricular failure and worsens the situation. This relationship is known as ventricular dependence or ventricular interaction, and can be appreciated readily with the increasing use of TEE in pulmonary transplantation (Figures 14-7 and 14-8).[61,123,124] The final step of this circuitous process is failure to perfuse the

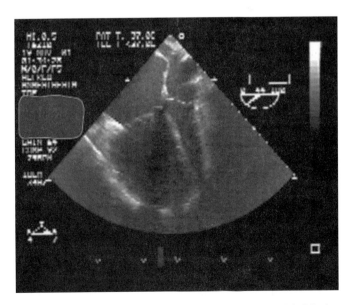

FIGURE 14-7 Acute right ventricular dilatation with septal shift, following pulmonary artery clamping during bilateral sequential lung transplantation. Midesophageal four-chamber view.

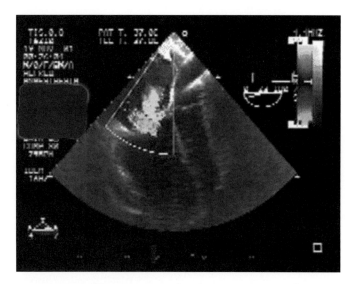

FIGURE 14-8 Acute right ventricular failure and severe tricuspid regurgitation. Midesophageal four-chamber view. (See also Color Plate 6.)

sinoatrial node, which leads to severe bradycardia and cardiac arrest. These processes can occur quickly and demand urgent identification and treatment. Appreciation of this concept and knowledge of the principles of how this process can be circumvented are crucial for anesthesiologists involved in pulmonary and cardiac transplantation (Table 14-3).

These principles include identification of those at risk, vigilance and invasive monitoring, maintenance of intravascular volume and myocardial contractility, and judicious use of vasoactive agents.[9,121,125-133] Acute rises in PVR occur after induction of anesthesia, during institution of OLV, and most - dramatically, during pulmonary artery ligation and clamping.[6-9] At each of these times, pulmonary hypertension is made worse by hypoxia, hypercarbia, and metabolic acidosis.[45,65,66,134,135]

The anesthesiologist should closely monitor pulmonary arterial and central venous pressure (CVP). An increase in CVP is a simple and reliable measure of right ventricular dysfunction. The right ventricle can also be directly observed via the surgical incision; right ventricular dysfunction is usually noted by the surgeon. Other monitoring (continuous cardiac output, right ventricular ejection fraction, mixed venous oximetry), but especially TEE, can be of assistance.[48,122,136]

Optimal right ventricular preload has been determined, at least in patients with right ventricular myocardial infarction. Berisha et al found that a CVP of 10 to 14 mmHg was associated with a better cardiac output in these patients.[131] Fluid loading should be used cautiously, however, because right ventricular function can deteriorate rapidly.[121,122,128] Increases in preload beyond a CVP of 15 mmHg have an adverse effect on right ventricular function in the presence of pulmonary hypertension.[124] This could be due to a relatively marked increase in RV wall tension and reduction in right-sided myocardial perfusion.

Right ventricular function can be improved with inotrope and pulmonary vasodilator therapy—for example, epinephrine, 20 to 200 ng/kg/min and sodium nitroprusside, 0.2 to 1.0 μg/kg/min, or epoprostenol, 2 to 10 ng/kg/min.[17,119,121,127-133] Alternatively, a milrinone infusion, 0.125 to 0.375 μg/kg/min may be used. This regimen is usually successful in those patients with moderate elevations in PVR, but care should be exercised in those with more severe pulmonary hypertension and right ventricular failure. Unfortunately, all currently available intravenous pulmonary vasodilators can result in unacceptable systemic hypotension, necessitating a reduction in infusion rate and possibly a concomitant increase in inotrope requirement (which can actually increase PVR). In these cases, the most reliable method of avoiding what might become an irretrievable situation is to treat systemic hypotension with a vasoconstrictor (e.g., metaraminol 0.5 to 2.0 mg, or a norepinephrine infusion 20 to 200 ng/kg/min).[6,47,121,124,125,128,132]

TABLE 14-3

Management of Right Ventricular Dysfunction Associated with Pulmonary Vasoconstriction or Pulmonary Artery Clamping

GENERAL PRINCIPLES

1. Preoperative evaluation	For identification of at-risk patients
2. Monitoring	Pulmonary artery catheter
	Transesophageal echocardiography
3. Avoid pulmonary vasoconstriction	Hypoxia, hypercarbia and acidosis
	Reflex response to light anesthesia

SPECIFIC TREATMENT OF MILD-TO-MODERATE PULMONARY HYPERTENSION

4. Pulmonary vasodilator therapy	Sodium nitroprusside, 0.2-2 μg/kg/min
	Epoprostenol, 2-15 ng/kg/min
5. Inotrope therapy	Epinephrine, 20-200 ng/kg/min
	Dobutamine, 5-20 μg/kg/min
	Milrinone, 0.125-0.375 μg/kg/min
6. Inhaled nitric oxide	NO, 20–40 ppm

TREATMENT OF ACUTE RIGHT VENTRICULAR FAILURE ASSOCIATED WITH SEVERE PULMONARY HYPERTENSION

7. Inhaled nitric oxide	NO, 40 ppm
8. Systemic vasoconstrictor therapy	Norepinephrine, 20–200 ng/kg/min
9. If unresponsive...	Initiate cardiopulmonary bypass

From Myles PS: *Semin Cardiothorac Vasc Anesth* 2:140, 1998.

This treatment increases systemic perfusion pressure and so improves right ventricular perfusion.[47,121,132] Although enhancement of right ventricular perfusion obviously contradicts the usual recommendation of using a pulmonary vasodilator, in those patients with acute RV failure, such enhancement is essential because of ventricular interaction. The increased systemic vascular resistance (left ventricular afterload) shifts the interventricular septum towards the right, which can assist left ventricular filling and contractility.

Whether a pulmonary vasodilator or a systemic vasoconstrictor is more beneficial for any particular patient depends on the specificity of these agents—how much systemic hypotension is caused by the pulmonary vasodilator or how much pulmonary vasoconstriction is caused by the systemic vasoconstrictor. This is difficult to predict at any particular time during the operation, so a trial of one or the other is required. Administration of a vasoconstrictor via a left atrial catheter has also been described, aiming to bypass the pulmonary circulation and reduce PVR, although a recent double-blind trial failed to demonstrate any benefit from this technique early after cardiac transplantation.[130,137] As suggested above, mild-to-moderate elevations in PVR are usually best treated initially with a vasodilator, and more severe elevations in PVR, especially if they are associated with acute right ventricular dysfunction, are best treated with a vasoconstrictor such as norepinephrine.

Myles and Venema were able to reverse an acute deterioration during BSLTx and avoid cardiopulmonary bypass using inhaled NO at 40 ppm.[14] Inhaled NO does not result in systemic hypotension and usually allows a reduction in inotrope requirement. This is an extremely useful addition to the armamentarium, as it allows concomitant use of systemic vasoconstrictors, thus maintaining right ventricular and vital organ perfusion. If the described interventions fail, then cardiopulmonary bypass is indicated.

Transesophageal Echocardiography

Use of TEE during cardiac surgery has increased dramatically in the last ten years and is also being used during cardiac and pulmonary transplantation. Routine assessment of cardiac structures and function, with a particular emphasis on right ventricular function and assessment of the pulmonary arterial and venous anastomoses, is becoming routine in many transplant centers. Nevertheless, TEE assessment of the right ventricle can be difficult. The right ventricle has complex morphology and prominent trabeculations, which can make volume estimations problematic.[45,136] In most patients, it is a very distensible chamber prone to alterations in shape according to volume status and phases of the respiratory cycle. Right-side ventricular systolic function can be assessed by right ventricle fractional area change and free wall excursion.[45,136] The configuration of the interventricular septum is also a useful guide to right ventricular function—pressure or volume overload leads to flattening of the septum towards the left ventricle.[122]

Schenk et al used transthoracic echocardiography to measure right ventricle dimensions prior to pulmonary transplantation. They found good correlations with magnetic resonance imaging assessment of right ventricular end-diastolic and end-systolic areas and so were able to estimate right ventricle frac-

tional area change ($r = 0.84$, $P < 0.001$). Imaging quality was poorer in patients with COPD.[136]

Vizza et al reviewed records of 434 patients with end-stage pulmonary disease who had undergone evaluation for pulmonary transplantation.[44] Right-side ventricular dysfunction, defined as a right-side ventricular ejection fraction less than 45% calculated from radionuclide ventriculography, was present in 267 patients (67%), including 94% of those with pulmonary vascular disease. Left-side ventricular dysfunction was uncommon (6%), except in those who had pulmonary hypertension (20%), suggesting a degree of ventricular interaction. The prevalence of moderate or severe tricuspid regurgitation on echocardiography was related to right-side ventricular function: 23% if right ventricular dysfunction was present compared with 3% if right-side ventricular function was normal. Both right-side ventricular and left-side ventricular dysfunction generally improved following transplantation.[44] A similar study was done by Florea et al in 103 patients with cystic fibrosis awaiting pulmonary transplantation. They found that right-side ventricular dysfunction (but not left-side ventricular dysfunction) was common in their population. Right-side ventricular dysfunction was associated with the degree of hypoxemia and hypercapnia and was probably secondary to increased PVR.[45]

Right-side ventricular diastolic dysfunction can be assessed using transtricuspid valve and hepatic vein flows and estimations of relaxation time, E- and A-wave velocities, and E-wave deceleration time, as with the left ventricle.[138] It should be noted that these can be affected by respiratory variations to a greater extent than can left ventricular diastolic assessment.

An important issue in pulmonary transplantation is whether the patient has a patent foramen ovale (PFO).[139] Such patients are at risk of right-to-left shunt, leading to hypoxia and systemic embolism. The factors determining the clinical significance of a PFO include the following[139]:

- Its size
- The pressure gradient between the right atrium and left atrium
- The direction of inferior vena cava (IVC) flow

Factors increasing PVR, such as coughing, mechanical ventilation, pulmonary vasoconstriction, and other causes of increased CVP such as cardiac tamponade, can increase the degree of shunt markedly. An interesting study was conducted by Cujic et al, who compared the effect of 10 cm PEEP on shunt fraction in seven patients who had a PFO with 39 patients who did not. The investigators found an increased shunt fraction in those with a PFO, whereas shunt fraction decreased in those without a PFO.[140] Thus it appears that PEEP could be detrimental in patients with a PFO; this has direct relevance to patients undergoing pulmonary transplantation. The direction of IVC flow can change during surgery and, with alteration in geometry, can increase flow through a PFO.[139]

On some occasions, there is unexplained poor gas exchange or postimplantation pulmonary edema following allograft implantation, which might be due to restricted pulmonary venous drainage at the site of anastomosis (Figures 14-9 and 14-10). Both the pulmonary arterial and venous anastomoses can be identified using TEE in most cases.[19,141,142] Cherqui et al evaluated the pulmonary arterial and venous anastomoses in 18 patients during pulmonary transplantation. All of the

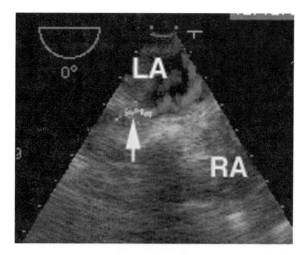

FIGURE 14-9 Color Doppler echocardiography showing a mosaic pattern of right lower pulmonary vein inflow *(arrows)* where it enters the left atrium (LA) and revealing severe obstruction of its anastomosis. (From Huang YC, Cheng YJ, Lin YH, et al: *Anesth Analg* 91:558, 2000. (See also Color Plate 7.)

pulmonary arterial (n = 13) anastomoses were visualized; one had a moderate stenosis that did not require reoperation. Of the 22 pulmonary venous anastomoses, 16 were considered normal, with a diameter greater than 0.5 cm and peak systolic flow velocity less than 100 cm/sec. In five cases, the anastomoses were not considered normal but did not require reoperation. In one case—a patient with early allograft dysfunction—severe pulmonary vein stenosis was identified that led to reoperation.[141] Others have reported similar experiences.[19,142] Huang et al suggest that a pulmonary vein diameter of less than 0.25 cm represents a critical threshold for allograft failure.[19] Unilateral allograft pulmonary edema should prompt TEE evaluation of the pulmonary venous anastomoses. Prompt detection of pulmonary vein stenosis can lead to surgical correction before the patient leaves the operating room.

Clamping and Unclamping of the Pulmonary Artery

Ligation or clamping of the pulmonary artery improves oxygenation during OLV but also increases pulmonary arterial pressure, which can lead to acute right ventricular failure. This is less likely to occur in patients with mild-to-moderate pulmonary hypertension, particularly if they have a degree of right ventricular hypertrophy. Patients with severe pulmonary hypertension cannot tolerate pulmonary artery clamping and so in most cases require cardiopulmonary bypass.

After completion of the pulmonary allograft anastomoses, the pulmonary venous-left atrial clamp is released in order to allow retrograde flow and removal of residual pneumoplegia, metabolites, and air from the allograft circulation. At the same time, gentle inflation of the allograft is commenced, and the pulmonary artery clamp is then removed.

Reperfusion of the allograft is sometimes associated with profound hypotension.[8,47] This has several possible causes, all of which can occur simultaneously. Causes include coronary artery air embolism (particularly to the right coronary artery due to its superior anatomic location), systemic release of residual allograft pneumoplegia and epoprostenol delivered during procurement, and possibly release of a variety of inflammatory mediators generated during reperfusion (Figure 14-11). It is not uncommon to observe marked ECG ST-segment elevation and/or ventricular arrhythmias, even in those with documented normal coronary arteries. Hence, hypotension might be secondary to both systemic vasodilation and right ventricular ischemia and once again is best treated with a vasoconstrictor (e.g., incremental metaraminol or phenylephrine) or a norepinephrine infusion. The initial dose required to treat hypotension at this stage can be very high (e.g., norepinephrine 100 to 2,000 ng/kg/min), but this usually reduces rapidly over a period of 5 to 15 minutes. Prolonged hypotension suggests

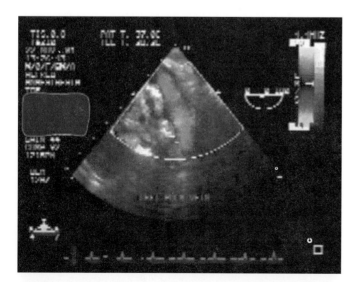

FIGURE 14-10 Color Doppler echocardiography of an acceptable left upper pulmonary vein anastomosis with pulmonary transplantation. (See also Color Plate 8.)

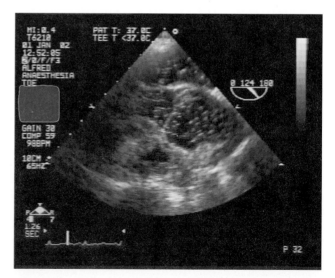

FIGURE 14-11 Aortic air embolism following unclamping of the pulmonary artery during bilateral sequential lung transplantation. Note the propensity of air bubbles to collect around the orifice of the right coronary artery. Midesophageal aortic valve long-axis view.

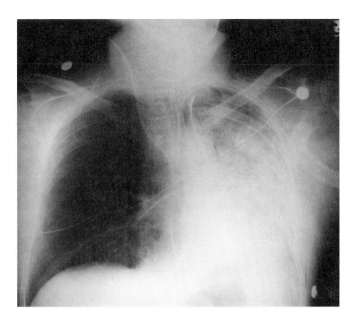

FIGURE 14-12 Postoperative chest x-ray of a single-lung transplant recipient with emphysema. The pulmonary allograft has patchy infiltrates, possibly due to edema and/or reperfusion injury. There is marked mediastinal shift due to native lung hyperinflation.

other problems, such as allograft dysfunction leading to persistent hypoxia, hypercapnia, elevated PVR and RV failure.[7,19] Ongoing hemodynamic support could require systemic vasoconstriction, inotropes, and/or inhaled NO. Reinstitution of two-lung ventilation might further relieve the situation, as PVR reduces and gas exchange improves.

Pulmonary Allograft Reinflation and Assessment

Ischemic reperfusion injury is a major cause of early allograft failure after transplantation.[13,111,112,115,143,144] Stimulation of oxygen-free radicals, followed by activation of inflammatory mediators, can lead to acute lung injury and impaired gas exchange. Administration of inhaled NO at the time of harvest could improve early allograft function, possibly by attenuating oxidant injury during storage and reperfusion.[34] Benefit might also occur with administration of NO postimplantation.[108-111,145] The known adverse effects of rapid lung reexpansion leading to pulmonary edema should be appreciated.[146] The allograft is particularly prone to edema and reperfusion injury and should always be considered to be at risk of acute lung injury. Therefore gentle, low-pressure manual reinflations should be accompanied by direct inspection of the allograft, aiming to avoid hyperinflation and limiting airway pressure to less than 30 cmH$_2$O. "Protective" mechanical ventilation strategies should then be employed.[72,87-89]

PEEP is commonly prescribed as part of the ventilator management of most critically ill patients, as it promotes alveolar recruitment and so enables a reduction in FIO$_2$.[87-89] The resultant increase in pulmonary compliance also leads to a reduction in intraalveolar pressure, in this way reducing another possible cause of pulmonary injury.[72,89,145,147] Many institutions employ low levels of PEEP to the allograft after implantation.[6,7]

Because of the reasons outlined previously, PEEP may not be suitable for patients with COPD who are undergoing SLTx after reestablishment of two-lung ventilation because the newly implanted pulmonary allograft has a much lower compliance than the native lung; this reduced compliance can result in asymmetric distribution of tidal volume, leading to native lung hyperinflation, mediastinal shift, and circulatory collapse (Figures 14-12 through 14-14). This problem can be addressed by adjusting ventilator management and sometimes requires differential lung ventilation with a DLT.[70,148-151] In such cases, the native emphysematous lung is ventilated as described earlier (maximizing expiratory time) and the pulmonary allograft is ventilated with reduced FIO$_2$ and low levels of PEEP. This obviously requires two ventilators and might need to be continued for some time postoperatively.[149]

Successful allograft implantation and pulmonary function can be assessed almost immediately. The lung should appear pink after reperfusion, and the airway anastomoses can be checked with fiberoptic bronchoscopy. There should be a dramatic reduction in PA pulmonary arterial pressures and an improvement in right ventricular function. There should also be an improvement in CO$_2$ clearance and oxygenation, allowing a reduction in FIO$_2$ and minute ventilation. A reduction in airway pressure is common. The pulmonary vascular anastomoses can be checked by TEE.[19,141] If there is doubt about any of these, they should be refashioned. In particular, pulmonary venous obstruction can lead to pulmonary edema and hypoxia.[19] Surgical retraction of the heart or an atrial clamp can transiently

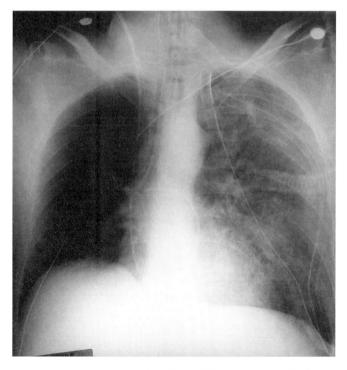

FIGURE 14-13 Correction of mediastinal shift with placement of a double-lumen tube and independent differential lung ventilation. The native lung is emphysematous and prone to hyperinflation, so ventilator settings are adjusted to maximize expiratory time (see also Figure 14-4). The pulmonary allograft is edematous and noncompliant and is ventilated with more typical ventilator settings that include positive end-expiratory pressure.

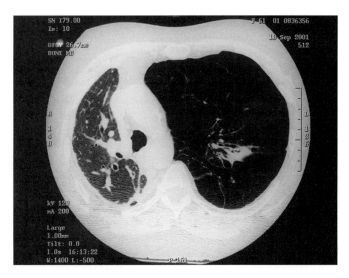

FIGURE 14-14 Postoperative CT scan of a single lung.

cause the same problem. Further objective assessments can also be made. Both the arterial end-tidal CO_2 gradient (an indicator of alveolar deadspace) and the alveolar-arterial oxygen gradient (an indicator of gas transfer and ventilation:perfusion matching) should decline.[8,152] Pulmonary compliance and resistance can also be measured with side-stream spirometry.[153]

Avoiding Cardiopulmonary Bypass

The benefits of CPB include improved surgical access and avoidance of the hemodynamic instability associated with pulmonary artery clamping. Patients could be exposed to fewer episodes of pulmonary hypertension, hypotension, DHI, hypoxia, hypercapnia, hypothermia, and acid-base disturbances. They are at increased risk of coagulopathy, however, which can lead to excessive postoperative bleeding and blood transfusion; they are also at increased risk of a greater positive fluid balance, leading to pulmonary edema.[6,22,23,154] CPB might be associated with increased pulmonary allograft dysfunction.[21-23]

The need for CPB is dependent on preoperative and intraoperative factors. Some patient conditions cannot be managed without CPB; these include severe pulmonary hypertension, persistent hypoxia, and acidosis. CPB is used for all patients undergoing HLTx, and some institutions routinely employ CPB for patients undergoing BSLTx, either generally or selectively.[6-8,12] There is some evidence that outcome might be improved if CPB can be avoided, though if the recipient is grossly unstable during the procedure, CPB should be considered.[6,8,41]

In general, patients with severe pulmonary hypertension and/or congenital heart disease usually require CPB, whereas those with suppurative pulmonary disease, restrictive pulmonary disease, or emphysema do not.[6] For patients undergoing BSLTx, the lung with the lowest perfusion should generally be replaced first, as replacement minimizes pulmonary hypertension and impaired gas exchange and could reduce the need for CPB.[27] Several attempts at predicting the need for CPB have been described.[24,41,42] Although useful as guidelines, these criteria have not been validated, particularly according to

recent practices with which inhaled NO is now available, DHI is better understood, and the tolerability of permissive hypercapnia is recognized. The need for CPB also depends on the experience and skills of the surgical and anesthetic teams.

Aeba et al, in a retrospective review of all pulmonary transplants, compared 55 patients who had their procedure done with CPB with 45 who did not. The CPB group had poorer oxygenation, more pulmonary infiltrates, and a longer period of mechanical ventilation. Mortality at 1 month was lower in the non-CPB group than in the CPB group (4% vs. 18%, $P = 0.033$).[22] A later study from the same group restricted to BSLTx compared 37 patients who had their procedure done with CPB with 57 who did not. Once again, the CPB group had poorer oxygenation, more pulmonary infiltrates, and a longer period of mechanical ventilation. They also found a lower 30-day mortality rate in the non-CPB group (7% vs. 14%), but this was not statistically significant ($P = 0.30$).[154] In contrast, Triantafillou et al did not find any effect of CPB on duration of mechanical ventilation or ICU stay in a series of 162 pulmonary transplant recipients.[24]

Although most patients undergoing SLTx and BSLTx can undergo their procedures without CPB, they remain at risk of hypoxia, hypercapnia, hypotension, and arrhythmias during various stages (as described in the foregoing discussion). Severe unresponsive deterioration in gas exchange and hemodynamic status demands urgent CPB. Surgical access can also be compromised by pulmonary tissue, adhesions, or small thoracic cavity size, particularly during BSLTx, and so CPB may be requested. Poor allograft function after implantation of the first lung during BSLTx might require CPB for implantation of the remaining lung.[6,8] In the author's institution, increasing experience shows that the requirement for CPB has decreased significantly, to less than 20% of BSLTx procedures.[6] CPB is rarely required for SLTx.

The introduction of heparin-bonded circuits and extracorporeal membrane oxygenation (ECMO) may be a useful advance in pulmonary transplantation.[148,155] Ko et al described their experience of ECMO in 15 patients undergoing pulmonary transplantation. The advantages of using femoral ECMO rather than conventional CPB in pulmonary transplantation include better surgical exposure (because the operative field is not disturbed by the bypass cannulae), stable cardiopulmonary function, reduced blood loss, and reduced transfusion requirements. Red blood cell transfusion requirements with SLTx were similar in 10 adult patients undergoing uncomplicated SLTx with ECMO support and in eight patients undergoing SLTx without any extracorporeal circulatory support.[155] ECMO support made postoperative critical care easier in recipients with graft lung edema, in that ECMO could be weaned off and removed at the bedside with no major complications.

Risks and Benefits of Epidural Analgesia

Patients undergoing SLTx have an extensive thoracotomy incision at the level of the fifth or sixth intercostal space, with adjacent rib resection. Most of those undergoing BSLTx have a "clam-shell" incision extending horizontally across both thoracic cavities at the lower end of the sternum.[27] Both these incisions result in significant postoperative pain, which impairs ventilation and sputum clearance. Use of postoperative opioids can further impair respiratory function and aggravate CO_2 retention, to the extent that ventilator weaning and extubation can be delayed. For this reason, postoperative epidural analgesia is frequently provided for these patients.[6,8,47] HLTx recipients have a midline sternotomy incision that is associated with less pain postoperatively and does not necessitate epidural analgesia. Patients with severe pulmonary hypertension are usually receiving long-term anticoagulation, so neuraxial blockade is contraindicated for them.

Although epidural techniques can reduce general anesthetic requirements (and perhaps reduce the risk of intraoperative awareness), the potential for hypotension and ultimately a further reduction in depth of anesthesia could be counterproductive. Some anesthesiologists avoid use of epidural local anesthetic intraoperatively if major blood loss and hemodynamic instability are a possibility.[156] Another approach is to use high-dose remifentanil, 0.4 to 1.0 µg/kg/min, to provide intraoperative stress ablation and hypnotic-sparing effect, and to commence the epidural infusion at the end of the procedure.[156]

Another major concern with thoracic epidural anesthesia is the risk of epidural hematoma because most patients are given heparin intraoperatively—routinely 5000 units before PA clamping, or full heparinization if CPB is required. Nevertheless, epidural anesthesia is considered safe if performed at least one hour before heparin administration.[6,8,158] There is some evidence that the risk of epidural abscess could be as high as 1:1930 after epidural block in a broad variety of surgical procedures. Wang et al remarked that additional risk factors for abscess formation included long duration of catheterization (3 days or longer), immunosuppression, and low-dose anticoagulation.[159] Thus the pulmonary transplant population can be considered to be at increased risk, and extra vigilance is required perioperatively.

The benefits of improved postoperative analgesia are persuasive despite these concerns. There is recent evidence from systematic reviews of randomized trials that conclude that major regional techniques improve outcome in many types of surgery.[160,161] Furthermore, two recent large trials investigating the effects of epidural anesthesia and analgesia in major abdominal surgery suggest that epidural analgesia reduces the risk of postoperative respiratory failure.[162,163] Rigg et al clearly demonstrated that epidural analgesia was associated with lower pain scores during the first three postoperative days (see Chapter 20).[163]

Fluid Management and Blood Transfusion

The pulmonary allograft is at increased risk of pulmonary edema because of the possibility of reexpansion pulmonary edema, reperfusion injury, and absence of lymphatic drainage.[8,9,144,164-166] Pulmonary transplantation (especially HLTx and BSLTx) can be a prolonged procedure, with significant blood loss and requiring large amounts of fluid administration.[6,23] This is particularly the case if the patient has undergone previous thoracic surgery whereby vascular pleural adhesions may be present, or if CPB is required. The recommended fluid management regimen remains uncertain, but it appears logical to avoid excessive crystalloid administration

and favor fluid restriction in order to minimize the risk of pulmonary edema.[167] Fluid restriction is favored in the current management of ARDS.[87]

Patients undergoing pulmonary transplantation with CPB generally have a larger positive fluid balance, leading to pulmonary edema and impaired gas exchange.[6,22,23,154] In contrast, there are some situations where, for technical reasons, pulmonary venous drainage can be improved by stopping mechanical ventilation and completing the implantation with CPB or ECMO; this procedure might reduce pulmonary edema formation.[12,27,155]

The need for blood transfusion is dictated by the patients' preoperative hemoglobin concentration (which is often high in this population because of chronic hypoxia) and by their intraoperative course. Regular patient assessment can guide rational fluid administration.[168] Recent evidence suggests that a restrictive approach to red-cell transfusion in critical-care patients could be associated with reduced mortality.[169] If indicated, fresh-frozen plasma and platelet transfusion might also be required. Homologous transfusion can be reduced with intraoperative autologous red-cell salvage, which is particularly useful in those patients who have extensive vascular adhesions.[170] In these cases, early administration of an antifibrinolytic agent might also be helpful.[171,172] Aprotinin has been shown to be the most effective agent in cardiac surgery and might offer additional benefits in pulmonary transplantation.[173,174]

Other Drug Therapy

Patients undergoing pulmonary transplantation receive a variety of drugs. These include anesthetic, vasoactive, and antibiotic agents. Routine immunosuppressant medications include oral cyclosporine, 3 to 5 mg/kg, oral or intravenous azathioprine, 1 to 4 mg/kg, and intravenous methylprednisolone—500 mg at commencement of the procedure and a further 500 mg following allograft implantation. These medications are continued postoperatively, with their dosages adjusted according to serum levels (cyclosporine), renal function (cyclosporine), and white blood cell count (azathioprine).

Cyclosporine acts by inhibiting T-cell function, lymphokine production, and T-cell growth factors, all of which suppress cell-mediated immunity. It appears to have no effect on hemopoeisis and phagocyte function, and so it has minimal impact on the risk of infection. Cyclosporine can cause renal and liver toxicity as well as seizures and neurotoxicity; hypertension is common with chronic administration. It can prolong the action of nondepolarizing neuromuscular blocking drugs, but in clinical practice this could be offset by the antagonistic effect of azathioprine at the neuromuscular junction.[175,176]

Azathioprine is converted to 6-mercaptopurine, an antimetabolite that blocks DNA metabolism and cell proliferation. Antithymocyte globulin, or a monoclonal antibody known as OKT3, can provide additional anti–T cell immunosuppression in the early phase after transplantation and so might be indicated for recipients at higher risk of early allograft rejection. Other immunosuppressant drugs are being developed for solid organ transplantation.[177] For example, sirolimus might have a role in patients with recurrent acute rejection, particularly if such rejection is associated with other immunosuppressant drug intolerance.[177,178]

Prophylactic antibiotic therapy is routine and can be tailored to local practice. Patients with infective pulmonary diseases such as cystic fibrosis and bronchiectasis require individualization of antibiotic administration to cover resistant organisms such as *Pseudomonas* and multidrug-resistant *Enterococci* and *Staphylococci*. Some recipients might have been recently hospitalized for respiratory failure and so could harbor resistant organisms as well. Discussion with a microbiologist or the treating respiratory physician should clarify the best antibiotic regimen for such patients. A typical order could include vancomycin, 10 mg/kg, or ticarcilllin, 3.1 gm, and tobramycin, 3 mg/kg. For all antibiotics, repeat dosing could be required intraoperatively, and this possibility should not be overlooked.

Patients with cyanotic congenital heart disease and those with severe pulmonary hypertension are usually receiving long-term warfarin anticoagulation. This can be reversed at the commencement of surgery with intravenous vitamin K, 5 to 10 mg, and fresh-frozen plasma transfusion.

Many patients undergoing pulmonary transplantation have a reversible component to their obstructive airways disease; for these patients, preoperative bronchodilator therapy should be continued intraoperatively if SLTx is undertaken. Bronchodilator therapy can reduce the risks of hypoxia, hypercapnia, and DHI and might also reduce the need for CPB.

Postoperative Care

Immediate tracheal extubation in the operating room can be achieved in selected cases, particularly for those patients undergoing SLTx. The advantages of immediate extubation include avoiding exchanging a DLT for a single-lumen tube, optimizing cough and sputum clearance, avoiding mechanical ventilation leading to anastomotic leak or other barotrauma, and early awakening and mobilization. Nevertheless, most pulmonary transplant recipients require a period of stabilization in the ICU before allowing awakening and tracheal extubation, yet this can occur within six hours if there are no complications.[47,53]

Early evaluation of allograft function includes ABG assessment of gas exchange and chest x-ray, and, if indicated, can include repeat bronchoscopy and pulmonary biopsy as well.

Postoperatively, adequate ventilation and clearance of secretions are assisted by effective pain relief. Multimodal analgesic techniques using opioid-sparing agents such as paracetamol and tramadol, and regional anesthesia constitute an important advance in such patients.[159,160,179] These measures allow a reduction in opioid administration and can reduce respiratory depression. Nonsteroidal antiinflammatory drugs (NSAIDs) are generally contraindicated in view of the concern regarding cyclosporine-induced nephrotoxicity. Patient agitation or respiratory distress could signal underlying surgical complications such as pneumothorax, hemothorax, or pulmonary collapse, in which case an immediate chest x-ray is warranted. The functional status of the epidural block, if used, should be confirmed and optimized with supplementary dosing (see Chapter 20).

The presence of infiltrates on chest x-ray is almost universal after pulmonary transplantation.[144,164,169] The causes include ischemic reperfusion injury associated with alveolar endothelial leakage and impaired interstitial fluid clearance due to absence of lymphatic drainage. These might or might not be associated with impaired gas exchange. Other causes include infection and rejection; these usually occur later and can be associated with prolonged stay in the ICU and hospital.

Boujakis et al analyzed their institutional SLTx data, comparing the chest radiographic scores of postoperative pulmonary infiltrates in those patients with pulmonary hypertension and emphysema. Pulmonary blood flow distribution should be more uneven in pulmonary hypertension, as the allograft receives preferential flow. The investigators could not find any evidence that pre-existing pulmonary hypertension in the native lung was associated with reperfusion injury as indicated by the extent of pulmonary infiltrates.[144]

Patients with COPD undergoing SLTx are at risk of their remaining native lung being subject to hyperinflation because of its high compliance.[70,148-150] This situation can lead to mediastinal shift and hemodynamic disturbances during and after surgery, particularly if the allograft is edematous and noncompliant (Figures 14-12 and 14-13). In these circumstances, it is prudent to leave the DLT in situ and employ differential lung ventilation.[151]

Postoperative oxygen therapy needs to be individualized in patients with severe pulmonary disease. The pulmonary allograft lacks stretch-receptor innervation, and the recipient is particularly prone to CO_2 retention in the weeks after transplantation. Patients with chronic CO_2 retention could be at risk of significant respiratory depression if their respiratory drive is dependent on hypoxia-stimulated chemoreceptors. Measurement of preoperative ABGs can guide an appropriate postoperative oxygen saturation target; in many cases, a level of 87% to 92% is sufficient and can be accurately achieved by using Venturi mask oxygen delivery.[87]

Common causes of early postoperative mortality include infection, rejection, hypoxic-ischemic encephalopathy secondary to severe hypotension or cardiac arrest, and ischemic reperfusion injury.[20] Other significant postoperative complications include excess bleeding, acute right ventricular failure, neurologic injury (brain, phrenic nerve, brachial plexus), drug toxicity (immunosuppressants, antibiotics, sedatives) and muscle weakness (myopathy, neuropathy, malnutrition).[3,10,22,27,29,69,110,111,143,148,180-183]

Subsequent Anesthesia for the Pulmonary Transplant Recipient

Advances in pulmonary transplantation have seen 55% of recipients survive at least 5 years after transplantation.[1] Many recipients require surgery or other procedures in the years after transplantation.[5] This finding might be due to complications associated with immunosuppression (infection, tumor, coronary artery disease, renal failure, osteonecrosis) or rejection (bronchiolitis obliterans). Common procedures include bronchoscopy for biopsy or dilatation and possibly stenting of bronchial stenosis, open lung biopsy, drainage of abscess or osteomyelitis, tumor excision, and other unrelated surgical conditions.

Most transplant recipients can be managed according to routine practice that includes optimal perioperative respiratory care, along with maintenance of immunosuppression. The emphasis in patient assessment should be on inquiring about dypsnea or oxygen dependence, exercise capacity, sputum production, current drug therapy, and details of recent hospitalizations. Details of any recent episodes of allograft rejection or infection should be scrutinized. The likelihood of subglottic stenosis, which is common after prolonged tracheal intubation or tracheostomy, can be identified by hoarseness or stridor, or noted on chest x-ray, CT scan, or previous bronchoscopy. Results of recent ABG estimations and pulmonary function testing are key information.

SLTx recipients with native-lung emphysema require special attention. They have a marked imbalance in pulmonary compliance, whereby the native lung is highly compliant and is at risk of DHI, and the transplanted lung has normal compliance, or (if affected by infection or rejection) low compliance. Thus, consideration should be given to use of a DLT if the surgical procedure requires tracheal intubation and mechanical ventilation. These patients can be managed according to a differential ventilation model: reduced minute ventilation to the native lung, allowing maximal expiratory time and thus a reduction in DHI, and standard ventilator settings (±PEEP) for the transplanted lung.[148-151] If OLV is required, it should be noted that the allograft generally receives the majority of pulmonary blood flow, and hypoxia is more likely to occur with ipsilateral surgery.

Summary

Advances in anesthesia for pulmonary transplantation have evolved from an increased understanding of the pathophysiology of end-stage pulmonary disease, pulmonary hypertension, and right ventricular dysfunction. The technical expertise required for intravascular and epidural catheterizations, insertion of a DLT and management of OLV, and selective use of TEE, multiple vasoactive drugs, and inhaled NO, provide unique challenges to the transplant anesthesiologist.

There are several anesthetic interventions that can reduce the need for CPB, facilitate early tracheal extubation, and result in marked and immediate improvement in patient status during and after transplantation. Surgery and anesthesia are no longer contraindicated in patients with end-stage pulmonary disease.

REFERENCES

1. Hosenpud JD, Bennett LE, Keck BM, et al: The registry of the International Society for Heart and Lung Transplantation: seventeenth official report –2000, *J Heart Lung Transplant* 19:909, 2000.
2. Zollinger A, Zaugg M, Weder W: Video-assisted thoracoscopic volume reduction surgery in patients with diffuse pulmonary emphysema: gas exchange and anesthesiological management, *Anesth Analg* 84:845, 1997.
3. Smith PC, Slaughter MS, Petty MG: Abdominal complications after lung transplantation, *J Heart Lung Transplant* 14:44, 1995.
4. Buettner A, McRae R, Myles PS, et al: Anaesthesia for bilateral lung volume reduction surgery, *Anaesth Intens Care* 27:503, 1999.
5. Haddow GR, Brock-Utne JG: A non-thoracic operation for a patient with single-lung transplantation, *Acta Anaesthesiol Scand* 43:960, 1999.
6. Myles PS, Weeks AM, Buckland MR: Anesthesia for bilateral sequential lung transplantation: experience of 64 cases, *J Cardiothorac Vasc Anesth* 11:177, 1997.
7. Bracken CA, Gurkowski MA, Naples JJ: Lung transplantation: historical perspectives, current concepts, and anesthetic considerations, *J Cardiothorac Vasc Anesth* 11:220, 1997.
8. Raffin L, Michel-Cherqui M, Sperandio M: Anesthesia for bilateral lung transplantation without cardiopulmonary bypass: Initial experience and review of intraoperative problems, *J Cardiothorac Vasc Anesth* 6:409, 1992.
9. Conacher ID: Isolated lung transplantation: A review of problems and a guide to anaesthesia, *Br J Anaesth* 61:468, 1988.
10. Carere R, Patterson GA, Liu P: Right and left ventricular performance after single- and double-lung transplantation, *J Thorac Cardiovasc Surg* 102:115, 1991.
11. Myles PS, Ryder IG, Weeks AM: Diagnosis and management of dynamic hyperinflation during lung transplantation, *J Cardiothorac Vasc Anesth* 11:100, 1997.
12. Marczin N, Royston D, Yacoub M: Pro: Lung transplantation should be routinely performed with cardiopulmonary bypass. *J Cardiothorac Vasc Anesth* 14:739, 2000.
13. Myles PS, Weeks AM: Alpha 1-antitrypsin deficiency: circulatory arrest following induction of anaesthesia, *Anaesth Intens Care* 20:358, 1992.
14. Myles PS, Venema H: Avoidance of cardiopulmonary bypass during bilateral sequential lung transplantation using inhaled nitric oxide, *J Cardiothorac Vasc Anesth* 9:571, 1995.
15. Quinlan JJ, Buffington CW: Deliberate hypoventilation in a patient with air trapping during lung transplantation, *Anesthesiology* 78:1177, 1993.
16. Horan BF, Cutfield GR, Davies IM: Problems in the management of the airway during anesthesia for bilateral sequential lung transplantation performed without cardiopulmonary bypass, *J Cardiothorac Vasc Anesth* 10:387, 1996.
17. Myles PS, Hall JL, Berry CB: Primary pulmonary hypertension: prolonged cardiac arrest and successful resuscitation following induction of anesthesia for heart-lung transplantation, *J Cardiothorac Vasc Anesth* 8:678, 1994.
18. Hohn L, Schweizer A, Morel DR, et al: Circulatory failure after anesthesia induction in a patient with severe primary pulmonary hypertension, *Anesthesiology* 91:1943, 1999.
19. Huang YC, Cheng YJ, Lin YH, et al: Graft failure caused by pulmonary venous obstruction diagnosed by intraoperative transesophageal echocardiography during lung transplantation, *Anesth Analg* 91:558, 2000.
20. Zander DS, Baz MA, Visner GA, et al: Analysis of early deaths after isolated lung transplantation, *Chest* 120:225, 2001.
21. Fullerton DA, McIntyre RC, Mitchell MB: Lung transplantation with cardiopulmonary bypass exaggerates pulmonary vasomotor dysfunction in the transplanted lung, *J Thorac Cardiovasc Surg* 109:212, 1995.
22. Aeba R, Griffith BP, Kormos RL: Effect of cardiopulmonary bypass on early graft dysfunction in clinical lung transplantation, *Ann Thorac Surg* 57:715, 1994.
23. Williams TJ, Snell GI, Hall MJ: Transplantation in cystic fibrosis: heart lung vs. bilateral sequential lung transplantation. *Aust NZ J Med* 24:484, 1994.
24. Triantafillou AN, Pasque MK, Huddleston CB, et al: Predictors, frequency, and indications for cardiopulmonary bypass during lung transplantation in adults, *Ann Thorac Surg* 57:1248, 1994.
25. Myles PS: Lessons from lung transplantation for everyday anesthesia. In Slinger P (ed): *Thoracic anesthesia,* St. Louis, 2001, Mosby.
26. Luft HS, Garnick DW, Mark DH: Hospital volume, physician volume, and patient outcomes: assessing the evidence, Ann Arbor, 1990, *Health Administration Press Perspectives.*
27. Esmore DS, Brown R, Buckland MR: Techniques and results in bilateral sequential single-lung transplantation, *J Card Surg* 9:1, 1994.
28. Griffiths BP, Hardesty RL, Armitage JM: A decade of lung transplantation, *Ann Surg* 218:310, 1993.
29. Kramer MR, Marshall SE, Starnes VA: Infectious complications in heart-lung transplantation. Analysis of 200 episodes, *Arch Intern Med* 153:2010, 1993.
30. Van Norman GA: A matter of life and death: what every anesthesiologist should know about the medical, legal, and ethical aspects of declaring brain death, *Anesthesiology* 91:275, 1999.
31. Griffith BP, Zenati M: The pulmonary donor, *Clin Chest Med* 11:217, 1990.
32. Dujardin KS, McCully RB, Wijdicks EF, et al: Myocardial dysfunction associated with brain death: clinical, echocardiographic, and pathologic features, *J Heart Lung Transplant* 20:350, 2001.
33. Buckley T: Management of the multiorgan donor. In Oh TE (ed): *Intensive care manual,* ed 4, Sydney, 1997, Butterworth-Heinemann.
34. Fujino S, Nagahiro I, Triantafillou AN, et al: Inhaled nitric oxide at the time of harvest improves early lung allograft function, *Ann Thorac Surg* 63:1383, 1997.

35. Snell GI, Rabinov M, Griffiths A, et al: Graft ischaemic time is an important predictor of survival post-lung transplantation. *J Heart Lung Transplant* 15:160, 1996.

36. Ueno T, Snell GI, Williams TJ, et al: Impact of graft ischemic time on outcomes after bilateral sequential single-lung transplantation, *Ann Thorac Surg* 67:1577, 1999.

37. Wisser W, Deviatko E, Simon-Kupilik N, et al: Lung transplantation following lung volume reduction surgery, *J Heart Lung Transplant* 19:480, 2000.

38. Munro PE, Bailey M, Esmore DS, et al: Surgical management of severe emphysema in Australia: lung transplant and lung volume reduction surgery, *J Heart Lung Transplant* 20:218, 2001.

39. Smith C: Patient selection, evaluation, and preoperative management for lung transplant candidates, *Clin Chest Med* 18:183, 1997.

40. Thaik CM, Semigran MJ, Ginns L, et al: Evaluation of ischemic heart disease in potential lung transplant recipients, *J Heart Lung Transplant* 14:257, 1995.

41. Hirt SW, Haverich A, Wahlers T: Predictive criteria for the need of extracorporeal circulation in single-lung transplantation, *Ann Thorac Surg* 54:676, 1992.

42. de Hoyos A, Demajo A, Snell G: Preoperative prediction for the use of cardiopulmonary bypass in lung transplantation, *J Thorac Cardiovasc Surg* 106:787, 1993.

43. Snell GI, Richardson M, Griffiths A, et al: Coronary artery disease in potential lung transplant recipients aged over 50: the role of coronary intervention, *Chest* 116:874, 1999.

44. Vizza CD, Lynch JP, Ochoa LL, et al: Right and left ventricular dysfunction in patients with severe pulmonary disease, *Chest* 113:576, 1998.

45. Florea VG, Florea ND, Sharma R, et al: Right ventricular dysfunction in adult severe cystic fibrosis, *Chest* 118:1063, 2000.

46. Yeatman M, McNeil K, Smith JA: Lung transplantation in patients with systemic diseases: an 11-year experience at Papworth hospital, *J Heart Lung Transplant* 15:144, 1996.

47. Myles PS: Aspects of anesthesia for lung transplantation, *Semin Cardiothorac Vasc Anesth* 2:140, 1998.

48. Hines R, Barash P: Intraoperative right ventricular dysfunction detected with a right ventricular ejection fraction catheter, *J Clin Monit* 2:206, 1986.

49. Thys DM, Cohen E, Eisenkraft JB: Mixed venous oxygen saturation during thoracic anesthesia, *Anesthesiology* 69:1005, 1988.

50. Ventakesh B, Clutton Brock TH, Hendry SP: A multiparameter sensor for continuous intra-arterial blood gas monitoring: a prospective evaluation, *Crit Care Med* 22:588, 1994.

51. Kurz A, Kurz M, Poeschl G: Forced-air warming maintains intraoperative normothermia better than circulating-water mattresses, *Anesth Analg* 77:89, 1993.

52. Kurz A, Sessler DI, Lenhardt R: Perioperative normothermia to reduce the incidence of surgical-wound infection and shorten hospitalization, *N Engl J Med* 334:1209, 1996.

53. Westerlind A, Nilsson F, Ricksten SE: The use of continuous positive airway pressure by face mask and thoracic epidural analgesia after lung transplantation. Gothenburg Lung Transplant Group, *J Cardiothorac Vasc Anesth* 13:249, 1999.

54. Gan TJ, Glass PS, Windsor A, et al: Bispectral index monitoring allows faster emergence and improved recovery from propofol, alfentanil, and nitrous oxide anesthesia, *Anesthesiology* 87: 808, 1997.

55. Song D, Joshi GP, White PF: Titration of volatile anesthetics using bispectral index facilitates recovery after ambulatory anesthesia, *Anesthesiology* 87:842, 1997.

56. Riegle EV, Otto AA, Krucylak CP: Recall of intraoperative events during pediatric lung transplantation, *Anesth Analg* 82:S380, 1996.

57. Leonard I, Myles P: Target-controlled intravenous anaesthesia with bispectral index monitoring for thoracotomy in a patient with severely impaired left ventricular function, *Anaesth Intens Care* 28: 318, 1999.

58. Brown RH, Wagner EM: Mechanisms of bronchoprotection by anesthetic induction agents: propofol versus ketamine, *Anesthesiology* 90:822, 1999.

59. Rooke GA, Choi J-H, Bishop MJ: The effect of isoflurane, halothane, sevoflurane, and thiopental/nitrous oxide on respiratory system resistance after tracheal intubation, *Anesthesiology* 86:1294, 1997.

60. Anonymous Editorial: Preoxygenation: science and practice, *Lancet* 339:31, 1992.

61. Katz WE, Gasior TA, Quinlan JJ, et al: Immediate effects of lung transplantation on right ventricular morphology and function in patients with variable degrees of pulmonary hypertension, *J Am Coll Cardiol* 27:384, 1996.

62. Pepke-Zaba J, Higenbottam TW, Dinh-Xuan AT: Inhaled nitric oxide as a cause of selective pulmonary vasodilation in pulmonary hypertension, *Lancet* 338:1173, 1991.

63. Kieler-Jensen N, Ricksten SE, Stenqvist O: Inhaled nitric oxide in the evaluation of heart transplant candidates with elevated pulmonary vascular resistance, *J Heart Lung Transplant* 13:366, 1994.

64. Haraldsson A, Kieler-Jensen N, Nathorst-Westfelt U, et al: Comparison of inhaled nitric oxide and inhaled prostacyclin in the evaluation of heart transplant candidates with elevated pulmonary vascular resistance, *Chest* 114:780, 1998.

65. Snell GI, Salamonsen RF, Bergin P, et al: Inhaled nitric oxide used as a bridge to heart-lung transplantation in a patient with end-stage pulmonary hypertension, *Am J Respir Crit Care Med* 151:1263, 1995.

66. Davis WB, Rennard SI, Bitterman PB: Pulmonary oxygen toxicity. Early reversible changes in human alveolar structures induced by hyperoxia, *N Engl J Med* 309:878, 1983.

67. Klein J: Normobaric pulmonary oxygen toxicity, *Anesth Analg* 70:195, 1990.

68. Schulte-Sasse Y, Hess W, Tarnow J: Pulmonary vascular response to nitrous oxide in patients with normal and high pulmonary vascular resistance, *Anesthesioloy* 57:9,1982.

69. Schwarz RE, Pham SM, Bierman MI: Tension pneumoperitoneum after heart-lung transplantation, *Ann Thorac Surg* 57:478, 1994.

70. Popple C, Higgins TL, McCarthy P, et al: Unilateral auto-PEEP in the recipient of a single-lung transplant, *Chest* 103:297, 1993.

71. Conacher ID: Dynamic hyperinflation—the anaesthetist applying a tourniquet to the right heart, *Br J Anesth* 81:116, 1998.

72. Zapol WM: Volotrauma and the intravenous oxygenator in patients with adult respiratory distress syndrome, *Anesthesiology* 77:847, 1992.

73. Tuxen DV, Lane S: The effects of ventilatory pattern on hyperinflation, airway pressures and circulation in mechanical ventilation of patients with severe air-flow obstruction, *Am Rev Respir Dis* 136:872, 1987.

74. Tuxen DV: Permissive hypercapnic ventilation, *Am J Respir Crit Care Med* 150:870, 1994.

75. Williams TJ, Tuxen DV, Scheinkestel CD: Risk factors for morbidity in mechanically ventilated patients with acute severe asthma, *Am Rev Respir Dis* 146:607, 1992.

76. Tan IKS, Bhatt SB, Tam YH: Effects of PEEP on dynamic hyperinflation in patients with airflow limitation, *Br J Anaesth* 70:267, 1993.

77. Ducros L, Moutafis M, Castelain MH, et al: Pulmonary air trapping during two-lung and one-lung ventilation, *J Cardiothorac Vasc Anesth* 13:35, 1999.

78. Gay PC, Rodarte JR, Hubmayr RD: The effects of positive expiratory pressure on isovolume flow and dynamic hyperinflation in patients receiving mechanical ventilation, *Am Rev Respir Dis* 139:621, 1989.

79. Pepe PE, Marini JJ: Occult positive end-expiratory pressure in mechanically ventilated patients with airflow obstruction, *Am Rev Respir Dis* 126:166, 1982.

80. Hoffman RA, Ershowsky P, Krieger BP: Determination of auto-PEEP during spontaneous and controlled ventilation by monitoring changes in end-expiratory thoracic gas volume, *Chest* 96:613, 1989.

81. Perel A, Segal E: Systolic pressure variation—a way to recognize dynamic hyperinflation, *Br J Anaesth* 76:168, 1996.

82. Conacher ID, McMahon CC: Pathognomonic pulse oximetry paradox, *Lancet* 346:448, 1995.

83. Normandale JP, Feneck RO: Bullous cystic lung disease. Its anaesthetic management using high-frequency jet ventilation, *Anaesthesia* 40:1182, 1985.

84. McCarthy G, Coppel DL, Gibbons JR: High-frequency jet ventilation for bilateral bullectomy, *Anaesthesia* 42:411, 1987.

85. Conacher ID: Prolonged interval jet ventilation. An alternative ventilation technique for patients with problematic cardiopulmonary pathophysiology, *Anaesthesia* 50:518, 1995.

86. Myles PS, Evans AB, Madder H: Dynamic hyperinflation: comparison of jet ventilation versus conventional ventilation in patients with severe end-stage obstructive lung disease, *Anaesth Intens Care* 25:471, 1997.

87. Artigas A, Bernard GR, Carlet J, et al: The American-European consensus conference on ARDS, Part 2. Ventilatory, pharmacologic, supportive therapy, study design strategies and issues related to recovery and remodelling, *Intensive Care Med* 24:378, 1998.

88. Acute Respiratory Distress Syndrome Network: Ventilation with lower tidal volumes as compared with traditional tidal volumes for acute lung injury and the acute respiratory distress syndrome, *N Engl J Med* 2(342):1301, 2000.

89. Amato MBP, Barbas CSV, Medeiros DM, et al: Effect of a protective-ventilation strategy on mortality in the acute respiratory distress syndrome, *N Engl J Med* 338:347, 1998.

90. Capan LM, Turndorf H, Chandrakant P: Optimization of arterial oxygenation during one-lung anesthesia, *Anesth Analg* 59:847, 1980.

91. Hurford WE, Kolkar AC, Strauss HW: The use of ventilation/perfusion lung scans to predict oxygenation during one-lung anesthesia, *Anesthesiology* 67:841, 1987.

92. Slinger P, Suissa S, Adam J, et al: Predicting arterial oxygenation during one-lung ventilation with continuous positive airway pressure in the nonventilated lung, *J Cardiothorac Anesth* 4:436, 1990.

93. Tugrul M, Camci E, Karadeniz H, et al: Comparison of volume-controlled with pressure-controlled ventilation during one-lung anaesthesia, *Br J Anaesth* 79:306, 1997.

94. Benumof JL, Augustine SD, Gibbons JA, et al: Halothane and isoflurane only slightly impair arterial oxygenation during one-lung ventilation in patients undergoing thoracotomy, *Anesthesiology* 67:910, 1987.

95. Karzai W, Haberstroh J, Priebe HJ: Effects of desflurane and propofol on arterial oxygenation during one-lung ventilation in the pig, *Acta Anaesthesiol Scand* 42:648, 1998.

96. Abe K, Shimizu T, Takashina M, et al: The effects of propofol, isoflurane, and sevoflurane on oxygenation and shunt fraction during one-lung ventilation, *Anesth Analg* 87:1164, 1998.

97. Fradj K, Samain E, Delefosse D, et al: Placebo-controlled study of inhaled nitric oxide to treat hypoxaemia during one-lung ventilation, *Br J Anaesth* 82:208, 1999.

98. Moutafis M, Dalibon N, Cokhen A, et al: Improving oxygenation during bronchopulmonary lavage using nitric oxide inhalation and almitrine infusion, *Anesth Analg* 89:302, 1999.

99. Anggard E: Nitric oxide: mediator, murderer, and medicine, *Lancet* 343:1199, 1994.

100. Gómez-Jiménez J, Salgado A, Mourelle M, et al: L-arginine: nitric oxide pathway in endotoxemia and human septic shock, *Crit Care Med* 23:253, 1995.

101. Hibbs JR, Westenfelder C, Taintor R, et al: Evidence for cytokine-inducible nitric oxide from L-arginine in patients receiving interleukin-2 therapy, *J Clin Invest* 89:867, 1992.

102. Tsujino M, Hirata Y, Imai T, et al: Induction of nitric oxide synthase gene by interleukin-1β in cultured rat cardiocytes, *Circulation* 90:375, 1994.

103. Burgner D, Rockett K, Kwiatkowski D: Nitric oxide and infectious diseases, *Arch Dis Child* 81:185, 1999.

104. Rich GF, Lowson SM, Johns RA: Inhaled nitric oxide selectively decreases pulmonary vascular resistance without impairing oxygenation during one-lung ventilation in patients undergoing cardiac surgery, *Anesthesiology* 80:57, 1994.

105. Fierobe L, Brunet F, Dhainaut JF: Effect of inhaled nitric oxide on right ventricular function in adult respiratory distress syndrome, *Am J Respir Crit Care Med* 151:1414, 1995.

106. Dellinger RP, Zimmerman JL, Taylor RW, et al: Effects of inhaled nitric oxide in patients with acute respiratory distress syndrome: results of a randomized phase II trial. Inhaled Nitric Oxide in ARDS Study Group, *Crit Care Med* 26:15, 1998.

107. Payen D, Vallet B, Genoa Group: Results of the French prospective multicentric randomized double-blind placebo-controlled trial on inhaled nitric oxide in ARDS, *Intensive Care Med* 25:S166, 1999.

108. Bacha EA, Herve P, Murakami S: Lasting beneficial effects of short-term inhaled nitric oxide on graft function after lung transplantation, *J Thorac Cardiovasc Surg* 112:590, 1996.

109. Okabayashi K, Triantafillou AN, Yamashita M: Inhaled nitric oxide improves lung allograft after prolonged storage, *J Thorac Cardiovasc Surg* 112:293, 1996.

110. Adatia I, Lillehei C, Arnold JH: Inhaled nitric oxide in the treatment of postoperative graft dysfunction after lung transplantation, *Ann Thorac Surg* 57:1311, 1994.

111. Macdonald P, Mundy J, Rogers P: Successful treatment of life-threatening acute reperfusion injury after lung transplantation with inhaled nitric oxide, *J Thorac Cardiovasc Surg* 110:861, 1995.

112. Murakami S, Bacha EA, Herve P, et al: Prevention of reperfusion injury by inhaled nitric oxide in lungs harvested from nonheart-beating donors. Paris-Sud University Lung Transplantation Group, *Ann Thorac Surg* 62:1632, 1996.

113. Date H, Triantafillou AN, Trulock EP, et al: Inhaled nitric oxide reduces human lung allograft dysfunction, *J Thorac Cardiovasc Surg* 111:913, 1996.

114. Della RG, Coccia C, Pugliese F, et al: Inhaled nitric oxide in patients with cystic fibrosis during preoperative evaluation and during lung transplantation, *Eur J Pediatr Surg* 8:262, 1998.

115. Kemming GI, Merkel MJ, Schallerer A, et al: Inhaled nitric oxide (NO) for the treatment of early allograft failure after lung transplantation. Munich Lung Transplant Group, *Intensive Care Med* 24:1173, 1998.

116. Barbera JA, Roger N, Roca J, et al: Worsening of pulmonary gas exchange with nitric oxide inhalation in chronic obstructive pulmonary disease, *Lancet* 347:436, 1996.

117. Haraldsson A, Kieler-Jensen N, Ricksten S-E, et al: The additive pulmonary vasodilatory effects of inhaled prostacyclin and inhaled milrinone in postcardiac surgical patients with pulmonary hypertension, *Anesth Analg* 93:1439, 2001.

118. Conte JV, Gaine SP, Orens JB, et al: The influence of continuous intravenous prostacyclin therapy for primary pulmonary hypertension on the timing and outcome of transplantation, *J Heart Lung Transplant* 17:679, 1998.

119. Jones K, Higgenbottam T, Wallwork J: Pulmonary vasodilation with prostacyclin in primary and secondary pulmonary hypertension, *Chest* 96:784, 1989.

120. Bemis CE, Serur JR, Borgenhagen D: Influence of right ventricular filling pressure on left ventricular filling pressure and dimension, *Circ Res* 34:498, 1972.

121. Stobierska-Dzierzek B, Awad H, Michler RE: The evolving management of acute right-sided heart failure in cardiac transplant recipients, *J Am Coll Cardiol* 38:923, 2001.

122. Agata Y, Hirashi S, Misawi H, et al: Two-dimensional echocardiographic determinants of interventricular septal configurations in right or left ventricular overload, *Am Heart J* 110:819, 1985.

123. Stojnic BB, Brecker SJ, Xiao HB, et al: Left ventricular filling characteristics in pulmonary hypertension: a new mode of ventricular interaction, *Br Heart J* 19:84, 1992.

124. Prewitt RM, Ghignone M: Treatment of right ventricular dysfunction in acute respiratory failure, *Crit Care Med* 11:346, 1983.

125. Vlahakes GJ, Turley K, Hoffman JIE: The pathophysiology of failure in acute right ventricular hypertension: hemodynamic and biochemical correlations, *Circulation* 63:87, 1981.

126. Salisbury PF: Coronary artery pressure and strength of right ventricular contraction, *Circ Res* 3:633, 1955.

127. Dagher E, Dumont L, Chartrand C: Additive effects of amrinone and dobutamine in experimental pulmonary hypertension, *Pediatric Res* 25:23A, 1989.

128. Ghignone M, Girling L, Prewitt RM: Volume expansion versus norepinephrine in treatment of a low cardiac output complicating an acute increase in right ventricular afterload in dogs, *Anesthesiology* 60:132, 1984.

129. Mathru M, Dries DJ: Is levophed lethal? *Chest* 95:1177, 1989.

130. Haider W, Zwolfer W, Hiesmayr M: Improved cardiac performance and reduced pulmonary vascular constriction by epinephrine administration via a left atrial catheter in cardiac surgical patients, *J Cardiothorac Vasc Anesth* 7:684, 1993.

131. Berisha S, Kastrati A, Goda A, et al: Optimal value of filling pressures in the right side of the heart in acute right ventricular infarction, *Br Heart J* 63:98, 1990.

132. Martin C, Perrin G, Saux P, et al: Effects of norepinephrine on right ventricular function in septic shock patients, *Intensive Care Med* 20:444, 1994.

133. Jenkins IR, Dolman J, O'Connor JP, et al: Amrinone versus dobutamine in cardiac surgical patients with severe pulmonary hypertension after cardiopulmonary bypass: a prospective, randomized double-blind trial, *Anaesth Intens Care* 25:245, 1997.

134. Euson Y, Giuntini C, Lewis ML: The influence of hydrogen ion concentration and hypoxia on the pulmonary circulation, *J Clin Invest* 43:1146, 1964.

135. Barer GR, Howard P, Shaw JW: Stimulus-response curves for the pulmonary vascular bed to hypoxia and hypercapnia, *J Physiol* 211:139, 1970.

136. Schenk P, Globits S, Koller J, et al: Accuracy of echocardiographic right ventricular parameters in patients with different end-stage lung diseases prior to lung transplantation, *J Heart Lung Transplant* 19:145, 2000.

137. Myles PS, Leong CK, Weeks AM: Early hemodynamic effects of left atrial administration of epinephrine after heart transplantation, *Anesth Analg* 84:976, 1997.

138. Nishimura RA, Tajik AJ: Evaluation of diastolic filling of left ventricle in health and disease: Doppler echocardiography is the clinician's Rosetta stone, *J Am Coll Cardiol* 30:8, 1997.

139. Sukernik MR, Mets B, Bennet-Guerrero E: Patent formaen ovale and its significance in the perioperative period, *Anesth Analg* 93:1137, 2001.

140. Cujic B, Polasek P, Mayers I, et al: Positive end-expiratory pressure increases the right-to-left shunt in mechanically ventilated patients with paten-foramen ovale, *Ann Intern Med* 119:887, 1993.

141. Michel-Cherqui M, Brusset A, et al: Intraoperative transesophageal echocardiographic assessment of vascular anastomoses in lung transplantation. A report on 18 cases, *Chest* 111:1229, 1997.

142. Leibowitz DW, Smith CR, Michler RE, et al: Incidence of pulmonary vein complications after lung transplantation: a prospective transesophageal echocardiographic study, *J Am Coll Cardiol* 24:671, 1994.

143. Glassman LR, Keenan RJ, Fabrizio MC: Extracorporeal membrane oxygenation as an adjunct treatment for primary graft failure in adult lung transplant recipients, *J Thorac Cardiovasc Surg* 110:723, 1995.

144. Boujoukis AJ, Martich GD, Vega JD, et al: Reperfusion injury in single-transplant recipients with pulmonary hypertension and emphysema, *J Heart Lung Transplant* 16: 439, 1997.

145. Petersen C, Baum M, Hormann C: Selecting ventilator setting according to variables derived from the quasi-static pressure/volume relationship in patients with acute lung injury, *Anesth Analg* 77:436, 1993.

146. Trachiotis GD, Vricella LA, Aaron BL, et al: Reexpansion pulmonary edema, *Ann Thorac Surg* 63:1206, 1997.

147. Dreyfuss D, Soler P, Baset G: High inflation pressure pulmonary edema, Am J Respir Dis 137:1159, 1988.

148. Badesch DB, Zamora MR, Jones S: Independent ventilation and ECMO for severe unilateral pulmonary edema after SLT for primary pulmonary hypertension, Chest 107:1766-1770, 1995.

149. Gavazzeni V, Iapichino G, Mascheroni D: Prolonged independent lung respiratory treatment after single-lung transplantation in pulmonary emphysema, *Chest* 103:96, 1993.

150. Smiley RM, Navedo AT, Kirby T: Postoperative independent lung ventilation in a single-lung transplant recipient, *Anesthesiology* 74:1144, 1991.

151. Adoumie R, Shennib H, Brown R, et al: Differential lung ventilation. Applications beyond the operating room, *J Thorac Cardiovasc Surg* 105:229, 1993.

152. West JB: Blood flow to the lung and gas exchange, *Anesthesiology* 41:124, 1974.

153. Bund M, Seitz W, Uthoff K, et al: Monitoring of respiratory function before and after cardiopulmonary bypass using side-stream spirometry, *Eur J Anaesthesiol* 15:44, 1998.

154. Gammie JS, Lee JC, Pham SM, et al: Cardiopulmonary bypass is associated with early allograft dysfunction but not death after double-lung transplantation, *J Thorac Cardiovasc Surg* 115:990, 1998.

155. Ko WJ, Chen YS, Lee YC: Replacing cardiopulmonary bypass with extracorporeal membrane oxygenation in lung transplantation operations, *Artif Organs* 25:607, 2001.

156. Bonica JJ, Kennedy WF, Akamatsu TJ: Circulatory effects of peridural block. III: Effects of acute blood loss, *Anesthesiology* 36:219, 1972.

157. Howie MB, Cheng D, Newman MF, et al: A randomized double-blinded multicenter comparison of remifentanil versus fentanyl when combined with isoflurane/propofol for early extubation in coronary artery bypass graft surgery, *Anesth Analg* 92:1084, 2001.

158. Odoom JA, Sih IL: Epidural analgesia and anticoagulation therapy. Experience with one thousand cases of continuous epidurals, *Anaesthesia* 38:254, 1983.

159. Wang LP, Hauerberg J, Schmidt JF: Incidence of spinal epidural abscess after epidural analgesia. A national 1-year study, *Anesthesiology* 91:1928, 1999.

160. Ballantyne J, Carr DB, deFerranti S, et al: The comparative effects of postoperative analgesia therapies on pulmonary outcome: cumulative meta-analysis of randomized, controlled trials, *Anesth Analg* 86:598, 1998.

161. Rodgers A, Walker N, Schug SA, et al: Reduction of postoperative mortality and morbidity with epidural or spinal anaesthesia: results from an overview of randomised trials, *BMJ* 321:1493, 2000.

162. Park WY, Thompson JS, Lee KK: Effect of epidural anesthesia and analgesia on perioperative outcome: a randomized, controlled Veterans Affairs cooperative study, *Ann Surg* 234:560, 2001.

163. Rigg JRA, Jamrozik K, Myles PS, et al: Epidural anaesthesia and analgesia and outcome of major surgery: a randomised trial, *Lancet* 359:1276, 2002.

164. Murray JG, McAdams HP, Erasmus JJ: Complications of lung transplantation: radiological findings, *Am J Roentgenology* 166:1405, 1996.

165. Theodore J, Jamiesson SW, Burke CM: Physiologic aspects of human heart-lung transplantation: pulmonary function status of the post-transplanted lung, *Chest* 86:349, 1984.

166. Anderson DC, Glazer HS, Semenkovich JW, et al: Lung transplant edema: chest radiography after lung transplantation—the first 10 days, *Radiology* 195:275, 1995.

167. Slinger P: Perioperative fluid management for thoracic surgery: the puzzle of postpneumonectomy pulmonary edema, *J Cardiothorac Vasc Anesth* 9:442, 1995.

168. Levy PS, Chavez RP, Crystal GJ: Oxygen extraction ratio: a valid indicator of transfusion need in limited coronary vascular reserve? *J Trauma* 32:769, 1992.

169. Hebert PC, Wells G, Tweeddale M, et al: Does transfusion practice affect mortality in critically ill patients? Transfusion Requirements in Critical Care (TRICC) Investigators and the Canadian Critical Care Trials Group, *Am J Respir Crit Care Med* 155:1618, 1997.

170. Scott WJ, Kessler R, Wernley JA: Blood conservation in cardiac surgery, *Ann Thorac Surg* 50:843, 1990.

171. Hardy JF, Desroches J: Natural and synthetic antifibrinolytics in cardiac surgery, *Can J Anaesth* 39:353, 1992.

172. Jaquiss RD, Huddleston C, Spray T: Use of aprotinin in pediatric lung transplantation, *J Heart Lung Transplant* 15:243, 1996.

173. Levi M, Cromheecke ME, de Jonge E, et al: Pharmacological strategies to decrease excessive blood loss in cardiac surgery: a meta-analysis of clinically relevant endpoints, *Lancet* 354:1940, 1999.

174. Roberts RF, Nishanian GP, Carey JN, et al: Addition of aprotinin to organ preservation solutions decreases lung reperfusion injury, *Ann Thorac Surg* 66:225, 1998.

175. Wood GG: Cyclosporine-vecuronium interaction, *Can J Anaesth* 36:358, 1989.

176. Dretchen KL, Morgenroth VH, Standaert FG, et al: Azathioprine: effects on neuromuscular transmission, *Anesthesiology* 45:604, 1976.

177. Briffa N, Morris RE: New immunosuppressive regimens in lung transplantation, *Eur Respir J* 10:2630, 1997.

178. Snell GI, Levvey BJ, Chin W, et al: Rescue therapy: a role for sirolimus in lung and heart transplant recipients, *Transplant Proc* 33:1084, 2001.

179. Vickers MD, O'Flaherty D, Szekely SM, et al: Tramadol: pain relief by an opioid without depression of respiration, *Anaesthesia* 47:291, 1992.

180. Maziak DE, Maurer JR, Kesten S: Diaphragmatic paralysis: a complication of lung transplantation, *Ann Thorac Surg* 61:170, 1996.

181. Berkowitz N, Schulman LL, McGregor C: Gastroparesis after lung transplantation. Potential role in postoperative respiratory complications, *Chest* 108:1602, 1995.

182. Sheridan PH, Cheriyan A, Doud J: Incidence of phrenic neuropathy after isolated lung transplantation, *J Heart Lung Transplant* 14: 684, 1995.

183. Kirshborn PM, Tapson VF, Harrison JK, et al: Delayed right heart failure following lung transplantation, *Chest* 109:575, 1996.

Thoracic Trauma 15

Bernard B. Baez, MD
Jeffrey T. Smok, MD
Brendan T. Finucane, MD
Kenneth J. Abrams, MD, MBA

THORACIC injuries are rarely isolated; they are often associated with other serious injuries and, in many cases, death. Patients presenting with these multiple injuries require emergency care and are a great challenge to all who care for them. A thorough knowledge of physiology and therapeutic options is required. The management of thoracic trauma, with its insults to the airway, ventilation, and hemodynamics, makes it ideally suited to the anesthesiologist.

Trauma is a very serious health problem in the United States today. Unfortunately, trauma continues to be a leading cause of death in the first four decades of life. The epidemiology of trauma patients displays a bimodal peak, the first occurring at around age 20. This peak is represented chiefly by males who are injured through violence or motor vehicle crashes. The second peak occurs around age 80 and is represented predominantly by women injured through falls or motor vehicle crashes. It is worth noting that motor vehicle crashes and falls alone make up some 68% of all injuries. Injuries due to violence (gunshots, stabbings, and fights) make up another 14%. The highest mortality rate of all injuries is from gunshot wounds.[1]

The development of emergency medicine as a specialty has also focused much more attention on trauma, both at the scene of the accident and in emergency departments. In results from the National Trauma Data Bank Report 2001, 161,438 patients were involved in some form of trauma and received care in an emergency department. Of these patients, 97% were resuscitated and transferred out of the emergency department for further care. Fifty-three percent of these patients went to regular hospital floors, 20% to the intensive care unit (ICU), and 24% to the operating room.[1] From these numbers it is easy to see that the emergency room is a first line of defense when it comes to trauma.

The financial burden of trauma on society is enormous. In the United States, there were 2.5 million hospitalizations due to injury alone in 1996 and 1997. These accounted for approximately 8% of total hospital discharges.[2] In the National Trauma Data Bank study of the 161,438 patients involved, medical care cost an estimated $3 billion. The hospital charges varied widely, ranging from stab wounds not requiring ICU care (average cost $6373), to major burns requiring ICU care (average cost $49,600).[1] In a recent Canadian report, the Canadian National Trauma Registry found that trauma accounts for $14 billion annually or 11% of medical spending in Canada.[3] In the United States, it has been estimated that trauma care accounts for approximately 2.3% of the gross national product.[4]

Statistics directly related to chest trauma are scant, but studies suggest that approximately 20% to 25% of trauma deaths are attributable to thoracic injuries.[5] The majority of chest injuries result from blunt trauma secondary to motor vehicle accidents and penetrating injuries secondary to gunshot wounds and stabbings. The spectrum of injuries ranges from simple rib fractures to vital organ trauma. In the western population, blunt trauma from motor vehicle accidents accounts for 70% to 80% of thoracic injuries.[5] Although the chest is often injured, most patients with chest trauma can be attended to with simple procedures; only a minority require surgery. Less than 10% of blunt trauma injuries require thoracotomy, while approximately 15% to 30% of penetrating wounds require a thoracotomy.[6]

With the aid of sophisticated audiovisual communications and telemetry, decision making by physicians can be brought to the scene of the accident. One of the major corrective actions required to improve the care of the seriously injured patient is regionalization of trauma care. Not every hospital has the equipment or personnel to deal with these patients; therefore, trauma care activity should be confined to those hospitals that do. This reorganization would result in a significant reduction in mortality among trauma victims and monetary benefits to the U.S. health care system.

This chapter focuses first on the patterns of injury, followed by discussions of medical problems that typically arise and therapeutic modalities available to maximize outcome following thoracic injury.

Types of Injury

In general, thoracic injuries are classified into two broad categories: penetrating and blunt (Table 15-1).

Penetrating Injuries

Penetrating injuries to the chest are usually the result of gunshot wounds or stabbings. Gunshot wounds, as mentioned previously, are far more likely than other injuries to be fatal. Gunshots cause more destruction due in part to their velocity on impact and to their ability to cause destruction over a wide

TABLE 15-1

Classification of Thoracic Injuries

Penetrating injuries	Gunshot	
	Stabbing	
Blunt injuries	Deceleration	Impact
	Direct impact	Momentum
	Compression (crush)	Anteroposterior
		Lateral

area. The amount of destruction occurring secondary to gunshot wounds is related to the kinetic energy transmitted to the tissues. This can be mathematically expressed as

$$KE = WV^2/2G$$

$$W = Weight$$

$$V = Velocity$$

$$G = Acceleration\ of\ gravity$$

With the wide range of ammunition available and their differing weights, as well as the multiple velocities from weapons of differing firepower, it becomes apparent why penetrating wounds secondary to gunshots can be so destructive. Stabbings, on the other hand, are less complex. The damage is usually confined to the structures directly underlying the point of contact. These wounds are less likely to be fatal and are easier to treat.

Blunt Injuries

The vast majority of chest injuries seen in practice today are a result of blunt trauma to the chest secondary to motor vehicle accidents. Injuries can range from simple rib fractures to severe destruction of tissues (such as the rupture of thoracic viscera). The more serious the injury, the greater the likelihood of rib fractures. Furthermore, fractures of the upper five ribs are usually associated with more serious injuries. In children, greater force is required to produce fractures than in adults because of the relatively greater flexibility of the juvenile thoracic cage.[7]

The exact mechanisms that produce visceral injury within the thoracic cavity following decelerating injuries are poorly understood, but, generally, the extent of injury depends on the mass of the offending object, the physical characteristics of the resulting shock wave, and the ability of the target tissue or tissues to dissipate this shockwave. Deceleration injuries can be divided into *momentum* and *impact* injuries. Momentum is energy that an object carries by virtue of its mass and velocity. Impact, on the other hand, is defined by the forcible striking of one body against another. The impact injury usually results in fractures to the sternum and ribs, with minimal damage to underlying structures. Momentum injuries occur to those organs that are suspended within the thoracic cage, such as the heart, lungs, and aorta. When the body is suddenly brought to a grinding halt on impact, these structures continue to move. The amount of destruction is proportional to the shearing forces imparted to the organ(s) involved. Rupture of the descending aorta at the isthmus occurs commonly in severe deceleration injuries, such as airline crashes. Other serious injuries that occur following blunt trauma include cardiac contusions and rupture, tracheal and bronchial tears, lung contusions, and diaphragmatic and esophageal injuries.

Direct-impact injuries by blunt objects—also called *direct-blow* injuries—can cause localized fractures of ribs, sternum, or scapula while also injuring the underlying parenchyma of the heart and lungs. Compression injuries of the chest are further divided into anteroposterior and lateral crush injuries. The anteroposterior compression injuries cause rib fractures with possible disruption of the bronchi and contusions of the heart. Lateral compression injuries cause ipsilateral fractures and possible contralateral fractures, with or without damage to the underlying structures.

Injuries to the thoracic cage are among the most common. The injury could range from a simple fracture of one or two ribs to the more complex flail chest injury. The one factor common to all rib fractures, simple or complex, is that they cause a disproportionate degree of pain. To the young, healthy adult, this is usually of no consequence; however, to the heavy smoker with advanced chronic obstructive pulmonary disease, there can be serious consequences. In the conscious patient, the diagnosis can be made clinically. Patients can usually pinpoint, with great accuracy, the exact location of the fracture or fractures. A chest radiograph should always be performed, not necessarily to confirm the diagnosis, but to rule out pneumothorax or atelectasis.

Classification of Injuries

Thoracic Injuries

FLAIL CHEST

Flail chest is one of the major thoracic injuries affecting breathing in the trauma patient. It can be recognized in the primary survey by the paradoxic movement of the chest wall during spontaneous respiration. The paradoxic movement is the outcome of multiple rib fractures (three adjacent ribs in two or more places). This injury is most commonly associated with blunt trauma to the chest wall and typically involves the anterolateral aspect of the chest. The posterior wall is heavily fortified with muscle and, therefore, it is rarely involved. On inspiration, the injured segment tends to encroach on the lung, which leads to impairment of ventilation and oxygenation. Injury to the upper ribs usually signifies serious trauma. The flail chest injury is rarely isolated and is usually an ominous sign, indicating serious underlying injuries to intrathoracic and/or intraabdominal organs.[8] The thoracic cage in older age groups is more calcified and brittle and, therefore, more susceptible to flail chest and other serious injuries. In contrast, the thoracic cage in pediatric patients is extremely elastic and resilient, affording much greater protection to underlying structures.

This condition may go unnoticed for hours and, in some cases, it is sometimes overshadowed by more overt injuries. The diagnosis is particularly difficult when the upper thoracic cage is involved. Chest radiography might not reveal fractures unless films are overpenetrated and oblique views are taken.[9] Radiologic signs of parenchymal damage to the lung might not be evident in the early stages; however, the presence of mediastinal air can signify bronchial or tracheal injury.[9] Serial blood gas measurements can be very helpful in establishing the diagnosis. The primary pathophysiologic defect associated with flail chest injury is inadequate oxygenation. Repetitive clinical assessment of patients with blunt trauma is the key to early detection of flail chest.

The management of this condition is controversial.[10-12] The goals of treatment are directed toward stabilization of the injured segment, maintenance of adequate ventilation, and effective pain relief. All patients with a flail chest should be admitted to a surgical ICU. Temporary stabilization of the flail segment should be carried out as soon as possible by using either sandbags or pillows until a decision about definitive treatment has been made. The treatment varies with the severity of the injury, ranging from simple supportive therapy (such as oxygen enrichment, physical therapy, and pain management) to full ventilatory support.[13] The latter is now considered to be the most effective treatment for patients who develop respiratory failure. Another treatment that has been used is external stabilization of the flail segment by traction on the injured segment. Currently, there are few indications for this mode of treatment. Moore and his colleagues have stabilized the chest wall in selective cases by intramedullary pinning of fractured ribs.[13]

Clinical observation, sequential arterial blood gas analysis, and assessment of the vital capacity and inspiratory force over a period of time usually determine the need for endotracheal intubation (Table 15-2). These criteria should be used in conjunction with close clinical observation. Any one component alone might not be sufficient grounds for committing a patient to ventilation, but certainly two or more in any one patient would make a strong case for doing so.[14]

PNEUMOTHORAX

By the nature of the injury, pneumothoraces fall into three categories: closed, open, and tension. A closed pneumothorax is defined by the presence of gas in the pleural space. In the trauma patient, this can result from blunt or penetrating trauma to the chest wall. Clinical signs in patients with a pneumothorax result from hypoxemia due to atelectasis and an intrapulmonary shunt. Venous return can also be impaired by positive pressure and mediastinal shift. Patients might complain of chest pain that is accentuated by deep breathing. Cyanosis can be evident, and the trachea can be deviated with larger pneumothoraces. Percussion of the chest reveals a tympanic sound, and breath sounds might be diminished or absent. Radiologic examination is the best diagnostic aid available, and all films should be taken during expiration.[15,16] The presence of rib fractures or subcutaneous emphysema should provide a clue to the diagnosis. Pneumothoraces with a volume more than 10% should be treated by tube thoracostomy in trauma patients.

Open pneumothoraces occur as a result of penetration of the chest wall and lung by sharp objects such as bullets, knives, ice picks, or rib fragments. An open pneumothorax is caused by a

---

TABLE 15-2

Criteria for Intubation

Pao_2 <70 mmHg with O_2 enrichment
Pao_2 >50 mmHg
pH <7.25
Tachypnea >30/min
Vital capacity <15 mL/kg
Negative inspiratory force <–20 cmH$_2$O

TABLE 15-3

Cardinal Signs of Tension Pneumothorax

Cyanosis
Marked decrease in pulmonary compliance
Rapid deterioration of vital signs
Diminished or absent breath sounds
Tracheal deviation

---

large defect in the chest wall, which equalizes intrapleural pressure with the atmosphere. The diagnosis of the "sucking" chest wound is fairly obvious from the clinical observation. The immediate treatment of this condition is to occlude the defect. Definitive treatment also involves insertion of a chest tube and repair of the defect.

Tension pneumothorax occurs when air enters the pleural cavity and cannot escape. This most commonly occurs during mechanical ventilation with positive pressure. Nevertheless, it can result from blunt or penetrating trauma, or from placement of a central-access catheter. In conscious patients, rapid deterioration is noted. Breath sounds are barely perceptible, and the trachea is markedly deviated. Cyanosis and cardiovascular collapse can follow (Table 15-3). This condition can easily be confused with pericardial tamponade, myocardial infarction, or shock secondary to hypovolemia.[17] During general anesthesia, a dramatic decrease in respiratory compliance with hemodynamic collapse should alert the anesthesiologist to the problem.[18] Nitrous oxide should be discontinued as soon as possible, as it accentuates the size of the pneumothorax.[19]

As soon as a tension pneumothorax is suspected, a large-bore needle should be inserted into the second intercostal space in the midclavicular line on the affected side. If the diagnosis is correct, rapid improvement is noted. This is a surgical emergency, and valuable time should not be wasted seeking radiologic confirmation. Figure 15-1 shows a portable radiograph of a patient with a large tension pneumothorax.

ACUTE TRAUMATIC HEMOTHORAX

Hemothorax occurs in approximately 70% of all major chest injuries. Massive hemothorax is defined by the rapid accumulation of more than 1500 mL of blood in the chest cavity. This life-threatening hemothorax most commonly results from a penetrating wound that lacerates the major thoracic vessels. It could also be the result of a sudden deceleration injury or blunt trauma. In the majority of cases, the source of bleeding is the pulmonary vessels, which normally have low perfusion pressures and, therefore, limited blood loss. More persistent bleeding can occur from an injury to the systemic vessels or the heart. The diagnosis of hemothorax is made on the basis of the nature of the injury and clinical examination of the chest. Clinically, massive hemothorax can be suspected when symptoms of shock are associated with diminished breath sounds on auscultation. A chest tube should be inserted as soon as possible in the sixth intercostal space in the midaxillary line on the injured side and connected to suction at a negative pressure of approximately –15 cmH$_2$O. If 1500 mL of blood is removed, it is likely that the patient will require a thoracotomy for further management of blood loss. Hypovolemia from blood loss is the

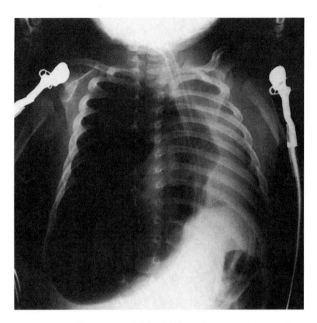

FIGURE 15-1 Chest x-ray of right-sided tension pneumothorax. (Courtesy Westchester County Medical Center Department of Radiology.)

most common presenting problem in patients with significant chest injury. Therefore the immediate treatment should be directed toward restoring blood volume. Central venous pressure monitoring is invaluable in both the diagnosis and management of patients with a hemothorax. Oxygen therapy is mandatory in those patients who have mechanical interference with ventilation. In most situations, there is sufficient time to allow the thoracotomy to be performed in the operating room.

TRACHEAL AND BRONCHIAL INJURIES

Tracheal and bronchial injuries, although uncommon, are some of the most serious injuries caused by trauma.[20,21] Most patients will die at the scene of the accident. Patients who arrive at the emergency department frequently present with dyspnea, cough, hemoptysis, subcutaneous emphysema, cyanosis, or atelectasis following blunt or penetrating trauma to the neck or upper chest.[21] Auscultation of the heart could reveal a crunching sound associated with pericardial air (Hamman's sign). Bertelsen and Howitz reviewed autopsy findings in approximately 1220 patients who succumbed to blunt chest trauma and found a 2.8% incidence of tracheobronchial rupture.[23] Approximately 80% of tracheobronchial injuries occur within 2.5 cm of the carina.[21,24] Tension pneumothorax can occur, especially if the tracheal wound communicates with the pleural cavity.[25] In some cases, a persistent air leak might be evident during attempts to ventilate the patient, and such a leak also suggests tracheobroncheal injury. All patients with suspected tracheal or bronchial injury require diagnostic bronchoscopy as soon as they are stable. Tracheobronchial injuries are often associated with other serious injuries, including cervical spine, esophageal, or diaphragmatic injury, or cardiac and pulmonary contusions. Pulmonary contusions can result in respiratory failure over time rather than instantaneously.

Small tracheal wounds with good apposition can be treated by endotracheal intubation, with the cuff of the endotracheal tube placed below the wound site.[20] More distal wounds could require the placement of a double-lumen endotracheal tube to provide better oxygenation. Fiberoptic bronchoscopy is a useful technique for more accurate positioning of endotracheal tubes in tracheobronchial injuries.[22] A small tracheal wound should heal within 48 hours.[26] Other clinicians recommend tracheostomy in this situation. Tracheostomy is indicated when there is extensive injury to the larynx and the cervical trachea or when endotracheal intubation cannot be performed. More extensive injuries involving complete separation of the trachea or bronchi require open surgical treatment. The distal trachea might retract retrosternally and require sternotomy and cardiopulmonary bypass for life support.

TRAUMATIC RUPTURE OF THE DIAPHRAGM

Traumatic rupture of the diaphragm usually occurs secondary to blunt trauma to the chest and abdomen.[27,28] A patient with this injury can be asymptomatic or might present with respiratory distress. If the diagnosis is suspected, it can be confirmed by chest radiography and by performing a diagnostic pneumoperitoneum.[29] Patients with chronic rupture usually present with symptoms of intestinal obstruction.[29] Diaphragmatic injuries are quite often associated with fractured ribs and a flail chest and, therefore, they frequently require mechanical ventilation for several days. In most circumstances, the intraabdominal pressure exceeds that of the thoracic cavity. This pressure difference is greater during inspiration; therefore, when a deficit occurs in the diaphragm, there is a tendency for abdominal viscera to enter the thoracic cavity.[30] Herniation of abdominal contents does not always take place immediately. Incarceration and strangulation are more likely to occur with small tears.

The anesthesiologist should be aware of this condition, which must be suspected when unexplained changes in pulmonary compliance occur intraoperatively in patients who have sustained serious chest injury. Patients with significant migration of viscera into the chest cavity also appear to be at greater risk from aspiration pneumonitis. The treatment of this condition, once diagnosed, is operative as soon as the patient's condition permits. The optimal approach to repair this injury is through the thoracic cavity, which requires the placement of a double-lumen endotracheal tube for surgical exposure.

Cardiac Injuries

Penetrating cardiac injuries as a result of gunshot or knife wounds frequently lead to immediate decompensation and death because of massive hemorrhage or cardiac tamponade. The right ventricle, which occupies the largest area beneath the sternum, is most commonly penetrated.[31] Nonpenetrating trauma caused by the impact of the chest against the steering wheel can cause serious injury without any external signs of thoracic trauma (Table 15-4). Cardiac contusion is the most common injury.

CARDIAC TAMPONADE

Cardiac tamponade follows a penetrating or blunt cardiac injury with disruption of the cardiac vessels. If 100 to 200 mL of fluid accumulates rapidly in the pericardium, an outflow obstruction could be created. Fluid within the pericardium also limits diastolic filling, giving the patient a reduced stroke volume. If this condition is not recognized and treated promptly, it can be fatal.[32]

Heavy reliance is placed on clinical impression in patients with cardiac tamponade. It should always be suspected in

TABLE 15-4

Cardiac Injuries Resulting from Severe Blunt Trauma

Cardiac contusion
Rupture of a chamber
Tears of valves and connecting arteries
Coronary artery injuries
Rupture of pericardium
Left ventricular aneurysm

TABLE 15-5

Diagnosis of Cardiac Tamponade

Site of wound
Beck's triad
Pulsus paradoxus
ECG
Shock and increased CVP

patients with wounds in the vicinity of the neck, precordium, or upper abdomen.[32] The classic signs are not always present (Table 15-5). Patients might appear restless, cyanotic, or clearly in shock. The symptomatology can be misleading in intoxicated patients. Beck's triad, consisting of distended neck veins, hypotension disproportional to blood loss, and muffled heart sounds, is difficult to perceive in a busy emergency room. Pulsus paradoxus, which is a decline in systolic blood pressure of 10 mmHg or more on inspiration, could be noted, although it is difficult to appreciate without continuous arterial pressure monitoring. Echocardiography is the diagnostic modality of choice and should be done if the patient's condition allows.[33] The ECG might be normal in some patients; it could have nonspecific ST-segment or T-wave abnormalities. Occasionally, it will show electrical alternans, which is suggestive of tamponade (Figure 15-2).

Pericardiocentesis can be used to relieve the tamponade in rapidly deteriorating patients. This is a temporizing measure, however, as blood rapidly reaccumulates in the pericardial sac. Surgical intervention is required for definitive treatment.

Pericardiocentesis should be carried out in a semi-sitting position. A 16- or 18-gauge metal needle is inserted into the subxiphoid region at an angle of 35 degrees and advanced towards the left shoulder. The hub of the needle can be connected to a V-lead of the ECG, and ECG monitoring can be carried out while the needle is advanced toward the pericardial sac. Accidental encroachment of the needle on the ventricular wall will be evident as ST-segment elevation. Removal of 30 to 60 mL of blood could result in dramatic improvement. If a plastic catheter is used for aspiration, it should be secured to allow repeated drainage.

Time will dictate the degree of monitoring to be carried out on patients with cardiac tamponade. In many situations, basic monitoring techniques are used. Whenever possible, the CVP should be monitored, allowing interpretation of the waveform while providing continuous pressure readings. In pericardial tamponade or effusion, the classic waveform is a pronounced systolic X descent with minimal Y descent (Figure 15-3).

Central venous pressure monitoring is not only useful in the diagnosis but also can be used as a guide to volume replacement after pericardial decompression. High central venous pressures (in the vicinity of 15 to 20 cmH$_2$O) should be maintained until the tamponade is relieved.[34]

The patient with tamponade functions with limited diastolic filling. Anesthetic management should center on maintaining a high heart rate, minimizing myocardial depression, and avoiding decreases in system vascular resistance (SVR) to preserve perfusion pressures. Agents should be selected with these goals in mind (Table 15-6). Induction with a sympathomimetic such as ketamine would be a desirable choice to provide analgesia, amnesia, and unconsciousness. Hemodynamic instability can be managed with inotropes and fluids. Mechanical ventilation decreases preload and cardiac output. If possible, the patient should be allowed to breathe spontaneously until the tamponade is decompressed. If controlled ventilation is necessary, high rates and low tidal volumes are acceptable, with the avoidance of positive end-expiratory pressure.

CORONARY ARTERY INJURIES

Division of a coronary artery invariably leads to hemorrhage and tamponade and, depending on the size of the vessel, can cause myocardial infarction. Most injuries involve the left coronary artery or its branches. The right coronary artery is protected by the sternum and for that reason is rarely injured. These injuries are usually discovered at the time of surgery, and lacerations of larger arteries are reanastomosed if possible. Saphenous vein grafts from the aorta to a coronary artery distal to the injury have been described.[35] Blunt injuries can result in occlusion of a coronary artery, eventually leading to myocardial infarction. From an anesthetic standpoint, provided a tamponade is not impending, these patients should be managed similarly to patients with acute myocardial infarctions.

CARDIAC CONTUSIONS

Blunt trauma to the chest wall resulting in cardiac contusions can occur in a variety of ways (Table 15-7). On sudden impact, the heart strikes the inner aspect of the chest wall with great force, often resulting in cardiac contusion and more serious injuries. The patient commonly complains of chest discomfort which, in light of the traumatic event, could be

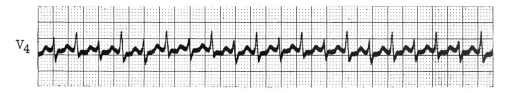

FIGURE 15-2 Electrocardiograph showing electrical alternatives in a patient with a cardiac tamponade.

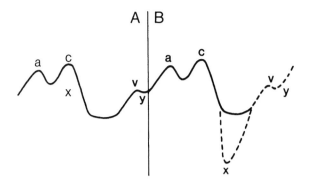

FIGURE 15-3 **A,** Normal a, c, and y waves with the x and y descents. **B,** Pronounced x descent seen in cardiac tamponade.

TABLE 15-7
Causes of Cardiac Contusion
Steering wheel injury
Fist
Club
Ball
Puck
Kick
Fall
Blast

interpreted as a chest wall contusion or a fracture of the sternum.

Rhythm disturbances are among the most common presenting signs in patients with cardiac contusion.[36] Conduction disturbances are more commonly associated with injuries to the right atrium and ventricle (Table 15-8).

Typical signs of injury might not appear for several hours after the initial trauma. There should be a high index of suspicion in patients presenting with rhythm or conduction disturbances and hypotension. Most routine and sophisticated tests have proved unreliable. Enzyme studies are of little help. Two-dimensional echocardiography has proven useful in diagnosis of regional wall motion abnormalities.[36,37] Patients with these injuries should be handled in the same manner as patients presenting with myocardial infarctions.[38]

INJURIES TO THE GREAT VESSELS

Hemorrhage resulting from injury to the great vessels is usually devastating, allowing only approximately 15% of patients to reach a medical facility alive.[39-40] Those patients who do survive transport to the hospital have been found to have a traumatic dissection of the aorta.[41-43] The hematoma is typically contained within the adventitia. Containment of the hematoma is short-lived, and surgical intervention must be prompt.

In the majority of cases, patients complain of a "ripping" chest pain to the back. On clinical examination, blood pressure is elevated, and there are symptoms of shock. The gold standard for diagnosis is the angiogram. Other radiologic findings that might raise the suspicion of a traumatic dissection include the following[44]:

● Mediastinal widening
● Hemothorax
● Tracheal or esophageal deviation
● A widened paratracheal stripe

Transesophageal echocardiography is useful for visualization of the aorta. Computed tomography in general is not employed because of time consumption and failure to provide a definitive diagnosis.[45] Caval injuries are among the most difficult to deal with surgically and are associated with an extremely high mortality rate.[46]

Because of the potential for massive blood loss, appropriate intravenous access should be established, and rapid-transfusion devices should be present and ready. While managing the patient with major thoracic vessel injuries, the anesthesiologist must be careful to avoid extremes in blood pressure, which can be controlled with beta-blockers and vasodilators.[47] The adventitia, which has contained the hematoma, cannot withstand the same wall pressure as the intact aorta. Only rarely is cardiopulmonary bypass needed in major thoracic injuries; however, the perfusionist must be ready at a moment's notice to proceed to bypass if necessary. Standard monitors—including arterial and central venous pressure catheters—should be applied.

Hemorrhagic Shock

Shock can be defined as a clinical syndrome resulting from inadequate blood and oxygenated tissue perfusion. In patients who have suffered trauma, hemorrhage is the presumed cause of shock. Clinicians must be able to distinguish shock due to hemorrhage from shock caused by tamponade, tension pneumothorax, or spinal cord injury. Hemorrhagic shock can be divided into four distinct classifications depending on the overall blood loss. The following classifications, proposed by the American College of Surgeons, are based on multiple physical characteristics displayed by the patients and do not rely wholly on blood pressure.[48]

● Class I is hemorrhage that encompasses 0% to 15% of total blood volume. In the absence of compounding factors, only heart rate will be increased, with a delay in capillary refill. There is usually no change in blood pressure or pulse pressure.

TABLE 15-6
Ideal Anesthetic Agent in the Presence of Cardiac Tamponade
Positive inotropic and chronotropic action
Peripheral vasoconstriction
Antiarrhythmic action
Anesthetic properties

TABLE 15-8
Signs of Cardiac Contusion
Pain
Dyspnea
Hypotension and tachycardia
Rhythm disturbances
Conduction abnormalities

- Class II refers to blood loss of 15% to 30%. Clinically, increases in heart rate and respiratory rate, a decrease in pulse pressure, cool, clammy skin, and delayed capillary refill can be seen. The pulse pressure decreases as a result of catecholamine release, which causes constriction of the peripheral vasculature and an increase in diastolic pressure.
- Class III is loss of 30% to 40% of blood volume. There are more impressive increases in heart rate and respiratory rate. Systolic blood pressure falls, and the patient becomes oliguric. Additional signs and symptoms appear neurologically; the patient could appear confused or agitated.
- Class IV represents loss of more than 40% of blood volume. At this point, there is a marked decrease in systolic blood pressure, urine output falls more or ceases to exist, and mental status deteriorates further. Hemorrhagic arrest occurs with more than 80% blood loss.

Patients invoke a number of responses to blood loss if it occurs over sufficient time. The most important compensatory mechanism is a redistribution of blood from the skin, muscle, and splanchnic vessels to the heart and brain. Normally, approximately 70% of the total blood volume is harbored in the venous capacitance vessels. This blood is redistributed rapidly to vital organs. Redistribution of blood is brought about by an elevation in serum catecholamines. Fluid migrates from the interstitial space to the intravascular space as a result of a decline in hydrostatic pressure in the capillaries, and serum lactate levels increase in response to the change to anaerobic metabolism. In the final stages of untreated shock, cardiac decompensation occurs. This could be related to the release of a specific myocardial depressant factor or to increased pulmonary vascular resistance. Animal studies suggest that cardiac decompensation does occur in hemorrhagic shock, but that it is a late event.

Anesthetic Considerations

In the trauma situation, time and opportunity for obtaining a standard anesthetic preoperative evaluation are often limited. Facts are frequently limited, too, and data must be obtained from other sources such as family, emergency room, and emergency medical service personnel.[49] Information important in the preoperative setting includes allergies, past medical and surgical history, and events surrounding the trauma.

The airway status of a trauma patient is a dynamic situation that requires the utmost vigilance by the anesthesiologist.[50,51] Patients often arrive with an endotracheal tube in place, but placement of the tube should be confirmed immediately clinically, and radiologically if time allows. When the patient is not intubated, a secure airway should be ensured. If the situation calls for it, endotracheal intubation should take place under controlled conditions. There are two levels of urgency for endotracheal intubation: emergent and urgent. Emergent situations include, but are not limited to apnea, hypoventilation, significant head injuries, and cyanosis. These scenarios require immediate control of ventilation. If intubation in the classic manner is unsuccessful, then a surgical airway should be attempted. Patients with burns, maxillofacial trauma, and distorted cervical anatomy are all prone to developing upper airway obstruction. Their ventilatory status is tenuous and could

require intubation in an urgent manner. Patients with unknown cervical spine status are frequently encountered. It is generally agreed that if intubation is required in these patients, "in-line stabilization" is the standard of care. This maneuver has been found to decrease cervical spine movement during orotracheal intubation.

The necessities of a proper intubation include the following:
- Preoxygenation
- A variety of intubating devices (blades/handles)
- Endotracheal tubes of various sizes
- Oral and nasal airways
- A CO_2 analyzer
- Access to a fiberoptic scope/tracheostomy equipment

Unless otherwise stated, standard ASA monitors should be in place at all times, if possible.

The choice of induction technique depends on the patient's overall status and should be tailored to meet the patient's individual needs. All trauma patients are considered to have a full stomach and should receive a rapid-sequence induction or liberal use of cricoid pressure during induction. The variety of induction agents are numerous but, overall, medications should be chosen that will achieve the goal of a hemodynamically smooth induction and intubation. Once the patient is intubated, the tube location should be definitively confirmed and then secured.

A question sure to arise is whether or not succinylcholine should be employed as the neuromuscular blocker in trauma patients. Succinylcholine provides adequate intubating conditions within a short period. Its pharmacodynamics are ideal for emergent intubations. Its drawbacks lie in its propensity to cause hyperkalemia and increased intragastric and intracranial pressures, and its status as a possible triggering agent for malignant hyperthermia. These eventualities must be weighed against the necessity for emergent controlled ventilation. It is up to the individual anesthesiologist and his or her clinical judgment whether succinylcholine or a nondepolarizing neuromuscular blocker should be used.

Patient Evaluation

Evaluation of the trauma patient requires the ability to identify and initiate treatment in an organized fashion to optimize patient outcome. Management strategies coordinating initial assessment of the trauma patient have been developed and taught to medical staff by the Medical College of Surgeons in its course on advanced trauma life support (ATLS). The approach has been broken down into the following four components:
- The primary survey
- Resuscitation of vital functions
- The secondary survey
- Definitive care

The goals are described in the following discussion; further details can be found within the ATLS guidelines.

The goal of the primary survey is to recognize life-threatening injuries (Table 15-9). As with all forms of emergency life support, it begins with the ABC's: airway, breathing, and circulation. As major injuries are encountered, they should be dealt with promptly. Large-bore intravenous access is established for restoration of intravascular volume while the primary survey is underway. A patient's airway should be protected, and

TABLE 15-9

Life-Threatening Injuries Picked Up During Primary Survey

Airway obstruction
Tension pneumothorax
Open pneumothorax
Flail chest
Massive hemothorax
Cardiac tamponade
Severe hypothermia

supplemental oxygenation should be supplied. If the patient is apneic, immediate endotracheal intubation is crucial, though this could be made more difficult in the case of a cervical spine injury. The mouth and oropharynx should be inspected and all foreign objects removed. The patient's chest and neck should be inspected to assess major injuries that affect breathing. Attention should be paid to respiratory movement, frequency, and quality. Injuries affecting circulation can be assessed by palpation of the patient's pulse for rate, rhythm, and quality. Neck veins should be observed for distention. A cardiac monitor, blood pressure cuff, and pulse oximeter should be placed for continuous monitoring of ECG activity, peripheral pressure, and oxygenation.

In the situation in which the patient has arrived at the emergency department with pulseless electrical activity (PEA) secondary to penetrating chest trauma, an immediate resuscitative thoracotomy could be indicated. Only a qualified physician can determine the need for this maneuver. When indicated, the patient is immediately intubated and mechanically ventilated. PEA secondary to blunt trauma is not an indication for thoracotomy.

The objective of the secondary survey is to uncover injuries that are not immediately life-threatening and to create a surgical priority list. This is done through a detailed physical examination, withdrawal of blood for review of laboratory values and arterial blood gases, and an upright chest x-ray if the patient is stable. Monitors placed during the primary survey are followed continuously. These findings are then reviewed and managed as needed. By the nature of the injuries, a differential list of suspected internal injuries is generated.

Management

The goals for fluid management of the trauma patient are to maximize oxygen delivery, control blood loss, and resuscitate with fluid. One of the keys to successful resuscitation of seriously traumatized patients is the ability to rapidly infuse fluids. At a minimum, two large-bore intravenous catheters should be placed. Antecubital veins are suitable for this purpose. Intravenous access can also be placed through central veins or by a cut-down technique if necessary. A central venous catheter may be inserted into the internal jugular vein quite safely, with minimal risk of pneumothorax. However, the subclavian route could be preferable in the shock state because its patency is maintained by its bony attachments to the first rib and clavicle. It is also more accessible because cervical collars frequently restrict access to jugular veins. A urinary catheter should be inserted as soon as possible after the diagnosis of shock has

been made. The optimal treatment of patients in hemorrhagic shock is a combination of blood products with crystalloids or colloids.

Volume Resuscitation

A number of options are available for volume resuscitation that can be divided into two categories: colloids and crystalloids.[52-57] The debate over colloids and crystalloids is beyond the scope of this chapter. What follows is a simple overview of volume resuscitation. Colloids include albumin, dextrans, and hetastarch. Albumin, a blood-derived colloid, is provided in 5% and 25% solutions.[55] Albumin is a desirable choice because its physiologic half-life is 15 to 20 days. Dextran may be used as a plasma expander in the presence of shock, as it remains within the intravascular space for approximately 12 hours. Hypersensitivity reactions to this agent have been reported. It can cause an increased bleeding time by interfering with platelet function when more than 1 L is infused. Dextran causes rouleaux formation and for this reason might interfere with cross-matching techniques. Hetastarch can also be used as a plasma expander in the presence of shock. A 6% solution has osmotic properties similar to those of human albumin. Hetastarch is less likely than dextran to cause anaphylaxis or coagulopathy. As a general rule, colloids are used in a 1:1 replacement scheme.

Crystalloids are the most common fluids used for intravascular fluid replacement. Because fluid losses by the trauma patient are isotonic, it is common to replace these losses with a comparable isotonic crystalloid solution. The choice of fluid can be based on a desire to maintain electrolyte and acid/base hemostasis or to avoid possible electrolyte derangements.

CELL-SAVER TECHNIQUES AND RAPID-INFUSION DEVICES

Cell-saver techniques involve the collection of blood which, after appropriate preparation and filtration, is returned to the donor.[56] Autotransfusion should not be used when the blood is soiled by fecal material. Various methods of anticoagulation are used, including citrate-phosphate-dextrose preservative or heparinization. Heparinization should not be used in patients with suspected intracranial bleeding. Autotransfusion is frequently associated with damage to the various blood components, which can result in a decreased red blood cell mass, an elevated bilirubin level, and hemoglobinuria. When massive quantities of blood are autotransfused (more than 5000 mL), coagulopathies frequently develop. Ionized calcium levels should be monitored, as hypocalcemia can develop due to the preservatives in the processed blood. During massive hemorrhage, valuable time could be lost preparing blood for retransfusion. Rapid-infusion devices have been developed that are capable of infusing as much as 2 L of fluid or blood in 1 minute. A heat exchanger is incorporated within the device to prevent hypothermia. Precautions must be taken to avoid air entrainment with these devices.

BLOOD COMPONENT REPLACEMENT

It is the role of the anesthesiologist to continually evaluate current and ongoing blood loss of the trauma patient. Blood loss can be estimated directly through blood contained in suction canisters and lap pads, or indirectly by physiologic responses to blood loss (decreasing hematocrit, mean arterial pressure, central venous pressure, and urine output). The American Society of Anesthesiologists created a task force to review the literature and provide guidelines for the use of blood component therapy. An algorithm was created to reduce the inappropriate use of blood component therapy, thereby avoiding exposure to the adverse effects of transfusions and limiting costs of transfusion.

Red Blood Cells. Current indications for transfusion of red blood cells are based on both hemoglobin triggers and surgical factors affecting the patient's oxygenation. For example, transfusion is rarely indicated for hemoglobin between 7 to 10 g/dL unless there is excessive blood loss (current and ongoing) and oxygen consumption. Other factors, such as atherosclerotic heart disease, will lower the threshold for transfusion. Each unit of packed red blood cells increases the hematocrit by approximately 3%.[57]

Platelets. Platelets may be given for thrombocytopenia (dilutional or absolute) or platelet dysfunction secondary to concurrent drug therapy. Platelet transfusions attempt to correct these deficits and thereby minimize surgical blood loss. For the surgical patient, transfusion is indicated when the count is below 50 $\times 10^9$ in the presence of microvascular bleeding, which manifests as oozing from wound edges, mucus membranes, and IV insertion sites. If there is known platelet dysfunction, transfusion may begin with the presence of microvascular bleeding. Typically, platelet transfusion of five single-donor units or one pooled unit will increase the platelet count by 5000 to 10,000.

Fresh-frozen plasma. Fresh-frozen plasma (FFP) can also be used to minimize surgical bleeding. The prothrombin time (PT) and partial thromboplastin time (PTT) are useful for measuring a coagulopathy that can be corrected with FFP. Laboratory values greater than 1.5 times normal secondary to dilution, consumption, or warfarin therapy indicate an appropriate time to begin FFP therapy. In the trauma setting, the physician can choose to initiate FFP therapy without waiting for coagulation studies when the patient is being massively transfused and has evidence of microvascular bleeding; processing of PT/PTT can take as long as 20 minutes. Correction of coagulopathy can be achieved with the administration of 10 to 15 mL/kg. of FFP. It should be noted that five platelet concentrates contain a quantity of coagulation factors that is similar to one unit of FFP.

Cryoprecipitate. Cryoprecipitate, which contains concentrated factor VIII, fibrinogen, fibronectin, and factor XIII, is also used to achieve hemostasis through correction of coagulopathies. Patients with genetic deficiencies in those coagulation factors should receive cryoprecipitate to control blood loss. In the trauma patient, consumptive coagulopathy leads to a decreased fibrinogen level, resulting in microvascular bleeding. Fibrinogen levels below 80 to 100 mg/dL are an indication for cryoprecipitate therapy. Once again, the physician may initiate therapy when fibrinogen levels are not readily available. Cryoprecipitate is given as 1 unit per 10 kg to raise fibrinogen by 50 mg/dL.

COMPLICATIONS OF TRANSFUSION THERAPY

Serious hazards are associated with the administration of blood component therapy to patients; the most acute complications result from administration of a mismatched unit (Table 15-10).[58] Immediate transfusion reactions, mediated by the recipient's antibodies to donor cells, can be fatal. In the anesthetized patient, the reaction can be apparent through a sud-

TABLE 15-10

Disturbances Caused by Massive Transfusion

Metabolic	Hyperkalemia
	Citrate toxicity
	Hypomagnesemia
	Acidosis/alkalosis
Physiologic	Hypothermia
	Coagulopathy

den rise in temperature, tachycardia disproportionate to surgical conditions, hypotension, hemoglobinuria, and diffuse oozing in the surgical field. Should this be suspected, the transfusion must be stopped immediately and a new type and crossmatch sent to the laboratory. The most common cause of significant transfusion reactions remains administration of a mismatched unit. Thus methodic scrutiny of the necessary documentation and patient identification is absolutely necessary for each unit given.

Although donated blood is screened for infectious agents, it is still possible to expose the patient.[59] The most common agent transmitted is cytomegalovirus, which, in most cases, leads to a subclinical infection. The risk of being exposed to hepatitis C is 0.03% per unit of blood given.[59,60] The risk of exposure to HIV ranges between 1:450,000 to 1:660,000.[60] Blood might also be contaminated with bacteria, resulting in sepsis. Contamination can be avoided if the unit is delivered in less than 4 hours.

Massive blood transfusion may be defined as replacement of one or more blood volumes (approximately 10 to 20 units) in a 24-hour period. In the exsanguinating trauma patient, one blood volume can be replaced in a matter of hours or minutes. The first and foremost concern is maintaining adequate oxygen delivery and volume. Complications from massive transfusion stem from hemodilution and can result in coagulopathy, hypothermia, hypocalcemia, hyperkalemia, and acidosis.

Coagulopathy. Dilutional coagulopathy is a direct result of blood and volume replacement.[61-64] Packed red blood cells do not contain coagulation factors. As stated before, the anesthesiologist must use both clinical observations from the surgical field and laboratory values to guide proper blood component replacement. The most common cause of a coagulopathy is thrombocytopenia. Disseminated intravascular coagulation (DIC) must be included in the differential diagnosis in any patient presenting with a bleeding diathesis. This typically occurs in patients receiving large quantities of stored blood. It is characterized by an initial tendency toward coagulation, which is followed rapidly by deficiencies in the clotting mechanism.

Hypothermia. The patient who requires large amounts of volume expanders and blood components is at risk for hypothermia.[62] Through inhibition of enzyme activity and platelet dysfunction, hypothermia can lead to coagulopathies. Oxygen delivery will also be impaired by lower temperature through a left shift in the hemoglobin-oxygen saturation curve. At temperatures below 30° C, hypothermia also can lead to cardiac arrhythmias and decreased renal function. The patient's core temperature should be monitored and warming devices placed on all access lines to maintain normothermia.

Hypocalcemia. Stored blood products contain a preservative-anticoagulant, citrate-phosphate-dextrose adenine (CPDA-1).

CPDA-1 preserved blood can be stored for up to 35 days. Shelf life of blood products can be extended to 42 days with the addition of Adsol, Nutricel, or Optisolit. When CPDA-1 blood products are infused in large quantities, the citrate will bind with calcium. With normal rates of infusion, changes in the ionized calcium level are minimal; however, when infusion rates exceed 1.5 mL/kg/min, symptoms and signs of hypocalcemia may appear.[61-64] These include hypotension, elevation of the central venous pressure, and tetany. The ECG might show evidence of a prolonged QT interval. Hyperventilation causes a decrease in ionized calcium levels and, therefore, should be carefully avoided during rapid infusions of stored blood. With ongoing transfusion, serial ionized calcium level should be recorded and treated.

Hyperkalemia. With time, the extracellular concentration of potassium in banked blood gradually increases. Concentration of extracellular potassium ranges from 4 on day one to 23 mEq/L by day 21.[64] Hyperkalemia is usually not a problem during normal rates of infusion. Even during rapid infusions, potassium from stored blood enters donor cells or is excreted by the kidneys. Hyperkalemia occurs in adults only when the rates of infusion exceed 100 mL/min or in patients with preexisting renal dysfunction; however, infants and children are more prone to this problem than are adults.

Metabolic acidosis. The trauma patient is often acidotic secondary to anaerobic metabolism from decreased tissue perfusion. Each unit of stored blood is typically acidic because of citrate and the accumulation of red cell metabolites. Although acidic, stored blood will be buffered in vivo by conversion of citrate to bicarbonate. The most common acid-base abnormality following massive transfusion is metabolic alkalosis. Once normal tissue perfusion has been restored, lactate and the citrate from blood component therapy are converted metabolically to bicarbonate.

In summary, the transfusion of massive quantities of blood induces several biochemical, physiologic, and metabolic changes, which, if not corrected, can cause serious morbidity and mortality.

Inotropes and Vasopressors in Shock

According to the Advanced Trauma Life Support recommendations, vasopressors have no place in the long-term treatment of shock due to hemorrhage. This is because the primary pathophysiologic defect is inadequate tissue perfusion secondary to blood loss; therefore, the primary treatment should be directed toward replenishing fluid and blood losses. Occasionally, it becomes necessary to use vasopressors (e.g., epinephrine) in patients presenting in extremis. Vasopressor support is of vital importance in this situation. Those drugs with predominant α-stimulating properties appear to be the most beneficial, and drugs with predominant β-stimulating effects the least. Dopamine, a precursor of norepinephrine, has been used in clinical practice for many years and has some interesting properties.[65] In low doses (1 to 3 µg/kg/min), it acts on the dopaminergic receptors, causing renal vasculature to dilate and a corresponding diuresis. In doses of 3 to 8 µg/kg/min, β_1-stimulation increases myocardial contractility, heart rate, and cardiac output. At doses of 8 to 20 µg/kg/min, α_1-receptor effects predominate. There is a large increase in systemic vascular resistance and a fall in renal blood flow. Dopamine also displays indirect effects (because of release of norepinephrine) at doses more than 20 µg/kg/min. Therefore this vasopressor might be of some definite benefit to patients in shock.[66] It is important, however, to replace blood and fluid losses while employing this therapy. In the terminal stages of shock, dopamine also might provide some inotropic support. Dopamine should always be infused through a central vein.

Epinephrine, a β- and α-agonist, is an important drug in emergency conditions. β_1-stimulation increases cardiac output, heart rate, and contractility. Epinephrine's β_2-stimulation vasodilates skeletal muscle and relaxes bronchial smooth muscle. The α properties increase coronary and cerebral perfusion pressure at the expense of splanchnic and renal blood flow. Epinephrine is commonly used in bolus doses of 0.05 to 1 mg and infusion rates of 0.05 to 0.3 µg/kg/min. Epinephrine's indications in ACLS are widely known; its use in trauma is more of a stabilizer until proper fluid resuscitation is achieved.

Renal Failure

A discussion of thoracic trauma would be incomplete without reference to renal failure. Although posttraumatic renal failure is uncommon, with an incidence of approximately 3%, it is associated with a 60% mortality rate.[67] The etiology of renal failure in the trauma setting is predominantly secondary to acute tubular necrosis.[68] Intense renal vasoconstriction accompanying hypovolemic shock accounts for the majority of cases of renal failure in trauma victims. Patients with serious muscle injuries also can develop renal failure secondary to myoglobulinuria. Finally, some patients develop renal failure secondary to drug toxicity in the course of treatment. Aminoglycosides and cephalosporins are known nephrotoxic substances, and radiographic contrast materials are also nephrotoxic.[69,70]

Oliguria, defined as a volume of more than 500 mL of urine in 24 hours or 0.5 mL/kg/hr or less of urine output during that period, is the most common sign of renal failure following major trauma. The cause of oliguria is uncertain but could involve renal tubular obstruction, passive backflow of the glomerular filtrate, or intense prerenal vasoconstriction. The predominant effects of filtration failure are the retention of creatinine, urea, and some electrolytes. In complete failure, the serum creatinine rises by approximately 1.5 mg/dL per day; however, these biochemical changes in blood or urine are of minimal help to the anesthesiologist during surgery. It is mandatory to measure the urine output in all patients presenting with significant blood loss or blunt trauma, and the urine output should be recorded on an hourly basis. The most likely cause of oliguria in the surgical setting is inadequate fluid or blood replacement. Should oliguria occur in the course of a surgical procedure, the most rational approach to the problem is to first rule out any technical problems with the catheter. A urine sample should be sent to the laboratory to measure urine electrolytes. Patients should be given a fluid challenge. Infusion of 300 to 500 mL of a balanced saline solution is recommended. Measurement of the central venous pressure is an invaluable tool in the assessment of the volume status in traumatized patients. If there is no response to this approach after approximately 30 minutes, sufficient cardiac output to the kidneys should be assessed. If cardiac output needs augmentation, then

TABLE 15-11

Indications for Emergency Thoracotomy

Penetrating trauma with cardiac electrical activity
Rapid collection of >1500 mL blood from a chest tube

a second bolus may be used. If oliguria persists despite adequate cardiac output and a maximized fluid status, the possibility of other causes should be entertained. These include renal artery or vein occlusion, ureteral obstruction, acute tubular necrosis, or inappropriate antidiuretic hormone secretion. Dopamine is the only vasopressor recommended in renal failure. Infusions should be monitored carefully. Doses in the range of 1 to 5 µg/kg/min have a favorable effect on the dopaminergic receptors in the renal vessels, causing dilatation. Acute renal failure is an important entity occurring in patients with serious trauma, and the anesthesiologist, who is usually first to detect the onset of this condition, must treat oliguria in these patients aggressively.

Summary

The anesthesiologist plays a highly important role in the management of patients with serious thoracic trauma. In the majority of cases, the anesthesiologist is confronted with patients who have serious physical and physiologic insults. It is important for physicians to remain focused on their immediate goals despite all the activity surrounding the patient. Constant attention must be paid to the possibility of performing a thoracotomy (Table 15-11). A combined coordinated effort by the entire medical staff is needed to elicit a successful outcome.

REFERENCES

1. American College of Surgeons: *National trauma data bank—report 2001, data for period 1994-1999,* www.facs.org/trauma/ntdb.html.
2. National Center for Health Statistics: *Injury report series 13,* 131:1996/1997.
3. National Trauma Registry: *1999 hospital admission report-1998-99. Canadian institute for health information (CIHI),* www.cihi.ca/facts/ntrindex.html.
4. Munez E: Economic cost of trauma in the United States, *J Trauma* 24:237, 1984.
5. Locicero J, Matter K: Epidemiology of chest trauma, *Surg Clin North Am* 69:15, 1989.
6. American College of Surgeons: Advanced trauma life support, 147, 1997.
7. Bloomer W: Chest trauma as affected by age and preexisting disease. In Daughtry DC (ed): *Thoracic trauma,* Boston, 1980, Little Brown.
8. Swan K, Swan B, Swan K: Deceleration thoracic injury, *J Trauma* 51:970, 2001.
9. Collins, J: Chest wall trauma, *J Thorac Imag,* 15:112, 2000.
10. Symbas PN: *Cardiothoracic trauma,* Philadelphia, 1998, WB Saunders.
11. Calhoon J: Chest trauma. Approach and management, *Clin Chest Med* 13:55, 1992.
12. Tanaka H, Tajimi K, Endoh Y, et al: Pneumatic stabilization for flail chest injury. an 11-year study, *Surg Today* 31:12, 2001.
13. Moore B: Operative stabilization of non-penetrating chest injuries, *J Thorac Cardiovasc Surg* 70:619, 1975.
14. Pierson D: Indications for mechanical ventilation in adults with acute respiratory failure, *Resp Care* 47:249, 2002.
15. Murphy C, Murphy M: *Radiology for anesthesia and critical care,* New York, 1987, Churchill Livingstone.
16. Hall F: Radiographic diagnosis of pneumothorax, *Radiology* 188:583, 1993.
17. Werne C, Sands M: Left tension pneumothorax masquerading as anterior myocardial infarction, *Ann Emerg Med* 14:164, 1985.
18. Barton E, Rhee P, Hutton K, et al: The pathophysiology of tension pneumothorax in ventilated swine, *J Emerg Med* 15: 147, 1997.
19. Old S: Management of trauma. nitrous oxide dangerous in pneumothorax, *BMJ* 5:1539, 1993.
20. Gabor S, Renner H, Pinter H, et al: Indications for surgery in tracheobronchial ruptures, *Eur J Cardiothorac Surg* 20:399, 2001.
21. Kiser A, O'Brien S, Detterbeck F: Blunt tracheobronchial injuries. treatment and outcomes, *Ann Thorac Surg* 71:2059, 2000.
22. Chen D, Han L, Hu Y, et al: Diagnosis and treatment of bronchial rupture from blunt thoracic trauma, *Chin Med J* (Engl) 114:540, 1998.
23. Bertelsen S, Howitz P: Injuries of the trachea and bronchi, *Thorax* 27:188, 1972.
24. Lloyd J, Heydinger D, Klassen K, et al: Rupture of the main bronchi in closed chest injury, *Arch Surg* 77:597, 1958.
25. Symbas P, Hatcher C, Boehm G: Acute penetrating tracheal trauma, *Ann Thorac Surg* 26:199, 1978.
26. Ramzy A, Rodriguez A, Turney S: Management of major tracheobronchial ruptures in patients with multiple system trauma, *J Trauma* 28:1353, 1988.
27. Ogle J, Klofas E: Tension pneumoperitoneum after blunt trauma, *J Trauma* 41:909, 1996.
28. Cupitt J, Smith M: Missed diaphragm rupture following blunt trauma, *Anaesth Intens Care* 29:292, 2001.
29. Wieneck R, Wilson R, Steiger Z: Acute injuries of the diaphragm. An analysis of 165 cases, *J Thorac Cardiovasc Surg* 92:989, 1986.
30. Reina A, Vidana E, Soriano P, et al: Traumatic intrapericardial diaphragmatic hernia. Case report and literature review, *Injury* 32:153, 2001.
31. Symbas PN, Harlaftis N, Waldo WJ: Penetrating cardiac wounds. A comparison of different therapeutic methods, *Ann Surg* 183:377, 1976.
32. Crawford R, Kasem H, Bleetmen A: Traumatic pericardial tamponade. Relearning old lessons, *J Accid Emerg Med* 14:252, 1997.
33. Tsang T, Oh J, Seward J, et al: Diagnostic value of echocardiography in cardiac tamponade, *Herz* 25:734, 2000.
34. Shabetai R, Fowler N, Guntheroth W: The hemodynamics of cardiac tamponade and constrictive pericarditis, *Am J Cardiol* 26:480, 1970.
35. Espada R, Whisennand H, Matter K, et al: Surgical management of penetrating injuries to the coronary arteries, *Surgery* 78:755, 1975.
36. Kaye P, O'Sullivan I.: Myocardial contusion. Emergency investigation and diagnosis, *Emerg Med J* 19:8, 2002.
37. Weiss R, Brier J, O'Connor W, et al: The usefulness of transesophageal echocardiography in diagnosing cardiac contusions, *Chest* 109: 73, 1996.
38. Christensen M, Sutton K: Myocardial contusion. New concepts in diagnosis and management, *Am J Crit Care* 2:28, 1993.
39. Parmly L, Mattingly T, Marion W: Nonpenetrating traumatic injury of the aorta, *Circulation* 17:1086, 1958.
40. Williams J, Graff J, Uku J, et al: Aortic injury in vehicular trauma, *Ann Thorac Surg* 57:726, 1994.
41. Daily P, Trueblood HW, Stinson FB, et al: Management of acute aortic dissections, *Ann Thorac Surg* 10:237, 1970.
42. Schmidt CA, Jacobson J: Thoracic aortic injury, *Arch Surg* 119:1244, 1984.
43. Greendyke RM: Traumatic rupture of the aorta, *JAMA* 195:119, 1966.
44. Fabian TC, Richardson J, Croce M, et al: Prospective study of blunt aortic injury. Multicenter trial of the American Association for the Surgery of Trauma, *J Trauma* 42:374, 1997.
45. Graham A, McManus K, McGuigan J, et al: Traumatic rupture of the thoracic aorta. Computed tomography may be a dangerous waste of time, *Ann R Coll Surg Engl* 77:154, 1995.
46. Bricker D, Morton J, Okies J, et al: Surgical management of injuries to the vena cava. Changing patterns of injury and newer techniques of repair, *J Trauma* 11:725, 1971.
47. Gammie J, Shah A, Hattler B, et al: Traumatic aortic rupture. Diagnosis and management, *Ann Thorac Surg* 66:295, 1998.
48. American College of Surgeons: *Committee on trauma and advanced trauma life support program for physicians,* Chicago, 1998, American College of Surgeons.
49. Kingsley C: Perioperative anesthetic management of thoracic trauma, *Anesth Clin North Am* 7:183, 1999.
50. Thierbach A: Airway management in trauma patients, *Anesth Clin North Am* 17:63, 1999.
51. Rodricks M: Emergent airway management—indications and methods in face of confounding conditions, *Crit Care Clin* 16:389, 2000.

52. Orlinsky M: Current controversies in shock and resuscitation, *Surg Clin North Am* 81:1217, 2001.

53. Rosenthal MH:. Intraoperative fluid management–what and how much? *Chest* 115:106s–112s, 1999.

54. McCunn M.: Nonblood fluid resuscitation—more questions than answers, *Anesth Clin North Am* 17: 1999.

55. Albumin therapy—your link to the latest clinical resources, www.albumintherapy.com, April 2002.

56. Landers DF: Vascular access and fluid resuscitation in trauma–issues of blood and blood products, *Anesth Clin North Am* 17:125, 1999.

57. Wiesen AR, Hospenthal DR, Byrd JC, et al: Equilibration of hemoglobin concentration after transfusion in medical inpatients not actively bleeding, *Ann Intern Med* 121:278, 1994.

58. Linden J, Tourault M, Schribner C: Decrease in frequency of transfusion fatalities, *Transfusion* 37:243, 1997.

59. Schreiber GB, Busch MP, Kleinman SH, et al: The risk of transfusion-transmitted viral infections, *N Engl J Med* 334:1685, 1996.

60. Lackritz EM, Satten GA, Aberle-Grasse J, et al: Estimated risk of transmission of the human immunodeficiency virus by screened blood in the United States, *N Engl J Med* 333:1721, 1996.

61. McFarland J: Perioperative blood transfusions. Indications and options, *Chest* 115:113s, 1999.

62. Eddy V: Hypothermia, coagulopathy, and acidosis, *Surg Clin North Am* 80:845–854, 2000.

63. Drummon J: The massively bleeding patient. *Anesth Clin North Am* 19:633, 2001.

64. Crosby E: Perioperative haemotherapy II. Risks and complications of blood transfusion, *Can J Anaesth* 39:822, 1992.

65. Mikhail MS, Morgan GE: Adrenergic agonist and antagonists. In (ed): *Clinical anesthesiology,* ed 2, 1992.

66. Schleien C: Postresuscitation management, *Ann Emerg Med* 37: 182, 2001.

67. Baek S, Makabali G, Shoemaker W: Clinical determinants of survival from postoperative renal failure, *Surg Gynecol Obstet* 140:685, 1975.

68. Wilson W: Oliguria a sign of renal success or impending renal failure? *Anesth Clin North Am* 19:841, 2001.

69. Silverblatt FJ: Antibiotic nephrotoxicity—a review of pathogenesis and prevention, *Urol Clin North Am* 557, 1975.

70. Ansari Z, Baldwin D: Acute renal failure due to radiocontrast agents, *Nephron* 17:28, 1976.

Pediatric Thoracic Surgery* 16

Guy M. Lerner, MD
Carol L. Lake, MD, MBA, MPH

PERIOPERATIVE management of neonates, infants, and children for thoracic, noncardiac procedures is demanding and challenging. Children undergoing these procedures generally are considered high-risk. Their young age and immature organ systems, the disease process, and the invasiveness of the surgery all may affect the outcome. In caring for these children, the anesthesiologist not only must appreciate the anatomic and physiologic differences from adults but also must have sufficient knowledge of other disciplines, such as neonatology. Furthermore, the anesthesiologist cannot work in isolation because cooperation among all specialties (e.g., surgery, anesthesiology, neonatology, critical care medicine, and nursing) is essential for reducing morbidity and mortality.

The focus of this chapter is to address anesthetic considerations when providing care for neonates, infants, and children undergoing thoracic, noncardiac surgery. After a general discussion of the relevant issues in pediatric anesthesia, management of the most common disease entities is discussed. A more complete summary of pediatric thoracic pathology is provided in the Appendix to this chapter. For management of cardiovascular procedures in pediatric patients, the interested reader is referred to standard textbooks such as Lake (*Pediatric Cardiac Anesthesia*) or Greeley (*Perioperative Management of the Patient with Congenital Heart Disease*).

Uniqueness of the Pediatric Patient

Knowledge of the anatomic and physiologic differences between children and adults is essential for the safe conduct of anesthesia. Some of these important differences are summarized in Table 16-1. The anesthesiologist must consider carefully these age- and size-related variables, as well as factors related to the specific disease process being treated, the operation being performed, the level of postoperative care available, and the preferences of the individual surgeon. Indeed, anesthetic management of the premature infant is virtually a spe-

cialty in itself.[1] As the child grows, matures, and passes into an "age of awareness," psychologic factors play an increasingly important role in anesthetic management if the trauma associated with hospitalization, fear, pain, and separation of child and parents is to be minimized.

Fetal to Neonatal Transition

The fetus has intrauterine renal, hepatic, endocrine, hematopoietic, and neural function. Maternal organ systems may assist fetal function to some extent by placental exchange, but for the most part, these systems are functional at birth, requiring no great transition. The gastrointestinal and neuromuscular systems continue to develop after birth, but they are usually capable of immediately meeting the infant's needs. The greatest changes required in adapting to extrauterine life involve the cardiovascular and respiratory systems.

FETAL RESPIRATION

Fetal respiration takes place at the capillary interfaces of the placenta. Maternal oxygen diffuses across the placenta to the fetal blood because of the gradient that exists between mother's arterial blood ($Po_2 = 90–100$ mmHg) and that of the fetus ($Po_2 = 30–35$ mmHg). Fetal carbon dioxide diffuses similarly by the Haldane and Bohr effects, respectively.[2] Obviously, fetal lungs contain no air. Pulmonary blood flow is limited before birth because the lungs are performing no ventilatory function.

FETAL CIRCULATION

During intrauterine life, the fetus depends on three arterial-venous communications, or "shunts," that are not normally present after birth—the ductus venosus, foramen ovale, and ductus arteriosus. Each of these communications plays a vital role in maintaining efficient fetal circulation in utero and in allowing the fetal blood to bypass the nonaerated lungs. Relatively oxygenated placental blood ($Po_2 = 60$ mmHg) flows from the low-pressure side of the placenta through the fetal umbilical vein to the fetal liver, through which it enters the inferior vena cava through the ductus venosus. This oxygenated blood mixes with fetal inferior vena caval blood and, to a lesser degree, with superior vena caval blood, resulting in blood with a Po_2 of approximately 35 to 40 mmHg that flows into the right atrium. The anatomic characteristics of the atrial septum with the "trap-door" flap of the foramen ovale (FO) direct most of this oxygen-rich blood across the FO to the left atrium (LA).

*The authors acknowledge the extensive use of material from the excellent chapter of Bland, Brosius, Mancuso, et al, "Anesthesia for Pediatric and Neonatal Thoracic Surgery," from the second edition of this book.

TABLE 16-1
Normal Values

Age		Heart Rate (bpm)	Blood Pressure (mmHg)	Respiratory Rate (breaths/min)	Hematocrit (%)	Blood Volume (mL/kg)	Maintenance Fluids mL/kg/24 hr	Caloric Requirements (cal/kg/24 hr)
Premature (<2000 g)	Preterm	140-160	50/30	40-60	40-50	100	100-120	120
Neonate	0-28 days	120-140	60/40	40-60	40-60	100	80-100	100
Infant	28 d-1 yr	80-120	60-90	30-50 40-60	30-40	8-80	8-80	80-100
Child	1-10 yr	80-100	80-120 40-70	20-30	30-40	70	60-80	40-80
Young adult	11-16 yr	60-90	90-140 50-80	10-20	35-45	60-70	60	40-60

The higher pressure in the right atrium keeps the foramen ovale open prior to birth; reversal of this pressure gradient at birth allows functional closure of the foramen ovale even though it might not close anatomically for many years. Left atrial blood then mixes with the small amount of pulmonary venous blood, crosses the mitral valve into the left ventricle, and is pumped into the aorta and systemic circulation. The brachiocephalic and coronary vessels receive the relatively well-saturated arterial blood.

Venous blood from the superior vena cava enters the right atrium, mixing minimally with blood from the inferior vena cava and placenta before crossing the tricuspid valve into the right ventricle (RV). A small percentage of the blood ejected by the RV goes to the lungs. The lower Po_2 of this blood results in pulmonary vasoconstriction and increased PVR. This small fraction of the right ventricular output that goes to the lungs mixes with blood from the bronchial arteries and drains into the LA. The remaining blood pumped from the RV follows the path of least resistance, passing from the pulmonary artery into the aorta through the ductus arteriosus to perfuse the lower portion of the systemic vascular bed and the fetal portion of the placenta through two umbilical arteries. Because of the streaming of caval blood in the right atrium, the blood in the lower body is not as well oxygenated as that of the aortic arch and brachiocephalic vessels.

In contrast to the extrauterine circulation, the arterial side of the fetal circulation is the low-pressure, low-resistance circuit due to the runoff into the low-resistance placenta. Pulmonary vascular resistance (PVR) greatly exceeds systemic vascular resistance until the first breath is taken and the umbilical cord is clamped. These two actions cause a simultaneous decrease in PVR and an increase in systemic vascular resistance. As the arterial Po_2 increases, PVR decreases further, and left-to-right (aortic-to-pulmonary arterial) shunting may occur across the still-patent ductus arteriosus. With further increases in Po_2, the ductus arterius begins to close and systemic vascular resistance increases, effectively closing the FO by increasing the left atrial pressure. PVR continues to decrease over a period of approximately 7 days, but normal values for PVR may not be achieved for several weeks after birth because the pulmonary vessels become more compliant.[3,4]

THE TRANSITIONAL CIRCULATION
In utero, the placenta is the organ of gas exchange, and the lungs are filled with amniotic fluid. A healthy, full-term newborn has successfully made the transition from intrauterine life to extrauterine life, with the lungs receiving the entire output from the RV and performing gas exchange. This change, although necessarily sudden at birth, is neither functionally nor anatomically permanent until at least several days after birth. The pulmonary vasculature is very reactive to many stimuli, and PVR may increase dramatically in response to hypoxemia, acidemia, hypercarbia, hypoglycemia, anemia, polycythemia, sepsis, and hypothermia.[5] Even in the healthy newborn, PVR is higher than in adults and only gradually decreases during the first few months of life, but it might not reach adult levels for several years.[6]

The transitional nature of the circulation in neonates is important to the anesthesiologist. If a baby has hypoxemia, hypercarbia, or acidemia, and if PVR increases with a resulting decrease in pulmonary blood flow, gas exchange will worsen and a downward spiral may occur, with blood flow returning to a pattern similar to that seen during fetal life. The foramen ovale will open, as will the ductus arteriosus (DA), and pulmonary blood flow will markedly diminish; however, now there is no placenta. This condition, variously called *persistent fetal circulation* (PFC) or persistent pulmonary hypertension of the newborn (PPHN)[7,8], is very difficult to treat, often requiring infusions of pulmonary vasodilators and catecholamines, along with vigorous efforts to correct the precipitating factor(s) (e.g., hypoxemia, hypercarbia, acidemia). It is preferable to prevent this syndrome with careful attention to arterial blood gases, pH, and patient temperature as well as careful administration of adequate anesthesia to blunt the increased sympathetic tone associated with surgical stress. Persistent fetal circulation may be associated with infection, polycythemia, diaphragmatic hernia, hypoglycemia, hypocalcemia, meconium aspiration, fetal asphyxia, or central nervous system (CNS) abnormalities. Differentiation of PFC from congenital heart disease may require the use of echocardiography and, in some cases, cardiac catheterization and cineangiography.

Maturational Changes
NEONATAL HEPATIC FUNCTION
Neonatal hepatic function is, for all practical purposes, intact at birth. The capacity of the neonate's liver to metabolize bilirubin, however, is almost equal to the normal load of hemoglobin presented. The result is that any stress that impedes metabolism or increases hemolysis may exceed the liver's capacity to conjugate bilirubin, with resulting hyperbilirubinemia. The glucuronyl transferase system requires a period of 6 to 7 days

to reach full functional capacity. Elevated levels of unconjugated bilirubin may result in bilirubin encephalopathy (kernicterus). When bound to albumin, unconjugated bilirubin tends not to enter the CNS; therefore, any condition that increases the presence of unbound bilirubin increases the possibility of permanent brain damage from kernicterus. Those conditions most commonly seen and most preventable are hypoalbuminemia, acidosis, hypoglycemia, hypoxia, hypothermia, and competition for or displacement from albumin binding sites by drugs such as salicylates. Less preventable are sepsis and hemolysis.

Neonates undergoing surgery should always be considered to be at risk for bleeding resulting from vitamin K deficiency. At birth, factors II, VII, IX, and X (the vitamin K-dependent factors) are 20% to 60% of adult values; the values are even lower in preterm infants. Consequently, the prothrombin time is prolonged.[9] Vitamin K_1 is usually given to newborn infants in the United States to prevent hemorrhagic disease. Because synthesis of these coagulation factors occurs in the relatively immature liver, even administration of vitamin K_1 may have minimal impact. Increased synthetic function might not be seen for several weeks. Nonetheless, giving vitamin K_1 at birth is still routine. If the neonate is undergoing surgery, this issue should certainly be addressed before the operation. During the procedure, the surgical field should be carefully observed for any bleeding tendencies. Maternal use of anticonvulsant drugs, warfarin, rifampin, and isoniazid could increase the risk of neonatal bleeding diasthesis.[10]

NEONATAL RENAL FUNCTION

The neonatal kidney is functionally suited for antenatal life and shares responsibility with the placenta and the mother's kidneys for removal of metabolites. After birth there is a period of maturation when the kidney assumes greater functional capacity and growth by the increased workload. Glomerular filtration rate doubles soon after birth, continues to rise, and quadruples when the infant is fully mature. The period of renal maturation is much longer than the period for hepatic maturation. By the age of 1 year, however, renal maturation is nearly complete and reaches its peak capacity at 2 to 3 years of age.[11] Traditionally, the neonatal kidney has been thought to be unable to excrete sodium loads or to concentrate urine to a significant degree. More recently, this theory has been modified to state that because of the higher extracellular fluid volume in the neonatal period and reduced solute loads (e.g., urea and sodium), the neonatal kidney appears not to concentrate.[12,13] For the healthy neonate who is unstressed and not undergoing surgery, the large extracellular fluid volume provides the necessary electrolytes to maintain normal serum sodium concentrations in the first week of life, while the excess extracellular fluid is passed as dilute urine. It is for this reason that salt-free fluids are frequently given to the newborn. The neonatal surgical candidate, however, may translocate fluids the same as any other patient and needs electrolyte replacement. Therefore salt-containing fluids should be given and electrolytes measured regularly.

FLUID, ELECTROLYTE, AND CALORIC REQUIREMENTS

Maintenance requirements for fluids and calories are summarized in Table 16-1. Sodium, potassium, and chloride requirements are all similar to those of adults, at 1 to 3 mEq/kg/24 hr. It must be stressed that these are accepted maintenance requirements and should be used only as guidelines. Adjustments should be made for third-space losses, the presence of congestive heart failure, existing deficits, changes in insensible losses, and drainage losses during surgery. Babies undergoing phototherapy for hyperbilirubinemia or exposed to infrared warmers for temperature maintenance may have as much as a 20% increase in fluid requirements because of increased evaporative losses.[14]

Glucose requirements are 2 to 6 mg/kg/min under normal circumstances and may be reduced when the neonate is under anesthesia. The basic glucose requirement is fulfilled by using 5% dextrose in H_2O, but higher concentrations of glucose may be needed. Caution must be exercised in conditions in which large volumes of fluid are administered (e.g., replacement of intraoperative volume loss) to avoid administering an excess of glucose because hyperosmolarity will result. Hyperosmolarity secondary to hyperglycemia or hypernatremia may play a part in the pathogenesis of intraventricular hemorrhage in neonates.[15,16] It cannot be overemphasized that premature infants, term newborns, and infants undergoing major thoracic procedures need careful monitoring of glucose, sodium, potassium, and calcium. The administration of hypotonic fluids in excess of maintenance volumes (e.g., 5% dextrose in 0.225% saline) may result in significant hyponatremia and should be avoided.[17]

AIRWAY ANATOMY

Anatomically, the child—and especially the infant—is different enough from the adult to make intubation more difficult (Table 16-2). The head is larger in proportion to the rest of the

---

TABLE 16-2

Unique Features of the Infant Airway

Relatively large head (occiput more prominent)

Short neck

Relatively large tongue

Small nares easily obstructed by secretions; infants are obligate nose breathers until approximately 2 months of age and will not open mouth to breathe even if nares are totally obstructed for any reason (e.g., secretions, edema, choanal atresia)

At term the infant larynx is more cephalad than that of the older child or adult; the lower border of the cricoid cartilage is located opposite the middle of C_6

Narrowest portion of the infant's airway is the subglottic area at the level of the cricoid cartilage, so edema greatly diminishes the cross-sectional diameter of airway and can result in stridor or varying degrees of airway obstruction

Epiglottis is relatively long and usually rather stiff, ω-shaped, and extends from the base of the tongue 45 degrees posteriorly

Trachea is short (approximately 4 cm); thus carina is more cephalad (T_3), making endobronchial intubation more likely

The angles formed by the main bronchi with the trachea vary considerably in infants: 10–35 degrees on the right and 30–50 degrees on the left

Thorax is relatively small; sternum soft, ribs are horizontally placed; diaphragms are relatively high; accessory muscles of respiration are weak

body, sometimes making it less stable; however, this disparity, particularly of the occiput, can be used to advantage during intubation by affording a natural "sniffing" position. In a healthy newborn infant, the neck is short in comparison with the adult. The tongue, like the head, is relatively larger in children than in adults and may cause obstruction during induction as well as ventilation by mask. The larynx is more cephalad in the child, lying approximately at the level of C_{2-3}, compared with C_5 in adults. The larynx is not, however, more anterior in the child, although it may seem so because of its cephalad placement and the large tongue. Beyond the larynx, the trachea-to-carina distance is only 4 cm in the infant. Extreme caution must be taken to pass a tracheal tube only 1.5 to 2.0 cm past the vocal cords to avoid bronchial intubation. The epiglottis projects cephalad at approximately 45° from the anterior wall of the larynx. This positioning often makes the epiglottis easier to visualize but more difficult to displace to allow intubation. Finally, the air passages themselves—the nose, nasopharynx, and trachea—must be considered. Being small, but not out of proportion to the infant, they may be easily obstructed owing to the presence of mucus, edema, nasogastric tubes, tape, or endotracheal tubes, for example. Care to prevent inadvertent obstruction must be exercised at all times.

In certain thoracic procedures, having a good understanding of pediatric airway anatomy is highly beneficial. Choosing an endotracheal tube of the right size and attaining the correct placement of that tube are often critical steps in the operative procedure. For example, improper placement of an endotracheal tube in a child with tracheoesophageal fistula can have disastrous consequences. The technique of one-lung ventilation, if required to improve the surgical exposure in the thorax, is an important skill for the pediatric thoracic anesthesiologist.

THERMOREGULATION

Hypothermia in the newborn and in the small child undergoing surgery continues to be a problem, particularly in major surgery of the chest, in which a large surface area is exposed to the air, thus allowing high evaporative and convective heat loss. Both the anesthesiologist and the surgeon should attempt to prevent the heat loss rather than try to correct it after it occurs. The consequences of unintentional hypothermia of the newborn (including 90% mortality in newborns whose temperatures were allowed to fall to 32° C) is well known.[18] It has been shown that not only the degree of hypothermia but also the frequency of deviation from normothermia—even without extreme temperature changes—contribute significantly to morbidity and mortality in the newborn period.[19]

Thermoneutrality is a delicate balance between heat production and heat conservation. The newborn and the small child have a limited ability to produce heat, mostly through the metabolism of brown fat. Premature infants have reduced stores of brown fat. To maintain thermoneutrality, the premature infant, newborn, and small child must depend heavily on heat conservation. Because of greater alveolar ventilation, the rate of heat lost to unheated, dry anesthetic gases by an infant is greater than that of an adult, which means that hypothermia can develop quite rapidly. Anesthesia ablates the body's response to cold stress, making heat conservation in the operating room essential if the morbidity of hypothermia is to be avoided.

Accepted warming techniques include raising the ambient temperature of the operating room, warming and humidifying anesthetic gases, using only warm scrub and irrigation solutions, using forced air warming, providing protection from wetting, using nonionizing heat lamps or thermal mattresses, and warming of all intravenous fluids.[20] Forced air convection is the most effective warming method because it actively transfers heat to the patient. The importance of using as many of these heat conservation methods as possible cannot be overemphasized if thermoneutrality is to be preserved. In children, oxygen consumption has been shown to double in the immediate postoperative period if the child is allowed to emerge from anesthesia in a hypothermic state.[21] If respiratory function is even mildly depressed by narcotics, relaxants, or intrinsic disease, the child may not be able to meet oxygen demands and can deteriorate rapidly. If unintentional hypothermia does occur during surgery, it must be corrected before removal of respiratory support. Equally important is maintenance of temperature during transport to and from the operating room. Portable heated isolettes and open beds equipped with warming lights or radiant heaters are available for this purpose.

THE PREMATURE INFANT

Infants of 37 weeks' gestation or less are classified as premature. Because these infants have not had the time to fully develop, all organ systems are immature and therefore not as ready for extrauterine life. Additionally, because premature infants are even smaller (sometimes much smaller) than term infants, access to them is very limited once draping and positioning have occurred. For this reason, the endotracheal tube, vascular catheters, and all monitors must be carefully secured before surgery begins. In addition to gestational age, newborns may be classified according to the birth weight for a given gestational age (i.e., appropriate, large, or small for gestational age). This is especially important for small gestational age (SGA) premature infants. Because SGA infants are usually subject to extraordinary stress during gestation, liver glycogen stores, iron stores, and muscle mass will be less than for other premature infants of the same gestational age. Often, pulmonary development is accelerated in SGA infants, so that the degree of respiratory distress they exhibit is less than expected. Morbidity and mortality figures increase dramatically in neonates weighing less than 2000 g and of less than 37 weeks' gestation.[22] Reducing these figures and providing a better quality of life for those who survive are the aims of the neonatal intensivists and others, including anesthesiologists caring for those infants. Consequently, the appearance of "prematures" in the operating rooms has become more commonplace and requires anesthetic expertise that gives consideration to their unique problems.

Respiratory Distress Syndrome

Respiratory distress syndrome (RDS), also known as *hyaline membrane disease*, is a disease of atelectasis caused by the deficiency or dysfunction of surfactant normally secreted by type II alveolar cells. Surfactant reduces surface tension in the alveolus, allowing for expansion during respiration. A detailed discussion of the medical management of RDS is beyond the scope of this chapter, and the interested reader is referred to a text of pediatric critical care. Some of these infants may be seen for thoracic procedures, however, so a brief discussion of this subject is in order.

Infants born prematurely have pulmonary disease resulting from both a decreased amount of and an immature form of surfactant. As a result of this lack of surfactant, surface tension in the alveoli is increased, which leads to widespread atelectasis. This decrease or loss of functional residual capacity (FRC) is the important pathophysiologic problem in RDS. The FRC can be partially reestablished with the application of end-expiratory pressure (the end-expiratory grunting done by infants with mild RDS is a form of self-administered positive end-expiratory pressure [PEEP]). For cases of more severe RDS, CPAP and mechanical ventilation with PEEP and increased FIO_2 are used as treatments. It is important to continue mechanical ventilation in the operating room in the same manner as was being done in the intensive care nursery. Ventilators on anesthesia machines may not be flexible enough to accomplish this, so it may be necessary for the infant's own ventilator to be brought into the operating room. Of course, if these infants are to undergo a thoracic procedure, the inspired oxygen concentration, as well as some ventilator parameters, may require adjustment to maintain optimal gas exchange.

Therapies for RDS include mechanical ventilation with PEEP, liquid ventilation with perfluorocarbons, use of surfactant, high-frequency oscillation, and extracorporeal membrane oxygenation. Inhaled nitric oxide (discussed later in this chapter) has also been used effectively to improve oxygenation in these infants.[23] (See the section in this chapter regarding mechanical ventilation of infants during anesthesia.)

The long-term outcome after respiratory distress syndrome may be complicated by the development of bronchopulmonary dysplasia (BPD). Infants with BPD are prone to increased reactivity of the airways, increased risk of pulmonary infection, hyperinflation, and development of emphysema or bullae with the risk of pneumothorax. Their pulmonary compliance may be reduced by the development of interstitial fibrosis. Some infants may be oxygen dependent and require steroids and diuretics to manage their increased airway resistance and fluid retention. Subglottic stenosis can also result after prolonged intubation or tracheostomy.

Pulmonary Hypertension

DEFINITION

Pulmonary hypertension is defined as a mean pulmonary artery pressure greater than 25 mmHg at rest or greater than 30 mmHg during exercise. Pulmonary vascular resistance (PVR) is usually considered in terms of the relationships between pulmonary transvascular pressure changes (P_{pa} to P_{la}) and the flow (F or cardiac output) through the lungs. If the pressure differences are plotted against flow, a curvilinear relationship results in which pulmonary vascular resistance is high at low flow and progressively diminishes with increasing flow.

Pulmonary hypertension may be caused by congenital heart disease or disease affecting the structure and function of the lung. It results from changes in the distensibility of the vasculature such as those occuring with pulmonary vasoconstriction, vascular remodeling, or loss of intrinsic nitric oxide–cyclic guanosine monophosphate vasodilation. This model, however, is applicable only to patients with the right and left sides of the heart in a series configuration. If the right and left sides of the heart are parallel, the output to the pulmonary and systemic circuits depends on the resistance in each.

PATHOPHYSIOLOGY

Pulmonary hypertension may result from increased flow (hyperkinetic type, where $P = r \times F$) or from increased resistance (pulmonary vascular obstruction or pulmonary venous hypertension where $P = R \times f$). If there is no abnormality in the left side of the heart, the pulmonary wedge pressure is normal. If there is obstruction or dysfunction of the left ventricle, however, pulmonary venous hypertension may be present. When the PVR is increased, the following two alterations in the pressure/flow relationship occur:

1. The rate of change of pressure per unit change in flow is greater than with normal PVR.
2. The pressure at a given flow is higher than with normal PVR.

Increased pulmonary blood flow and increased shear forces in the pulmonary vasculature may adversely affect the pulmonary vascular endothelium and its intrinsic production of nitric oxide.[24]

DIAGNOSIS

Confirmation of pulmonary hypertension usually requires direct measurement of pulmonary pressure during catheterization of the right side of the heart. Noninvasive determination of right-sided heart and pulmonary pressure, however, is possible in 95% of patients of all ages (excluding children with complex congenital heart disease).[25] In children with congenital heart disease, Ebeid and coworkers demonstrated a correlation of 0.87 between PVR and the right ventricular preejection period/velocity time integral (RVPEP/VTI). This noninvasive parameter had 97% accuracy, 100 % sensitivity, and 92% specificity in detecting patients with PVR less than 3 Wood unit M^2 when pulmonary hypertension was present.[26] In neonates with severe hypoxemia and cyanosis unresponsive to oxygen, echocardiographic demonstration of a right-to-left shunt through the DA or foramen ovale confirms the presence of PPHN (high pulmonary vascular resistance and low pulmonary blood flow).

THERAPY

Therapies for pulmonary hypertension depend upon cause. In pediatric patients, therapy is initially directed at the cause, and additional therapy is directed toward the residual pulmonary hypertension. Pharmacologic vasodilators may also be used to determine the degree of pulmonary vasoreactivity before a surgical procedure for congenital heart disease to determine its feasibility. General measures include oxygen, ventilation to an alkalotic pH, and control of PCO_2. Supplemental oxygen clearly attenuates pulmonary hypertension in patients with chronic pulmonary parenchymal disease. Oxygen may be helpful during exercise or sleep in some children with pulmonary hypertension. It is of less benefit in patients with Eisenmenger physiology. An increased inspired concentration of oxygen is mandatory during surgical procedures. Mechanical ventilation to maintain an alkalotic pH may help to control pulmonary vascular tone in neonates with PPHN or congenital heart disease.

SURFACTANT THERAPY

Surfactant is a mixture of surfactant-specific proteins and phospholipids. It can be separated into two subtypes: small aggregates and large aggregates. The surface-active component is the large aggregates and is the metabolic precursor of the small aggregates. Alveolar surfactant is synthesized by type II alveolar epithelial cells. It facilitates mucus clearance, protects against infection (antimicrobial functions), has antiinflammatory properties, and decreases surface tension in the alveoli through its concentration of dipalmitoylphosphatidylcholine.[27] Natural preparations extracted from animals, synthetic preparations, and recombinant (primarily containing dipalmitoylphosphatidylcholine) are available. Surfactant use in the prophylaxis of infant respiratory distress syndrome to improve pulmonary compliance is well documented.[28] Use of surfactant therapy during pediatric thoracic surgery outside the neonatal period has not been described. However, its benefits of improving small airway patency with inflammatory lung disease, pneumonia, bronchiolitis, or acute respiratory failure should encourage use in older children. Surfactant therapy, combined with high PEEP, improves oxygenation in an adult animal acute lung injury model (see Chapter 6).[29]

VASODILATORS

The goal of pulmonary vasodilator therapy is to achieve even a small reduction in right ventricular afterload caused by the pulmonary hypertension. The reduction in pulmonary artery pressure and increase in right ventricular output, however, must be achieved without systemic hypotension. Although dipyridamole produces pulmonary vasodilation through the cyclic guanosine monophosphate pathway, it has not been demonstrated to decrease pulmonary artery pressure effectively in pediatric patients.[30] Nitroglycerin and nitroprusside also produce pulmonary vasodilation but are associated with significant systemic hypotension. Short-acting agents (such as intravenous prostacyclin or inhaled nitric oxide) are used both during right-side heart catheterization to assess pulmonary vasoreactivity and for longer term therapy.

INTRAVENOUS PROSTACYCLIN

Prostacyclin and its analogs are endothelial-derived vasodilators that reduce pulmonary vascular resistance through increasing cyclic adenosine monophosphate. Chronic intravenous prostacylin may remodel the pulmonary vascular bed, resulting in reversibility of apparently irreversible pulmonary vascular obstructive disease.[31] The prostacyclin analog ciloprost, given intravenously, induces significant pulmonary vasodilation in animals but adversely affects systemic pressures more than nitric oxide.[32] Nevertheless, long-term intravenous (IV) prostacyclin has been used to improve pulmonary hemodynamics in children with congenital heart disease-induced pulmonary hypertension.[33] Inhalation of prostacyclin reduces pulmonary artery pressure and intrapulmonary right-to-left shunting, but during long-term administration, systemic absorption of prostacyclin causes systemic vasodilation following a few hours of administration.[34]

INHALED NITRIC OXIDE

Nitric oxide (NO) is formed endogenously when nitric oxide synthase (NOS) catalyzes the hydroxylation of the amino acid L-arginine to L-citrulline. The actions of NO are mediated through its activation of soluble guanylate cyclase, which catalyzes the conversion of guanosine triphosphate to cyclic guanosine monophosphate (cGMP)—a process that relaxes vascular smooth muscle. The production of cGMP is controlled by its degradation by cGMP-specific phosphodiesterases. Concomitant administration of phosphodiesterase inhibitors such as zaprinast or dipyridamole has been demonstrated to potentiate and prolong the pulmonary vasodilating effect of NO without altering its pulmonary vascular selectivity.[35]

NOS exists in two forms in human airways: as constitutive NOS (cNOS) and as inducible NOS (iNOS). Constitutive NOS has two subforms: neuronal NOS and endothelial NOS.[36] Inducible NOS is calmodulin independent and calcium independent and is induced by cytokines from inflammatory cells to enhance the response to infection. In sepsis, iNOS produces large amounts of NO for long periods of time and results in the profound systemic vasodilation seen in the systemic inflammatory response syndrome. Constitutive NOS is calmodulin dependent and calcium dependent and causes release of small amounts of NO for short periods of time. Its subtype, eNOS is an important modulator of pulmonary vascular resistance. Blockade of the endogenous production of NO can be accomplished in animal models by agents that compete with L-arginine, such as L-NMMA (N^G-mono-methyl-L-arginine) or L-NAME (N^G-nitro-L-arginine methyl ester). When given by inhalation, the half-life is a few seconds because it is bound to oxyhemoglobin, which subsequently is reduced back to hemoglobin with release of NO_3^-. Other metabolic pathways include interaction with dissolved oxygen in blood to form NO_2^- and combination with deoxyghemoglobin to form stable nitrosohemoglobin, or with carrier molecules to form S-nitrosothiols.[37]

Administration. Commercially, NO is produced by oxidation of ammonia over platinum, or reaction of sodium nitrite with sulfuric acid or sulfur dioxide with nitric acid. It is stored in aluminum alloy tanks. Toxic nitrogen dioxide (NO_2) is also formed during commercial production of NO and can react with water to form nitric acid. Attempts to scavenge NO_2 with soda lime, noXon (Hoechst AG, Frankfurt, Germany)—a polymeric polyphenylsulphide—or Zeolite (Grace, Worms, Germany)—a tetrahedron framework of AlO_4 and SiO_2 supporting naturally occurring and synthetic minerals—have been unsuccessful.[38] Acute overdosage produces nitrogen dioxide, pulmonary edema and hemorrhage, hypoxemia, severe methemoglobinemia, and death.[36]

Safe delivery of inhaled NO requires the following[39]:
- A safe, simple, reliable system
- Accurate monitoring of NO delivery
- Limited production of NO_2
- Scavenging of NO
- Measurement of oxygen concentration downstream from the point of entry
- Continuous analysis of delivered concentration
- Frequent calibration of monitoring equipment
- Analysis of methemoglobin levels in patients
- Administration of the lowest effective concentration

NO can be delivered in the operating room using the Ohmeda INOvent (Ohmeda, Madison, WI) or via a nitrous oxide flowmeter attached to a tank of nitric oxide connected to the anesthesia machine by a specially fitted pressure hose.[40] The INOvent's features include the following:
- Inspiratory gas sampling downstream (just proximal to the Y piece) from the point of injection (just distal to the inspiratory valve)

- Electrochemical analysis
- Displays of FiO_2, NO, and NO_2, multiple alarms
- Capability for use with a manual bag ventilation system for transport

When used with a critical care ventilator, NO is injected between the ventilator output and the humidifier in an amount proportional to the ventilator flow.

The INOvent setup, however, requires use of a fresh gas flow from the anesthesia machine that is equal to or greater than the minute volume of ventilation.[40,41] If a lower fresh gas flow is used, the inhaled concentration of NO will be approximately twice that set on the INOvent. Because high fresh gas flows carry the added disadvantage of increased heat and moisture loss from the patient and increased risk of environmental pollution if scavenging devices are ineffective, use of a standard neonatal ICU ventilator may be easier, even though it precludes administration of volatile anesthetics. Special systems that deliver pulses of nitric oxide into the inhaled gas at the beginning of a breath have been used in experimental settings.[42]

Pharmacologic Effects. Nitric oxide has been shown as effective treatment for persistent pulmonary hypertension of the newborn (PPHN), pulmonary hypertension secondary to hypoxic respiratory failure in neonates, and other neonatal conditions, such as diaphragmatic hernia or meconium aspiration[43,44-46]. Its physiologic effects include the following:

- Dose-dependent selective pulmonary arterial and venous vasodilation
- Decreased mean pulmonary artery pressure (when abnormally increased)
- Improved right ventricular performance, enhanced ventilation/perfusion matching
- Increased oxygenation by improvement in shunt
- Mild bronchodilation

When combined with oxygen (which produces a similar decrease in pulmonary vascular resistance alone), NO produced significantly greater pulmonary vasodilation.[47] In two studies in infants, use of nitric oxide reduced the need for extracorporeal membrane oxygenation (ECMO) (40% of NO patients compared with 71% of control infants required ECMO) but did not change mortality in PPHN.[48,49] In 53% of infants, NO doubled systemic oxygenation, and long-term NO therapy sustained systemic oxygenation.[49]

NO may tend to increase blood flow to well-ventilated areas of the lung. In acute lung injury models inducing ventilation-perfusion mismatching, however, the response is inconsistent with both increases and decreases in ventilation-perfusion mismatching reported.[50,51] The responsiveness of the neonatal lung to NO depends on gestational age and pulmonary vascular maturity. The advantages of nitric oxide over ECMO are considerable; it is cheaper, simpler to administer, and requires no special centers for use.

Toxic effects of NO include methemoglobinemia, production of NO_2, and cellular toxicity. These effects have not been reported in pediatric patients, however, with the exception of two infants in whom nitrotyrosine residues were detected in airway secretions.[52] Potential adverse effects of NO are the development of increased left ventricular filling secondary to increased pulmonary blood flow, platelet dysfunction, decreased surface tension of surfactant, and rebound pulmonary

hypertension on discontinuation. NO oxidizes ferrous ion (Fe^{++}) to ferric ion (Fe^{+++}) to create methemoglobin. The development of methemoglobinemia is dose-related and unlikely at doses of less than 20 ppm. NO should not be administered to patients with reduced ventricular function in whom pulmonary edema and heart failure may result. NO has been shown to reduce peak contractile performance of the left ventricle by hastening the onset of myocardial relaxation in adult humans.[53] Although NO inhibits platelet aggregation and agglutination by increasing platelet cyclic GMP and increases bleeding time in animal studies, increased bleeding has not been observed in human infants.[54] NO has been reported to reduce surfactant protein A gene expression by distal respiratory epithelial cells[55] and to decrease surface tension of surfactant recovered from bronchoalveolar lavage fluid.[55,56] Rebound pulmonary hypertension may result from suppressed endogenous production of NO in the airways (down regulation). This phenomenon is controlled by slow weaning of the dose down to 5 ppm, allowing sufficient time for recovery of pulmonary function before weaning is attempted, increasing the FiO_2 to 0.65 before discontinuation, and using pharmacologic methods (e.g., milrinone) or other phosphodiesterase inhibitors (e.g., sildenafil) to control PVR.[57,58] Rebound typically begins as a slow increase in pulmonary artery pressure beginning several minutes following discontinuation of NO and lasting for only 5 to 10 minutes.[59] It is not usually accompanied by systemic hypotension or hypoxia. Rebound can be distinguished from inability to wean from NO by its transient nature. Finally, it must be recognized that not all patients will respond to NO because of high endogenous levels of NO (as in sepsis) or in blood groups B and AB.[60,61]

COMBINATION OF VASODILATORS WITH NITRIC OXIDE

NO can also be combined with other vasodilators not dependent upon guanylyl cyclase to produce additional selective pulmonary vasodilation. In experimental animal models with pulmonary vasoconstriction produced by U46619 (acute) or monocrotaline (chronic), adenosine and prostacyclin further decreased pulmonary artery pressures.[62] In human trials comparing inhaled iloprost (a stable prostacyclin analog) with inhaled NO, both drugs were equally efficacious in reducing pulmonary vascular resistance but did not demonstrate increased efficacy in combination.[63]

OTHER POSSIBILITIES

ECMO can be used to provide systemic oxygenation while other therapies are used to treat the primary lung disease responsible for hypoxia. Endothelin receptor blockers, oral or intravenous L-arginine (NO precursor), and thromboxane synthase inhibitors/receptor blockers may prove eventually to alleviate pulmonary hypertension. Currently available phosphodiesterase inhibitors such as sildenafil can selectively dilate the pulmonary circulation but do not prolong the pulmonary vasodilator action of NO in animal models.[64] Whether sildenafil can augment the pulmonary vasodilator response to NO may depend on use of the combination in animal models (no augmentation) vs. human clinical situations (increased response).[64,65] Because of the risk of thrombotic events in patients with pulmonary hypertension, if pulmonary vasodilation can be achieved with NO or prostacyclin, oral calcium channel blockers may benefit children with pulmonary hypertension.[66] Anticoagulation may increase survival rates in adults with pulmonary hypertension; however, the benefits of anticoagulation have not been documented in children.[66,67]

Retrolental Fibroplasia or Retinopathy of Prematurity

The newborn, especially the premature infant of less than 34 weeks' gestational age and weighing less than 1000 g, is at risk for retinopathy of prematurity (ROP). The immature retinal vasculature vasoconstricts in response to a variety of stresses and stimuli including hyperoxia, hypoxia, sepsis, blood transfusions, and various arterial carbon dioxide tensions.[68] It has been seen in infants who have never been exposed to oxygen therapy.[69] With the advances seen in neonatology, ROP has increased. Infants at greatest risk for ROP are most likely to have surgery. The role of intraoperative oxygen administration in the etiology of ROP is open to debate, as studies have not shown a correlation between specific arterial oxygen tensions and the development of ROP. The dilemma that the anesthesiologist faces when caring for children at risk for ROP is balancing the need for oxygenation of endo-organs (e.g., heart and brain) against the damaging effects of hyperoxia on the immature retina. Every attempt should be made to avoid more oxygen than is needed to maintain adequate Pao_2 tensions. An infant is thought to be at risk for ROP until about 44 weeks' gestational age, at which time the retina should be mature. Intraoperative strategies used to lower the risk of this complication are the following:

1. Use the lowest possible oxygen concentration to maintain oxygen saturation between 93% to 95% and avoid hyperoxia.[70]
2. Delay elective surgery to a gestational age of greater than 44 weeks.
3. Monitor oxygen saturation from a preductal site (e.g., right upper extremity, nose, earlobe).
4. Maintain preductal Pao_2 in the 40 to 70 mmHg range.

Apnea of Prematurity

Premature and former premature infants who undergo surgery are at risk for postanesthetic apnea, periodic breathing, and bradycardia. The incidence of apneic episodes (i.e., cessation of breathing for more than 15 seconds) is inversely related to both postconceptual age and gestational age.[71] (Postconceptual age is the sum of gestational age plus postnatal age. Because the majority of patients undergoing thoracic procedures will be monitored in a special care unit after surgery, this potential complication should be noticed easily. Nonetheless, it is important to discuss respiratory function and the effects of anesthetics and surgery on respiratory mechanics and control in the neonate.

Respiratory function in the neonate and premature infant having surgery is of concern because central respiratory control is immature. Anesthetics have a dose-dependent, depressant effect on the central, medullary control centers as well as on the peripheral muscles involved in respiration. When exposed to a hypoxic gas mixture, neonates and premature infants show a biphasic response. Initially, they show a hyperventilatory response, which is then followed by a decrease in ventilation.[72] In the healthy, term neonate, this response follows the adult pattern by 3 weeks of age, when there is a sustained hyperventilatory response to hypoxemia. Why the premature infant is unable to mount a

sustained response is unknown. In addition, the neonatal response to hypercapnia is also abnormal, as the neonate and premature infant can increase ventilation only to four times baseline values. In contrast, the older infant's response would be tenfold to twentyfold. Narcotic and inhalation anesthetics have been shown to depress the centrally mediated response to carbon dioxide in adults. Furthermore, studies in adults have shown that even small amounts of residual halothane can ablate the response to hypoxia.[73] Although little data are available, it can be surmised that neonates and premature infants would be especially sensitive to the depressant effects of anesthetics.

Anesthetics acting peripherally, as well, depress muscle tone. Upper-airway obstruction from decreased pharyngeal tone may lead to labored breathing, fatigue, and apnea. A decrease in intercostal muscle tone may lead to a decrease in functional residual capacity and to the development of hypoxemia.[74] The diaphragm of the neonate has more fatigue-prone muscle fibers, which also increases the risk of respiratory embarrassment with anesthetic agents. Other factors that might predispose the patient to apnea include hypothermia, sepsis, metabolic derangements such as hypoglycemia and acidosis, congenital anomalies, or central nervous system disease. Coté and coworkers, in a meta-analysis of recent literature, showed that continued apnea at home and anemia (hematocrit less than 30%) were independent risk factors for the development of apnea in premature infants.[71]

Infants who are most at risk for postoperative apnea are neonates, premature infants, and former premature infants up to 60 weeks' postconceptual age. Liu et al and Malviya et al suggested that the risk of apnea significantly declines by 46 and 44 weeks postconceptual age, respectively.[75,76] At the other extreme, Kurth reported that apnea persisted in children over 60 weeks' postconceptual age.[77] It should be noted that the detection of apnea might be a function of the level of monitoring. Studies using nursing observation and impedance pneumography were less likely to detect apneic episodes than studies with more technologically sophisticated, continuous monitoring.

Although there still appears to be controversy regarding the home-readiness of these patients after outpatient surgery, these issues are not germane to the discussion of the neonate or former premature infants undergoing a thoracic surgical procedure. These patients will probably be monitored postoperatively in an intensive care setting. Nonetheless, the anesthesiologist should be aware of factors that may predispose the infants to apnea and increased morbidity. The practitioner certainly should avoid metabolic derangements, hypothermia, and anemia. The use of regional anesthesia might be beneficial because it not only reduces intraoperative anesthetic and postoperative analgesic requirements, but also could facilitate postoperative respiratory function. The use of caffeine (10 mg/kg as a single dose) might prevent apneic episodes in high-risk infants, premature infants, and neonates for several days.[78] In older children, the pharmacokinetics of caffeine suggest a half-life of 5 hours.

Hypoglycemia

Hypoglycemia is defined as a blood glucose of less than 30 mg/dL during the first 72 hours of life, and less than 40 mg/dL after 72 hours. The occurrence of hypoglycemia in the newborn period is quite common. In SGA infants, it is the most common form of morbidity, approaching 67%.[79,80] Lower blood glucose values are accepted as normal in infants. In low-birthweight infants (i.e., term infants with weights less than 2500 g), hypoglycemia is defined as a blood glucose level of less than 20 mg/dL.

Before delivery, both the fetal and the maternal pancreases regulate the blood sugar with some degree of placental crossover. At birth, the interruption of this interdependence may manifest itself as a delayed assumption of normal glucose metabolism in the newborn. The most common example is that of the infant of a diabetic mother. Fetal insulin production is quite high in an attempt to make up for maternal hypoinsulinism and hyperglycemia. At birth, insulin output is still high—or at least, the response to increases in blood sugar is greater than normal—resulting in severe hypoglycemia.

Other conditions that contribute to the incidence of hypoglycemia in the newborn period are the following:

- Perinatal distress of any kind
- Toxemia
- Twinning
- Erythroblastosis fetalis
- Sepsis
- Asphyxia
- CNS defects
- Hypothermia
- Hypocalcemia
- Congenital heart disease
- Maternal medications
- Endocrine deficiency (hypothyroidism)
- Adrenal hemorrhage
- Polycythemia
- Hyperbilirubinemia
- Abrupt withdrawal of glucose

A history of any of these conditions should make the anesthesiologist aware of the possibility of hypoglycemia and the need to determine blood glucose levels in the perioperative period. Normal glucose requirements for prematures and other newborns are 2 to 6 mg/kg/min, and these values might need to be considerably higher under stressful conditions. If hypoglycemia is present before anesthesia, the occurrence of hyperglycemia and the dangers of hyperosmolarity must be prevented once the child is anesthetized because the anesthesia may reduce glucose requirements. It could be difficult to predict blood glucose levels during anesthesia.

The stress response should not be relied upon to maintain normoglycemia. Serial analysis of blood glucose should be performed. In particular, the neonate's immature hepatic function might make it prone to hypoglycemia, to the development of intraventricular hemorrhage secondary to hyperosmolarity from hyperglycemia, and to osmotic diuresis. Hyperglycemia may also affect wound healing and infection.

Hypocalcemia

Neonatal hypocalcemia is related to low parathyroid hormone activity and decreased stores of available calcium.[81] Parathyroid hormone activity in the term infant is normal after approximately 3 days, but in the premature infant it might not become normal for up to several weeks.[82,83] Hypocalcemia may also be seen with massive and rapid transfusion of blood products,

especially whole blood and fresh-frozen plasma. These blood products contain sodium citrate, which binds to ionized calcium, causing the hypocalcemia. Packed red blood cells also contain sodium citrate but, because of the small plasma volume, hypocalcemia is less likely to occur under conditions of a rapid transfusion and more likely when both blood loss and transfusion with pRBCs have been excessive. Infusion rates exceeding 1.5 to 2.0 mL/kg/min should be monitored closely for electrocardiographic evidence of hypocalcemia. Such evidence may include a widening QRS complex, a prolonged QT interval, and a flattened or peaked T wave. Hypotension from decreased cardiac contractility may be evident clinically.

Although hypocalcemia may be seen in all newborns, it is most prevalent in stressed infants, prematures, infants of diabetic mothers, sepsis cases, asphyxiated infants, and infants with RDS. As with hypoglycemia, awareness on the part of the anesthesiologist should be the rule, and treatment should be available. Either calcium gluconate or calcium chloride can be used to treat hypocalcemia. Calcium gluconate should be administered at three times the amount of calcium chloride because the gluconate salt contains one-third less ionized calcium. Maintenance therapy should start at 250 mg/kg/24 hr of calcium chloride or 750 mg/kg/24 hr of calcium gluconate. Signs of hypoglycemia and hypocalcemia may be masked during anesthesia when muscle relaxants are used with artificial ventilation.

Stress Response of Neonates to Surgery

The neural structures necessary for processing proprioceptive information are present in the newborn, and various measures of cortical function suggest that the sensory cortex is very active in neonates.[84,85] It is clear that noxious stimuli evoke a whole spectrum of responses in the newborn infant, and these are characterized collectively as the *stress response to surgery*. The CNS and structures required for long-term memory are well developed during the neonatal period. There is not yet firm evidence, however, that neonates remember early painful experiences. Given the strong evidence regarding the profound influence that noxious stimuli have on neonates' behavior, changes in cardiorespiratory function, and metabolic alterations, it is incorrect to assume that neonates neither experience nor record painful events. There are no indications that warrant a surgical procedure being performed on a neonate without adequate anesthesia.

Stress results in marked changes in cardiorespiratory variables.[86,87] Both heart rate and blood pressure increase during noxious procedures such as blood drawing, but these increases can be blunted by the prior administration of local anesthesia. Palmar sweating has been measured in neonates and has been correlated with the state of arousal; marked changes are noted during heelstick blood drawing.[88] Hormonal and metabolic responses of neonates to surgical stimulation are well known; marked increases in serum cortisol have been documented.[89,90] In preterm and full-term infants, Anand et al found marked alteration in levels of many hormones, as well as significant effects on metabolism that sometimes persisted for significant periods beyond the surgical procedure.[91,92] In neonates who had minimal anesthesia, there appeared to be increased protein breakdown.[93] Clinically, a group of neonates who underwent surgery with fentanyl/O_2/N_2O anesthesia had significantly fewer postoperative complications than a similar group who underwent surgery with O_2/N_2O anesthesia.[94]

Preoperative Assessment

All too often, the amount of preoperative information available to the anesthesiologist is inversely related to the severity of the disease being treated. The critically ill, cyanotic newborn may be transferred from another facility and must be evaluated quickly by the receiving physicians to establish a diagnosis. Investigative procedures such as radiographs, echocardiography, cardiac catheterization, and laboratory evaluation must be accomplished quickly so that life-saving measures can be taken.

Evaluation of the cyanotic newborn infant poses special problems because multiple causes can result in arterial desaturation. Congenital heart defects must be considered, but other causes of hypoxemia include congenital diaphragmatic hernia, tracheoesophageal fistula with aspiration pneumonia, other pneumonias, sepsis, pneumothorax, congenital pulmonary space-occupying defects, and upper airway obstruction (Figure 16-1).

Older children scheduled for elective thoracic operations are now rarely admitted more than 1 day in advance of surgery and might even arrive on the morning of surgery. Thus, consultations with pulmonologists, cardiologists, or other specialists may be performed on an outpatient basis or simply might not be available until just before the operation. It is of particular importance for the anesthesiologist to obtain a careful and thorough history and physical examination. Because elective thoracic procedures, the presence of upper respiratory infections, contagious childhood diseases, febrile episodes, or gastrointestinal symptoms are of special concern.

When dealing with congenital anomalies such as tracheoesophageal fistula or certain forms of congenital heart disease, the anesthesiologist should always be aware that other associated anomalies may be present.[95,96] Such defects should be discussed with parents, and their expected influence on the immediate and later outcome of the proposed operation should be considered. Nutritional status should be elucidated by the history and by the anesthesiologist's physical examination. The upper airway and the mobility of the mandible and the cervical spine should be examined. Pulmonary function may be evaluated by careful auscultation of the lungs, observation of the child's breathing pattern, and the results of arterial and/or capillary blood gases, the chest radiograph, and any indicated pulmonary function tests. The need for ventilatory support following thoracic operations can usually be determined during the preoperative visit.

Cardiac function can be estimated from the history and physical examination recorded by the referring physician. The degree of compensation for congestive heart failure can be judged by the ability of the child to eat, the presence of excessive sweating, and overall growth, especially in response to medical therapy. The extent and duration of cyanosis are usually proportional to the hematocrit, except when nutritional problems intervene to prevent compensatory polycythemia. The anesthesiologist's own examination of the precordium,

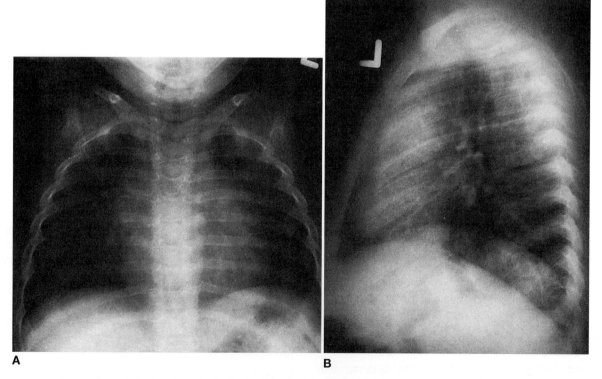

FIGURE 16-1 A, Normal infant's chest radiograph showing widening of mediastinum due to normal thymic shadow, horizontal ribs, and relatively high diaphragm. The buckling of the trachea toward the right is normal with expiration. **B,** The lateral radiograph shows retrosternal fullness, also due to the normal thymic shadow.

peripheral pulses, perfusion, color, and general habitus of the patient will also be helpful. Hepatic and renal function may be affected by the presence or absence of cardiac dysfunction. Palpation of the liver edge and careful review of significant laboratory data—including blood urea nitrogen, creatinine, and liver enzymes—may help to elucidate the status of these organs.

Whenever possible, a patient's previous anesthetic history should be evaluated by noting the response during previous hospitalizations if surgery was performed, and by discussing the patient's past history with parents. Important also is the determination of any family history suggesting problems associated with anesthesia, including such entities as malignant hypothermia or pseudocholinesterase deficiency.

An understanding of the details of the planned surgical procedures is essential for the anesthesiologist caring for any patient. In thoracic operations, which are frequently complex, the information is best obtained by direct communication with the attending surgeon. It is also helpful to ascertain the status of the nonoperative lung.

The preoperative visit by the anesthesiologist with the patient and the family is extremely important in the overall management of any operation, but especially for thoracic surgery. Besides obtaining the needed information concerning the patient, the anesthesiologist's preoperative visit is helpful in allowing the parents and patient to ask questions, to express fears and anxieties, and to understand more clearly what is planned. An explanation is given to the parents as to the plan for premedicant drugs, induction techniques, expected time for surgery, the need for intensive care unit or respiratory support, and postoperative pain management modalities. A discussion of anticipated anesthetic risk with the parents (and patient, if appropriate) is necessary for informed consent. This should serve to reassure rather than frighten.

Preoperative Preparation

The Anesthesiologist

When a child presents for thoracic surgery, the anesthesiologist's initial responsibility is twofold. First, the anesthesiologist must assess his or her own competency and skill to provide a safe anesthetic; and second, the caring institution must have the necessary resources and personnel to provide subspecialty care. It should be recognized that the majority of American children having surgery do so outside the setting of a children's hospital. Macario's demographic survey of hospitals in Northern California showed that approximately 80% of the institutions cared for children from age zero to 6 years.[97] Nonetheless, the essential question is: does subspecialty care, for example the presence of a pediatric anesthesiologist, improve outcome in children presenting for major surgery including surgery in the thorax? This is not to imply that those anesthesiologists caring for children on a casual basis do not have the competency or skills. The focus of this discussion is not the need for subspecialty care for all children but only for such care for those at greatest risk for an adverse outcome. There is compelling evidence that a certain subset of children could be better served by anesthesiologists more proficient in their care.

Based upon studies from Keenan et al, there is the suggestion that infants (defined as age less than 1 year) with ASA status more than three having extensive (i.e., thoracic) surgery or emergency surgery may benefit from the expertise of a subspecialist.[98] Looking at the anesthetic records of more than 4000 infants and neonates undergoing surgery from 1983 to 1990, Keenan et al looked for the frequency of cardiac arrests. There were four anesthesia-related cardiac arrests in the group of patients cared for by nonpediatric anesthesiologists and none in the pediatric anesthesiologist group. These authors suggested that the use of pediatric anesthesiologists might decrease morbidity. Another retrospective chart review from this same group looked for the frequency of bradycardia in infants and children, its associated causes and morbidity, and factors influencing its frequency.[99] Evaluating almost 8000 noncardiac anesthetic records from children aged zero to four, they used bradycardia (HR less than 100) to define an adverse event. The frequency of bradycardia was 1.27% in infants and 0.16% at 4 years of age. This decline in frequency of bradycardia with age was statistically significant. Causes of bradycardia included the patient's disease, the surgical procedure, anesthetic overdose, and hypoxemia. Interestingly, approximately 80% of the anesthetic overdoses were in healthy patients under the care of a nonpediatric anesthesiologist. Associated factors for increasing frequency of bradycardia were ASA status III to V, longer surgical times, and whether the supervising anesthesiologist was a pediatric subspecialist. Bradycardia was less than half as likely when the attending was a pediatric anesthesiologist. These authors concluded that bradycardia was more frequent in infants, more likely in sicker patients presenting for major surgery, and less likely when a pediatric anesthesiologist was involved in the care.

Other studies looking at pediatric morbidity and mortality but not at the role of the caregiver support similar conclusions.[100-102] Tiret et al found that the incidence of complications was nine times higher in infants than in children; risk factors for complications were decreasing age and ASA status.[103] Cohen et al also concluded that age less than 1 year and increasing ASA status were risk factors for complications.[104] Data from pediatric and adult anesthesia closed malpractice claims showed that infants younger than 6 months of age represented the single largest group to experience an adverse outcome.[105] More specifically, looking at closed claim data from the Pediatric Perioperative Cardiac Arrest (POCA) registry, two thirds of the cardiac arrests occurred in ASA III-V patients, and 95% of the deaths occurred in this sicker subgroup. Infants accounted for 55% of the arrests.[106]

Is subspecialty care necessary and does subspecialty care improve outcome for children presenting for major surgery?[107] These questions are difficult to answer given the rarity of the event and types of numbers involved to prove a significant difference. Nonetheless, more than two decades' worth of data would suggest that the youngest, sickest children having major surgery are at highest risk for complications. This essentially is a profile of the patient presenting for thoracic surgery. The anesthesiologist caring for such patients should recognize these issues and act accordingly.

Patient and Parent Preparation

Reducing parent and patient anxiety and enhancing cooperation are goals that all anesthesiologists should have when dealing with children.[108-114] Frequently, newborns and previously healthy children are the patients who present for thoracic surgery. In either case, the shock of a child having major surgery can be quite a frightening experience. The anesthesiologist often is the last member of the team to meet the patient and family prior to surgery, yet this fact should not diminish the importance of their role. Many concerns that parents have are in the anesthesiologist's domain. Death during surgery and "Is my child going to be in pain?" are issues often discussed at a preoperative visit. Litman et al showed that a majority of parents were pleased that a risk of death was discussed even in front of the child.[115] Postoperative pain control, through the use of neuraxial narcotics and local anesthetic infusions, is an area that can have a tremendous impact on patient and parent satisfaction, and these plans should be discussed with the parents as well. In any case, the importance of gaining the confidence of both parent and child should not be understated, and a policy of openness is highly recommended.

Although reducing preoperative anxiety is important, it is not clear whether there are any serious long-term consequences if this goal is not met.[110,116-120] Behavioral changes such as sleep and eating disturbances may persist for several weeks, and it has been suggested that increased anxiety at the time of induction may delay gastric emptying and increase gastric pH. Nonetheless, separation from the parents and a smooth induction should be part of the anesthetic plan. Risk factors for preoperative anxiety include the following[110,112]:

1. Age range of 1 to 5 years
2. Parental anxiety
3. Prior medical encounters of poor quality
4. Shy and inhibited children
5. Children of divorced parents

Pharmacologic or behavioral interventions to reduce anxiety are acceptable and have their proponents. Parental presence in the operating room at the time of anesthetic induction and/or preoperative hospital visitation is practiced at some hospitals. Whether these programs reduce preoperative anxiety and its sequelae is unclear.[121-131] The most widely accepted method to reduce preoperative anxiety is pharmacologic.[114,132]

Preoperative Orders and Premedication

Preoperative Fasting

Guidelines for preoperative fasting in children have been reevaluated over the past decade.[133-137] Although concerns for aspiration of gastric contents are always paramount, the practice of "NPO after midnight" has come under increasing scrutiny. In part, this change has been driven by knowledge concerning gastric emptying but also by parents and anesthesiologists who have to deal with hungry, irritable children who are prone to hypoglycemia following fasts of more than 8 hours. When deciding whether a child is properly fasted for surgery, the anesthesiologist must consider the type of food ingested, the patient's age, and comorbid conditions.

There is no absolute definition as to what constitutes a solid food. Foods can be defined based on their appearance in the stomach. For example, gelatin is a solid in appearance but is considered by practitioners as a liquid because it liquefies in the stomach after ingestion; on the other hand, cow's milk is a

liquid that breaks down into liquid and solid states once in the stomach. The physiologic evidence of gastric emptying would suggest that liquids and solids empty independently of each other, that liquids can empty in the absence of gastric motility, and that liquids empty quickly from the stomach.[138] Digestion of solids is slow, with lipid meals digesting more slowly than carbohydrate meals, which in turn digest more slowly than protein-based meals.[139] Essentially, food content is the most significant factor when considering gastric emptying.[133]

More specifically, looking at gastric emptying of infant formula and human breast milk in full-term and premature infants, Cavell found that most infants had no gastric residual volume after 2 hours.[140,141] Several infants did have large residuals, however. Their conclusions were that breast milk emptied faster than formula and that both required more than 2 hours for complete emptying. Similarly, in van der Walt's study of 62 healthy infants age younger than 3 months given human milk or formula 3 to 4 hours before surgery, several patients had gastric residuals greater than 0.4 mL/kg.[142] Litman et al compared breastfed infants with those given clear liquids up to 2 hours before surgery. These investigators stopped their study, as many of the breastfed infants had large gastric aspirates. The data from these studies suggest at least a 3-hour fast after ingestion of either breast milk or formula is necessary to assure complete gastric emptying.[143] Cow's milk is considered a solid food substance because it separates into liquid and curd phases once in the stomach.

The ingestion of clear liquids before surgery has been well studied in infants. Using a variety of liquids and volumes, these studies would suggest that healthy children could safely ingest an unlimited amount of clear fluids up to 2 hours before surgery.[143-151] Similar investigations in adults also suggest that this practice is safe in adolescents.[152-154]

Overall gastric aspiration is a rare event, yet this risk should be balanced against the benefits of a more "liberal" fasting policy. Improved parent and patient satisfaction, increased gastric pH, increased caloric intake, and decreased incidence of hypoglycemia are some of the benefits of preoperative ingestion of clear fluids. Comorbid conditions such as gastroesophageal reflux, bowel disease, trauma, and emergency surgery need to be considered. Based upon the available evidence and the past decade of clinical practice, this practice is both safe and effective.

In summary, clear fluids may be taken up to 2 hours before surgery; breast milk and formula may be ingested up to 3 to 4 hours before surgery. Although there are no data to support an optimal time frame, there should be a mandatory fast of 6 to 8 hours after solid food intake. It may be desirable to suggest that NPO times be "time prior to arrival at the hospital" in case surgical schedules change and patients have their surgery sooner than expected.

Premedication

Premedication for children should reduce patient and parental anxiety and enhance cooperation at the time of induction. It should be individualized to the specific patient and his or her disease. It is now common practice in many centers to use only oral premedication for children in whom there is no vascular access. Almost every premedication is successful in 80% of patients and fails to produce a calm child in only 20% of cases (Table 16-3).[155]

Anesthetic Premedication

Drug	Dose	Timing Before Induction
ORAL PREMEDICATION		
Fentanyl (oral/transmucosal)	5-15 ug/kg	30-45 minutes
Midazolam	0.5-0.75 mg/kg (max 15-20 mg)	20-30 minutes
Ketamine 3-10 mg/kg + atropine 0.02-0.04 mg/kg	10-15 minutes	
NASAL PREMEDICATION		
Midazolam	0.2-0.3 mg/kg	10 minutes
Sufentanil 0.3-3 ug/kg	10 minutes	
Ketamine 1-5 mg/kg	5-15 minutes	
RECTAL PREMEDICATION		
Midazolam	0.3-1 mg/kg	20-30 minutes
Methohexital	25-30 mg/kg	9-11 minutes
INTRAMUSCULAR PREMEDICATION		
Pentobarbital	2 mg/kg (max 100 mg)	60 minutes
Morphine 0.1 mg/kg (max 10 mg)		
Atropine (above three are given together)	0.01 mg/kg (max 0.4 mg)	
Midazolam	0.05-0.15 mg/kg	
Ketamine 3-4 mg/kg	10-15 minutes	
Midazolam	0.05-0.15 mg/kg	
Atropine (Above three are given together)	0.02 mg/kg	
INTRAVENOUS PREMEDICATION		
Midazolam	0.05-0.15 mg/kg	1-2 minutes
Ketamine 0.25-0.5 mg/kg	1-2 minutes	

Oral, nasal, intravenous, and rectal routes are used, with the choice of administration mode dependent on the patient, the surgical procedure, and the anesthesiologist.

The ideal premedicant drug should include the following[132,156]:

1. Readily accepted by all patients
2. Have a rapid onset
3. Have a rapid offset so as not to delay recovery
4. Be without serious side effects
5. Be cost-effective

Although no one drug meets all these criteria, midazolam is the most widely used preoperative medication. Despite a bitter taste, midazolam can be flavored with apple juice or cherry syrup; concentrated formulations keep the ingested volume to a minimum. Acetaminophen or ibuprofen elixir can also disguise the taste. Midazolam can be given by the following routes:

- Oral (0.5 to 0.75 mg/kg, maximum 15 mg)
- Nasal (0.2 to 0.3 mg/kg)
- Sublingual (0.2 to 0.3 mg/kg)
- Rectal (1 mg/kg)
- IM (0.15 mg/kg)
- IV (0.1 mg/kg)

With oral midazolam, the time to separation from the parent is reported to be as early as 10 minutes after drug administration.[157-160] The nasal route has an even quicker onset, with the rectal route comparable to the oral route.[161] The duration of pharmacodyanamic effect of this drug is about 45 minutes. Midazolam does not delay discharge, and a lingering postoperative effect should not be of concern after thoracic surgery. It can decrease the incidence of emergence delirium—a condition of increased excitation commonly seen in preschool-age boys following surgery (but not necessarily following anesthesia).[162,163] Midazolam is most suitable for children between the ages of 10 months to 5 years. At 10 months of age, separation anxiety may be apparent, and beyond 5 years of age, children should be able to cope with new situations.

SPECIFIC PREMEDICANT DRUGS

Anticholinergic Agents. The anticholinergic agents are often omitted in patients who have a relatively fixed cardiac output (e.g., those experiencing aortic stenosis, pulmonary stenosis, or mitral stenosis) and in whom a significant increase in heart rate is undesirable. Atropine can be given by many routes and is beneficial for drying secretions in the pediatric population undergoing thoracic surgery. Atropine effectively blocks the action of the cardiac vagus nerve and may obviate the decrease in cardiac output seen with induction doses of halothane and other volatile agents.[164] Atropine probably should be administered to patients who receive ketamine for induction of anesthesia. It probably should not be given to children who have a history of a recent significant elevation of body temperature. Intramuscular and intravenous doses are 20 μg/kg.

Ketamine. Ketamine (3 to 6 mg/kg) is a useful alternative that can be administered by a variety of routes.[165-170] Oral (6 mg/kg), intramuscular (2 to 6 mg/kg), and rectal (6 mg/kg) ketamine produces the desired effects of a good premedication—namely, separation from the parents and acceptance of the face mask. Nasal ketamine (3 mg/kg), like midazolam, has been shown to be neurotoxic when applied to neural tisssues in animals.[171] Therefore with all the other choices for administration, the nasal route may not be the best. Adding midazolam might eliminate some of the unpleaseant, psychotropic emergence reactions seen with the use of ketamine. Ketamine might increase oral secretions, which in turn might increase the risk of laryngospasm on induction. Atropine (0.02 mg/kg) can be added to the "cocktail" for its antisialagogue effect. Oral ketamine would be useful in the patient whom prior oral sedation with midazolam had failed. Intramuscular ketamine is usually reserved for the combative patient in whom intravenous access, mask induction, or oral intake is not possible.

Fentanyl. Orally administered fentanyl (the Fentanyl Oralet) in doses of 10 to 15 µg/kg produces reliable sedation.[172-174] Absorption is through the oral mucosa, and swallowing the drug is effective, but there is high first pass metabolism in the liver. Concerns about preoperative desaturation, nausea, and vomiting can be minimized by taking the patient to the operating room shortly after completion of the oralet. The incidence of these side effects in some studies has been high, however. Interestingly, fentanyl blood levels continue to rise for 10 to 20 minutes after completion of the oralet. This may provide some degree of postoperative analgesia after brief procedures.

EMLA Cream. If an intravenous catheter must be inserted for administration of premedication or induction drugs (in cases of rapid-sequence induction or critically ill patients), a eutectic mixture of local anesthetic (lidocaine 2.5% and prilocaine 2.5% EMLA) should be applied topically to the anticipated site of venipuncture.[175] For adequate analgesia, the EMLA cream must be applied at least 1 hour before the placement of the catheter and should be covered with an occlusive dressing. The cream should be applied to more than one site in the event that the initial cannulation is unsuccessful. It can also be applied by a parent before arrival at the hospital. The dorsum of the hand and the antecubital fossa are desirable sites for EMLA application. Dosing guidelines should be followed. EMLA is contraindicated in infants younger than 1 month of age.

Anesthetic Management

In general, the pathologic condition prompting the need for surgery, as well as the physical status of the patient, determines the choice of the anesthetic technique to be used. According to American Society of Anesthesiologists (ASA) categories, infants and children requiring thoracic operations may be physical status I or II (e.g., an asymptomatic patent ductus arteriosus), but more often than not, young patients for thoracic operations will be ASA physical status III or IV. That is, their disease is systemic in nature such that it limits normal growth and development (III) or is a constant threat to life (IV).

Induction Techniques

Induction techniques depend on the patient, the parents, the procedure, the overall anesthetic plan, the condition being treated, and the skills of the anesthesiologists. Intravenous, intramuscular, and inhalation induction techniques are used (as described later) for specific thoracic procedures. Sicker patients will usually come to the operating room with intravenous catheters and monitoring devices in place. This often facilitates the induction of anesthesia because the administration of narcotics and muscle relaxants can be titrated to desired effect.

Monitoring During Thoracic Operations

The monitoring selected by the anesthesiologist depends on the following factors:

1. The physical status of the patient
2. The operation anticipated
3. The expected postoperative course

Even the simplest operation in the very sick infant or child may warrant extensive monitoring. Many children undergoing thoracic surgery require accurate and reliable monitoring in both the operating room and the intensive care unit. Correct interpretation by the anesthesiologist of the provided data is also essential. Even the most sophisticated monitoring systems available today fail to tell what is really necessary to know: the presence of pain, the accurate assessment of regional perfusion, and the metabolic changes occurring within the cell. The anesthesiologist is the "ultimate" monitor; the instruments used, either simple or complex, are only data-collecting devices that enable the anesthesiologist to receive, process, and assimilate data and to respond appropriately.

If no direct monitoring devices are in place on arrival of the patient in the OR, the essential monitoring instruments are applied before or during induction. These include the following types of devices:

1. The precordial stethoscope applied so that both heart sounds and breath sounds are audible
2. A blood pressure cuff (usually an oscillometric type)
3. Multilead ECG
4. A pulse oximeter

Table 16-4 lists the monitoring devices that should be considered for use in patients undergoing thoracic operations.

ELECTROCARDIOGRAPHY

ECG leads should be placed so as to demonstrate clearly any atrial depolarization (P wave), ventricular depolarization (QRS), and the repolarization complex (T wave), so that

---

TABLE 16-4

Monitoring of the Pediatric Patient Undergoing Thoracic Surgery

Preinduction

Precordial stethoscope
ECG
Nerve stimulator
Temperature
Pulse oximeter
Blood pressure cuff (usually oscillometric)

Postinduction, before start of operation

Intraarterial catheter
Central venous pressure catheter or pulmonary artery catheter
Urinary bladder catheter
Rectal temperature thermistor probe (or esophageal or nasopharyngeal)
Esophageal stethoscope (often with temperature)
Nerve stimulator (determine twitch, tetanus, and train-of-four responses before administering neuromuscular blocking agents)
Transesophageal echocardiography

Before closure of surgical incisions

Right or left atrial or pulmonary arterial catheters in selected patients

arrhythmias arising from atrium or ventricle and changes in repolarization due to drug effect or electrolytes (K^+ or Ca^{++}) can be appreciated. Lead placement should also take into account the planned surgical field and patient position to avoid contamination and injury. Although the ECG is a valuable source of information concerning the cardiovascular system, it must be remembered that it is only an electrical signal and provides no information about cardiac function.

The resting heart rate of the infant or child is normally more rapid than that of the adult. Therefore, the definitions of significant tachycardia and bradycardia are different for the two age groups.[176] In infants, a heart rate greater than 180 beats/min or less than 100 beats/min should be evaluated carefully.

PULSE OXIMETRY

When an infant or child has a disease that is already compromising cardiac and/or pulmonary function and these structures are manipulated or retracted during the course of an operation, life-threatening arterial hypoxemia is a common occurrence (Figure 16-2).

Previously, hypoxia-induced bradycardia was the earliest monitor of hypoxia during procedures such as bronchoscopy, repair of diaphragmatic hernia, and aortopulmonary shunt creation. A functioning pulse oximeter allows both the anesthesiologist and the surgeon to appreciate any degree of hypoxemia.

In a single-blind study of pediatric patients, Coté et al demonstrated the clinical efficacy of pulse oximetry.[177] One group of anesthesiologists had availability of oximetry data and alarms, while the other group was blinded and unable to hear alarms. There were twice as many desaturations (defined as saturations 85% or less for 30 seconds or more) in the blinded group. In addition, the anesthesiologist was relatively slow at detecting desaturations when compared with the oximeter, and this was regardless of experience. Major desaturations often occur in the absence of clinical signs (especially bradycardia), and higher-risk infants were more likely to have a desaturation episode than ASA 1 or ASA 2 infants. Finally, visual correlation of cyanosis and desaturation was poor. Clearly, the routine use of pulse oximetry has changed anesthetic practice for the better. It is better than the clinician at detecting oxygen desaturation and possible impending hypoxia.

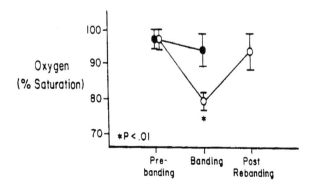

FIGURE 16-2 Although the pulse oximeter is a standard monitor during all anesthetics, it has particular value in pediatric thoracic anesthesia, as shown in this demonstration of inadequate pulmonary blood flow associated with partial occlusion of the pulmonary artery during a pulmonary banding procedure. (From Casthely PA et al: *J Cardiothorac Anesth* 1:297, 1987.)

Probe placement is critical. Probe position should reflect the oxygen saturation of the blood that is perfusing vital organs such as the brain and the heart. For example, if a severe coarctation or interruption of the aortic arch is present, venous blood will perfuse the lower body and perhaps the left arm through the patent ductus arteriosus. A probe placed on the lower extremities or on the left upper extremity will record the oxygen saturation of both arterial blood and shunted venous blood. In this situation, the probe should be placed on the right upper extremity or on an earlobe because one of these locations will best reflect the oxygen saturation of arterial blood. During thoracic surgery, the loss of the pulse oximeter signal should be respected and the cause should be sought immediately. Often, the probe has been dislodged, or ambient light or electrocautery interferes with the signal. Other, more serious causes (including hypoxemia and decreased perfusion) need to be addressed promptly. The oximeter probe sensor may not be able to detect a peripheral pulse during hypovolemia, vasoconstriction from hypothermia, or decreased cardiac output. It should be noted that in the data from the Pediatric Cardiac Arrest Registry, an abnormality of oxygen saturation as measured by pulse oximetry occurred in almost 50% of the cardiac arrests.[106] This abnormality was heralded most often by loss of pulse oximetry signals.

CAPNOMETRY

Monitoring of expired levels of carbon dioxide has also proven extremely valuable for the same reasons found for pulse oximetry.[178] Capnometry is useful in detecting a kinked or plugged endotracheal tube, circuit disconnection, esophageal intubation, accidental extubation, malignant hyperthermia, air embolism, and bronchospasm. Capnometry also provides information regarding quantity of pulmonary blood flow in children with right-to-left shunts.[179] If right-to-left shunting is extreme (or if a newly created aortopulmonary shunt is inadequate), a large discrepancy exists between the normal or elevated arterial carbon dioxide and a low end-expiratory value (Figure 16-3). Appropriate interventions to reduce the extent of shunting will narrow this gap. Most important, capnometry allows for real-time adjustments in ventilation and assessment of the efficacy of that maneuver, correlated to the surgery and disease state of the child. Although this benefit is important in all operations, in thoracic surgery this is especially true when manipulation of intrathoracic structures alters pulmonary compliance and ventilation-perfusion relationships.

ARTERIAL BLOOD PRESSURE

The systemic arterial pressure is determined by blood volume, cardiac output, peripheral resistance, elasticity of the arterial wall, proximal patency of the artery, and the characteristics of the recording system. Systemic arterial pressure and organ perfusion are related through vascular resistance. Blood flow to any given organ may be adequate even when there is relative hypotension; conversely, organ flow may be inadequate when the blood pressure is normal or even elevated. Nevertheless, the accurate measurement and recording of systemic blood pressure, either directly or indirectly using oscillometric or Doppler devices, are important in assessing adequacy of cardiac function.

Most, but not all, thoracic operations require the insertion of intraarterial catheters for direct pressure measurement. If intraarterial pressure monitoring is not considered necessary,

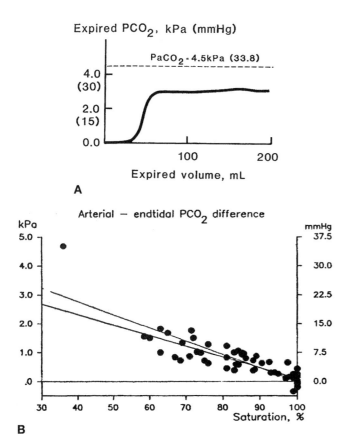

A

B

FIGURE 16-3 **A,** This single-breath, expired carbon dioxide waveform demonstrates the increase in alveolar dead space (the area between the line representing arterial carbon dioxide and the expired carbon dioxide waveform) in a child with congenital heart disease and right-to-left shunt. **B,** In children with congenital heart disease, there is a curvilinear negative correlation between the arterial-to-end-tidal carbon dioxide gradient and arterial oxygen saturation, and there is a positive correlation with hemoglobin concentration and respiratory quotient. (From Fletcher RL: *Anesthesiology* 72:210, 1991.)

an oscillometric system (e.g., Dinamapp) is used. The cuff should be placed on an extremity opposite that in which intravenous infusions are being given, as the time required for inflations and deflations of the cuff interferes with fluid and drug administration. If intraarterial monitoring is used, the cannula is placed in a location convenient to the anesthesiologist to allow frequent arterial blood sampling for measurements of blood gases, hematocrit, serum electrolytes, blood glucose, and other necessary parameters. The radial artery is usually selected for percutaneous catheterization just proximal to the volar carpal ligament. Stopcocks should not be used at the hub of the 22-gauge, 1-inch plastic cannula. A T-connector with a rubber diaphragm may be used instead of the stopcock to reduce the risk of inadvertent injection of air, frequent motion and arterial trauma produced by turning the stopcock handle, and bacterial contamination from the open end of the stopcock. The rubber diaphragm of the T-connector can be used for sampling by puncturing it with a small-bore needle and allowing a few drops of blood to drip out to clear the cannula of flush solution. Little or no negative pressure need be applied to the syringe

during sampling, as it will fill from the force of the intraarterial pressure. Negative pressure tends to collapse the very small pediatric radial artery and leads to thrombogenic trauma, spasm, and early loss of the monitoring catheter.

When the radial artery on either side is not patent or otherwise not available, alternative sites of cannulation must be considered. The left radial artery should not be used for monitoring during operations for repair of vascular rings because the left subclavian artery may be clamped during the repair and the radial artery trace lost. An alternative site is the axillary artery, cannulated either directly or with a modified Seldinger technique.[180] This site is accessible to the anesthesiologist and comfortable for the patient, and it provides excellent sampling and waveforms because of the large size of the artery. Excellent collateral circulation around the shoulder provides safety from vascular compromise. No neurologic damage to the brachial plexus has been found.[180] Careful flushing to avoid central arterial embolization, as with all arterial catheters, is advised. Superficial temporal artery cannulation is another alternative. Direct femoral arterial cannulation may be necessary in cases in which radial and temporal arteries have already been used, but this is quite inconvenient because blood sampling must be done from the leg.[181]

Umbilical arterial catheters are useful if present in the neonate undergoing an intrathoracic operation.[182] Position of the catheter tip should be checked radiographically before its use. The catheter can be placed either above or below the renal arteries at the L_1 level. A proximally placed catheter at the level of the diaphragm may predispose the infant to an increased risk of embolization to the mesenteric and renal vessels. A distally placed catheter should be at the aortic bifurcation at the L_3 to L_4 level. In this position, the catheter could slip into one of the iliac vessels, causing ischemia.[183] Blood sampling for blood gases from an umbilical arterial catheter, in the presence of increased PVR and a patent ductus arteriosus, might be misleading. In such a case, blood shunted right-to-left through the ductus will cause the PaO_2 below the ductus to appear falsely low. Blood leaving the heart and perfusing the retinal arteries may have a dangerously high PaO_2, placing the susceptible patient at risk for retrolental fibroplasia.[184]

CENTRAL VENOUS PRESSURE

Central venous pressure (CVP) measurement is indicated when the volume status of the child is unstable or likely to change rapidly, as would be expected when massive blood or third-space loss is anticipated. Central venous catheters provide a useful route for the injection of irritating medications such as calcium, vasopressors, or blood products.

Central venous catheters can also be inserted through the internal or external jugular veins or through the subclavian, femoral, axillary, or antecubital veins in children. A 20-gauge, 1.25-inch intravenous catheter is introduced into an external jugular vein, through which a J wire is passed and manipulated into the chest. The CVP catheter is then placed over the J wire and advanced into the central circulation. Percutaneous internal jugular vein catheterization can also be accomplished easily in pediatric patients undergoing thoracic operations. A low incidence of complications is reported by advocates of this technique.[185,186] Approaching the internal jugular vein (IJV) at a point high in the neck is advisable in children to avoid the lung.

The use of Doppler to locate the IJV improves the success of cannulation.[187] The subclavian vein may also be used via an infraclavicular approach for CVP catheter insertion.[188]

Extreme caution should be exercised in the care of centrally placed catheters and, indeed, all venous catheters in children with cyanotic congenital heart disease. Even very small air bubbles in any intravenous catheter, tubing, or connectors pose potentially lethal hazards because of the possibility of an air embolus to the brain, the coronary arteries, or other vital organs. In the acyanotic child, air in the venous system may also reach the systemic circulation through a patent foramen ovale, atrial or ventricular septal defect, or patent ductus arteriosus during coughing, a Valsalva maneuver, or positive pressure ventilation.

TRANSESOPHAGEAL ECHOCARDIOGRAPHY

Single and biplane transesophageal echocardiographic (TEE) transducers are available in sizes for imaging patients as small as 1400 g.[189] Tracheal or bronchial obstruction or compression by the transesophageal transducer has been reported.[190] During thoracic surgical procedures, transesophageal echocardiography is a valuable adjunct to monitor the direction and volume of shunting through septal defects, ventricular function, and valvular regurgitation when cardiac malformations are known to be present. TEE is also helpful during surgery for division of vascular rings or ligation of a patent ductus arteriosus. Beause the details of TEE are beyond the scope of this chapter, the interested reader is referred to a textbook of pediatric cardiac anesthesia for details. It should be noted, however, that interpretation of echocardiograms in congenital heart disease requires extensive training and experience.

TEMPERATURE

The importance of monitoring and maintaining normothermia in children during surgery and anesthesia is well documented.[191] Changes in body temperature during anesthesia may result from exposure to a cold environment, physiologic responses to anesthesia, infusion of cold intravenous fluids or blood, vasoconstriction, or vasodilatation. Uncontrolled hypothermia is undesirable in any patient, but in the neonate and premature infant it produces metabolic acidosis and myocardial and respiratory depression. Hyperthermia is also dangerous because it causes oxygen consumption to increase significantly.[192]

Temperature should be monitored in every pediatric patient undergoing thoracic surgery, and the choice of site depends on the anesthetic and surgical procedure. Temperature monitoring sites can be representative of either core or peripheral sites. Core sites, which are prefereable, include tympanic membrane, pulmonary artery, rectal, nasopharyngeal, and esophageal. In anesthetized children, these temperatures are similar. If an esophageal probe is used, it should be positioned in the distal third of the esophagus near the great vessels of the heart. Because there is minimal insulation between the trachea and esophagus at this point, gas flow in the trachea may influence the readings.[193] A nasopharyngeal probe is positioned posterior to the soft palate. Inaccurate readings may occur in the presence of an air leak around an uncuffed endotracheal tube. Rectal probes may be inaccurate because insulation from feces or cooler blood in the lower extremities. Tympanic probes require proper insertion so as not to injure the tympanic membrane.[194]

URINARY OUTPUT

Urinary output during surgery is one of the most reliable signs of adequate hydration, blood volume, and cardiac output. Almost all patients undergoing complex intrathoracic procedures should have a urinary bladder catheter placed for accurate, timed measurements of urine volume and, at times, specific gravity and osmolarity. In short procedures, such as ligation of a patent ductus, urinary catheters are often safely omitted. The urethral meatus of the newborn or premature infant may be too small to accept even the smallest Foley catheter. If this is the case, a small infant feeding tube (8 Fr) can be inserted just beyond the point of the first urine drainage and fixed in place to the skin either with a suture or using benzoin and adhesive tape. Adequate urine production is considered to be 1 mL/kg body weight/h.

ARTERIAL BLOOD GASES, ELECTROLYTES, HEMOGLOBIN, AND GLUCOSE

Blood obtained from an arterial cannula is periodically analyzed for blood gases, sodium, potassium, hemoglobin/hematocrit, glucose, and ionized calcium. No particular interval between these samples is recommended, the frequency being determined by the hemodynamic stability of the patient and the intraoperative course. It is important to make some or all of these determinations shortly after induction of anesthesia to determine acid-base status, adequacy of ventilation, and baseline serum electrolytes and glucose.

ASSESSMENT OF BLOOD LOSS

Accurate estimation of blood loss is difficult, at best; however, careful attention must be paid to this aspect of thoracic operations in patients of all ages, especially in a very young infant. This is best accomplished by the following:
1. Close observation of the operative field
2. Careful monitoring of pulse rate, estimation of pulse volume, and frequent measurement of blood pressure (the systolic blood pressure is a reliable indicator of blood volume in the infant)
3. Weighing of all sponges and pads before they begin to dry out, and subtracting known dry weight from weight of bloody sponges or laps
4. Measuring blood suctioned from the surgical field in low-volume graduated suction bottles easily visible or accessible to the anesthesiologist
5. Keeping an accurate record of irrigation used in the surgical field to avoid confusion with actual blood loss on sponges or in a suction container
6. Estimation of blood on drapes

A running total of estimated blood loss should be recorded on the anesthesia record at appropriate intervals, and the final total as well as the amount replaced should be reported to the surgeon and to the nurse caring for the patient postoperatively.

Intubation of the Trachea

For children undergoing intrathoracic surgical procedures, the choice of nasal vs. oral intubation is relatively easy. Any child who is expected to need postoperative ventilatory support may benefit from nasotracheal intubation. A nasotracheal tube may be placed initially in some patients, or an orotracheal tube may be replaced by a nasal tube after the surgical procedure is completed. Nasal tubes are easier to secure and tolerated better with less chewing and gagging, and the need for an uncomfortable oral airway is eliminated. If heparin is used during surgery, caution must be exercised during insertion of the nasotracheal tube to avoid bleeding from the nasal mucosa. Nasotracheal intubation should be performed well before anticoagulation or deferred until heparin has been antagonized.

In preparation for intubation, all needed equipment should be tested and at hand. The low oxygen reserves of the premature newborn allow little time for intubation, and not enough time for stopping to obtain equipment. The choice of laryngoscope blades depends on personal preference. Anatomic considerations (e.g., the short neck and bulky tongue) make the use of straight blades generally more desirable in the newborn and small child. Most premature and SGA infants require a Miller 0 or Guedel 1 blade; the Miller 1 is more suitable for full-term infants. Beyond the age of two years, curved blades become an equally acceptable choice. In all cases, more than one size of blade should be on hand should the primary choice prove unsuitable.

Choice of appropriate tube size and type should be based on the patient's age and size (Table 16-5). Other considerations, such as a previous recent intubation, history of prolonged intubation, or previous surgery, may modify the selection of the expected tube size. Traditionally, anesthesiologists used uncuffed endotracheal tubes for children younger than 8 years of age. Reasons for this included the fact that a cuff would necessitate using a smaller endotracheal tube, which increases airway resistance and the work of breathing. Cuffs may increase mucosal injury, and seals with uncuffed tubes can easily be obtained at the cricoid ring, provided the appropriate size tube is chosen. Nonetheless, there are advocates of cuffed endotracheal tubes in children, and this practice might have several advantages. Cuffed endotracheal tubes can be adjusted, and thus multiple attempts at laryngoscopy to find the right size are not necessary. The risk of aspiration may be reduced when the trachea is completely sealed. Finally, end-tidal gas monitoring might be more accurate in the presence of a cuffed endotracheal tube. Khine et al showed that the use of cuffed endotracheal tubes is a safe practice.[195]

There are several indications for awake intubation without neuromuscular blockade or assisted ventilation—for example,

tracheoesophageal fistula, where gas introduced under pressure may pass from the trachea into the distal esophagus and distend the stomach. For the most part, there is really no one correct method, and the method of intubation depends on the skill and experience of the anesthesiologist as well as on the disease of the patient. Advantages to the awake approach are that the patient maintains his or her own airway and the airway is "protected" if gastric contents are regurgitated. Concerns seen with an awake intubation are increases in intracranial pressure, uncontrolled hypoxemia, bradycardia, and stress to the neonate. However, Stow et al showed that anterior fontanelle pressures, seen as a measure of intracranial pressure, are similar in the crying neonate to that of the neonate having an awake intubation.[196] Tracheal intubation performed with the patient under general anesthesia has the advantages of an unresponsive patient. Reflexes are obtunded and ventilation can be controlled if necessary.

Preoxygenation plays a critical role in the safety of intubation in the infant and small child. These patients are already at a disadvantage by having increased oxygen demands (4 to 6 mL/kg/min) and proportionately less alveolar surface through which to absorb oxygen. Their alveolar ventilation is normally twice that of an adult. Thus, it is understandable why the time elapsed between loss of oxygen supply or alveolar ventilation and the onset of hypoxemia is very short. When other disease exists, such as congestive heart failure, pneumonia, or respiratory distress of the newborn, borderline hypoxemia may already exist and can be dangerously exaggerated during intubation if preoxygenation is not used. Preoxygenation before intubation should be done in most children, using 100% oxygen. An exception to this practice is in the premature infant who is at risk for developing retrolental fibroplasia and in whom an oxygen concentration no more than 10% greater than that which is the therapeutic level before the surgery should be used for preoxygenation.

Once intubated, proper anchoring of the endotracheal tube is essential because the patient may be virtually inaccessible during thoracic surgery. Nasal intubation requires anchoring that will prevent the in-and-out motion of the tube and avoid compression of the nares. Oral intubation requires both lateral stabilization and prevention of the in-and-out motion. Tincture of

TABLE 16-5

Selection of Endotracheal Tubes

GUIDELINES FOR SELECTION OF ENDOTRACHEAL TUBE, MEASURED IN MILLIMETERS OF INTERNAL DIAMETER

Premature or small for gestational age	2.5-3.0 mm
Healthy term newborn	3.5 mm
6 mo to 2 yr	4.0-4.5 mm
Greater than 2 yr	[age (yr) + 18]/4

GUIDELINES FOR PROPER DEPTH OF INSERTION OF ENDOTRACHEAL TUBES (APPROXIMATE)

Age (yr)/2 + 12 = cm depth of insertion at teeth

	Oral	Nasal
Newborn	9.5 cm	Crown-heel length × 0.21 cm
6 mo	10.5-11 cm	Crown-heel length × 0.16 + 2.5 cm
>1 yr	age + 12 cm	Crown-heel length × 0.16 + 2.5 cm

benzoin can be applied to the face and to the tube before taping, as saliva dissolves most adhesives. If the patient will be positioned so that secretions will drain out of the mouth onto the endotracheal tube, a bite block made of an absorbent material may be placed in the mouth to prevent secretions from reaching the tape. Newborn infants have a waxy layer of material on the skin, known as *vernix caseosa*. This material can interfere with adhesives (e.g., tape, ECG, and grounding pads), and should be removed with mild soap or alcohol before surgery. After the endotracheal tube is well anchored, the stomach should be aspirated to remove any air or other material contents.

Maintenance of Anesthesia

After induction of anesthesia has been accomplished, intravenous and monitoring catheters are established, the trachea has been intubated, and the tracheal tube has been secured, the appropriate level of anesthesia is usually maintained with a combination of NO/oxygen and sevoflurane or isoflurane in low concentrations, along with a nondepolarizing neuromuscular blocking drug. In higher-risk patients, the potent anesthetics may be omitted and a narcotic substituted.

In most pediatric thoracic operations, a sump-type nasogastric tube is inserted into the stomach to avoid gastric distention intraoperatively from swallowed air or from anesthetic gases that may leak around the endotracheal tube. Gastric distention may interfere with the surgical exposure (especially during operations in the left hemithorax) and can cause reflex bradycardia and hypotension. An esophageal stethoscope is placed with its tip in the midesophagus to monitor heart sounds and breath sounds during surgery. In thoracic procedures, the surgeon should always be informed of the presence of an esophageal stethoscope because palpation of the instrument in the esophagus may cause the surgeon to believe the esophagus is the trachea (see the discussion of tracheoesophageal fistula that follows).

It is important that the anesthesiologist have a clear view of the operative field to be able to correlate hemodynamic changes with surgical manipulations and to view the progress of the operation. The intrathoracic exposure can be improved by hypoventilation during crucial surgical maneuvers and ventilating adequately after these measures are accomplished. Ventilation should be decreased or stopped during placement of pericostal sutures to prevent puncture or laceration of the lung parenchyma. During the placement of chest tubes, and especially during the puncture of pleura, ventilation should likewise be temporarily interrupted.

The maintenance of a patent airway (endotracheal tube) during thoracic operations is the primary responsibility of the anesthesiologist. The use of humidified anesthetic gases decreases the likelihood of obstruction because of secretions or small amounts of blood that can enter the tracheobronchial tree during surgery. The judicious use of small amounts of normal saline as irrigation (0.5 to 2.0 mL) followed by gentle suctioning at an appropriate point in the operation might prevent catastrophic obstruction of the airway.

MECHANICAL VENTILATION

Mechanical ventilation is used during thoracic operations, but manual ventilation is necessary for the detection of subtle or gross changes in compliance. Many anesthesiologists use semiclosed circle systems for the ventilation of infants during thoracic surgery. In many infants or children with thoracic surgery, the use of a critical care ventilator such as the Siemens Servo 900 C (Siemens Medical Systems, Danvers, Mass.) may be preferable to modifying an anesthesia ventilator to fit an infant. Pressure-controlled ventilation, rather than volume-limited ventilation, may be needed. The actual delivered ventilation when using an adult circle system and anesthesia ventilator, however, depends primarily on peak inspiratory pressure, rate, and lung compliance.[197]

Both Ohmeda (Ohmeda, Madison, Wis.) and North American Drager (Telford, Penn., USA) [NAD] produce anesthesia machine ventilators with both pressure control and volume control capability. Studies of these ventilators reveal that all tend to overshoot the set inspiratory pressures, and the Ohmeda Aestiva, in particular, delivers a tidal volume of about 19 mL less than does the Servo 900.[198] The tidal volume from the NAD was only approximately 6 mL less than that delivered by the Servo 900. All ventilators (Siemens, NAD, and Ohmeda) measured expiratory volume to be greater than actual delivered tidal volume.

Another alternative is the NAD Narkomed 6000 ventilator system. It includes a piston-driven ventilator functioning similarly to the Narkomed GS during time-cycled, pressure-limited ventilation. If time-cycled, volume-limited ventilation is needed, however, the 6000 system can be set easily to achieve the small tidal volumes required for infants.[199] Therefore in order to have the convenience of delivering volatile anesthetics, the anesthesiologist may need to adjust inspiratory times and pressures to deliver the desired tidal volume when an Ohmeda or NAD Narkomed GS anesthesia machine ventilator is used in infants with lung disease. The clinical importance of these differences in delivered tidal volume has been questioned, and many pediatric anesthesiologists, rather than accepting a preset pressure limit, adjust the ventilator to produce adequate chest movement in infants with low-compliance lungs.[200]

TERMINATION OF OPERATION, IMMEDIATE POSTOPERATIVE MEASURES, AND TRANSPORT TO THE INTENSIVE CARE UNIT

Once the planned operation is complete, and before chest closure, an attempt should be made to correct any atelectasis that may have occurred because of lung compression. This should be done gently, gradually, and under direct vision, so that excessive pressures are not applied to the airways, which could result in pneumothorax on the contralateral side. If the chest tube is to be removed in the operating room and not left in place during the immediate postoperative period (as with an uncomplicated patent ductus arteriosus ligation), it is usually placed directly through the incision and the pericostal sutures are pulled together tightly around it. It can safely be removed after several positive pressure breaths are given. A chest radiograph in the operating room is taken to confirm reexpansion of the lung on the affected side.

EXTUBATION

Extubation can be accomplished in the operating room in uncomplicated thoracic procedures or delayed for postoperative ventilation in the intensive care unit. In either situation, the minimum criteria for extubation listed in Table 16-6 must be met before extubation occurs. A postextubation chest radiograph is

Minimum Criteria For Extubation

Inspired oxygen	≤40%
IMV	≤2
CPAP or PEEP	≤4 cmH$_2$O
Stable blood gases	Pao$_2$ 80–100 mmHg
	Paco$_2$ 35–45 mmHg
	pH 7.30–7.40
Cardiovascular stability	Minimal or no vasopressors
Metabolism or reversal of muscle relaxants and respiratory depressants	
CNS stability	No active seizure disorder or progressive coma
Electrolyte balance	Including glucose and calcium

usually indicated after any thoracic surgical procedure because right upper-lobe atelectasis is quite common after prolonged intubation in children. Competency of the glottic structures to prevent aspiration may not be regained for as long as 8 hours after extubation; therefore cautious feedings of clear liquids should be given initially and progressed only as tolerated (see Appendix 16-1).

PATIENT TRANSPORT

It is important that a well-defined system for transfer of the patient to the care of the intensive care unit nurses from that of the anesthesia personnel be clearly understood by both parties to ensure a safe and effective transition. In critically ill children, a battery-powered monitor should be used to display the arterial pressure, ECG, and Spo$_2$ during transport. On arrival in the intensive care unit, the arterial pressure monitoring system is transferred to the intensive care unit equipment from the transport monitor. The venous or atrial monitoring catheters are then connected to the appropriate transducers. While this is being done, the anesthesiologist or respiratory therapist should continue to ventilate the patient's lungs by hand, and not until after the pressure monitors are connected and displayed should manual ventilation be discontinued and the patient undergo mechanical ventilation. The ventilator can be preset by a respiratory therapist before the patient arrives in the intensive care unit, after communication with the anesthesia personnel in the operating room. Examination by the anesthesiologist and respiratory therapist after institution of mechanical ventilation should be done to ensure adequate chest expansion, presence of bilateral breath sounds, the need for suctioning of the tracheal tube, and the rate of actual ventilation. Blood gas values should be obtained to determine the adequacy of ventilation at an appropriate time after arrival in the intensive care unit.

The anesthesiologist should give a detailed report to the intensive care unit nurse and physician intensivist responsible for the patient as soon as both think that the patient is stable. This report should include the procedure performed, anesthetic technique used, total amount of drugs, fluids, and blood administered, drugs reversed at the end of surgery (e.g., neuromuscular blocking drugs, heparin), problems encountered during the case, urine output, and any anticipated postoperative difficulties.

Postoperative Pain Management

In the past decade, anesthesiologists have sought to push the scope of their practices beyond the traditional operating room environment.[201] Acute postoperative pain management programs have been spearheaded by the efforts of anesthesiologists. Caring for pediatric patients after thoracic surgical procedures is an excellent opportunity for those with the skills and knowledge to offer services and extend their care beyond the day of surgery. Besides the issues of being a "perioperative" physician, there are ethical and physiologic concerns that suggest a more active approach in treating postoperative pain. Historically, children have been undertreated for pain.[202] For the most part, this has been due to a lack of understanding of the pharmacodynamic and pharmacokinetic profiles of the drugs most often used in pain management. Furthermore, fears among physicians and parents that all children would be at risk for respiratory depression and addiction certainly have limited the use of narcotics. If narcotics were used at all, it was most often as an IM shot, which is ineffective for the treatment of postoperative pain and especially noxious for children, who "fear the needle." It should now be widely accepted that neonates and infants respond to painful stimuli, and that suppression of painful stimuli intraoperatively and postoperatively may have beneficial effects by reducing the neuroendocrine stress response, decreasing tissue catabolism, and improving pulmonary mechanics (Table 16-7).[203] Possible interventions and a plan for postoperative pain management should be discussed with both parents and surgeon before the surgical procedure. Thoracic surgery lends itself to a variety of techniques, including the use of central neuraxial blocks with local anesthetics and opioids, intrapleural catheters, peripheral nerve blocks performed by the surgeon, and intravenous opioid infusions. The technique chosen should be appropriate for the patient's chronologic and developmental age. Necessary postoperative assessment and monitoring for the chosen technique should be available.

Intravenous Opioids

Opioids are the most common medications used for moderate-to-severe postoperative pain. Morphine is the most frequently administered drug.[204] Continuous opioid infusions have the advantage of providing more consistent and predictable therapeutic blood levels. Continuous infusions avoid the "ups and downs"—the "in pain or oversedated" phenomenon—associated with intermittent administration. Patients given continuous infusions still need monitoring because the drug can accumulate, leading to respiratory depression. Age-related differences in the clearance of morphine are worth noting. Preterm infants have prolonged clearances, which are inversely related to the postconceptual age of the infant.[205,206] Clearance in full-term neonates is one third less than in older children.[207] After 1 month of age, clearance exceeds adult levels until adolescence. Whether neonates are more "sensitive" to the respiratory depressant effects of narcotics is a matter of debate.[208] The lack of maturational development of the central respiratory centers and the decreased metabolic function of the liver may contribute to this phenomenon more than the immature blood-brain barrier of the neonate.[204] Although age may affect dosing

TABLE 16-7

Postoperative Analgesics

Drug	Route of Administration	Dose Range
Acetaminophen	PO	10–15 mg/kg q 4 hr
Ibuprofen	PO	3–30 mg/kg q 6 hr
Morphine	PO	0.2–0.6 mg/kg q 4 hr
	IV	0.05–0.1 mg/kg q 3-4 hr
	PCA	0.01–0.02 mg/kg with lockout interval of 6-10 min
Meperidine	PO	1–1.5 mg/kg/4 hr
	IV	1 mg/kg q 4 hr
Methadone	PO	0.1–0.2 mg/kg q 8-12 hr
	IV	0.05–0.1 mg/kg q 4-6 hr
Fentanyl	IV	1–3 ug/kg hr
Sufentanil	IV	0.1–0.3 μg/kg/hr

regimens and, subsequently, blood levels, what really ensures the success and safety of continuous opioid infusions are frequent assessment and monitoring. The method of assessment should match the developmental age of the child, and staff should understand the behavioral and physiologic responses to pain.[209] Respiratory depression, the most feared complication of opioid infusions, is not an all-or-none phenomenon. Respiratory depression is usually preceded by many hours of an overly sedated patient. Monitors should not be used as a substitute for frequent assessment.

Other medications used for continuous infusions are fentanyl, hydromorphone, and meperidine. Fentanyl may be suitable in the hemodynamically unstable patient. As with morphine, reduced clearance remains an issue in the neonate, while infants have increased clearance greater than that of adults. At an age of 1 year or greater, clearance is similar to adults.[204] Hydromorphone is five times more potent than morphine, and its advantage is related to less intense or even the absence of the morphine-related side effects of nausea, dysphoria, pruritus, and urinary retention. Meperidine has one tenth the potency of morphine. Despite its clinical use for years, meperidine's active metabolite, normeperidine, has a long half-life and could accumulate (excreted through the kidneys), especially with prolonged infusions. Normeperidine is a central nervous stimulant that may produce seizures in susceptible individuals.[210]

Patient-Controlled Analgesia

Patient-controlled analgesia (PCA) is appropriate for most children over the age of 7, but this modality has also been used in patients as young as 5 years of age. Parent and patient teaching is essential for the successful use of PCA.[211,212] Parents should understand that not only are safeguards built into the PCA pump algorithm, but also that there is an inherent safety in PCA itself.[213] Increasing boluses generally leads to increased sedation and less patient use. Patients should not be afraid to bolus themselves postoperatively in anticipation of painful procedures, and they should understand that they should not wait until pain is severe to push the button. PCA has proven to be safe, and it is most attractive because the child has control over his or her own pain medicine. Psychologically, this may be beneficial because the child can titrate the medication to balance pain control with possible side effects. Morphine, fen-

tanyl, and hydromorphone are all acceptable for PCA use. Dosing guidelines should take into consideration an initial bolus dose, the PCA dose, possibly a basal infusion rate, an hourly maximum dose, and a lockout time.[204]

Central Neuraxial Blockade

Epidural analgesia through the lumbar, thoracic, and caudal approaches has become the standard of care for postoperative pain management in patients undergoing thoracic procedures. Although epidurals are commonly done while under anesthesia, there are concerns that nerve root and spinal cord damage could occur during placement of the block. Yet, clinical experience attests to the safety of these blocks.[214-216] The benefits of a well-done neuraxial block far outweigh the potential of a possibly rare complication. Absolute contraindications to neuraxial blockade include parent refusal, systemic infection, local infection at the site, coagulopathy, and thrombocytopenia. Anatomic anomalies, such as myelodysplasia and sacral dysgenesis, may preclude neuraxial blockade because the epidural space may not be accessible. Alone or together, local anesthetics and opioids are the most common agents used; newer agents like clonidine and ketamine may show some promise but currently are not widely utilized.

CAUDAL ANALGESIA

A "single-shot" caudal is the easiest and most reliable block to perform in children.[214] The failure rate is low in patients under the age of 7, and major complications are rare.[217] Preservative-free morphine, however, is the only suitable drug to provide analgesia in the thoracic dermatomes from a single injection. Local anesthetics are prohibitive because of the large volumes (and potential toxicity) required to reach thoracic levels and because the duration of analgesia from a single injection is limited. Caudal morphine has been used with good success in children of all ages, including neonates. Morphine has hydrophilic properties, and once in the epidural space, morphine slowly penetrates the dura, passing into the cerebrospinal fluid (CSF). Being hydrophilic, morphine stays in the aqueous CSF, traveling to higher dermatomes and spinal receptors. Approximately 4 hours after injection, the drug reaches the fourth ventricle and higher respiratory centers. Morphine's interaction with receptors in this area is responsible for the potential side effects from this therapy. Respiratory depression is the most feared complication. In a retrospective review,

Valley and Bailey looked at caudal morphine in 138 patients with doses of 0.070 mg/kg.[218] Seventy-five percent of patients had no additional requirements for about 10 hours. Eleven patients had significant respiratory depression (i.e., requiring an intervention); 10 of these 11 patients were less than 1 year of age and weighed less than 9 kg. Seven of the 11 patients had systemic narcotics during their operations, and the remaining 4 patients received their doses via caudal catheters. The average time to respiratory depression was approximately 4 hours. Mayhew et al, using doses of 0.030 mg/kg, had no incidences of respiratory depression in 500 patients, 23 of whom were less than one month of age.[219] Krane et al stated that the optimal dose of caudal morphine was 0.030 mg/kg provided the patient was monitored for 24 hours after administration.[220] Overall, caudal morphine is an effective and safe (albeit limited) therapy provided that the risks of respiratory depression are appreciated. As with systemically administered narcotics, neonates and infants appear to be at the highest risk. Patients who receive systemic narcotics during their operations may be particularly susceptible. Monitoring and frequent assessment in the immediate postoperative period are critical to the success of this intervention.

Catheter techniques provide the greatest flexibility and ease of use. Continuous infusions of local anesthetics alone or in combination with narcotics can provide uninterrupted pain relief over several days.

THORACIC EPIDURAL TECHNIQUE

Entry to the epidural space can be through the caudal, lumbar, or thoracic routes. A continuous epidural technique is the gold standard for analgesia after thoracic surgery. An epidural catheter-threaded cephalad from the caudal canal to the thoracic dermatomes is a reliable and easily performed technique that is suitable for neonates, infants, and children to the age of 6.[221,222] The loose and gelatinous fat and the lack of a well-developed vascular plexus in the child's epidural space allow a styleted catheter to reach the thoracic dermatomes. There is often resistance and coiling of the catheter around the T_{10} level. Catheter tip placement can be confirmed by radiographic imaging. Removal of a coiled or knotted catheter does not appear to be a problem.

A lumbar epidural can be performed in any age group.[223] For analgesia to penetrate the thoracic dermatomes, the catheter needs to be threaded cephalad or a medication (such as morphine) that has rostral spread must be used. Because of the large volumes required to reach higher levels, local anesthetics would be prohibitive.

Thoracic epidural analgesia is the most ideal for thoracic surgery. Catheter tips can be reliably placed at the median level of the incision, and it can be expected that minimal drugs would be required to produce selective segmental analgesia. Clinical reports have demonstrated the safety and efficacy of this modality, but most would agree that this procedure should be reserved for those practitioners with significant experience in regional blockade.[224]

Not only does adequate postoperative analgesia improve deep breathing and allow earlier mobilization, but it also may have a beneficial effect on respiratory mechanics.[225-230] Diaphragmatic dysfunction that follows chest surgery is thought to be the result of reflex inhibition of phrenic nerve activity. A thoracic epidural with local anesthesia will block this diaphragmatic reflex and increase chest wall compliance. These changes are independent of the analgesic effect and may improve postoperative diaphragmatic function.[231-234] In a study looking at various modes of neuraxial analgesia in children undergoing cardiopulmonary bypass, Peterson et al favored the thoracic epidural approach. The incidence of complications such as transient postoperative paresthesias was lower in the thoracic epidural group. This difference might be due to the shorter catheter threading distance for thoracic epidurals when compared with catheters passed from the lumbar and caudal areas.[235]

PERIDURAL DRUGS

Many dosing regimens are available to treat postoperative pain.[204] Flexibility in approach, frequent assessment, vigilance in monitoring, and recognition of potential complications are important to ensure the success of whichever modality is chosen. Bupivacaine, alone or in combination with preservative-free morphine or fentanyl, is the most common medication used in continuous epidural infusions. If the catheter tip is placed at the dermatomal level of the incision, bupivacaine alone may suffice. In neonates and infants, bupivacaine so administered would be ideal because the risk of respiratory depression from opioids is a concern. In this age group, however, bupivacaine infusions alone need to be carefully monitored, as there have been case reports of bupivacaine toxicity from prolonged infusions.[236-238] In the serum, bupivacaine is bound to α1-acid glycoprotein. This protein is lower in infants compared to older children, leading to an increase in the half-life of bupivacaine. Because of the analgesic synergism that may exist between epidural local anesthetics and opioids, adding fentanyl to bupivacine should allow the use of a more dilute solution of local anesthetic.

Fentanyl is a lipophilic opioid that quickly penetrates the dura. Once in the CSF, it travels only a short distance in the CSF before passing back through the dura into the epidural fat. Thus, fentanyl produces analgesia only in those dermatomes where it interacts with spinal cord receptors. Fentanyl, like all opioids, causes respiratory depression. Unlike morphine, however, the respiratory depression is thought not to be from rostral spread in the CSF but from systemic absorption of the drug from the epidural space.

The choice of local anesthetic and narcotic combination is determined by the type of surgery, the location of the catheter tip, the ability to add adjunct medications, and the patient's monitoring environment. For example, a full-term neonate, with a caudally placed epidural catheter with the tip at a T_{10} level, is status postthoracotomy for repair of a tracheoesophageal fistula. The patient is extubated, and avoidance of respiratory depression precludes use of neuraxial narcotics. A dilute local anesthetic solution (0.125% bupivacaine) infusing through the epidural catheter, "prn" orders for intravenous morphine, and rectal acetaminophen may be sufficient.

The local anesthetics ropivacaine and levobupivacaine have recently been introduced for use in epidural analgesia.[239,240] Potential benefits, when compared with bupivacaine, include a higher threshold for cardiac and neurologic toxicity. Ropivacaine produces a differential nerve blockade with less motor block. In children, studies comparing equal doses of ropivacaine to bupivacaine for caudal blockade have shown similar profiles with regard to onset, duration of analgesia, and motor blockade. In infants younger than 6 months of age, the pharmacokinetic profile is similar to bupivacaine. There are decreased clearance and significantly higher free plasma concentrations and free fractions due to both immature organ function and decreased protein binding capacity.[241] Until further data are available, it is recommended to use reduced doses and limit infusion times to less than 48 hours in this age group.

Clonidine and ketamine are two adjuncts that can be added to local anesthetics to prolong the block and quality of analgesia. These drugs hold promise as possible replacements for opioids, as they are free of the opioid side effects. Clonidine is an α_2- agonist that has an antinociceptive effect (most likely at the spinal cord level) and potentiates the effects of epidurally administered narcotics and local anesthetics. Clonidine can prolong analgesia twofold to threefold.[242,243] Moderate hypotension (that responds to crystalloid infusion) and drowsiness are reported concerns with epidural clonidine usage. S(+)-Ketamine is an N-methyl-D-aspartate (NMDA) receptor antagonist, and blockade of the NMDA receptor in the substantia gelatinosa of the spinal cord reduces noxious stimulus-induced allodynia and hyperalgesia.[244] S(+)-Ketamine is the (+)-enantiomer of racemic ketamine, and it has three times the analgesic potency of the racemate. S(+)-Ketamine is preservative free and is therefore suitable for neuraxial blockade.[245] S(+)-Ketamine, in higher doses (1 mg/kg), has been shown to produce analgesia equivalent to bupivacaine with 1:200,000 epinephrine when given in caudals for pediatric herniorrhaphy.[246] At lower doses (0.5 mg/kg), S(+)-ketamine prolongs the analgesic effect of local anesthetics twofold to threefold. Psychomimetic side effects do not appear to be a problem at these doses.[246]

Intrapleural Analgesia

Continuous intrapleural administration of local anesthetics has been used successfully in children after thoracic surgery. Although the intrapleural space can be entered percutaneously as though performing a thoracentesis, the catheter is most easily placed by the surgeon at the time of surgery before wound closure. An epidural kit contains the essential equipment. Systemic absorption and toxicity from local anesthetics are of concern, as the pleural space has a large surface that promotes uptake of these drugs. Bupivacaine, 0.25% with epinephrine 1:200,000, should be used to prolong the drug's effect and decrease absorption. The mechanism by which intrapleural analgesia works is not well understood, but there does appear to be a gravitational effect in that the patient must be positioned with the operative side up to get the drug into the paravertebral gutters. Because of concerns about toxicity, bupivacaine infusion rates should not exceed 0.5 mg/kg/hr.[247] The effect that a chest tube "to suction" has on this modality is not known.

Intercostal Nerve Blocks

Intercostal nerve blocks performed by the surgeon before closure and under direct vision are a safe and effective method that should provide from 6 to 12 hours of postoperative pain relief. The amount injected depends on the size and age of the child. Before injecting, the toxic dose should be calculated. Caution should be exercised because absorption is rapid.[248] A long-acting preparation, such as bupivacaine, should be used, and epinephrine should be added to decrease drug absorption and prolong the block.

Analgesic Adjuvants

Nonsteroidal antiinflammatory drugs (NSAIDs) and acetaminophen are two nonopioid medications that are widely used as pain relievers but often overlooked as effective adjuncts to treat postoperative pain. Studies suggest that these medications are effective at reducing the narcotic and local anesthetic requirements in the pediatric patient.[249,250] Ketorolac tromethamine is an NSAID that is used to treat moderate-to-severe postoperative pain. Analgesic efficacy is similar to that of commonly used opioids. Ketorolac, however, lacks the opioid side effects of pruritus, sedation, nausea, and respiratory depression. Being an NSAID, ketorolac does impair platelet function, and there is the potential for gastrointestinal bleeding or even increased bleeding following surgery. Ketorolac may also precipitate acute renal failure in patients with preexisting renal impairment. Initial and maintenance dosing of ketorolac is 0.5 mg/kg given intravenously every 6 hours. This regimen has been shown to produce therapeutic blood concentrations in children and adults.[251,252]

Acetaminophen is a very common medication used in the pediatric population. The oral dose is 15 mg/kg, and its cherry flavor is often used to disguise the bitter taste of the premedication, midazolam. Recent literature would suggest that rectal dosing guidelines have been inadequate and that an initial rectal dose of 30 to 40 mg/kg, followed by 15 to 20 mg/kg orally or per rectum every six hours is more appropriate.[253-256] Total daily dosing should not exceed 100 mg/kg/day in children and 60 mg/kg/day in neonates.[257] Absorption of the drug from the rectal vault is erratic.[253] Peak blood levels take an average of 2 hours to achieve, but clinical reports have demonstrated an analgesic effect and opioid-sparing effect after short outpatient procedures.[258,259] It should be mentioned that there is no known analgesic level. Even at the higher rectal doses, blood levels have consistently been in the antipyretic range.[258,259]

Postoperative Ventilatory Support

The need for postoperative ventilatory support should be anticipated preoperatively, discussed with the parents, and explained to the patient if he or she is of an appropriate age. The requirement for such support is based on the preoperative condition of the patient, the specific operation planned, the anesthetic technique used, and the expected postoperative course. In very small infants and in almost all newborn babies undergoing thoracic operations, the tracheal tube is left in place, and mechanical ventilation is used for several hours to days, depending on the general condition of the patient. Weaning is begun as soon as hemodynamic and respiratory parameters appear stable.

Management of Postoperative Complications

Infants and children undergoing thoracic surgical procedures are subject to serious postoperative complications involving the lungs, airway, heart, and great vessels. Most of these complications can be prevented by meticulous attention to intraoperative detail on the parts of both surgeon and anesthesiologist.

Morbidity and mortality from intrathoracic operations can be further reduced by systemic postoperative assessment and the application of a few simple principles of general postoperative support.

Pneumothorax

Pneumothorax is an accumulation of air outside the lung, but within the pleural cavity and/or mediastinum, which occupies space needed for full lung inflation and cardiac filling. Air may remain in the chest after any intrathoracic operation, or it may accumulate postoperatively from an air leak in the lung or tracheobronchial tree. A rubber or plastic tube is usually left in the pleural cavity after thoracotomy, or in the mediastinum when a median sternotomy incision is used. This tube is connected to a collection and drainage system that allows air, blood, and fluid to escape while preventing air from entering the chest. Most drainage systems use the water-seal principle. Some surgeons, however, prefer not to leave a chest tube in place after relatively simple intrathoracic procedures in which the lung itself has not been incised and bleeding is negligible. In such cases, air is evacuated from the chest as the ribs and muscle are approximated, and positive pressure is maintained on the airways by the anesthesiologist until the chest is completely closed. A radiograph is obtained immediately after completion of the operation to be sure that no air remains. A small residual pneumothorax will usually resolve spontaneously in a few hours without causing difficulty, but careful follow-up is required.

Two specific problems related to pneumothorax deserve special consideration. First, the development of a tension pneumothorax in which air continues to leak from the lung or tracheobronchial tree into the undrained pleural space or mediastinum requires the immediate insertion of a chest tube to prevent compression of the lung, shift of the mediastinum, and life-threatening hypoxia, hypercarbia, and low cardiac output. A tension pneumothorax can occur from the rupture of the lung surface or rupture of a small bleb due to excessive positive pressure, coughing, intraoperative trauma, or agitation in a patient receiving mechanical ventilation. It is diagnosed by clinical deterioration in the patient's vital signs (hypertension followed by hypotension, tachycardia followed by bradycardia, and respiratory distress), acute reduction in breath sounds, decreased pulmonary compliance, displacement of the cardiac point of maximal impulse, and by hypoxemia, hypercarbia, and acidosis as reflected in the arterial blood gases. A chest radiograph can be used to confirm the diagnosis.

The second important problem relates to the development of a pneumothorax in the unoperated pleural cavity, where a chest tube is not likely to be in place. This problem is dangerous and so likely to be overlooked that some surgeons open and drain both pleural cavities in addition to the mediastinum in critically ill patients who undergo certain intrathoracic operations, particularly when a median sternotomy is performed. Chest tubes are left in place for 24 to 48 hours postoperatively after a median sternotomy. They are "stripped" frequently to avoid the accumulation of a blood clot that might prevent adequate drainage of air or blood. The tubes are not removed if there is evidence of a continued air leak within the chest. At the time of removal, precautions need to be taken to avoid entry of the air

into the chest through the opening in the chest wall or through the holes in the tubes themselves. A chest radiograph is obtained shortly after removal of the tubes to confirm that no pneumothorax remains. The patient is observed carefully for the next few hours for signs of respiratory distress or deterioration in vital signs that might suggest a recurrent pneumothorax. Occlusive dressings are placed over the chest tube tracts. In small infants with thin chest walls, a suture can be placed around the chest tube and tied down to occlude the wound as the tube is withdrawn. Even a small residual pneumothorax increases the chances for blood and fluid accumulation within the pleural cavity and may lead to postoperative empyema.

Hemothorax and Hemomediastinum

Blood loss and postoperative bleeding are quite variable during and after intrathoracic operations. In cases of lung biopsy, lobectomy, or patent ductus arteriosus ligation, for example, virtually no blood loss is expected. In contrast, massive bleeding and prolonged postoperative drainage may be encountered during and after reoperation for a complex congenital heart defect. Chest drainage tubes are inserted after an operation within the chest or mediastinum in which even minimal postoperative bleeding is expected. Excessive bleeding requires evaluation of hemostatic variables by measurement of platelets, PT, PTT, and ACT. Before reexploration of the chest, all possible measures should be taken to restore normal coagulation, including the administration of fresh-frozen plasma, platelets, and protamine. In selected patients, antifibrinolytic agents, fresh whole blood, platelets, plasma, cryoprecipitate, and vitamin K may be indicated. Acceptable rates for postoperative bleeding as a function of the size of the patient have been published by Kirklin et al.[260] Rates of bleeding in excess of these limits may require reexploration in the absence of hemostatic abnormalities.

Serious complications may occur as a result of waiting too long in the hope that conservative measures and time will take care of the bleeding. Chest tubes are of only limited effectiveness in draining blood from the pleural cavities and mediastinum. Proper position, suction, and "stripping" are important; however, once clots begin to collect within the chest, tube function deteriorates, and the likelihood of reexploration for evacuation of the clot and control of bleeding increases. Accumulation of blood within the chest seriously compromises pulmonary function and cardiac output. Cardiac arrhythmias and tamponade occur quickly in children and may even require urgent reopening of the incision in the intensive care unit to prevent death.

Normal body temperature should be restored as quickly as possible postoperatively to enhance hemostasis. PEEP (5 to 10 cm) can be tried to reduce postoperative intrathoracic bleeding.[261] Agitation and hypertension should be controlled pharmacologically. In spite of all these potentially useful measures, a very low threshold for reexploration to control postoperative bleeding and to evacuate a hemothorax or hemomediastinum is the best insurance for a subsequent complication-free recovery.

Atelectasis

Postoperative atelectasis is, to a greater or lesser degree, an almost universal occurrence after intrathoracic operations in infants and small children. Surgical manipulation of the small, fragile, and often congested lung, associated with postoperative incisional pain and the child's instinctive reluctance to cooperate with even the most skillfully designated program for pulmonary toilet, often complicate recovery. Children with congenital cardiac defects are frequently weak and debilitated, and increased pulmonary blood flow or pulmonary venous congestion from left ventricular failure further complicates the problem.

Management of atelectasis in the older child should begin during the preoperative orientation, when the child is taught to cooperate with nurses and respiratory therapists during the conduct of chest percussion, deep breathing, coughing, and suctioning. Incentive spirometry is particularly effective in the older children, especially when one of the clown like or ball-containing "game" devices is used during preoperative training.

When postoperative fever, tachycardia, tachypnea, and diminished breath sounds suggest atelectasis, a chest radiograph usually confirms the presence of areas of uninflated lung. If vigorous chest physical therapy and incentive spirometry fail to eliminate the atelectasis, nasotracheal aspiration is used. In patients who are still intubated, irrigation and positive pressure ventilation usually reexpand the atelectatic segment, unless the tube itself is obstructing one or more bronchi; the right upper lobe is particularly susceptible to obstruction by an improperly placed endotracheal tube. Reintubation with endotracheal suctioning and positive pressure ventilation can be used for a few hours in infants with persistent atelectasis. Bronchoscopy may be required to examine each bronchial orifice and directly extract obstructing mucus plugs or blood clots. It is particularly useful following an episode of vomiting and suspected aspiration and can be done at the bedside in the intensive care unit.

Children with neuromuscular disorders, scoliosis, small airways, cardiac disease, chronic debilitation, and cystic fibrosis pose particularly troublesome problems and may require a tracheostomy to manage persistent or recurrent postoperative atelectasis. If atelectasis is not prevented or promptly corrected, pneumonitis and life-threatening sepsis may develop within a few days.

Upper-Airway Obstruction

Upper-airway obstruction after extubation of the infant or child is far more common than in the adult. The likelihood of such obstruction is increased by a difficult intubation, multiple attempts at intubation, overhydration, congestive heart failure, and prolonged intubation. If the child has been agitated or overly active while awakening from anesthesia, trauma to the vocal cords and trachea can produce edema that may result in some degree of upper-airway obstruction following extubation. Small infants with large tongues and short necks are particularly at risk, especially those with craniofacial anomalies involving the upper airway.

To minimize the likelihood of postextubation upper-airway obstruction, the intubated child should be heavily sedated and receive humidified gases. In those children particularly at risk of obstruction, dexamethasone (0.1 mg/kg) should be given 30 minutes before extubation, and all equipment necessary for prompt reintubation should be kept at the bedside until a satisfactory upper airway is assured. When prolonged ventilatory support is required, a tracheostomy should be considered to minimize trauma to the vocal cords and to eliminate the pressure and potential necrosis with subsequent stenosis at the level of the narrow subglottic cricoid ring. With meticulous care, however, infants can be ventilated for many weeks using endotracheal intubation.

Anesthesia for Specific Pediatric Thoracic Procedures

The most common pediatric thoracic procedures are bronchoscopy, congenital diaphragmatic hernia, tracheoesophageal fistula, mediastinal masses, and ligation of patent ductus arteriosus. Other, less common, procedures are detailed in Appendix 16-1.

Bronchoscopy and Bronchography

BRONCHOSCOPY. Therapeutic and diagnostic bronchoscopy in the pediatric patient are not uncommon procedures. It requires skill and cooperation between the endoscopist and anesthesiologist because the airway must be "shared," and each must understand and appreciate the problems of the other. The development of the pediatric magnifying bronchoscope has greatly enhanced the safety and effectiveness of bronchoscopy in infants and children. This system provides sheaths of varying sizes and lengths to be used on even the smallest infants, although ventilation is more difficult with the 3.0-mm instrument because of the resistance of the system itself when the light source and magnifying lens are in place. The larger instruments furnish adequate ventilating capabilities and allow the surgeon to continue the visual examination while the patient is being ventilated via the 15-mm sidearm attached to the anesthesia system. With these larger instruments, small biopsy forceps can be passed through the instrument channel while ventilation is maintained with the telescope in place. If larger forceps are needed, the telescope must be removed and biopsy or foreign body extraction accomplished without optical magnification via the main channel on the bronchoscope.[262] Indications for diagnostic bronchoscopy in children include the following[263]:

- Determination of the cause of stridor, such as laryngotracheomalacia, laryngeal webs, or postintubation or posttracheotomy stenosis
- Determination of the origin of hemoptysis
- The investigation of persistent pneumonia or atelectasis
- The workup of tracheoesophageal fistula
- Mediastinal mass

With current advances in neonatal medicine, many premature infants with a history of respiratory distress syndrome and prolonged intubation are undergoing diagnostic bronchoscopy.

Therapeutic bronchoscopy in children is usually done to remove aspirated foreign bodies. Children under the age of 3 are the most likely to inhale foreign bodies. The foreign body most likely will be inhaled into the tracheobronchial tree, where it will be impacted and cause a local inflammatory reaction. Distal collapse of bronchi and pneumonia often ensue. Removal of foreign bodies may be especially treacherous, depending on the size and nature of the aspirated material. Fragmentation can occur, producing glottic, tracheal, or bilateral mainstem obstruction. In some cases, the endoscopist may be forced to push the foreign material down into the right or left mainstem bronchus to allow ventilation of the unobstructed air passages. If the foreign body is impacted in the bronchus, a Fogarty catheter may be slipped past the object with the balloon deflated; once it is beyond the foreign body, the balloon is inflated and pulled toward or even into the bronchoscope.

The anesthetic technique for rigid bronchoscopy is tailored to the condition of the patient and the indication for the procedure. Before the anesthetic and surgical procedure, the case should be discussed with the surgeon. It is important to know why the bronchoscopy is being done because the rationale should determine the proper anesthetic technique. If it is a diagnostic bronchoscopy for laryngotracheomalacia, then spontaneous ventilation is appropriate, as dynamic motion of the airway is necessary for the diagnosis. If stenosis is suspected, muscle paralysis and positive pressure ventilation may be sufficient; being prepared with a smaller-than-normal-size endotracheal tube may also be helpful. A good rule of thumb is that if the lesion is fixed, paralysis should suffice; for dynamic lesions, including a foreign body, spontaneous ventilation is the best option. Atropine or glycopyrrolate may be given intravenously as an antisialagogue to help control secretions. Some have suggested using atropine to prevent vagal reflexes during the procedure; however, provision of an adequate depth of anesthesia is usually sufficient. If the patient has an intravenous catheter, this may used for induction, keeping in mind that respiration might have to be controlled. Before insertion of the bronchoscope, an atomizer that sprays a mist of local anesthetic (lidocaine 2% or 4%, 4 mg/kg) into the oropharyngeal cavity may be used. The spray may lessen anesthetic requirements and blunt the response to the bronchoscopy. Alternatively, the anesthesiologist can perform direct laryngoscopy and spray the trachea and vocal cords with local anesthetic solution (lidocaine 2% or 4%, 4 mg/kg). Care should be taken not to apply the local anesthetic when the patient is "light," as this may induce laryngospasm. Volatile anesthetic agent in 100% oxygen should be used for maintenance. Halothane or sevoflurane are the agents least irritating to the airways, and sevoflurane may be preferable in that a greater depth can be obtained without risk of cardiovascular depression.[264] After the bronchoscope is inserted through the vocal cords, ventilation occurs through the side port of the bronchoscope. Because of the leaks around the bronchoscope, ventilation often is inadequate. High fresh gas flow rates and high inspired volatile agent concentrations are often required to compensate for this problem. After the examination, the patient may be reintubated before awakening; however, this choice is solely a function of how the anesthesiologist chooses to manage the airway (see Chapter 9).

Bronchoscopic or laryngoscopic instrumentation of the upper airway carries with it the possibility of significant laryngeal or subglottic edema, especially in smaller infants and children. Management of this complication includes postoperative humidification of inspired gases, adequate hydration, intermittent positive pressure breathing, racemic epinephrine (0.5 mL of racemic epinephrine diluted with 3.5 mL of normal saline every 2 to 3 hours), and dexamethasone (0.5 mg/kg up to

10 mg). Endotracheal intubation may be required if these measures do not suffice.[265]

Cystic Fibrosis. Flexible fiberoptic bronchoscopy for cystic fibrosis deserves special mention. Bronchoscopy and bronchial lavage in patients with cystic fibrosis are performed to open airways obstructed by thick, inspissated secretions. These patients are often quite ill, with borderline or overt respiratory failure, superimposed pneumonia, and cor pulmonale. The anesthetic management must take into account all of these factors. The uptake of the inhalation agents is slow because of the lung disease. At this institution, management of these patients is with a laryngeal mask airway (LMA) with the patients under general anesthesia. An adapter is connected to the LMA that allows insertion of the flexible bronchoscope while remaining connected to the anesthesia circuit. As the LMA sits above the vocal cords, it will often be easier for the endoscopist to guide the scope into the airway. As the patient is breathing spontaneously, depth of anesthesia can be easily regulated. Narcotics may be used and titrated to the respiratory rate. After the procedure, the patient's airways are often irritated, and the narcotics may also help with cough suppression. Because of its effect on airway secretions, atropine is relatively contraindicated in cystic fibrosis.

Postoperative Complications. Bronchoscopic and laryngoscopic instrumentation of the upper airway always carry with them the risk of significant laryngeal or subglottic edema, especially in smaller infants and children. Management of this complication includes postoperative humidification of inspired gases, adequate hydration, intermittent positive pressure breathing or racemic epinephrine (0.5 mL of racemic epinephrine diluted with 3.5 mL of normal saline) every two to three hours, and dexamethasone.[265] Endotracheal intubation may be required if these measures do not suffice.

BRONCHOGRAPHY
Bronchography may be necessary to define the extent of certain parenchymal diseases of the lung, such as segmental bronchiectasis. Contrast material is introduced with a catheter passed via the bronchoscope or an endotracheal tube, depending on the ease with which the catheter can be placed into the desired area of the bronchial tree. This procedure is usually done in the radiology department to use fluoroscopy, and the patient may need to be turned into several positions to obtain adequate diagnostic films. After the necessary radiographs are obtained, as much of the contrast material as possible is suctioned from the bronchial tree. Anesthesia should be sufficiently deep to prevent coughing when the contrast is introduced, as coughing can spread the material and result in poor-quality radiographs.

Anesthesia for bronchography is similar to that for bronchoscopy. An intravenous induction and sevoflurane or halothane/oxygen maintenance or an inhalation induction is used as described previously. If an endotracheal tube instead of a bronchoscope is used to pass the contrast catheter, a curved 15-mm connector with a removable cap is used so that ventilation can be maintained while manipulation of the catheter is under way.

Esophagoscopy
Indications for upper gastrointestinal tract endoscopy include management of acquired or congenital esophageal stricture,

evaluation of the extent and degree of caustic or acid burns of the esophagus, removal of foreign bodies, determination of the extent of reflux esophagitis in patients with dysfunction of the gastroesophageal sphincter, identification and treatment of esophageal varices, and evaluation of a tracheoesophageal fistula in conjunction with bronchoscopy. The flexible fiberoptic esophagogastroscope is sometimes used in children; however, rigid instruments are usually used, especially for the removal of foreign bodies and the management of esophageal strictures, which constitute the most common reasons for esophagoscopy in the pediatric patient.

Because patient cooperation is necessary, general anesthesia is almost always required in the pediatric age group. The exception to this may be for the removal of coins in the esophagus, which can sometimes be accomplished using light sedation and insertion of the Foley catheter into the esophagus through the nose. Under fluoroscopic visualization, the coin is pulled from the esophagus by inflating the balloon tip as it lies beyond the coin.[266]

For many patients undergoing esophagoscopy, a rapid-sequence induction using preoxygenation, thiopental, succinylcholine, and cricoid pressure is probably the safest method of anesthesia, especially if there is known to be esophageal dilatation above a stricture with the possibility of retained material. A few small infants may require awake intubation (see the discussion on tracheoesophageal fistula). Elective esophagoscopy for other conditions can be done safely using an inhalation induction. Maintenance of anesthesia after intubation of the trachea is accomplished with deep levels of inhalation agents because light levels of anesthesia that allow coughing or movement could result in esophageal or pharyngeal perforation and must be avoided.

In very small infants, the esophagoscope may impinge on the endotracheal tube and cause obstruction. This complication, as well as the possibility of accidental extubation during the procedure, must be managed carefully. Stridor can also result after esophagoscopy and should be managed as outlined in the section on bronchoscopy. Sharp foreign bodies may perforate small or major blood vessels, and significant bleeding may require blood replacement.

Video-Assisted Thoracic Surgery and One-Lung Anesthesia

First introduced as a surgical technique in 1991, video-assisted thorascopic surgery (VATS) has numerous advantages compared with open thoracotomy.[267-269] Because the surgery is done through the use of miniaturized thoracoscopes and video cameras, incisions are small, and tissue disruption (i.e., rib spreaders are not used) is minimized. Consequently, there is less pain postoperatively and better pulmonary function. Postoperative recovery should be more rapid, and patients can be discharged from the hospital earlier.[268,270,271] Preliminary reports have suggested these potential benefits with this new procedure. VATS has been performed in infants weighing less than 1 kg, and it has been used in the surgical treatment of pulmonary lesions as well as for the correction of certain congenital cardiac defects.[267-269,272]

Anesthetic management for VATS most often involves one-lung ventilation (OLV).[273-275] OLV provides better surgical exposure during the procedure. Currently, VATS is the most common indication for selective lung separation. Other indications are isolation of a healthy lung from the contaminated material in a diseased lung, bronchiectasis, and bronchopleural fistula. Double-lumen tubes are not available in pediatric sizes, but selective mainstem intubation and bronchial blockade using a Fogarty catheter have been used to achieve one-lung ventilation in infants and smaller children.[277] In larger children and adults, the standard of care for OLV would be the use of a double-lumen endotracheal tube (ETT). The smallest double-lumen ETT available is a 26 Fr (Rusch, Duluth, Ga.), which has an outer diameter of 8.7 mm and corresponds to a 6.5-mm internal diameter standard single-lumen ETT. With a popular formula ([age+16]/4) to calculate the appropriate endotracheal tube size in children, it can be seen that placing a standard double-lumen tube in a child younger than 8 years of age would be difficult. Fortunately, over the past decade, several methods to provide OLV in small children and infants have been described.

MAINSTEM BRONCHIAL INTUBATION

The most basic method is to blindly pass a single-lumen ETT into the appropriate bronchus, thus providing selective lung ventilation.[274,278] In left-sided surgery, for example, the ETT should be passed into the right mainstem bronchus. The ETT will preferentially pass into the right mainstem bronchus because of its more proximal takeoff from the carina. For the ETT to be positioned in the left mainstem bronchus, a styleted tube or direct visualization and guidance with a flexible fiberoptic bronchoscope (FOB) might be necessary. In either case, confirmation of correct placement is by auscultation of breath sounds and direct visualization with the flexible FOB. Because the airways narrow distally, some have suggested using an ETT 1.5 to 2.0 mm smaller than what would normally be calculated by the above formula for intubation of the trachea.[279] Using a smaller ETT may make ventilation more difficult, however, as airway resistance is increased, and there is a greater leak of fresh gases around the cricoid ring. Also, monitoring of anesthetic gases may be impaired. With the use of a smaller ETT, there is the possibility of an inadequate seal in the bronchus. Failure of the operative lung to collapse or contamination of the healthy lung is possible. For an ETT placed in the right mainstem bronchus, there is the possibility that the takeoff to the right upper-lobe bronchus may become obstructed, leading to collapse of that segment. Some have suggested cutting a "second" Murphy eye into the ETT to ensure proper ventilation of this lobe.[280] A cuffed ETT may be used, and this may better isolate the nonoperative lung from contaminants. Proper placement must be ensured, however, so that the inflated cuff is not obstructing the bronchus to the right upper lobe. A familiarity with airway anatomy and dimensions is essential when performing OLV in children.[276,281,282] Other issues have been raised regarding this most basic technique. Because this is only a single-lumen method, differential lung ventilation cannot be applied. If hypoxemia were to occur during the procedure and while under single-lung ventilation conditions, CPAP could not be applied to the operative lung. The only method to correct the hypoxemia would be ventilation of both lungs, with the ETT repositioned above the carina.

BRONCHIAL BLOCKERS

A second method utilizing an endotracheal tube and a balloon-tipped bronchial blocker is well described by Hammer et al.[275]

The child is initially intubated with an age-appropriate ETT while under anesthesia. The ETT is passed into the bronchus of the operative side. This is confirmed by auscultation of breath sounds and by flexible fiberoptic bronchoscopy. A guidewire is passed through the lumen of the ETT into the bronchus, and the ETT is removed. A bronchial blocker, which is a balloon-tipped catheter with an end hole, is passed over the wire into the bronchus. The age-appropriate ETT is reinserted adjacent to the bronchial blocker and placed above the carina. An FOB is used to confirm correct placement of the bronchial blocker; the bronchial blocker is then secured to the side of the ETT. Complications with this technique are infrequent but potentially serious. The major disadvantage to the bronchial blocker technique is that the catheter could become dislodged and obstruct ventilation to both lungs at the level of the carina. There also has been a case report of bronchial rupture, and this was thought to be due to overdistention of the low-volume, high-pressure balloon on a Fogarty embolectomy catheter.[283] Advantages to the use of the bronchial blocker technique include the following:

1. Differential lung ventilation and the application of CPAP or insufflation of oxygen to the operative, nondependent lung through the lumen of the bronchial blocker
2. Suctioning of the operative side via the lumen of the bronchial blocker
3. Isolation of the operative lung from the nonoperative lung.

Hammer recommends 5-Fr bronchial blockers for children younger than 5 to 6 years of age and 6-Fr catheters for older children.[276]

UNIVENT TUBES

A variation on the use of a single-lumen tube with bronchial blockers is the Univent ETT (Fuji Systems Corporation, Tokyo, Japan). The Univent tube is a conventional ETT with a small, attached second lumen containing a bronchial blocker. The bronchial blocker lumen is open to air and can be used for suctioning and insufflation of oxygen. The balloon has low-volume, high-pressure characteristics.[276] With the Univent tube positioned above the carina, a flexible fiberoptic bronchoscope is used to visualize the balloon-tipped cuff of the blocker being advanced by an assistant into the appropriate bronchus on the operative side. The pediatric Univent tube comes in a size as small as 3.5-mm internal diameter. In smaller tubes, the bronchial blocker takes up a larger proportion of the cross-sectional area of the tube's lumen and may increase resistance to gas flow.

Although there have been technologic advances in the anesthetic and surgical management of children having thoracic surgery, very little is known about OLV in this age group. In particular, the effect of OLV and CO_2 insufflation during VATS on the hemodynamics of children with shunt lesions is not known. In Lavoie's study, 75% of the patients had intracardiac or extracardiac shunts.[271] In infants, oxygenation during OLV in the lateral decubitus position is comparatively less than it would be in the adult.[279] This discrepancy between adults and infants occurs because infants have an easily compressible rib cage that does not support the underlying lung. For this reason, functional residual capacity is close to residual volume in infants undergoing OLV. Airway closure and atelectasis in the dependent, nonoperative lung are more likely to occur.

Furthermore, the action of hydrostatic pressure in shunting blood from the operative lung to the dependent lung is less operative in the infant than in the adult; this is due to the size differences between the two age groups. Because oxygen consumption in the infant is increased and because the lateral decubitus position exacerbates hypoxemia, infants and children undergoing OLV are at risk for hypoxemia.

Congenital Diaphragmatic Hernia

Congenital diaphragmatic hernia (CDH) presenting in the immediate newborn period is one of the most life-threatening, yet surgically correctable, conditions encountered by the anesthesiologist. The incidence of CDH is approximately one in 2400 live births.[284-286] Despite advances in surgical, anesthetic, and neonatal intensive care, the survival for infants with CDH is institution-specific and ranges from 60% to 80%.[287-290] Survival is largely dependent on the degree of pulmonary hypoplasia and associated congenital heart disease (Figure 16-4).[287-296] The introduction of extracorporeal membrane oxygenation (ECMO) in the late 1970s appears to have improved survival, but this therapy is generally reserved for the most critically ill infants. Attempts to save a number of these high-risk neonates who previously would not have been candidates for any form of treatment have been at the expense of overall survival rates and an increase in long-term morbidity.

Congenital diaphragmatic hernia is classified according to the anatomic location of the diaphragmatic defect (Figure 16-5). Herniation of abdominal viscera may occur at any of three diaphragmatic locations: the posterolateral foramen of Bochdalek, the anterior foramen of Morgagni, or the esophageal hiatus. Unilateral Bochdalek hernias account for more than 80% of all defects and are most likely to present with severe symptoms in the neonatal period. Left-sided defects are four to five times more frequent than right-sided defects, and bilateral defects are rare. Another 2% to 4% of hernias are of the Morgagni type. These are anteriorly located, tend to be small, and typically present well beyond the neonatal period. Symptoms are usually mild, and diagnosis is occasionally made as an incidental finding on chest radiograph. Hiatal hernias account for the remainder and also typically present beyond the newborn period, with gastrointestinal rather than pulmonary findings.[285,287]

Embryologically, the earliest precursor of the diaphragm is septum transversum, formed at approximately 4 weeks' gestation from mesenchyme located between the heart and coelomic cavity. It is joined by the dorsal mesentery of the foregut to form the central tendon of the developing diaphragm. At this time, the pleuroperitoneal cavity exists as a single, undivided space. From the developing central tendon and from the posterolateral coelomic wall, pleuroperitoneal folds develop and gradually extend medially to divide the cavity into distinct pleural and peritoneal compartments. An ingrowth of mesenchyme between the layers of the pleuroperitoneal membrane provides the muscular component.

Closure is usually complete by the ninth week of gestation, the posterolateral portions of the diaphragm being the last to close and the right side closing earlier than the left. Coincident with development and closure of the diaphragm, the developing midgut undergoes rapid elongation in the umbilical stalk

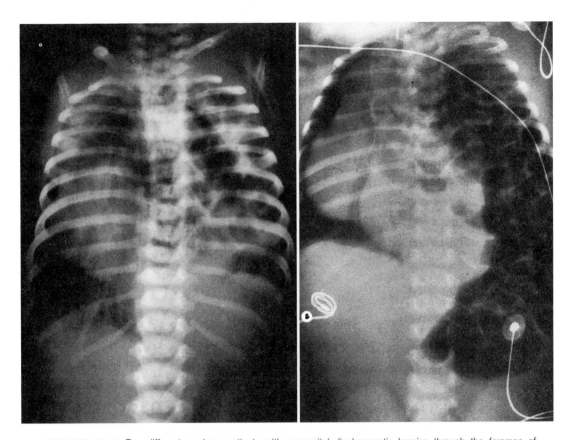

FIGURE 16-4 Two different newborn patients with congenital diaphragmatic hernias through the foramen of Bochdalek. Preoperative chest radiographs show intestinal organs mostly within the left hemithorax and herniation of the mediastinal structures into the right side. There is absence of most gas shadows from the abdomen, except for a small amount in the stomach and descending colon.

and returns to the peritoneal cavity. If either the gut returns prematurely or diaphragmatic closure is delayed, herniation of abdominal viscera into the pleural cavity may occur.[285,287,297,298]

The presence of abdominal viscera within the fetal pleural space results in a maturational disturbance of the developing lung. Necropsy specimens of lungs of infants dying of CDH are remarkable for a decrease in total lung mass, a severe reduction in the number of airway generations, and a parallel reduction in alveolar number. The ipsilateral lung, especially the ipsilateral lower lobe, is more severely affected than the contralateral. Associated abnormalities are present within the pulmonary vascular tree. The main pulmonary arteries are small in proportion to the reduced lung mass, and there is a reduction in vascular tree branching generations. Also, there is muscular hypertrophy of the media, with the presence of smooth muscle within the walls of small-diameter vessels that are normally devoid of a muscular component.[292,299-301]

Infants born with the common, left-sided Bochdalek hernia frequently have the classic triad of cyanosis, dyspnea (respiratory distress), and cardiac dextroposition. Physical findings may include tachypnea, nasal flaring, suprasternal and subcostal retractions, an abnormally scaphoid abdomen, and diminished breath sounds either unilaterally or bilaterally. Audible peristaltic sounds over the affected hemithorax may be present, but this is an inconsistent finding. Anteroposterior chest radiographs demonstrate a shift of mediastinal structures to the side opposite the hernia, as well as air-filled bowel loops

within the thoracic cavity. The abdomen generally shows a paucity of gas, and a nasogastric tube placed for gastrointestinal decompression may be found to have the tip located within the thorax. If the diagnosis remains unclear, air or radiopaque contrast material may be instilled through the nasogastric tube to better delineate the location of the gastrointestinal tract.[285,287] Both age at presentation and the severity of symptoms have prognostic significance. Mortality is correspondingly greater for those infants who present in the delivery suite in immediate distress, who have CPR shortly after birth, and who have cardiac anomalies. Infants presenting beyond 18 to 24 hours of age have less severe anatomic and physiologic derangements and can be expected to have near 100% survival.[291,302] Interestingly, infants diagnosed prenatally have a greater mortality rate. This may be due to the fact that larger hernias and associated lethal nonpulmonary malformations are more easily seen by ultrasonographic examination.

Associated congenital anomalies occur in approximately 10% to 30% of infants with CDH (Table 16-8).[291,293] The incidence of other anomalies is approximately two times as frequent among infants with right-sided (as opposed to left-sided) defects. A wide range of associated malformations affecting virtually every organ system has been reported, and such malformations may occur in isolation or as a part of multiple anomalies within a single patient. As might be expected, mortality is increased in the presence of major associated anomalies.[293,303] This is particularly true when the cardiovascular

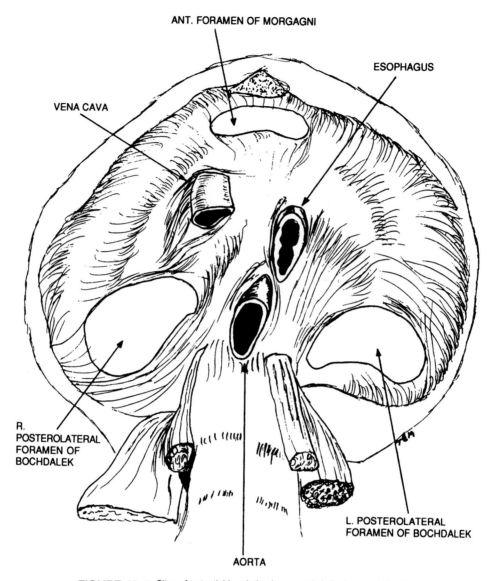

FIGURE 16-5 Sites of potential herniation in congenital diaphragmatic hernia.

system is involved. In Greenwood et al's series of 48 infants, 23% had associated cardiovascular abnormalities.[303] Mortality in this group was 73%, in contrast to 27% mortality in infants without cardiac abnormalities. Table 16-8 provides a representative inventory of reported anomalies categorized by organ system.[291,293]

TABLE 16-8

Associated Anomalies in Patients with Congenital Diaphragmatic Hernia

Organ System	Malformation
Cardiovascular	Any form of cyanotic or acyanotic defect
Gastrointestinal	TE fistula, malrotation, various atresias, omphalocoele
Genitourinary	Hypospadius, hydronephrosis, renal dysplasia
Central nervous system	Spina bifida defects, hydrocephalus, cerebral dysgenesis
Musculoskeletal	Syndactyly, amelias
Chromosomal	Trisomy 18, trisomy 21

The pathophysiologic derangements produced by CDH are a consequence both of pulmonary parenchymal hypoplasia and abnormalities in structure and function of the pulmonary vasculature. Affected infants can be classified into the following three broad physiologic categories:

1. The first group comprises those infants who have experienced severe compression of fetal lung buds, producing profound bilateral hypoplasia that prohibits extrauterine survival regardless of therapeutic interventions.

2. On the other extreme are those infants who have only mild ipsilateral pulmonary hypoplasia and near-normal pulmonary vascular hemodynamics and in whom near 100% survival is anticipated.

3. Comprising the third group are those infants with more severe pulmonary maldevelopment accompanied by a persistence of the transitional circulation.[304] Survival of infants in this group is to a large degree influenced by proper therapeutic management, although overall mortality remains at approximately 60%.

Figure 16-6 summarizes the pathophysiologic alterations accompanying large Bochdalek hernias. Functionally, the lungs of affected infants are noncompliant because of the severe reduction in lung mass and a relative deficiency of surfactant (Figure 16-7).[305] These deficiencies result in altered gas exchange leading to hypercarbia and hypoxemia. Supranormal inflating pressures and respiratory rates to provide adequate tidal volume and minute ventilation often result in significant barotraumas, and contralateral pneumothorax is not uncommon.[293]

Pulmonary vascular hypertension (PVR) occurs as a consequence of reduced total cross-sectional area of the pulmonary vascular bed, abnormal muscularity of pulmonary vessels, and abnormal hypersensitivity of the vessels to vasoconstrictor stimuli (principally hypercarbia and hypoxia). Acidosis, hypothermia, and elevated airway pressures also may contribute to sustained elevations in PVR.[292,299,306,307] With patency of the ductus arteriosus, the parallel arrangement of the pulmonary and systemic circulations that is characteristic of the fetal circulatory pattern persists. The magnitude and direction of flow of right ventricular output will depend on the relative resistance to flow within the two vascular beds: pulmonary via the pulmonary artery and systemic via the ductus arteriosus. In the face of significantly increased PVR, flow will be preferentially directed right-to-left across the ductus arteriosus, further contributing to systemic hypoxemia. A right-to-left shunt also could occur at the atrial level because right ventricular and right atrial pressures increase owing to elevated right ventricular afterload. Left atrial pressure may decrease coincidentally because of decreased pulmonary venous return, further contributing to an atrial pressure gradient that favors right-to-left shunting of blood. Primary myocardial dysfunction occurs as a consequence of elevated afterload, persistent hypoxemia, and acidosis. Left ventricular hypoplasia, perhaps due to in utero mediastinal compression, may also be present in infants with CDH.[308]

The combined effects of these pathophysiologic alterations result in the establishment of a vicious cycle of hypoxemia,

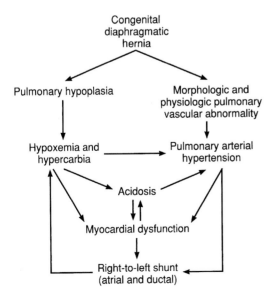

FIGURE 16-6 Cycle of pathophysiologic events that occur in infants with severe congenital diaphragmatic hernias.

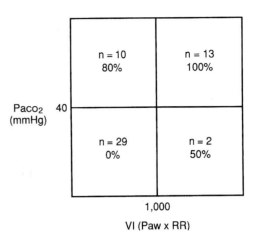

FIGURE 16-7 Relationship between ventilatory index (VI), $Paco_2$, and expected mortality in infants with congenital diaphragmatic hernia receiving conventional therapy. %, Expected mortality. (From Bohn D, Tamura M, Perrin D, et al: *J Pediatr* 111:423, 1987.)

hypercarbia, pulmonary hypertension, myocardial dysfunction, and right-to-left shunting of blood through persistent fetal channels. If uninterrupted, this sequence of events ultimately proves fatal. The goal of preoperative stabilization and subsequent intraoperative anesthetic management is to interrupt this cycle. The focus of management is the reduction of PVR and associated right-to-left shunts. This is accomplished through a combination of optimized ventilation, support for myocardial function, and correction of metabolic derangements (acidosis, electrolytes, glucose, temperature).

A standard of practice for the treatment of CDH does not exist. As most of the published literature originates from single institutions with limited numbers of patients, there appears to be variability in treatment protocols and differences in the adoption of new technologies.[309] Infants with small defects and without other anomalies should have a low mortality rate. Care should be relatively straightforward. High-risk patients with large defects and other anomalies may require risky and novel therapies for survival. Identification of this group of patients who would benefit from such interventions has remained elusive. For the intermediate-risk patient, therapy is tending toward delaying surgery, passive ventilatory support, and cardiovascular stabilization. The components of conventional therapy differ somewhat from institution to institution, but generally include the following:

1. Conventional mechanical ventilatory support to produce respiratory alkalosis
2. Support of intravascular volume and correction of metabolic derangements (acidosis, electrolytes)
3. Inotropic support as indicated
4. Various combinations of sedatives, narcotics, and neuromuscular blocking agents
5. Appropriate interventions for barotraumas
6. Possibly a trial of pulmonary vasodilatators

Identification of patients who are unlikely to survive with conventional support becomes important because extracorporeal membrane oxygenation (ECMO) has been used successfully in this subgroup and has reduced overall mortality. Conversely, because ECMO is associated with significant risks, it should possibly be reserved for this group of high-risk patients.[310,311]

Once the diagnosis of CDH is made, all patients should be placed in an oxygen-enriched atmosphere. A large-gauge nasogastric tube (10–14 Fr) should be inserted to decompress the stomach and prevent further accumulation of air, which will affect ventilatory mechanics adversely. If respiratory distress and cyanosis persist, endotracheal intubation should be accomplished after preoxygenation with 100% oxygen. Neuromuscular blockade and intravenous narcotics may be used to facilitate intubation, but positive pressure ventilation by mask should be minimized so that no further gastrointestinal distention occurs. Also, for this reason, awake intubation by skilled personnel may be preferable to intubation under general anesthesia. Neuromuscular blockade is usually advisable to facilitate ventilation and to avoid wide swings in blood pressure that could adversely affect pulmonary hemodynamics. Past efforts to hyperventilate patients to produce a respiratory alkalosis with the goal of decreasing pulmonary vascular resistance have come under scrutiny. Kays et al have shown an improved survival rate by eliminating hyperventilation and accepting both higher $Paco_2$ and lower Pao_2.[289] Wung showed similar results.[290,312] These and other investigators are willing to accept $Paco_2$ values more than 65 mmHg, postductal saturations as low as 60%, and preductal saturations no less than 85% provided that the patient remains hemodynamically stable. Blood pH less than 7.20 is treated with $NaHCO_3$. Ventilatory management involves strictly limiting peak inspired pressures to 28 cmH_2O or less. Oxygen is weaned as tolerated. After this protocol, improved survival rates are thought to be because of reductions in both ventilator-induced lung injury and the incidence of pneumothorax. Postmortem studies in babies with CDH and studies evaluating mechanical ventilation with high airway pressures have shown various degrees of lung injury, including ruptured alveoli, torn alveolar basement membranes, alveolar hemorrhage, and edema. These can lead to atelectasis, decreased compliance, and impaired gas exchange and may be a precursor to pneumothorax.[313-315] In these reports of passive ventilation the premise is that pulmonary hypertension will resolve despite the presence of hypercarbia and acidosis. It is noteworthy that in the study by Kays et al, the use of passive ventilation did not decrease the need for ECMO, but the survival for patients receiving ECMO was improved.[289]

Nonetheless, despite these reports, hyperventilation may still be the norm. In 1997, the Neonatal Inhaled Nitric Oxide Study Group reported that approximately 80% of CDH patients were treated with hyperventilation and alkalosis therapy. If hyperventilation is the accepted course of therapy, then it should be recognized that a pH above 7.5 is often required to induce pulmonary vasodilatation of a degree sufficient to reduce right-to-left shunting.[316] Ventilatory parameters necessary to achieve this goal obviously will vary according to the degree of pulmonary hypoplasia. Indeed, in the most severely affected infants, hypocarbia may not be attainable despite high airway pressures and respiratory rates. Prognostically, this is a very ominous sign. An additional risk directly related to the severity of pulmonary hypoplasia and the magnitude of ventilatory support is the development of a contralateral pneumo-

thorax, which should be suspected whenever an acute deterioration in oxygenation or hemodynamics occurs.[293] Prompt therapy is mandatory because the attendant hypoxemia, acidosis, and hemodynamic compromise can result in abrupt increases in PVR and a return to a fetal circulatory pattern that may have been corrected previously. The development of a pneumothorax in the perioperative period is associated with a high mortality rate (75% to 80%), and early use of neuromuscular blockade appears to reduce its incidence. Some centers advocate placement of a prophylactic chest tube in the contralateral hemithorax before or at the time of repair to prevent this potentially catastrophic complication.

Although ventilatory management is the primary focus of preoperative stabilization, several other points should be addressed. A warm environment is essential, and the temperature of the environment and infant should be monitored throughout the perioperative period because of the adverse effects of hypothermia on oxygen consumption and acid-base balance. Metabolic acidosis should be treated judiciously with intravenous $NaHCO_3$ as an adjunct to elevating pH to a level beneficial for the pulmonary vasculature and myocardial performance.

Theoretically, selective dilatation of the pulmonary vasculature would result in a reduction in pulmonary artery pressure, an increase of pulmonary blood flow, and correction of right-to-left shunting at the ductal and atrial levels. Unfortunately, no specific pulmonary vasodilator exists. A variety of vasodilating agents have been used in the setting of primary pulmonary hypertension.[304] Inhaled NO, the latest agent to be tried, appears to be attractive, but a prospective study of 53 patients with CDH showed no decrease in mortality or need for intervention with ECMO.

Traditional wisdom has dictated that severely symptomatic infants with CDH undergo surgical repair as early as possible. This approach is based on the assumption that surgical decompression of the herniated viscera will result in prompt improvement in pulmonary mechanics and gas exchange. The premise is that mechanical compression of the lung is the major factor in pulmonary dysfunction of CDH. This traditional approach is currently undergoing reevaluation, however.[289,290,317-323] Several investigators have demonstrated that the condition of many infants is substantially improved before operative repair if a longer period of preoperative stabilization is allowed; this finding may be associated with a significant decrease in early mortality. Preoperative stabilization is continued until no further improvements in metabolic, pulmonary, or hemodynamic condition can be achieved—an end point that is generally attainable within 4 to 18 hours of arrival in a tertiary-care facility. This approach is particularly advocated for those infants with the most severe derangements of cardiorespiratory function, to optimize their condition before operative intervention. None of the studies have shown a detrimental effect on mortality by using this strategy. In support of this view is the work of Bohn, who studied pulmonary compliance preoperatively and postoperatively in infants with CDH. Not only did operative reduction of the hernia fail to improve this measure of pulmonary function, but it actually had a detrimental effect on compliance in seven of nine infants studied.[294]

Routine intraoperative monitoring should be used for all neonates undergoing operative repair of CDH. Additional monitoring, however, is nearly always required for these infants because of the severity of their illness and the peculiar pathophysiology derangements characteristic of their disease. Breath sounds should be continuously monitored with a precordial stethoscope placed over the contralateral hemithorax. An arterial catheter is indicated for frequent sampling of arterial blood gases as well as continuous blood pressure monitoring. Right radial artery cannulation is preferred because this supplies a measure of preductal blood perfusing the cerebral circulation. Umbilical artery catheters with their tips in the postductal aorta provide good assessment of the total magnitude of the right-to-left shunt (atrial and ductal). Although two arterial catheters (preductal and postductal) might be ideal, a reasonable alternative is to place a pulse oximeter probe on an extremity with a ductal location opposite to that of the arterial catheter (i.e., preductal if the arterial catheter is postductal, or vice versa). Reliable venous access is essential for the administration of blood products, fluids, and medications. Peripheral intravenous catheters are best placed in the upper extremities, as abdominal closure following reduction of the hernia carries the potential for compromise of lower-extremity venous return. Central venous catheter insertion via an internal jugular vein will provide reliable venous access. Additionally, it can provide useful information regarding right-sided filling pressures and venous oxygen saturation. A urinary catheter should also be used for continuous monitoring of urine volume and intermittent assessment of urinary chemistries and concentration. The latter measurements may have greater importance postoperatively because it has been demonstrated recently that CDH infants sometimes develop a syndrome consistent with symptoms of inappropriate secretion of antidiuretic hormone (SIADH) in the postoperative period.[324]

Surgical repair of a diaphragmatic hernia is usually carried out through an abdominal approach, with the patient in the supine position. The hernia is reduced by gentle traction on the intestine, and the diaphragmatic defect is closed by direct suture. Before diaphragmatic closure, a chest tube is placed in the ipsilateral pleural space and connected to waterseal. Large defects may require the use of a prosthetic graft to achieve closure. If the patient's condition permits, Ladd's procedure is performed for correction of associated malrotation. Abdominal closure follows, which also may require incorporation of prosthetic material depending on the severity of cardiorespiratory compromise associated with this part of the procedure.

Anesthetic management of the infant undergoing repair of CDH primarily consists of intraoperatively continuing those therapeutic maneuvers used during preoperative stabilization. Sufficient depth of anesthesia is required to minimize sympathetic responses to surgical stimulation that could adversely affect pulmonary vascular resistance. A stable systemic and pulmonary hemodynamic state needs to be maintained. This can usually be provided with a basic narcotic-oxygen-relaxant anesthetic technique. NO should be avoided for the following three reasons:

1. Nitrous oxide increases the potential for overdistention of the bowel, leading to further respiratory embarrassment.
2. Use of nitrous oxide in significant concentrations by necessity limits the concentration of delivered oxygen. In the most severely affected neonates, 100% oxygen is almost required because of its beneficial effect of lowering PVR.

3. There is the theoretic concern that nitrous oxide, independent of its effect of lowering on F_{IO_2}, may have pulmonary vasoconstrictive properties.

In premature neonates at risk for retinopathy of prematurity who are maintaining PaO_2 in excess of 100 mmHg, air may be added to the inspired gas to achieve a safe reduction in F_{IO_2}.

Fentanyl, in a total dose of 10 to 50 µg/kg, usually provides adequate depth of anesthesia while maintaining stable hemodynamics. Fentanyl is administered in 2 to 5 µg/kg boluses, assessing hemodynamic response between doses. A minimum of 10 µg/kg is usually administered prior to initial surgical incision. If surgical stimulation results in an excessive increase of pulse or blood pressure, or if there is evidence of increasing right-to-left shunt, further incremental doses of narcotic are administered until stability is restored. Small concentrations of one of the volatile agents may be used as an adjunct to narcotics in the more stable patients undergoing repair.

Neuromuscular blockade is a necessary adjunct to the chosen anesthetic. Paralysis facilitates surgical repair of the defect, especially where diaphragmatic and abdominal closure are concerned. Additionally, paralysis minimizes fluctuation in airway pressure that could adversely affect PVR and increase the likelihood of a contralateral pneumothorax.

Intraoperatively, it is probably preferable to control ventilation manually rather than mechanically. Most pediatric anesthesiologists recommend maintaining peak inspiratory pressures below 30 cmH$_2$O to avoid adverse effects on pulmonary blood flow and to reduce the potential for pneumothorax. Rapid rates of 60 to 120 breaths/min may be required. The goal is to produce hypocarbia at the lowest feasible peak and mean airway pressures. Any sudden change in either compliance or oxygen saturation could indicate a contralateral pneumothorax, which should be investigated and treated immediately. After reduction of the herniated viscera, vigorous attempts to inflate the hypoplastic ipsilateral lung should be avoided because they are usually futile and increase the potential for contralateral pneumothorax. During abdominal closure, it is important to pay close attention to changes in compliance and hemodynamics. Excessive elevations of intraabdominal pressure associated with closure of the abdominal wall could impede both ventilation and venous return from the lower half of the body. Creation of a ventral hernia by closing only skin without fascial closure is one option. Silastic prostheses, such as those used for repair of abdominal wall defects, may be required in extreme cases.

Throughout the intraoperative course, frequent sampling of arterial blood for measurement of blood gases, glucose, electrolytes, and hematocrit is necessary. Maintenance fluid consists of 10% dextrose in water supplemented with sodium chloride. Third-space losses can potentially be high (5 to 10 mL/kg/hr) and are replaced with isotonic fluid as indicated by pulse, blood pressure, CVP, and urine volume. Blood loss is usually small, but blood should be available and administered to maintain a hematocrit of 40% or greater.

At the termination of surgery, infants are transported to the neonatal intensive care unit with an endotracheal tube in place. Ventilation with 100% oxygen is continued; neuromuscular blockers are not reversed, and narcotic administration at a dosage of 2 to 5 µg/kg/h of fentanyl is maintained. Provisions for proper temperature maintenance and monitoring should be made for transport. Therapy directed at alleviating PFC is continued in the intensive care unit. The duration of ventilatory assistance and choice of other therapeutic modalities depend on the infant's response in the early postoperative period.

As stated earlier, CDH infants fall into one of three general categories based on the severity of their disease states. One group is characterized by mild pathophysiologic derangements, has minimal pulmonary hypoplasia, does not revert to a fetal circulatory pattern, and requires little special postoperative management. Occasionally, these patients may even be candidates for tracheal extubation at the end of the operative procedure. A second group of patients is characterized by such severe bilateral pulmonary hypoplasia that survival is impossible, despite the use of all currently available means of support. The CDH in the remaining group of infants is intermediate in severity, and survival is to a large degree dependent on proper therapeutic management. Most of these infants will experience a brief postoperative period of adequate oxygenation (the "honeymoon" period). Ventilatory and pharmacologic therapy aimed at reducing PVR may sustain oxygenation, allowing for gradual weaning of support and ultimate survival. In others, the honeymoon period is transient, followed by reversion to a fetal circulatory pattern and attendant severe hypoxemia. Finally, some infants who are potentially salvageable may never experience a honeymoon period. Severe pulmonary vascular hypertension, right-to-left shunting, and persistent hypoxemia are manifest in the immediate postoperative period and are not amenable to conventional therapy.

ECMO is generally reserved for the most critically ill infants in whom standard ventilatory measures fail or in whom initial gas exchange suggests inadequate lung parenchyma for long-term survival. Selection criteria for ECMO typically include one or more of the following:

1. Demonstrating inadequate oxygenation on conventional therapy (Pao_2 less than 40 to 60, A-aDO_2 more than 500 to 600 mmHg)
2. An acute deterioration in cardiorespiratory status (abrupt decrease in Pao_2, unresponsive acidosis, hemodynamic instability)
3. Unrelenting barotraumas

Exclusionary criteria typically include the following[311,325-326]:

1. Serious coexisting anomaly (chromosomal, cardiac, or neurologic)
2. More than 7 to 10 days of ventilatory support
3. Birth weight less than 2 kg or gestational age less than 35 weeks
4. Preexisting intracranial hemorrhage

Complications are significant and mainly relate to the need for systemic anticoagulation. Significant bleeding problems—approximately half of which are fatal—occur in approximately 25% to 40% of CDH patients treated with ECMO. In spite of its drawbacks, ECMO has been used successfully in infants who would likely have died if treated with conventional therapies. Redmond et al reported a 50% long-term survival in ECMO-treated infants whose predicted mortality according to Bohn et al's original criteria was 100%.[325] Similarly, Heiss et al found an 83% survival in a group of ECMO-treated infants who were predicted by Bohn et al to have a 50% mortality rate.[311] The overall survival

in ECMO-treated patients is conservatively 50% for a population whose expected survival is less than 25% with conventional therapy. Repair of the hernia on ECMO may be associated with higher complication rates resulting from bleeding.[302,311,325,326] However, refinements in surgery, such as the use of fibrin glues and synthetic patches, minimize this complication.

Follow-up studies of patients with repaired diaphragmatic hernias are generally encouraging, although most series report a variety of subtle abnormalities. It appears that there is a persistent reduction of the number of branches of both bronchi and pulmonary arteries on the affected side, resulting in decreased ventilation and perfusion.[297,327,328] Plain chest radiographs are frequently normal but may reveal a decrease in vascularity on the affected side.[329] Lung scans may confirm the hypoperfusion suggested on plain film.[330] Measurements of lung volumes are usually normal, although some investigators suggest that this may be due to overexpansion of existing alveoli rather than to growth in alveolar number, as normally occurs.[328-330] An asymptomatic preemphysematous state may exist in older individuals.[329] Despite these abnormalities, it appears that patients surviving repair of CDH develop sufficient lung function to allow normal activity without symptoms, at least into adolescence and early adulthood.

The long-term outcomes of patients with neonatal respiratory failure treated with ECMO have been encouraging as well. The overall incidence of significant neurologic or pulmonary sequelae appears to be similar in ECMO and conventionally treated patients.[331-333] At follow-up, approximately 30% of patients in each treatment group have readily detectable neurologic sequelae, although asymptomatic electroencephalographic abnormalities may be somewhat higher in ECMO-treated patients. Infants with congenital diaphragmatic hernia represent a small percentage of patients in these series.[334-336]

With regard to the management of CDH, there have been three eras.[288] The difference between the second therapeutic period and the first is the addition of ECMO to the clinician's armamentarium. The additional option of delayed surgical repair is the primary difference between the second and third eras. As can be seen from the discussion, results are variable and institution-specific. Some have claimed that ECMO increases survival, whereas others have not found it to affect outcome.[337,338] What is clear is that infants who normally would not have had a chance at surviving now have that possibility. This outcome is associated with higher mortality rates and greater morbidity in those who do survive.

Finally, recognizing the severity of this disease process and the relatively poor outcomes in CDH, several investigators have taken to repairing these defects in utero.[339-343] Whether intrauterine repair proves to be a viable alternative and fresh approach to the severe anatomic pathophysiologic derangements seen in CDH remains to be seen. If anything, the efforts by these investigators speak to the difficulties in treating patients with CDH.

Esophageal Atresia and Tracheoesophageal Fistula

Esophageal atresia (EA) with or without a tracheoesophageal fistula (TEF) is a common congenital anomaly. The incidence of these related defects is approximately one in 3000 live births.[344] In about 50% of the cases, EA with or without TEF may present with other anomalies.[303,345,346] Cardiovascular defects such as ventricular septal defect, tetralogy of Fallot, coarctation of the aorta, patent ductus arteriosus, and atrial septal defect may occur in as many as 25% of the cases. Anomalies of the VATER association (vertebral defects, tracheoesophageal fistula, radial and renal dysplasia) are seen. In any patient who has EA and TEF, other anomalies should be suspected. Factors that decrease survival in patients with EA with or without TEF are the following:

- Prematurity
- Low birth weight
- Presence of cardiac anomalies
- Pulmonary complications

Among patients with EA and/or TEF, 30% to 40% are premature, and mean birth weight is low when compared with that of the general population. Smith reported that the incidence of prematurity or birth weight less than 2500 g is 50% in patients with EA/TEF.[347] In the absence of these risk factors, survival should be 100%. In evaluating 303 patients over a 10-year period, Spitz was able to show that coexisting congenital heart disease combined with birth weight below 1500 g decreased survival from 97% to 22%.[348]

The presence of polyhydramnios during pregnancy may indicate some form of intestinal obstruction in the fetus; if it is present, the diagnosis of esophageal atresia can be made at the time of delivery or shortly afterward by carefully attempting to insert a soft radiopaque catheter in the stomach either nasally (which, if successful, could also rule out the presence of choanal atresia) or through the mouth. If atresia is present, posteroanterior and lateral chest films will reveal the catheter coiling in the upper blind pouch of the atretic esophagus. The abdomen will be distended and tympanitic if there is a fistula between the esophagus and the trachea. Respiratory embarrassment may occur if gastric distention is significant enough to cause impairment of diaphragmatic excursion. If the diagnosis is not made in utero, it is often suspected after the first feeding, when coughing, choking, and cyanosis may occur. Further radiographic studies of the abdomen should show air in the abdomen if both EA and TEF are present; absence of air in the gastrointestinal tract could indicate EA without TEF.

There are several anatomic variants of EA and TEF[349] (Figure 16-8):

- EA with the fistula between the distal esophagus and the distal trachea (the most common type, 87% of occurrences)
- EA without TEF (8%)
- TEF without EA, also known as "H type" (4%), usually presents later in infancy. These children often have abdominal distention, choking with feedings, and recurrent pneumonias. Bronchoscopy is often required for diagnosis.

Once the diagnosis has been established, efforts should be made to prevent pulmonary complications and to delineate any other anatomic anomalies, especially cardiac. As stated above, these factors contribute to increased morbidity and mortality. Aspiration of secretions or feedings from the proximal esophageal segment almost always results in atelectasis or pneumonitis of the right upper lobe. Regurgitation of gastric contents through the fistula results in chemical pneumonitis that resists treatment. Pulmonary complications might be avoided or minimized by withholding feedings, inserting a suction system into the upper pouch of the atretic esophagus to remove secretions, and nursing the infant in a 45-degree head-up position. As the operation is not an emergency, antibiotic treatment for pneumonia (if present) can be initiated. Furthermore, a delay in the operation allows the infant to make a better transition from a fetal to a neonatal circulation and allows time for a more thorough workup. Early intubation for airway protection may be useful in esophageal atresia without TEF, but it is of no use when there is a communication between the trachea and distal esophagus, because most of the ventilator gas will travel into the stomach rather than the lungs.

Before definitive repair, a gastrostomy for feeding may be performed under local anesthesia, especially if lung function is compromised from respiratory disease syndrome (RDS) or pneumonitis.[350] This procedure might allow more time for treatment of the patient's pulmonary problems. In a contrary point of view, some investigators have suggested that severe RDS with noncompliant lungs might be an indication for early ligation of the TEF and surgical correction by primary anastomosis.[351-355] The premature infant with EA with or without TEF is at risk not only for RDS but also for pneumonia secondary to aspiration. Aspiration of gastric contents contributes significantly to the morbidity and mortality in this patient population, and the sooner the TEF is closed, the less likely aspiration is to occur. Furthermore, placement of a gastrostomy tube might

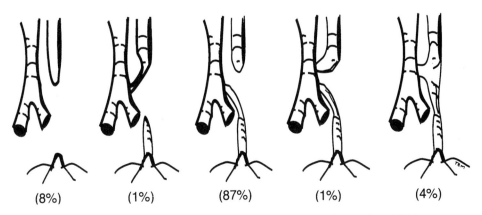

(8%)   (1%)   (87%)   (1%)   (4%)

FIGURE 16-8 Drawing showing the most common types of tracheoesophageal fistulas.

provide only a low-resistance route of escape for fresh anesthetic gases under positive pressure. This would be particularly apparent in the neonate with poor lung compliance requiring significant ventilatory assistance. In this instance, a fresh gastrostomy would serve as a "pop-off." The path of least resistance for fresh gas to flow would be away from the lungs and through the TEF toward the lower-resistance gastrointestinal tract. There are reports of various maneuvers to control the potential air leak through the gastrostomy, including placement of the open end of the gastrostomy tube underwater and occlusion of the esophageal end of the fistula by retrograde placement of a Fogarty balloon-tipped catheter.[356-358] On the other hand, if a gastrostomy is not placed beforehand, severe gastric distention could occur when positive pressure ventilation is initiated. Cardiac arrest and gastric rupture have been reported to occur in this situation. Regardless of the approach, there has been a tendency for earlier intervention to ligate the fistula and prevent aspiration.

ANESTHETIC AND PERIOPERATIVE MANAGEMENT

The monitoring technique is usually dictated by the general condition of the infant: the sicker the infant, the more complex the monitoring regimen. Standard monitors plus an arterial line and two peripheral intravenous lines should be sufficient in most cases. Central venous access generally is not necessary, although a urinary catheter can be helpful in guiding fluid resuscitation. Measures to preserve the patient's body heat should be instituted. An esophageal probe cannot be placed for temperature monitoring or auscultation of breath sounds and heart tones. If anal atresia is present, a nasopharyngeal probe might be the next best alternative. A precordial stethoscope is placed in the left axilla because the patient will be positioned for a right thoracotomy. This could well be the most important monitor because during much of the operation, the right lung receives little ventilation, as it is retracted out of the surgeon's way. If breath sounds are lost from the left axillary stethoscope, it could be indicative of a possible right mainstem intubation or an endotracheal tube that has been obstructed because of surgical manipulation, secretions, or a clot in the tube's lumen.[359]

Intraoperative management of patients with EA/TEF requires great skill and patience from both the surgeon and the anesthesiologist. Developing a plan for airway management with the surgeon is critical for success. Placement of the endotracheal tube and isolation of the respiratory tract from the gastrointestinal tract are the initial goals in airway management. The endotracheal tube needs to be positioned above the carina and below the fistula to ensure ventilation of both lungs while simultaneously preventing gas flow through the fistula.[353] Because the most common place for the fistula to enter the trachea is 1 to 2 cm above the carina, there is little margin for error. Whether the endotracheal tube is placed with the patient awake or anesthetized depends solely on the expertise of the anesthesiologist and the infant's comorbid conditions. Prior to either scenario, suctioning the upper esophageal pouch and preoxygenation should be performed. In the awake patient, atropine (20 µg/kg) may be given to prevent a vagal response to direct laryngoscopy. Correct placement of the endotracheal tube requires advancing the tube into the right mainstem bronchus; it is then withdrawn until bilateral breath sounds are heard. As

an alternative approach, the surgeon, after the induction of general anesthesia, performs rigid bronchoscopy and places a Fogarty embolectomy catheter in the fistula.[356,360,361] The airway is then managed by the anesthesiologist, who places an endotracheal tube as described previously. This routine has the advantage of completely isolating the respiratory and gastrointestinal tracts from one another and delineating the patient's anatomy and possible variants, and by having a rigid catheter in the TEF, the surgeons can more easily identify the fistula. Once the airway is secure, gentle positive pressure ventilation is attempted. If gastric inflation does not occur, a muscle relaxant may be administered safely and positive pressure ventilation continued. The patient is placed in the left lateral decubitus position for a right thoracotomy. Adequacy of ventilation and the position of the endotracheal tube are again rechecked.

No particular anesthetic technique has been shown to be superior. The choice of anesthetic should be tailored to the patient's condition. If the patient has an epidural catheter, it may be used intraoperatively. Breath sounds should be monitored continuously. Suctioning of the trachea should be frequent because blood and secretions can cause obstruction of the endotracheal tube. The use of a humidification system in the anesthetic circuit is useful in preventing inspissation of secretions in the endotracheal tube, and it has the added advantage of reducing heat loss via the lungs.

Postoperative care in infants with EA/TEF is determined by coexisting anomalies, pulmonary dysfunction, and gestational age. The surgeon may request that the patient remain intubated and sedated to avoid stress to the esophageal anastomosis. If early intubation is indicated, neuraxial blockade may be appropriate.

Mediastinal Masses

Mediastinal masses may involve anterior (lymphomas, thymomas, teratomas, thyroid tumors, vascular tumors, and germ cell tumors), middle (bronchogenic or esophageal cysts, aortic aneurysms, pericardial cysts), or posterior (paragangliomas, neurofibromas, Schwannomas, ganglioneuromas) mediastinum.[362-363] Unfortunately, the usual laboratory studies—blood counts, bone marrow aspiration, and serial chemistries—might fail to provide an adequate pathologic diagnosis.[364] Although radiation therapy has been suggested before general anesthesia and biopsy of some types of mediastinal masses, radiation could interfere with pathologic diagnosis. Surgical biopsy or excision may be the treatment of choice, either alone or in combination with radiation therapy or chemotherapy, and such children usually require general anesthesia.

Mediastinal masses produce the following four areas of compromise of importance to anesthesiologists:

- Obstruction of the superior vena cava (SVC)
- Respiratory compromise
- Cardiopulmonary compromise (pericardial, myocardial) and compression of the pulmonary artery
- Neurologic impairment resulting from spinal cord involvement by posterior mediastinal masses

SUPERIOR VENA CAVA OBSTRUCTION

Venous return is compromised by superior vena caval obstruction, usually from malignant masses on the right side, such as lymphoma. The SVC syndrome—the clinical presentation of SVC obstruction—is more severe if the tumor is fast growing or below the azygous vein because collateral circulation cannot develop.[365] Three stages of the SVC syndrome have been described[366]:

1. SVC obstruction
2. Venous pressure increase up to 40 mmHg distal to the obstruction
3. Development of venous collaterals via the azygous, vertebral, internal mammary, and lateral thoracic veins, accompanied by edema of the head, neck, and upper extremities, with cyanosis caused by venous stasis

Respiratory symptoms often accompany SVC syndrome. Laryngeal edema that results from SVC obstruction may make tracheal intubation more difficult. The venous congestion may first become apparent or worsen during induction or during emergence from anesthesia, as coughing and bucking on the tracheal tube occur.[366] Venous congestion can be severe enough to cause acute airway obstruction. Head-up position and judicious fluid administration are helpful. Although excessive fluid may worsen the symptoms of SVC syndrome, a decrease in preload, leading to hypotension in association with compromised venous return, is equally undesirable.

SVC obstruction also compromises cerebral venous drainage. Cerebral perfusion pressure can be decreased by acute exacerbations of venous obstruction. Head-up position is recommended to facilitate cerebral venous drainage. Additional therapies include radiation therapy, chemotherapy, steroids, and diuretics. For the anesthesiologist, the compromised SVC circulation limits the speed with which drugs injected into the veins of the upper extremity will reach the systemic circulation. Drugs should be given into the inferior vena cava circulation, if possible, or additional time should be allowed for the decreased circulation time to avoid overdose. Central venous access, if required, should be placed via the femoral route. Vascular thrombosis in the compromised SVC circulation is also likely. Drugs with irritating potential injected into partially obstructed venous channels may elicit phlebitic reactions or even extravasate into tissues. Obstruction of the SVC also can distort the surgical field and enhance bleeding, so provision for massive blood loss is important in resections of mediastinal masses.

RESPIRATORY PROBLEMS

Respiratory signs such as wheezing, bronchitis, croup, stridor, decreased breath sounds, retractions, cough, and dyspnea are common indicators of mediastinal masses in children. Mediastinal masses may first be noted on a chest x-ray taken for various reasons. Because these masses can grow rapidly, all x-ray studies should be recent, but because a plain chest x-ray can be very misleading with regard to airway obstruction and is of limited value in the assessment of cardiovascular compromise, other laboratory studies are indicated before beginning anesthesia. Such studies include a respiratory flow/volume loop (if the patient will cooperate), chest and upper airway computed tomography (CT) scan, and, occasionally, awake fiberoptic bronchoscopy (Figure 16-9).[368] Tracheal obstruction and compression are determined by dividing the smallest AP tracheal diameter on the CT scan by the AP diameter of the normal trachea at the thoracic inlet and then multiplying by 100. If the trachea is more than 50% obstructed on CT scan, airway

obstruction during anesthetic induction or emergence is likely.[369] There is no clear consensus regarding the preoperative diagnostic laboratory studies necessary for a child with a mediastinal mass found on chest x-ray film who shows no signs or symptoms of cardiorespiratory compromise before general anesthesia is induced. Children with mediastinal masses can be divided into two categories based on the risk of airway obstruction or cardiovascular collapse during general anesthesia: high risk and moderate risk (Table 16-9).

CARDIAC PROBLEMS

Pericardial tamponade-like symptoms, pulmonary artery compression, and direct myocardial involvement can result from mediastinal masses. Keon reported a patient with mediastinal lymphoma whose cardiovascular compromise was similar to pericardial tamponade or constrictive pericarditis and caused death when a halothane induction further depressed myocardial function.[370] Evaluation for signs of pericardial tamponade such as pulsus paradoxus, ECG evidence, or echocardiographic findings should be done before anesthesia. Direct myocardial involvement by mediastinal tumors may also occur.[371] Arrhythmias during anesthesia have been attributed to myocardial or pericardial involvement.[363] Compression of the pulmonary artery by a mediastinal mass can cause outflow obstruction of the right ventricle and severely limit pulmonary venous return to the left side of the heart.[372,373]

ANESTHETIC MANAGEMENT

In addition to the usual history, it is important to ask the child and the parents specifically about the presence of syncope and dyspnea, as well as intolerance of, or preference for, any certain anatomic position; the information thus gleaned may indicate airway compromise or impairment of venous return or stroke volume. In the physical examination of the cardiorespiratory system, evidence of superior vena cava syndrome (e.g., stridor, facial cyanosis, distention of neck veins, head and neck edema) should be sought.

Even in children, local anesthesia, superficial cervical plexus block (if major superior vena cava syndrome is absent), or ketamine sedation can be used to obtain a biopsy for diagnosis of the type of mediastinal mass. The anesthesiologist might first encounter the patient with a mediastinal mass when consulted to provide anesthesia for the CT scan, which is requested by the oncologist as part of a preoperative workup. A flow/volume loop may demonstrate intrathoracic airway obstruction, but not all children will cooperate for this test.[374] Awake fiberoptic bronchoscopy may be used for both airway evaluation and intubation, but it should be performed only by a skilled pediatric bronchoscopist. Some investigators report that fiberoptic bronchoscopy is not useful and is possibly hazardous.[375]

There are numerous reports of catastrophies involving patients with mediastinal masses during all phases of general anesthesia (induction, maintenance, and emergence), including cardiovascular collapse secondary to pulmonary artery obstruction, direct cardiac involvement, or partial or complete airway obstruction.[376,377] When the vital structures contained within the anterior and middle mediastinum (the heart, pericardium, great vessels, trachea, and the recurrent laryngeal nerve) are considered, it is surprising that so many children with mediastinal masses undergo general anesthesia without difficulty

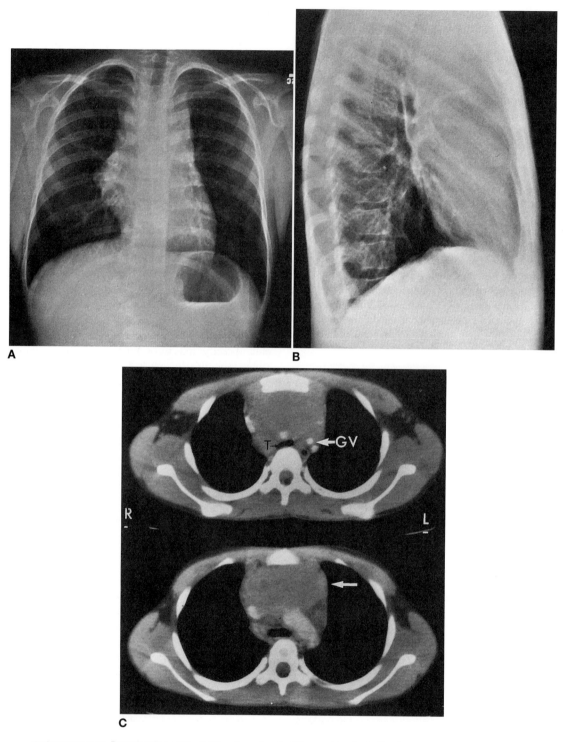

FIGURE 16-9 Posterior **(A)** and lateral **(B)** radiographs of a 15-year-old patient with a large anterior mediastinal mass showing posterior displacement and some narrowing of the tracheal lumen. CT scan **(C)** demonstrates the mass *(lower arrow)* displacing and compressing the great vessels (GV) and the trachea (T).

and that many evidence few or no cardiorespiratory signs or symptoms preoperatively.[375] Ferrari et al described 163 pediatric patients younger than 18 years of age who received general anesthesia before radiation therapy without significant morbidity or mortality.[378] In their series, two patients experienced airway difficulties on induction of anesthesia and were tracheally intubated using a rigid bronchoscope. Two other patients whose respiratory compromise occurred during anesthetic maintenance were improved by changing position.

Securing the airway with an adequately sized tube or rigid bronchoscope is the ultimate goal. Multiple attempts with tracheal tubes or bronchoscopes may produce total obstruction of a partially obstructed trachea or bronchus. Although awake oral or nasotracheal intubation might be used for the older child or

TABLE 16-9
Mediastinal Mass on Chest X-Ray

High Risk	Moderate Risk
SYMPTOMS AND SIGNS Positive history and physical examination	**SYMPTOMS AND SIGNS** Children without signs and symptoms of cardiorespiratory compromise and whose diagnostic studies are within normal limits
Computed tomographic scan with tracheal lumen narrowed by >35% Abnormal flow/volume loop Abnormal airway seen during awake fiberoptic bronchoscopy	
MANAGEMENT Biopsy peripheral lymph node with local anesthesia Needle biopsy (CT directed) lymph node if possible Presumptive treatment with radiation and/or steroid to decrease tumor size; perform indicated procedure (biopsy or excision) with general anesthesia when patient at lower risk	**MANAGEMENT** If possible, perform peripheral lymph node biopsy with local anesthesia
If general anesthesia absolutely necessary for diagnosis, place all monitors preinduction, have femoral-femoral bypass available, use inhalation induction with sevoflurane, avoid neuromuscular blockade, induce anesthesia with child in most comfortable position, be able to change position easily and quickly, and have flexible and rigid bronchoscopes available	If administering general anesthesia, inhalation induction, maintain spontaneous ventilation, avoid neuromuscular blocking agents, be able to change patient's position quickly, have rigid bronchoscopy available

teenager, it may not be possible for younger children. One approach for younger children is maintenance of spontaneous ventilation using either a tracheal tube or laryngeal mask airway.[379] Controlled ventilation and general anesthesia may unmask airway compression that is absent in the awake patient. Controlled ventilation under neuromuscular blockade and anesthesia decreases chest wall tone, relaxes bronchial smooth muscles (increasing the compressibility of the airways), reduces the caudal movement of the diaphragm, and eliminates the active inspiratory effort that supports the airway.

A creative, rapidly changeable anesthetic technique is essential for the child who has a mediastinal mass. The recent use of thoracoscopy, Chamberlain procedures, and mediastinoscopy does not change the anesthetic management problems.[380] The conclusions of Ferrari and Bedford about the safety of general anesthesia in pediatric patients with mediastinal masses have been questioned when applied in institutions or by anesthesiologists who have less experience with such patients.[378,381]

Respiratory problems may also be present in the postoperative period. Laryngomalacia, tracheomalacia, or bronchomalacia may be present after tumor resection. Extubation should be performed under controlled circumstances, with immediate provision for reintubation. Prolonged intubation may be necessary

until radiation therapy or chemotherapy for the tumor can be performed or until postsurgical edema subsides. Serial chest radiographs postoperatively can demonstrate diminution in tumor size and airway obstruction. It is also important to provide adequate postoperative pain relief to avoid pain and anxiety that would cause tachypnea and increased airflow velocity through a partially obstructed tracheobronchial tree.

Tracheostomy

Fortunately, the need for urgent tracheostomy in infants and children is rare. Endotracheal intubation is usually possible, even in cases of relatively severe acute epiglottitis.[382] Tracheostomy can be a difficult and dangerous procedure in the small infant with a short, fat neck, especially when the child is agitated and struggling. Every effort should be made to gain satisfactory control of the airway by tracheal intubation and/or bronchoscopy and to perform the tracheostomy under the ideal circumstances of the operating room and general anesthesia with controlled ventilation.

Tracheostomy is considerably simplified by the presence of a ventilating bronchoscope in the trachea. The rigid instrument can be manipulated by the anesthesiologist to displace the trachea directly anteriorly beneath the skin. Major arteries and veins thus fall to either side, whereas good ventilation is assured. Supplemental local-infiltration anesthesia can be used to allow a "light" level of general anesthesia. The electrocautery is used to dissect and control bleeding, as even minimal postoperative bleeding can be dangerous and difficult to control. Tracheostomy tubes of several appropriate sizes should be available in the operating room, and proper adaptors for the ventilation system should be tested for compatibility. Cuffed tracheostomy tubes are usually not necessary in children, and their use is discouraged because mucosal erosion, necrosis, and subsequent tracheal stenosis are more likely when cuffed tubes are used. Because the carina is very high in the infant and small child, it is often necessary to shorten the tracheostomy tube to ensure good ventilation of both lungs. A tracheostomy tube resting on or very near the carina will also be difficult to suction and will provoke paroxysms of coughing. Postoperatively, a chest radiograph is obtained and the child is observed carefully in the intensive care unit. Many children having tracheostomies will require controlled positive pressure ventilation postoperatively because of the underlying disease that necessitated the procedure. Even those seemingly healthy children who required tracheostomy for acute upper airway obstruction (epiglottitis) must be observed very carefully. Accidental removal or obstruction of the tube must be detected immediately if life-threatening hypoxemia is to be prevented. Humidified air with the desired F_{IO_2} should be delivered to the tracheostomy. Removal of a tracheostomy tube that has been in place for several weeks or more should be preceded by a diagnostic bronchoscopy to ensure that the upper airway is patent and that there is no obstructing granuloma at the site of the tracheostomy (see Appendix 16-1).

Patent Ductus Arteriosus

Persistent patency of the ductus arteriosus in infants born prematurely is well documented.[383] If the circulation of the newborn fails to complete the transition from the fetal form to the adult form, patency of the ductus arteriosus may be present. Prematurity, maternal exposure to rubella virus, respiratory distress syndrome, and some forms of congenital cardiac lesions increase the likelihood of ductal patency. The vasoconstrictor response of the ductus to an increase in the partial pressure of oxygen during early neonatal life is proportional to gestational age: the lower the gestational age, the greater the likelihood of patency of the ductus.[384] Forty-two percent of babies who weigh less than 1000 g and 20.2% of those weighing less than 1750 g will have clinical evidence of patency of the ductus.[385,386] As is seen in other varieties of left-to-right shunts, the clinical findings depend on the size of the ductus and the relationship between pulmonary and systemic resistances.

Because many infants born prematurely have RDS, the severity of the disease determines the degree of left-to-right shunting. In more severe RDS, pulmonary resistance remains higher in relation to systemic resistance and results in less shunting. In the most severe forms of RDS, pulmonary resistance exceeds systemic resistance, and right-to-left shunting through the ductus results in a decrease in Pao_2 distal to the ductal connection to the aorta. As RDS improves and pulmonary resistance falls below systemic resistance, more and more left-to-right shunting may take place and congestive heart failure may ensue, requiring pharmacologic maneuvers to attempt to cause the ductus to close. Medical measures to manage congestive heart failure in the preterm infant with RDS and a patent ductus include fluid restriction and diuretics. These therapies may allow time for the infant to mature and the ductus to close spontaneously. Indomethacin, a prostaglandin inhibitor, can be given enterally or intravenously in a dose of 0.1 to 0.3 mg/kg to facilitate closure of the ductus. When these therapies fail, however, an interventional catheterization procedure or surgical closure of the ductus may be required.

Patency of the ductus is diagnosed by echocardiography and by the physical finding of a continuous murmur at the first or second intercostal space. Chest radiograph and electrocardiographic findings depend on the size of the ductus. Large shunt flows through the ductus cause left ventricular hypertrophy or left atrial enlargement on ECG, and on a chest radiograph, enlargement of the left side of the heart with increased pulmonary vascular markings are seen.

PREMATURE INFANTS

The perioperative management of a premature neonate with RDS requiring ductus ligation is quite different from that of an older child who is asymptomatic and is undergoing ductus ligation to prevent the complications of heart failure, pulmonary hypertension, or subacute bacterial endocarditis. Management of the neonate is usually a continuation of the preoperative management except for the need for administration of volume because of prior fluid restriction. In some institutions, ligation of the ductus is performed in a special treatment room in the neonatal intensive care unit. In others, the infant is transported to the operating room for the procedure. In either instance, the infant must be maintained in a thermoneutral environment. Intraarterial and intravenous catheters already in place should be used for pressure monitoring and blood sampling. If an intraarterial catheter is not in place, however, placement is not usually attempted, owing to the briefness of the surgical procedure and the ability to use oximetric and noninvasive blood

pressure measurements. If narcotic infusions are already being given, these may be supplemented with additional narcotics, such as fentanyl and neuromuscular blocking agents for anesthetic management. Mechanical ventilation, either manual or with the help of an infant ventilator, should be used to maintain acceptable ventilatory parameters as indicated by oximetry and capnometry, taking into account the right lateral decubitus position. One-lung ventilation, achieved by direct surgical compression of the left lung during open thoracotomy, may be poorly tolerated by the very sick premature infant. Because retinopathy of prematurity has a multifactorial etiology, with hyperoxia being one contributing factor, the saturation measured by the pulse oximeter should be between 93% and 95% if the infant is less than 44 weeks' gestation. In the neonate, the ductus arteriosus may be quite large and nearly the size of the aorta or the pulmonary artery. For that reason, placement of the pulse oximeter on the lower extremity and of the noninvasive blood pressure cuff on the right upper extremity allows the anesthesiologist and surgeon to assess flow in the ascending and descending aorta during test occlusion of the vessel to be ligated. A decrease in arterial saturation and a decrease, followed by an increase, in end-tidal carbon dioxide, indicate occlusion of the pulmonary artery rather than of the ductus. In the preterm infant, simple ligation of the ductus is the surgical procedure of choice. When the ductus is ligated, there should be an increase in diastolic arterial pressure and loss of the continuous murmur. Postoperative management of the preterm infant should be similar to preoperative management until the infant's heart failure and respiratory distress improve and respiratory weaning can begin. Adequate analgesia with intravenous narcotics or other techniques should be given in the postoperative period.

DUCTAL CLOSURE IN OLDER CHILDREN

In older children, nonsurgical closure with interventional catheterization techniques (such as placement of Gianturco coils or other occlusion devices) is often possible and eliminates the need for intrathoracic surgery. Deep sedation with propofol, midazolam, fentanyl, ketamine, or other narcotics in combination is preferred over general anesthesia. For details on these techniques, the interested reader is referred to texts on pediatric cardiac anesthesia and pediatric anesthesia. Nonetheless, the presence of an anesthesiologist in the catheterization laboratory during these procedures ensures that the airway is secure and that emergencies, such as bleeding or the need for transesophageal echocardiography, can be managed quickly. If thoracoscopy or open thoracotomy is needed for surgical division of the ductus in the older child, a combined general plus regional anesthetic technique is often used effectively. An intraarterial catheter for pressure monitoring and blood sampling may be placed, although in children with minimal symptoms, noninvasive monitoring of oxygen, carbon dioxide, and arterial pressure will suffice. An epidural catheter permits postoperative analgesia with a continuous infusion of local anesthetics and narcotics.

Vascular Rings

Vascular rings are a group of anomalies of the great vessels and their branches that produce airway obstruction. True vascular rings are either of the following:

- A double aortic arch
- A right aortic arch with a left-sided ligamentum arteriosum that compresses the trachea and esophagus

An anomalous origin of the innominate artery may also produce compression.

The incidence of vascular rings is small, and a great number of these lesions are asymptomatic. Embryologically, vascular rings result from the persistence of embryonic structures in the aortic arches. The most common type of complete ring is the double aortic arch, in which both right and left aortic arches remain patent. The second most common type is a right aortic arch with a retropharyngeal right subclavian artery and a left-sided ductus arteriosus. A third type is the right aortic arch with mirror-image branching and a left ligamentum arteriosum. This last type is frequently associated with cyanotic congenital heart disease.

Incomplete vascular rings include innominate artery compression, pulmonary artery sling, and retropharyngeal right subclavian artery. Congenital heart disease is frequently associated with incomplete rings, as anomalous pulmonary arteries result in pulmonary artery slings.

Infants with vascular rings become symptomatic early in life, evidencing cyanosis, wheezing, dysphagia, or respiratory distress as soon as the first day of life. By 3 months of age, most infants with vascular rings are symptomatic, although a few can present as late as 1 year of age. Symptoms include inspiratory stridor, chronic cough, bronchopneumonia, noisy respirations, feeding difficulties, and dysphagia.

Studies to establish the correct diagnosis include a lateral chest radiograph that demonstrates flattening of the trachea and a barium swallow that shows posterior indentation by the vascular structure. If bronchus suis (origin of the right upper-lobe bronchus from the trachea) is present, the chest radiograph shows differential atelectasis in various lobes. Bronchoscopy may be a helpful diagnostic tool for the child with an anomalous innominate artery because a pulsatile mass is seen in the trachea. Computed tomography, magnetic resonance imaging, and echocardiography, in conjunction with chest radiograph and barium swallow, provide an accurate diagnosis of most types of vascular rings.

Perioperative management of children with vascular rings depends on the complexity of the vascular anatomy. For rings producing only mild airway obstruction, adequate vascular access, standard noninvasive anesthetic monitors, and a standard single-lumen tracheal tube may be sufficient. More complex lesions and severe airway compromise necessitate use of an intraarterial catheter, a central venous catheter, and large-bore intravenous access. Intraoperative monitoring of airway resistance and flow-volume loops are helpful to ensure that obstruction is relieved by surgery.[387] An inhalation induction should be performed and the airway ensured before neuromuscular blockers are administered. Multiple sizes of tracheal tubes should be available, as the tracheal lumen may be severely compressed. In anomalous pulmonary arteries, OLV might be needed and can be provided by the placement of two smaller tubes, with one tube extending past the obstruction and the second tube in the trachea or with a bronchial blocker. Most vascular rings are approached surgically via a left posterolateral thoracotomy with an open or thoracoscopic

technique. For patients with a left-sided arch and a right-sided ligamentum arteriosum, a right thoracoscopy or thoracotomy is performed. Anomalous innominate artery is approached through a median sternotomy or an anterior thoracotomy.

Postoperative tracheomalacia or laryngomalacia may be present and may necessitate prolonged postoperative ventilation. Measurement of a flow-volume loop can be helpful for timing of extubation. Extubation at the conclusion of surgery is desirable if no airway compromise is expected. If respiratory distress is the presenting symptom of the vascular ring, postoperative ventilation may be required for several days to weeks owing to tracheomalacia. Judicious fluid management, steroids, humidified oxygen, and racemic epinephrine are helpful adjuncts following extubation if a compromised tracheal segment is likely to be present. Good postoperative analgesia is also helpful to minimize excessive airflow through stenotic airway segments associated with agitation and pain. Postoperative respiratory function can also be affected by surgical complications such as injury to the phrenic nerve, recurrent laryngeal nerve, or thoracic duct.

Prevention of Bacterial Endocarditis During Diagnostic or Therapeutic Surgical Procedures

Certain patients requiring thoracic surgery may also have rheumatic or congenital heart defects that necessitate the administration of appropriate antibiotics to prevent endocarditis. During the preoperative evaluation, the anesthesiologist should be aware of the incumbent risks of endocarditis (if prophylaxis is omitted), the types of procedures and the defects for which antibiotic coverage is recommended, and the dosage and time of administration of the appropriate antimicrobial medications. It should be remembered that even hemodynamically insignificant defects (e.g., mild rheumatic mitral valve insufficiency, small ventricular septal defects, or mild pulmonic or aortic valve stenosis, which may include a congenital bicuspid valve) require antibiotic administration during certain procedures to prevent this very serious complication of heart disease. The Committee on Rheumatic Fever and Bacterial Endocarditis of the Council on Cardiovascular Disease in the Young of the American Heart Association recommends that procedures requiring antibiotic prophylaxis include the following[388]:

- All dental procedures that are likely to induce gingival bleeding (Simple adjustment of orthodontic devices and shedding of deciduous teeth are not included.)
- Diagnostic or therapeutic procedures of the upper or lower respiratory tract, including tonsillectomy, adenoidectomy, rigid bronchoscopy, esophagoscopy, or other operations that could cause disruption of the respiratory mucosa (Laryngoscopy and endotracheal intubation for anesthesia via the oral route are excluded if trauma to the oral, pharyngeal, or glottic structures does not occur. Nasotracheal intubation is an indication for prophylaxis.)
- Genitourinary tract surgery or instrumentation, including cystoscopy, urethral catheterization, prostatic surgery, and bladder surgery
- Gastrointestinal and gallbladder surgery or instrumentation, including esophagoscopy, esophageal dilation, sclerotherapy

TABLE 16-10

Pediatric Antibiotic Prophylaxis Against Subacute Bacterial Endocarditis

During oral, dental, esophageal, or respiratory tract procedures

Standard general prophylaxis		
	Amoxicillin	50 mg/kg orally 1 hour before procedure
	Ampicillin	50 mg/kg IM or IV 30 minutes before procedure if unable to take orally
Penicillin-allergic patients	Clindamycin	20 mg/kg orally 1 hr before procedure
	Cephalexin or cefadroxil	50 mg/kg orally 1 hr before procedure
	Azithromycin or clarithromycin	15 mg/kg orally 1 hr before procedure
Unable to take oral medications AND allergic to penicillin	Clindamycin	20 mg/kg IV 30 minutes before procedure
	Cefazolin	25 mg/kg IM or IV 30 minutes before procedure

During genitourinary/gastrointestinal (excluding esophageal) procedures

High risk patients (prosthetic heart valves, previous history of endocarditis, complex cyanotic congenital heart disease, surgically created systemic-pulmonary shunts or conduits)		
	Ampicillin + gentamicin	Ampicillin, 50 mg/kg IV/IM (not exceeding 2 gms. + gentamicin, 1.5 mg/kg within 30 minutes before procedure. Six hours later, give ampicillin 25 mg/kg or amoxicillin 25 mg/kg orally
High risk patients allergic to ampicillin/amoxicillin		
	Vancomycin + gentamicin	20 mg/kg IV over 1–2 hours 1.5 mg/kg IM/IV with completion of infusion within 30 minutes of start of procedure
Moderate risk patients (uncorrected PDA, VSD, primum ASD, aortic coarctation, bicuspid aortic valve, rheumatic valvular disease, hypertrophic cardiomyopathy)		
	Amoxicillin or Ampicillin	Amoxicillin, 50 mg/kg orally 1 hr before procedure or ampicillin, 50 mg/kg IM/IV within 30 minutes of start of procedure
Moderate risk patients allergic to penicillin		
	Vancomycin	20 mg/kg IV over 1-2 hr, completing the infusion within 30 minutes of start of procedure

From Dajani AS, Taubert KA, Wilson W, et al: *Circulation* 277:1794, 1997.

for varices, rectal and colon procedures (including colonoscopy and proctosigmoidoscopic biopsy), and upper gastrointestinal endoscopy

• Surgery of the heart and great vessels, including patent ductus arteriosus ligation, systemic-to-pulmonary-artery shunting procedures, pulmonary artery banding, and all "open heart" operations

• Surgical procedures involving any infected or contaminated tissues (e.g., incision and drainage of abscesses and circumcision)

• Patients with long-term indwelling catheters (e.g., hyperalimentation)

• Subsequent cardiac surgery for any of the above listed types of surgery, excepting patients with uncomplicated atrial septal defects of the secundum variety closed with direct suturing without a prosthetic patch and patients who have had ligation or division of a patent ductus arteriosus more than 6 months before the present procedure

• Any patient with a documented previous episode of endocarditis, even if there is no clinically detectable heart defect

Endocarditis associated with most cardiac operations is usually because of *Staphylococcus aureus,* coagulase-negative staphylococci, or diphtheroids. Streptococci, gram-negative bacteria, and fungi are less common sources of infection. Prophylaxis, therefore, should be directed primarily against staphylococci and is best only for a short duration. Penicillinase-resistant penicillins, such as the first-generation cephalosporins, are usually given, although the choice of drug should be based on each hospital's antibiotic susceptibility profile.

The patient taking ordinary rheumatic fever prophylactic antibiotics is not covered adequately for prevention of endocarditis for the surgical and diagnostic procedures in the foregoing list. The planned operation determines the antibiotic regimen to be followed for the prevention of endocarditis. Thoracic operations, including bronchoscopy and esophagoscopy, require the administration of appropriate doses of penicillin, ampicillin, or amoxicillin given orally or parenterally (Table 16-10), and sometimes gentamicin as well. Penicillin-sensitive patients may be given oral erythromycin or vancomycin. The parenteral administration of vancomycin should be done with extreme caution, as rapid intravenous injection can result in significant untoward reactions.

REFERENC6ES

1. Cook DR, Marcy JH (eds): *Neonatal anesthesia*, Pasadena, Cal., 1989, Appleton-Davis.
2. Smith CA, Nelson NM (eds): *The physiology of the newborn infant*, Springfield, Ill., 1976, Charles C. Thomas.
3. Rudolph AM: Fetal circulation and cardiovascular adjustments after birth. In Rudolph AM (ed): *Pediatrics*, ed 18, p 1219, East Norwalk Conn., 1987, Appleton and Lange.
4. Rudolph AM: The changes in the circulation after birth: their importance on congenital heart disease, *Circulation* 41: 343, 1970.
5. Hickey PR, Hansen DD: Anesthesia and cardiac shunting in the neonate: ductus arteriosus, transitional circulation and congenital heart disease, *Semin Anesth* 3:106, 1984.

6. Bohn D: Anomalies of the pulmonary valve and pulmonary circulation. In Lake CL (ed): *Pediatric cardiac anesthesia*, ed 3, p 373, East Norwalk, Conn., 1998, Appleton and Lange.
7. Hickey PR, Crone RK: Cardiovascular physiology and pharmacology in children: normal and diseased pediatric cardiovascular systems. In Ryan JF, Todres ID, Cote CJ, et al (eds): *A practice of anesthesia for infants and children*, p 173, Philadelphia, 1986, WB Saunders.
8. Reid LM: Structure and function in pulmonary hypertension, *Chest* 89:279, 1986.
9. Shapiro AD, Jacobson LJ, Armon ME et al: Vitamin K deficiency in the newborn infant: prevalence and perinatal risk factors, *J Pediatr* 109:675, 1986.
10. Mountain KR, Hirsh J, Gallus AS: Neonatal coagulation defect due to anticonvulsant drug treatment in pregnancy, *Lancet* 1:265, 1970.
11. Martyn JAJ: Pediatric clinical pharmacokinetics: principles and concepts. In Ryan JF, Todres ID, Cote CJ, et al (eds): *A practice of anesthesia for infants and children*, p 65, Philadelphia, 1986, WB Saunders.
12. Arant BS: The newborn kidney. In Rudolph AM (ed): *Pediatrics*, ed 18, p 1143, East Norwalk Conn., 1987, Appleton and Lange.
13. Bennett EJ: *Fluids for anesthesia and surgery in the newborn and the infant*, Springfield, IL, 1975, Charles C Thomas.
14. Williams PR, Oh W: Effect of radiant heaters on insensible water loss in newborn infants, *Am J Dis Child* 128:511, 1974.
15. Volpe JJ: Neonatal periventricular hemorrhage: past, present, and future, *J Pediatr* 92:693, 1978.
16. Simmons MA, Adcock EW, Bard H, et al: Hypernatremia and intracranial hemorrhage in neonates, *N Engl J Med* 291:6, 1974.
17. Dabbagh S, Ellis D: Regulation of fluids and electrolytes in infants and children. In Motoyama EK, Davis PJ (eds): *Smith's anesthesia for infants and children*, ed 5, p 118, St. Louis, 1990, Mosby.
18. Oliver TK Jr: Temperature regulation and heat production in the newborn, *Pediatr Clin North Am* 12:765, 1966.
19. Pearlstein PH, Edwards NK, Atherton MD, et al: Computer assisted newborn intensive care, *Pediatrics* 57:494, 1976.
20. Kurz A, Kurz M, Pieschl G, et al: Forced-air warming maintained intraoperative normothermia better than circulating-water mattresses, *Anesth Analg* 77:89, 1993.
21. Roe CF, Santulli TV, Blair CS: Heat loss in infants during general anesthesia and operations, *J Pediatr Surg* 1:266, 1976.
22. Lubchenco LO: The high-risk infant. In Lubchenco LO (ed): *Major problems in clinical pediatrics*, vol 14, p 294, Philadelphia, 1976, WB Saunders.
23. Skimming JW, Bender KA, Hutchison AA, et al: Nitric oxide inhalation in infants with respiratory distress syndrome, *J Pediatr* 130:225, 1997.
24. Wessel DL, Adatia I, Giglia TM, et al: Use of inhaled nitric oxide and acetylcholine in the evaluation of pulmonary hypertension and endothelial function after cardiopulmonary bypass, *Circulation* 88:2128, 1993.
25. Borgeson DD, Seward JB, Miller FA, et al: Frequency of Doppler measurable pulmonary artery pressures, *J Am Soc Echocardiogr* 9:832, 1996.
26. Ebeid MR, Ferrer PL, Robinson B, et al: Doppler echocardiographic evaluation of pulmonary vascular resistance in children with congenital heart disease, *J Am Soc Echocardiogr* 9:822, 1996.
27. Bennett NR: Paediatric intensive care, *Br J Anaesth* 83:139, 1999.
28. Yee WF, Scarpetti EM: Surfactant replacement therapy, *Pediatr Pulmonol* 11:65, 1991.
29. Hartog A, Gommers D, Haitsma JJ, et al: Improvement of lung mechanics by exogenous surfactant: effect of prior application of high positive end-expiratory pressure, *Br J Anaesth* 85:752, 2000.
30. Ziegler JW, Ivy DD, Wiggins JW, et al: Effects of dipyridamole and inhaled nitric oxide in pediatric patients with pulmonary hypertension, *Am J Respir Crit Care Med* 158:1388, 1998.
31. McLaughlin VV, Genthner DE, Panella MM, et al: Reduction in pulmonary vascular resistance with long-term epoprostenol (prostacyclin) therapy in primary pulmonary hypertension, *N Engl J Med* 334:296, 1996.
32. Van Obbergh LJ, Charbonneau M, Blaise G: Combination of inhaled nitric oxide with IV nitroglycerin or with a prostacyclin analogue in the treatment of experimental pulmonary hypertension, *Br J Anaesth* 77:227, 1996.
33. Rosenzweig EB, Kerstein D, Barst RJ: Long-term prostacyclin for pulmonary hypertension with associated congenital heart defects, *Circulation* 99:1858, 1999.
34. Pappert D, Busch T, Gerlach H, et al: Aerosolized prostacyclin vs. inhaled nitric oxide in children with severe acute respiratory distress syndrome, *Anesthesiology* 82:1507, 1998.
35. Ichinose F, Adrie C, Hurford WE, et al: Prolonged pulmonary vasodilator action of inhaled nitric oxide by zaprinast in awake lambs, *J Appl Physiol* 78:1288, 1995.
36. Steudel W, Hurford WE, Zapol WM: Inhaled nitric oxide: basic biology and clinical applications, *Anesthesiology* 91:1090, 1999.
37. Troncy E, Francoeur M, Blaise G: Inhaled nitric oxide: clinical applications, indications, and toxicology, *Can J Anaesth* 44:973, 1997.
38. Lindberg L, Rydgren G: Evaluation of nitrogen dioxide scavengers during delivery of inhaled nitric oxide, *Br J Anaesth* 81:404, 1998.
39. Branson RD, Hess DR, Campbell RS, et al: Inhaled nitric oxide delivery systems and monitoring, *Respir Care* 44:281, 1999.
40. Ceccarelli P, Bigatello LM, Hess D, et al: Inhaled nitric oxide delivery by anesthesia machines, *Anesth Analg* 90:482, 2000.
41. Tobias JD, Grueber RE: Nitric oxide administration using an operating room ventilator, *Am J Anaesthesiol* 27:137, 2000.
42. Katayama Y, Higenbottam TW, Cremona G, et al: Minimizing the inhaled dose of NO with breath-by-breath delivery of spikes of concentrated gas, *Circulation* 98:2429, 1998.
43. Leveque C, Hamza J, Berg AE, et al: Successful repair of a severe left congenital diaphragmatic hernia during continuous inhalation of nitric oxide, *Anesthesiology* 80:1171, 1994.
44. Young JD: Inhaled nitric oxide in acute respiratory failure, *Br. J Anaesth* 79:695, 1997.
45. Neonatal Inhaled Nitric Oxide Study Group: Inhaled nitric oxide and hypoxic respiratory failure in infants with congenital diaphragmatic hernia, *Pediatrics* 99:838, 1997.
46. Hoffman GM, Ross GA, Day SE, et al: Inhaled nitric oxide reduces the utilization of extracorporeal membrane oxygenation in persistent pulmonary hypertension of the newborn, *Crit Care Med* 25:352, 1997.
47. Atz AM, Adatia I, Lock JE, et al: Combined effects of nitric oxide and oxygen during acute pulmonary vasodilator testing, *J Am Coll Cardiol* 33:813, 1999.
48. Neonatal Inhaled Nitric Oxide Study Group: Inhaled nitric oxide in full-term and nearly full-term infants with hypoxic respiratory failure, *N Engl J Med* 336:597, 1997.
49. Roberts JD, Fineman JR, Morin FC, et al: Inhaled nitric oxide and persistent pulmonary hypertension of the newborn, *N Engl J Med* 336:605, 1997.
50. Putensen C, Rasanen J, Downs JB: Effect of endogenous and inhaled nitric oxide on the ventilation-perfusion relationships in oleic-acid lung injury, *Am J Respir Crit Care Med* 150:330, 1994.
51. Hopkins SR, Johnson EC, Richardson RS, et al: Effects of inhaled nitric oxide on gas exchange in lungs with shunt or poorly ventilated areas, *Am J Respir Crit Care Med* 156:484, 1997.
52. Hallman M, Bry K, Turbow R, et al: Pulmonary toxicity associated with nitric oxide in term infants with severe respiratory failure, *J Pediatr* 132:827, 1998.
53. Paulus WJ, Vantrimpont PJ, Shan AM: Acute effects of nitric oxide on left ventricular relaxation and diastolic distensibility in humans. Assessment by bicoronary sodium nitroprusside infusion, *Circulation* 89:2070, 1994.
54. Hogman M, Frostell C, Arnberg H, et al: Prolonged bleeding time during nitric oxide inhalation in the rabbit, *Acta Physiol Scand* 151:125, 1994.
55. Ayad O, Wong HR: Nitric oxide decreases surfactant protein A gene expression in H441 cells, *Crit Care Med* 26:1277, 1998.
56. Robbins CG, Davis JM, Merritt TA, et al: Combined effects of nitric oxide and hyperoxia on surfactant function and pulmonary inflammation, *Am J Physiol* 269:L545, 1995.
57. Hess D: Adverse effects and toxicity of inhaled nitric oxide, *Respir Care* 44:315, 1999.
58. Atz AM, Wessel DL: Sildenafil ameliorates effects of inhaled nitric oxide withdrawal, *Anesthesiology* 91:307, 1999.
59. Kovalchin JP, Mott AR, Rosen KL, et al: Nitric oxide for the evaluation and treatment of pulmonary hypertension in congenital heart disease, *Tex Heart Inst J* 224:308, 1997.
60. Holzmann A, Bloch KD, Sanchez LS, et al: Hyporesponsiveness to inhaled nitric oxide in isolated, perfused lungs from endotoxin-challenged rats, *Am J Physiol* 271:L981, 1996.
61. Weimann J, Bauer H, Bigatello L, et al: ABO blood group and inhaled nitric oxide in acute respiratory distress syndrome, *Lancet* 351:1786, 1998.

62. Aranda M, Bradford KK, Pearl RG: Combined therapy with inhaled nitric oxide and intravenous vasodilators during acute and chronic experimental pulmonary hypertension, *Anesth Analg* 89:152, 1999.

63. Rimensberger PC, Spahr-Schopfer I, Berner M, et al: Inhaled nitric oxide versus aerosolized iloprost in secondary pulmonary hypertension in children with congenital heart disease, *Circulation* 103:544, 2001.

64. Weimann J, Ulrich R, Hromi J, et al: Sildenafil is a pulmonary vasodilator in awake lambs with acute pulmonary hypertension, *Anesthesiology* 92:1702, 2000.

65. Bigatello LM, Hess D, Dennehy KC, et al: Sildenafil can increase the response to inhaled nitric oxide, *Anesthesiology* 92:1827, 2000.

66. Rich S, Kaufman E, Levy PS: The effect of high doses of calcium channel blockers on survival in primary pulmonary hypertension, *N Engl J Med* 327:76, 1992.

67. Barst RJ, Maislin G, Fishman AP: Vasodilator therapy in primary pulmonary hypertension in children, *Circulation* 99:1197, 1999.

68. Bossi E, Koerner F: Retinopathy of prematurity, *Intens Care Med* 21:241, 1995.

69. Kalina RE, Hodson WA, Morgan BC: Retrolental fibroplasias in a cyanotic infant, *Pediatrics* 50:765, 1972.

70. Bucher HU, Fanconi S, Baeckert P, et al: Hyperoxemia in newborn infants: detection by pulse oximetry, *Pediatrics* 84:226, 1989.

71. Coté CJ, Zaslavsky A, Downes JJ, et al: Postoperative apnea in former preterm infants after inguinal herniorrhaphy: a combined analysis, *Anesthesiology* 82:809, 1995.

72. Welborn LG, Ramirez N, Oh TH, et al: Postanesthetic apnea and periodic breathing in infants, *Anesthesiology* 65:658, 1986.

73. Knill RL, Gelb AW: Ventilatory responses to hypoxia and hypercapnia during halothane sedation and anesthesia in man, *Anesthesiology* 49:244, 1978.

74. Tusiewicz K, Bryan AC, Froese AB: Contributions of changing rib cage:diaphragm interactions to the ventilatory depression of halothane anesthesia, *Anesthesiology* 47:327, 1977.

75. Liu LMP, Coté CJ, Goudsouzian NG, et al: Life-threatening apnea in infants recovering from anesthesia, *Anesthesiology* 59:506, 1983.

76. Malviya S, Swartz J, Lerman J: Are all preterm infants younger than 60 weeks postconceptual age at risk for postanesthetic apnea? *Anesthesiology* 78:1076, 1993.

77. Kurth CD, LeBard SE: Association of postoperative apnea, airway obstruction, and hypoxemia in former premature infants, *Anesthesiology* 78:1076, 1993.

78. Welborn LG, DeSoto H, Hannallah RS, et al: The use of caffeine in the control of postanesthetic apnea in former premature infants, *Anesthesiology* 68:796, 1988.

79. Lubchenco LO, Bard H: Incidence of hypoglycemia in newborn infants classified by birth weights and gestational age, *Pediatrics* 47:831, 1971.

80. Cowett RM, Anderson GE, Maguire CA, et al: Ontogeny of glucose homeostasis in low-birth-weight infants, *J Pediatr* 112:462, 1988.

81. Bakwin H: Tetany in newborn infants: relation to physiologic hypoparathyroidism, *J Pediatr* 14:1, 1939.

82. Tsang RC, Chen I, Friedman MA, et al: Neonatal parathyroid function: role of gestational age and postnatal age, *J Pediatr* 83:728, 1973.

83. Schediwie HE, Odell WD, Risher DA, et al: Parathormone and perinatal calcium homeostasis, *Pediatr Res* 13:1, 1979.

84. Rivzi T, Wadhwa S, Bijlan V: Development of spinal substrate for nociception, *Pain* 4:195(S), 1987.

85. Humphrey T: Some correlations between the appearance of human fetal reflexes and the development of the nervous system, *Prog Brain Res* 4:43, 1964.

86. Williamson PS, Williamson ML: Physiologic stress reduction by a local anesthetic during newborn circumcision, *Pediatrics* 71:36, 1983.

87. Holve RL, Bromberger PJ, et al: Regional anesthesia during newborn circumcision, *Clin Pediatr* 22:813, 1983.

88. Harrin VA, Rutter H: Development of emotional sweating in the newborn infant, *Arch Dis Child* 57:691, 1982.

89. Srinivasan G, Jarn R, Pildes R, et al: Glucose homeostasis during anesthesia and surgery in infants, *J Pediatr Surg* 21:718, 1986.

90. Obara H, Sugiyama D, Tanaka O, et al: Plasma cortisol levels in pediatric anesthesia, *Can Anaesth Soc J* 31:24, 1984.

91. Anand KJS, Brown MJ, Causon R, et al: Can the human neonate mount an endocrine and metabolic response to surgery? *J Pediatr Surg* 20:41, 1985.

92. Anand KJS, Brown MJ, Bloom S, et al: Studies on the hormonal regulation of fuel metabolism in the human neonate undergoing anesthesia and surgery, *Hormone Res* 22:115, 1985.

93. Anand KJS, Hickey PR: Pain and its effects in the human neonate and fetus, *N Engl J Med* 317:1321, 1987.

94. Anand KJS, Hickey PR: Halothane-morphine compared with high-dose sufentanil for anesthesia and postoperative analgesia in neonatal cardiac surgery, *N Engl J Med* 326:1, 1992.

95. Noonan JA: Association of congenital heart diseases with other defects, *Pediatr Clin North Am* 25:797, 1978.

96. Greenwood RD, Rosenthal A, Nadas AS: Cardiovascular abnormalities associated with diaphragmatic hernia, *Pediatrics* 57:92, 1976.

97. Macario A, Hackel A, Gregory GA, et al: The demographics of inpatient pediatric anesthesia: implications for credentialing policy, *J Clin Anesth* 7:507, 1995.

98. Keenan RL, Shapiro JH, Dawson K: Incidence of anesthetic cardiac arrest in infants: effect of pediatric anesthesiologists, *J Clin Anesth* 3:433, 1991.

99. Keenan RL, Shapiro JH, Kane FR, et al: Bradycardia during anesthesia in infants: an epidemiologic study, *Anesthesiology* 80:76, 1994.

100. Beecher HK, Todd DP: A study of the deaths associated with anesthesia and surgery, *Ann Surg* 140:1, 1954.

101. Rackow H, Salnitre E, Green LT: Frequency of cardiac arrest associated with anesthesia in infants and children, *Pediatrics* 28:697, 1961.

102. Olsson GL, Hallen B: Cardiac arrest during anesthesia: a computerized study in 250,543 anaesthetics, *Acta Anaesthesiol Scand* 32:653, 1988.

103. Tiret L, Nivoche Y, Hatton F, et al: Complications related to anaesthesia in infants and children, *Br J Anaesth* 61:263, 1988.

104. Cohen MM, Cameron CB, Duncan PG: Pediatric anesthesia morbidity and mortality in the perioperative period, *Anesth Analg* 70:160, 1990.

105. Morray JP, Geiduschek JM, Caplan RA, et al: A comparison of pediatric and adult anesthesia closed malpractice claims, *Anesthesiology* 78:461, 1993.

106. Morray JP, Geiduschek JM, Ramamoorthy C, et al: Initial findings of the pediatric perioperative cardiac arrest registry, *Anesthesiology* 93:6, 2000.

107. Morray JP: Implications for subspecialty care of anesthetized children, *Anesthesiology* 80:969, 1994.

108. McGraw T: Preparing children for the operating room: psychological issue, *Can J Anaesth* 41:1094, 1994.

109. Kain Z, Mayes L: Anxiety in children during the perioperative period. In Borestein M, Genevro J (eds): *Children development and behavioral pediatrics*, p 85, Mahwah NJ, 1996, Lawrence-Erlbaum Associates.

110. Kain ZN, Mayes LC, O'Connor TZ, et al: Preoperative anxiety in children. Predictors and outcomes, *Arch Pediatr Adol Med* 150:1238, 1996.

111. Burton L: Anxiety relating to illness and treatment. In Verma V (ed): *Anxiety in children*, p 151, New York, 1984, Metheun Croom Helm.

112. Vetter T: The epidemiology and selective identification of children at risk for preoperative anxiety reactions, *Anesth Analg* 77:96, 1993.

113. Schwartz BH, Albino JE, Tedesco LA: Effects of psychological preparation on children hospitalized for dental operations, *J Pediatr* 102:634, 1983.

114. Zuckerberg AL: Perioperative approach to children, *Pediatri Clin North Am* 41:15, 1983.

115. Litman RS, Perkins FM, Dawson SC: Parental knowledge and attitudes toward discussing the risk of death from anesthesia, *Anesth Analg* 77:256, 1993.

116. Kotiniemi L, Ryhanen P: Behavioral changes and children's memories after intravenous, inhalation and rectal induction of anaesthesia, *Paediatr Anaesth* 6:201, 1996.

117. Kotiniemi LH, Ryhanen PT, Moilanen IK: Behavioral changes following routine ENT operations in two-to-ten-year-old children, *Paediatr Anaesth* 6:45, 1996.

118. Kotiniemi LH, Ryhanen PT, Moilanen IK: Behavioral changes in children following day-case surgery: a 4-week follow-up of 551 children, *Anaesthesia* 52:970,1997.

119. Kotiniemi LH, Ryhanen PT, Valanne J, et al: Postoperative symptoms at home following day-case surgery in children: a multicentre survey of 551 children, *Anaesthesia* 52:963, 1997.

120. Vernon DT, Schulman JL, Foley JM: Changes in children's behavior after hospitalization, *Am J Dis Child* 111:581, 1966.

121. O'Bryne K, Peterson L, Saldana L: Survey of pediatric hospitals' preparation programs: evidence of the impact of health psychology research, *Health Psychol* 16:147, 1997.

122. Pruitt S, Elliott C: Paediatric procedures. In Johnston M, Wallace L (eds): *Stress and medical procedures*, Oxford, 1990, Oxford University Press.

123. Melamed BG, Ridley-Johnson R: Psychological preparation of families for hospitalization, *Dev Behav Pediatr* 9:96, 1988.

124. American Academy of Pediatrics CoHC: Child life programs, *Pediatrics* 91:671, 1993.
125. Vernon D, Foley J, Sipowicz R, et al: The psychological responses of children to hospitalization and illness, Springfield, Ill., 1965, Charles C Thomas.
126. Kain Z, Caramico L, Mayes L, et al: Preoperative preparation programs in children: a comparative study, *Anesth Analg* 87:1249, 1998.
127. Gauderer WM, Lorig JL, Eastwood DW: Is there a place for parents in the operating room? *J Pediatri Surg* 24:705, 1989.
128. Bevan JC, Johnston C, Haig MJ, et al: Preoperative parental anxiety predicts behavioral and emotional responses to induction of anesthesia in children, *Can J Anaesth* 37:177, 1990.
129. Kain Z, Mayes L, Wang S, et al: Parental presence during induction of anesthesia vs sedative premedication: which intervention is more effective? *Anesthesiology* 89:1147, 1998.
130. Kain ZN, Mayes LC, Caramico LA, et al: Parental presence during induction of anesthesia. A randomized controlled trial, *Anesthesiology* 84:1060, 1996.
131. Hickmoitt KC, Shaw EA, Goodyer I, et al: Anaesthetic induction in children: the effect of maternal presence on mood and subsequent behaviour, *Eur J Anaesthesiol* 6:145, 1989.
132. Kain ZN, Mayes LC, Bell C, et al: Premedication in the United States: a status report, *Anesth Analg* 84:427, 1997.
133. Splinter WM, Schreiner MS: Preoperative fasting in children, *Anesth Analg* 89:80, 1999.
134. Coté CJ: NPO after midnight for children—a reappraisal, *Anesthesiology* 72:589, 1990.
135. Fasting S, Soreide E, Raeder JC: Changing preoperative fasting policies. Impact of a national consensus, *Acta Anaesthesiol Scand* 42:1188, 1998.
136. Green CR, Pandit SK, Schork MA: Preoperative fasting time: is the traditional policy changing? Results of a national survey, *Anesth Analg* 83:123, 1996.
137. Practice guidelines for preoperative fasting and the use of pharmacologic agents to reduce the risk of pulmonary aspiration: application to healthy patients undergoing elective procedures: a report by the American Society of Anesthesiologists Task Force on Preoperative Fasting, *Anesthesiology* 90:896, 1999.
138. Andres JM, Mathias JR, Clench MH, et al: Gastric emptying in infants with gastroesophageal reflux, *Dig Dis Sci* 33:393, 1988.
139. Moukarzel AA, Sabri MT: Gastric physiology and function: effects of fruit juices. *M J Am Coll Nutr* 15:185, 1996.
140. Cavell B: Gastric emptying in preterm infants, *Acta Paediatr Scand* 68:725, 1979.
141. Cavell B: Gastric emptying in infants, *Acta Paediatr Scand* 60:370, 1971.
142. van der Walt JH, Foate JA, Murrell D, et al: A study of preoperative fasting in infants aged less than three months, *Anaesth Intens Care* 18:527, 1990.
143. Litman RS, Wu GL, Quinlivan JK: Gastric volume and pH in infants fed clear liquids and breast milk prior to surgery, *Anesth Analg* 79:482, 1994.
144. Splinter WM, Stewart JA, Muir JG: The effects of preoperative apple juice on gastric contents, thirst, and hunger in children, *Can J Anaesth* 36:55, 1989.
145. Sandhar BK, Goresky GV, Maltby JR, et al: Effect of oral liquids and ranitidine on gastric fluid volume and pH in children undergoing outpatient surgery, *Anesthesiology* 71:327, 1989.
146. Splinter WM, Stewart JA, Muir JG: Large volumes of apple juice preoperatively do not affect gastric pH and volume in children, *Can J Anaesth* 37:36, 1990.
147. Splinter WM, Schaefer JD, Zunder IH: Clear fluids three hours before surgery do not affect the gastric fluid contents of children, *Can J Anaesth* 37:498, 1990.
148. Crawford M, Lerman J, Christensen S, et al: Effects of duration of fasting on gastric fluid pH and volume in healthy children, *Anesth Analg* 71:400, 1990.
149. Miller BR, Tharp JA, Issacs WB: Gastric residual volume in infants and children following a three hour fast, *J Clin Anesth* 2:301, 1990.
150. Schreiner MS, Triebwasser A, Keon TP: Ingestion of liquids compared with preoperative fasting in pediatric outpatients, *Anesthesiology* 72:593, 1990.
151. Splinter WM, Schaefer JD: Unlimited clear fluid ingestion two hours before surgery in children does not affect volume or pH of stomach contents, *Anesthes Intens Care* 18:522, 1990.
152. Maltby JR, Lewis P, Martin A, et al: Gastric fluid volume and pH in elective patients following unrestricted oral fluid until three hours before surgery, *Can J Anaesth* 38:425, 1991.
153. Read MS, Vaughan RS: Allowing preoperative patients to drink: effects on patients' safety and comfort of unlimited oral water until 2 hours before anesthesia, *Acta Anaesthesiol Scand* 35:591, 1991.
154. Phillips S, Hutchinson S, Davidson T: Preoperative drinking does not affect gastric contents, *Br J Anaesth* 70:6, 1993.
155. Coté CJ: Preoperative preparation and premedication, *Br J Anaesth* 83:16, 1999.
156. Coté CJ: Sedation for the pediatric patient. A review, *Pediatr Clin North Am* 41:31, 1994.
157. Levine MF, Spahr-Schopfer IA, Hartley E, et al: Oral midazolam premedication in children: the minimum time interval for separation from parents, *Can J Anaesth* 40:726, 1993.
158. McMillan CO, Spahr-Schopfer IA, Sikich N, et al: Premedication of children with oral midazolam, *Can J Anaesth* 39:545, 1992.
159. Feld LH, Negus JB, White PF: Oral midazolam preanesthetic medication in pediatric outpatients, *Anesthesiology* 73:831, 1990.
160. Weldon BC, Watcha MF, White PF: Oral midazolam in children: effect of time and adjunctive therapy, *Anesth Analg* 75:51, 1992.
161. Davis PJ, Tome JA, McGowan FX Jr, et al: Preanesthetic medication with intranasal midazolam for brief pediatric surgical procedures: effect on recovery and hospital discharge times, *Anesthesiology* 82:2, 1995.
162. Davis PJ, Greenberg JA, Gendelman M, et al: Recovery characteristics of sevoflurane and halothane in preschool-aged children undergoing bilateral myringotomy and pressure equalization tube insertion, *Anesth Analg* 88:34, 1999.
163. Lapin SL, Auden SM, Goldsmith LJ, et al: Effects of sevoflurane anaesthesia on recovery in children. A comparison with halothane, *Paediatr Anaesth* 9:299, 1999.
164. Eger EI, Kraft ID, Keasling HH: A comparison of atropine, or scopolamine, plus pentobarbital, meperidine, or morphine as pediatric preanesthetic medication, *Anesthesiology* 22:962, 1961.
165. Gutstein HB, Johnson KL, Heard MB, et al: Oral ketamine preanesthetic medication in children, *Anesthesiology* 76:28, 1992.
166. Alderson PJ, Lerman J: Oral premedication for paediatric ambulatory anaesthesia: a comparison of midazolam and ketamine, *Can J Anaesth* 41: 221, 1994.
167. Warner DL, Cabaret J, Velling D: Ketamine plus midazolam, a most effective paediatric oral premedicant, *Pediatr Anaesth* 5:293, 1995.
168. Cioaca R, Canavea I: Oral transmucosal ketamine: an effective premedication in children, *Paediatr Anaesth* 6:361, 1996.
169. Diaz JH: Intranasal ketamine preinduction of paediatric outpatients, *Pediatri Anaesth* 7:273, 1997.
170. Weksler N, Ovadia L, Muati G, et al: Nasal ketamine for paediatric premedication, *Can J Anaesth* 40:119, 1993.
171. Malinovsky JM, Cozian A, Lepage JY, et al: Ketamine and midazolam neurotoxicity in the rabbit, *Anesthesiology* 75:91, 1991.
172. Dsida RM, Wheeler M, Birmingham PK, et al: Premedication of pediatric tonsillectomy patients with oral transmucosal fentanyl citrate, *Anesth Analg* 86:66, 1998.
173. Feld LH, Champeau MW, vanSteennis CA, et al: Preanesthetic medication in children: a comparison of oral transmucosal fentanyl citrate versus placebo, *Anesthesiology* 71:374, 1989.
174. Epstein RH, Mendelk HG, Witkowski TA, et al: The safety and efficacy of oral transmucosal fentanyl citrate for preoperative sedation in young children, *Anesth Analg* 83:1200, 1996.
175. Buckley MM, Benfield P: Eutectic lidocaine/prilocaine cream. A review of the topical anaesthetic/analgesia efficacy of a eutectic mixture of local anaesthetics (EMLA), *Drugs* 46:126, 1993.
176. Nadas AS, Fyler D: *Pediatric cardiology*, ed 3, p 191, Philadelphia, 1972, WB Saunders.
177. Coté CJ, Goldstein EA, Coté MA, et al: A single-blind study of pulse oximetry in children, *Anesthesiology* 68:184, 1988.
178. Schuller JL, Bovill JG: Severe reduction in end-tidal PCO_2 following unilateral pulmonary artery occlusion in a child with pulmonary hypertension, *Anesth Analg* 68:792, 1989.
179. Fletcher R: The relationship between the arterial to end-tidal PCO_2 differences and hemoglobin saturation in patients with congenital heart disease, *Anesthesiology* 75:210, 1991.
180. Lawless S, Orr R: Axillary arterial monitoring of pediatric patients, *Pediatrics* 84:273, 1989.
181. Glenski JA, Beynum FM, Brady J: A prospective evaluation of femoral artery monitoring in pediatric patients, *Anesthesiology* 66:227, 1987.
182. Vidayasagar D, Downes JJ, Boggs TR: Respiratory distress syndrome of newborn infants. II. Techniques of catheterization of umbilical artery and clinical results of treatment, *Clin Pediatr* 9:332, 1970.

183. Fletcher MA, Brown DR, Landers S, et al: Umbilical arterial catheter use: report of an audit conducted by the Study Group for Complications of Perinatal Care, *Am J Perinatol* 11:94, 1994.

184. Kinsey VE, Arnold HJ, Kalina RD, et al: PaO$_2$ levels and retrolental fibroplasias: a report of the cooperative study, *Pediatrics* 60:655, 1977.

185. Prince SR, Sullivan RL, Hackel A: Percutaneous catheterization of the internal jugular vein in infants and children, *Anesthesiology* 44:170, 1976.

186. Coté C, Jobes DR, Schwartz AJ, et al: Two approaches to cannulation of a child's internal jugular vein, *Anesthesiology* 50:371, 1979.

187. Alderson PJ, Burrows FA, Stemp LI, et al: Use of ultrasound to evaluate internal jugular vein anatomy and to facilitate central venous cannulation in paediatric patients, *Br J Anaesth* 70:145, 1993.

188. Pybus DA, Poole JL, Crawford MC: Subclavian venous catheterization in small children using a Seldinger technique, *Anaesthesia* 37:451, 1982.

189. Ungerleider RM, Greeley WJ, Kisslo J: Intraoperative echocardiography in congenital heart disease surgery: preliminary report on a current study, *Am J Cardiol* 63(S1):3F, 1989.

190. Gilbert TB, Panico FG, McGill WA, et al: Bronchial obstruction by trans-esophegeal echocardiography probe in a pediatric cardiac patient, *Anesth Analg* 74:156, 1992.

191. Lake CL: Monitoring of the pediatric patient. In Lake CL (ed): *Pediatric cardiac anesthesia*, ed 3, p 208, East Norwalk CT, 1998, Appleton and Lange.

192. LaFarge CG, Miettinen OS: The estimation of oxygen consumption, *Cardiovasc Res* 4:23, 1970.

193. Bissonnette B, Sessler DI, LaFlamme P: Intraoperative temperature monitoring sites in infants and children and the effect of inspired gas warming on esophageal temperature, *Anesth Analg* 69:192, 1989.

194. Wallace CT, Marks WE Jr, Adkins WY, et al: Perforation of the tympanic membrane, a complication of tympanic thermometry during anesthesia, *Anesthesiology* 41:290, 1974.

195. Khine HH, Corddry DH, Kettrick RG, et al: Comparison of cuffed and uncuffed endotracheal tubes in young children during general anesthesia, *Anesthesiology* 86:627, 1997.

196. Stowe PJ, McLeod ME, Burrows FA, et al: Anterior fontanelle pressure responses to tracheal intubation in the awake and anesthetized infants, *Br J Anaesth* 60:167, 1988.

197. Tobin MJ, Stevenson GW, Horn BJ, et al: A comparison of three modes of ventilation with the use of an adult circle system in an infant lung model, *Anesth Analg* 87:766, 1998.

198. Stayer SA, Bent ST, Skjonsby BS, et al: Pressure-control ventilation: three anesthesia ventilators compared using an infant lung model, *Anesth Analg* 91:1145, 2000.

199. Stevenson GW, Tobin M, Horn B, et al: A comparison of two ventilator systems using an infant lung model, *Anesthesiology* 93:285, 2000.

200. Stevenson GW, Horn B, Tobin M, et al: Pressure-limited ventilation of infants with low-compliance lungs: the efficacy of an adult circle system versus two free-standing intensive care unit ventilator systems using an in vitro model, *Anesth Analg* 89:638, 1999.

201. Saidman LJ: The 33rd Rovenstine lecture: what I have learned from 9 years and 9000 papers, *Anesthesiology* 83:191, 1995.

202. Mather L, Mackie J: The incidence of postoperative pain in children, *Pain* 15:271, 1983.

203. Anand KJ: Pain, plasticity, and premature birth: a prescription for permanent suffering, *Nat Med* 6:971, 2000.

204. Coté JC, Ryan JF, Todres DI, et al: A practice of anesthesia for infants and children, ed 3, Philadelphia, 2001, WB Saunders.

205. Scott CS, Riggs KW, Ling EW, et al: Morphine pharmacokinetics and pain assessment in premature newborns, *J Pediatr* 135:423, 1999.

206. Lynn AM, Slattery JT: Morphine pharmacokinetics and pain assessment in early infancy, *Anesthesiology* 66:136, 1987.

207. Hartley R, Levene MI: Opioid pharmacology in the newborn, *Bailliere's Clin Paediatr* 3:467, 1995.

208. Kupferberg HJ, Way HJ: Pharmacologic basis for the increased sensitivity of the newborn to morphine, *J Pharmacol Exp Ther* 141:105, 1063.

209. Morton NS: Prevention and control of pain in children, *Brit J Anaesth* 83:118, 1999.

210. Kussman BD, Sethna NF: Pethidine-associated seizures in a healthy adolescent receiving pethidine for postoperative pain control, *Pediatr Anaesth* 8:349, 1998.

211. Berde CB, Lehn BM, Yee JD, et al: Patient-controlled analgesia in children and adolescents : a randomized, prospective comparison with intramuscular administration of morphine for postoperative analgesia, *J Pediatr* 118:460, 1991.

212. Gillespie J, Morton NS: Patient-controlled analgesia for children: a review, *Pediatr Anaesth* 2:51, 1992.

213. Kotzer AM, Coy J, LeClaire AD: The effectiveness of a standardized educational program for children using patient-controlled analgesia, *J Soc Pediatr Nurs* 3:117, 1998.

214. Brown TCK, Eyres RL, McDougal RJ: Local and regional anesthesia in children, *Brit J Anesth* 83:65, 1999.

215. Bromage PR, Benumof JL: Paraplegia following intracord injection during attempted epidural anaesthesia under general anaesthesia, *Reg Anaesth Pain Med* 23:104, 1998.

216. Krane EJ, Dalens BJ, Murat I, et al: The safety of epidurals placed during general anaesthesia, *Reg Anaesth Pain Med* 23:433, 1998.

217. Dalens B, Hasnaui A: Caudal anesthesia in pediatric surgery: success rate and adverse effects in 750 consecutive patients, *Anesth Analg* 68:83, 1989.

218. Valley RD, Bailey AG: Caudal morphine for postoperative analgesia in infants and children: a case report of 500 cases, *J Clin Anesth* 7:640, 1995.

219. Mayhew JF, Brodsky RC, Blakey D, et al: Low-dose caudal morphine for postoperative analgesia in infants and children. A case report of 500 cases, *J Clin Anesth* 7:640, 1995.

220. Krane EJ, Tyler DC, Jacobson LE: The dose-response of caudal morphine in children, *Anesthesiology* 71:48, 1989.

221. Bosenberg AT, Bland BA, Sculte-Steinberg O, et al: Thoracic epidural anesthesia via caudal route in infants, *Anesthesiology* 69:265, 1988.

222. Gunter JB, Eng C: Thoracic epidural anesthesia via the caudal approach in children, *Anesthesiology* 76:935, 1992.

223. Dalens B, Tanguy A, Haberer JP: Lumbar epidural anesthesia for operative and postoperative pain relief in infants and young children, *Anesth Analg* 65:1069, 1986.

224. Tobias JD, Lowe S, O'Dell N: Thoracic epidural anaesthesia in infants and children, *Can J Anaesth* 40:879, 1993.

225. Hendolin H, Lahtinen J, Lansimies E, et al: The effect of thoracic epidural analgesia on respiratory function after cholecystectomy, *Acta Anaesthesiol Scand* 31:645, 1987.

226. Rawal N, Sjostrand U, Christoffersson E, et al: Comparison of intramuscular and epidural morphine for postoperative analgesia in the grossly obese: influence on postoperative ambulation and pulmonary function, *Anesth Analg* 63:583, 1984.

227. Cuschieri RJ, Morran CG, Howie JC, et al: Postoperative pain and pulmonary complications: comparison of three analgesic regimens, *Br J Surg* 72:495, 1985.

228. Sydow FW: The influence of anesthesia and postoperative analgesic management on lung function, *Acta Chir Scand* 550(S):159, 1988.

229. Bromage PR, Camporesi E, Chestnut D: Epidural narcotics for postoperative analgesia, *Anesth Analg* 59:473, 1980.

230. Guinard JP, Mavrocordato P, Chiolero R, et al: A randomized comparison of intravenous versus lumbar and thoracic epidural fentanyl for analgesia after thoracotomy, *Anesthesiology* 77:1108, 1992.

231. Pansard JL, Mankikian B, Bertrand M, et al: Effects of thoracic extradural block on diaphragmatic electrical activity and contractility after upper abdominal surgery, *Anesthesiology* 78:63, 1993.

232. Ford G, Whitelaw W, Rosenal T, et al: Diaphragm function after upper abdominal surgery in humans, *Am Rev Respir Dis* 127:431, 1987.

233. Simmonneau G, Vivien A, Saberne R, et al: Diaphragm dysfunction induced by upper abdominal surgery: role of postoperative pain, *Am Rev Respir Dis* 128:899, 1983.

234. Fratacci MD, Kimball WR, Wain JC, et al: Diaphragmatic shortening after thoracic surgery in humans, *Anesthesiology* 79:654, 1993.

235. Peterson KL, DeCampli WM, Pike N, et al: A report of two hundred twenty cases of regional anesthesia in pediatric cardiac surgery, *Anesth Analg* 90:1014, 2000.

236. McCloskey JJ, Haun SE, Deshpande J: Bupivacaine toxicity secondary to continous caudal epidural infusion in children, *Anesth Analg* 75:231, 1996.

237. Luz G, Innerhofer P, Bachmann B, et al: Bupivacaine plasma concentrations during continuous epidural anesthesia in infants and children, *Anesth Analg* 82:231, 1996.

238. Larsson BA, Lonnquist PA, Olsson GL: Plasma concentrations of bupivacaine in neonates after continous epidural infusion, *Anesth Analg* 84:501, 1997.

239. Morton NS: Ropivacaine in children, *Brit J Anesth* 85:344, 2000.

240. McClure: Ropivacaine, *Brit J Anesth* 76:300, 1996.
241. Hansen TG, Ilet KF, Lim SI, et al: Pharmacokinetics and clinical efficacy of long-term postoperative epidural ropivacaine infusion in children, *Br J Anaesth* 85:347, 2000.
242. Anzai Y, Nishikawa T: Thoracic epidural clonidine and morphine for postoperative pain relief. Report of investigation, *Can J Anaesth* 42:292, 1995.
243. Ivani G, DeNegri P, Conio A, et al: Ropivacaine-clonidine combination for caudal blockade in children, *Acta Anaesth Scand* 44:446, 2000.
244. Abdel-Ghaffar ME, Abdulatif M, Al-Ghamdi A, et al: Epidural ketamine reduces postoperative epidural PCA consumption of fentanyl/bupivacaine, *Can J Anesth* 45:99, 1998.
245. Sandler AN, Schmid R, Katz J: Epidural ketamine for postoperative analgesia, *Can J Anaesth* 45:99, 1998.
246. Marhofer P, Krenn CG, Plochl W, et al: S(+)-ketamine for caudal block in paediatric anaesthesia, *Brit J Anaesth* 84:341, 2000.
247. Berde CB: Convulsions associated with pediatric regional anesthesia, *Anesth Analg* 75:164, 1992.
248. Bricker SRW, Telford RJ, Booker PD: Pharmacokinetics of bupivacaine following intraoperative intercostal nerve block in neonates and in infants aged less than 6 months, *Anesthesiology* 70:942, 1989.
249. Watcha MF, Jones MB, Lagueruela RG, et al: Comparison of ketorolac and morphine as adjuvants during pediatric surgery, Anesthesiology 76:368, 1992.
250. Buckley MM, Brogden RN: Ketorolac: a review of its pharamacodynamic and pharmacokinetic properties, and therapeutic potential, *Drugs* 39:86, 1990.
251. Olkkola KT, Maunuksela EL: The pharmacokinetics of postoperative intravenous ketorolac tromethamine in children, *Br J Clin Pharmacol* 31:182, 1991.
252. Dsida RM, Wheeler M, Birmingham PK, et al: Age-stratified pharmacokinetics of ketorolac tromethamine in pediatric surgical patients, *Anesth Analg* 94:266, 2002.
253. Birmingham PK, Tobin MJ, Henthorn TK, et al: Twenty-four hour pharmacokinetics of rectal acetaminophen in children, *Anesthesiology* 87:244, 1997.
254. Birmingham PK, Tobin MJ, Fisher DM, et al: Initial and subsequent dosing of rectal acetaminophen in children, *Anesthesiology* 94:385, 2001.
255. Montgomery CJ, McCormack JP, Reichart CC, et al: Plasma concentrations after high-dose (45 mg/kg) rectal acetaminophen in children, *Can J Anaesth* 42:982, 1995.
256. Anderson BJ, Holford NH: Rectal acetaminophen pharmacokinetics, *Anesthesiology* 88:1131, 1998.
257. Lin YC, Sussman HH, Benitz WE: Plasma concentrations after rectal administration of acetaminophen in preterm neonates, *Paediatr Anaesth* 7:457, 1997.
258. Rusy LM, Houck CS, Sullivan LJ, et al: A double-blind evaluation of ketorolac tromethamine versus acetaminophen in pediatric tonsillectomy: analgesia and bleeding, *Anesth Analg* 80:226, 1995.
259. Korpela R, Korvenoja P, Meretoja OA: Morphine-sparing effect of acetaminophen in pediatric day-case surgery, *Anesthesiology* 91:442, 1999.
260. Kirklin JW, Karp RB, Bargeron LA: Surgical treatment of ventricular septal defect. In Sabiston DC, Spencer FC (eds): *Surgery of the chest*, ed 3, p 1044, Philadelphia, 1976, WB Saunders.
261. Ilabaca PA, Ochsner JL, Mills NL: Positive end-expiratory pressure in the management of the patient with a postoperative bleeding heart, *Ann Thorac Surg* 30:281, 1980.
262. Johnson DG: Bronchoscopy. In Welch KJ, Randolph JG, Ravitch MM, et al (eds): *Pediatric surgery*, ed 4, p 619, Chicago, 1986, Year Book Medical Publishers.
263. Benumof JL: *Anesthesia for thoracic surgery*, ed 2, p 688, Philadelphia, 1995, WB Saunders.
264. Lerman J, Davis PJ, Welborn LG, et al: Induction, recovery, and safety characteristics of sevoflurane in children undergoing ambulatory surgery. A comparison with halothane, *Anesthesiology* 84:1332, 1996.
265. Jordan WS, Graves CL, Elwyn RA: New therapy for postintubation laryngeal edema and tracheitis in children, *JAMA* 212:585, 1970.
266. Campbell JB, Quattromani FL, Foley LC: Catheter technique for removal of foreign bodies: experience with 100 cases, *Pediatr Radiol* 11:174, 1981.
267. Lewis RJ, Caccavale RJ, Sisler GE: Special report: video endoscopic thoracic surgery, *N Engl J Med* 88:473, 1991.
268. Laborde F, Noirhomme P, Karan J, et al: A new video-assisted thoracoscopic surgical technique for interruption of patent ductus arteriosus in infants and children, *J Thorac Cardiovasc Surg* 105:278, 1993.

269. Burke RP, Wernovsky G, van der Velde M, et al: Video-assisted thoracoscopic surgery for congenital heart disease, *J Thorac Cardiovasc Surg* 109:499, 1995.
270. Hazelrigg SR, Landreneau RJ, Boley TM: The effect of muscle-sparing versus standard posterolateral thoracotomy on pulmonary function, muscle strength, and postoperative pain, *J Thorac Cardiovasc Surg* 101:394, 1991.
271. Lavoie J, Burrows FA, Hansen DD, et al: Video-assisted thoracoscopic surgery for the treatment of congenital cardiac defects in the pediatric population, *Anesth Analg* 82:563, 1996.
272. Ryckman FC, Rodger BM: Thoracoscopy for intrathoracic neoplasia in children, *J Pediatr Surg* 17:521, 1982.
273. Horswell JL: Anesthetic techniques for thoracoscopy, *Ann Thorac Surg* 56:624, 1993.
274. Rowe R, Andropolous D, Heard M, et al: Anesthetic management of pediatric patients undergoing thoracoscopy, *J Cardiothorac Vasc Anesth* 8:563, 1994.
275. Hammer GB, Manos SJ, Smith BM, et al: Single-lung ventilation in pediatric patients, *Anesthesiology* 84:1503, 1996.
276. Hammer GB, Fitzmaurice BG, Brodsky JB: Methods of single-lung ventilation in pediatric patients, *Anesth Analg* 89:1426, 1999.
277. Rao CC, Krishna G, Grosfeld J, et al: One-lung pediatric anesthesia, *Anesth Analg* 60:450, 1977.
278. Kubota H, Kubota Y, Toshiro T, et al: Selective blind endotracheal intubation in children and adults, *Anesthesiology* 67:587, 1987.
279. Patankar SS, Hammer GB, Brodsky JB: Single-lung ventilation in young children: practical tips on using conventional cuffed endotracheal tubes for VATS, *Anesth Analg* 91:248, 2000.
280. Tan PP, Chu J-J, Ho AC, et al: A modified endotracheal tube for infants and small children undergoing video-assisted thoracoscopic surgery, *Anesth Analg* 86:1212, 1998.
281. FASEB: *Respiration and circulation (biological handbooks)*, p 105, Bethesda MD, 1971, Federation of American Societies for Experimental Biology.
282. Griscom NT, Wohl MEB: Dimensions of the growing trachea related to age and gender, *Am J Roentgenol* 146:233, 1986.
283. Borchardt RA, LaQuaglia MP, McDowell RHG, et al: Bronchial injury during lung isolation in a pediatric patient, *Anesth Analg* 87:324, 1998.
284. Holder TM, Ashcraft KW: Congenital diaphragmatic hernia. In Ravich MM (ed): *Pediatric surgery*, ed 3, p 432, Chicago, 1979, Year Book Medical Publishers.
285. Harrison MR, Bjorda RI, Langmark F, et al: Congenital diaphragmatic hernia: the hidden mortality, *J Pediatr Surg* 13:227, 1978.
286. Cullen ML, Klein MD, Philippart AI: Congenital diaphragmatic hernia, *Surg Clin North Am* 61:1115, 1985.
287. Skari H, Bjornland K, Haugen G, et al: Congenital diaphragmatic hernia: a meta-analysis of mortality factors, *J Pediatr Surg* 35:1187, 2000.
288. Weber TR, Kountzman B, Dillon PA, et al: Improved survival in congenital diaphragmatic hernia with evolving therapeutic strategies, *Arch Surg* 133:498, 1998.
289. Kays DW, Langham MR, Ledbetter DJ, et al: Detrimental effects of standard medical therapy in congenital diaphragmatic hernia, *Ann Surg* 230:340, 1999.
290. Wung JT, Sahni R, Moffitt ST, et al: Congenital diaphragmatic hernia: survival treated with very delayed surgery, spontaneous respiration, and no chest tube, *J Pediatr Surg* 30:406, 1999.
291. Reynolds M, Luck SR, Lappen R: The critical neonate with diaphragmatic hernia: a 21-year perspective, *J Pediatr Surg* 19:364, 1984.
292. Dibbins AW: Congenital diaphragmatic hernia-hypoplastic lung and pulmonary vasoconstriction, *Clin Perinatol* 5:93, 1978.
293. Hansen J, James S, Burrington J, et al: The decreasing of pneumothorax and improving survival of infants with congenital diaphragmatic hernia, *J Pediatr Surg* 19:385, 1984.
294. Bohn D, Tamura M, Perrin D, et al: Ventilatory predictors of pulmonary hypoplasia in congenital diaphragmatic hernia, confirmed by morphologic assessment, *J Pediatr* 111:423, 1987.
295. Bohn D, Jame I, Filler R, et al: The relationship between $PaCO_2$ and ventilation parameters in predicting survival in congenital diaphragmatic hernia, *J Pediatr Surg* 19:666, 1984.
296. O'Rourke PP, Vacanti JP, Crone RK, et al: Use of the postductal PaO_2 as a predictor of pulmonary vascular hypoplasia in infants with congenital diaphragmatic hernia, *J Pediatr Surg* 23:904, 1988.
297. Wells LJ: Development of the human diaphragm and pleural sacs, *Contrib Embryol* 35:109, 1954.

298. Wesselhoeft CW, DeLuca FG: Neonatal septum transversum defects, *Am J Surg* 147:481, 1984.

299. Geggel RL, Reid LM: The structural basis of PPHN, *Clin Perinatol* 3:525, 1984.

300. Kitagawa M, Hislop A, Boyden EA, et al: Lung hypoplasia in congenital diaphragmatic hernia, *Br J Surg* 58:342, 1971.

301. Reale FR, Esterly JR: Pulmonary hypoplasia: a morphometric study of the lungs of infants with diaphragmatic hernia, anencephalia and renal malformations, *Pediatrics* 51:91, 1973.

302. Wiener ES: Congenital posterolateral diaphragmatic hernia: new dimensions in management, *Surgery* 92:670, 1982.

303. Greenwood RD, Rosenthal A, Nadas AS: Cardiovascular abnormalities associated with congenital diaphragmatic hernia, *Pediatrics* 57:92, 1976.

304. Ein SH, Barker G, Olley P, et al: The pharmacologic treatment of newborn diaphragmatic hernia—a 2-year evaluation, *J Pediatr Surg* 15:384, 1980.

305. Sakai H, Tamura M, Hosokawa Y, et al: Effect of surgical rapair on respiratory mechanics in congenital diaphragmatic hernia, *J Pediatr* 111:432-438, 1987.

306. Peckham GJ, Fox WW: Physiologic factors affecting pulmonary artery pressure in infants with persistent pulmonary hypertension, *J Pediatr* 93:1005, 1978.

307. Ehrlich FE, Salzberg AM: Pathophysiology and management of congenital posterolateral diaphragmatic hernias, *Amer Surg* 44:26, 1978.

308. Siebert JR, Haas JE, Beckwith JB: Left ventricular hypoplasia in congenital diaphragmatic hernia, *J Pediatr Surg* 19:567, 1984.

309. Congenital Diaphragmatic Hernia Study Group: Estimating disease severity of congenital diaphragmatic hernia in the first 5 minutes of life, *J Pediatr Surg* 36:141, 2001.

310. Krummel TM, Greenfield LJ, Kirkpatrick BV, et al: Clinical use of an extracorporeal membrane oxygenator in neonatal pulmonary failure, *J Pediatr Surg* 17:525, 1982.

311. Heiss K, Manning P, Oldham KT, et al: Reversal of mortality for congenital diaphragmatic hernia with ECMO, *Ann Surg* 209:225, 1989.

312. Wung JT, James LS, Kilchevsky E, et al: Management of infants with severe respiratory failure and persistence of the fetal circulation, without hyperventilation, *Pediatrics* 76:488, 1985.

313. Kolobow T, Moretti MP, Fumagalli R, et al: Severe impairment in lung function induced by high peak airway pressure during mechanical ventilation. An experimental study, *Am Rev Respir Dis* 135:312, 1987.

314. Tsuno K, Prato P, Kolobow T: Acute lung injury from mechanical ventilation at moderately high airway pressures, *J Appl Physiol* 69: 956, 1990.

315. Wilson JM, Lund DP, Lillehei CW, et al: Congenital diaphragmatic hernia—a tale of two cities: the Boston experience. *J Pediatr Surg* 32:401, 1997.

316. Drummond WH, Gregory GA, Heymann MA, et al: The independent effects of hyperventilation, tolazoline, and dopamine on infants with persistent pulmonary hypertension, *J Pediatr* 98:603, 1981.

317. Wilson JM, Lund DP, Lillehei CW, et al: Delayed repair and preoperative ECMO does not improve survival in high-risk congenital diaphragmatic hernia, *J Pediatr Surg* 27:368, 1992.

318. de la Hunt MN, Madden N, Scott JE, et al: Is delayed surgery really better for congenital diaphragmatic hernia? A prospective randomized clinical trial, *J Pediatr Surg* 31:1554, 1996.

319. Reickert CA, Hirshl RB, Schumacher R, et al: Effect of very delayed repair of congenital diaphragmatic hernia on survival and extracorporeal life support use, *Surgery* 120:766, 1996.

320. Wung JT, Sahni R, Moffitt ST, et al: Congenital diaphragmatic hernia: survival treated with very delayed surgery, spontaneous respiration, and no chest tube, *J Pediatr Surg* 30:406, 1995.

321. Frenckner B, Ehren H, Granholm T, et al: Improved results in patients who have congenital diaphragmatic hernia using preoperative stabilization, extracorporeal membrane oxygenation, and delayed surgery, *J Pediatr Surg* 32:1185, 1997.

322. Breaux CW, Rouse TM, Cain WAS, et al: Improvement in survival of patients with congenital diaphragmatic hernia utilizing a strategy of delayed repair after medical and/or extracorporeal membrane oxygenation stabilization, *J Pediatr Surg* 26:333, 1991.

323. West KW, Bengston K, Rescorla FJ, et al: Delayed surgical repair and ECMO improves survival in congenital diaphragmatic hernia, *Ann Surg* 216:454, 1992.

324. Rose MI, Smith SD, Chen H: Inappropriate fluid response in congenital diaphragmatic hernia: first report of a frequent occurrence, *J Pediatr Surg* 23: 1147, 1988.

325. Redmond C, Heaton J, Calix J, et al: A correlation of pulmonary hypoplasia, mean airway pressure, and survival in congenital diaphragmatic hernia treated with extracorporeal membrane oxygenation, *J Pediatr Surg* 22:1143, 1987.

326. Johnston PW, Bashener B, Liberman R, et al: Clinical use of extracorporeal membrane oxygenation in the treatment of persistent pulmonary hypertension following surgical repair of congenital diaphragmatic hernia, *J Pediatr Surg* 23:908, 1988.

327. Thurlbeck WM, Kida K, Langston C, et al: Postnatal lung growth after repair of diaphragmatic hernia, *Thorax* 34:338, 1979.

328. Wohl M, Griscom NT, Stnede DJ, et al: The lung following repair of congenital diaphragmatic hernia, *J Pediatr* 90:405, 1977.

329. Reid IS, Hutcherson RJ: Long-term follow-up of patients with congenital diaphragmatic hernia, *J Pediatr Surg* 11:939, 1976.

330. Chatrath RR, el-Shafie M, Jones RS: Fate of hypoplastic lungs after repair of congenital diaphragmatic hernia, *Arch Dis Child* 46:633, 1971.

331. van Murs KP, Robbins ST, Reed VL, et al: Congenital diaphragmatic hernia: long-term outcome in neonates teated with extracorporeal membrane oxygenation, *J Pediatr* 122:893,1993.

332. Naik S, Greenaugh A, Zhang YX, et al: Prediction of morbidity during infancy after repair of congenital diaphragmatic hernia, *J Pediatr Surg* 31:1651, 1996.

333. D'Agostino JA, Bernbaum JC, Gerdes M, et al: Outcome for infants with congenital diaphragmatic hernia requiring extracorporeal membrane oxygenation: the first year, *J Pediatr Surg* 30:10, 1995.

334. Andrews AF, Nixon CA, Cilley RE et al: One- to three-year outcome for 14 neonatal survivors of extracorporeal membrane oxygenation, *Pediatrics* 78:692, 1986.

335. Krummel TM, Greenfeld LJ, Kirkpatrick BV, et al: The early evaluation of survivors after extracorporeal membrane oxygenation for neonatal pulmonary failure, *J Pediatr Surg* 19:585, 1984.

336. Towne BH, Lott IT, Hicks DA, et al: Long-term follow-up of infants and children treated with extracorporeal membrane oxygenation (ECMO), *J Pediatr Surg* 20:410, 1985.

337. Lessin MS, Thompson IM, Deprez M, et al: Congenital diaphragmatic hernia with or without extracorporeal membrane oxygenation: are we making progress? *J Am Coll Surg* 181:65, 1995.

338. Wilson JM, Lund DP, Lillhei CW, et al: Delayed repair and preoperative ECMO does not improve survival in high-risk congenital diaphragmatic hernia, *J Pediatr Surg* 27:368,1992.

339. Harrison MR, Langer JC, Adzick NS, et al: Correction of congenital diaphragmatic hernia in utero, V. initial clinical experience, *J Pediatr Surg* 25:47, 1990.

340. Harrison MR, Adzick NS, Flake AW, et al: Correction of congenital diaphragmatic hernia in utero: VI. hard-earned lessons, *J Pediatr Surg* 28:1411, 1993.

341. Hedrick MH, Estes JM, Sullivan KM, et al: Plug the lung until it grows (PLUG): a new method to treat congenital diaphragmatic hernia in utero, *J Pediatr Surg* 31:1335, 1996.

342. Skarsgard ED, Meuli M, VanderWall KJ, et al: Fetal endoscopic tracheal occlusion (Fetendo-PLUG) for congenital diaphragmatic hernia, *J Pediatr Surg* 31:1335, 1996.

343. Harrison MR, Mychaliska GB, Albanese CT, et al: Correction of congenital diaphragmatic hernia in utero IX: fetuses with poor prognosis (liver herniation) can be saved by fetoscopic temporary tracheal occlusion, *J Pediatr Surg* 33:1017, 1998.

344. Waterston DJ, Bonham-Carter RE, Aberdeen E: Congenital tracheoesophageal fistula in association with esophageal atresia, *Lancet* 2:55, 1963.

345. Barry JE, Auldist AW: The VATER association: one end of a spectrum of anomalies, *Am J Dis Child* 128:769, 1974.

346. Rittler M, Paz JE, Castilla EE: VACTERL association, epidemiologic definition and delineation, *Am J Med Gen* 63:529, 1996.

347. Smith RM: *Anesthesia for infants and children,* ed 4, St Louis, Mo. 1980, Mosby.

348. Spitz L, Kiely EM, Morecroft JA, et al: Oesophageal atresia: at risk groups for the 1990s, *J Pediatr Surg* 29:723, 1994.

349. Myers NA, Aberdeen E: Congenital esophageal atresia and tracheoesophageal fistula. In Ravitch MM, Welch KJ, Benson CD, et al (eds): *Pediatric surgery,* p 446, Chicago, 1979, Year Book Publishers.

350. Templeton JM, Templeton JJ, Schnaufer L, et al: Management of esophageal atresia and tracheoesophageal fistula in the neonate with severe respiratory distress syndrome, *J Pediatr Surg* 20:394, 1985.

351. Abrahamson J, Shandling B: Esophageal atresia in the underweight baby. A challenge, *J Pediatr Surg* 7:608, 1972.
352. Dryden GE: Gastric distention during tracheoesophageal fistula repair, *J Indiana Med Assoc* 62:46, 1969.
353. Salem MR, Wong AY, Lin YH, et al: Prevention of gastric distention during anesthesia for newborns with tracheoesophageal fistulas, *Anesthesiology* 38:82, 1973.
354. Jones TB, Kirchner SG, Lee F, et al: Stomach rupture associated with esophageal atresia, tracheoesophageal fistula and ventilatory assistance, *AJR* 134:675, 1980.
355. Pohlson EC, Schaller RT, Tapper D: Improved survival with primary anastomosis in the low-birth-weight neonate with esophageal atresia and tracheoesophageal fistula, *J Pediatr Surg* 23:418, 1988.
356. Reeves ST, Burt N, Smith CD: Is it time to reevaluate the airway management of tracheoesophageal fistula? *Anesth Analg* 81:866, 1995.
357. Myers CR, Love JW: Gastrostomy as a gas vent in repair to tracheoesophageal fistula, *Anesth Analg* 47:119, 1968.
358. Karl HW: Control of life-threatening air leak after gastrostomy in an infant with respiratory distress syndrome and tracheoesophageal fistula, *Anesthesiology* 62:670, 1985.
359. Buchino J, Keenan WJ, Pretsch JB, et al: Malposition of the endotracheal tube in infants with tracheoesophageal fistula, *J Pediatr* 109:524, 1986.
360. Block ED, Filston HC: A thin fiberoptic bronchoscope as an aid to occlusion of the fistula in infants with tracheoesophageal fistula, *Anesth Analg* 67:791, 1988.
361. Filston HC, Chitwood WF, Schkolne B, et al: The Fogarty balloon catheter as an aid to management of the infant with esophageal atresia and tracheoesophageal fistula complicated by severe RDS or pneumonia, *J Pediatr Surg* 17:149, 1982.
362. Northrip DR, Bohman BK, Tsueda K: Total airway occlusion and superior vena cava syndrome with anterior mediastinal tumor, *Anesth Analg* 65:1079, 1986.
363. Mackie AM, Watson CB: Anaesthesia and mediastinal masses, *Anaesthesia* 34:899, 1984.
364. Miller RM, Simpson JS, Ein SH: Mediastinal masses in infants and children, *Pediatr Clin North Am* 26:677, 1979.
365. Yellin A, Rosen A, Reichert N, et al: Superior vena cava syndrome. the myth—the facts, *Am Rev Respir Dis* 141:1114, 1990.
366. Dwieck H: The patient with an anterior mediastinal mass, *Anesth News* May:26-31, 1995.
367. Riley RH, Harris LA, Davis, NJ, et al: Superior vena cava syndrome following general anesthesia, *Anaesth Intens Care* 20:229, 1992.
368. Kirks DR, Fram EK, Vock P, et al: Tracheal compression by mediastinal masses in children: CT evaluation, *AJR* 141:647, 1983.
369. Shamberger RC, Hozman RS, Griscom NT, et al: CT-guided quantitation of tracheal cross-sectional area as a guide to the surgical and anesthetic management of children with anterior mediastinal masses, *J Pediatr Surg* 26:138, 1991.

370. Keon TP: Death on induction of anesthesia for cervical node biopsy, *Anesthesiology* 55:471, 1981.
371. Neumann GG, Weignarten AE, Abramowitz RM, et al: The anesthetic management of the patient with an anterior mediastinal mass, *Anesthesiology* 60:144, 1984.
372. Halpern S, Chatten J, Meadows AT, et al: Anterior mediastinal masses: anesthesia hazards and other problems, *J Pediatr* 102:407, 1983.
373. Johnson D, Hurst T, Cujec B, et al: Cardiopulmonary effects of an anterior mediastinal mass in dogs, *Anesthesiology* 74:725, 1991.
374. Prakash VBS, Abel MD, Hubmayr RD: Mediastinal mass and tracheal obstruction during general anesthesia, *Mayo Clin Proc* 63:1004, 1988.
375. Azizkhan RG, Dudgeon DL, Buck JR, et al: Life-threatening airway obstruction as a complication of the management of mediastinal masses in children, *J Pediatr Surg* 20:816, 1985.
376. John RE, Narang VPS: A boy with an anterior mediastinal mass, *Anaesthesia* 43:864, 1988.
377. Narang S, Harte BH, Body SC: Anesthesia for patients with a mediastinal mass, *Anesth Clin North Am* 19:559, 2001.
378. Ferrari LR, Bedford RF: General anesthesia prior to treatment of anterior mediastinal masses in pediatric cancer patients, *Anesthesiology* 72:991, 1990.
379. Sibert KS, Biondi JW, Hirsch NP, et al: Spontaneous respiration during thoracotomy in a patient with a mediastinal mass, *Anesth Analg* 66:904, 1987.
380. Cirino LM, Milanez de Campos JR, Fernandez A, et al: Diagnosis and treatment of mediastinal tumors by thoracoscopy, *Chest* 117:1787, 2000.
381. Tinker TD, Crane DL: Safety of anesthesia for patients with anterior mediastinal masses, *Anesthesiology* 73:1060, 1990.
382. Sweeney DB, Allen TH, Steven IM: Acute epiglottitis: management by intubation, *Anesth Intensive Care* 1:526, 1973.
383. Thibault DW: Patent ductus arteriosus complicating the respiratory distress syndrome in preterm infants, *J Pediatr* 86:120, 1975.
384. McMurphy DM, Heyman MA, Rudolph AM, McImon KL: Developmental change in constriction of the ductus arteriosus: response to oxygen and vasoactive substances in the isolated ductus arteriosus of the fetal lamb, *Pediatr Res* 6:231, 1972.
385. Ellison RC, Peckham GJ, Lang P, et al: Evaluation of preterm infant for patent ductus arteriosus, *Pediatrics* 71:364, 1983.
386. Rosen DA, Rosen KR: Anomalies of the aortic arch and valve. In Lake CL (ed): *Pediatric cardiac anesthesia*, ed 3, p 453, East Norwalk, Conn., 1998, Appleton and Lang.
387. Hishitani T, Ogawa K, Hoshino K, et al: Usefulness of continuous monitoring of airway resistance and flow-volume curve in the perioperative management of infants with central airway obstruction: a case of vascular ring, *J Thorac Cardiovasc Surg* 122:1229, 2001.
388. Dajani AS, Taubert KA, Wilson W, et al: Prevention of bacterial endocarditis, *Circulation* 96:358, 1997.

Appendix 16-1 Anesthetic Considerations for Pediatric Patients Requiring Surgery for Thoracic Abnormalities

Achalasia

Description—Motor disturbance of the esophagus in which the cardia does not relax during swallowing, resulting in esophageal dilation, esophagitis, regurgitation, failure to thrive, and, often, aspiration pneumonitis.

Anesthetic and perioperative considerations—Preexisting chronic aspiration pneumonitis and poor nutritional status often necessitate postoperative mechanical ventilation and vigorous chest physiotherapy, and sometimes a regimen of total parenteral nutrition.

Agenesis, Aphasia, or Hypoplasia of Lung or Lobe(s)

Description—Embryologic defects; symptoms vary from none to severe respiratory insufficiency.

Anesthetic and perioperative considerations—Mediastinum may be markedly shifted toward affected side; trachea may be kinked; associated vascular hypoplasia and pulmonary arterial hypertension; therapeutic or diagnostic bronchoscopy is often necessary for severe respiratory infections.

Bronchiectasis

Description—Dilation of bronchi from inflammatory destruction of bronchial and peribronchial tissues; exudates often accumulate in dependent areas or in affected lung.

Anesthetic and perioperative considerations—Bronchoscopy and bronchography are often helpful in defining the extent of the process and in obtaining cultures directly from affected areas. If medical therapy fails, lobectomy is indicated.

Bronchobiliary Fistula

Description—A fistula connecting the right middle lobe bronchus and the left hepatic duct.

Anesthetic and perioperative considerations—Bronchoscopy and bronchography for diagnosis and surgical excision of the intrathoracic portion of the fistula. Severe recurrent respiratory infections and atelectasis dictate vigorous preoperative and postoperative chest physiotherapy and often-repeated therapeutic bronchoscopy.

Bronchopulmonary Dysplasia

Description—Chronic lung disease occurring in preterm infants with hyaline membrane disease who require long-term artificial ventilation. Results from a combination of factors, including barotrauma, oxygen, infection, and scarring. Patients usually manifest hypoxemia, hypercarbia, and increased pulmonary vascular resistance. Cor pulmonale and congestive heart failure may also be present.

Anesthetic and perioperative considerations—Effects of bronchopulmonary dysplasia may persist well beyond the first year of life. Infants frequently undergo chronic bronchodilator and diuretic therapy, which may require adjustment in the perioperative period. Careful attention to electrolytes and fluid administration is necessary. Nitrous oxide, as a part of the anesthetic regimen, may be contraindicated because of emphysematous airtrapping. Ventilatory patterns during anesthesia should be designed to allow for adequate expiratory time and to avoid excessive airway pressure so that the possibility of pneumothorax is minimized. Postoperative apnea monitoring and pulse oximetry are usually indicated for up to 24 hours or longer.

Chylothorax

Description—Chylous pleural effusion that could be due to a congenital abnormality of the thoracic duct or trauma, especially after palliative cardiovascular procedures involving a left thoracotomy.

Anesthetic and perioperative considerations—Conservative management usually suffices (repeated aspiration and insertion of thoracostomy tube connected to underwater seal). Persistent drainage (longer than 3 or 4 weeks) after appropriate conservative measures may be treated surgically by ligation of the thoracic duct just above the diaphragm. Loss of protein often results in severe nutritional problems, and hyperalimentation is usually required.

Corrosive or Caustic Burns of the Esophagus

Description—Chemical burns of mucosa.

Anesthetic and perioperative considerations—Initially, esophagoscopy is usually done to determine the extent of damage. Burns of epiglottic and laryngeal mucosa can compromise the airway and make intubation difficult.

Cystic Adenomatoid Malformation

Description—Malformed bronchi lead to irregular aeration. Air accumulates in the potential cystic structures.

Anesthetic and perioperative considerations—Sudden massive blood loss can result during removal from avulsion of vessels arising from the aorta and entering cystic areas. Preoperative arteriography should define the extent and location of blood supply. May mimic congenital diaphragmatic hernia on chest x-ray.

Cystic Fibrosis

Description—Multisystem disease of exocrine cells affecting lungs and pancreas.

Anesthetic and perioperative considerations—This chronic lung disease leads to pulmonary insufficiency in many patients. Pulmonary complications include pneumothorax and massive hemoptysis from erosion of enlarged thin-walled bronchial vessels. Bronchoscopy for therapeutic bronchial lavage or for location of bleeding site with subsequent resection or embolization of bleeding bronchial vessels may be necessary. For selected patients with more localized lung disease, pulmonary resection may be performed. Respiratory support with tracheal intubation and mechanical ventilation during infectious exacerbations are not uncommon.

Cystic Hygroma

Description—A cystic tumor arising along the course of the primitive lymphatic sacs.

Anesthetic and perioperative considerations—Most commonly seen in the neck region. They may be very large and impinge on normal airway structures and result in obstruction of the upper airway, making intubation difficult; occasionally, they extend into the mediastinum.

Diaphragmatic Hernias

Foramen of Bochdalek hernia

Description—Posterolateral (usually left) diaphragmatic defect allowing herniation of abdominal contents into thoracic cavity, with compression of the ipsilateral lung and shift of the mediastinum toward the contralateral side.

Anesthetic and perioperative considerations—Often, the most serious of all neonatal surgical problems because of rapidly progressive respiratory failure and early death if not corrected quickly. Resuscitative measures (intubation, ventilation, and treatment of metabolic and respiratory acidosis) must be instituted immediately. Extracorporeal membrane oxygenation may be beneficial in neonates with severe respiratory compromise.

Foramen of Morgagni Hernia

Description—Retrosternal herniation of portion of bowel. Usually presents later and less dramatically than Bochdalek hernia.

Anesthetic and perioperative considerations—May be asymptomatic. Surgical repair is indicated when diagnosed because of the risk of incarceration. May occur in pericardium, resulting in compromise of cardiac output.

Ectopic Bronchus (Epiarterial Bronchus, "Pig Bronchus")

Description—Origin of right upper-lobe bronchus from trachea.

Anesthetic and perioperative considerations—Tracheal intubation may block right upper-lobe bronchus, resulting in atelectasis; ectopic bronchus may be associated with chronic right upper-lobe infection and bronchiectasis.

Empyema

Description—Accumulation of pleural space, often associated with staphylococcal pneumonia.

Anesthetic and perioperative considerations—Large empyemas can compress the lung and compromise respiratory function; they are usually managed with a thoracostomy tube placed under local anesthesia. Chronic empyema may require decortication of the fibrinous covering on parenchymal and pleural surfaces to reexpand the affected lung.

Erb-Duchenne Palsy

Description—Injury (usually birth trauma) to the upper brachial plexus (fifth and sixth cervical nerves) resulting in loss of ability to abduct the arm from the shoulder, externally rotate the arm, or supinate the forearm. Muscle function of the hand is retained.

Anesthetic and perioperative considerations—This and other forms of brachial plexus injuries may be associated with phrenic nerve injuries and paralysis of the diaphragm on the involved side.

Esophageal Duplication (Enteric Cyst)

Description—Spherical or tubular posterior mediastinal structures with muscular walls and lining of any type of gastrointestinal epithelium or cileated epithelium. Associated anomalies include hemivertebrae of upper thoracic spine and intraabdominal enteric cysts. These usually do not communicate with the lumen of the esophagus but may be connected to the small bowel.

Anesthetic and perioperative considerations—Large cysts can compress the lung. Because they frequently contain acid-secreting gastric mucosa, peptic ulceration may occur and erode into lung, bronchus, or esophagus with resulting hemorrhage.

Esophageal Perforation

Description—Usually traumatic, caused by instrumentation for preexisting disease. May occur in newborn (usually on the right side) from birth trauma; presents as a sudden respiratory collapse accompanied by hydropneumothorax.

Anesthetic and perioperative considerations—Esophagoscopy for preexisting disease (stricture of esophagus from corrosive burns or tracheoesophageal fistula) is a common procedure in pediatric patients. Anesthesia must be appropriately deep to prevent coughing while the esophagoscope is in place. In newborns presenting with hydropneumothorax from esophageal perforation, immediate aspiration is necessary, followed by thoracotomy and repair of the perforation.

Esophageal Stenosis

Description—Rarely, a congenital defect associated with tracheoesophageal fistula without esophageal atresia, or as isolated congenital stenosis in which the esophageal wall contains tissues of respiratory tract origin, including ciliated epithelium and cartilage. More commonly, this condition is acquired and associated with esophageal reflux.

Anesthetic and perioperative considerations—Excision is required if ectopic tissue is present. Repeated esophageal dilations are indicated, either with esophagoscope or by bougienage, to alleviate restenosis due to scar tissue formation. Esophageal perforation is always a possible complication. Infants are often malnourished and require total parenteral nutrition.

Esophageal Stricture

Description—The result of trauma to the esophagus from several possible causes: tracheoesophageal fistula repair, corrosive burns of esophagus, or congenital esophageal stenosis.

Anesthetic and perioperative considerations—Requires repeated dilations, with perforation always a possible complication. Colon interposition (or other visceral esophageal bypass) may be necessary.

Esophagitis

Description—In infants, this could be the result of gastroesophageal reflux with or without hiatal hernia and may subside spontaneously by 12 months of age if no hiatus hernia is associated. May present as recurrent apnea or failure to thrive from recurrent vomiting during early infancy, and respiratory infections from repeated aspirations could be quite severe. If symptoms cannot be controlled by propping the baby in infant seat to prevent reflux, some form of antireflux procedure may be indicated. Anemia can result fiom chronic blood loss. (See *gastroesophageal reflux* later.)

Eventration of the Diaphragm

Description—Congenital defect of the muscular layer of the diaphragm allowing (usually) minor herniation of part of abdominal organs into the chest, usually right-sided. The condition may be asymptomatic or, rarely, it may present similarly to a Bochdalek hernia. Respiratory symptoms depend on the extent of herniation of the abdominal contents and range from minimal to severe; gastric volvulus can result when there is significant eventration of the left hemidiaphragm.

Anesthetic and perioperative considerations—On chest x-ray, there is usually a smooth dome-shaped elevation of the diaphragmatic shadow on the affected side with loss of lung volume. Small asymptomatic eventrations should be corrected whether or not they are symptomatic. If respiratory infection is present, appropriate medical therapy with antibiotics, chest physiotherapy, and even therapeutic bronchoscopy is usually indicated prior to correction.

Gastroesophageal Reflux (Chalasia)

Description—Results from dysfunction of esophagogastric junctions; may or may not be associated with hiatus hernia.

Anesthetic and perioperative considerations—Vomiting, malnutrition, failure to thrive, recurrent respiratory infections, and chronic anemia characterize these infants. Condition may clear spontaneously by 12 to 18 months of age with conservative treatment (frequent feedings and propping baby in infant seat). Hyperalimentation is often necessary. Indications for

antireflux procedure include esophagitis, esophageal stricture, significant hiatus hernia, and recurrent and unresponsive pulmonary problems resulting from aspiration. Ventilatory support after repair is often required because of the poor general condition of the patient as well as to preexisting pulmonary infection.

Hemothorax and Hemopneumothorax

Description—Usually the result of trauma induced either accidentally or surgically. Coexisting pneumothorax is common.

Anesthetic and perioperative considerations—The hemothorax or hemopneumothorax must be drained with thoracostomy tubes, usually employing local anesthesia. Blood loss into chest cavity can be massive; portions of the lung may become trapped by clotted blood that will not drain through a thoracostomy tube, in which case open thoracotomy could be required to remove clotting and reexpand the lung. Traumatic left-sided hemothoraces are more commonly associated with injuries to the great vessels, whereas those on the right are usually due to injury to the pulmonary hilum. Respiratory support may be necessary during recovery.

Hiatal Hernia

Description—Herniation of the upper part of the stomach into the left hemithorax; the sliding type is more common than the paraesophageal type.

Anesthetic and perioperative considerations—See *gastroesophageal reflux* and *esophagitis* above. Treatment is usually directed at associated gastroesophageal reflux. Chronic aspiration and pulmonary disease may be significant.

Hyaline Membrane Disease

Description—Idiopathic respiratory distress syndrome primarily seen in premature newborns as a result of surfactant deficiency. May occur in infants of diabetic mothers at a greater gestational age or those born by cesarean section or under other stressful conditions during labor and delivery. Hypoaerated and poorly compliant lungs are typical; long-term ventilatory support may be required. Damage to upper airway may result in subglottic stenosis. Ligation of patent ductus arteriosus may be required during the course of treatment. Bronchopulmonary dysplasia (chronic lung disease) is a common sequela.

Kartagener's Syndrome

Description—Situs inversus totalis, paranasal sinusitis, bronchiectasis.

Anesthetic and perioperative considerations—May require excision of the bronchiectatic segment of lung.

Lobar Emphysema, Congenital

Description—Obstructive emphysema, usually of one of the upper lobes (the left upper lobe, most commonly). May be the result of defective bronchial cartilage to the affected lobe.

Anesthetic and perioperative considerations—May cause severe respiratory symptoms in newborn period requiring immediate surgical intervention, or may not become symptomatic for up to 5 to 6 months. Lobectomy is the treatment of choice. Intubation and positive pressure ventilation can further overinflate the lobe and compromise respiratory exchange in other parts of the lung. During induction of anesthesia, spontaneous ventilation should preserved until the chest is opened and the emphysematous lobe is brought out of the operative site. Nitrous oxide should not be used until after lobectomy is accomplished. After the lobectomy is accomplished, the remaining tissue should be gently reexpanded under direct vision before beginning closure of the thoracotomy incision.

Lobar Emphysema, Acquired

Description—Usually the result of localized obstruction from foreign bodies, inflammatory reaction, extrinsic compression of the bronchus or of a bronchiole by lymph nodes, or a tumor in the mediastinum. (Extrinsic bronchial compression usually results in atelectasis, but emphysema results only rarely.)

Anesthetic and perioperative considerations—Bronchoscopy is usually required for diagnosis and is therapeutic in the instance of a suspected or known foreign body. (See the section of this chapter on bronchoscopy.) Anesthetic considerations are similar to those for congenital lobar emphysema.

Lung Abscess

Description—In infants and children, this condition usually results from aspiration of infected material when pulmonary defense mechanisms are overwhelmed or when there is serious systemic disease or immunosuppression.

Anesthetic and perioperative considerations—Bronchoscopy may be diagnostic as well as therapeutic. Long-term medical therapy with large doses of intravenous antibiotics plus intermittent bronchoscopy to promote drainage usually suffice. Although resection is difficult in children, it can be accomplished using a balloon-tipped Fogarty catheter placed in the bronchus during bronchoscopy (see the section of this chapter on bronchoscopy).

Lung Cysts, Bronchogenic

Description—Usually unilobar and thick-walled structures lined with respiratory epithelium; may be located within the lung, mediastinum, or pericardial sac adjacent to main bronchi. Only occasionally communicates with bronchus.

Anesthetic and perioperative considerations—May not be seen on x-ray, but may produce compression of trachea or bronchus. May be difficult to find and to dissect, especially if within the mediastinum. Injury to the phrenic nerve or to other mediastinal structures can complicate the postoperative course.

Lung Cysts, True Congenital

Description—May be unilobar or multilobar, with extensive compromise of adjacent lung tissue and other intrathoracic structures.

Anesthetic and perioperative considerations—Communications with bronchial air passages make infection almost inevitable. Appropriate antibiotics and therapeutic bronchoscopy may be indicated prior to excision of cystic lobe, but

significant compromise of lung function (either from compression or infection) may make excision urgent. Postoperative ventilator support, especially in the chronically ill and malnourished infant or child, may be necessary.

Mediastinal Emphysema (Pneumomediastinum)

Description—Air in mediastinum.

Anesthetic and perioperative considerations—Often associated with RDS of premature infants and in children with respiratory distress from any cause. Usually associated with pneumothorax, which can necessitate drainage through catheter or thoracotomy tube. May be seen after tracheotomy and esophageal or tracheal perforation. A tension pneumothorax or large pneumopericardium resulting in tamponade requires immediate treatment to remove air. Nitrous oxide should not be used as part of anesthetic management in patients with pneumomediastinum or pneumothorax.

Mediastinal Masses, Cysts, and Tumors

Description—Epithelium-lined cystic masses of enteric, neurogenic, bronchogenic, or coelomic origin, or solid vascular or granulomatous tumors, malignant or benign, primary or metastatic.

Anesthetic and perioperative considerations—May be asymptomatic, even when quite large. Clinical manifestations appear from expanding, space-occupying structure and depend on location. Tracheal or bronchial compression may result in respiratory distress, making thoracotomy urgent. Intubation can be difficult if tracheal deviation is present, and appropriate measures to cope with difficult intubation—including preparation for bronchoscopy and tracheostomy—should be taken before anesthesia is begun. May present with respiratory (shortness of breath, positional dyspnea, etc.), cardiovascular (caval compression, positional intolerance, etc.), or pericardial (tamponade) symptoms. Induction of anesthesia might result in acute airway obstruction and inability to ventilate or in cardiovascular collapse. Ventilatory support may be necessary postoperatively owing to tracheomalacia or bronchomalacia.

Mediastinitis

Description—Severe systemic infection of mediastinal structures. May follow pharyngeal, esophageal, or tracheal perforation from any cause; thoracic or cervical operations complicated by wound infection; or rupture of infected mediastinal lymph nodes.

Anesthetic and perioperative considerations—Incision, drainage, and massive antibiotic therapy are required. May also require intermittent instillation of bacteriocidal solutions (such as povidone iodine) through mediastinal drainage tubes. A plastic surgical procedure involving a rectus flap transfer graft is effective in many cases of severe mediastinitis following sternotomy. Ventilatory support is usually necessary postoperatively.

Myasthenia Gravis

Description—Autoimmune disorder in which acetylcholine receptors in muscle are affected, resulting in weakness. May be seen in pediatric patients even in neonatal period and should always be suspected in infants of mothers with myasthenia. Infant may be receiving cholinesterase inhibitor therapy.

Anesthetic and perioperative considerations—In an infant born of a mother with myasthenia gravis, the condition can be transient or persistent and may require ventilatory support in the newborn. Muscle relaxants as adjunctive anesthetic agents are rarely, if ever, needed in myasthenic patients. Thymectomy may be indicated in patients unresponsive to medical management, and postoperative ventilatory support after thymectomy may be necessary. Cholinesterase inhibitor therapy should be part of the anesthetic considerations.

Pectus Deformities

Pectus Excavatum

Description—Funnel chest; severity varies from very mild (usually not requiring early surgical correction) to severe, requiring early surgical intervention. Usually sporadic incidence, but familial occurrence not rare; may often be seen in patients with Marfan syndrome. Frequently progressive.

Anesthetic and perioperative considerations—Usually thought to be "aymptomatic" in infancy and childhood, but subtle cardiac and pulmonary abnormalities have been shown to be present in many patients and are related to displacement and compression of the heart and to a decrease in intrathoracic volume. Besides the psychologic, cosmetic, and orthopedic reasons for correction, these pathophysiologic changes can become severe with progression over time. Anesthetic considerations during and after repair include the possibility of pneumothorax, the production of a "flail chest" if surgical dissection is extensive, and postoperative atelectasis from splinting due to pain.

Pectus Carinatum

Description—Pigeon breast; usually not apparent at birth, but becomes evident at 3 or 4 years of age. May be seen in patients with Marfan syndrome or congenital heart disease.

Anesthetic and perioperative considerations—The more severe forms can cause compression and displacement of the heart and reduction of intrathoracic volume, as is seen in pectus excavatum deformities. The same perioperative considerations apply as for pectus excavatum.

Pericardial Problems

Partial Absence of the Pericardium

Description—Can be total or partial; left (most common), right, or diaphragmatic. Can be associated with congenital diaphragmatic hernia or heart disease. Arises from defective formation of the pleuropericardial membrane or of the septum transversum.

Anesthetic and perioperative considerations—Total absence of the pericardium usually does not require surgical correction. Partial defects on the left can result in herniation of ventricles or left atrial appendage with strangulation. Right-sided defects may result in obstruction of the superior vena cava. Surgical treatment includes either enlargement of the defect to prevent strangulation or closure using a portion of the mediastinal pleura. When associated with diaphragmatic hernia or congenital heart disease, clinical findings usually are primarily due to the associated defect.

Pericardial Cysts

Description—Coelomic cyst, rare in childhood.

Anesthetic and perioperative considerations—Usually asymptomatic. Surgical removal is usually done to establish the diagnosis.

Pericarditis (Acute)

Description—May be primary (e.g., viral, rheumatic, bacterial, postpericardiotomy) or a secondary manifestation of systemic disease.

Anesthetic and perioperative considerations—Except for bacterial (purulent) pericarditis, the condition is usually self-limiting and rarely requires surgical intervention except for removal of fluid if signs of cardiac tamponade are present. Purulent pericarditis is usually secondary to a severe infectious process such as pneumonitis, osteomyelitis, or meningitis. *Staphlyococcus aureus* and *Haenophilus influenza* are the most common agents. Purulent pericarditis requires surgical drainage, vigorous antibiotic therapy, and general postoperative support measures with close monitoring.

Chronic Constrictive Pericarditis

Description—Rare in childhood; the etiology is usually unknown, but it may follow purulent or viral pericarditis.

Anesthetic and perioperative considerations—Radical pericardiectomy via median sternotomy may be required, with extensive resection of visceral and parietal pericardium from atria, cavae, and ventricles. Intraopertive and postoperative monitoring should include arterial and pulmonary artery catheters and urinary output. Postoperative ventilatory support is usually required.

Pericardial Effusion with Cardiac Tamponade

Description—Unusual in childhood, except after cardiovascular surgical procedures, including non–open heart operations.

Anesthetic and perioperative considerations—Cardiac tamponade occurs when blood, fluid, or air within the pericardium interferes with ventricular filling during diastole and reduces stroke volume and cardiac output. It is most commonly seen after surgery and must be considered first in differential diagnosis if a low cardiac output state exists in such patients. Treatment of acute tamponade in postoperative patients includes immediate opening of the chest incision to relieve compression and to control bleeding; tamponade in other situations (rheumatic, viral, or bacterial infections) may be treated initially by echocardiographically guided needle drainage in emergent situations, but almost always requires surgical drainage (see above). Cardiac-depressant drugs such as thiopental and the potent inhalation anesthetics should be avoided during anesthesia, but the principal problem is decreased ventricular volume.

Pneumomediastinum

Description—Air in mediastinum.

Anesthetic and perioperative considerations—See *mediastinal emphysema*, above.

Pneumopericardium

Description—Air in the pericardium.

Anesthetic and perioperative considerations—May be associated with pneumothorax and pneumomediastinum in premature newborns with RDS. Sufficient quantities of air, like quantities of blood or other fluids, may result in cardiac tamponade and require removal by pericardiocentesis.

Pneumothorax

Description—Air in the pleural space.

Anesthetic and perioperative considerations—May occur during anesthesia, especially in patients requiring high inflation pressure to expand lungs because of any cause (e.g., infants with idiopathic respiratory distress or congenital diaphragmatic hernia). Treatment of significant pneumothorax (probably greater than 30%) involves needle aspiration or thoracostomy tube so that the lung can be expanded. The presence of a pneumothorax precludes the use of nitrous oxide during anesthesia, at least until the chest is opened or a thoracotomy tube is inserted. Tension pneumothorax (see below).

Pneumatocele

Description—Emphysematous blebs or cysts resulting from rupture of alveoli so that single or multilocular cavities occur; the condition is usually the result of *S. aureus* pneumonia, but it may be congenital (bullous emphysema).

Anesthetic and perioperative considerations—Pneumatoceles in patients with *S. aureus* pneumonia may require thoracostomy drainage to treat respiratory distress or tension pneumothorax. These complications can occur suddenly and without warning.

Phrenic Nerve Palsy

Description—Traumatic origin.

Anesthetic and perioperative considerations—Trauma to either phrenic nerve from birth injury (e.g., breech delivery) or surgical trauma (e.g., Blalock-Taussig or Blalock-Hanlon operation) results in upward displacement and decreased movement of the ipsilateral diaphragm. Lung volume is decreased and ventilatory exchange is impaired. Phrenic nerve palsy must be differentiated from eventration of diaphragm or diaphragmatic hernia. Spontaneous recovery can occur, but occasionally plication of the diaphragm on the affected side is necessary to improve respiratory function.

Poland's Syndrome

Description—A spectrum of defects, usually unilateral, in which there is absence of the pectoralis minor and part of pectoralis major muscles, along with defects of costal cartilages and ribs at the sternal insertions, hypoplasia of subcutaneous tissue, and upward displacement and hypoplasia of the nipple and breast on the affected side. Hand deformities may also be associated.

Anesthetic and perioperative considerations—Paradoxic movement with respirations is seen in larger defects. Usually asymptomatic, but it may be surgically corrected to prevent progressive deformity of chest wall, as well as for psychologic and cosmetic reasons. After correction of larger defects, ventilatory support may be required as with more extensive pectus repairs (see above).

Pulmonary Artery Sling

Description—Anomalous left pulmonary artery arising from the right pulmonary artery and coursing towards the left side over the right mainstem bronchus and behind the lower trachea between the trachea and esophagus.

Anesthetic and perioperative considerations—One of the most severe types of vascular malformations that compresses the trachea and esophagus. Compression of right mainstem bronchus can result in obstructive emphysema and/or atelectasis of the right lung. Hypoplasia of the distal trachea and right bronchus along with defective tracheal and bronchial cartilages make ventilatory management difficult. There is a high incidence of associated congenital cardiac defects (see the section of this chapter on vascular rings).

Pulmonary Arteriovenous Fistula

Description—Fistulous and often aneurysmal connection between pulmonary artery and vein; may be single but often is multiple. There is a high incidence in patients with Osler-Weber-Rendu hereditary hemorrhagic telangiectasia.

Anesthetic and perioperative considerations—Signs and symptoms depend on the size and extent of shunting of unsaturated blood into the systemic circulation. Cyanosis and polycythemia can be severe. Brain abscess, hemoptysis, or hemorrhage into the pleural space can occur. Congestive heart failure is rare. Surgery is indicated in most cases unless there are multiple fistulae involving both lungs. Anesthetic considerations are the same as with any patient with a right-to-left shunt. Postoperative ventilatory support might be necessary if the dissection is extensive.

Pulmonary Sequestration

Description—The accessory lower lobe is almost always located in the left hemithorax. There is nonfunctioning pulmonary tissue, usually with no connection to the airway system or to the pulmonary arterial tree; blood supply is from the systemic circulation.

Anesthetic and perioperative considerations—May be asymptomatic or may present as recurrent pneumonia in the region of the left lower lobe. Surgery is indicated because of a high incidence of infection in sequestered lobes. Aortography to determine origin of the blood supply is helpful in avoiding significant blood loss during surgical removal.

Right Middle Lobe Syndrome

Description—Extrinsic compression and obstruction of the right middle-lobe bronchus resulting in pneumonitis, atelectasis, and eventually, bronchiectasis. Compression is usually due to mediastinal lymph nodes.

Anesthetic and perioperative considerations—Diagnostic and therapeutic bronchoscopy are often required. Persistent or recurrent right middle-lobe collapse often makes lobectomy necessary.

Scimitar Syndrome

Description—Anomalous venous return from the right lung to the inferior vena cava with an intact atrial septum.

Anesthetic and perioperative considerations—Correction requires cardiopulmonary bypass. Physiology and hemodynamics are similar to those found in secundum arial septal defects. There may be abnormalities of the lung parenchyma as well as of the right pulmonary arterial tree.

Sternal Clefts

Description—May vary from small V-shaped defects in the upper sternum to complete separation of the sternum, with the heart outside the pericardium and the chest wall (ectopia cordis).

Anesthetic and perioperative considerations—With larger clefts, the heart and great vessels are covered only by skin and subcutaneous tissue. Direct closure may compress the heart and lungs. May be associated with diaphragmatic and abdominal wall defects. True ectopia cordis is very rare and carries a grave prognosis, as severe anomalies of the inside of the heart and of the great vessels are invariably present.

Subcutaneous Emphysema

Description—Air in the subcutaneous tissues.

Anesthetic and perioperative considerations—Usually due to the rupture of alveoli into mediastinal structures, with subsequent dissection of air into the mediastinum and into subcutaneous tissues of the chest, neck, and face. May occur after tracheostomy or be associated with pneumothorax and pneumomediastinum in RDS. Treatment is directed at the underlying cause.

Subglottic Stenosis

Description—Narrowing of the cricoid area of the upper airway.

Anesthetic and perioperative considerations—May be congenital, but usually results from trauma due to instrumentation or endotracheal intubation for prolonged periods; usually granulomatous or due to cartilagenous defects. Bronchoscopy is often required to determine extent of stenosis, and tracheostomy may also be required. Endoscopic resection with laser ablation of granulomatous lesions can result in relief of obstruction, but stenosis can recur.

Tension Pneumothorax

Description—Air under pressure in the pleural space.

Anesthetic and perioperative considerations—When the amount of air in the pleural space is great enough to cause the intrapleural pressure to exceed atmospheric pressure, the collapsed lung, the heart, and other mediastinal structures shift to the opposite side, compressing the other lung. In addition, venous return is impaired, and torsion on the great vessels can markedly impair cardiac function; circulatory collapse can occur. Immediate aspiration, followed by insertion of a chest tube, is mandatory. This may occur during anesthesia or mechanical ventilation.

Thymus Conditions

Description—The thymus normally occupies the anterior-superior mediastinum and can give the impression of cardiac enlargement or mediastinal widening on chest x-ray films of young children.

Anesthetic and perioperative considerations—Thymic tissue may extend into the neck, and thymic cysts may occur in these areas, as well as in the mediastinum. Thymic cysts may enlarge rapidly and produce symptoms. Thymic tumors are rare but are sometimes seen in infancy and childhood.

Tracheal Stricture (Acquired)

Anesthetic and perioperative considerations—Abnormal mediastinal strictures of many varieties can produce significant tracheal (or bronchial) compression and result in severe respiratory distress. Endotracheal intubation or tracheostomy may not relieve the obstruction, and selective right or left mainstem bronchial intubation or instrumentation with a rigid bronchoscope may be necessary.

Tracheomalacia

Description—Partial or nearly complete collapse of trachea during inspiration.

Anesthetic and perioperative considerations—Common cause of stridor and partial upper-airway obstruction in infants and small children. The condition is due to incomplete formation or weakness of the tracheal wall, especially of cartilagnous rings. Laryngomalacia produces similar symptoms and is due to weakness or incomplete formation of rigid laryngeal structures. Bronchoscopy and laryngoscopy are often necessary to make the diagnosis and to rule out other causes of upper-airway obstructive symptoms (e.g., foreign body, subglottic stenosis, vocal cord paralysis).

Vocal Cord Paralysis

Description—Can result from birth trauma or recurrent laryngeal nerve damage during surgical procedures involving the chest or neck, or as part of the Arnold-Chiari malformation.

Anesthetic and perioperative considerations—Laryngoscopy with the patient breathing spontaneously is necessary to diagnose vocal cord paralysis. The condition is a common cause of stridor following transcervical approach for the division of a tracheoesophageal fistula or cervical esophagostomy for esophageal atresia. It can also follow ligation of a patent ductus arteriosus or of a Blalock-Taussig shunt.

Acknowledgment

Radiographs are courtesy of Turner Ball, MD, Brit Gay, MD, and Ellen Patrick, MD, Department of Radiology, Henrietta Egleston Hospital for Children, Emory University School of Medicine, Atlanta, GA. Diagrams are by Mr. Terry E. Morris, MMSc.*

Postthoracotomy Complications 17

Thomas L. Higgins, MD, FACP, FCCM

PATIENTS undergoing thoracic surgery are considered high risk by virtue of age, concurrent medical problems, debilitation due to cancer or malnutrition, or the presence of underlying lung disease from smoking, occupational exposure, or their primary disease processes. Even a well-performed surgical procedure can fail because of complications, which can occur in the operating room or subsequently in the postanesthesia recovery unit (PACU), intensive care unit (ICU), or surgical ward. Whereas thoracic surgical patients were once routinely admitted to ICUs for immediate postoperative monitoring and therapy, the recent trend has been to manage many patients in lower-acuity settings—often surgical "step-down" units that primarily differ from medical-surgical wards in terms of nursing orientation and staffing ratios. Anesthesiologists and critical-care specialists will be concerned with complications of the cardiovascular, respiratory, or nervous systems but also must be aware of surgical complications that can precipitate acute decompensation or require urgent return to the operating room.

The location for immediate postoperative care depends both on the degree of patient illness and on the ability of a particular hospital unit to provide postoperative ventilation support and/or hemodynamic monitoring. The nursing staff should be trained to recognize postoperative events specific to thoracic surgery and should be especially familiar with the mechanics of chest tube drainage and suction. Increasingly, patients undergoing bronchoscopy, mediastinoscopy, esophageal dilatation, esophagoscopy, laryngoscopy, pleuroscopy, or scalene node biopsy spend just a short time in the PACU and are then transferred to a regular room only if an overnight stay is necessary. Patients undergoing lobectomy, segmental or wedge pulmonary resections, hiatal hernia repairs, or Heller myotomy can generally be recovered in the PACU, but they might require overnight monitoring in either the PACU or another critical-care unit. Patients undergoing esophagectomy, esophagogastrectomy, and pneumonectomy are likely to have ongoing monitoring and intervention needs, are at risk for requiring postoperative ventilation, and are usually managed in an intensive care setting.

Identification of the High-Risk Patient

Preoperative assessment and management are covered in Chapter 1. Surgical entry to the chest, even without tissue resection, produces changes to forced vital capacity (FVC) and functional residual capacity (FRC). Lateral thoracotomy is associated with greater postoperative impairment than is median sternotomy. FVC and FRC can decrease to less than 60% of their preoperative values on the first postoperative day, with a delay of up to 2 weeks before baseline values are recovered. The decline in FRC is especially important, because the resulting atelectasis causes physiologic shunting and hypoxemia.

In patients with severe chronic obstruction, the best predictors of postoperative ventilation requirements are arterial PO_2 less than 70% of predicted for age and the presence of dyspnea at rest.[1] The risk of postoperative pneumonia is highest in patients with low admission serum albumin concentrations, higher scores on the ASA physical status classification, a history of smoking, prolonged preoperative stay, longer operative procedures, and surgical sites involving the thorax or upper abdomen[2].

Obese patients tend to cough poorly, retain secretions, and develop basilar atelectasis. In this population, expiratory reserve volume (ERV) frequently drops to values below the lung's closing volume, resulting in perfused, unventilated segments of lung and a widened (A-a) PO_2 gradient. Cigarette smoking contributes to perioperative morbidity through impaired mucus secretion and clearance, along with small-airway narrowing. Patients who have recently quit smoking (within 8 weeks of surgery) appear to have an increased risk of postoperative pulmonary complications, possibly due to transient increases in sputum volume.[3]

Shapiro et al developed a system for risk classification following thoracic and abdominal procedures (Table 17-1).[4] Blood gas and spirometric abnormalities, concurrent illness, and expectations for postoperative ambulation generate point values that are summed to indicate level of risk. Low-risk patients do not generally require oxygen therapy after discharge from the recovery room. Moderate-risk patients require observation, whether in an ICU or a lower-activity area. The high-risk patient usually requires postoperative monitoring and interventions.

Immediate Postoperative Issues

Routine postoperative monitoring includes blood pressure determination (either manually, by automated sphygmomanometer, or through an indwelling arterial pressure catheter), continuous ECG monitoring, and continuous pulse oximetry. Selected patients could require use of central venous pressure or pulmonary artery catheters to assess hemodynamic states.

Most patients undergoing thoracotomy have chest tubes placed to drain the surgical site. In patients undergoing pneumonectomy, chest tubes are generally avoided because of risk of

TABLE 17-1

Calculating The Risk of Pulmonary Complications of Thoracic and Abdominal Procedures

Category	Points*
EXPIRATORY SPIROGRAM	
Normal (%FVC and %FEV$_1$/FVC >150% of predicted)	0
%FVC and %FEV$_1$/FVC = 100 – 150% of predicted	1
%FVC and %FEV$_1$/FVC < 100% predicted	2
Preoperative FVC <20 mL/kg	3
Postbronchodilator FEV$_1$/FVC <50% of predicted	3
CARDIOVASCULAR SYSTEM	
Normal	0
Controlled hypertension, myocardial infarction without sequelae for more than two years	0
Dyspnea on exertion, orthopnea, paroxysmal nocturnal dyspnea, dependent edema, congestive heart failure, angina	1
ARTERIAL BLOOD GASES	
Acceptable	0
Paco$_2$ >50 mmHg or Pao$_2$ <60 mmHg on room air	1
Metabolic pH abnormality >7.50 or <7.30	1
NERVOUS SYSTEM	
Normal	0
Confusion, obtundation, agitation, spasticity, uncoordination, bulbar malfunction	1
Significant muscular weakness	1
POSTOPERATIVE AMBULATION	
Expected ambulation (minimum, sitting at bedside) within 36 hours	0
Expected complete bed confinement for at least 36 hours	1

*From Shapiro BA, Harrison RA, Kacmarek RM, et al: *Clinical application of respiratory care*, ed 3, Chicago, 1985, Year Book.
0 Points = low risk, 1–2 Points = moderate risk, 3 Points = high risk.

infection unless there is a need for postoperative monitoring of the pneumonectomy space. Chest tubes should not be clamped during patient transport; the risk is that bleeding will not be recognized or that tension pneumothorax could occur. Patients arriving in the PACU or ICU should have a focused examination that includes review of vital signs, auscultation for breath sounds, and visual inspection of monitoring catheters and chest tube connections. Chest tubes, aside from those in a pneumonectomy space, are typically connected to a vacuum regulator to provide –20 cm H_2O of suction. A chest radiograph confirms correct placement of endotracheal, nasogastric, and chest tubes and can help identify pneumothorax, mediastinal shift, or significant atelectasis.

Chest tube drainage systems provide calibrated drainage chambers, mechanisms to limit excess positive pressure, and a system to regulate the amounts of negative pressure (suction) applied. Packaged commercial systems can be best understood as incorporating the features of traditional three-bottle systems (Figure 17-1). Although the physical locations might vary among manufacturers, all such units incorporate a calibrated drainage chamber, a water-seal chamber, and a negative pressure regulator. Postoperative management protocols generally dictate hourly charting of chest tube output and surgical notification if drainage is more than 100 mL/hr for more than 4 hours, or more than 200 mL in any 1 hour observation period. Total expected drainage in the first 24 hours is roughly 300 to 600 mL and should taper to less than 200 mL by the second postoperative day. The fluid level in the water-seal chamber should fluctuate with respirations if there is no air leak; if no fluctuations are seen, tube patency should be checked. Air bubbles should be expected in the chamber that limits the amount of applied suction, but air bubbles in the water-seal chamber represent an active leak. Most pulmonary resection

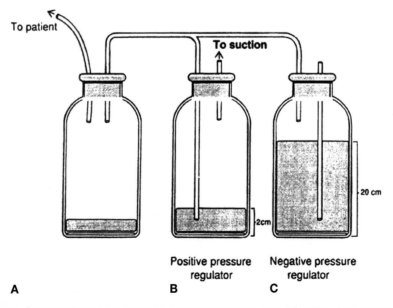

FIGURE 17-1 Commercially available chest tube drainage systems are essentially a three-bottle system. **Bottle A** is the collection chamber. **Bottle B** provides a water seal and escape mechanism for extrapleural/intrathoracic air. **Bottle C** is a safety device to limit the amount of negative pressure that can be applied.

patients have small air leaks, which should resolve as the underlying lung parenchyma expands to fill the pleural space completely. A significant air leak in a ventilated patient will be apparent as bubbling through the water seal and may also be apparent as a discrepancy between inspired and exhaled tidal volume on the ventilator. Leaks might occur only above a threshold inflation pressure, and ventilation techniques—such as smaller volumes at higher rates or pressure-controlled ventilation—can minimize air loss and allow a seal to develop. Once all air leaks have resolved and drainage is minimal (<100 mL/24 hr), chest tubes may be removed while the patient performs a Valsalva maneuver or during the expiratory phase of mechanical ventilation. Routine chest x-rays are not necessary after uncomplicated removal of chest tubes, and the decision to reinsert a chest tube can be based on the patient's clinical examination.[5]

Extubation and Airway Concerns

When possible, the goal is to extubate the patient in the operating room, thus avoiding positive pressure ventilation or coughing or bucking on the endotracheal tube. Specific considerations, such as concurrent cardiac instability, developing acute lung injury, inability to protect against aspiration, or an open-chest condition, could require continued ventilation support and intubation. In high-risk patients, silent aspiration of gastric contents is an important complication after pulmonary resection, and maintenance of endotracheal intubation for 24 hours postoperatively has been shown to decrease both the occurrence of pneumonia and the operative mortality rate in this subset.[6] Lung separation techniques (Chapter 8) are commonly required in the operating room but are generally unnecessary in the postoperative period. Double-lumen endotracheal tubes (DLTs) are large and more likely to cause airway trauma and edema. They are also likely to shift position with patient motion and are more difficult to suction through, owing to lumens that might not admit a standard-size suction catheter. For these reasons, the DLT will usually be removed at the end of the operation and replaced by a single-lumen tube if continued mechanical ventilation is required. Specific indications for continued selective endobronchial intubation (Table 17-2) might include protection against lung soilage with pus or blood, or the need to provide differential ventilation or positive end-expiratory pressures when the lungs have differing compliance.[7]

TABLE 17-2
Indications for Use of Endobronchial Intubation

Absolute	To prevent soilage of contralateral lung with pus, blood, or secretions
	To control distribution of ventilation with bronchopleural fistula, cystic lesions, or conditions of differential lung compliance
	For unilateral bronchopulmonary lavage
	For unilateral lung transplantation
Relative	Surgical exposure—pneumonectomy and thoracic aneurysm
	Surgical convenience—esophageal resection and lobectomy

From Rice TW, Higgins TL, Kirby TJ: Management of the general thoracic surgical patient. In Sivak ED, Higgins TL, Seiver A (eds): *The high-risk patient: management of the critically ill*, Baltimore, 1995, Williams & Wilkins.

Extubation criteria will differ between immediate postoperative patients and those who have required prolonged ICU ventilatory support. For "fresh" postoperative patients, the patient ideally should be fully reversed from neuromuscular blockade, awake and following instructions, demonstrating adequate airway protection and cough reflexes, and oxygenating and ventilating well on minimal or no ventilator support. Measurements of maximal inspiratory pressure (generally more than –25 cmH$_2$O) and respiratory rate to tidal volume (f/Vt) ratio (generally <100) are not required, but they can be reassuring.

Specific reasons to delay extubation would include airway compromise due to edema or bleeding, inadequate pulmonary reserve, compromised myocardial function or perioperative infarction, an expectation of large fluid shifts with thoracoabdominal procedures, severe neurologic impairment, or continued bleeding with high likelihood of a return to the operating room. Esophageal surgery patients are at particularly high risk for reflux and aspiration, and extubation may reasonably be delayed until the first postoperative day to assure that airway reflexes have recovered fully.

Intubation and manipulation of the airway can result in laryngeal and glottic edema. Substantial edema is present if the patient cannot move air around the endotracheal tube with the cuff down but the lumen occluded. Corticosteroids and elevation of the head of the bed might be helpful, but time is usually most important in resolving this problem. If there is any doubt about airway patency, the endotracheal tube should be removed only under direct laryngoscopic or fiberoptic observation, with a surgical tracheostomy instrument tray immediately at hand to provide airway access should reintubation be impossible because of airway edema.

Postoperative Fluid Management

Loss of pulmonary capillary integrity is common after long procedures, significant lung retraction, pulmonary resections, lung transplantation, or aspiration of gastric contents. Acute lung injury can progress to Acute Respiratory Distress Syndrome (ARDS). Ideal fluid management has not been determined (an NIH-funded study is currently underway to examine this issue), so fluid administration should be individualized based on patient needs. If the patient is hemodynamically stable and producing adequate urine, minimizing fluid administration could limit accumulation of lung water and subsequent difficulty with oxygenation. Patients who have had considerable dissection and mobilization of tissue planes (esophagectomy, esophagogastrectomy, excision of large mediastinal tumors) can require large volumes of fluid replacement (typically many liters) to support adequate cardiac preload as intravascular fluid escapes to the "third space." This fluid will usually mobilize spontaneously beginning on the second or third postoperative day, which can create problems with intravascular fluid overload in patients with cardiac or renal compromise. High-risk patients thus might require continued ICU-level monitoring and intervention with inotropes, vasopressors, fluids, and diuretics. Colloids (albumin, hetastarch, plasma) remain in the intravascular compartment longer than crystalloids and substantially reduce the total volume required; but in the presence of capillary leak, even colloids will enter the "third-space" and subsequently exert oncotic pressure out of the intravascular compartment and into tissues. Considerable controversy exists regarding ideal postoperative hemoglobin values. In most patients, a restrictive blood cell transfusion strategy (allowing transfusion only when hemoglobin levels were less than 7%) is as least as safe as, and possibly superior to, a more liberal approach (transfusing for hemoglobin less than 10%)[8]. In a subset of patients with cardiac disease, there is a trend toward increased mortality when hemoglobin values are less than 9.5%. Hebert et all found that patients with anemia, an APACHE II score over 20, and a cardiac diagnosis had a significantly lower mortality rate when transfused.[9] More recently, a randomized study by the same group suggests that hemodynamically stable, critically ill patients with cardiovascular disease (with the possible exception of patients with acute myocardial infarction or unstable angina) may safely be maintained at hemoglobin concentrations of 7% to 9%.[10]

Nutritional Support

Oral intake can be resumed by most patients undergoing routine pulmonary resections within the first 24 hours. Pneumonectomy patients are generally kept NPO for 24 to 48 hours because mediastinal shift, diaphragmatic elevation, alteration of the esophageal hiatus, and possible damage to the vagus and recurrent laryngeal nerves make aspiration more likely. Aspiration is a life-threatening complication in any patient, but particularly in the pneumonectomy patient; thus, evaluation for an intact swallowing mechanism and adequate gag reflex is recommended before oral feeding. In complex patients with hemodynamic instability, ventilator dependency, preoperative cachexia, or those expected to be NPO for more than 48 hours, early nutrition should be established via enteral or parenteral routes. Preoperative dysphagia is associated with severe malnutrition and a requirement for prolonged parenteral nutritional support.[11]

Difficulties with Postoperative Ventilation

In patients with otherwise healthy lungs, ventilatory support can be delivered at tidal volumes of 8 to 10 mL/kg with a ventilator rate sufficient to avoid hypercapnea. If acute lung injury (ALI) or ARDS develops, a lung-protective ventilatory strategy becomes important.[12] Such a strategy places limits on lung inflation pressures (typically less than 35 cmH$_2$O) and volumes (typically less than 6 mL/kg) and may accept hypercapnea as a consequence. Increasing the inspiratory time promotes lung expansion in atelectatic areas. The normal inspiratory-to-expiratory (I:E) ratio is about 1:2; as this ratio approaches 1:1 or inverts, or as inspiratory times become longer than 1 second, problems with patient tolerance and auto-PEEP may occur. Increased sedation and addition of neuromuscular blockade may be necessary when inverting I:E ratios. Bronchodilators and careful titration of inspiratory and expiratory times using waveform monitoring on the ventilator can help reduce auto-PEEP.

High-frequency jet ventilation (HFJV) is frequently used in the operating room during laryngoscopy, bronchoscopy, microlaryngeal procedures, and airway surgery. The role of HFJV in the ICU, particularly for management of hypoxemic respiratory failure, is poorly defined aside from utility in ventilating patients with bronchopleural fistulae and large leaks. Under these specific circumstances, a patient's required minute ventilation can sometimes be better attained at lower airway pressures with HFJV than with conventional ventilation. The reduction in airway pressures is thought to minimize the amount of air passing through the fistula. Healing is promoted by allowing adjacent tissues to approximate and seal the fistula. In the face of decreased pulmonary compliance (which occurs with ARDS, for example), the beneficial effect of HFJV in lowering airway pressures is questionable.[13]

Independent Lung Ventilation

Unilateral lung disease is unusual, but it results in a situation in which application of sufficient pressure to ventilate the diseased lung produces overdistention and ventilation/perfusion (V/Q) mismatching in the other lung. Some commercially available ventilators can be linked together in a master-slave combination allowing a synchronized respiratory cycle with independent control of CPAP, tidal volume, and pressure limits for each lung. A single ventilator can also be used to ventilate one lung while a small amount of CPAP is applied to the other lung. Disadvantages of independent lung ventilation techniques include the following:

- The risk of placing and maintaining the DLT in a patient with existing lung disease and
- Difficulty with suctioning and bronchoscopy through the narrower individual lumens of the DLT.

Ventilation techniques such as pressure-controlled inverse-ratio ventilation (PC-IRV) can sometimes achieve reexpansion of atelectatic segments even when there are substantial differences in lung segment compliances.

Postthoracotomy Complications

Postthoracotomy complications can be divided into general complications (Table 17-3) and complications specific to certain procedures (Table 17-4). Complications can also be categorized as primarily affecting the airway, parenchyma, pleura and chest wall, or cardiovascular system.

Airway Issues
RETAINED SECRETIONS AND BLOOD IN THE AIRWAY
Retained secretions and blood are especially common if the airway was opened, as, for example, during a bronchoplastic procedure or closure of a bronchial stump. Flexible fiberoptic bronchoscopy helps to clear obstructions if there have been excessive or bloody secretions in the airway. Mechanical airway obstruction secondary to secretions can be further aggravated by bronchospasm, the likelihood and frequency of which are reduced with bronchodilators and (occasionally) corticosteroids.
LARYNGEAL EDEMA
Laryngeal edema, which may manifest as stridor, is common after prolonged intubation with large tubes or DLTS, the passage of rigid bronchoscopes, or multiple reintubations. Treatment includes placing the patient in an upright or sitting position and the use of intravenous corticosteroids and inhaled racemic epinephrine. A critical airway may be improved by the

TABLE 17-3

Complications of Noncardiac Thoracic Surgery

Airway complications

Arytenoid dislocation
Airway edema/stridor
Aspiration of gastric contents
Retained secretion

Pulmonary complications

Atelectasis
Bronchospasm
Tracheobronchial obstruction
Mediastinal shift
Air leakage
Lung torsion and infarction
Bronchopleural fistula
Pleural effusion, emphysema, chylothorax
Pneumothorax
Reexpansion, pulmonary edema, and
    postpneumonectomy

Chest wall problems

Paradoxical motion
Mediastinal and subcutaneous emphysema
Hematoma
Wound dehiscence
Pain

Hemorrhage

Postoperative bleeding into the pleura
Bleeding into the tracheobronchial tree

Cardiac complications

Arrhythmias (especially atrial fibrillation)
Pulmonary hypertension, right heart failure
Cardiac herniation
Pulmonary thromboembolism
Myocardial infarction, congestive failure
Tension pneumothorax

Nerve injuries

Intercostal nerves
Phrenic nerve
Vagus nerve
Recurrent laryngeal nerve
Brachial plexus injury

General

Acute pain and splinting
Postthoracotomy pain
Respiratory failure
Nutritional depletion
Anesthetic complications

administration of heliox, a helium and oxygen mixture.[14] Helium, being denser and less viscous than nitrogen, allows laminar flow to occur through the critically swollen upper airway. Delayed resolution of airway edema might require prolonged endotracheal intubation or temporary tracheostomy. Intermittent noisy inspiration and painful swallowing should raise the suspicion of arytenoid dislocation, which can cause postextubation respiratory failure, though rarely.[15] Treatment consists of surgical reduction using gentle pressure with a laryngeal spatula; this must be accomplished before the cricoarytenoid joint becomes fibrosed out of normal position.

VOCAL CORD INJURY

Vocal cord injury may result from direct trauma or indirectly, by means of damage to the recurrent laryngeal nerves. The right recurrent laryngeal nerve arises in the right chest apex and then travels around the right subclavian artery to return to the larynx. The left recurrent laryngeal nerve is more susceptible to injury because of its course around the aortic arch. Excessive traction, aggressive dissection surrounding these nerves, or surgical sacrifice of these nerves can precipitate postoperative vocal cord palsy. Mediastinoscopy, anterior mediastinotomy, left pulmonary resection with subaortic exenteration, and resections of mediastinal tumors are procedures during which the recurrent laryngeal nerve could be damaged. If airway and laryngeal edema also occur, the vocal cords might function for the first few days after extubation, and serious injury might not be noted until the patient returns from the ward to the ICU with suspected aspiration pneumonia. Patients with vocal cord paralysis are initially managed with aggressive chest physiotherapy and withholding oral feeding. If there is permanent damage or division of the recurrent laryngeal nerve, then surgical repair of the vocal cord might be necessary.

Parenchymal Issues

ATELECTASIS

Atelectasis is very common after thoracic surgery because of the surgical procedure, splinting of the thoracic cage, inadequate cough, hypoventilation, retained secretions, or inadequate control of new or preexisting bronchospasm. In patients with marginal pulmonary reserve, atelectasis and its associated increase in the work of breathing along with impaired gas exchange can eventually result in respiratory failure and reintubation. Retained bronchial secretions and colonization of the airway promote pneumonia, particularly in patients with underlying COPD. Clinical findings with significant atelectasis include tachypnea, tachycardia, arrhythmias, and hypoxemia. Atelectasis by itself does not generally cause fever unless there is concurrent infection.[16] Clinical percussion or auscultation could reveal signs of a consolidated lung segment. The chest x-ray may show "platelike" atelectasis, or segmental, lobar, or total atelectasis of the lung. Although the operative side is more frequently involved, contralateral lung and bilateral involvement might be seen. Treatment includes adequate pain control, incentive spirometry, chest physiotherapy, and inhalation therapy aimed at expanding the collapsed lung and clearing the airway of retained secretions. Physiotherapy and postoperative suctioning are most important in patients after left upper lobectomy, because as the left lower lobe rises to fill the left hemithorax, the long left bronchus tends to kink as it passes under the aortic arch. Routine bronchoscopy is not necessary in most cases, but it does have a role in helping to clear established atelectasis.[17]

MEDIASTINAL SHIFT

Mediastinal shift can occur when the mediastinum compensates for volume loss after removal of pulmonary tissue by shifting toward the involved hemithorax. This compensatory process should normally obliterate empty space without affecting functioning lung. Changes are most marked after

TABLE 17-4

Complications of Specific Thoracic Procedures

Procedure	Complications
Anterior mediastinotomy (Chamberlain)	Damage to recurrent laryngeal nerve (particularly left-side)
Bronchoscopy/mediastinoscopy	Bleeding from major vessels if torn, air leak with biopsy of bronchus
Bronchopleural fistula repair	Persistent leak, dehiscence
Bronchopulmonary lavage	Respiratory distress/contralateral spillage
Bullectomy	Tension pneumothorax, air leak
Chest wall reconstruction	Blood loss, altered chest wall compliance, unstable chest, infection from prosthetic material
Clagett window	Air leak
Collis Belsey	Gastric leak, splenic injury
Decortication	Blood loss, air leak(s)
Esophageal dilatation	Esophageal perforation, pleural effusion, airway obstruction
Esophagoscopy	Esophageal perforation
Esophagogastrectomy	"Third-spacing" of fluids, anastomotic leak, gastric devasculatization, splenic injury, gastric torsion
Heller myotomy	Esophageal tear
Lobectomy	Bronchial leak, lobar collapse, lobar torsion
Lung transplant	Rejection (day 5), reperfusion injury, infection, overdistention of native lung, dehiscence
Mediastinal tumor excision	Airway obstruction with sedation/anesthesia, damage to recurrent laryngeal nerve
Nissen fundoplication	Esophageal obstruction (with tight wrap), splenic injury
Pectus repair	Costrochondritis, unstable sternum
Pleuroscopy	Pharyngeal laceration, air leak
Pneumonectomy	Atrial arrhythmias (atrial fibrillation, MAT), mediastinal shift, cardiac torsion, air embolism, disrupted bronchus
Thoracic aortic aneurysm	Paraplegia, bleeding, aortobronchial fistula, esophageal injury
Thymectomy	In myasthenics, possible weakness and respiratory failure
Tracheal resection	Fixed neck flexion postoperatively, dehiscence, air leak

From Higgins TL: Selected issues in postoperative management. In American College of Chest Physicians, *The ACCP critical care board review*, Northbrook, Ill, 1998, American College of Chest Physicians.

pneumonectomy, in which the remaining lung expands and pushes the mediastinum to the operated side; elevation of the diaphragm and narrowing of the interspaces of the empty hemithorax also occur. Serosanguinous fluid then fills the postpneumonectomy space at a rate of about two rib spaces per day.[18] Figure 17-2 demonstrates the progressive mediastinal shift in the days *(A)*, months *(B)*, and years *(C)* after pneumonectomy.

Excessive mediastinal shift in the immediate postoperative period following segmental or lobar resection suggests loss of volume on the operated lung due to atelectasis. Less commonly, fluid accumulation or pneumothorax on the contralateral (nonoperative) side might also cause an exaggerated mediastinal shift.

LOBAR COLLAPSE

Lobar collapse occurs after right upper lobectomy when altered geometry results in atelectasis. The horizontal fissure rises and rotates to a more perpendicular position, resulting in twisting and kinking of the long and narrow middle-lobe bronchus. Early bronchoscopy is necessary to rule out torsion, and repeat bronchoscopy might be required to remove retained secretions.

LOBAR TORSION

Lobar torsion occurs after resection of pulmonary tissue when the vessels of a remaining lobe or segment become twisted as the lung expands. Torsion occurs most commonly after right upper lobectomy because the loss of anchoring attachments allows mobile pulmonary parenchyma to twist around its remaining hilar attachment. Lobar torsion can also occur after bilobectomy on the right with torsion of the remaining upper or lower lobe, or after left-side lobectomy with torsion of the remaining lobe. Typically, the pulmonary and bronchial arteries remain open; however, the lower-pressured pulmonary

veins collapse, compromising venous outflow. Engorgement causes massive enlargement of the lung area drained by the involved veins. The patient could be asymptomatic or could demonstrate significant atelectasis on the early postoperative chest x-ray. Later, the x-ray might demonstrate complete "white out" of the involved segment or lobe. Early intervention is essential to prevent progression to lung infarction. Biochemical signs of tissue necrosis can be seen as ischemia progresses, and expectorated secretions will be bloody, purulent, and malodorous. Similar drainage can occur from chest tubes.[19] Bronchoscopy will reveal abrupt occlusion or a twisted appearance of the airway, but it might be possible to pass the bronchoscope distally. Pulmonary angiography and perfusion scans might demonstrate lack of flow to the involved portion of lung but are not always diagnostic. Treatment of torsion is immediate with attempts to detorsion. Lobectomy is necessary if lung tissue has already become nonviable.

REEXPANSION PULMONARY EDEMA

Reexpansion pulmonary edema can occur after rapid removal of a large pleural effusion or after reexpansion of a pneumothorax. The unilateral alveolar pulmonary edema generally resolves rapidly.[20]

POSTPNEUMONECTOMY PULMONARY EDEMA

Postpneumonectomy pulmonary edema is a form of noncardiogenic edema that presents as progressive hypoxemic respiratory distress hours to days after otherwise uncomplicated lung resection. A combination of increased filtration gradients across the pulmonary microvasculature plus hyperpermeability have been suggested as the causes, although the pathophysiology is not yet fully understood.[21] Avoidance of aggressive perioperative fluids is recommended; treatment is supportive but

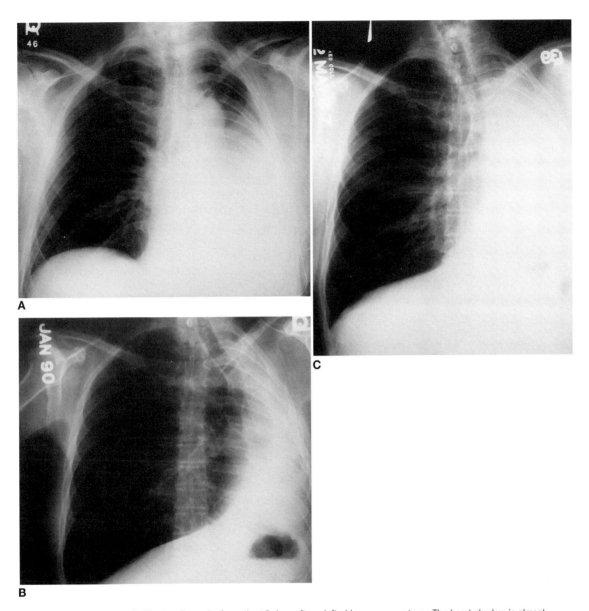

FIGURE 17-2 A, Chest radiograph of a patient 3 days after a left-side pneumonectomy. The heart shadow is almost completely in the left hemothorax. The space normally filled with the left lung is largely opaque because of heart shadow and accumulated fluid. Note also that the intercostal spaces are narrower on the left than on the right. **B,** The same patient 1 month after left-side pneumonectomy. Note the flattened right hemidiaphragm and further mediastinal shift (with tracheal deviation) as a result of further expansion of the remaining lung. **C,** The same patient nearly 3 years after left-side pneumonectomy. Dramatic tracheal deviation toward the operative side is seen. The mediastinum completely fills a very diminished left hemithorax.

requires differentiation from cardiogenic and infectious causes or diffuse pneumonitis (see Chapter 11).

Pleural and Chest Wall Issues

POSTOPERATIVE AIR LEAKS are common and expected. They usually result from small distal fistulae between tiny bronchioles or respiratory units and the pleural cavity. One of the main functions of the chest tubes is to evacuate air from these small air leaks and assure complete expansion of the lung and adherence of the cut surface of the lung to the parietal pleura. Two chest tubes placed in the pleura at the level of the diaphragm

going to the apex—one anteriorly and one posteriorly—should drain blood, pus, and air effectively and allow the lung to expand fully.[22] With complete expansion of the lung, small air leaks will seal. Repositioning of the chest tubes or insertion of further chest tubes into undrained spaces, adequate suction applied to the pleural cavity, and full expansion of the lung with vigorous chest physiotherapy all help to close small distal fistulae. A significant bronchopleural fistula will cause both a persistent air leak from the chest tube and incomplete expansion of the lung in the pleural cavity. In the first postoperative week, bronchopleural fistulae result from technical problems, such as failure of the anastomosis, disruption of a bronchial closure, or retained secretions or foreign bodies. Major bronchopleural fistulae are associated with a mortality rate of greater than 20%.[23] In a patient undergoing pneumonectomy, an early bronchopleural fistula is a surgical emergency requiring immediate diagnostic bronchoscopy to assess stump integrity; reoperation is also likely to be required. Expectoration of large amounts of pink, frothy sputum could be misdiagnosed as pulmonary edema. The patient should be positioned with the operated or pneumonectomy side down to trap remaining fluid in the pneumonectomy space and protect against drowning and spillage of possibly infected material to healthy lung. A chest tube will usually be needed and should be placed high in the midaxillary line, as significant shift of the mediastinum and diaphragm can occur.

Bronchopleural fistulae that present later in the perioperative period are less of an emergency but also more difficult to correct. After the first week, the fistula is frequently due to an empyema or local peribronchial abscess. The late occurrence of a bronchopleural fistula—usually more than 6 months after the operation—is often associated with recurrent lung carcinoma.

PNEUMOTHORAX

Pneumothorax can occur even in the absence of an obvious air leak. Initial steps include inspection of the drainage system to ensure that tubes are patent and that the underwater seal is adequate. A loculated pneumothorax that does not communicate with the drainage system must be distinguished from large bullae. A persistent pneumothorax not associated with an air leak or signs of sepsis can be observed clinically and might respond to increased suction on the present system. A persistent pneumothorax associated with an air leak indicates an established bronchopleural fistula.

MEDIASTINAL AND SUBCUTANEOUS EMPHYSEMA

Mediastinal and subcutaneous emphysema result from air—driven by positive pressure ventilation or patient coughing—that dissects through subcutaneous tissue planes. Air from disrupted alveoli and small bronchi can dissect along the pulmonary vessels and bronchial tree and enter the mediastinum. Air in the pleural space also can gain access to the mediastinum through surgically created disruptions in the pleura. Air then dissects along the mediastinal structures and enters the subcutaneous tissues of the neck, chest, and head.

Pneumoperitoneum sometimes follows pneumothorax.[24] Air in the mediastinum dissects distally into the retroperitoneum, ruptures into the peritoneal cavity, and presents on the radiograph as free air under the diaphragm.

Subcutaneous emphysema can be identified clinically by crepitus, by visible accumulation of air in the patient's neck and face (particularly around the eyes), and on chest x-ray. The problem is generally self-limiting unless there is associated pneumothorax or bronchopleural fistula. The patient should receive a careful assessment for the presence of a persistent pulmonary air leak and for the possibility of leakage from nonpulmonary structures such as the esophagus, which could have been injured during surgery. On rare occasions, massive air collections can compromise the airway and require urgent intubation or tracheostomy. It might be necessary to evacuate paratracheal air to facilitate intubation. Otherwise, treatment includes placing pleu-

ral chest tubes for suctioning, and reassuring the patient and family members that the problem is temporary.

PARADOXICAL CHEST WALL MOTION

Paradoxical chest wall motion is seen in postoperative, spontaneously breathing patients when bony elements of the thorax have been resected. The extent of paradox is related to the amount of chest wall support removed, but its influence on a patient's spontaneous ventilation will depend on the patient's preoperative physiologic reserve. Patients with chronic pulmonary disease will tolerate less paradox than those with normal preoperative pulmonary function. The state of the mediastinum also plays a role in determining the amount of paradox. Less paradoxical air movement occurs in patients whose mediastinum is fixed by fibrosis from preexistent pleural pathology, such as tuberculosis.

Surgical methods of stabilizing the chest wall include musculocutaneous chest wall flaps, plastic mesh, and metal struts.[25-27] By stabilizing the chest, paradox is minimized, and the function of remaining lung improves.

Initial postoperative management of patients requiring chest wall resection includes continued tracheal intubation and mechanical ventilation, perhaps with some PEEP. Within 48 hours, stabilization of the chest wall is usually sufficient to allow removal of ventilatory support.

BLEEDING INTO THE TRACHEOBRONCHIAL TREE

Bleeding into the tracheobronchial tree presents as hemoptysis. Spontaneous massive hemoptysis was once a common complication of advanced tuberculosis but is now rare. Significant bleeding into the tracheobronchial tree can be seen as a complication of bronchoscopic biopsy of an adenoma or vascular malignancy. Rarely, a bronchoscopist can enter a bronchial artery or pulmonary vessel. Pulmonary artery rupture can also occur as a complication of pulmonary artery catheterization. Although rare, massive hemoptysis is both frightening and rapidly lethal if uncorrected.

Treatment includes control of bleeding, keeping the airway clear, and maintaining adequate ventilation. With a rigid bronchoscope, it might be possible to tamponade the bleeding site with pledgets soaked with vasoconstrictors. If this fails, immediate thoracotomy is required, preferably using a DLT to permit ventilation of the healthy lung while bleeding is controlled and clots are drained from the opposite side. If double-lumen intubation is not feasible, then blockade of the involved bronchus with packing or with a Fogarty catheter can be attempted (Figure 17-3).

BLOOD LOSS

Blood loss into the pleural space is expected but should not exceed 500 to 600 mL in 24 hours. Ongoing blood loss of 100 to 200 mL per hour is an indication for reexploration with clot removal and control of the bleeding site. Bleeding after the first 24 hours following thoracotomy is unusual. Erosion by infection of a vessel at the point of suture or pressure from a rib or chest tube can precipitate late bleeding and requires emergency thoracotomy.

FLUID AND AIR

Fluid and air collections can require insertion of additional, appropriately sized chest tubes. Locating these collections with two-dimensional portable chest x-ray can be difficult; success is often achieved with surface ultrasound or CT scanning to better define proposed chest tube locations.

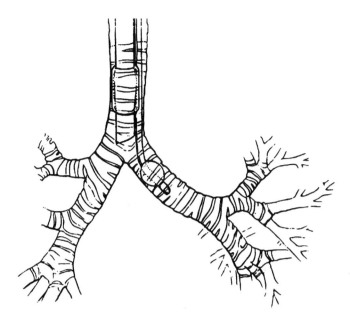

FIGURE 17-3 Forgarty embolectomy catherter used as a bronchial blocker. Under emergency conditions, the catheter could be inserted through a pediatric bronchoscopic swivel adapter through the endotracheal tube lumen. (From Rice TW, Higgins TL, Kirby TJ: Management of the general thoracic surgical patient. In Sivak ED, Higgins TL, Seiver A [eds]: *The high-risk patient: management of the critical ill,* Baltimore, 1995, Williams & Wilkins.)

PERSISTENT PLEURAL FLUID DRAINAGE

Persistent pleural fluid drainage should be evaluated with chemistry, cell count, and culture samples. Transudative effusions are often due to extrathoracic causes (hypoalbuminemia, congestive failure) and can be drained via thoracentesis if necessary. Exudative pleural effusions raise the suspicion of pneumonia or empyema, even if organisms are not cultured from the fluid.

EMPYEMA

Empyema is initially treated with closed-tube drainage and antibiotic therapy. Once the patient has been stabilized and any bronchopleural fistula has been identified and treated, drainage of the empyema cavity is converted from closed- to open-tube drainage. A chest-x-ray is then taken to determine whether the mediastinum is fixed or has shifted and compressed the contralateral remaining lung. If the mediastinum is stable, then drainage of the cavity may be permanently converted to open drainage. This can take the form of rib resection and marsupialization of the pneumonectomy cavity (Clagett window or Eloessor flap). With time, the pneumonectomy cavity shrinks in size, and the window or flap may be closed.

WOUND INFECTIONS

Wound infections are uncommon with the appropriate use of prophylactic (antistaphylococcal) antibiotics in the perioperative period. The incidence of thoracic wound infections is higher in procedures where pus is drained, or when the gastrointestinal tract has been opened (drainage of empyema, lung abscess, mediastinitis, or perforated esophagus).

CHYLOTHORAX

Chylothorax can complicate any thoracic procedure, particularly if there has been dissection around the aorta, near the esophagus, or in the posterior mediastinum resulting in injury to the thoracic duct. Damage to the thoracic duct can result in a fistula with drainage volumes of 1 to 3 L per day. Analysis of the fluid reveals a high protein content, lymphocytosis, and elevated levels of fat and chylomicrons. Chyle is bacteriostatic and sterile, so infection is infrequent. Symptoms might not become apparent until chest tubes are removed and the patient is fed. Dyspnea and recurrent effusion—often a thick creamy drainage—are noted. Management includes keeping the patient NPO (to keep the thoracic duct at rest) and complete drainage of the pleural space to promote full expansion of the lung. Nutritional support can be accomplished with intravenous hyperalimentation or medium-chain triglyceride (MCT) formulas through the enteral route. In most cases, drainage stops within 1 to 2 weeks. If the chylothorax does not resolve, then thoracotomy with ligation of the thoracic duct is indicated to prevent continuous loss of fat and fat-soluble vitamins. Contrast lymphangiogram or nuclear lymphangiogram using technetium-99m antimony colloid can be helpful in defining the site of injury.[28]

Cardiovascular Complications
MASSIVE POSTOPERATIVE HEMORRHAGE

Significant hypotension at the time of patient transfer to the recovery room or ICU can indicate massive postoperative hemorrhage. Emergency operation is usually required, and findings can include slipped ties from the pulmonary vein or, less commonly, from the pulmonary artery. Bleeding is almost always from the systemic circulation—often from vessels in the chest wall or in the mediastinum, from branches of the azygous system, or from branches of the bronchial arteries.[29]

Slower postoperative hemorrhage is more commonly the result of small bleeding arteries or veins in the mediastinum or chest wall. Reoperation may be required for control of bleeding; evacuation of the hemothorax prevents future fibrothorax and restrictive lung disease.

CARDIAC HERNIATION

Cardiac herniation can occur after a large pericardial defect is created, usually following intrapericardial pneumonectomy. Although rare, cardiac herniation is lethal if unrecognized, and overall mortality is approximately 50%.[30,31] Events that can precipitate this complication, usually at the end of the operation or in the immediate postoperative period, include coughing, change in patient position, positive pressure ventilation, or excessive negative pressure in the pneumonectomy space. The heart becomes displaced and entrapped within a pericardial defect, altering the geometry and obstructing the vena cavae and cardiac outflow tracts.[32-34] The edges of the defect compress the myocardium, typically at the level of the atrioventricular groove, leading to myocardial ischemia, arrhythmias, and obstruction to ventricular outflow if the herniation is not promptly reduced.[35] Severe restriction in venous return and falling cardiac output are typical of herniation after right pneumonectomy.[36] Examination can reveal jugular venous distention, a displaced cardiac impulse, and cardiovascular collapse. The ECG might show abnormal rotation of the electrical axis, arrhythmias, and ST-T wave abnormalities. Chest x-rays are diagnostic in right-sided herniation (Figure 17-4), but left-sided herniation might not be apparent without a lateral chest film. Patient survival depends on immediate reoperation to reduce

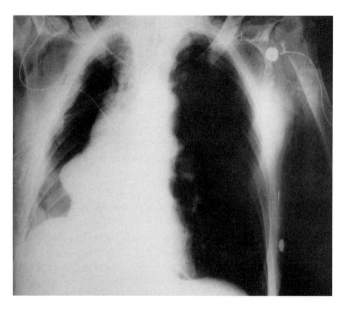

FIGURE 17-4 Partial cardiac herniation after right-side pneumonectomy. (From Brooks JW: Complications of thoracic and chest way surgery. In Greenfield LJ [ed]: *Complications of surgery and trauma*, ed 2, Philadelphia, 1990, JB Lippincott.)

the heart into the pericardial space. While the patient is being prepared and transported to the operating room, steps to reverse the pressure differential that favors herniation can be taken in an attempt to reduce the hernia even before the chest is opened. Suction of the operative pleural space should be discontinued; air injection into the empty hemithorax might be considered. Meanwhile, spontaneous ventilation of the intact lung is desirable; if positive pressure ventilation is used, ventilation should be rapid and shallow to minimize peak airway pressures. Placing the patient in the lateral position with the operated hemithorax uppermost allows gravity to contribute to the reduction.

LOW CARDIAC OUTPUT SYNDROME

Low cardiac output syndrome (LCOS) presents with hypotension, oliguria, mental status changes, metabolic acidosis, arterial hypoxemia, and low mixed venous oxygen saturation. The clinical findings represent failure to deliver adequate oxygen to tissues, with resulting organ dysfunction. The oxygen extraction ratio, or the ratio of oxygen consumption to oxygen delivery (normally 24–28%) is elevated as tissues attempt to extract available oxygen. In the absence of sufficient oxygen, glucose metabolism switches from aerobic to anaerobic metabolism. The Krebs cycle cannot function without oxygen, and as a result pyruvate accumulates and is converted to lactate, which contributes to systemic metabolic acidosis. Postoperative causes of LCOS include acute myocardial infarction, myocardial ischemia, right ventricular failure, cardiac arrhythmias, and cardiac tamponade. Excessive intrapleural pressure, which can occur with high levels of positive end-expiratory pressure (PEEP), can also restrict ventricular filling and reduce cardiac output. Hypoxemia and myocardial ischemia in the perioperative period can further compromise cardiac output in patients with preexisting cardiac failure. Other factors that contribute to perioperative LCOS include inadequate blood volume, anemia, hypocalcemia, and other electrolyte imbalances. Treatment should address factors that determine cardiac output: heart rate, cardiac rhythm, left and right ventricular preload, left and right ventricular afterload, and myocardial contractility. The early postoperative hypermetabolic state can be partly controlled by placing the patient in a 30° sitting position.[37] Because oxygen delivery is dependent on hemoglobin concentration and saturation, anemia and hypoxemia must also be corrected.

PULMONARY HYPERTENSION

This is common in patients with COPD, owing partly to progressive, irreversible fibrotic obliteration of alveolar-capillary units, and partly to hypoxic pulmonary vasoconstriction, which may be reversible. The pulmonary vascular bed loses its ability to expand in response to increased blood flow, such as occurs with exercise or the hypermetabolic states that occur postoperatively or with sepsis. As pulmonary artery pressure increases, right ventricular function deteriorates with a subsequent decrease in ejection fraction.[38,39] Experimentally, right ventricular contractility falls in association with increased pulmonary artery pressures.[40] Subendocardial ischemia occurs from ventricular wall stress as the chamber dilates.

Surgical resection of lung tissue acutely decreases the cross-sectional area of the pulmonary vasculature. Normally, the remaining pulmonary vasculature can compensate for the stress-induced increases in pulmonary blood flow. In patients with preexisting COPD, these compensatory mechanisms are limited, and severe pulmonary hypertension and right heart failure may result. Although preoperative testing should eliminate many high-risk patients as operative candidates, the extent of surgical resection and the postoperative response are not always perfectly predictable.[41] High-risk patients are frequently managed with a pulmonary artery catheter. Right-sided heart failure is defined by the constellation of a high right atrial pressure with normal pulmonary artery occlusion (wedge) pressure plus low cardiac output. Clinically, peripheral edema, hepatomegaly, and oliguria may occur.

Treatment should aggressively address reversible causes of pulmonary vasoconstriction (hypoxemia, acidosis) and increased blood flow (pain, fever). Attempts can be made to reduce pulmonary vascular resistance with pulmonary vasodilators and/or inotropic agents that are also pulmonary vasodilators (dobutamine, milrinone). Optimizing volume status may be difficult using pressure measurements alone, and echocardiographic assessment of right- and left-sided filling can help determine the need for fluid repletion. Although fluid restriction is generally recommended, improvements in cardiac output might be possible with judicious volume loading. Each patient's therapy must be individualized, guided by pressure or volume monitoring and by serial or continuous determinations of cardiac output and derived hemodynamic parameters.

PULMONARY EMBOLI

Pulmonary emboli can complicate any surgical procedure. Although thrombosis in the deep veins of the legs accounts for most cases, thrombi can also form in a long pulmonary artery stump after pulmonary resection and then enter into the contralateral pulmonary artery.[42,43]

Pulmonary emboli can be difficult to diagnose in the perioperative period, when the differential diagnosis of hypoxemia also includes atelectasis, sepsis, ARDS, and pneumonia. Radioisotope lung scans are of limited diagnostic value in postthoracotomy patients, in whom perfusion defects from atelectasis and preexisting chronic lung disease are expected. Pulmonary arteriography is considered the most accurate method of diagnosis but is invasive and requires dye injection. Spiral computed tomography of the chest is emerging as an alterative to standard angiography.

The initial presentation of a large pulmonary embolus may be sudden cardiovascular collapse leading to imminent death. Emergency pulmonary embolectomy with cardiopulmonary bypass can be lifesaving but is associated with a high mortality rate.[44] Uncontrollable intrapulmonary hemorrhage following restoration of flow is the most serious complication.[45] Thrombolytic approaches are generally contraindicated by recent surgery but might be possible in selected situations. If the patient survives the first hour, treatment is directed at stabilizing hemodynamics with inotropic drugs and preventing further episodes of embolization. Continuous intravenous heparin therapy is titrated to increase coagulation test results to greater than twice normal values. This can later be converted to oral anticoagulation or use of a low-molecular-weight heparin. Prophylaxis against venous thromboembolism is recommended for high-risk patients, which includes those older than 40 years who are obese, have malignant disease, or have a history of deep-vein thrombosis. Subcutaneous "mini-dose" heparin, low-molecular-weight heparin twice or thrice daily, and sequential pneumatic compression of the legs during and after surgery can be employed. Insertion of a vena cava filter can be considered if the source of emboli is thought to be from the pelvis or lower extremity, especially if there are contraindications to anticoagulation.[46] The caval filter can be inserted through a transvenous approach under local anesthesia.[47]

POSTOPERATIVE ARRHYTHMIAS

Postoperative arrhythmias are common in patients undergoing thoracic surgery. The frequency and severity of supraventricular tachyarrhythmias increase with patient age and magnitude of the procedure. Factors that contribute to arrhythmias include underlying cardiac disease, increased pulmonary vascular resistance, effects of anesthetic and cardiovascular agents, hypovolemia, and electrolyte shifts that might be influenced by the ventilatory pattern. For example, hyperventilation from normal values to a $Paco_2$ of 30 or 20 mmHg is associated with decreases in serum potassium from normal (4.03 mEq/L) to 3.64 and 3.12 mEq/L, respectively[48]. Irritation of the right side of the heart and pulmonary veins from surgery, inflammation, and mediastinal shift also plays a role.

Almost half of all high-risk patients undergoing noncardiac surgery have frequent ventricular ectopic beats or nonsustained ventricular tachycardia, but these patients do not require treatment in the absence of other signs or symptoms[49]. Significant perioperative arrhythmias include supraventricular tachycardias (paroxysmal atrial tachycardia, atrial flutter, atrial fibrillation with rapid ventricular response); ventricular tachycardia or fibrillation; and high-grade conduction disturbances, including atrioventricular dissociation and complete heart block. Pharmacologic and mechanical choices for each of these arrhyth-

mias are outlined in Table 17-5. If there is severe circulatory compromise, electrical cardioversion should be considered for acute arrhythmias. Other less-threatening arrhythmias can be managed pharmacologically. Narrow-complex, supraventricular tachycardias can be differentiated from ventricular tachyarrhythmias by vagal stimulation (carotid sinus massage) or intravenous adenosine. Intravenous amiodarone is particularly useful, as it corrects atrial and ventricular arrhythmias, even with impaired cardiac function.[50] It is now recommended as the drug of choice for junctional tachycardias and as an alternative to calcium channel blockers for the treatment of paroxysmal supraventricular tachycardias and ectopic or multifocal atrial tachycardias. β-Adrenergic blockade accelerates the conversion of postoperative supraventricular arrhythmias.[51] Diltiazem may be preferable to other calcium channel blockers in patients whose ventricular function is compromised (ejection fraction less than 40%). Digoxin is widely used perioperatively to lessen the incidence and severity of arrhythmias and often is effective for postpneumonectomy atrial fibrillation and flutter. Intravenous verapamil, propranolol, or esmolol can also be used. Nonspecific factors, such as pain and fever, should also be addressed and corrected.

Other Considerations
MYASTHENIA GRAVIS

Myasthenia gravis (MG) can respond to surgical removal of a thymoma or to thymectomy even in the absence of tumor. Most myasthenic patients can be extubated in the operating room or shortly after arrival in the ICU if neuromuscular function is adequate and conventional tests of ventilatory reserve are met. One of 10 patients will require postoperative mechanical ventilation, usually for less than 3 days.[52] Predictors of the need for postoperative mechanical ventilation include a history of chronic respiratory disease (unrelated to the myasthenia), disease of a duration greater than 6 years, daily use of more than 750 mg of pyridostigmine, and preoperative vital capacity of less than 2.9 L (see Chapter 13).

LEAKAGE OF ESOPHAGEAL CONTENTS

Leakage of esophageal contents from the site of esophageal surgery, myotomy, or hiatal hernia repair is fairly common. After transhiatal esophagectomy, one large study found a leak rate of 11%, aspiration in 4%, and gastric perforation in 1.5%.[53] Initial management of esophageal perforation includes thoracotomy, reinforced closure with a pedicle wrap, and drainage. The esophagus is kept at rest, usually with a nasogastric tube, but occasionally with esophagostomy and gastrostomy. Surgical manipulation of the esophagus releases all three isoenzymes of creatine kinase (CPK), compromising the utility of CPK-MB for diagnosis of perioperative myocardial infarction.

INTERCOSTAL NERVE INJURY

Intercostal nerve injury can occur after lateral thoracotomy. Direct interruption, crushing with retractors, laceration by fractured rib ends, stretching of nerve roots, and inclusion in sutures during closure can all occur. The patient may notice an area of numbness or hypersthesia over the area of the fifth or sixth thoracic dermatome. Normally, this does not result in disability, but in some cases a chronic pain syndrome can result.

POSTTHORACOTOMY PAIN

Pain after thoracotomy is a persistent or recurrent pain along the route of a thoracotomy scar that has not resolved within two

TABLE 17-5

Treatment of Perioperative Arrhythmias

Rhythm	Initial Choices	Other Choices
Ventricular fibrillation **Ventricular tachycardia** VF and pulseless VT should be treated with cardioversion first Hemodynamically stable VT can be treated pharmacologically, followed by synchronized cardioversion if necessary	DC cardioversion—200 J; increase energy as required Follow up stable rhythm with either **Amiodarone** 300 mg IV bolus over 10 minutes, then infusion as per package insert; or **Lidocaine** 1.0–1.5 mg/kg initial IV bolus followed by infusion of 1-4 mg/min IV	**Vasopressin** 40 μg IV **Epinephrine** to convert fine to coarse VF before cardioversion **Magnesium** 1-2 g IV, specific treatment for *torsades de pointes* only **Bretylium** 5-10 mg/kg IV **Procainamide** IV 17 mg/kg over 1 hour, then 2-6 mg/min for stable VT only
Atrial fibrillation (new, acute) **Atrial flutter** Treatment may not be needed if hemodynamics are stable. Rate control is next priority if blood pressure is stable. Anticoagulation needed; risk of thromboemboli if duration >48 hr Chronic atrial fibrillation might not convert	**Ibutilide** (Corvert) 0.01 mg/kg IV to total 1 mg (1 vial) over 10 minutes or **DC synchronized cardioversion** 50–100 j; increase as needed Or **Diltiazem** 0.25–0.3 mg/kg IV followed by infusion for rate control	Intravenous beta-blockade: **Esmolol** 5-10 mg IV bolus, beware of bronchospasm **Atenolol** 5-10 mg IV **Metoprolol** 5 mg IV **Procainamide** (see above) **Amiodarone** (see above) **Verapamil** 2.5-5 mg IV **Digoxin** load with 0.5 mg IV then 0.25 mg q 8hr to 1.0 mg total
Ectopic or multifocal atrial tachycardia	Address underlying lung problem Check fluid status	IV β-Blockers or IV calcium channel blockers with EF ≥40%; amiodarone or diltiazem with CHF or EF <40% No DC cardioversion!
Atrioventricular nodal reentrant tachycardia (AVNRT)	Vagal maneuvers, carotid sinus massage, valsalva as initial Rx IV **Adenosine** (6, 6,12 mg) Cardioversion if hemodynamically unstable	**Phenylephrine** 50-100 μg IV to raise BP and convert via carotid sinus reflex IV **Diltiazem** 0.25-0.3mg/kg IV β-**Blockers** Possibly IV digoxin with markedly decreased ejection fraction Intravenous β-Blockade: beware of bronchospasm **Esmolol** 5-10 mg IV bolus **Atenolol** 5-10 mg IV **Metoprolol** 5 mg IV
Sinus tachycardia Adenosine helpful to distinguish supraventricular from sinus tachycardia Carotid sinus massage will slow rate, then return to baseline	Check fluid balance, temperature, and pain control and correct; often no treatment required unless patient is at risk for myocardial ischemia	
Premature ventricular contractions: Treat if associated with R-on-T phenomenon or inadequate perfusion, otherwise no treatment needed	**Lidocaine** 1.0-1.5 mg/kg initial IV bolus followed by infusion of 1-4 mg/min IV	**IV beta-blocker** (see under sinus tachycardia) **Procainamide** IV 17 mg/kg over 1 hour then 2-6 mg/min, maximum rate 20 mg/min
Sinus bradycardia	Does not require treatment unless hypoperfusion is present	**Atropine** 0.5-2.0 mg IV **Isoproterenol** 1-4 μg/min **Dopamine** 5 μg/kg/min
Heart block 1° AV block 2° AV block: Mobitz I 2° AV block: Mobitz I	No treatment required No treatment required Close monitoring; transcutaneous or temporary transvenous pacing for HR <40 or if unstable	
Complete heart block 3° AV block	Atropine 0.5-1.0 mg IV Transcutaneous or temporary transvenous pacing	**Isoproterenol** 1-4 μg/min **Dopamine** 5+ μg/kg/min

months after surgery. The pain may be myofascial or a form of deafferentation pain. Myofascial pain presents as soreness of the incisional site aggravated by movement, often with "trigger-point" areas of sensitivity. Myofascial pain usually responds to physical therapy and injection of the trigger points with local anesthetics. Deafferentation pain presents with causalgia-like symptoms, including sensory loss, burning, and evidence of sympathetic hyperactivity over the distribution of the nerve involved.[54] Treatment includes sympathetic or local nerve block-

ade with local anesthetics, transcutaneous electrical stimulation, and medication with antidepressant drugs. Surgical resection and cryoneurotomy have been attempted with only occasional success.[55] Interruption of the neural pathway proximal to the lesion could actually worsen deafferentation pain in some patients.

SYSTEMIC TUMOR EMBOLIZATION

Systemic tumor embolization can complicate resection of primary lung tumors[56,57] or pulmonary manifestations of a metastatic sarcoma. Although rare, this complication tends to occur with large tumors that invade the pulmonary vein, or when it is reported that there was difficulty in obtaining an adequate venous resection margin. The presence and location of peripheral emboli can be confirmed by arteriography. Unless subsequent embolectomy is indicated, it can be difficult to distinguish between tumor embolization and the more usual thromboemboli. Immunocytochemistry and molecular detection by reverse transcriptase polymerase chain reaction (RT-PCR) have been used to detect disseminated tumor cells from nonhematologic malignancies.[58] Visceral malignancies have also been reported to produce rapidly evolving pulmonary hypertension and respiratory failure of unknown cause by means of a thrombotic pulmonary microangiopathy.[59]

INTENSIVE CARE UNIT

Unplanned admissions or readmissions to the ICU occur as a result of respiratory decompensation, as a result of fluid overload, aspiration, atelectasis, or retained secretions. Pain relief must be adequate to permit deep breathing and effective use of the incentive spirometer. Selected patients may require inhaled bronchodilators, corticosteroids, and/or mucolytics such as N-acetylcysteine. Chest percussion, postural drainage, and nasotracheal suctioning may be required to mobilize thick secretions and correct refractory atelectasis. Respiratory failure might be reversible when due to a treatable complication such as infection, fluid overload, aspiration, pulmonary edema, pulmonary embolus, or pneumothorax. Unfortunately, respiratory insufficiency is sometimes irreversible when surgical resection has resulted in inadequate pulmonary reserve. Failure to wean from ventilatory support requires arrangements for tracheostomy, enteral feeding, and long-term ventilator support.

REFERENCES

1. Nunn JF, Miledge S, Chen D, et al: Respiratory criteria for fitness for surgery and anesthesia, *Anaesthesia* 43:543, 1988.
2. Garibaldi RA, Britt MR, Coleman ML, et al: Risk factors for postoperative pneumonia, *JAMA* 70:677, 1981.
3. Warner MA, Offord KP, Warner ME, et al: Role of preoperative cessation of smoking and other factors in postoperative pulmonary complications: a blinded, prospective study of coronary artery bypass patients, *Mayo Clin Proc* 64:609, 1989.
4. Shapiro BA, Harrison RA, Kacmarek RM, et al: *Clinical application of respiratory care,* ed 3, Chicago, 1985, Year Book.
5. Palesty JA, McKelvey AA, Dudrick SJ: The efficacy of x-rays after chest tube removal, *Am J Surg* 179:13, 2000.
6. DeHaven CB, Hurst JM, Branson RD: Evaluation of two different extubation criteria: attributes contributing to success, *Crit Care Med* 14:92, 1986.
7. Adoumie R, Shennib H, Brown R, et al: Differential lung ventilation. Applications beyond the operating room, *J Thor Cardiovasc Surg* 105:229, 1993.
8. Hebert PC, Well G, Blajchman MA, et al: A multicenter, randomized, controlled clinical trial of transfusion requirements in critical care, *N Engl J Med* 340:409, 1999.
9. Hebert PC, Wells G, Tweeddale M, et al: Does transfusion practice affect mortality in critically ill patients? *Am J Respir Crit Care Med* 155:1618, 1997.
10. Hebert PC, Yetisir E, Martin C, et al: Is a low transfusion threshold safe in critically ill patients with cardiovascular diseases? *Critical Care Med* 29:227, 2001.
11. Stizman JV: Nutritional support of the dysphagic patient: methods, risks, and complications of therapy, *Parenteral Nutrition* 14:60, 1990.
12. Ullrich R, Lorber C, Röder G, et al: Controlled airway pressure therapy, nitric oxide inhalation, prone position, and extracorporeal membrane oxygenation (ECMO) as components of an integrated approach to ARDS, *Anesthesiology* 91:1567, 1999.
13. Baumann MH, Sahn SA: Medical management and therapy of bronchopleural fistulas in the mechanically ventilated patient, *Chest* 97:721, 1990.
14. Skrinskas GJ, Hyland RH, Hutcheon MA: Using helium-oxygen mixtures in the management of acute upper airway obstruction, *Can Med Assoc J* 128:555, 1983.
15. Castella X, Gilabert J, Perez C: Arytenoid dislocation after tracheal intubation: an unusual cause of acute respiratory failure? *Anesthesiology* 74:613, 1991.
16. Marik P: Fever in the ICU, *Chest* 117:855, 2000.
17. Marini JJ, Pierson DJ, Hudson LD: Acute lobar atelectasis: a prospective comparison of fiberoptic bronchoscopy and respiratory therapy, *Am Rev Respir Dis* 119:971, 1979.
18. Kopec SE, Irwin RS, Umali-Torres CB, et al: The postpneumonectomy state, *Chest* 114:1158, 1998.
19. Mulin MJ, Zumbro GL, Fishback ME, et al: Pulmonary lobar gangrene complicating lobectomy, *Ann Surg* 175:62, 1972.
20. Humphreys RL, Berne AS: Rapid re-expansion of pneumothorax: a cause of unilateral pulmonary edema, *Radiology* 96:509, 1970.
21. Shapira OM, Shahian DM: Postpneumonectomy pulmonary edema, *Ann Thorac Surg* 56:190, 1993.
22. Symbas PN: Chest drainage tubes, *Surg Clin North Am* 69:41, 1989.
23. Hankins JR, Miller JE, Allar S, et al: Bronchopleural fistula: thirteen-year experience with 77 cases, *J Thorac Cardiovasc Surg* 76:755, 1978.
24. Glauser FL, Bartlett RA: Pneumoperitoneum in association with pneumothorax, *Chest* 66:536, 1974.
25. Bjork VO: Thoracoplasty. A new osteoplastic technique, *J Thorac Cardiovasc Surg* 28:194, 1954.
26. Graham J, Usher FC, Perry JL, et al: Marlex mesh as a prosthesis in the repair of thoracic wall defects, *Ann Surg* 151:469, 1960.
27. LeRoux BT, Stemmler P: Maintenance of chest wall stability. A further report, *Thorax* 26:424, 1971.
28. Rice TW, Kirsh JC, Schacter IB, et al: Simultaneous occurrence of chylothorax and subarachnoid pleural fistula after thoracotomy, *Can J Surg* 30:256, 1987.
29. Peterffy A, Henze A: Hemorrhagic complications during pulmonary resections: a retrospective review of 1428 resections with 113 hemorrhagic episodes, *Scand J Thorac Cardiovasc Surg* 17:283, 1983.
30. Deiraniva AK: Cardiac herniation following intrapericardial pneumonectomy, *Thorax* 29:545, 1974.
31. Rodgers BM, Moulder PV, Delaney: Thoracoscopy: new method of early diagnosis of cardiac herniation, *J Thorac Cardiovasc Surg* 78:623, 1979.
32. Deiraniva AK: Cardiac herniation following intrapericardial pneumonectomy, *Thorax* 29:545, 1974.
33. Dippel WF, Ehrenhaft JL: Herniation of the heart after pneumonectomy, *J Thorac Cardiovasc Surg* 65:207, 1973.
34. Gates GF, Setle RS, Cope JA: Acute cardiac herniation with incarceration following pneumonectomy, *Radiology* 94:561, 1970.
35. Yacoub MH, Williams WG, Ahmad A: Strangulation of the heart following intrapericardial pneumonectomy, *Thorax* 23:261, 1968.
36. McKleven JR, Urgena RB, Rossi NP: Herniation of the heart following radical pneumonectomy: a case report, *Anesth Analg* 51:680, 1972.
37. Brandt LS, Bertolini R, Janni A, et al: Energy metabolism of thoracic surgical patients in the early postoperative period. Effect of posture, *Chest* 109:630, 1996.
38. Berger HJ, Matthay RA: Noninvasive radiographic assessment of cardiovascular function in acute and chronic respiratory failure, *Am J Cardiol* 47:950, 1981.
39. Matthay RA, Berger HJ, Davies R, et al: Right and left ventricular exercise performance in chronic obstructive pulmonary disease: radionuclide assessment, *Ann Intern Med* 93:234, 1980.
40. Cassidy SS, Robertson CH, Pierce AK, et al: Pulmonary hypertension in sepsis. Measurement of the pulmonary artery diastolic-pulmonary wedge pressure gradient and the influence of passive and active factors, *Chest* 73:583, 1980.
41. Olsen GN: The evolving role of exercise testing prior to lung resection, *Chest* 95:218, 1989.
42. Arciniegas E, Coates EO: Massive pulmonary arterial thrombosis after pneumonectomy, *J Thorac Cardiovasc Surg* 61:487, 1971.
43. Chaung TH, Dooling JA, Conally JM, et al: Pulmonary embolization from vascular stump thrombosis following pneumonectomy, *Ann Thorac Surg* 2:290, 1966.
44. Sautter KD, Myers WO, Ray JF, et al: Pulmonary embolectomy: review and current status, *Prog Cardiovasc Dis* 17:371, 1975.
45. Brown S, Muller D, Buckberg G: Massive pulmonary hemorrhagic infarction following revascularization of ischemic lungs, *Arch Surg* 108:795, 1974.

46. Greenfield LJ: Complications of venous thrombosis and pulmonary embolism, In Greenfield LJ (ed): *Complications in surgery and trauma*, ed 2, p 430, New York, 1990, JB Lippincott.

47. Greenfield LJ, Stewart JR, Crute S: Improved techniques for Greenfield vena caval filter insertion, *Surg Gynecol Obstet* 156:217, 1983.

48. Edwards R, Winnie AL, Ramamurthy S: Acute hypocapnic hypokalemia: an iatrogenic anesthetic complication, *Anesth Analg* 56:786, 1977.

49. O'Kelly B, Brownder WS, Massie B, et al: Ventricular arrhythmias in patients undergoing noncardiac surgery, *JAMA* 268:217, 1992.

50. Clemo HF, Wood MA, Gilligan DM, et al: Intravenous amiodarone for acute heart rate control in the critically ill patient with atrial tachyarrhythmias, *Am J Cardiol* 81:594, 1998.

51. Balser JR, Martinez EA, Winters BD, et al: Beta-adrenergic blockade accelerates conversion of postoperative supraventricular tachyarrhythmias, *Anesthesiology* 89:1052, 1998.

52. Eisenkraft JB, Papatestas AE, Kahn CH, et al: Predicting the need for postoperative mechanical ventilation in myasthenia gravis, *Anesthesiology* 65:79, 1986.

53. Agha EP, Orringer MB, Amendola MA: Gastric interposition following transhiatal esophagectomy: radiographic evaluation, *Gastrointest Radiol* 10:17, 1985.

54. Carlsson CA, Persson K, Peletieri L: Painful scars after thoracic and abdominal surgery, *Acta Chir Scand* 151:309, 1985.

55. Conacher ID: Percutaneous cryotherapy for post-thoracotomy neuralgia, *Pain* 25:227, 1986.

56. Starr DS, Lawrie GM, Morris GC Jr: Unusual presentation of bronchogenic carcinoma: care report and review of the literature, *Cancer* 47:398, 1981.

57. Xiromeritis N, Klonaris C, Papas S, et al: Recurrent peripheral arterial embolism from pulmonary cancer. Care report and review of the literature, *Int Angiol* 19:79, 2000.

58. Goeminne JC, Guillaume T, Symann M: Pitfalls in the detection of disseminated non-hematological tumor cells, *Ann Oncol* 11:785, 2000.

59. Pinckard JK, Wick MR: Tumor-related thrombotic pulmonary microangiopathy: review of pathologic findings and pathophysiologic mechanisms, *Ann Diagn Path* 4:154, 2000.

Postoperative Respiratory Failure and Treatment

18

James G. Ramsay, MD

Marshall Murphy, MD

RESPIRATORY failure after thoracic surgery is a significant cause of morbidity and mortality in this high-risk patient population. The incidence of major postthoracotomy pulmonary complications reported in recent literature—for example, pneumonia, lobar atelectasis, or the need for mechanical ventilation for more than 24 hours—ranges from 22% to 25%, whereas the incidence of respiratory failure (requiring mechanical ventilation for more than 48 hours after surgery) following thoracic surgery ranges from about 3% to 10%.[1-5] In most reports, respiratory failure accounts for approximately half of the mortality within the first 30 days after surgery. The reported incidence of respiratory failure and the overall mortality rate for several thoracic procedures are given in Table 18-1. Respiratory failure and mortality are greater after right-sided pneumonectomy than after left-sided pneumonectomy and likewise greater after extrapleural as opposed to intrapleural pneumonectomy.[6] The addition of chest wall resection to intrathoracic surgery also adds to the incidence of respiratory failure and mortality.[1] Preexisting pulmonary disease and other concomitant disease processes increase the risk of postoperative respiratory insufficiency and failure. Anticipation and early recognition are essential to provide the best possible outcome for the patient in respiratory failure (see Chapter 17).

Definition

Respiratory failure is the inability of the respiratory system to provide sufficient gas exchange to prevent life-threatening hypoxemia or hypercapnia. The clinical picture suggests the diagnosis, and the arterial blood gas analysis is confirmatory (Table 18-2). Respiratory failure can be purely hypoxemic, in which case there is inadequate arterial partial pressure of oxygen in the blood but normal or low arterial partial pressure of carbon dioxide. Physiologic causes of hypoxemic respiratory failure include hypoventilation, ventilation-perfusion mismatch, right-to-left intrapulmonary or intracardiac shunts, abnormalities in alveolar oxygen diffusion, and low fraction of inspired oxygen.[7] Failure to oxygenate the blood after thoracic surgery is usually the result of a severe mismatch of perfusion and ventilation (V/Q mismatch), with the result that pulmonary blood flows through poorly ventilated or edematous lung and there is inadequate time or alveolar exposure for absorption of O_2. Increased pulmonary water from direct surgical injury, capillary leak, or fluid overload can cause V/Q mismatch, as can focal areas of consolidation from collections (air, blood), infection, inflammation, or atelectasis. The most severe form of V/Q mismatch is true shunting of pulmonary blood without any absorption of O_2, as might occur with a completely atelectatic or consolidated segment or lobe.

Hypoventilation alone might result in hypoxemia. The simplified form of the alveolar gas equation estimates the partial pressure of oxygen in the alveoli based on the inspired partial pressure of oxygen and the partial pressure of arterial carbon dioxide:

$$P_{AO_2} = P_{IO_2} - P_{aCO_2}/R$$

where P_{AO_2} is the alveolar partial pressure of oxygen, P_{IO_2} is the partial pressure of inspired oxygen, and P_{aCO_2} is the arterial partial pressure of carbon dioxide (R represents the respiratory exchange ratio). Severe hypoventilation, with a resultant rise in P_{aCO_2}, would therefore be expected to result in some degree of hypoxemia. The degree of hypoxemia caused by pure hypoventilation can usually be overcome by supplemental oxygen, however.[8]

Intracardiac shunt with right-to-left-sided blood flow causes arterial desaturation somewhat independent of pulmonary disease. The condition in which this most commonly occurs in the adult is patent foramen ovale (PFO), which is present—at least in a probe-patent form—in approximately 25% of the population.[9] Short of actual closure of the shunt, the treatment requires reducing the gradient for blood flow from right to left—either reducing the right-sided pressure or increasing the left atrial pressure. In the presence of a PFO, application of

---

TABLE 18-1

Respiratory Failure* and 30-Day Mortality after Major Thoracic Surgery Procedures

	Respiratory Failure	Overall Mortality
LUNG RESECTION		
Wedge Resection	(not reported)	0.8%–1.4% (1,2)
Lobectomy	3.2%–6.6% (3,5)	1.2%–4% (1–5)
Pneumonectomy	6.9%–9.3% (3,5)	3.2%–11.5% (1–5)
ESOPHAGOGASTRECTOMY	2.1% (43)	2.1%–6.7% (43-45)
LUNG VOLUME REDUCTION SURGERY	29% (37)	2.3%–16% (37–39)

From Busch E, Verazin G, Antkowiak JG, et al: *Chest* 105:760, 1994 and Stephan F, Boucheseiche S, Hollande J, et al: *Chest* 118:1263, 2000.
*Defined as the need for mechanical ventilation for more than 48 hours after surgery.
In two reports, lobectomy was not separated from pneumonectomy. In one report, the incidence of trachestomy was 14%; in the other, the incidence of respiratory failure was 6%.

TABLE 18-2

TABLE 18-2

Diagnosis of Acute Respiratory Failure

Clinical

Central nervous system	Agitation, restlessness, diaphoresis from distress
	Headache, confusion from hypercarbia or hypoxemia
	Dizziness, focal twitching from hypercarbia
	Insomnia, personality change from hypoxemia
	Stupor, confusion, coma from severe hypercarbia or severe hypoxemia
	Seizures from severe hypoxemia
Cardiovascular system	Tachyarrhythmias from hypoxemia or hypercarbia
	Bradyarrhythmias from severe hypoxemia
	Systemic hypertension from hypoxemia or hypercarbia
	Pulmonary hypertension from hypoxemia or hypercarbia
	Hypotension/cardiac failure from severe hypoxemia or hypercarbia
Respiratory system	Intact respiratory drive: tachypnea, labored respirations, dyspnea, intercostal retractions
	Impaired respiratory drive: bradypnea or apnea
	Cheyne-Stokes respirations

Laboratory

Oxygenation*:	Arterial Po_2 < 50–60 mmHg
	Peripheral arterial saturation (pulse oximetry) <90%
Carbon dioxide†:	Arterial Pco_2 > 50–60 mmHg

*Respiratory "failure" due to hypoxemia might not require mechanical ventilatory support if it is responsive to supplemental oxygen therapy
†Chronic elevations in arterial Pco_2 are accompanied by retention of bicarbonate and relatively normal arterial pH and do not necessarily indicate respiratory "failure." Hypercarbia associated with acidosis always indicates respiratory failure and usually requires mechanical ventilatory support.

increasing levels of positive intrathoracic pressure (positive end-expiratory pressure, or PEEP) can worsen arterial oxygenation.[10] Positive intrathoracic pressure can increase impedance to ejection by the right ventricle, resulting in an elevation in the central venous pressure (CVP). This, in turn, can increase the flow of blood across the atrial septum from right to left.

Hypercapnic respiratory failure occurs when ventilation of the lungs is insufficient to maintain an adequate arterial partial pressure of carbon dioxide. Hypercapnic respiratory failure can occur with structural or functional abnormalities of the chest wall and muscles of respiration. Decreased function of the muscles of respiration can be seen with residual neuromuscular blockade and with surgical disruption. Structural or mechanical problems with the chest wall induced by surgery can lead to hypoventilation by affecting the normal decrease in intrathoracic pressure seen during inspiration. Such problems include pneumothorax, pulmonary contusion leading to decreased distensibility of the lung tissue, and flail chest. These types of hypercapnic failure are associated with respiratory distress and usually tachypnea: the patient is trying to achieve a normal

arterial Pco_2 but cannot. Decreased central respiratory drive can also result in hypoventilation. Decreased central drive is sometimes seen with residual anesthesia or postoperative sedation, or with central nervous system disease (e.g., perioperative stroke). Conditions associated with chronic carbon dioxide retention (e.g., obstructive airway disease, obesity-hypoventilation syndrome) can be exacerbated by depressant medications or structural changes induced by surgery.

Although pure hypoxemic or pure hypercapnic respiratory failure may be seen, most surgical patients with postoperative respiratory failure exhibit a mixed picture. Chest wall and parechymal injury, edema, retained secretions or blood, and atelectasis interfere with gas exchange and increase the work of breathing. Surgical injury to the chest wall and pain also interfere with normal mechanical function, decreasing the effectiveness of the respiratory effort and increasing the work of breathing.

Preoperative Predictors of Postoperative Respiratory Failure

Although conflicting results in the available medical literature make it difficult to establish precise criteria for determining which patients are most at risk for postoperative respiratory failure, the history, physical examination, and specific investigations of the patient enable the surgeon and anesthesiologist to estimate risk and identify processes that can be treated or improved before surgery. Preoperative factors associated with an increased incidence of postoperative respiratory failure are summarized in Table 18-3 (see Chapter 1).

History

Preexisting conditions that have been associated with increased risk of respiratory dysfunction and failure in the general surgery patient population include advanced age (over 70 years), chronic pulmonary disease, smoking, cardiac dysfunction, and neuromuscular diseases that affect the muscles of respiration or glutition.[11] Arozullah et al recently published a multifactorial index for predicting postoperative respiratory failure, which includes chronic obstructive pulmonary disease (COPD) age, dependent functional status, and surgical site as independent risk factors for patients in the general surgical population.[12] Patients who report dyspnea at rest, with light exercise (walking on a level surface 100 yards) or with activities of daily living (dressing, talking) have an approximately twofold increase in respiratory complications after thoractomy.[13]

A history of smoking has long been associated with postoperative pulmonary complications. In general, smokers have a relative risk factor for having postoperative pulmonary complications of up to 4.3 when compared with nonsmokers.[14] Patients with COPD related to smoking have a relative risk of postthoracotomy respiratory complications of 4.7 when compared with nonsmokers.[14]

Although carboxyhemoglobin levels return to normal levels in as few as 12 hours after smoking cessation and red blood cell mass becomes normal within a week, a reduction in the risk of perioperative respiratory dysfunction has only been demonstrated in patients who quit smoking a minimum of 8 weeks before surgery.[15] Conversely, a retrospective study showed that

Preoperative Factors Associated with Increased Risk of Postoperative Respiratory Failure

History

Age >70 years
Smoking history with chronic obstructive pulmonary disease
Cardiac dysfunction
Neuromuscular disease
Poor functional status/dyspnea with light exertion

Physical Findings

Increased baseline work of breathing
Preoperative wheezing (not controlled by bronchodilators)
Lower extremity edema/jugular venous distention (suggestive of right-side heart dysfunction)
Obesity
Cachexia

Laboratory

Pco_2 >45 mmHg
Po_2 <50 mmHg
ppoFEV$_1$ <40% predicted
ppoDLco <40% predicted
RV/TLC >30%
VO$_2$max <15 mL/kg/min

ppo, Predicted postoperative; *DLCO,* diffusion capacity for carbon monoxide; *FEV$_1$,* forced expiratory volume in one second; *RV,* residual volume; *TLC,* total lung capacity; *VO$_2$max,* maximum oxygen consumption.

patients who continue to smoke within 1 month of pneumonectomy are at increased risk for having a major postoperative respiratory complication, including respiratory failure.[16]

Asymptomatic asthma does not seem to be associated with any increase in the incidence of pulmonary complications or need for postoperative mechanical ventilation after thoracotomy. If the patient is free from wheezing in the immediate preoperative period and FEV$_1$ by spirometry is greater than 80% of the predicted value, there is no increased risk of bronchospasm or other pulmonary complications.[17] On the other hand, a patient with asthma who has had recent episodes of bronchospasm and wheezing should be treated cautiously and might benefit from prophylactically administered corticosteroids before anesthesia and surgery. Steroids can be administered orally or by inhalation. An advantage of inhaled steroid preparations is a reduced systemic side-effect profile. A substantial amount of these drugs, however, can enter the systemic circulation via the respiratory tract and also from the gastrointestinal tract secondary to medication that deposits in the oropharynx and is swallowed. Patients with asthma should remain on their routine bronchodilator and antiinflammatory medications until the time of surgery.

Physical Examination

Examination directed at the pulmonary status begins with simple observation of the patient's breathing pattern. Tachypnea or signs of increased work of breathing, such as intercostal retractions on inspiration, indicate severe disease either of the airways or of lung parenchyma. Wheezing heard during auscultation indicates obstruction to outflow through narrowed bronchioles, which could be associated with an exacerbation of asthma or COPD. Increased anterior-to-posterior diameter of the chest is indicative of hyperinflation of the lungs, such as is seen in COPD. Clubbing of the digits suggests chronic hypoxemia.

Patients with COPD can develop evidence of right ventricular enlargement and dysfunction (cor pulmonale). This is due to increased pulmonary artery pressure resulting from loss of capillaries in the pulmonary vascular bed and chronic hypoxic pulmonary vasoconstriction. Clinical evidence of right-side ventricular failure, such as lower-extremity edema and jugular venous distention, should prompt an evaluation of the patient's right ventricular function, including echocardiography and catheterization of the right side of the heart.

The nutritional status of the patient should also be assessed. Malnourished states, including both undernourishment and obesity, have been associated with postoperative pulmonary complications and difficulty in weaning from mechanical ventilation in the postoperative period. Patients who undergo thoracotomy for excision of bronchogenic carcinoma and patients with severe COPD can have associated malnourishment, including frank cachexia. These patients tend to experience delayed healing and are at increased risk of infection during the postoperative period.

Although obesity alone has not been associated with an increased risk of postoperative pulmonary complications, obese patients are predisposed to development of conditions that could increase their risk for pulmonary complications following thoracic surgical procedures.[14] Obesity is associated with reductions in total lung capacity, functional residual capacity (FRC), and vital capacity by up to 30%. Obese patients might therefore have significant baseline V/Q mismatch and are at increased risk for having atelectasis in the postoperative period. The reduction in FRC in these patients is attributed primarily to a decrease in expiratory reserve volume.[18] Obesity is a major risk factor for the development of obstructive sleep apnea (OSA).[19] Patients with OSA may have elevated systemic, pulmonary artery, and pulmonary artery occlusion pressures. The elevated pulmonary artery pressures in turn can lead to right-side heart dysfunction. These patients are, therefore, at increased risk for having postoperative cardiac complications as well as atelectasis and hypoxemia in the postoperative period.

Laboratory Evaluation

Arterial blood gas analysis, chest roentgenogram, and pulmonary function testing (PFT) are three tests commonly performed before thoracic surgery to help with risk stratification. Although there are no specific radiographic findings that are predictive of respiratory failure, severe hypoxemia (arterial Po_2 less than 50 mmHg on room air), carbon dioxide retention, and a predicted postoperative (ppo) FEV$_1$ less than 0.7 L or less than 40% are associated with a significant risk.[20] Evidence clearly establishing a relationship between hypercarbia alone and postoperative respiratory dysfunction is lacking, however.

Preoperative spirometry has not been shown to have a predictive value for postoperative respiratory failure in nonthoracic surgery, but it does appear to be predictive in the patient undergoing thoracotomy.[20-22] Spirometric PFT might help characterize the severity of disease and allow determination of perioperative change from baseline function. It could also demonstrate which patients will benefit from bronchodilator therapy. In a study from the mid-1980s, Nakahara et al found that patients with a ppoFEV$_1$ more than 40% of predicted normal values had no major postoperative pulmonary complications, whereas all patients with a ppoFEV$_1$ less than 30% of predicted normal required postoperative mechanical ventilatory support.[23]

Prediction of the postoperative FEV$_1$ is based on a calculation of the amount of functional lung tissue remaining after resection, which is then multiplied by the preoperative measured value to yield the ppoFEV$_1$. In patients with minimal baseline respiratory dysfunction, an estimate of functional lung tissue remaining after resection is acceptable for calculating ppoFEV. One method of calculation assumes a total of 42 lung subsegments with a breakdown of 6 subsegments in the right upper lobe, 4 subsegments in the right middle lobe, 12 subsegments in the right lower lobe, and 10 subsegments in each of the left lobes.[24] For example, a patient with a preoperative FEV$_1$ of 2.3 L who is to undergo a right lower lobectomy would have an estimated ppoFEV$_1$ as follows:

Fractional contribution of right lower lobe: 12/42 = 0.285
Functional lung tissue remaining after resection: 1 − 0.285 = 0.715
ppoFEV1: 2.3 × 0.715 = 1.64 L

A more accurate assessment of the contribution of segmental regions of the lung can be obtained by radiolabeled, macroaggregated albumin lung scanning. In patients with significant baseline pulmonary disease, lung scanning offers a relatively precise method for predicting the postoperative pulmonary function.[25] When lung scanning is inaccurate, it usually has underestimated postoperative function. This underestimation could be related to an overestimation of the contribution of diseased lung tissue to the total ventilation-perfusion of the lungs. Resection of the diseased area surrounding a bronchogenic tumor mass, for example, could actually improve the ventilation of the surrounding healthier lung parenchyma and, in the long run, improve ventilation-perfusion matching.

The predicted postoperative diffusion capacity for carbon monoxide (DLCO) has also been correlated with postoperative respiratory status after lung resection. Measurement of the DLCO is often included with preoperative PFT, and the predicted postoperative value (ppoDLCO) can be calculated in a manner analogous to ppoFEV$_1$. Ferguson et al found an increased incidence of both pulmonary and cardiac complications in patients with a ppoDLCO less than 40% of predicted values.[26]

In a small study, Uramoto et al found three independent risk factors that correlated with an increased incidence of postoperative pulmonary complications in patients undergoing lobectomy for non–small cell carcinoma of the lung. The factors were the following[27]:

- A serum lactate dehydrogenase (LDH) level more than 230 U/L
- A residual volume to total lung capacity (RV/TLC) more than 30%
- A baseline Pao$_2$ less than 80 mmHg

Recently, more focus has been placed on studies involving exercise testing for prospective candidates for lung resection. Exercise testing has the potential advantage of simultaneously assessing the cardiovascular and pulmonary systems and their interaction. A simple but clinically useful test is symptom-limited stair climbing. The patient is asked to climb as many flights of stairs as possible at his/her own pace but without stopping. In a study of patients undergoing thoracotomy, sternotomy, or upper abdominal surgery, Girish et al found that 89% of patients unable to climb one flight of stairs and 82% of patients unable to complete two flights developed a postoperative cardiopulmonary complication.[28] No patient able to complete seven flights experienced a postoperative cardiopulmonary complication.

More formal and reproducible exercise testing, such as standardized cycle or treadmill ergometry, can be used to obtain an accurate measurement of the maximum measured oxygen uptake (VO$_2$max). In a study by Bolliger et al, a VO$_2$max less than 10 mL/kg/min was associated with 100% mortality after lung resection, suggesting this parameter as an absolute cutoff value for lung resection candidates.[29] On the other hand, patients who fail to meet other criteria for lung resection may be deemed acceptable candidates if they are capable of performing exercise testing and demonstrate a VO$_2$max more than 15 mL/kg/min.[30]

Although there is conflicting evidence surrounding the predictive value of routine preoperative testing for partial lung resection, the patient undergoing total pneumonectomy represents a unique situation in which pulmonary function testing is considered essential in the effort to avoid disastrous postoperative pulmonary insufficiency. Tests involved are used to estimate the adequacy of pulmonary function of the remaining lung as well as ability of the remaining pulmonary vasculature and the right ventricle to handle the total pulmonary blood flow after occlusion and ligation of the pulmonary artery on the operative side. Initial evaluation consists of routine spirometric pulmonary function studies. If the preoperative forced expiratory volume in one second (FEV$_1$) is more than 1.6 L, the maximum voluntary ventilation is more than 55% of predicted, or the predicted postoperative diffusing capacity (DLCO) is more than 10 mL/min/mmHg, the patient can be expected to tolerate pneumonectomy.[26,31,32] Failure to meet these criteria will necessitate further studies, such as split-lung (single-lung) function studies. In split-lung function testing, ventilation and perfusion of the nonoperative lung are determined. A calculated FEV$_1$ more than 800 mL for the nonoperative lung should be adequate to allow contralateral pneumonectomy. Measurement of pulmonary artery pressure while temporarily occluding pulmonary artery flow to the operative lung can also be performed. If, on occlusion, the PA pressure rises above 35 mmHg or if hypoxemia ensues, pneumonectomy would be expected to lead to significant postoperative respiratory and cardiac dysfunction.[33]

Procedure and Extent of Resection

THORACOTOMY FOR LUNG RESECTION

The extent of resection during thoracotomy for lung cancer is related to the incidence of postoperative pulmonary complications and 30-day mortality (Table 18-1). In addition, Busch et al reported an 82% incidence of postoperative pulmonary complications in patients who required extended resection (including chest wall). This compared with an overall incidence of 39% in their study of patients undergoing thoracotomy.[1] On the other hand, a review of the muscle-sparing thoracotomy approach (where the latissimus dorsi and serratus anterior muscles are not severed) vs. standard thoracotomy found no morbidity or mortality benefit.[34] Not surprisingly, older studies and more recent reports have found increasing age to be a major risk factor for the development of serious pulmonary complications, including respiratory failure and mortality.[4,5,35]

LUNG VOLUME REDUCTION SURGERY

Lung volume reduction is a surgical strategy to improve ventilation-perfusion matching in patients with severe emphysema. Prospective candidates usually have an FEV_1 of less than 30% of predicted and poor exercise tolerance resulting from dyspnea. The concept of the procedure is to reduce lung volume (by up to 30% in some patients) with an improvement in the function of the remaining lung tissue. The lung parenchyma is removed from less well-ventilated and perfused apical segments, with improvement in function believed to be related to improved chest wall mechanics allowing greater elastic recoil with the reduced lung volume.[36] In one report, the incidence of postoperative acute respiratory failure was 29%, with a mortality of 33% in this group of patients.[37] Overall, the reported mortality after lung volume reduction surgery ranges from a low of 2.3% to up to 16% in the highest-risk patients.[38,39]

TRANSSTERNAL THYMECTOMY

Transsternal thymectomy remains a viable treatment option for patients with myasthenia gravis who have worsening symptoms despite maximal medical therapy with anticholinesterase medications and corticosteroids. Thymectomy has been shown to improve symptoms in up to 75% of patients.[40] In the perioperative period, the myasthenic patient may show exquisite sensitivity to nondepolarizing neuromuscular blocking medications and may have increased sensitivity to medications that cause respiratory depression, such as opioids. In the past, these patients remained intubated after surgery and were extubated only after careful assessment and reinstitution of preoperative anticholinesterase medications. As medical management has improved, many of these patients now present for surgery with their disease well controlled, and with careful anesthetic management, they can be extubated immediately after the procedure. Historically, preoperative predictors of the need for postoperative ventilatory support include duration of the disease for longer than 6 years, concomitant chronic lung disease, a daily dose of pyridostigmine more than 750 mg (or its equivalent), and a preoperative vital capacity less than 2.9 L.[41] In a series of 71 patients undergoing resection of thymoma, the incidence of postoperative respiratory complications was 13%, with only one death due to respiratory failure.[42] An increase in the use of thoracoscopic techniques for this procedure might reduce the incidence of postoperative respiratory complications.

ESOPHAGOGASTRECTOMY

The incidence of adenocarcinoma of the distal esophagus has increased over the past several decades, with risk factors including a history of tobacco use and alcohol consumption.[43] Esophagogastrectomy offers the only hope of cure. Esophagogastrectomy for carcinoma at or near the gastroesophageal junction may be performed via a transhiatal approach (without thoracotomy) or via a transthoracic approach (Ivor Lewis procedure). Pulmonary complications occur in 15% to 25% of patients, with pneumonia and/or respiratory failure comprising about half of this incidence. The in-hospital mortality rate following transthoracic esophagogastrectomy ranges from 2.1% to 6.7%.[43-45]

LUNG TRANSPLANTATION

Lung transplantation is increasingly performed for end-stage lung disease from a variety of causes; transplantation opportunities are limited to a large degree by donor availability. After reperfusion of the donor lung, more than half of the patients exhibit some degree of noncardiogenic pulmonary edema, and postoperative mechanical ventilation for at least 24 hours is the norm. This is discussed in a later section of this chapter concerning pulmonary edema.

Specific Etiologies of Respiratory Failure: Their Prevention and Treatment

Table 18-4 summarizes the common conditions leading to acute postoperative respiratory failure. Similar to the diagnosis itself, the cause is seldom single or simple; more often, it represents a combination of postoperative factors with predisposing physiology or underlying conditions.

Atelectasis

Surgery on the thorax and upper abdomen leads to some degree of postoperative pulmonary dysfunction and atelectasis, which can persist for days or weeks. Changes in the mechanics of breathing that occur in the postthoracotomy patient include decreases in inspiratory capacity (IC) and vital capacity (VC) and a lesser decrease in the functional residual capacity (FRC).

TABLE 18-4

Acute Causes of Respiratory Failure After Thoracic Surgery

Atelectasis/retained secretions	
Pneumonia	
Pulmonary embolus	
Pulmonary edema	Postpneumonectomy pulmonary edema
	Pulmonary reimplantation response
Acute respiratory distress syndrome	
Pneumothorax	
Bronchopulmonary fistula	
Torsion of residual lobe	
Neurologic injuries	Phrenic nerve
	Recurrent laryngeal nerves

Although the relative decrease in FRC is less than the decreases in IC and VC, the clinical repercussions are significant. The reduced FRC allows pleural pressure in the dependent portions of the lung to exceed atmospheric pressure, resulting in a negative transpulmonary pressure. This leads to narrowing or actual closure of small airways not supported by cartilage. The pressure at which these small airways close is defined as the closing capacity.[46] The reduced ventilation of the alveoli distal to these airways results in atelectasis and ventilation-perfusion mismatch or shunt. The reduction in chest wall compliance associated with the pressure of the abdominal contents against the diaphragm in the supine position leads to a reduction in FRC in the supine patient. Closing capacity, unlike FRC, is not affected by position; however, closing capacity rises with age. By the seventh decade of life, most patients have a closing capacity that exceeds FRC even when they are in an upright position.[47]

Although some degree of atelectasis occurs in almost all postthoracotomy patients, the severity and clinical implications vary widely. Mild atelectasis usually requires little treatment—other than supplemental oxygen administration in the postanesthesia care unit—and resolves as the patient awakens and increases depth of breathing. A more severe form of atelectasis, lobar atelectasis, occurs in approximately 5% of patients after pulmonary resection. Lobar atelectasis is defined roentgenographically by complete lobar collapse and mediastinal shift. Risk factors include male sex, advanced age, and reduced preoperative FEV_1.[48] This extreme form of atelectasis usually requires bronchoscopy, might require mechanical ventilatory support, and can lead to longer lengths of stay both in the intensive care unit (ICU) and in the hospital.

Prevention and treatment of atelectasis have traditionally consisted of cough and deep breathing exercises, incentive spirometry, and chest physiotherapy (Table 18-5). Although coughing and deep breathing help clear secretions and potentially reopen atelectatic areas of lung, the ability of surgical patients to cough is significantly impaired after thoracic surgery. The maximal intrapleural pressures produced during voluntary coughing are reduced to as low as 29% of preoperative values and may remain as low as 50% of the preoperative value 3 weeks after surgery.[49] Cough effort can be improved with the patient in the sitting position and with manually assisted compression of the chest wall. In a study of patients after abdominal surgery, simply mobilizing patients from sitting in bed to sitting in a chair improved FRC by an average of 17%.[50]

Incentive spirometry (IS) is a simple, inexpensive method of helping patients obtain maximal inspiratory effort.[51]

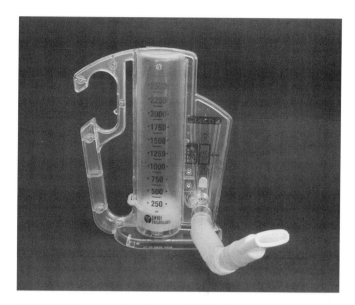

FIGURE 18-1 Incentive spirometer (DHD Healthcare Corp.). The patient makes a sustained inhalation effort through the mouthpiece, guided by an effort indicator on the right side of the device. This causes a floating marker (inside the graduated cylinder) to be drawn up to the appropriate "target" volume, indicated by the external white marker.

Figure 18-1 shows a typical single-patient use of an incentive spirometry device. Incentive spirometry can also be followed as a bedside test for evaluation of postoperative pulmonary function after lung surgery. The performance on IS correlates well with inspiratory reserve volume and forced vital capacity.[52] Decline in a patient's abililty to perform IS can be an early indicator of an acute worsening of the patient's pulmonary status. Although IS is widely accepted as a tool to help prevent atelectasis, this has not been established clearly in clinical studies. A review of the medical literature by Overend et al failed to find supporting evidence for the routine use of IS after cardiac or upper abdominal surgery.[53] Although the goal of IS is to encourage deep inspiration—which could promote coughing and clearing of secretions—an alternative approach is to focus on maintaining airway patency during expiration. This is termed *positive expiratory pressure* (PEP) *therapy* and has been shown to improve clearance of secretions (Figure 18-2).[54] The patient uses this device for several breaths, then makes coughing or "huffing" efforts. Yet another type of device is the "flutter valve," which causes fluttering of the expiratory airway pressure, thus aiding the mobilization of secretions.

Either positive pressure breathing (i.e., positive inspiratory pressure) through a mouthpiece or face mask or continuous positive airway pressure (CPAP) delivered by nasal or face mask can be beneficial in maintaining lung volume and recruiting lung volume that has been lost to atelectasis.[55] Biphasic (also called *bilevel*) positive airway pressure (BiPAP) has also been used to support patients with hypoxema in the postanesthesia care unit.[56] Figure 18-3 illustrates the nasal mask used for BiPAP or CPAP. The role of nasal BiPAP in prevention or treatment of acute respiratory failure is discussed later in this chapter.

Pain is a major factor contributing to the reduction in patients' cough efforts and deep breathing after thoracotomy.

TABLE 18-5

Prevention of Atelectasis

Cough and deep breathing exercises
Incentive spirometry
Positive expiratory pressure devices
Noninvasive positive-pressure breathing devices
Continuous positive airway pressure
Bilevel positive airway pressure
Adequate analgesia

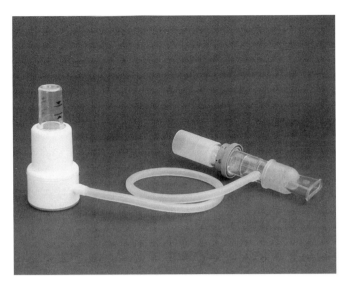

FIGURE 18-2 Positive expiratory pressure (PEP) device (DHD Healthcare Corp.). The patient performs a submaximal inspiration, then exhales through a respiratory resistance set at a preset target level. During exhalation, a floating marker appears between the arrows on the cylinder.

Adequate control of postoperative pain, including use of epidural analgesia, has been shown to improve maximal cough pressures in postthoracotomy patients.[57] Although the use of opioid infusions through either lumbar-level or thoracic-level epidural catheters can provide adequate postthoracotomy analgesia, only analgesia provided by thoracic-level catheters was demonstrated to decrease mortality in a recent meta-analysis of postoperative outcomes.[58] Various infusions can be used, including an opioid alone or, for a thoracic-level catheter, a combination of an opioid and a local anesthetic. The combination of an opioid and a local anesthetic has been shown to be synergistic and permits a lower dose of each than if either were used alone.[59] Other modalities of regional anesthesia to provide

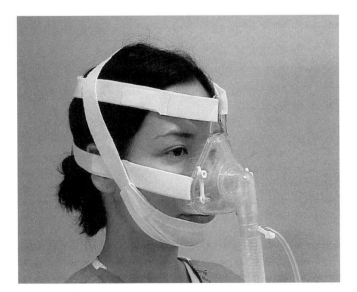

FIGURE 18-3 Nasal mask used to provide mask CPAP and/or mask BiPAP (Respironics Inc). An air-filled, soft sealing rim provides an occlusive seal around the nose; head straps keep the mask in place.

postthoracotomy analgesia include intrapleural administration of local anesthetic and intercostal nerve blocks. Intercostal nerve blocks can be performed by the anesthesiologist preoperatively or postoperatively or by the surgeon during the procedure. The blocks can be performed with local anesthetic or, for a more protracted duration of analgesia, with phenol. Intraoperative cryoablation of intercostal nerves has also been used to provide an extended period of analgesia.

Bronchospasm

In patients with known bronchospastic disease or who were shown to have improved after the use of bronchodilators during preoperative spirometry, postoperative airway constriction could contribute to respiratory failure. Increased airways resistance contributes to increased work of breathing and also can create the "auto-PEEP" effect. This occurs when terminal airways/alveoli do not fully empty through narrowed airways during expiration, resulting in positive pressure rather than zero pressure at end-expiration distal to the obstruction. For flow to be generated into these alveoli during inspiration, this positive pressure must first be overcome, creating a further increase in the work of breathing.[60] Inhaled bronchodilating agents should be considered in all patients who exhibit respiratory distress after thoracic surgery. Inhaled β-adrenergic agonists, which enhance bronchodilatation through increasing intracellular levels of cyclic AMP through stimulation of adenylate cyclase, include albuterol, metaproterenol, and racemic epinephrine. Racemic epinephrine might also reduce respiratory mucosal edema through its α-adrenergic effects on mucosal vasculature. Anticholinergic medications, such as atropine and ipratropium, are also effective bronchodilators, mediating their activity by decreasing intracellular levels of cyclic GMP. Steroidal compounds are also available for inhalation administration and serve a useful role in preventing inflammatory-mediated bronchospasm, although they are not indicated for acute bronchospasm (see Chapter 6).

Retained Secretions

A patient's inability to clear secretions contributes to atelectasis and pulmonary infections. Dehydration of the tracheobronchial mucosa occurs with use of nonhumidified oxygen, which can lead to mucociliary dysfunction and drying of secretions. The ensuing decrease in a patient's ability to mobilize and clear secretions can contribute to the formation of atelectasis; humidification of oxygen is therefore recommended. Patients with tenacious secretions might benefit from inhaled agents that decrease the viscosity of secretions, such as N-acetylcysteine or dornase alfa (Pulmozyme, Genetech, Inc.) Dornase is a recombinant human DNAse that has been demonstrated to decrease viscosity of respiratory secretions in patients with cystic fibrosis and to help reexpand atelectatic lobes in this population.[61] Efficacy in patients with chronic bronchitis has not been demonstrated for long-term use but has been suggested in acute exacerbations.

Inhaled medications can be delivered by handheld nebulizers or by metered-dose inhalers (MDI). The MDI allows the patient to self-deliver the inhaled medication, although the patient must be able to coordinate actuation of the device with deep inspiration. Combinations of medications with additive

TABLE 18-6

Adjuvants to Routine Postoperative Respiratory Care

Chest physiotherapy	
	Percussion/vibration
Nasotracheal suctioning	
Fiberoptic bronchoscopy	
	Therapeutic
	Diagnostic
Minitracheostomy	

effects, such as albuterol with ipratropium (Combivent, Boehringer Ingelheim), can also be packaged in MDI.[62]

For the patient who does not respond to deep-breathing exercises, IS, and PEP therapy, along with inhaled bronchodilators or mucolytics, there are several adjuvant therapies that can be used to improve the patient's status (Table 18-6). Modalities of chest physiotherapy include postural drainage, percussion and vibration over the affected lung segments, and incentive to cough. Postural drainage is performed by positioning the patient with the lung segments to be drained in a superior position. Drainage is most effective when combined with percussion and vibration, but proper positioning might be limited by the patient's condition. Percussion is performed throughout the respiratory cycle and is followed by vibration during the exhalation phase.

Tracheal suctioning can be used to remove secretions from the trachea mechanically and to induce deep breathing and coughing. In the nonintubated patient, tracheal suctioning is usually performed by a blind nasal technique. Suctioning should be performed after preoxygenation of the patient with a high FIO_2 and might be better tolerated through a nasal airway or "trumpet." The catheter should be advanced without suction and removed from the trachea with intermittent suction. Frequent or aggressive suctioning can cause mucosal damage and could induce bronchospasm, laryngospasm, and cardiac rhythm disturbances.

An alternative to blind nasotracheal suctioning is placement of a minitracheotomy (a small, uncuffed endotracheal tube through an incision in the cricothyroid membrane) to facilitate suctioning of secretions. This procedure is safe and effective in decreasing the need for other interventions (such as chest physiotherapy); it also could decrease postoperative respiratory complications.[63-65] Potential complications are rare but include bleeding into the trachea, infection, and tracheal occlusion by granuloma formation.[66] Minitracheotomy is not intended to provide a means for positive pressure ventilation and is not a replacement for endotracheal intubation when indicated.

Fiberoptic bronchoscopy (FOB), in addition to its diagnostic role in the patient with an acute worsening of respiratory function, can be used for more aggressive clearance of secretions or blood in the tracheobronchial tree. Under direct visualization, tenacious secretions can be suctioned from affected airways. A review of the practice of FOB in a large teaching hospital confirmed the safety of the procedure with a major complication rate of 0.5% and a minor complication rate of 0.8%.[67] Complications include laryngospasm, bronchospasm,

pneumothorax, and pulmonary hemorrhage. In the awake, nonintubated patient, FOB requires topical anesthesia of the upper airway and sedation.

Pneumonia

Decreased mucociliary clearance and persistent atelectasis place the thoracic surgical patient at increased risk for postoperative nosocomial pneumonia. After thoracotomy, patients also have altered systemic and lung host defenses, which increase susceptibility to postoperative pneumonia.[68] The occurrence of pneumonia, especially after lung resection, significantly increases the patient's risk for respiratory insufficiency and need for mechanical ventilation. Nosocomial pneumonia is the single most important risk factor for mortality in the postthoracotomy patient.[4] The incidence of nosocomial pneumonia ranges from 6.4% to 20%.[2] Overall, mortality rates for nosocomial pneumonia range from 20% to 80%, with gram-negative bacilli and *Staphylococcus aureus* being the most common pathogens.[68]

The diagnosis of postoperative pneumonia is suggested by fever, leucocytosis, purulent secretions, and a new or expanding infiltrate on the chest radiograph. The diagnosis can be confirmed by sputum cultures, although multiple organisms are often identified because of contamination with oral and skin flora. Also, the use of perioperative antibiotic prophylaxis can confound culture results. Bronchoalveolar lavage (BAL) or protected specimen brush by FOB can be used to obtain a culture sample to more positively identify the pathogenic organism. Initiation of therapy should not be delayed for the results of these tests, however. Mortality has been shown to be reduced with appropriate empiric antibiotic therapy rather than delaying until BAL is performed.[69] For suspected pneumonia occurring early in the postoperative period in a patient who was not in the hospital preoperatively, community-acquired organisms such as *Streptococcus pneumonia* and *Hemophilus influenza* should be targeted. For a patient who has been in the hospital preoperatively, or in whom pneumonia is suspected more than 48 hours after surgery, empiric antibiotic therapy should target hospital-acquired organisms such as *Pseudomonas aeruginosa, Acinetobacter,* and *Klebsiella* species, as well as methicillin-resistant *S. aureus.* Ventilator-associated pneumonia is discussed later in this chapter.

Pulmonary Embolism

In a study of 77 patients after thoracotomy but before the use of subcutaneous heparin prophylaxis, the incidence of deep venous thrombosis was 19%, with pulmonary embolism occurring in 5%.[70] In a large series of lung resection patients (1735 patients), early fatal acute cardiorespiratory failure occurred in 26. Autopsy in 20 of these patients demonstrated pulmonary embolism in 19.[71] In patients with shock due to massive pulmonary emboli, the mortality rate is in excess of 30%.[72] Because thoracic surgery patients usually have at least two major risk factors for deep venous thrombosis (malignancy and major surgery), prophylaxis should include both sequential compression devices applied to the calves and low-dose, subcutaneous heparin or low-molecular-weight heparin.

Signs and symptoms of pulmonary embolism include dyspnea, tachypnea, arterial hypoxemia, pulmonary hypertension, right ventricular failure, and shock. Lung perfusion scanning with technetium 99m–labeled albumin, when combined with ventilation scanning with xenon 133, can demonstrate areas of ventilation-perfusion mismatch, although this test is of limited use when there is preexisting lung disease or recent lung surgery. Spiral computed tomography (CT) can demonstrate pulmonary emboli and is quicker and easier to perform than ventilation-perfusion scanning.[73,74] Although the gold standard for detection of pulmonary emboli is pulmonary angiography, in many centers spiral CT has essentially eliminated the need for this more invasive test. Postoperative patients are not candidates for thrombolytic therapy, but therapeutic heparinization is safe if initiated at least 24 to 48 hours after surgery. Massive embolism could require surgical embolectomy.[72]

Pulmonary Edema

The etiology of pulmonary edema after thoracic surgery can be cardiogenic or noncardiogenic. Increased hydrostatic pressure in the pulmonary vasculature, which might be associated with left ventricular dysfunction or excessive intravenous fluid administration, can lead to cardiogenic pulmonary edema. Increased permeability of the alveolar capillary membranes, such as that occurring with acute respiratory distress syndrome (ARDS), leads to noncardiogenic pulmonary edema.

Postpneumonectomy pulmonary edema (PPE) is a particularly severe form of pulmonary edema that can occur after pneumonectomy and is associated with a high mortality rate. Resections of lesser amounts of lung tissue are not associated with this entity.[75] Risk factors that have been associated with PPE include the side of operation (with right-side pneumonectomy having a higher risk than left-side), perioperative fluid overload, the use of fresh frozen plasma intraoperatively, and, paradoxically, excessive diuresis in the first 24 hours postoperatively. A variety of etiologies for PPE have been proposed, with most focusing on potential causes of increased pulmonary capillary endothelial permeability. An increase in endothelial permeability has been demonstrated by measuring the pulmonary accumulation of intravenously administered technetium 99m–labeled albumin after pneumonectomy.[76] Inflammatory-mediated damage of the pulmonary endothelium seems to be a common denominator in the development of PPE. The use of high inspired oxygen concentration during one-lung ventilation, along with ischemia/reperfusion injury, could induce oxidative damage of the alveolar capillary endothelium.[77] Intraoperative intravenous fluid administration of 2000 mL or more also has been associated with development of PPE.[78]

The development of pulmonary edema after lung transplantation has been termed the *pulmonary reimplantation response* (PRR). Although PRR has not been shown to affect survival of transplant patients, its occurrence does cause increased duration of ventilator support and ICU stay. Contrary to what might be expected, Kahn et al were not able to demonstrate that prolonged ischemic time of the donor lung or the presence of pulmonary hypertension was independently associated with the development of PRR.[79] The use of cardiopulmonary bypass during the transplant procedure was shown to be an independent risk factor, however. Treatment has been primarily supportive, but recently researchers have been focusing on treatment

modalities that could decrease the injury caused to the donor lung by reperfusion. In a sheep model, inhibiting adherence of polymorphonuclear leukocytes to activated endothelium through the blocking of L- and E-selectins by specific antibodies demonstrated a reduced incidence of PRR.[80] A recent study of daclizumab, an interleukin-2 antagonist, demonstrated no significant differences in immediate clinical or radiographic manifestations of PRR, however.[81]

Pneumothorax

After thoracotomy, the surgeon usually places two chest tubes into the operative hemithorax. One chest tube is placed inferiorly to preferentially drain blood and fluids, whereas a second tube is placed superiorly to preferentially vent air. Pneumothorax can develop postoperatively if a chest tube is inadvertently kinked, clamped off, or dislodged. Although a small leak might cause few or no symptoms, a large, undrained air leak can result in tension pneumothorax, with a shift of the trachea and mediastinum to the contralateral side. The increase in intrathoracic pressure causes a decrease in venous return to the right heart and can result in cardiovascular collapse. Pneumothorax can also occur on the nonoperative side as the result of rupture of a pulmonary cyst or bulla if excessive airway pressures develop during mechanical (especially one-lung) ventilation. Inadvertent and unrecognized surgical entry into the pleura of the nonoperative side can cause pneumothorax, as can inadvertent lung puncture during placement of central venous catheters, or placement of intrapleural catheters for postoperative analgesia.

Definitive treatment for a pneumothorax is placement of a chest tube, usually in the fourth or fifth intercostal space between the anterior and midaxillary lines. In the case of tension pneumothorax, if a delay in the placement of a chest tube is anticipated and the patient's condition is deteriorating, a needle thoracostomy can be performed by placing a large-bore (e.g., 14-gauge) venous catheter above the third rib in the midclavicular line. This measure effectively converts the tension pneumothorax to a simple pneumothorax.

Bronchopulmonary Fistula

Bronchpulmonary fistula occurs when there is disruption of a bronchial stump or tracheobronchial anastomosis associated with a large air leak from the lung. The initial sign is often a dramatic increase in air leak noticed in the chest tube drainage chamber. If the air leak exceeds the capacity of the chest tube to evacuate the air, there will be a persistent pneumothorax. Respiratory insufficiency can ensue in the mechanically ventilated patient secondary to loss of tidal volume into the pleural space and chest tube.

Although definitive treatment is surgical correction, temporary ventilator management might include placement of a double-lumen endotracheal tube (DLT) to allow differential lung ventilation. Alternatively, a bronchial blocker can be used on the affected side to limit flow to that side.

Aspiration of Gastric Contents

In the thoracic surgery population, the risk of aspiration of gastric contents is increased in patients presenting with esophageal disease. Intraoperative aspiration can lead to a pulmonary injury causing edema and inflammation and, eventually, hypoxemia. Aspiration pneumonitis is one of the causes of ARDS the management of which is discussed in a subsequent section of this chapter.

Torsion of Residual Lobe

Torsion of a residual lobe of the lung around its bronchus can complicate lobectomy. The loss of lung tissue on the surgical side could allow abnormal movement of the residual lung tissue, most commonly the right middle lobe and the lingula. In addition to the intrapulmonary shunt that develops as a result of occlusion of the affected bronchus, blood supply to the affected lobe is compromised and can lead to infarction.

The diagnosis can be suspected by the onset of respiratory distress or failure in association with the appearance of a collapsed or abnormal lobe on the chest radiograph, which does not respond to the usual therapies for atelectasis. The diagnosis can then be confirmed by bronchoscopy. Definitive therapy consists of surgical correction of the torsion, which should be performed urgently if infarction of the lobe is to be prevented.

Neurologic Injuries

Although neurologic injuries occur only rarely after thoracic surgery, they can lead to pulmonary insufficiency in the postoperative period. Damage to a phrenic nerve can occur after thoracotomy, especially if extensive dissection into the mediastinum is necessary to remove tumor. Unilateral phrenic nerve palsy can be tolerated by a patient with good pulmonary reserve. In a patient with baseline compromised pulmonary status, which is possible with advanced chronic obstructive disease, unilateral phrenic nerve paralysis leads to difficulty in weaning from mechanical ventilation. Bilateral phrenic nerve paralysis leads to pulmonary insufficiency in any patient. The diagnosis is suggested by an elevated hemidiaphragm on postoperative chest film. It can be confirmed by observing paradoxic motion of the affected hemidiaphragm under fluoroscopy.

Recurrent laryngeal nerve injury can be seen after extensive hilar lymph node dissection. The left recurrent laryngeal nerve is at greater risk of injury due to its more caudal course. Unilateral injury is generally well tolerated, but bilateral injury can cause significant stridor after extubation as a result of spasm of the vocal cord adductor muscles.

Mechanical Ventilation after Thoracic Surgery

Table 18-7 summarizes the common reasons to continue mechanical ventilation into the postoperative period after thoracic surgery. Many of these relative indications are common to major surgery of all types and reflect planning to "stabilize" an often elderly patient after major stress. Preoperative and intraoperative discussion with the surgical team allow for appropriate arrangements to be made in advance regarding care in the postanesthesia care unit (PACU) or ICU.

Two major issues in early postoperative mechanical ventilation after thoracic surgery are the following:
1. Concern for bronchial anastomoses after lung resection

TABLE 18-7

Relative Indications for Mechanical Ventilation after Thoracic Surgery

Preoperative	Preoperative mechanical ventilation
	Predicted low postoperative FEV_1 (<30% predicted)
	Esophagogastrectomy or thoracoabdominal aneurysm repair
Intraoperative	Prolonged intraoperative course
	Massive fluid administration or transfusion
	Hypothermia
	Cardiac failure
	Surgical complication
	Need for postoperative lung isolation (air leak, drainage)
	Need for postoperative chest wall immobilization/stabilization
Immediate postoperative	Incomplete recovery of neuromuscular function
	Inadequate respiratory drive (excessive opioid administration)
	Requirement for ≥50% FiO_2
	Visible respiratory distress

2. Leaving tracheal tubes that are designed for intraoperative lung isolation

Regarding bronchial anastomoses, there is always a concern that positive airway pressures might expose the patient to increased risk of bronchial anastomotic leaks or disruption. This concern must be balanced with the need for oxygenation (which could require PEEP) and adequate minute ventilation for elimination of CO_2. The clinical goal is to avoid elevated airway pressures by reducing the delivered tidal volume or by using pressure-limited modes of ventilation when possible (see subsequent discussions later in this chapter). There are no publications defining the "safe" upper limit of positive airway pressure after lung resection; however, common sense dictates that lower airway pressures are safer.

Double lumen or Univent (Fuji Systems Corporation, Tokyo, Japan) tracheal tubes have small inner diameters related to their outer diameter, making tracheal/airway toilet difficult and imposing additional work of breathing when this is demanded of the patient. In addition, PACU and ICU nurses and respiratory therapists are usually unfamiliar with such tubes. Unless there is a need to continue lung isolation postoperatively (e.g., a persistent large air leak or draining infection), it is desirable to replace such specialty tubes with single-lumen tubes before leaving the operating room. In those patients with difficult airways or those who have or are expected to have oral or airway edema, clinical judgment must be used; the aforementioned problems could be a necessary evil in the face of potential loss of the airway. Although long tube-exchanging devices for DLTs are available (Figure 18-4), use of these does not guarantee the ability to readvance a single-lumen tube through a very edematous or difficult airway. It might be prudent to plan to change the tube at a later time.

Preoperative Indications for Postoperative Mechanical Ventilation

Patients arriving in the operating room who are already ventilated for any reason are unlikely to tolerate extubation immediately after their procedure. Withdrawal of mechanical

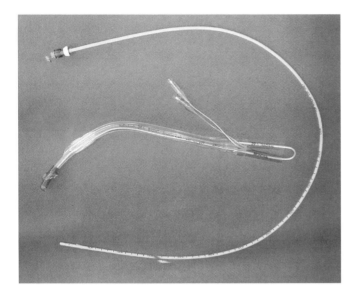

FIGURE 18-4 Long tube changer for use with double-lumen tracheal tubes (Cook Critical Care, Bloomington, Illinois). A 39F left double-lumen tube is illustrated, with the tube changer curved around it. The changer is hollow, and the adaptor (shown on the lower tip of the changer) permits attachment to a standard anesthesia circuit oxygen supply.

ventilation should be done in a gradual, controlled manner, and the operating room is not a suitable place for this process. As discussed previously, patients with poor predicted postoperative FEV_1 (less than 30% of predicted) are at the highest risk for immediate postoperative respiratory failure.[19-20] These patients might benefit from a staged withdrawal of mechanical ventilation while other physiologic functions (cardiac, endocrine, renal) is ensured to be optimal and while normothermia and analgesia are achieved. Specific major procedures that are usually associated with elective postoperative mechanical ventilation for at least 24 hours include esophagectomy or esophagogastrectomy and thoracic or thoracoabdominal aortic aneurysm repair.[82-84] Apart from the extent and duration of surgery, these latter procedures are associated with extended periods of one-lung ventilation, and the operative-side lung is often contused or partially atelectatic despite having been reinflated at the end of surgery. This leads to hypoxemia and increased work of breathing. Reporting on 100 consecutive thoracoabdominal aneurysm repairs, Money et al found the mean duration of intubation to be 5.8 days, with a 21% incidence of respiratory failure.[83] An earlier report from Crawford's group suggested an incidence of respiratory failure in patients with chronic pulmonary disease of 58% and a mortality rate of 43% in this group.[85]

Intraoperative Indications for Postoperative Mechanical Ventilation

Unanticipated operative complications can lead to circumstances that are unfavorable to immediate postoperative extubation. Foremost among these indications are any complications or conditions that lead to difficulty in obtaining adequate intraoperative oxygenation or CO_2 elimination. Other factors that need to be considered in relation to the list in Table 18-1 are: underlying comorbid conditions, age, and time of day. A period of

elective postoperative mechanical ventilation permits stabilization of organ systems (e.g., volume status, cardiac function, coagulation/hemostasis control) while oxygenation and ventilation are ensured. Withdrawal of mechanical ventilation can be done in a staged and controlled manner without the pressure of time that exists in the operating room. The list of relative indications in Table 18-1 must be tempered with clinical judgment throughout and at the end of the procedure; continued discussion of the plan with the surgical team can facilitate a smooth transition from the operating room to the PACU or ICU.

Immediate Postoperative Indications for Mechanical Ventilation

At the end of thoracic surgery, circumstances that prevent extubation might arise or become evident. Foremost among these are inadequate neuromuscular function (as assessed objectively by nerve stimulation or clinically by weakness) and inadequate spontaneous respirations (low respiratory rate in association with high end-tidal or arterial CO_2 concentration). Although these complications must be resolved before extubation, of greater concern are problems with oxygenation (e.g., requirement of 50% or more FIO_2 to achieve an O_2 saturation of 90% or more), ventilation (inadequate CO_2 elimination despite tachypnea), and visible respiratory distress. Uncontrolled pain can contribute to these findings, but they also could represent a physiologic derangement likely to require more than a few minutes for resolution. Specific blood gas criteria or respiratory measurements are frequently quoted as indicating a need for mechanical ventilation; however, in the rapidly changing situation at the end of surgery, it is difficult to apply such criteria. A clinical judgment must be made to assist or control ventilation for an additional period, usually requiring that the patient also be (re)sedated. At this time, a call to the PACU or ICU should be made with a request for a mechanical ventilator and sedative infusion(s). A chest radiograph and arterial blood gas analysis should be performed at the earliest opportunity.

In addition to permitting the administration of high, known concentrations of oxygen, positive pressure ventilation assists oxygenation by elevating the mean airway pressure throughout the respiratory cycle. This positive pressure keeps open or expands partially collapsed alveoli and perhaps opens some fully collapsed ones. PEEP improves oxygenation in pulmonary edema and acute lung injury both by these mechanisms and by redistributing (but not reducing) lung water.[86,87] Increasing the fraction of inspired oxygen (FIO_2) improves arterial oxygenation by increasing transport in those areas that are absorbing O_2. True shunt will respond only to reexpansion of collapsed segments or to reduction in the size of the shunt. This could require bronchoscopy and can be aided by PEEP. Thus failure of oxygenation is treated by increasing the FIO_2 or mean airway pressure.

Usually, work by the respiratory muscles to ventilate the lungs requires only a small percentage of total body oxygen consumption, but this percentage can be several times higher in the postoperative patient and higher still in acute respiratory failure.[88] Mechanical ventilation also takes over the work of breathing for the patient in distress and guarantees alveolar ventilation. Thus, mechanical ventilation with PEEP treats both components of acute respiratory failure.

Ventilatory Modes

Modern mechanical ventilators used in critical care are sophisticated microprocessor-controlled devices that sense and interact with the patient. This is in stark contrast to the traditional anesthesia ventilator that has three controls: respiratory rate, tidal volume, and inspiratory flow rate. The clinician sets the tidal volume; therefore this traditional anesthesia ventilator delivers volume-cycled, controlled mandatory ventilation (CMV). Short of disconnect and high-pressure alarms, the only sensors for the patient are the watchful eyes and ears of the anesthesiologist. Patients who might require an extended period of mechanical ventilation tend to have abnormal (e.g., noncompliant) and changing lungs, share their primary caregiver—the ICU nurse—with at least one other patient, and are awake and making respiratory efforts. These patients need a ventilator with sophisticated alarms, sensors, and response modes.

CONTINUOUS POSITIVE AIRWAY PRESSURE

Lungs are ventilated by drawing in gas with the respiratory muscles. During inspiration, airway pressure (P_{aw}) is negative with respect to the atmosphere, and during expiration, P_{aw} is positive (Figure 18-5). The only mode of "ventilation" that truly mimics this pattern is continuous positive airway pressure (CPAP): breathing spontaneously at elevated airway pressure (Figure 18-6). Strictly speaking, this is not a mode of ventilation because there is no inspiratory assist. This mode of ventilation is usually used to improve oxygenation in patients who do not have ventilatory failure because it helps increase the FRC and reduces atelectasis. It can allow spontaneous breathing to occur at a more compliant part of the pressure-volume relationship of the thorax, reducing the work of breathing (Figure 18-7).[89] CPAP can be provided by a continuous high-flow circuit, or it can be delivered through a microprocessor-controlled ventilator that senses effort (airway pressure or flow) and responds accordingly. In the former case, the airway pressure varies slightly during the respiratory cycle, but the high level of flow and built-in reservoir prevent large swings in pressure. In the latter case, the flow is delivered in response to

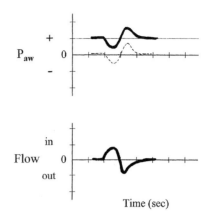

FIGURE 18-6 Airway pressure and gas flow during spontaneous breathing through a continuous positive airway pressure (CPAP) circuit. The pressures and flows mirror those for a spontaneous breath *(dashed line),* but the baseline pressure is elevated. P_{aw}, Airway pressure.

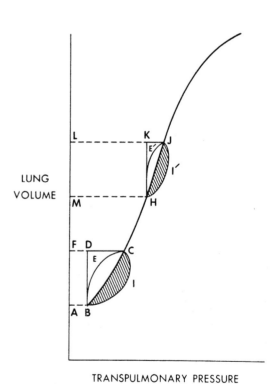

FIGURE 18-7 Pressure-volume diagram of elastic and resistive (nonelastic) work done on the lungs during spontaneous breathing in postoperative patients with atelectasis. *(A)* Breathing at ambient airway pressure (e.g., via "T-tube"). *(B)* Breathing with CPAP. *Solid-line BCHJ* is the elastic pressure-volume curve for the lung, determined by measuring transpulmonary pressures at the instant of zero flow. Hatched areas represent nonelastic work *(BIC and HIJ).* Measured elastic work is represented by *BCD and HJK.* A component of elastic work done on the lung is not considered. In the absence of CPAP, this component is normally small *(ABDF);* about half of the work is done by the inspiratory muscles and half by elastic recoil of the chest wall. These contributions both diminish with CPAP, so that most or all of *MHKL* represents work done by the CPAP system (From Katz JA, Marks JD: *Anesthesiology* 63:598, 1985.)

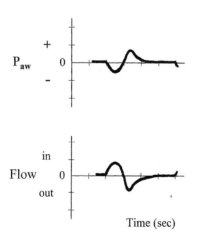

FIGURE 18-5 Airway pressure and gas flow during normal spontaneous breathing. Relative to atmospheric pressure, the airway pressure decreases by a few centimeters of water during inspiration, and during expiration it increases by a few centimeters of water. During normal breathing, there is a period of no pressure or of flow change between breaths. P_{aw}, Airway pressure.

the sensor, attempting always to meet the patient's demands and to achieve the preset level of CPAP.

The device that keeps the airway pressure positive in a CPAP circuit is the PEEP valve: a device on the expiratory limb that permits gas to escape only if the airway pressure remains above the preset level. When the patient is receiving inspiratory assist (i.e., all the modes discussed in the sections that follow), the positive airway pressure at end-expiration is referred to as PEEP rather than CPAP. In most postoperative patients, a minimum level of 5 cm H_2O is used.

PRESSURE-SUPPORT VENTILATION

Although perhaps easy to understand as inspiratory-assisted CPAP, pressure-support ventilation (PSV) is a mode that is quite complex to deliver. As illustrated in Figure 18-8, PSV supports spontaneous inspiratory airway pressure to an elevated, constant level. The patient initiates an effort, and the ventilator—sensing either flow or pressure—delivers flow at a high rate to achieve the preset level of support. Once this level is reached, the delivered flow rate *decelerates* as the inspiratory effort declines, then transitions into expiration when a low level of inspiratory flow is reached. For these tasks to be accomplished, the ventilator requires sensitivity, adaptation, and speed of response. The flow delivered varies between respiratory efforts: a large effort results in a large flow rate (i.e., the machine is trying to reach a positive pressure while the patient is creating a negative airway pressure by effort), while a small effort results in a small flow. The duration of inspiration is determined by the patient's effort as well. Thus, PSV is a patient-initiated mode of ventilation in which airway pressure is the independent (i.e., set) factor, whereas tidal volume is the dependent factor.

Pressure support, with its high initial flow rate, can be viewed as a mechanism to help the patient overcome the work of breathing imposed by the tracheal tube. Fiastro et al have demonstrated elegantly how increasing levels of PSV over-

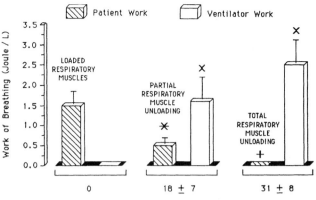

FIGURE 18-9 Work of breathing performed by an intubated patient decreases significantly as pressure support is increased from 0 (loaded respiratory muscles) to 18 cmH_2O (partial respiratory muscle unloading) to 31 cmH_2O (total respiratory muscle unloading). Partial unloading allows the patient to breathe at a nonfatiguing level, while with total unloading, the ventilator provides essentially all the work of breathing. Data are mean ± SD. (From Banner MJ, Gabrielli A, Layon AJ: *Chest* 106:1835, 1994)

come the pressure work imposed by decreasing sizes of tubes and/or increasing inspiratory flow demands.[90] In most circumstances (i.e., adults with 7.5- to 8.5-mm internal diameter tubes), 5 to 10 cmH_2O of PSV overcomes the externally imposed work of breathing. Increasing levels of PSV provide increasing amounts of ventilatory support; at high levels, PSV supports most, if not all, of the work of breathing (Figure 18-9). Although PSV is often viewed as a supplemental form of mechanical ventilation (either in addition to volume ventilation or for use during weaning), it can be used as the principal form of ventilation even in patients with lung injury.[91] As the flow is delivered to match the demand of the patient, it can be better tolerated than fixed flows and volumes and can result in a reduced need for sedation.[92]

Patients with obstructive sleep apnea often use a device during sleep that delivers CPAP or PSV to keep the airway open. This is the same or similar apparatus referred to previously in the discussion on the prevention and treatment of atelectasis. The assisted ventilation is delivered through a tightly applied face mask, or more commonly through a nasal mask (Figure 18-2); the patient learns to occlude the mouth or glottis, preventing the escape of gas. The most common mode is referred to as BiPAP, meaning that there is a positive baseline airway pressure (CPAP or PEEP), and inspiration is assisted to reach a higher positive pressure, that is, PSV. Some devices alternate at fixed intervals between two levels of expiratory pressure, allowing spontaneous breathing at both levels. So-called noninvasive ventilation was first described for use in patients with acute exacerbations of chronic obstructive airways disease; more recently, it has been studied in acute respiratory failure in both medical and surgical settings.[93] The goal is avoidance of intubation, with some studies suggesting such an approach can reduce the risk of nosocomial infections and even mortality.[94,95] Because BiPAP requires a conscious, cooperative patient, is

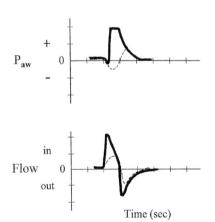

FIGURE 18-8 A pressure-supported, spontaneous breath *(heavy line)*. The dashed line represents a normal spontaneous breath (as in Figure 18-4, *A*). At the start of the inspiratory effort by the patient, the ventilator gives a burst of flow to achieve the preset level of airway pressure (i.e., the pressure-support level). The remainder of inspiratory flow is "decelerating" to keep the airway pressure at the preset level. When the decelerating flow reaches a predetermined level (which differs among ventilators), expiration begins. P_{aw}, Airway pressure.

difficult to use with a nasogastric tube and cannot be used if there are excessive secretions; if the patient is "in extremis," BiPAP is of limited use in the immediate postoperative period. In a small study of 20 patients 5 hours after thoracic resections, Aguilo et al found that nasal BiPAP with an F_{IO_2} of 21% improved oxygenation while the mask was in place and was well tolerated apart from inducing a pleural air leak in one of 10 patients.[96] In another recent study, Auriant et al suggest that the use of noninvasive ventilation (i.e., mask CPAP or BiPAP) for acute respiratory failure after lung resection could reduce mortality when compared with tracheal intubation.[97] This report in 24 patients awaits confirmation by other studies.

PRESSURE-CONTROLLED VENTILATION

Pressure-controlled ventilation (PCV) uses the same principle as PSV; the clinician determines the airway pressure (the independent variable), and the volume delivered is the dependent variable. Because this is a controlled mode of ventilation, each breath is initiated by the ventilator, and the duration of flow delivery is also controlled. This mode of ventilation is used in deeply sedated (and often paralyzed) patients for whom the goal is to control airway pressure, even if this means that the tidal volume could change with the lung disease. The most common use of this form of ventilation is in acute lung injury or ARDS (see the pertinent sections of this chapter).

VOLUME-CONTROLLED VENTILATION MODES

Common to all volume-controlled ventilation modes is the delivery of clinician-designed breaths of a known volume. This is in contrast to PSV and PCV, in which the clinician sets the airway pressure, knowing that the tidal volume will not be constant or ensured. In all the volume-controlled modes, the clinician decides how big the tidal volume will be and at what rate the flow will be delivered. Figure 18-10 illustrates a volume-controlled breath. In this example, a flow rate of 60 L/min is delivered for 1 second, delivering a tidal volume of 1 L. The airway pressure that is reached will depend on the airway resistance and on the compliance of the respiratory system, but unless the pressure is so high that the alarm limit is reached, the volume will

be delivered. The clinician also determines the respiratory rate (i.e., how many breaths per minute will be delivered).

Controlled Mandatory Ventilation (CMV). This is the mode of ventilation delivered by the traditional anesthesia ventilator, and all breaths appear as in Figure 18-10. If the patient makes efforts over and above what the machine is delivering, there is no mechanism for response (i.e., the airway pressure might decline when the patient makes an effort, but the machine has no sensor to respond to the effort).

Assist-Controlled Ventilation (ACV). In the ACV mode, the patient receives the preset tidal volumes as determined by the clinician, but now the machine has a sensor activated that allows it to respond to a patient effort. The response is fixed: the machine delivers another of the preset volumes. Thus, if a patient is receiving 10 breaths per minute but wants another four, each of the four efforts will result in a full preset volume being delivered. Figure 18-11 illustrates the response in the ACV mode to a patient effort. It is important to note here that the patient continues to make a respiratory effort throughout inspiration, even while the ventilator is delivering the predetermined volume. This causes the airway pressure to be lower than it would have been for a breath delivered in the absence of a patient effort.

Intermittent Mandatory Ventilation (IMV). As in CMV or ACV, the clinician sets the number of breaths, as well as the tidal volume and inspiratory flow rate for the mandatory breaths. If the patient wants additional breaths, the sensor is activated and allows the patient to take spontaneous breaths between the preset tidal volume breaths. The airway pressure and flow for these spontaneous breaths are identical to those illustrated in Figures 18-5 (no PEEP) or 18-6 (CPAP). This mode of ventilation has traditionally been the most popular among surgical patients, as it was originally described for this indication. It permits the clinician to reduce the number of breaths provided

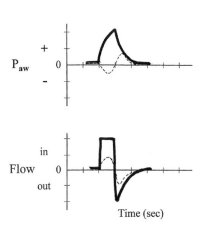

FIGURE 18-10 A volume-controlled breath initiated by the ventilator *(heavy line)*. The dashed line represents a normal spontaneous breath (as in Figure 18-4, *A*). A constant flow is given for a predetermined period that delivers the preset tidal volume. The airway pressure rises continually during inspiration because the flow is given at a constant rate.

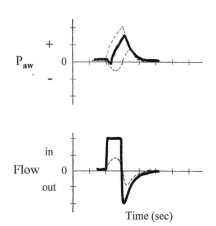

FIGURE 18-11 A patient-triggered, volume-controlled breath *(heavy line)*. The lower dashed line represents a normal spontaneous breath (as in Figure 18-4, *A*); the upper dashed line represents the airway pressure for a breath initiated by the ventilator (as in Figure 18-4, *D*). The patient makes an inspiratory effort throughout inspiration, so the airway pressure is a result of this effort and the positive pressure created by the flow delivered by the machine. This airway pressure pattern is seen in patient-triggered breaths in the assist-control mode, and in patient-triggered mandatory breaths in the IMV mode.

by the machine gradually because the patient breathes more on his or her own during weaning.

A common practice is to pressure-support the spontaneous breaths in the IMV mode (i.e., "IMV with PSV"). The preset volume-controlled breaths are unchanged: the patient will still receive a clinician-set number of breaths, each of which is given at a preset flow level to provide a known volume (i.e., CMV breaths). If the patient wants additional breaths, rather than spontaneous breaths (Figures 18-5 or 18-6) that would be received on the IMV setting, the spontaneous breaths are now pressure supported (Figure 18-8).

SYNCHRONIZATION

Modern ventilators synchronize all the mandatory breaths with patient efforts. For example, if a patient's lungs are being ventilated in the IMV mode at a rate of 10 breaths per minute, the mandatory breaths are given every 6 seconds. Synchronization ("SIMV") means that the ventilator allows the patient to trigger these 10 breaths and moreover that the ventilator will not deliver a mandatory breath on top of a spontaneous breath. Thus if the patient is making efforts, each of the mandatory breaths will look like a triggered AC breath (Figure 18-11). Other patient efforts will trigger spontaneous breaths (or PSV breaths, if this has been added to the SIMV).

One way of viewing synchronization is to consider the ventilator as having two clocks that initiate breaths. The first clock is set to trigger a breath at the preset rate—for a rate of 10 breaths per minute, a breath is triggered every 6 seconds. The second clock begins ticking at the start of each 6-second cycle, waiting for a patient effort. If an effort is made, this triggers the "synchronized" mandatory breath (Figure 18-11). If an effort is not made within a short period—a fraction of the cycle length—the machine will deliver the mandatory breath (Figure 18-10).

ALTERNATIVE MODES OF MECHANICAL VENTILATION

A variety of modifications to the foregoing "standard" ventilatory modes as well as entirely different modes have been described. Although small observational and descriptive studies have illustrated the use of many of these modes in specific circumstances, none has been shown to provide definitive benefits over the standard modes already described. As in other clinical contexts, how skilled clinicians use the tools they are familiar with is more important than the tools themselves. Table 18-8 lists some alternative ventilatory modes, their characteristics, and some circumstances in which they have been used or recommended.[98-104]

Postoperative Ventilation of the Thoracic Surgery Patient

The most common mode of ventilation used in surgical patients is SIMV with PSV. The IMV mode allows the clinician to give a guaranteed minute ventilation; the PSV assists the patient's spontaneous efforts in between the mandatory breaths. Based on studies performed in anesthetized patients, large tidal volumes have traditionally been recommended—in the range of 10 to 15 mL/kg (i.e., 700 to 1000 mL in a 70-kg patient). These volumes appeared to be required to prevent atelectasis and improve intrapulmonary gas distribution.[105] This practice should now be questioned in light of the remarkable findings

TABLE 18-8

Alternative Modes of Mechanical Ventilation

Mode	Special Feature	Recommended Use
Inverse ratio	Inspiratory time exceeds expiratory time. Requires heavy sedation/paralysis	Severe lung injury and hypoxemia
Airway pressure release	Ventilation occurs through transient releases of CPAP. Spontaneous breathing is possible, reducing need for sedation	Severe lung injury and hypoxemia
Independent lung	Requires double-lumen tube and two synchronized ventilators	Severe unilateral lung disease
High-frequency Jet	High pressure jet of low volume at high rate (e.g., 60/min) with entrainment	Thoracic surgery; bronchopleural fistula
High-frequency oscillation	Very high frequency oscillation of respiratory tract, plus bias flow	Refractory hypoxemia in ARDS

From Tharratt RS, Allen RP, Albertson TE: *Chest* 94:755, 1988; Garner W, Downs JB, Stock MC, et al: *Chest* 94:779, 1988; Parish JM, Gracey DR, Southern PA, et al: *Mayo Clin Proc* 59:822, 1984; Carlon GC, Ray C, Pierri MK, et al: *Chest* 81:350, 1982; Nevin M, Van Besouw JP, Williams CW, et al: *Ann Thorac Surg* 44:625, 1987; Butler WJ, Bohn DJ, Bryan AC, et al: *Anesth Analg* 59:577, 1980; and Ferguson ND, Stewart TE: *Crit Care Clin* 18:91, 2002.

not only from the "ARDSnet" trial (see discussion that follows) but also from many other studies demonstrating potential harm to diseased lungs from large volumes and pressures. In addition, most postthoracotomy patients will have undergone lung resection and will have reduced lung parenchyma. As an alternative to large tidal volumes, smaller volumes (5 to 8 mL/kg) should be considered, with PEEP of 5 cmH$_2$O to prevent atelectasis. Addition of 10 to 15 cmH$_2$O of PSV helps overcome the work of breathing imposed by the tracheal tube, especially if a double-lumen or Univent tube is still in place. Table 18-9 indicates suggested initial postoperative ventilator settings for a thoracic surgery patient. To limit airway pressure, the volume-cycled breaths should be discontinued as soon as possible.

The many possible causes of postoperative respiratory failure have been addressed in the foregoing discussions. In some circumstances, these inciting and predisposing factors can be

TABLE 18-9

Initial Ventilator Settings after Thoracic Surgery

Mode	SIMV with Pressure Support
Tidal volume	5-8 mL/kg
Respiratory rate	10-15/min*
Inspiratory flow	50-70 L/min†
PEEP	5 cmH$_2$O
Pressure support	5-15 cmH$_2$O
FiO$_2$	70% (adjust per O$_2$ saturation)

*Lower rate if the patient is making efforts; higher if not.
†Lower flow rate if airway pressure is high.

resolved or compensated for by the patient in the first hours or day after surgery because the acute stress of surgery subsides and effective analgesic techniques are in place. Mechanical ventilation can then be withdrawn rapidly and uneventfully. In a small percentage of patients, however, a severe form of respiratory failure can be incited by perioperative events. This severe form of failure is associated with a high mortality rate and a prolonged ventilator course.

Acute Lung Injury and Acute Respiratory Distress Syndrome

As defined by the American-European consensus conference on ARDS, acute lung injury or acute lung injury (ALI) is "a syndrome of inflammation and increased permeability that is associated with a constellation of clinical, radiologic, and physiologic abnormalities that cannot be explained by, but may coexist with, left atrial or pulmonary capillary hypertension."[106] Because this is a clinical syndrome with a spectrum of severity, ARDS is reserved for the "most severe end of this spectrum."[106] Table 18-10 indicates how the consensus conference differentiates between the severity of ALI and that of ARDS. In addition to the importance of this article in summarizing the state of knowledge of the syndrome originally described in 1967, the consensus clarified that it should be called "acute" rather than "adult" respiratory distress syndrome, consolidated the definition of the syndrome (Table 18-10), and helped initiate the process of designing multicenter outcome studies.[107] Defining the syndrome was critical in the design of therapeutic trials that have been reported in recent years and of other trials that are ongoing.

Acute lung injury or ARDS can be induced by direct insults to the lung, such as aspiration of gastric contents, pulmonary infection, or contusion, but more commonly it is associated with sepsis syndrome and severe trauma, pancreatitis, or massive transfusion. These latter initiating factors are viewed as indirect insults or "secondary" causes.[106] It is uncommon to see the diffuse infiltrates that characterize ALI and ARDS immediately after surgery; such a finding on the postoperative radiograph is more likely to represent hydrostatic edema due to fluid overload or left-sided cardiac failure. Hydrostatic pulmonary edema is radiographically indistinguishable from ALI and ARDS. The incompletely understood systemic process that is thought to cause ALI and ARDS is more likely to present a few days after surgery. This process is the result of an interaction among a primary injury to the lung or other organ system, the host response, and the therapy.

The current view is that a systemic inflammatory response is initiated by initial insult, resulting in the activation of many host defense systems that have deleterious effects on vital organs, including the lungs. The clinical presentation is shortness of breath and hypoxemia, requiring intubation and mechanical ventilation. CT scanning demonstrates lung consolidation and atelectasis, mostly in dependent zones, with relative sparing of other areas. Pathologic findings include diffuse alveolar damage, including inflammation in lung zones that appear normal on the chest radiograph.[108] The damaged lung is infiltrated with neutrophils, macrophages, and red blood cells, and its alveoli contain hyaline membranes and protein-rich edema fluid. Hundreds of publications have investigated the role of activated neutrophils, inflammatory cytokines, the complement system, and abnormal coagulation as inciting or aggravating factors in the development of ALI and ARDS. The reader is referred to a recent review of this topic.[109]

Direct injury to the lung as a result of surgery, or indirect effects from other organ system dysfunctions, trauma of surgery, or multiple transfusions can initiate the pathophysiology leading to ALI and ARDS in thoracic surgery patients. In a six-year (1991-1997) review of all pulmonary resections done at the Royal Brompton Hospital in London, England, the combined incidence of ALI and ARDS was 3.9%.[110] The overall mortality from ARDS is approximately 50%, although there is some suggestion that mortality has declined somewhat in recent years; in the review from the Royal Brompton Hospital, ALI/ARDS was associated with 72.5% of the mortality.[110,111] Patients with the syndrome typically go on to have other organ dysfunctions, developing the multiple organ dysfunction syndrome (MODS).[112] In fact, most patients who succumb do so from nonrespiratory organ failures.[113] The MODS syndrome occurs in approximately 15% of ICU patients and is responsible for 80% of ICU deaths.[114] Rather than the severity of gas exchange abnormality in ARDS, other patient-specific factors—such as preexisting organ system dysfunction, increasing age, and the presence of sepsis—are more predictive of mortality. As more systems become involved in the MODS, mortality increases exponentially. Patients who survive ARDS are likely to have relatively intact pulmonary function within 6 to 12 months, although health-related quality of life is reduced.[115] If the lung injury in ARDS does not resolve in 7 to 10 days, it can progress to fibrosis, and finally to obliteration of the pulmonary capillary bed with pulmonary hypertension.

Therapy

Despite more than 30 years of research into the causes and treatment of ALI and ARDS, these remain clinical syndromes with elusive etiologies. A great deal of progress has been made in understanding the pathophysiology; however, the earliest events that trigger the inflammation and damage of lung tissue are not yet fully understood. Therapies targeting early events have been disappointing; some of these are referred to in the discussion that follows. Current therapy is therefore support-

TABLE 18-10

Definitions of Acute Lung Injury (ALI) and Acute Respiratory Distress Syndrome (ARDS)

	Timing	Oxygenation	Chest X-ray	Pulmonary artery occlusion pressure
ALI	Acute onset	Pa_{O_2}/Fi_{O_2} ≤300 mmHg*	Bilateral infiltrates on frontal x-ray	≤18 mmHg or no clinical evidence of left atrial hypertension
ARDS	Acute onset	Pa_{O_2}/Fi_{O_2} ≤200 mmHg*	Bilateral infiltrates on frontal x-ray	≤18 mmHg or no clinical evidence of left atrial hypertension

From Bendixen HH, Hedley-White J, Laver MB: *N Engl J Med* 269:991, 1963.
*Regardless of PEEP

ive, attempting to provide vital organ support without further damaging the lungs and providing an environment for healing.

MECHANICAL VENTILATION WITH PEEP

Perhaps one of the most surprising outcomes of the intense research into ARDS has been the gradual realization that the mainstay of therapy itself, mechanical ventilation, could worsen—and even, in some animal models, actually cause—lung injury. More than 20 years ago, ventilation with high volumes and pressures was shown to cause pulmonary edema in animal models.[116] Further studies have documented such injury—in particular, the worsening of existing injury with high volumes—in a variety of animal models and settings. Recent publications have demonstrated that inflammatory markers are elevated when high volumes are used to ventilate the lungs of patients with ARDS, and that survival from the syndrome can be improved by using small (6 to 8 mL/kg vs. 10 to 12 mL/kg) tidal volumes.[117] The "ARDSnet" trial funded by the National Heart, Lung and Blood Institute in the United States, and performed by the "ARDS network" of institutions, documented a reduction in mortality from almost 40% to 31% simply by using a smaller tidal volume in association with a protocolized strategy for Fio_2, PEEP, and management of acid-base disorders.[118] This approach to ventilation has been termed *lung protective*. An overview of the protocol is given in Table 18-11 and can be found at www.ardsnet.org. This study is now widely quoted as definitive evidence that smaller tidal volumes should be used in patients with ARDS.

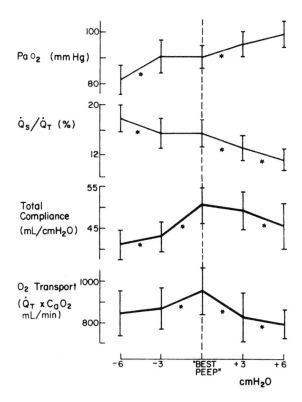

FIGURE 18-12 Mean values (± SEM) of arterial oxygen tension (Pao_2), intrapulmonary shunt (Q_S/Q_T), total static compliance, and oxygen transport, measured at the level of PEEP resulting in maximum oxygen transport ("Best PEEP"), compared with values obtained at 3 and 6 cmH_2O of PEEP below (−3, −6) and above (+3, +6) that level in 15 patients with acute pulmonary failure. Significant changes ($P < 0.05$) at each 3 cm of water increment of PEEP. (From Suter PM, Fairley HB, Isenberg MD: *N Engl J Med* 292:284, 1975.)

TABLE 18-11

Summary of Ventilator Management in the "ARDSNET" Trial (Patients Receiving Lower Tidal Volumes)

Ventilator mode	Volume assist-control
Initial tidal volume (mL/kg of predicted body weight)	6
Plateau pressure (cm of water)	≤30
Ventilator rate setting (breaths/min) to achieve pH 7.3-7.45	6-35
Ratio of duration of inspiration to expiration	1:1-1:3
Oxygenation goal	Pao_2 55-80 mmHg or Spo_2 88-95%
Allowable combinations of Fio_2 and PEEP (cm of water)*	0.3 and 5
	0.4 and 5
	0.4 and 8
	0.5 and 8
	0.5 and 10
	0.6 and 10
	0.7 and 10
	0.7 and 12
	0.7 and 14
	0.8 and 14
	0.9 and 14
	0.9 and 16
	0.9 and 18
	1.0 and 20
	1.0 and 22
	1.0 and 24
Weaning	By pressure support; required by protocol when Fio_2 ≤0.4

From the Acute Respiratory Distress Syndrome Network: *N Engl J Med* 342:1301, 2001.
*Further increases in PEEP to 34 cm of water are allowed but not required. See text for abbreviations.

In conjunction with the beneficial effect of tidal volumes smaller than the traditional 10 to 15 mL/kg, it has also become clear that collapse and reexpansion of alveoli with each respiratory cycle can cause injury, and that this risk can be reduced or prevented by adequate levels of PEEP.[119] Determining the optimal level of PEEP has concerned clinicians for more than 25 years and continues to be a dilemma. In 1975, Suter et al coined the phrase "best PEEP" in relating the PEEP level to oxygen delivery to the tissues (Figure 18-12).[120] These investigators found that although increasing levels of PEEP usually resulted in better oxygenation of the arterial blood, cardiac output (and hence, oxygen delivery) declined as the intrathoracic pressure rose above a certain level. In recent years, while taking this latter concept into consideration, there has been a greater interest in finding the level of PEEP that keeps the greatest number of alveoli open, ventilating only on the compliant portion of the pressure-volume relationship of the lung. The PEEP is increased so that ventilation occurs above the "lower inflection point" of the pressure-volume relationship as shown in Figure 18-13, with a tidal volume that is below the upper inflection point.[121] Unfortunately, there is no agreement on how to derive this point accurately at the bedside or whether this is indeed the correct strategy. Clinically, the most reasonable strategy is to follow the protocol used in the

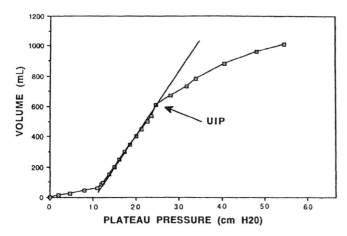

FIGURE 18-13 A pressure-volume curve of the respiratory system in a patient with ARDS. Note the lower inflection point at the bottom of the curve (the curve starts at the level of intrinsic PEEP in this patient). The upper inflection point (UIP) is the first point that departs from linearity. (From Roupie E, Dambrosio M, Servillo G, et al: *Am J Respir Crit Care Med* 152:121, 1995.)

ARDSnet trial, usually requiring between 10 and 15 cm H_2O of PEEP.

As the practice of using reduced tidal volumes has increased, two clinical problems have become apparent. The first is the need for high respiratory rates to achieve normal arterial CO_2 levels, and sometimes failing to achieve the latter. The phrase "permissive hypercapnia" has been coined, meaning that a higher-than-normal CO_2 level can be tolerated to protect the lung from high tidal volume ventilation.[122] Either the respiratory acidosis is tolerated, or a bicarbonate infusion can be used to restore the pH toward normal. In the ARDSnet trial, a pH of 7.30 was tolerated; in other studies, even lower pH levels have been accepted. The second problem is that despite relatively high PEEP levels, the use of small tidal volumes can result in gradual collapse of alveoli and worsened oxygenation. This has led to the investigation of "recruitment" maneuvers such as intermittent application of high levels of airway pressure, analogous to the old concept of sighs. Recent work suggests that such recruitment maneuvers can improve oxygenation in early ARDS, whether with pressure-support or volume-controlled ventilation.[123,124]

IMMUNE "MODULATION"

Despite a consensus that activated neutrophils and the release of cytokines appear to be immune manifestations of the pathophysiology of ARDS, therapies modulating the immune system have for the most part been disappointing.[125] A large, randomized clinical trial of high-dose methylprednisolone (30 mg/kg every 6 hours for 24 hours) given in early ARDS failed to show a benefit.[126] More recently, Meduri et al reported that 2 mg/kg of the same drug daily for 14 days, followed by slowly tapering dosing in late ARDS (7 to 10 days after onset), significantly improved survival.[127] The editorial accompanying this report questioned the analysis and conclusions that could be drawn from a study in such a small number of patients (24 total; 16 received steroids).[128] A multicenter study of this issue, funded by the National Institute of Health in the United States, is currently in progress.

Other types of "immune" therapies have been tried in ARDS, including antioxidants, pentoxifylline, and inhibitors of arachidonic acid metabolism. None of these substances has been effective. "Immunonutrition" has received considerable attention, especially after publication of a study demonstrating a modest benefit with use of a fish-oil derived, high-fat formula.[129] Although not specifically a study of patients with ARDS, a recent large trial demonstrated a survival benefit in septic patients who received activated protein C.[130]

Prone position. In 1974, Bryan proposed that during mechanical ventilation, the dorsal regions of the lung would receive improved ventilation in the prone position.[131] Since that time, a variety of publications have proved that he was correct. Both animal and human studies have demonstrated improved matching of ventilation to perfusion as well as overall better distribution of blood flow and transpleural pressure gradients.[132,133] An elegant study demonstrated, with serial CT scanning, the dramatic effects of prone positioning on regional lung density.[134] Although the majority of the more than 20 studies of the prone position in the setting of ALI and ARDS have demonstrated an improvement in oxygenation, outcome studies have been inconclusive or disappointing. The largest randomized trial in 304 patients failed to show a survival benefit.[135] In a post hoc analysis of this study, there did appear to be a trend toward improved short-term outcomes in the patients with highest severity scores. Use of the prone position in a critically ill patient can be a challenge to the clinical staff; however, it can be done with safety, as attested to by this recent trial. Although the current data do not indicate that prone positioning improves overall outcome in ARDS, this position does improve oxygenation in most patients. Further trials will delineate the circumstances in which prone positioning might be beneficial, and it remains an adjunctive therapy that warrants consideration.

SURFACTANT, INHALED NITRIC OXIDE, AND PARTIAL LIQUID VENTILATION

These three therapies have all been evaluated in clinical trials in ARDS patients. Surfactant is produced by type II pneumocytes, reducing surface tension and promoting stability of alveoli. In neonatal ARDS, deficient surfactant production plays a significant role, and surfactant replacement therapy is beneficial.[136] A multicenter trial in adults with sepsis-induced ARDS failed to show a benefit; however, there is some optimism that better delivery systems and newer synthetic molecules might make this therapy effective.[137,138] Inhaled nitric oxide has been shown repeatedly to improve arterial oxygenation and reduce pulmonary vascular pressures in patients with lung injury and ARDS.[139] Because this molecule is quickly absorbed and then inactivated by hemoglobin, it has minimal systemic effects and is therefore a "selective" pulmonary vasodilator, increasing blood flow to the alveoli to which it has been delivered. Despite this action and its reproducible clinical effect, outcome studies have failed to demonstrate a survival benefit in ARDS.[140,141] Partial liquid ventilation involves filling part or most of the airways with a perfluorocarbon liquid, and ventilating with a conventional gas ventilator. Limited trials have been performed in small numbers of newborns with respiratory failure, and a multicenter pilot study in adults was published recently. In the 65 patients who received the perfluorocarbon, only a post hoc analysis suggested a possible benefit in patients younger than 55 years.[142] It is possible that some combination of inhaled nitric oxide, surfactant, or partial liquid ventilation might eventually prove to be of benefit in ARDS, but the studies to date do not support the use of these therapies.

Complications of Mechanical Ventilation

Trauma to the Lungs or Tracheobronchial Tree

Damage to the lung parenchyma as a consequence of mechanical ventilation is discussed in earlier sections of this chapter. In thoracic surgery patients, the potential risk of suture line or bronchial stump disruption as a result of positive airway pressure has also been examined. Suture line disruption can cause catastrophic pneumothorax or respiratory failure or can result in chronic air leak, bronchopleural fistula, and infection. Although objective data regarding these latter complications are scarce, one report suggested a correlation of postoperative mechanical ventilation or pulmonary edema with bronchopleural fistula.[143] Avoidance of intubation and PPV are certainly desirable but not always possible. As discussed previously, use of pressure-limited modes of ventilation and use of small tidal volumes if volume-controlled modes are used might help avoid high pressures. Auriant et al suggested that noninvasive ventilation could reduce the mortality in acute respiratory failure after pneumonectomy.[97]

Ventilator-Associated Pneumonia

One of the most serious complications associated with mechanical ventilation is pneumonia. A number of reviews of this topic have been published recently, summarizing the incidence and severity of the problem and potential strategies for prevention, diagnosis, and therapy. Each of these strategies is controversial because of the difficulty in agreeing upon diagnostic criteria, the diverse patient populations, and preexisting antimicrobial therapy that most patients with ventilated lungs receive. There is little disagreement about the severity of the problem, however. The reported incidence varies from 8% to 28% of patients receiving mechanical ventilation for more than 48 hours, which is approximately threefold to tenfold the incidence of pneumonia in other hospitalized patients.[144-147] The mortality rate is reported to range from 24% to 50% and can be as high as 76% in specific settings with high-risk pathogens.[144-147]

DIAGNOSIS

The diagnosis of ventilator-associated pneumonia is usually made based on the clinical suspicion of a pulmonary infection (fever, leucocytosis, purulent sputum, and new pulmonary infiltrate) and confirmed by a positive sputum or positive sample from an invasive sampling technique (e.g., protected specimen brush or bronchoalveolar lavage). Early-onset pneumonia (within 4 days of the onset of mechanical ventilation) typically has a better prognosis because the disease tends to be less severe and the infecting pathogens less difficult to treat. The use of bronchoscopic techniques to obtain specimens has been a controversial topic for decades, and the debate continues. A very broad summary of the debate might be that whereas tracheal aspirates are simple to obtain, they often are contaminated by oropharyngeal organisms that might not be the true

pathogen. This circumstance can result in a course of broad-spectrum antibiotics that might lead to the emergence of a resistant organism or that might not treat the actual pathogen, and might prevent or delay further investigation of other significant causes of infection. The counterargument is that the published evidence for the more expensive bronchoscopic-based diagnostic techniques leading to an improved outcome is not strong. This debate is covered extensively by Chastre and Fagon.[146] Alternative, less invasive procedures such as blind "mini-BAL" could provide the benefit of the more expensive bronchoscopic BAL at a much lower cost.[148] The emergence of resistant pathogens has become a major issue worldwide, and nowhere is it more acute than in the mechanically ventilated patient. Published evidence does support improved outcomes if antimicrobial therapy is appropriately focused or targeted in this setting, but the best use of such therapy requires obtaining appropriate specimens. Figure 18-14 illustrates diagnostic and therapeutic strategies based on bronchoscopic techniques.

PREVENTION

Prevention of ventilator-associated pneumonia is marginally less controversial than diagnosis. Early administration (e,g., within the first week) of antibiotics is associated with a lower risk of pneumonia, but this protection disappears after 2 to 3 weeks, and prolonged antibiotic administration is associated with infection by resistant pathogens.[144,149] This finding highlights the need for a careful diagnostic and therapeutic strategy that is frequently reevaluated during the course of antimicrobial therapy. Specific antimicrobial therapy should be guided by gram stain and culture sensitivity reports, institutional experience, and protocols. There is some evidence that "rotation" of prescribing patterns (changing the antibiotic class or agent of first choice at scheduled intervals such as every 3 months) might reduce the incidence of ventilator-associated pneumonia as well as the emergence of resistant organisms.[150]

The use of H_2-blockers vs. sucralfate to prevent stress ulceration and the effect of this therapy on the incidence of ventilator-associated pneumonia have been evaluated in many studies, with conflicting results. The use of H_2-blockers raises the pH of the stomach contents, potentially allowing bacterial growth. Whether this high pH appreciably raises the risk of pneumonia is not clear. Sucralfate must be given frequently into the stomach to be effective in preventing ulcers and might not be quite as effective as the H_2-blocker ranitidine.[151] Similarly, the presence and type of nasogastric or nasojejunal tube have been evaluated, also with conflicting results. Use of the nasal route for tubes appears to be associated with an increased risk of radiographic sinusitis, but it is not clear whether the incidence of infectious sinusitis or related pneumonia is affected.[152]

Management of the respiratory circuit and secretions could affect the incidence of pneumonia. Accumulation of condensate in ventilator tubing is associated with the growth of pathogens, and spilling of this condensate into the lungs by manipulation of the tubing can innoculate the patient with a large infectious burden. Heated ventilator tubings reduce the amount of condensate but are expensive and have not been shown to reduce infection.[153] The use of heat and moisture exchangers rather than humidifiers dramatically reduces the condensate. This practice might reduce the incidence of

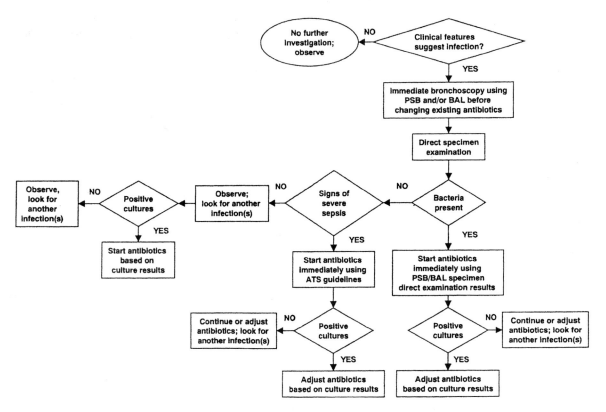

FIGURE 18-14 An "invasive" (i.e., requiring fiberoptic bronchoscopy) diagnostic and therapeutic strategy applied to patients with suspected ventilator-associated pneumonia. *PSB,* Protected specimen brush; *BAL,* bronchoalveolar lavage. (From Chastre J, Fagon JY: *Am J Respir Crit Care Med* 165:867, 2002.)

infection and is relatively inexpensive if the exchanger is changed every 48 hours. These devices may impose a small additional deadspace and resistive load, and so might not be appropriate for all patients. Ventilator tubing need not be changed more often than once weekly.

Suctioning of tracheal and oral secretions has been examined in a number of studies. Open tracheal suction systems (i.e., disconnection of the ventilator circuit with suction with a disposable catheter) have been compared to closed systems with varying results, as has a specialized tracheal tube that permits subglottic suctioning just above the cuff. A recent publication suggested that the latter device was effective at reducing the incidence of ventilator-associated pneumonia, but not the overall mortality rate.[154]

Monitoring the Consequences of Mechanical Ventilation

Monitoring of mechanical ventilation includes an examination of the physiologic effect on gas exchange, the systemic effects of positive intrathoracic pressure, and the mechanical effects on the lungs themselves.

Gas Exchange

Noninvasive monitoring of oxygen saturation with pulse oximetry (SpO_2) and alveolar ventilation with end-tidal CO_2 ($ETCO_2$) have enabled real-time monitoring and rapid adjustments in ventilator settings. Although very few conditions

invalidate the SpO_2 readings (e.g., inability to obtain a signal or abnormal hemoglobin populations such as methemoglobin), the gradient between $ETCO_2$ and the arterial CO_2 can vary widely between patients and within the same patient over time. This is especially true with abnormal lungs. The gas leaving the lungs at end-expiration should represent true alveolar gas, but there is always an effect from "deadspace" alveoli (i.e., ventilation but no perfusion) that makes $ETCO_2$ somewhat lower than the arterial value. Although capnometry can be used to guide ventilator management in patients with relatively normal lungs, in the patient with a large deadspace the arterial to end-tidal gradient can be very large (e.g., more than 20 mmHg) and can change with the disease process or ventilator setting changes.[155,156] Patients undergoing thoracic surgery are likely to have an element of underlying lung disease, making it important to establish the relationship between arterial and end-tidal values for CO_2 before relying on the latter as a monitor. When there is a change in the clinical status of the patient or an important therapeutic decision, it is advisable to verify the arterial CO_2 concentration. With severe lung disease, acute lung injury, and ARDS, $ETCO_2$ measurements should not be relied upon. Arterial blood gas analysis remains the gold standard for assessment of arterial oxygenation and ventilation.

Positive Intrathoracic Pressure

Positive intrathoracic pressure might have an impact on cardiac performance. With relatively compliant lungs, positive pressure created by the ventilator is transmitted to the entire thor-

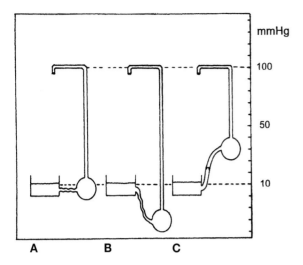

FIGURE 18-15 Diagrammatic representation of the effects of changing pleural (intrathoracic) pressure on right-side ventricular inflow and left-side ventricular outflow. **A,** Normal: the heart and lung are shown as a single-pump oxygenator filled from a venous reservoir at a pressure of 2 mmHg via collapsible tubes. The pump oxygenator expels blood into the systemic arteries to achieve a pressure head equivalent to 100 mmHg. **B,** Muller maneuver: reducing intrathoracic pressure to -30 mmHg is comparable to lowering the pressure within the heart-lung pump by an equivalent amount relative to that in the systemic and arterial reservoirs. The left-side ventricle must develop more force to "raise" the pressure of blood to the previous arterial pressure. Filling of the right-side ventricle is potentiated by the favorable venous return gradient. **C,** Valsalva maneuver: elevation of intrathoracic pressure to 30 mmHg has the opposite effect. The heart-lung pump is "raised" relative to the systemic reservoirs. Systolic ejection is facilitated, as less energy is required to raise aortic blood to the level of the previous arterial pressure. Venous return to the right side of the heart is impeded by the adverse gradient. (From McGregor M: *N Engl J Med* 301:480, 1979.)

acic cavity and could affect the preload and afterload to the heart. If cardiac function is normal, the predominant effect is a reduction in venous return leading to a decrease in cardiac output. This is illustrated in Figure 18-12, where the "best PEEP" was the level at which the increase in oxygenation of the blood was not offset by a reduction in cardiac output.[120] Where there is left-side ventricular dysfunction and elevated filling pressure, the reduction in preload could reduce ventricular distention and improve cardiac performance. In addition, making the intrathoracic cavity positive with respect to the rest of the body reduces the afterload to the left ventricle (Figure 18-15).[157]

Right ventricular function could be adversely affected by high levels of PEEP (e.g., more than 10 cmH$_2$O). The right-side ventricle is a thin-walled cavity that normally generates relatively low pressures (e.g., 25 mmHg systolic). High levels of PEEP that are required to oxygenate the blood might increase the impedance to right ventricular ejection, causing right ventricular dilatation and a decrease in contractility.[158] In patients who have undergone pulmonary resection (in particular, pneumonectomy), the right-side ventricle is already stressed by needing to pump the normal cardiac output through a reduced pulmonary vascular tree. Overdistention of the right ventricle could distort the interventricular septum, interfering with left ventricular filling.[159] Echocardiographic assessment of ventric-

ular function, pulmonary artery catheterization, or cardiac output measurement by stand-alone devices might be useful in determining the effect of mechanical ventilation on cardiac performance.

Another undesirable feature of PPV is the creation or worsening of autoPEEP, previously described. Application of external PEEP can "match" the auto-PEEP and reduce the patient effort required to initiate a spontaneous breath or trigger a machine breath. If, however, a rapid respiratory rate is set on the ventilator or if lung disease causes reduced expiratory flow rates not permitting the lung to fully empty with expiration, auto-PEEP can be worsened with PPV.

Pulmonary Mechanics

Bedside assessment of pulmonary mechanics can be used to help guide ventilator management. The airway pressure that is created by a mechanical ventilator is a function of ventilator factors (gas flow rate, gas flow pattern, inspiratory and expiratory time, and end-expiratory pressure [PEEP]) and patient factors (compliance of the lungs and thoracic cavity, resistance of the airways). The ventilator settings can be changed and the patient's pathologic condition can be recognized and treated, based on some simple bedside measures. Figure 18-16 illustrates the airway pressures and calculations that can be performed if an inspiratory hold maneuver is performed. Such a maneuver requires an unassisted (i.e., not a patient-assisted) breath, typically a volume-preset breath given at a relatively constant flow rate.

From the peak, "plateau," and end-expiratory pressures and the inspiratory flow rate, a reasonable clinical estimate of respiratory compliance and airways resistance can be made. These measurements can be followed over time to quantify the disease process and determine whether the ventilator settings are appropriate. For example, increasing or elevated airways resistance can be treated with bronchodilators, but the inspiratory flow rate should also be decreased. Close observation of the

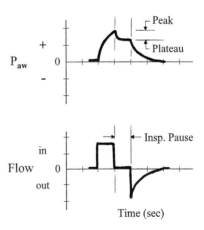

FIGURE 18-16 Airway pressures and gas flow during a ventilator-initiated, volume-controlled breath with an inspiratory "pause." The peak airway pressure is reached when the preset volume has been given; the plateau pressure is reached during the inspiratory pause, when there is no gas flow out of the patient. As a clinical approximation, the difference between the peak and plateau pressures divided by the inspiratory flow rate is the airway "resistance," whereas the difference between the plateau and end-expiratory pressures divided by the tidal volume is the "compliance" of the respiratory system. P_{aw}, Airway pressure.

expiratory flow pattern can also detect the presence of end-expiratory flow, indicating the presence of auto-PEEP.

Withdrawal of Mechanical Ventilation

Withdrawal or "weaning" from mechanical ventilation should begin at the earliest opportunity. Many factors play into the decision to withdraw ventilatory support, the first being adequate control or resolution of the condition that originally led to the need for ventilation. In the postoperative thoracic surgery patient, this could simply be correction of acute issues such as pain control, fluid status, and temperature. If gas exchange has been the principal issue, then ability of the patient to achieve acceptable pH, Pco_2, and Po_2 or saturation must be assessed. In general, requirement for more than 50% oxygen or 5 to 8 cmH$_2$O of PEEP to obtain a Po_2 of 60 mmHg or saturation of more than 90% with the aid of PPV suggests that oxygenation will not be adequate without such assistance. Similarly, elevated Pco_2 in association with decreased pH suggests either oversedation or inadequate ventilatory capacity. Medical problems that could contribute to respiratory failure (e.g., heart failure) should be stable or controlled, and the patient should be responsive and able to clear secretions. Requirement for frequent (e.g., more frequently than every 2 hours) suctioning, fever, or the requirement for significant inotropic or vasopressor therapy all suggest that the patient might not be ready for withdrawal of respiratory support. Table 18-12 lists criteria that should be fulfilled before patients can be considered for ventilator "weaning" or a spontaneous breathing trial as described in the discussions that follow.

A collective task force of the American College of Chest Physicians, American Association for Respiratory Care, and the American College of Critical Care Medicine recently published a series of evidence-based guidelines for withdrawal of ventilatory support.[160] This article and the accompanying series of reviews on the same topic are excellent resources for current thinking regarding ventilator weaning. Analogous to the startling revelation that a simple reduction in tidal volume leads to improved survival in ARDS, there is a clear, emerging consensus that daily (or at least frequent) trials of spontaneous breathing (i.e., through a T-piece or with low-level CPAP or pressure support) will identify a large number of patients who are ready to have the ventilator support withdrawn. Two large trials indicated that clinicians did not recognize that discontinuing support would be possible in more than two thirds of the patients who were successfully identified with a spontaneous breathing trial.[161,162] These studies found that such trials reduced the duration of mechanical ventilation when compared with other techniques, such as gradual withdrawal of IMV or pressure support. Spontaneous trials must be initiated with close observation, as some patients cannot tolerate even a few minutes of such a trial. Psychologic support, encouragement, and physical presence of a caregiver at the bedside are essential. Table 18-13 summarizes the evaluation of a patient during a spontaneous breathing trial.

Spontaneous breathing trials also identify patients who are not ready for withdrawal of ventilator support. When this occurs, the reasons for failure need to be examined carefully. They could include inadequate resolution of the primary or underlying problem, weakness (e.g., nutritional depletion), or inadequate recovery from sedation, for example. As these problems are being addressed, the task force strongly recommends continuing the spontaneous breathing trials on a daily basis and supporting the patient between the trials with "a stable, nonfatiguing, comfortable form of ventilatory support."[160] Partial support modes (IMV with or without pressure support) that respond to and assist patient efforts should be used rather than controlled modes (e.g., "assist-control"). Protocols should be developed to allow respiratory therapists and nurses to continually adapt the ventilator support to the patient's needs, as such adaption has been shown to reduce the duration of mechanical ventilation.[163,164]

Similar to the daily performance of spontaneous breathing trials, a large prospective study showed that daily interruptions of sedative infusions decreased the duration of mechanical ven-

---

TABLE 18-12

Criteria for Considering Ventilator Weaning*

Subjective

Resolution of the underlying cause(s) of respiratory failure
Resolution or control of contributing disease states
Clinical staff believe weaning should be considered
Secretions are controlled or decreasing
Patient can cough and cooperate

Objective

Oxygenation: Po_2 ≥60 mmHg with Fio_2≤50% and ≤8 cmH$_2$O PEEP
Minute ventilation requirement not excessive (<15 L/min)
No significant acidosis (pH ≥7.30)
Afebrile (temperature <38°C)
Cardiovascular status stable without significant support
Adequate oxygen delivery (hemoglobin, cardiac output)
Metabolic status stable

*From MacIntyre NR (Chair), Cook DJ, Ely EW Jr, et al: *Chest* 120(Suppl):375S, 2001.

TABLE 18-13

Evaluation of a Spontaneous Breathing Trial (30-120 min)*

Subjective clinical assessments indicating intolerance/failure

Change in mental status
Visible discomfort
Diaphoresis
Signs of increased work of breathing

Objective assessments indicating intolerance/failure

Decreasing oxygen saturation
Decreasing pH
Increasing Pco_2
Tachycardia/dysrhythmia
Hypertension
Tachypnea or irregular pattern

Objective measures associated with successful ventilator discontinuation

Respiratory rate ≤30/min
Tidal volume ≥4-6 mL/kg
Of/VT ratio† 60-105

*From MacIntyre NR (Chair), Cook DJ, Ely EW Jr, et al: *Chest* 120(Suppl):375S, 2001.
†Respiratory rate (f) divided by tidal volume (VT) in liters. Also known as the "rapid shallow breathing index."

tilation.[165] This study was performed in a medical ICU; however, the principles embodied in the strategy are applicable to surgical patients as well. It documents the common experience that patients are often oversedated, and that the tendency of the caregivers is to maintain a stable level rather than attempt to reduce the dose to the minimum required. Such reduction is best accomplished by use of a sedation protocol, which has also been shown to reduce the duration of mechanical ventilation.[166] More recently, two reviews of sedation in the ICU have been published, both coming to similar conclusions.[167,168] Both sedation and analgesia must be addressed, usually requiring separate drugs. Propofol is the agent most likely to permit a predictable recovery, and it should be used when this is a short-term goal. Drawbacks to this agent are its cost and the high triglyceride content, which might need to be monitored. Midazolam is useful for short-term sedation (e.g., less than 48 hours), but recovery becomes unpredictable after long-term infusions. Lorazepam should be given by intermittent dosing rather than as an infusion and is a good choice for long-term sedation, with the drawback that recovery could be prolonged. Withdrawal of sedation in anticipation of weaning or extubation can be accompanied by agitation; in some circumstances, this can be addressed by conversion from longer-acting drugs to propofol for 1 to 2 days.

Extubation

Separate from weaning and the requirement for ventilatory assistance, readiness for removal of a transoral or transnasal tube requires its own assessment. The patient must be awake, cooperative, and able to cough and clear secretions, and the airway must be patent. Although there is no perfect way of assessing airway patency, a "cuff leak" test can be performed in a subjective or objective manner. For the former, the clinician simply deflates the cuff on the tube and listens for audible air leak either during spontaneous breathing or with PPV. Absence of an audible leak suggests airway edema, and the potential for postextubation obstruction. This is more likely with prolonged intubation, trauma, obesity, or female gender.[160] The test can be quantified by measuring the volume lost during volume-controlled ventilation, although another group of investigators did not find the test useful in surgical patients.[169-170] If a cuff test of any kind suggests minimal or absent air leak but a decision is made to proceed with extubation, a "tube changer" should be used to allow urgent reintubation as needed.

Tracheotomy

When the period of mechanical ventilation is likely to be prolonged (e.g., more than 7 to 10 days), there are several reasons why tracheotomy is a favored approach. First (and possibly most important), tracheotomy allows for a much greater degree of comfort by removing the transoral or transnasal tube and associated holding device or tape. This alone can result in a reduced need for sedation. By introducing a permanent path into the airway, the need for physical restraint is reduced, and the patient can be mobilized (e.g., to a chair) with less risk and greater ease. In those patients who can tolerate periods without the ventilator, a one-way speaking valve ("Passey-Muir" valve) can permit the patient to speak, and the patient might be able to swallow liquid or solid food at an earlier stage. Finally, replacement of the relatively long transoral or transnasal tube with a much shorter tracheotomy tube reduces the imposed airways resistance and facilitates removal of secretions.[171] These benefits are certainly apparent to bedside clinicians; however, measurable benefits, such as reduction in the incidence of ventilator-associated pneumonia or duration of mechanical ventilation, have not been demonstrated convincingly.[172]

REFERENCES

1. Busch E, Verazin G, Antkowiak JG, et al: Pulmonary complications in patients undergoing thoracotomy for lung carcinoma, *Chest* 105:760, 1994.
2. Stephan F, Boucheseiche S, Hollande J, et al: Pulmonary complications following lung resection: a comprehensive analysis of incidence and possible risk factors, *Chest* 118:1263, 2000.
3. Herschler-Schulte CJW, Hylkema BS, Meyer RW: Mechanical ventilation for acute post-operative respiratory failure after surgery for bronchial carcinoma, *Thorax* 40:387, 1985.
4. Wada H, Nakamura T, Nakamoto K, et al: Thirty-day operative mortality for thoracotomy in lung cancer, *J Thorac Cardiovasc Surg* 115:70, 1998.
5. Harpole DH, DeCamp M, Daly J, et al: Prognostic models of 30-day mortality and morbidity after major pulmonary resection, *J Thorac Cardiovasc Surg* 117:969, 1999.
6. Harpole DH, Liptay, DeCamp MM: Prospective analysis of pneumonectomy: risk factors for major morbidity and cardiac dysrhythmias, *Ann Thorac Surg* 61:977, 1996.
7. Kane RD, Rasanen J: Hypoxemia. In Kirby RR, Gravenstein N (eds): *Clinical anesthesia practice*, Philadelphia, 1994, WB Saunders.
8. West JB: *Pulmonary pathophysiology, the essentials*, ed 3, Baltimore, 1977, Williams and Wilkins.
9. Hagen PT, Schulz DG, Edwards WD: Incidence and size of patent foramen ovale during the first ten decades of life: an autopsy study of 965 normal hearts, *Mayo Clin Proc* 59:17, 1984.
10. Dewan NA, Gayasaddin M, Angelillo VA, et al: Persistent hypoxemia due to patent foramen ovale in a patient with adult respiratory distress syndrome, *Chest* 89:611, 1986.
11. Vaughn GC, Downs JB: Perioperative pulmonary function, assessment and intervention, *Anesthesiol Rev* 17:19, 1990.
12. Arozullah AM, Daley J, Henderson WG, et al: Multifactorial risk index for predicting postoperative respiratory failure in men after major noncardiac surgery, *Ann Surg* 232:242, 2000.
13. Doles RE, Dionne G, Leech JA, et al: Preoperative prediction of pulmonary complications following thoracic surgery, *Chest* 104:155, 1993.
14. Smetana GW: Preoperative pulmonary evaluation, *N Engl J. Med* 340:937, 1999.
15. Warner MA, Divertie MB, Tinker JH: Postoperative cessation of smoking and pulmonary complications in coronary artery bypass patients, *Anesthesiology* 60:380, 1984.
16. Vaporciyan AA, Merriman KW, Ece F: Incidence of major pulmonary morbidity after pneumonectomy: association with time of smoking cessation, *Ann Thorac Surg* 73:420, 2002.
17. Epstein S, Daly B, Celli B: Predicting complications after pulmonary resection: preoperative exercise testing vs a multifactorial cardiopulmonary risk index, *Chest* 104:694, 1993.
18. Fox GS: Anesthesia for intestinal short circuiting in the morbidly obese with reference to the pathophysiology of gross obesity, *Can Anaesth Soc J* 22:307, 1975.
19. Boushra NN: Anaesthetic management of patients with sleep apnea syndrome, *Can J Anaesth* 43:599, 1996.
20. Reilly JJ: Evidence-based preoperative evaluation of candidates for thoracotomy, *Chest* 116(Suppl 6):474S, 1999.
21. Weissman C: Pulmonary function after cardiac and thoracic surgery, *Anesth Analg* 88:1272, 1999.
22. Markos J, Mullan BO, Hillman DR, et al: Preoperative assessment as a predictor of mortality and morbidity after lung resection, *Am Rev Resp Dis* 139:902, 1989.
23. Nakahara K, Ohno K, Hashimoto J, et al: Prediction of postoperative respiratory failure in patients undergoing lung resection for cancer, *Ann Thorac Surg* 46:549, 1988.

24. Nakahara K, Monden Y, Ohno K, et al: A method for predicting postoperative lung function and its relation to postoperative complications in patients with lung cancer, *Ann Thorac Surg* 39:260, 1985.

25. Reilly J, Mentzer S, Sugarbaker D: Preoperative assessment of patients undergoing pulmonary resection, *Chest* 103:342S, 1993.

26. Ferguson MK, Reeder LB, Mick R: Optimizing selection of patients for major lung resection, *J Thorac Cardiovasc Surg* 109:275, 1995.

27. Uramoto H, Nakanishi R, Fujino Y, et al: Prediction of pulmonary complications after a lobectomy in patients with non–small cell lung cancer, *Thorax* 56:59, 2001.

28. Girish M, Trayner E Jr, Damann O, et al: Symptom-limited stair climbing as a predictor of post-operative cardiopulmonary complications after high-risk surgery, *Chest* 120:1147, 2001.

29. Bolliger CT, Wyser C, Roser H, et al: Lung scanning and exercise testing for the prediction of postoperative performance in lung resection candidates at increased risk for complications, *Chest* 108:341, 1995.

30. Berchard D, Wetstein L: Assessment of exercise oxygen consumption as preoperative criterion for lung resection, *Ann Thorac Surg* 44:344, 1987.

31. Pate P, Tenholder M, Griffin J, et al: Preoperative assessment of the high-risk patient for lung resection, *Ann Thorac Surg* 61:1494, 1996.

32. Miller J: Physiologic evaluation of pulmonary function in the candidate for lung resection, *J. Thorac Cardiovasc Surg* 105:347, 1993.

33. Gal T: Pulmonary function testing. In Miller RD (ed): *Anesthesia*, ed 4, p 883, New York, 1994, Churchill Livingstone.

34. Landreneau RJ, Pigula F, Luketich JD: Acute and chronic morbidity differences between muscle-sparing and standard lateral thoracotomies, *J Thorac Cardiovasc Surg* 112:1346, 1996.

35. Ginsberg RJ, Hill LD, Egan RT, et al: Modern thirty-day operative mortality for surgical resections in lung cancer, *J Thorac Cardiovasc Surg* 86:654, 1983.

36. Cooper JD, Patterson GA, Sunderson RS, et al: Results of 150 consecutive bilateral lung volume reduction procedures in patients with severe emphysema, *J Thorac Cardiovasc Surg* 112:1319, 1996.

37. Chatila W, Furukawa S, Criner GJ: Acute respiratory failure after lung volume reduction surgery, *Am J Resp Crit Care Med* 162:1292, 2000.

38. Fujimoto R, Teschler H. Hillejan L, et al: Long-term results of lung volume reduction surgery, *Eur J Cardiothorac Surg* 21:483, 2002.

39. National Emphysema Treatment Trial Research Group: Patients at risk for death after lung volume research surgery, *N Engl J. Med* 345:1075, 2001.

40. Drachman DB: Myasthenia gravis, *N Engl J Med* 298:136, 1978.

41. Eisenkraft JB, Papatestas AE, Kahn CH, et al: Predicting the need for postoperative ventilation and myasthenia gravis, *Anesthesiology* 65:79, 1986.

42. Moore KH, McKenzie PR, Kennedy CW, et al: Thymoma: trends over time, *Ann Thorac Surg* 72:203, 2001.

43. Karl RC, Schreiber R, Boulware D, et al: Factors affecting morbidity, mortality, and survival in patients undergoing Ivor Lewis esophagogastrectomy, *Ann Surg* 231:635, 2000.

44. Ellis FH, Heatley GJ, Krasna MJ, et al: Esophagogastrectomy for carcinoma of the esophagus and cardia; a comparison of findings and results after standard resection in three consecutive eight-year intervals with improved staging criteria, *J Thorac Cardiovasc Surg* 113:83, 1997.

45. Alexiou C, Beggs D, Salama FD, et al: Surgery for esophageal cancer in elderly patients: the view from Nottingham, *J Thorac Cardiovasc Surg* 116:545, 1998.

46. Craig DB: Postoperative recovery of pulmonary function, *Anesth Analg* 60:46, 1981.

47. West JB: *Pulmonary pathophysiology*, ed 3, Baltimore, 1977, Williams and Wilkins.

48. Uzieblo M, Welsh R, Pursel SE, et al: Incidence and significance of lobar atelectasis in thoracic surgical patients, *Am Surg* 66:476, 2000.

49. Byrd RB, Burns JR: Cough dynamics in the post-thoracotomy state, *Chest* 67:654, 1975.

50. Meyers JR, Lembek L, O'Kane H, et al: Changes in functional residual capacity of the lung after operation, *Arch Surg* 110:576, 1975.

51. Shapiro BA, Peruzzi WT: Respiratory care. In Miller RD (ed): *Anesthesia*, ed 5, New York, 2000, Churchill Livingstone.

52. Bastin R, Moraine J, Bardocsky G, et al: Incentive spirometry performance: a reliable indicator of pulmonary function in the early postoperative period after lobectomy? *Chest* 111:563, 1997.

53. Overend TJ, Anderson CM, Lucy SD, et al: The effect of incentive spirometry on postoperative pulmonary complications, a systematic review, *Chest* 120:971, 2001.

54. Mahlmeister MJ, Fink JB, Hoffman GL, et al: Positive expiratory pressure mask therapy; theoretical and practical considerations and a review of the literature, *Respir Care* 36:218, 1991.

55. Stock MC, Downs JB, Gauer PK, et al: Prevention of postoperative pulmonary complications with CPAP incentive spirometry and conservative therapy, *Chest* 87:151, 1985.

56. Tobias JD: Noninvasive ventilation using bilevel positive airway pressure to treat impending respiratory failure in the postanesthesia care unit, *J Clin Anesth* 12:409, 2000.

57. Yamazaki S, Ogawa J, Shohzu A, et al: Intrapleural cough pressure in patients after thoracotomy, *J Thorac Cardiovasc Surg* 80:600, 1980.

58. Rogers A, Walker N, Schug S, et al: Reduction of postoperative mortality and morbidity with epidural or spinal anesthesia: results from an overview of randomized trials, *Br Med J* 321:1, 2000.

59. Mourisse J, Hasenbios AWM, Gielen JM, et al: Epidural bupivacaine, sufentanil or the combination for post-thoracotomy pain, *Acta Anaesth Scand* 36:70, 1992.

60. Pepe PE, Marin JJ: Occult positive end-expiratory pressure in mechanically ventilated patients with airflow obstruction, *Am Rev Resp Dis* 126:166, 1982.

61. Slattery DM, Waltz DA, Deham B, et al: Bronchoscopically administered recombinant human Dnase for labor atelectasis in cystic fibrosis, *Pediatr Pulmonol* 31:358, 2001.

62. The Combivent Inhalation Aerosol Study Group: In chronic obstructive pulmonary disease, a combination of ipratropium and albuterol is more effective than either agent alone: an 85-day multicenter trial, *Chest* 105:1411, 1994.

63. Quidaciouli F, Guasone F, Pastorino G, et al: Use of minitracheotomy in high-risk pulmonary resection surgery, *Minerva Chir* 49:315, 1994.

64. Issa MM, Healy DM, Maghur HA, et al: Prophylactic minitracheotomy in lung resections, *J Thorac Cardiovasc Surg* 101:895, 1991.

65. Balkan ME, Ozdulger A, Tastepe I, et al: Clinical experience with mini tracheotomy, *Scand J Thorac Cardiovasc Surg* 30:93, 1996.

66. Inagawa G, Suzuki J, Morimura N, et al: Tracheal obstruction caused by minitracheotomy, *Int Care Med* 26:1707, 2000.

67. Pugh A, Pachi E: Complications of fiberoptic bronchoscopy at a university hospital, *Chest* 107:430, 1995.

68. Ferdinand B, Shennib H: Postoperative pneumonia, *Chest Surg Clin N Am* 8:529, 1998.

69. Luna C, Vujacich P, Niederman M, et al: Impact of BAL data on therapy and outcome of ventilator-associated pneumonia, *Chest* 111:676, 1997.

70. Ziomek S., Read RC, Tobler HG, et al: Thromboembolism in patients undergoing thoracotomy, *Ann Thorac Surg* 58:603, 1994.

71. Kalweit G, Huwer H, Volkmer I, et al: Pulmonary embolism: a frequent cause of acute fatality after lung resection, *Eur J Cardiothorac Surg* 10:242, 1996.

72. Wood KE: Major pulmonary embolism, *Chest* 121:877, 2002.

73. Velmahos GC, Vassiliu P, Wilcox A, et al: Spiral computed tomography for the diagnosis of pulmonary embolism in critically ill surgical patients: a comparison with pulmonary angiography, *Arch Surg* 136:505, 2001.

74. Mullins MD, Becker DM, Hagspiel KD, et al: The role of spiral computed tomography in the diagnosis of pulmonary embolism, *ACP Journal Club* 133:32, 2000.

75. van der Werff YD, van der Houwen HK, Heijmans PJM, et al: Postpneumonectomy pulmonary edema, *Chest* 111:1278, 1997.

76. Waller DA, Keavey P, Woodfine L, et al: Pulmonary endothelial permeability changes after major lung resection, *Ann Thorac Surg* 61:1435, 1996.

77. Jordan S, Mitchell JA, Quinlan GJ, et al: The pathogenesis of lung injury following pulmonary resection, *Eur Resp J* 15:790, 2000.

78. Paquin F, Marchal M, Mehiri S, et al: Postpneumonectomy pulmonary edema: analysis and risk factors, *Eur J Cardiothoracic Surg* 10:929, 1996.

79. Khan SU, Salloum J, O'Donovan PB, et al: Acute pulmonary edema after lung transplantation, *Chest* 116:187, 1999.

80. Demertzis S, Langer F, Graeter T, et al: Amelioration of lung perfusion injury by L- and E-selectin blockade, *Eur J Cardiothorac Surg* 16:174, 1999.

81. Marom EM, Choi YW, Palmer SM, et al: Reperfusion edema after lung transplantation: effect of daclizumab, *Radiology* 221:508, 2001.

82. Schilling MK, Gasmann N, Sigurdsson GH, et al: Role of thromboxane and leukotriene B4 in patients with acute respiratory distress syndrome after oesophagectomy, *Br J Anaesth* 80:36, 1998.

83. Money SR, Rice K, Crockett D, et al: Risk of respiratory failure after repair of thoracoabdominal aortic aneurysms, *Am J Surg* 168:152, 1994.

84. Engle J, Safi HJ, Miller CC III, et al: The impact of diaphragm management on prolonged ventilator support after thoracoabdominal aortic repair, *J Vasc Surg* 29:150, 1999.

85. Svensson LG, Hess KR, Coselli JS, et al: A prospective study of respiratory failure after high-risk surgery on the thoracoabdominal aorta, *J Vasc Surg* 21:271, 1991.

86. Gattinoni L, D'Andrea L, Pelosi P, et al: Regional effects and mechanism of positive end-expiratory pressure in early adult respiratory distress syndrome, *JAMA* 269:2122, 1993.

87. Malo J, Ali J, Wood LDH: How does positive end-expiratory pressure reduce intrapulmonary shunt in canine pulmonary edema? *J Appl Physiol* 57:1002, 1984.

88. Field S, Kelly SM, Macklem PT: The oxygen cost of breathing in patients with cardiorespiratory disease, *Am Rev Resp Dis* 126:9, 1982.

89. Katz JA, Marks JD: Inspiratory work with and without continuous positive airway pressure in patients with acute respiratory failure, *Anesthesiology* 63:598, 1985.

90. Fiastro JF, Habib MP, Quan SR: Pressure support compensation for inspiratory work due to endotracheal tubes and demand continuous positive airway pressure, *Chest* 93:499, 1998.

91. Cereda M, Foti G, Marcora B, et al: Pressure support ventilation in patients with acute lung injury, *Crit Care Med* 28:1269, 2000.

92. Stewart KG: Clinical evaluation of pressure support ventilation, *Br J Anaesth* 63:362, 1989.

93. Hillberg RE, Johnson DC: Noninvasive ventilation, *N Engl J Med* 337:1746, 1997.

94. Massimo A, Conti G, Bufi M, et al: Noninvasive ventilation for treatment of acute respiratory failure in patients undergoing solid organ transplantation, *JAMA* 283:235, 2000.

95. Girou E, Schortgen F, Delclaux et al: Association of noninvasive ventilation with nosocomial infections and survival in critically ill patients, *JAMA* 284:2361, 2000.

96. Aguilo R, Togores B, Pons S, et al: Noninvasive ventilatory support after lung resection surgery, *Chest* 112:117, 1997.

97. Auriant I, Jallot A, Herve P, et al: Noninvasive ventilation reduces mortality in acute respiratory failure following lung resection, *Am J Respir Crit Care Med* 164:1231, 2001.

98. Tharratt RS, Allen RP, Albertson TE: Pressure-controlled inverse-ratio ventilation in severe respiratory failure, *Chest* 94:755, 1988.

99. Garner W, Downs JB, Stock MC, et al: Airway pressure release ventilation (APRV): a human trial, *Chest* 94:779, 1988.

100. Parish JM, Gracey DR, Southern PA, et al: Differential mechanical ventilation in respiratory failure due to severe unilateral lung disease, *Mayo Clin Proc* 59:822, 1984.

101. Carlon GC, Ray C, Pierri MK, et al: High-frequency jet ventilation: theoretical considerations and clinical observations, *Chest* 81:350, 1982.

102. Nevin M, Van Besouw JP, Williams CW, et al: A comparative study of conventional vs high-frequency jet ventilation with relation to the incidence of postoperative morbidity in thoracic surgery, *Ann Thorac Surg* 44:625, 1987.

103. Butler WJ, Bohn DJ, Bryan AC, et al: Ventilation by high-frequency oscillation in humans, *Anesth Analg* 59:577, 1980.

104. Ferguson ND, Stewart TE: New therapies for adults with acute lung injury: high-frequency oscillatory ventilation, *Crit Care Clin* 18:91, 2002.

105. Bendixen HH, Hedley-White J, Laver MB: Impaired oxygenation in surgical patients during general anesthesia with controlled ventilation. A concept of atelectasis, *N Engl J Med* 269:991, 1963.

106. Bernard GR, Artigas A, Brigham KL, et al: The American-European consensus conference on ARDS: definitions, mechanisms, relevant outcomes, and clinical trial coordination, *Am J Respir Crit Care Med* 149:818, 1994.

107. Ashbaugh DG, Bigelow DB, Petty TL, et al: Acute respiratory distress in adults, *Lancet* 2:319, 1967.

108. Pittet JF, MacKersie RC, Martin TR, et al: Biological markers of acute lung injury: prognostic and pathogenetic significance, *Am J Respir Crit Care Med* 155:1187, 1997.

109. Ware LB, Matthay MA: The acute respiratory distress syndrome, *N Engl J Med* 342:1334, 2000.

110. Kutlu CA, Williams EA, Evans TW et al: Acute lung injury and acute respiratory distress syndrome after pulmonary resection, *Ann Thorac Surg* 69:376, 2000.

111. Milberg JA, Davis DR, Steinber KP, et al: Improved survival of patients with acute respiratory distress syndrome (ARDS) 1983-1993, *JAMA* 273:306, 1995.

112. Khadaroo RG, Marshall JC: ARDS and the multiple organ dysfunction syndrome: common mechanisms of a common systemic process, *Crit Care Clin* 18:127, 2002.

113. Ferring M, Vincent JL: Is outcome from ARDS related to the severity of respiratory failure? *Eur Resp J* 10:1297, 1997.

114. Deitch EA: Multiple organ failure. Pathophysiology and potential future therapy, *Ann Surg* 216:117, 1992.

115. McHugh LG, Milberg JA, Whitcomb ME, et al: Recovery of function in survivors of the acute respiratory distress syndrome, *Am J Respir Crit Care Med* 150:90, 1994.

116. Webb HH, Tierney DF: Experimental pulmonary edema due to intermittent positive-pressure ventilation with high inflation pressures : protection by positive end-expiratory pressure, *Am Rev Resp Dis* 110:556, 1974.

117. Ranieri VM, Suter PM, Tororella C, et al: Effect of mechanical ventilation on inflammatory mediators in patients with acute respiratory distress syndrome, *JAMA* 282:54, 1999.

118. The Acute Respiratory Distress Syndrome Network: Ventilation with lower tidal volumes as compared with traditional tidal volumes for acute lung injury and the acute respiratory distress syndrome, *N Engl J Med* 342:1301, 2000.

119. Levy MM: Optimal PEEP in ARDS: changing concepts and current controversies, *Crit Care Clin* 18:15, 2002.

120. Suter PM, Fairley HB, Isenberg MD: Optimum end-expiratory airway pressure in patients with acute pulmonary failure, *N Engl J Med* 292:284, 1975.

121. Roupie E, Dambrosio M, Servillo G, et al: Titration of tidal volume and induced hypercapnia in acute respiratory distress syndrome, *Am J Respir Crit Care Med* 152:121, 1995.

122. Hickling KG: Permissive hypercapnia in ARDS: current concepts, *Int Care World* 12:121, 1995.

123. Patroniti N, Foti G, Cortinovis B, et al: Sigh improves gas exchange and lung volume in patients with acute respiratory distress syndrome undergoing pressure support ventilation, *Anesthesiology* 96:788, 2002.

124. Grasso S, Mascia L, Del Turco M, et al: Effects of recruiting maneuvers in patients with acute respiratory distress syndrome ventilated with protective ventilatory strategy, *Anesthesiology* 96:795, 2002.

125. Vincent JL: New management strategies in ARDS: immunomodulation, *Crit Care Clin* 18:69, 2002.

126. Bernard GR, Luce JM, Sprung CL; et al: High-dose corticosteroids in patients with the adult respiratory distress syndrome, *N Engl J Med* 317:1565, 1987.

127. Meduri GU, Headley AS, Golden E, et al: Effect of prolonged methylprednisolone therapy in unresolving acute respiratory distress syndrome, *JAMA* 280:159, 1998.

128. Wheeler A: Methylprednisolone for unresolving ARDS, *JAMA* 280:2074, 1998.

129. Gadek JE, DeMichele SJ, Karlstad MD, et al: Effect of enteral feeding with eicosapentaenoic acid, gamma-linolenic acid, and antioxidants in patients with acute respiratory distress syndrome. Enteral nutrition in ARDS study group, *Crit Care Med* 27:1409, 1999.

130. Bernard GR, Vincent JL, Laterre PF, et al: Efficacy and safety of recombinant human activated protein C for severe sepsis, *N Engl J Med* 344:699, 2001.

131. Bryan AC: Comments of a devil's advocate, *Am Rev Respir Dis* 110 (Suppl):143, 1974.

132. Mure M, Domino KB, Lindahl SG, et al: Regional ventilation-perfusion distribution is more uniform in the prone position, *J Appl Physiol* 88:1076, 2000.

133. Pappert D, Rossaint R, Slama K, et al: Influence of positioning on ventilation-perfusion relationships in severe adult respiratory distress syndrome, *Chest* 106:1511, 1994.

134. Gattinoni L, Pelosi P, Vitale G et al: Body position changes redistribute lung computed-tomographic density in patients with acute respiratory failure, *Anesthesiology* 74:15, 1991.

135. Gattinoni L, Tognoni G, Pesenti A, et al: Effect of prone positioning on the survival of patients with acute respiratory failure, *N Engl J Med* 345:568, 2001.

136. Long W, Thompson T, Sundell H: Effects of two rescue doses of a synthetic surfactant on mortality rate and survival without bronchopulmonary dysplasia in 700 to 1350 gram infants with respiratory distress syndrome, *J Pediatr* 118:5955, 1991.

137. Anzueto A, Baughman RP, Guntupalli KK, et al: Aerosolized surfactant in adults with sepsis-induced acute respiratory distress syndrome, *N Engl J Med* 334:1417, 1996.

138. Walmrath D, Gunther A, Ghofrani A, et al: Bronchoscopic surfactant administration in patients with severe adult respiratory distress syndrome and sepsis, *Am J Respir Crit Care Med* 154:57, 1996.

139. Klinger JR: Inhaled nitric oxide in ARDS, *Crit Care Clin* 18:45, 2002.

140. Dellinger RP, Zimmerman JL, Taylor RW, et al: Effects of inhaled nitric oxide in patients with acute respiratory distress syndrome: results of a randomized phase II trial, *Crit Care Med* 26:15, 1998.

141. Lundin S, Mang H, Smithies M, et al: Inhalation of nitric oxide in acute lung injury: results of a European multicenter study, *Intensive Care Med* 25:911, 1999.

142. Hirschl DB, Croce M, Gore D, et al: Prospective, randomized, controlled pilot study of partial liquid ventilation in adult acute respiratory distress syndrome, *Am J Respir Crit Care Med* 165:781, 2002.

143. Wright CD, Wain JC, Mathiessen DJ, et al: Postpneumonectomy bronchopleural fistula after sutured closure: incidence, risk factors, and management, *J Thorac Cardiovasc Surg* 112:1367, 1993.

144. Chastre J, Fagon J-Y: Ventilator-associated pneumonia, *Am J Respir Crit Care Med* 165:867, 2002.

145. Vincent JL, Bihari DJ, Suter PM, et al: The prevalence of nosocomial infection in intensive care units in Europe. Results of the European prevalence of infection in intensive care (EPIC) study. EPIC international advisory committee, *JAMA* 274:639, 1996.

146. Centers for Disease Control and Prevention: Monitoring hospital-acquired infections to promote patient safety: United States, 1990-1999, *MMWR* 49:149, 2000.

147. American Thoracic Society: Hospital-acquired pneumonia in adults: diagnosis, assessment of severity, initial antimicrobial therapy, and preventative strategies. A consensus statement. American Thoracic Society, November 1995, *Am J Respir Crit Care Med* 153:1711, 1996.

148. Grossman R (Chair): American College of Chest Physicians evidence-based assessment of diagnostic tests for ventilator-associated pneumonia, *Chest* 17:4 (Suppl 2):177S, 2000.

149. Cook DJ, Walter SD, Cook RJ, et al: Incidence of and risk factors for ventilator-associated pneumonia in critically ill patients, *Ann Intern Med* 129:433, 1998.

150. Grudson D, Hilbert G, Vargas F, et al: Rotation and restricted use of antibiotics in a medical intensive care unit. Impact on the incidence of ventilator-associated pneumonia caused by antibiotic-resistant gram-negative bacteria, *Am J Respir Crit Care Med* 162:837, 2000.

151. Cook D, Guyatt G, Marshall J, et al: A comparison of sucralfate and ranitidine for the prevention of upper gastrointestinal bleeding in patients requiring mechanical ventilation. Canadian critical care trials group, *N Engl J Med* 338:791, 1998.

152. Rouby JJ, Laurent P, Gonsnach M, et al: Risk factors and clinical relevance of nosocomial maxillary sinusitis in the critically ill, *Am J Respir Crit Care Med* 150:776, 1994.

153. Craven DE, Steger KA, Barber TW: Preventing nosocomial pneumonia : state of the art and perspectives for the 1990s, *Am J Med* 91:44S, 1991.

154. Smulders K, van der Hoeven H, Weers-Pothoff I, et al: A randomized clinical trial of intermittent subglottic secretion drainage in patients receiving mechanical ventilation, *Chest* 121:858, 2002.

155. Withington DE, Ramsay JG, Saoud T, et al: Weaning from ventilation after cardiopulmonary bypass: evaluation of a noninvasive technique, *Can J Anaesth* 38:15, 1991.

156. Hoffman RA, Kreiger BP, Kramer MR, et al: End-tidal carbon dioxide in critically ill patients during changes in mechanical ventilation, *Am Rev Resp Dis* 14:1265, 1989.

157. McGregor M: Pulsus paradoxus, *N Engl J Med* 301:480, 1979.

158. Biondi JW, Schulman DS, Soufer R: The effect of incremental positive end-expiratory pressure on right ventricular hemodynamics and ejection fraction, *Anesth Analg* 67:144, 1988.

159. Sibbald WJ, Driedger AA: Right ventricular function in acute disease states; pathophysiologic considerations, *Crit Care Med* 11:339, 1983.

160. MacIntyre NR (Chair), Cook DJ, Ely EW Jr, et al: Evidence-based guidelines for weaning and discontinuing ventilatory support, *Chest* 120(Suppl):375S, 2001.

161. Estaban A, Frutos F, Tobin MJ, et al: A comparison of four methods of weaning patients from mechanical ventilation: the Spanish lung failure collaborative group, *N Engl J Med* 332:345, 1995.

162. Brochard L, Rauss A, Benito S, et al: Comparion of three methods of gradual withdrawal from ventilatory support during weaning from mechanical ventilation, *Am J Respir Crit Care Med* 150:896, 1994.

163. Marelich GP, Murin S, Battistella F, et al: Protocol weaning of mechanical ventilation in medical and surgical patients by respiratory care practitioners and nurses: effect on weaning time and incidence of ventilator-associated pneumonia, *Chest* 118:459, 2000.

164. Kollef MH, Shapiro SD, Silver P, et al: A randomized, controlled trial of protocol-directed versus physician-directed weaning from mechanical ventilation, *Crit Care Med* 23:567, 1997.

165. Kress JP, Pohlman AS, O'Connor MF, et al: Daily interruptions of sedative infusions in critically ill patients undergoing mechanical ventilation, *N Engl J Med* 342:1471, 2000.

166. Brook AD, Ahrens TS, Schaiff R, et al: Effect of a nursing-implemented sedation protocol on the duration of mechanical ventilation, *Crit Care Med* 27:2609, 1999.

167. Ostermann ME, Keenan SP, Seiferling RA, et al: Sedation in the intensive care unit: an intensive review, *JAMA* 283:1451, 2000.

168. Jacobi J, Fraser GL, Coursin DB, et al: Clinical practice guidelines for the sustained use of sedatives and analgesics in the intensive care unit, *Crit Care Med* 30:119, 2002.

169. Miller R, Cole R: Association between reduced cuff leak volume and postextubation stridor, *Chest* 110:1035, 1996.

170. Engoren M: Evaluation of the cuff leak test in cardiac surgery patients, *Chest* 116:1029, 1999.

171. Lin MC, Huang CC, Yang CT, et al: Pulmonary mechanics in patients with prolonged mechanical ventilation requiring tracheostomy, *Anaesth Intens Care* 27:581, 1999.

172. Heffner JE: The role of tracheotomy in weaning, *Chest* 120(Suppl):477S, 2001.

Cardiovascular Adaptation to Lung Resection

Paul M. Heerdt, MD, PhD, FAHA

EACH year, approximately 60,000 noncardiac thoracic surgical procedures are performed in the United States, most for the treatment of cancer. Over the last 20 years, outcome after lung surgery has improved steadily; partly for this reason, even extensive resections are now being offered to patients with significant comorbidities or advanced age.[1-3] In addition, the development of procedures such as lung volume reduction surgery and transplantation has added the challenge of caring for severely compromised patients who previously would not have been regarded as surgical candidates.

Cardiac complications account for a large percentage of the perioperative morbidity associated with lung resection, in part because of a median age in excess of 65 years and the prevalence of concomitant coronary, vascular, or valvular heart disease.[1,4,5] Accordingly, specific clinical study of how lung resection influences short- and long-term cardiac performance is hampered by the complexities of dissociating primary sequelae from secondary events (e.g., induced ischemia). Furthermore, the common overlay of parenchymal lung disease only serves to heighten the physiologic complexity of these patients.

An important feature of postthoracotomy cardiovascular sequelae is that hemodynamically significant complications do not usually occur until after a 48- to 72-hour window of relative stability.[6] Most patients subsequently demonstrate a progressive functional improvement during convalescence, with eventual resumption of daily activities within the constraints of preexisting disease and the extent of lung resected. These observations suggest that the cardiopulmonary response to lung resection varies over time, with an initial acute "reactive phase" that is different from the "adaptive phase" apparent during a period of cellular and structural adaptation within the heart. The adaptive phase could, in turn, be different from the steady-state "compensated phase" achieved after stabilization of delayed processes extrinsic to the heart, such as secondary growth of remaining lung. This chapter reviews the perioperative cardiovascular response to lung resection, with subsequent consideration of secondary cardiopulmonary adaptation.

Endpoints for Quantifying Functional Adaptation to Lung Resection

In many ways, the acute alterations in cardiopulmonary function elicited by lung resection parallel those produced by progression of intrinsic parenchymal pulmonary disease. Ultimately, the efficacy of functional adaptation to or compensation for each process can be characterized in terms of oxygen uptake and peripheral extraction. It is important, however, to appreciate the fact that adaptation to alterations in oxygen transport is a coordinated, whole-body phenomenon involving multiple steps. Within this framework, disturbance of one step elicits adaptive changes in other steps in order to establish a new functional equilibrium.[7]

Fundamentally, oxygen transport is a sequential process of ventilation matched with blood flow, diffusion through lung and capillaries, chemical interaction with hemoglobin and myoglobin, and, ultimately, mitochondrial oxidative phosphorylation. In most subjects (e.g., individuals not physically trained), maximum oxygen uptake (VO_2max) is limited by maximum cardiac output and peripheral oxygen extraction, not by pulmonary diffusing capacity or maximum ventilation. Accordingly, augmenting maximum cardiac output and enhancing oxygen extraction with regular exercise markedly increases VO_2max, while increasing maximum ventilation or diffusing capacity has minimal effect.[7] In the perioperative period, as well as during subsequent postoperative convalescence, secondary processes such as physical deconditioning and anemia can augment the primary deficit created by lung removal or disruption of ventilation by chest wall dysfunction. Following recovery and assumption of a steady-state compensated phase, physical limitation is influenced by the extent of resection and magnitude of deconditioning, both within the context of preexisting disease. Ultimately, however, whether physical limitation after lung resection—often presenting not only as dyspnea but also as leg fatigue—is cardiac or pulmonary in origin remains somewhat controversial.

Two obvious considerations in the assessment of how lung resection alters exercise capacity are the extent of resection and the time frame over which data are acquired. Miyoshi et al measured VO_2max in a group of 16 patients (13 lobectomy, 3 pneumonectomy) both before surgery and 9 ± 2 and 26 ± 12 days after surgery.[8] When comparing postsurgical with preoperative values, they found, on average, a 27% decline in VO_2max at the first postoperative time point but only an 18% reduction at the later time point. Analysis of their data suggested that the early drop was both respiratory and circulatory in origin, with subsequent short-term improvement due to the augmented respiratory performance provided by recovery from the surgical insult and normalization of chest wall mechanics. In contrast, Nezu et al examined the initial loss and subsequent recovery of exercise capacity (characterized as VO_2max) 3 and 6 months after lobectomy or pneumonectomy.[9] Their data show the following:

- The initial decline in VO_2max was about twice as great in the pneumonectomy group.

- Six months after resection, there was modest improvement in the lobectomy group but no change in patients having pneumonectomy.

A subsequent report of pulmonary function up to 4 years after lung resection showed no major changes in comparison with data acquired after the first 4 to 6 months, with the exception of modest improvements in airway resistance and diffusing capacity.[10] It is noteworthy, however, that 80% of the patients exhibiting physical limitation 4 to 6 months postoperatively demonstrated long-term improvement in daily activity. Although multiple studies consistently find a close relationship between extent of resection and functional loss of exercise capacity, some investigators have failed to find direct correlations, thus raising the issue of other factors.[9,11-14] Because maximal cardiac output could be limited along with ventilatory capacity and pulmonary diffusing capacity, many authors believe that a postresection decline in VO_2max is primarily a circulatory phenomenon.[10,14-19] Other studies, however—including one that compared thoracotomy alone with limited resection and pneumonectomy—implicate a primary reduction in ventilatory reserve.[13,20]

Lung Resection and Cardiac Performance

Despite extensive clinical experience with lung resection, understanding of the subsequent direct effect—both acute and long term—on performance of the heart remains remarkably confused. In general, changes in cardiac pump function have been attributed to an acute increase in right ventricular (RV) afterload resulting from pulmonary arterial (PA) ligation. Although this simple paradigm of increased afterload leading to RV dilation, reduced ejection fraction, and dampened stroke volume is attractive, multiple experimental and clinical observations complicate universal application.

Theoretical and Experimental Considerations
THE CONCEPT OF AFTERLOAD

Central to understanding the mechanical interaction between the heart and circulation is an appreciation of the fact that multiple properties interact to influence ventricular afterload. Because the concept was derived from studies involving application of a constant weight to isolated muscle, afterload is difficult to quantify precisely in intact hearts because ejection is opposed by a variable hydraulic load. Clinically, ventricular afterload is commonly summarized as *vascular resistance* calculated as

Mean pressure/*mean* flow

Because the pressure and flow generated by the heart are not steady and continuous, but intermittent and pulsatile, ejection is opposed not only by steady-state resistive forces but also by elastic (large vessels are distended with each beat) and reflective (pressure and flow waves reflected backwards) forces. Accordingly, expression of afterload in terms of simple resistance is incomplete. Functional significance of this concept can be found in the fact that when the impact of increased PA pressure secondary to a primary change in resistance (e.g., vasoconstriction of small pulmonary vessels) is compared with a similar pressure response produced by a primary change in compliance (e.g., ligation of a large pulmonary artery), a

different functional alteration in RV hydraulic work is evident.[21] In order to incorporate all components, proximal aortic or PA pressure and flow characteristics can be resolved mathematically into individual frequency components (as each waveform actually represents summation and cancellation of forward and backward waves of multiple frequencies) and used to calculate *input impedance* (Z_{in}). This "frequency domain" analysis of pressure and flow throughout the entire cardiac cycle allows for creation of an *impedance spectrum* in which the pressure/flow amplitude and phase ratios over a range of frequencies are plotted.[22] Specific components of the input impedance spectrum can then be used to determine the location and magnitude of wave reflection and construct a three-element model of the circulation emulating an electrical circuit. This "lumped parameter" model contains a direct current (DC), frequency-independent component representing resistive, nonpulsatile load and characterized by Z at 0 frequency (Z_0); an alternating current (AC), frequency-dependent component representing pulsatile load and described by the "characterstic" Z (Z_C) defined as the average of values at 3 Hz and higher; and a capacitor (energy-storage element) characterized by the compliance of the proximal aorta or pulmonary artery which, through elastic recoil, transmits energy downstream during diastole. Conceptually, these ideas have been likened to a Windkessel model based on similarities with primitive systems that allowed air (or water for firehoses) to be pumped by hand (pulsatile work or AC component) into a distensible chamber (energy-storage element), which dampened the pulsations and discharged the air as a continuous stream (steady-state or DC component) (Figure 19-1).

THE CONCEPT OF CONTRACTILITY: APPLICATION TO THE RIGHT VENTRICLE OF PRINCIPLES DERIVED FOR THE LEFT-SIDE VENTRICLE

Contractility essentially reflects the ability of the myocyte to generate tension in the face of a specific load; when the relationship shifts so that tension develops more rapidly or to a greater degree for the load, contractility increases. Although contractility is relatively easy to quantify in isolated muscle systems or intact hearts beating isovolumically, this is not the case in the ejecting heart. Load-independent methods for assessing contractility in the intact heart have proven extremely valuable in experimental preparations, but clinical application is often complicated. In general, indices of contractility can be derived from the phase of isovolumic contraction, the phase of ventricular ejection, the end-systolic pressure-volume relationship (ESPVR), or the relationship between stroke work and end-diastolic volume.

One of the most common and useful indices of contractility is the first derivative of pressure development during isovolumic contraction (dP/dt). Although this index is sensitive for detecting acute alterations in contractility, easy to interpret, and relatively independent of afterload, precise measurement of dP/dt requires high-fidelity measurement of pressure (which can be distorted by ventricular wall properties and valve dysfunction) and is influenced by preload. Alternative approaches include ejection phase indices, the most common of which is ejection fraction. Calculated as stroke volume divided by end-diastolic volume, the normal RV ejection fraction is 45% to 50%. Although ejection fraction provides useful information

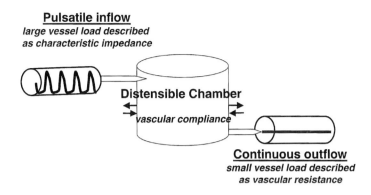

Pulsatile inflow
large vessel load described
as characteristic impedance

Distensible Chamber
vascular compliance

Continuous outflow
small vessel load described
as vascular resistance

FIGURE 19-1 The Windkessel model of the circulation, which dissociates pulsatile from nonpulsatile components of afterload.

about systolic pump performance and can be readily measured for both ventricles in the clinical setting, it is heavily influenced by afterload, which reduces its value as a specific index of contractility. The most load-independent indices of contractility are those derived from pressure-volume relationships. Suga and Sagawa first described the use of the ESPVR for characterizing ventricular contractility in a load-independent manner based on the concept of volume elastance (E) defined as $\Delta P/\Delta V$.[23] Conceptually, if the empty heart is considered to behave like an elastic sac, with filling there is an initial increase in volume without significant pressure change. Eventually a volume is reached (V_0) at which contents go from being unstressed (no pressure) to stressed (under pressure); pressure then begins to rise as volume increases. If the subsequent pressure-volume relationship is linear, then the slope of this line at any volume (V) is $P/V-V_0$, which represents E. Unlike an elastic sac, however, the heart actively increases wall tension during contraction. As the wall stiffens, the relationship between pressure and volume (and, therefore, the value of E) changes. As ejection occurs and volume falls relative to pressure, E increases to reach a maximum near the end of systole. In the intact heart, end-systolic elastance (E_{es}) can be determined by varying loading conditions to provide a range of pressures and volumes, and regressing the point of end-systole for each beat; the slope of this regression is E_{es}, and the x (or volume) intercept is V_0 (Figure 19-2). This method assumes that V_0 stays relatively constant and that the $P/V-V_0$ slope remains linear, which is valid under most physiologic conditions. Acute alterations in contractility, however (e.g., the negative inotropic effect of volatile anesthetics), can alter both the slope and volume intercept of the ESPVR, and nonlinear (monoexponential and quadratic) ESPVR relationships have been described. Furthermore, E_{es} can be influenced by how end-systole is defined, which becomes particularly important when applying the concept to the RV.[24] As shown in Figure 19-2, the LV pressure-volume loop tends to be rectangular and to have a relatively well-defined end-systolic point in the upper-left corner just before isovolumic relaxation. In contrast, the RV pressure-volume loop is more triangular, with little isovolumic relaxation and no clearly defined point of end-systole, thus complicating derivation of E_{es}.

An alternative to E_{es} is preload-recruitable stroke work (PRSW), which essentially represents a linearization of the Frank-Starling relationship.[25] To measure PRSW, venous return to the intact heart is decreased acutely and the area of each P/V loop, which represents the external work performed during the beat, is plotted as a function of the end-diastolic volume (Figure 19-3). The slope of this relationship determines how much work the heart is capable of at any given preload. When contractility increases or decreases, the slope rises or falls as the heart performs more or less work for a given preload. In the assessment of acute alterations in contractility, this technique appears to have less variation in the volume intercept and more shift in slope than E_{es}. Furthermore, because the RV

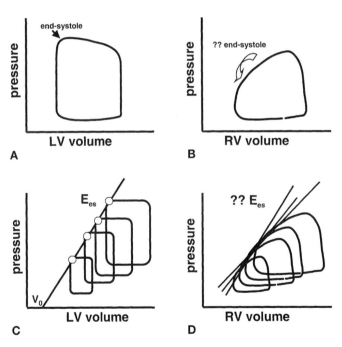

FIGURE 19-2 **A,** A left ventricular (LV) pressure-volume loop with the point of end-systole well defined in the upper-left corner. **B,** A right ventricular (RV) pressure-volume loop, which, in contrast to the LV, has a poorly defined end-systolic point. **C,** Representation of LV pressure-volume loops during an acute change in load. Slope of the regression of the end-systolic points for individual loops yields end-systolic elastance (E_{es}), and the x-intercept represents the volume at which pressure begins to rise (V_0). **D,** Representation of RV pressure-volume loops during an acute change in load. Poor definition of the end-systolic point for each loop complicates simple calculation of RV E_{es}.

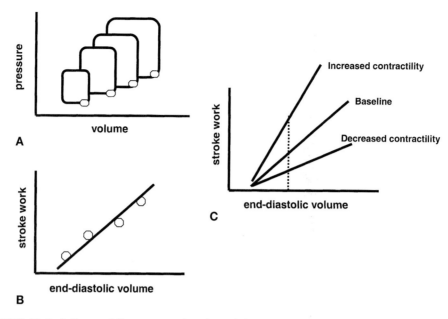

FIGURE 19-3 A, Representative pressure-volume loops during an acute reduction in preload. The dot in the lower-right corner designates end-diastole, while the area of each loop represents the stroke work for that beat. **B,** The slope of a line derived by plotting the area of each loop (stroke work) as a function of the end-diastolic volume, yielding preload-recruitable stroke work (PRSW). **C,** Variations in PRSW reflect conditions in which the chamber does more (increased contractility) or less (reduced contractility) stroke work for a given preload (end-diastolic volume).

end-diastolic point is relatively clear, application of PRSW to the RV is simpler and perhaps more precise than E_{es}.

VENTRICULAR-VASCULAR INTERACTION

With each beat, the heart expends a certain amount of energy for tension development to produce pressure and for myocyte shortening to produce flow. The balance between tension and shortening dictates performance and efficiency of the chamber as a pump and is influenced by both afterload and contractility. A number of methods have been described for characterizing ventricular-vascular interaction. By far the most common is ejection fraction, which provides general information about how well the heart can pump but not about how efficiently the heart is working. A relatively simple approach to this question is to examine the hydraulic work performed by the ventricle (the product of pressure and flow) over a range of loading conditions. At low afterload, hydraulic work is low because the pressure term is small; at high load, hydraulic work is low because the flow term is small. In between, if contractility is kept constant, there is a point where the pressure-flow product reaches a maximum and the afterload is said to be optimally matched with the contractility.[21] As noted previously, afterload is determined not only by steady-state resistance but also by pulsatile factors presented by the large elastic vessels. An extension of ventricular-vascular matching concepts based on the product of pressure and flow, therefore, considers pump performance in both nonpulsatile and pulsatile (oscillatory) terms. This conceptualization makes it possible to characterize how much power generated by the system (work per unit time) goes toward moving blood forward and how much is lost to pulsatility (i.e., goes toward distending the system).[26]

Power output (W) is calculated by multiplying instantaneous pressure and flow, with the area under the waveform for each cardiac cycle representing the total power (W_T) of that beat. These values are averaged over a series of beats. If the mean pressure and flow over the same sequence of beats are multiplied, steady-state power (W_{SS}) is derived. W_T represents the sum of W_{SS} and oscillatory power (W_{OS}—that which goes toward distending the system); thus, W_{OS} can be calculated by subtraction. Examining the distribution of W_T between steady-state and oscillatory components provides a convenient means for quickly assessing the nature of energy transfer from the ventricle to the circulation.

ANIMAL MODELS OF LUNG RESECTION

A large body of literature exists describing the response to lung surgery in animal models ranging from mice to nonhuman primates. Figure 19-4 depicts aspects of the hemodynamic response to left-side pneumonectomy in anesthetized, healthy swine. On the third day after surgery, modest increases in RV and PA pressures are evident along with a rise in both end-diastolic and end-systolic volumes within the RV. The changes in RV pressure and volume are manifest in a right-upward shift of the P/V relationship and a change in morphology of the P/V loop. As shown in Table 19-1, despite increases in RV and PA pressures and a fall in RV ejection fraction 3 days after pneumonectomy, cardiac output is maintained.

Effects on Afterload. Using basic pressure and blood flow data to calculate PVR (Table 19-1) indicates a modest increase (16%) in small-vessel load, whereas more in-depth analysis using input impedance spectra demonstrates a 50% rise in large-vessel load, as indexed by characteristic impedance. Close inspection of the timing for peak pressure development in both the RV and pulmonary artery provides a visual image of the impact of alterations in wave reflection produced by proximal vascular ligation. As shown in Figure 19-5, under controlled conditions, maximal RV pressure is attained early in systole; following pneumonectomy, it is attained late in systole.

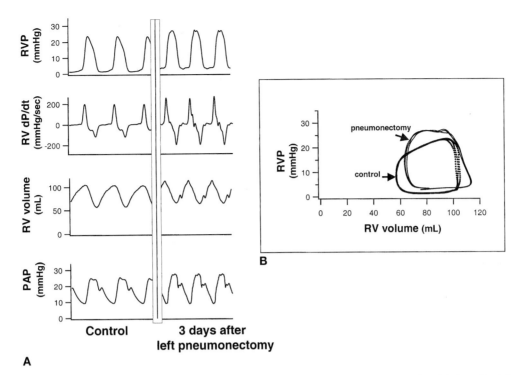

FIGURE 19-4 **A,** Representative tracings of hemodynamic variables obtained before (control) and 3 days after left pneumonectomy in domestic swine. **B,** Right ventricular (RV) pressure-volume loops obtained before (control) and three days after left-side pneumonectomy in domestic swine. A shift in location of the loop is evident, as is a change in morphology.

This phenomenon of "late-phase loading" has been observed in a variety of conditions associated with changes in the pulmonary vasculature and has been characterized as producing mechanically unfavorable loading of the still-ejecting chamber.[27] Although the example shown represents a relatively acute response, other investigators have reported maintenance of increased PVR and characteristic impedance years after left pneumonectomy in dogs, suggesting that facilitory adaptation within the pulmonary circulation does not occur to any great extent.[28]

Effects on Contractility and Ventricular-Vascular Coupling. As evident in Figure 19-4, after pneumonectomy RV dP/dt appears to increase slightly. Given the load-dependent nature of this contractile index, however, whether this response reflects an increase in inherent contractility or is a consequence of increased RV volume (preload) is uncertain. In contrast, as shown in Table 19-1, calculation of PRSW—a relatively load-independent index of contractility—indicates a modest (12%)

reduction. Calculating the ratio of oscillatory to total RV power (Table 19-1) indicates that after pneumonectomy, more of the hydraulic work done with each beat goes toward distending the system as opposed to providing forward flow. On the whole, these experimental observations underscore the potential complexity of clinically assessing the cardiac response to lung resection in the setting of limited access to multiple hemodynamic variables. Furthermore, they raise the importance of dissociating hemodynamic conditions at rest from those present during exercise or other stressors. Remarkably, experimental studies have demonstrated consistently that despite the doubling of blood flow to the remaining lung after pneumonectomy, there is actually minimal change in the slope of the PA pressure-flow relationship when cardiac output is increased by exercise or hypoxia.[29,30] These studies indicate that in experimental animals, the vascular reserve of the remaining lung is not exceeded by marked increases in cardiac output, and that

TABLE 19-1

Hemodynamic Variables in Experimental Animals with Prior Surgery (Control) or 3 Days After Left Pneumonectomy (PNM)

	CO (L/min)	RVEF (%)	mPAP (mmHg)	RVP Peak (mmHg)	Zc (dyn × s × cm⁻⁵)	PVR (dyn × s × cm⁻⁵)	PRSW work/ vol slope	Wos/WT (%)
Control (n = 3)	3.5 ± 0.2	49 ± 2	26 ± 2	16 ± 1	41 ± 4	254 ± 16	62 ± 0.2	30 ± 3
PNM (n = 4)	3.4 ± 0.3	41 ± 3	30 ± 2	18 ± 1	64 ± 6	295 ± 22	49 ± 0.3	40 ± 9

Control, No operation; *PNM,* left pneumonectomy; *CO,* cardiac output; *RVEF,* right ventricular ejection fraction; *RVP,* right ventricular pressure; *mPAP,* mean pulmonary artery pressure; *Zc,* characteristic input impedance, which reflects the contribution to afterload of large vessels; *PVR,* pulmonary vascular resistance; *PRSW,* preload-recruitable stroke work; W_{os}/WT, the ratio of oscillatory RV power to total power.

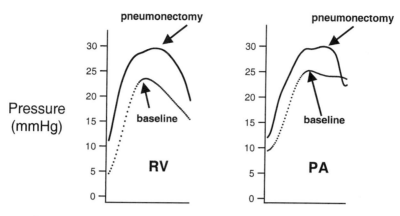

FIGURE 19-5 Comparison of the timing for peak pressure development within the right ventricle (RV) and pulmonary artery (PA) before (control) and three days after left pneumonectomy. Before lung removal, the highest RV and PA pressures occur early in systole. After pneumonectomy, the highest pressures occur late in systole, probably due to an alteration in the timing of wave reflection.

small increases in resting mean PA pressure and PVR after pneumonectomy are largely the passive result of diverting the entire cardiac output through one lung. Similar conclusions have not been universal within clinical studies, however.

Clinical Considerations

Given the inherent differences between healthy laboratory animals and patients with a spectrum of underlying cardiopulmonary disease and advanced age, it is not surprising that many clinical studies present a somewhat different picture of the cardiovascular response to lung resection. During the course of any intrathoracic procedure, there are a variety of physiologic stresses imposed which, while relatively insignificant in young healthy subjects, can have an acute influence—both individually and collectively—on cardiovascular function and challenge adaptive processes in patients with limited reserve.

ENTRANCE OF CHEST CAVITY

Simply opening the thorax stimulates primary (e.g., reflex) and secondary (e.g., elaboration of inflammatory mediators, pain and autonomic activity) events that can influence cardiovascular performance regardless of the magnitude of lung resected. These events probably influence ventilatory performance to an even greater extent because of chest wall disruption. Appreciation of this situation has helped foster the notion that minimally invasive lung resection might provide multiple levels of patient benefit, including improved postoperative cardiac performance. Although the data are limited and studies not well controlled, investigation has begun to suggest the potential for reduced atrial arrhythmia and enhanced RV mechanical function in high-risk elderly patients after video-assisted thoracoscopic surgery when compared with open thoracotomy.[3,31]

SINGLE-LUNG VENTILATION

During most thoracic surgical procedures, one lung is collapsed selectively to facilitate surgical exposure. Because of the acute changes in distending airway pressure, vascular reactive processes such as hypoxic vasoconstriction, and the mechanical consequences of physical atelectasis, cardiac loading conditions can change during single-lung ventilation. As shown in Figure 19-6, initiation of single-lung ventilation in healthy sub-

jects elicits a modest, progressive rise in pulmonary arterial pressure but little change in other hemodynamic variables. As shown in Figure 19-7, however, the imposition of single-lung ventilation in a patient with parenchymal lung disease and baseline pulmonary hypertension elicits a more pronounced rise in pulmonary arterial pressure, with concomitant change in central venous pressure but no reduction in systemic arterial pressure. In addition to the direct effects of lung collapse during single-lung ventilation, secondary physical and metabolic consequences can occur after reexpansion.[32,33]

LUNG MANIPULATION AND VASCULAR LIGATION

It is understood implicitly that even in limited lung resection, lung tissue must be grasped and retracted to facilitate access to the lesion as well as to vascular and bronchial structures. As shown in Figure 19-7, ligation of major branches of the pulmonary artery produces acute, sustained hemodynamic effects.

LYMPHATIC DISRUPTION AND PULMONARY CAPILLARY DYSFUNCTION

After thoracotomy and lung resection, approximately 5% of patients manifest radiographic and/or functional evidence of pulmonary edema—a phenomenon that is generally categorized as "postpneumonectomy pulmonary edema" regardless of whether an entire lung was removed.[34,35] Although this response was attributed initially to overhydration, more recent data have implicated a primary capillary injury resulting from processes, such as barotrauma, volutrauma, or reperfusion injury after single-lung ventilation.[32-34] Whatever the mechanism, the following three important features are evident:

1. First, the response is rarely acute; the vast majority of cases evolve over several days after surgery.
2. Second, there is a spectrum of severity ranging from largely asymptomatic diffuse pulmonary infiltrates to an acute lung injury picture (normal left heart filling pressures but a Pao_2/Fio_2 ratio less than 300) or fulminant ARDS (normal left heart filling pressures but a Pao_2/Fio_2 ratio less than 200).
3. Finally, and most important, there is the reported mortality rate—often due, at least in part, to heart failure—of 33% for acute lung injury and up to 100% for ARDS.[33-37]

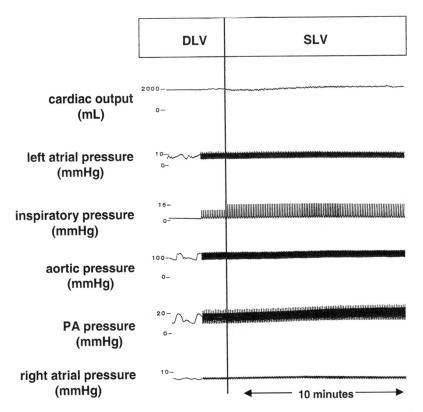

FIGURE 19-6 Representative tracings of hemodynamic variables and inspiratory pressure before and after initiation of single-lung ventilation in a normal subject. *PA,* Pulmonary artery; *DLV,* double-lung ventilation; *SLV,* single-lung ventilation.

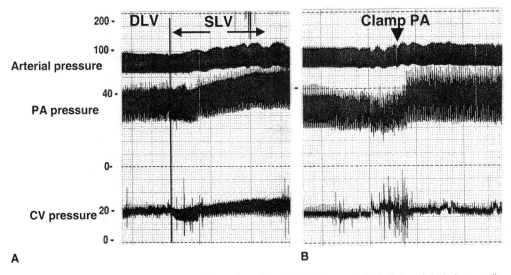

FIGURE 19-7 A, Representative tracings of hemodynamic variables before and after initiation of single-lung ventilation. **B,** Representative tracings before and after clamping the left pulmonary artery in a patient with preexisting pulmonary hypertension secondary to parenchymal lung disease. *DLV,* Double-lung ventilation; *SLV,* single-lung ventilation; *PA,* pulmonary artery; *CV,* central venous.

The Hemodynamic Response to Lung Resection

Multiple studies demonstrate that acute cardiovascular alterations after lung resection are largely (though not exclusively) influenced by the extent of resection and underlying disease. Interestingly, resting mean PA pressure and PVR tend to normalize after lung resection, although the magnitude of change is dependent on extent of resection (e.g., lobectomy vs pneumonectomy).[38,39] Despite relative normalization of PA pressure, however, RV ejection fraction continues to fall in the first few days after surgery, a trend that suggests that evolving reactive or adaptive processes influence this index of RV performance.[4,38,39] Other studies indicate that resting RV ejection fraction might then remain depressed indefinitely, despite the normal propensity for the heart to hypertrophy as compensation for increased load.[40] From a functional standpoint, however, resting hemodynamics alone do not provide a clear picture because they can be altered markedly by exercise. Furthermore, reported data must be interpreted in the context of how much lung was resected and how strenuous the exercise challenge was. For example, Okada et al examined hemodynamic variables—including thermodilution RV ejection fraction at rest and during submaximal exercise (sufficient to produce about 25% increase in heart rate)—before and 3 weeks after lobectomy or pneumonectomy.[39] With data from all patients combined, under resting conditions there were no significant preoperative vs. postoperative differences in heart rate, mean arterial pressure, pulmonary capillary wedge pressure, mean PA pressure, central venous pressure, RV volumes, or cardiac index. There were, however, modest reductions in both stroke volume index (48 ± 8 vs. 41 ± 8) and RV ejection fraction (43 ± 3 vs. 37 ± 6). As shown in Figure 19-8, during submaximal exercise both mean PA pressure and PVR rose to a much greater relative degree after lung resection than before. Despite these changes, however, there was not a marked difference in the RV ejection fraction response or that of stroke volume and cardiac output. Accordingly, unlike the preservation of PA pressure/flow slope evident after extensive lung resection in animal studies, this investigation indicates an increased slope following lung resection in humans. Nonetheless, the observation that the capacity to increase both stroke volume and cardiac output was preserved, if not enhanced, during submaximal exercise raises the question of whether the RV was truly dysfunctional despite the fall in RV ejection fraction. In contrast, another study examining more strenuous exercise in pneumonectomy patients up to 10 years after resection indicates that stroke volume eventually becomes fixed at some maximal value (i.e., it cannot rise with increasing work load) despite more than sufficient time for compensatory hypertrophy of the heart.[15] This study also highlighted two very important points. First, it clearly demonstrated that despite fixed ventilatory deficits and a ceiling on stroke volume and cardiac output, exercise training following pneumonectomy still improves VO₂max by enhancing peripheral oxygen extraction. Second, it reinforced the prospect that changes in cardiac performance after pneumonectomy (and possibly lesser resections) are not exclusively the result of altered RV afterload but could involve changes in left ventricular function as well.

In general, studies with PA catheterization or echocardiography have indicated preservation of left ventricular mechanical

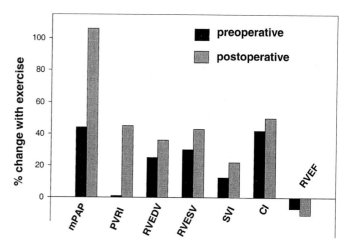

FIGURE 19-8 Hemodynamic response to submaximal exercise before and after lung resection. (From Okada M, Ota T, Okada M, et al: *J Thorac Cardiovasc Surg* 108:503, 1994.)

performance both at rest and during exercise after lung resection. One investigation with nuclear stethoscope technology, however, indicated reductions in stroke volume and left ventricular end-diastolic volume that could be explained by impaired RV function, but reductions in LV ejection fraction and ejection rate that could not.[41] Similar conclusions were reached in an animal study that assessed the hemodynamic response to exercise in dogs following pneumonectomy.[42] Although this study did not elucidate a specific mechanism, it raised the prospect of reorientation of the heart within the cardiac fossa, producing mechanical impairment of LV filling or ejection. A similar conclusion has been reached in clinical investigation based on the observation that pleuromediastinal adhesion and organized hemofibrothorax in combination with overexpansion of remaining lung might reduce compliance of the cardiac fossa and restrict the Starling mechanism on both sides of the heart.[15]

Lung Resection and Right Ventricular Pulmonary Vascular Coupling

Other studies support the prospect that more than just an acute increase in RV afterload influences cardiac performance after lung resection. Although mean PA pressure and PVR have been reported to be 20% to 27% lower in normal subjects than in pneumonectomy patients both at rest and during submaximal exercise, the highest PA pressure achieved in the pneumonectomy patients never exceeded that measured in healthy subjects at maximal exercise.[43,44] Furthermore, clinical studies have demonstrated the capacity of the heart to increase cardiac output continually up to a mean PA pressure of nearly 60 mmHg in healthy subjects exercising under hypoxic conditions.[45] In an effort to more closely characterize the relationship between postthoracotomy changes in RV afterload (characterized as PVR) and pump function in patients having lesser resections, Reed et al examined the influence of the relatively selective pulmonary vasodilator prostaglandin E₁ (PGE₁) on thermodilution-derived RV ejection fraction before and 48 hours after lobectomy.[38] Despite a modest decline in calculated PVR during PGE₁ under both conditions, these investigators were unable to demonstrate any augmentation of RV ejection fraction, regardless of whether lung had been removed. Nonetheless, RV ejection fraction was reduced by lung resection, suggesting that other factors such as depressed contractility contributed to the response. Accordingly, the authors of the study attempted to characterize contractility using an adaptation of the concept of preload-recruitable stroke work. Using rapid infusion of colloid to increase preload, these investigators found that although the starting point of the curve was different for lung resection patients (i.e., higher baseline end-diastolic volume), the slope of the relationship over a range of preload was the same. From these data, they concluded that changes in RV contractility also do not contribute to reduced RV ejection fraction after lung resection.

Although these conclusions need to be interpreted carefully because of a rather unorthodox application of the concept of preload-recruitable stroke work (which cannot exclude the influence of homeostatic reflexes), the suggestion of a dissociation between RV ejection fraction and both afterload and contractility after limited lung resection raises two major issues. The first issue relates to mechanism. Unlike the pneumonectomy patients in whom intrathoracic scarring was complete and a compensated state had been achieved, these subjects were studied in the immediate postoperative period, suggesting that reactive, nonphysical factors (e.g., limited compliance of the cardiac fossa) extrinsic to the individual myocyte—such as ventricular interaction or the synchrony of RV regional contraction—are influencing performance of the RV as a pump.[15] The second (and perhaps more fundamental) issue relates to the global significance of reduced RV ejection fraction, which will be discussed next.

Interpretation of Altered Right Ventricular Ejection Fraction Following Lung Resection

In the absence of concomitant parenchymal lung compromise, multiple studies conducted at rest have indicated RV dilation and significant reduction in RV ejection fraction but preserved stroke volume following major lung resection, findings that suggest adequate Frank-Starling compensation.[39,46] Indeed, one study demonstrated that a low perioperative RV ejection fraction, even in the presence of poor respirometric pulmonary function tests, is not generally predictive of perioperative morbidity.[40] When the RV, however, is challenged acutely by postoperative pulmonary embolism, pneumonia, acute lung injury, or frank ARDS, it will fail.[37] In the context of long-term outcome (e.g., 6 months or longer), exercise limitation has been conventionally regarded as a cardiac phenomenon, with dyspnea a manifestation of a fixed, maximal RV stoke volume. This concept is supported by increased long-term morbidity in patients with an RV ejection fraction less than 35% after pulmonary vascular ligation.[40] Recent data, however, demonstrate that in many postpneumonectomy patients, exercise limitation is actually respiratory, not cardiac, in origin—a finding that challenges application of the fixed stroke volume paradigm to all patients.[20] Assessment of RV pump function in the thoracic surgical population is often technically complex, and interpretation is subjective. For example, in two relatively large studies (*n* values of 39 and 22) using transthoracic echocardiography to assess RV function after pneumonectomy, both concluded that RV dilation occurred in the early postoperative

period, but only one study interpreted this response as indicative of significant RV dysfunction.[46,47] It is important that the two studies used different approaches to analyzing data; because of technical limitations with visualizing the RV proper (particularly in patients with obstructive lung disease), the study negative for RV dysfunction focused on regional wall motion, the velocity of any tricuspid regurgitation jet, and estimated peak RV pressure. In contrast, the positive study used a subtraction technique based on a hemiellipsoid model and the area-length method to calculate ejection fraction. Other investigations have used label imaging or fast-response thermodilution to measure RV ejection fraction directly. Thermodilution measurements in particular have been used widely in the perioperative setting and have the advantage of also supplying pressures within the right side of the heart because the technique requires placement of a pulmonary artery catheter. Unfortunately, the accuracy (and thus, the clinical utility) of these measurements might be diminished by tricuspid regurgitation, which is common in elderly patients (who constitute a large percentage of patients undergoing lung resection) and is exacerbated by acute increases in RV afterload.[48]

Right Ventricular Diastolic Function and Supraventricular Arrhythmias

Although pericardial restraint does not influence RV function under normal conditions, with the increased volumes that accompany increased afterload, the pericardium does become limiting, and diastolic compliance falls.[49] Consistent with this observation, echocardiographic assessment of biventricular diastolic function after lung resection has indicated a much greater impact on the RV than on the left-side ventricle.[50] Accordingly, the cardiac response to leg raising or loss of atrial contraction will be expected to be more pronounced after lung resection. The functional significance of these changes is heightened by the fact that supraventricular arrhythmias are the most common complication of thoracotomy, occurring in about 20% of patients.[51] Within this subset of patients, 64% exhibit atrial fibrillation (AF), 23% manifest supraventricular tachycardias, and 13% exhibit atrial flutter.[52] In general, the primary risk factors of supraventricular arrhythmias are over 70 years of age, extent of resection, and preexisting cardiac disease.[51,53,54] As with the progressive postoperative decline in RV ejection fraction, supraventricular arrhythmias generally do not develop for 48 to 72 hours, suggesting a reactive, inflammatory, or autonomic component that acts to initiate the arrhythmia (the arrhythmogenic stimulus), which is then facilitated or perpetuated by cellular or structural changes (the arrhythmogenic substrate) within the myocardium. Multiple lines of investigation suggest that atrial arrhythmogenesis in general can be linked to alterations in myocyte ion transients dictated by stretch-sensitive ion channels.[55-57] Thus a common perception is that distention of the right atrium resulting from impaired RV ejection is a primary stimulus for postpneumonectomy AF. Some clinical studies, however, have failed to find any association among RV distention, atrial size, and arrhythmia after pneumonectomy.[58] Analogous to ventricular tachycardia, AF is thought to be due to reentrant mechanisms, with the atria requiring areas of abnormal dispersion of refractoriness to initiate and maintain the reentrant circuit.[51] Accordingly, conditions that alter atrial effective refractory period (ERP) tend to be proarrhythmic. To date, the specific stimuli for initiating AF after lung resection are unknown, although factors such as sympathovagal imbalance, myocarditis, and pericarditis have been implicated along with myocyte stretch.[51,57] Alternatively, specific anatomic substrates, particularly atrial fibrosis, have been implicated consistently in the perpetuation of arrhythmia once initiated. Aging alone induces fibrosis and other degenerative changes in atrial anatomy that are accompanied by potentially proarrhythmic physiologic alterations, such as shorter ERP, longer sinoatrial and atrioventricular nodal conduction times, atrial stiffening, and splitting of the atrial excitation waveform by the pectinated trabeculae.[59,60]

Cardiopulmonary Structural Adaptation

Under most circumstances, the distortion of myocytes that accompanies increased pressure and volume within any heart chamber triggers a sequence of events (many of which are calcium-regulated) that eventually lead to adaptive hypertrophy of individual cells.[61] Whereas the major hypertrophic stimulus is probably physical stretch of the myocardium, this process also involves autonomic neurotransmitters and intracardiac paracrine/autocrine mediators. These individual factors coalesce to produce a cascade of immediate and, ultimately, prolonged molecular and cellular events that are mediated, in part, by altered expression of a variety of genes within both myocytes and noncontractile elements of the myocardium.[62] The clinical observation that most hemodynamically significant cardiac sequelae after lung resection occur after 48 to 72 hours raises the question of whether an evolving response to both the trauma of surgery and increased right heart volumes plays a part. Similarly, the acute increase in blood flow (and, possibly, in inspiratory volume) to the remaining lung are most likely sufficient to initiate a variety of secondary responses within the pulmonary parenchyma.

Cardiac Hypertrophy

Although the myocardial response to increased pressure or volume is generally linked to progressive alterations in myocyte size over weeks to months, multiple genes encoding for transcription factors and other proteins can be rapidly (within minutes to hours) influenced by acute changes in cardiac pressure and volume.[62,63] Remarkably, despite both experimental and clinical data demonstrating acute dilation of the right side of the heart after lung resection, there are limited data specifically examining either the time course or the magnitude of secondary molecular and structural myocardial remodeling. Studies in rats after right pneumonectomy have indicated the following three stages of RV reaction[64]:

1. Acute disturbances and initiation of secondary responses (0 to 10 days)
2. Steady hypertrophy of the RV (10 to 90 days)
3. A stage of decompensation (90 days and beyond)

Histologic analysis of the myocardium over this time frame revealed a progressive loss of cardiomyocytes and their nuclei. Other data from rats indicate up to a 72% increase in RV mass after right pneumonectomy.[65] Experimental studies in small dogs also have demonstrated hypertrophy (increases in both

length and width of myocytes) of the right atrium and RV that correlates with both the extent of lung resected and the postoperative period of observation and that is nonuniform within the heart—contributing, perhaps, to eventual decompensation.[66] In contrast, significant RV hypertrophy is not evident up to 70 days postresection after left pneumonectomy in sheep.[29]

How these experimental data relate to humans is unclear, particularly in light of the supervening influences of age and preexisting disease. Multiple lines of investigation indicate that when major lung resection is performed at a very young age, cardiopulmonary adaptation in general is more extensive and efficient.[67-69] For example, Murray et al studied the cardiovascular response to hypoxia in dogs 5 years after pneumonectomy performed at 6 to 10 weeks or 1 year of age.[67] They found that although both groups exhibited similar increases in PVR and pulmonary characteristic impedance while breathing a low F_{IO_2}, the RV response was clearly more hyperdynamic in animals undergoing pneumonectomy as puppies—a response attributed to an enhanced performance of the RV as a pump that was independent of afterload. Also evident within this study was the fact that although the animals undergoing surgery as adults failed to show as robust an RV response to hypoxia as those operated on as puppies, they did not mount a less dynamic response than nonoperated control animals and exhibited no sign of RV pump failure, despite a >60% rise in mean PA pressure.

At the opposite end of the age spectrum, senescence alters characteristics of myocardial systolic function and dampens the cardiac response to increased pressure-volume load. As a probable adaptation to generalized age-induced arterial stiffening, myocardial excitation-contraction coupling is lengthened, thus allowing individual cells to experience a prolongation of both the calcium-transient and force-bearing capacity.[70,71] This response, in turn, serves to enhance ventricular ejection into a stiff circulation. Age-related alterations in excitation-contraction coupling have been attributed largely to down-regulation of the gene encoding for the sarcoplasmic endoreticular calcium ATPase subtype 2a, which is responsible for calcium uptake into the sarcoplasmic reticulum from the cytosol.[70] Aging also dampens the chronotropic and inotropic responses to sympathetic stimulation, due to a decline in the ability of myocardial β-receptors to augment calcium influx through the L-type calcium channel.[70,71] Accordingly, the elderly heart maintains stroke volume during stress more by dilation ("in situ adaptation") than by marked increases in contractility. This observation could have particular importance in the post–lung resection RV, as aging alone produces chamber dilation in humans.[72] In the left-side ventricle, aging has been reported to diminish the hypertrophic response to exercise, both pressure and volume overload, and possibly to thyroid hormone stimulation.[73-76] Fundamental differences between the left and right ventricles, however, specifically in regard to embryology, structure, load, and growth with maturation, complicate direct extrapolation of data derived from one chamber to the other. For example, in both animals and humans, normal senescence produces an increase in mass of the LV but not of the RV.[70] Furthermore, the aging process produces greater cellular hypertrophy, fibrosis, myosin heavy-chain isoform shift, and prolongation in the duration of contraction in the LV than in the RV. To date, there are no reports of how myocardial hypertrophic remodeling secondary to increased RV pressure-volume load following lung resection is influenced by senescence. There are, however, data that clearly indicate age-related diminution of both cellular and biochemical indices of RV hypertrophy following pulmonary arterial banding.[77]

Not uncommonly, patients who require lung resection have underlying pulmonary parenchymal disease that already has elicited cardiac adaptation to chronic changes in cardiac loading. In particular, chronic obstructive pulmonary disease (COPD) can alter RV afterload by reducing the area of the pulmonary vascular bed, initiating regional hypoventilation with secondary hypoxic vasoconstriction, or simply compressing the vasculature by hyperinflation.[78] Alternatively, preload of both ventricles can be altered by lung hyperinflation and septal shift secondary to RV dilation. Compounding hemodynamic alterations is the possibility that the increased work of breathing associated with chronic lung disease (particularly restrictive disease) can lead to a "circulatory steal" phenomenon, whereby blood is diverted to the diaphragm and away from other skeletal muscles during exercise.[78] In most patients with COPD, resting PA pressures tend to be normal, and in those with elevated PA pressures, the increase is usually characterized as mild to moderate.[78,79] During exercise, however, PA pressures can rise rapidly, even in patients with normal pressures at rest, because of a combination of dynamic hyperinflation, regional hypoxic vasoconstriction, and structural changes in the pulmonary vascular bed. Although the maximal PA pressures attained do not usually exceed those observed in healthy subjects during strenuous exercise, they occur at much lower work rates and cardiac output, consistent with a prominent shift in the PA pressure-flow relationship. Accordingly, a level of preexisting (and perhaps even subclinical) COPD might contribute to the disparity between experimental and clinical observations regarding PA pressure-flow relationships after lung resection. Not surprisingly, RV ejection fraction has been reported to be reduced in patients with COPD and not to increase with exercise.[80] Nonetheless, COPD patients tend to exhibit a normal increase in cardiac output relative to VO_2max, probably due more to an augmented heart rate response than to increased stroke volume.[81] There are no available data describing how underlying lung disease specifically influences cardiac adaptation to lung resection. In a study of 20 patients with modest preexisting COPD and low-normal RV ejection fraction who underwent lung resection, however, Lewis et al could not demonstrate any correlation between perioperative PA pressure or PVR and RV ejection fraction, nor any value of RV ejection fraction in predicting short-term morbidity.[40] These investigators did demonstrate, however, that if RV ejection fraction declined to <35%, or if the RV ejection fraction/PVR ratio rose to >5 after ligation of the PA supply to the resected area, this response was predictive for long-term (>6 months) morbidity. Although not conclusive, this study suggests that although these patients had sufficient cardiac reserve to tolerate the acute insult of lung resection, a diminished capacity for long-term adaptation influenced eventual outcome.

Compensatory Lung Growth

It has long been known that following removal of lung tissue, the remaining lung expands. Functionality of this expanded lung, however, is not necessarily proportional to the increase in size. As with cardiac compensation, the magnitude of pulmonary adaptation appears to depend upon the extent of lung resected, age, and underlying disease. Furthermore, experimental data are influenced by species variation, with mice and rats in particular exhibiting a marked compensatory growth of remaining lung. In larger animals and human beings, adaptation to altered gas exchange has been characterized as occurring at three different levels[82]:

1. Recruitment of diffusing capacity reserves in remaining lung
2. Enlargement of remaining alveolar airspaces and thinning of the alveolar tissue barrier
3. Compensatory lung growth

In immature animals, pneumonectomy stimulates alveolar regeneration of sufficient magnitude to return lung volume, diffusing capacity, and extravascular septal tissue volume to normal.[82,83] Aspects of lung mechanical function remain abnormal, however, and regeneration of extraalveolar airways and blood vessels is limited. Similar responses appear to occur in human beings.[84] In mature animals, compensatory growth appears to occur only after removal of the left lung.[85] This finding suggests a threshold of resection below which the existing lung can adapt through physiologic recruitment and structural remodeling. Nonetheless, unlike immature animals, mature ones maintain long-term cardiopulmonary deficits regardless of which lung was removed.[82]

A variety of stimuli have been proposed to account for adaptive changes in the lung. Recent data examining the impact of mediastinal shift upon remaining lung after pneumonectomy have concluded that, although mechanical strain is a major stimulus for regenerative lung growth, other signals account for a significant amount of the compensatory response.[86-88] Also implicated has been the increased blood flow to remaining lung, as augmentation of shear forces within vessels elicits a variety of responses from vascular endothelial cells, with potential downstream effects.[89,90] Interestingly, unlike the marked pulmonary vascular remodeling that accompanies increased pulmonary blood flow from left-to-right shunts, pneumonectomy elicits only modest changes.[29]

REFERENCES

1. Reed CE: Physiologic consequences of pneumonectomy, *Chest Surg Clin NA* 9:449, 1999.
2. Tanita T, Hoshikawa Y, Tabata T, et al: Functional evaluations for pulmonary resection for lung cancer in octogenarians. Investigation from postoperative complications, *Jpn J Thorac Cardiovasc Surg* 47:253, 1999.
3. Mikami I, Koizumi K, Tanaka S: Changes in right ventricular performance in elderly patients who underwent lobectomy using video-assisted thoracic surgery for primary lung cancer, *Jpn J Thorac Cardiovasc Surg* 49:153, 2001.
4. Okada M, Okada M, Ishii, et al: Right ventricular ejection fraction in the perioperative risk evaluation of candidates for pulmonary resection, *J Thorac Cardiovasc Surg* 112:364, 1996.
5. Ommen SR, Odell JA: Atrial arrhythmias after cardiothoracic surgery, *N Engl J Med* 336:1429, 1997.
6. Amar D, Roistacher N, Burt M, et al: Effects of diltiazem versus digoxin on dysrhythmias and cardiac function after pneumonectomy, *Ann Thorac Surg* 63:1374, 1997.
7. Hsia CC: Coordinated adaptation of oxygen transport in cardiopulmonary disease, *Circulation* 104:963, 2001.

8. Miyoshi S, Yoshimasu T, Hirai T, et al: Exercise capacity of thoracotomy patients in the early postoperative period, *Chest* 118:384, 2000.

9. Nezu K, Kushibe K, Tojo T, et al: Recovery and limitation of exercise capacity after lung resection for lung cancer, *Chest* 113:1511, 1998.

10. Miyazawa M, Haniuda M, Nishimura H, et al: Long term effects of pulmonary resection on cardiopulmonary function, *J Am Coll Surg* 189(1):26, 1999.

11. Corris PA, Ellis DA, Hawkins T, et al: Use of radionuclide scanning in the preoperative estimation of pulmonary function after pneumonectomy, *Thorax* 42:285, 1987.

12. Bolliger CT, Jordan P, Soler M, et al: Pulmonary function and exercise capacity after lung resection, *Respir J* 9:415, 1996.

13. Pelletier C, Lapointe L, LeBlanc P: Effects of lung resection on pulmonary function and exercise capacity, *Thorax* 45:497, 1996.

14. DeGraff, AC Jr, Taylor HF, Ord JW, et al: Exercise limitation following extensive pulmonary resection, *J Clin Invest* 44:1514, 1965.

15. Hijazi OM, Ramanathan M, Estrera AS, et al: Fixed maximal stroke index in patients after pneumonectomy, *Am J Respir Crit Care Med* 15:1623, 1998.

16. Birath G, Malmberg R, Simonsson BG: Lung function after pneumonectomy in man, *Clin Sci* 29:59, 1965.

17. Johnson RL, Taylor HF, DeGraff AC: Functional significance of a low pulmonary diffusing capacity for carbon monoxide, *J Clin Invest* 44: 789, 1965.

18. Mossberg B, Bjork O, Holmgren A: Working capacity and cardiopulmonary function after extensive lung resections, *Scand J Thorac Cardiovasc Surg* 10:247, 1976.

19. Hsia CC, Ramanathan M, Estrera AS: Recruitment of diffusing capacity with exercise in patients after pneumonectomy, *Am Rev Respir Dis* 145:811, 1992.

20. Nugent AM, Steele IC, Carragher AM, et al: Effect of thoracotomy and lung resection on exercise capacity in patients with lung cancer, *Thorax* 54:334, 1999.

21. Elzinga G, Piene H, DeJong JP: Left and right ventricular pump function and consequences of having two pumps in one heart: a study on the isolated cat heart, *Circ Res* 46:564, 1980.

22. Piene H: Matching betrween right ventricle and pulmonary bed. In Yin FCP (ed): *Ventricular/vascular coupling*, p180, New York, 1987, Springer Verlag.

23. Sagawa K, Maughan L, Suga H, et al: *Cardiac contraction and the pressure volume relationship*, New York, 1988, Oxford University Press.

24. Heerdt PM, Dickstein ML: Assessment of right ventricular function, *Sem Cardiothorac Vasc Anesth* 1:215, 1997.

25. Matsuwaka R, Matsuda H, Nakano S, et al: A new method of assessing left ventricular function under assisted circulation using a conductance catheter, *ASAIO Trans* 35:449, 1989.

26. Heerdt PM, Dickstein ML, Gandhi CD: Disparity of isoflurane effects on left and right ventricular afterload and hydraulic power generation in swine, *Anesth Analg* 87:511, 1998.

27. Ha B, Lucas CL, Henry GW, et al: Effects of chronically elevated pulmonary arterial pressure and flow on right ventricular afterload, *Am J Physiol* 267:H155, 1994.

28. Lucas CL, Murray GF, Wilcox BR, et al: Effects of pneumonectomy on pulmonary input impedance, *Surgery* 94:807, 1983.

29. Smith M, Coates G, Kay JM, et al: The response of the pulmonary circulation to exercise during normoxia and hypoxia following pneumonecotmy in the adult sheep, *Can J Physiol Pharmacol* 67:202, 1989.

30. Hsia CC, Carlin JI, Cassidy SS, et al: Hemodynamic changes after pneumonectomy in the exercising foxhound, *J Appl Physiol* 69:51, 1990.

31. Neustin SM, Kahn P, Krellenstein DJ, et al: Incidence of arrhythmias after thoracic surgery: Thoracotomy versus video-assisted thoracoscopy, *J Cardiothorac Vasc Anesth* 12:659, 1998.

32. Jordan S, Mitchell JA, Quinlan GJ, et al: The pathogenesis of lung injury following pulmonary resection, *Eur Respir J* 15:790, 2000.

33. Lases EC, Duurkens VA, Gerritsen WB, et al: Oxidative stress after lung resection therapy, *Chest* 117:999, 2000.

34. Zeldin RA, Normandin D, Landtwing D, et al: Postpneumonectomy pulmonary edema, *J Thorac Cardiovasc Surg* 87:359, 1984.

35. Waller DA, Gebitekin C, Saunders NR, et al: Noncardiogenic pulmonary edema complicating lung resection, *Ann Thorac Surg* 55:140, 1993.

36. Kutlu CA, Williams EA, Evans TW, et al: Acute lung injury and acute respiratory distress syndrome after pulmonary resection, *Ann Thorac Surg* 69:376, 1999.

37. Mathisen DJ, Kuo EY, Hahn C, et al: Inhaled nitric oxide for adult respiratory distress syndrome after pulmonary resection, *Ann Thorac Surg* 66:1894, 1998.

38. Reed CE, Dorman BH, Spinale FG: Mechanisms of right ventricular dysfunction after pulmonary resection, *Ann Thorac Surg* 62:225, 1996.

39. Okada M, Ota T, Okada M, et al: Right ventricular dysfunction after major pulmonary resection, *J Thorac Cardiovasc Surg* 108:503, 1994.

40. Lewis JW Jr, Bastanfar M, Gabriel F, et al: Right heart function and prediction of respiratory morbidity in patients undergoing pneumonectomy with moderately severe cardiopulmonary dysfunction, *J Thorac Cardiovasc Surg* 108:169, 1994.

41. Fujisaki T, Gomibuchi M, Shoji T: Changes in left ventricular function during exercise after lung resection—study with a nuclear stethoscope, *Nippon Kyobu Geka Gakkai Zasshi* 40:1685,1992.

42. Hsia CCW, Carlin JI, Cassidy SS, et al: Hemodynamic changes after pneumonectomy in the exercising foxhound, *J Appl Physiol* 69:51, 1990.

43. Staňek VJ, Widimsky J, Hurych J, et al: Pressure, flow and volume changes during exercise within pulmonary vascular bed in patients after pneumonectomy, *Clin Sci* 37:11, 1969.

44. Johnson RL Jr, Hsia CCW, Cassidy SS, et al: A post-pneumonectomy comparison of cardiac output and gas exchange in humans and dogs during heavy exercise. In Sutton JR, Coates G, Remmers JE (eds): *Hypoxia: the adaptations*, Toronto, 1990, BC Decker.

45. Groves BM, Reeves JT, Sutton JR, et al: Operation Everest: II. elevated high-altitude pulmonary resistance unresponsive to oxygen,; *J Appl Physiol* 63:521, 1984.

46. Amar D, Burt ME, Roistacher N, et al: Value of perioperative Doppler echocardiography in patients undergoing major lung resection, *Ann Thorac Surg* 61:516, 1996.

47. Kowalewski J, Brocki M, Dryjanski T, et al: Right ventricular morphology and function after pulmonary resection, *Eur J Cardiothorac Surg* 15:444, 1999.

48. Heerdt PM, Blessios GA, Beach ML, et al: Flow dependency of error in thermodilution measurement of cardiac output during acute tricuspid regurgitation, *J Cardiothorac Vasc Anesth* 15:183, 2001.

49. Burger W, Straube M, Behne M, et al: Role of pericardial constraint for right ventricular function in humans, *Chest* 107:46, 1995.

50. Takaki A, Sugi K, Sano T, et al: Different responses of right and left ventricular diastolic function to pulmonary resection: echocardiographic study with leg elevation for preload augmentation, *J Cardiol* 36:241, 2000.

51. Ommen SR, Odell JA: Atrial arrhythmias after cardiothoracic surgery, *N Engl J Med* 336:1429, 1997.

52. Krowka MJ, Pairolero PC, Trastek VF, et al: Cardiac dysrhythmia following pneumonectomy. Clinical correlates and prognostic significance, *Chest* 91:490, 1987.

53. Amar D, Zhang HY, Leung DH, et al: Older age is the strongest predictor of postoperative atrial fibrillation 96:352, 2002.

54. Cardinale D, Martinoni A, Cipolla CM, et al: Atrial fibrillation after operation for lung cancer: clinical and prognostic significance, *Ann Thorac Surg* 68:1827, 1999.

55. Yue L, Feng J, Gaspo R, et al: Ionic remodeling underlying action potential changes in a canine model of atrial fibrillation, *Circ Res* 81:512, 1997.

56. Bode F, Katchman A, Woosley RL, et al: Gadolinium decreases stretch-induced vulnerability to atrial fibrillation, *Circulation* 101:2200, 2000.

57. Van Wagoner DR, Nerbonne JM: Molecular basis of electrical remodeling in atrial fibrillation, *J Mol Cell Cardiol* 32:1101, 2000.

58. Amar D, Roistacher N, Burt M, et al: Clinical and echocardiographic correlates of symptomatic tachydysrhythmias after non-cardiac thoracic surgery, *Chest* 108:349, 1995.

59. Spach MS, Dolber PC: Relating extracellular potentials and their derivatives to anisotropic propagation at a microscopic level in human cardiac muscle. Evidence for electrical uncoupling of side-to-side fiber connections with increasing age, *Circ Res* 58:356, 1986.

60. Wei JY: Age and the cardiovascular system, *N Engl J Med* 327:1735, 1992.

61. Calaghan SC, White E: The role of calcium in the response of cardiac muscle to stretch, *Prog Biophys Molec Biol* 71:59, 1999.

62. Swynghedauw B: Molecular mechanisms of myocardial remodeling, *Pharmacol Rev* 79:215, 1999.

63. Ogino K, Cai B, Gu A, et al: Factors contributing to pressure overload-induced immediate early gene expression in adult rat hearts in vivo, *Am J Physiol* 277:H380, 1999.

64. Bilich GL, Kiselev AA, Puzikov AO: Myocardial reaction of the right ventricle to lung resection, *Arkh Anat Gistol Embriol* 94:46, 1988.

65. Gnatiuk MS: Structural-functional changes in the myocardium of rats following pneumonectomy, *Patol Fiziol Eksp Ter* 4:39, 1991.

66. Gnatiuk MS: Morphometric research on the cardiomyocytes in cardiac hyperfunction, *Tsiologiia* 33:51, 1991.

67. Murray GF et al: Cardiopulmonary hypoxic response 5 years postpneumonectomy in beagles, *J Surg Res* 41:236, 1986.

68. Cagle PT, Thurlbeck WM: Postpneumonectomy compensatory lung growth, *Am Rev Respir Dis* 138:1314, 1988.

69. Cagle PT, Langston C, Thurlbeck WM: The effect of age on postpneumonectomy growth in rabbits, *Pediatr Pulmonol* 5:92, 1988.

70. Lakatta EG: Myocardial adaptations inn advanced age, *Basic Res Cardiol* 88(suppl 2):125, 1993.

71. Patel MB, Sonnenblick EH: Age associated alterations in structure and function of the cardiovascular system, *Am J Geriatr Cardiol* 7:15, 1998.

72. Boldt J, Zickmann B, Thiel A, et al: Age and right ventricular function during cardiac surgery, *J Cardiothorac Vasc Anesth* 6:29, 1992.

73. McCafferty WB, Edington DW: Skeletal muscle and organ weights of aged and trained male rats, *Gerontologia* 20:44, 1974.

74. Isoyama S, Wei JY, Izumo S, et al: Effect of age on the development of cardiac hypertrophy produced by aortic constriction in the rat, *Circ Res* 61:337, 1987.

75. Isoyama S, Grossman W, Wei JY: Effect of age on myocardial adaptation to volume overload in the rat, *J Clin Invest* 81:1850, 1988.

76. Florini JR, Saito Y, Manowitz EJ: Effect of age on thyroxine-induced cardiac hypertrophy in mice, *J Gerontol* 28:293, 1973.

77. Kuroha M, Isoyama S, Ito N, et al: Effects of age on right ventricular hypertrophic response to pressure-overload in rats, *J Mol Cell Cardiol* 23:1177, 1991.

78. Sietsma K: Cardiovascular limitations in chronic pulmonary disease, *Med Sci Sport Exerc* 33:S656, 2001.

79. Oswald-Mammosser M, Apprill M, Bachez P, et al: Pulmonary hemodynamics in chronic obstructive pulmonary disease of the emphysematous type, *Respiration* 58:304, 1991.

80. Matthay RA, Arroliga AC, Wiedemann HP, et al: Right ventricular function at rest and during exercise in chronic obstructive pulmonary disease, 101(5 Suppl):255S, 1992.

81. Light RW, Mintz HM, Linden GS, et al: Hemodynamics of patients with severe chronic obstructive pulmonary disease during progressive upright exercise, *Am Rev Respir Dis* 130:391, 1984.

82. Takeda SI, Ramanathan M, Estrera AS, et al: Postpneumonectomy alveolar growth does not normalize hemodynamic and mechanical function, *J Appl Physiol* 87:491, 1999.

83. Takeda S, Hsia CC, Wagner E, et al: Compensatory alveolar growth normalizes gas-exchange function in immature dogs after pneumonectomy, *J Appl Physiol* 86:1301, 1999.

84. Laros CD, Westermann CJ: Dilatation, compensatory growth, or both after pneumonectomy during childhood and adolescence. A thirty-year follow-up study, *J Thorac Cardiovasc Surg* 93:570, 1987.

85. Hsia CC, Herazo LF, Fryder-Doffey F, et al: Compensatory lung growth occurs in adult dogs after right pneumonectomy, *J Clin Invest* 94:405, 1994.

86. Hsia CC, Wu EY, Wagner E, et al: Preventing mediastinal shift after pneumonectomy impairs regenerative alveolar tissue growth, *Am J Physiol Lung Cell Mol Physiol* 281:L1279, 2001.

87. Landesberg LJ, Ramalingam R, Lee K, et al: Upregulation of transcription factors in lung in the early phase of postpneumonectomy lung growth, *Am J Physiol Lung Cell Mol Physiol* 281:L1138, 2001.

88. Dubaybo BA, Bayasi G, Rubeiz GJ: Changes in tumor necrosis factor in postpneumonectomy lung growth, *J Thorac Cardiovasc Surg* 110:396, 1995.

89. Leuwerke SM, Kaza AK, Tribble CG, et al: Inhibition of compensatory lung growth in endothelial nitric oxide synthase-deficient mice, *Am J Physiol Lung Cell Mol Physiol* 282:L1272, 2002.

90. McBride JT, Kirchner KK, Russ G, et al: Role of pulmonary blood flow in postpneumonectomy lung growth, *J Appl Physiol* 73:2448, 1992.

Pain Management

I.D. Conacher, MB, ChB, MRCP, FFARCS
Peter D. Slinger, MD, FRCPC

A MODERN philosophy of pain management for trauma and surgery must provide more than mere humanitarian succor to the distressed patient. A system for relieving pain not only must prove its positive influence on the processes of recovery but also should be measurable both in terms of patient satisfaction, and, scientifically, in terms of improved function and progressive effects on healing. Pain management must be prophylactic, integral to surgery, and proactive rather than reactive.

Lung volume reduction surgery is a good modern example of a procedure to which these principles apply.[1] Effective pain relief, along with a determination to return the patient to self-ventilation as early as possible, is vital to the success of lung volume reduction surgery and dictates the course of perioperative management. There has been a trend toward lower morbidity and mortality rates in thoracic surgery that has paralleled the development of postoperative analgesic techniques (Table 20-1).[2-5] Much of this improvement in outcomes seems to be related to better pain relief.

The modern patient is "empowered," armed with knowledge gathered from the Internet and with insights from consumer and patient organizations. They have the right to receive information about options and the balance of risk of analgesic techniques; to give informed consent; and to opt out of treatment if therapy is not meeting their expectations or if its complications are deemed worse than the discomfort. These realities show the shortcomings of much traditional teaching on thoracic analgesia. Some techniques are not patient friendly; some can be discarded as not effective; some have unacceptable rates of adverse effects; and still others do not stand up to evidence-based analysis. Cryotherapy, transcutaneous nerve stimulation, and acupuncture are gross examples; sublingual analgesia, intramuscular injection, subcutaneous catheters, single intercostal nerve injection, bolusing techniques, interpleural injec-

tion, and lumbar epidurals can be indicated on occasion but require further qualification.[6-12]

Some of the contemporary themes in pain management for thoracic analgesia have been examined from a perspective of dynamics that influence modern health care delivery systems. Essentially, these are driven by an impetus to ration personnel, time, or (principally) cost.[13] These resources are often beyond the control of anesthesiologists and are typically dictated by such circumstances as bed availability in an intensive care or high-dependency unit or by the number of patients on an operating schedule—not by the concerns of managing an anesthetized patient, nor by the more common and traditional limits of responsibility to an individual in pain who has undergone major surgery or had multiple trauma.

Delivery systems are controlled and exercised by acute pain services. So fundamental is the pain service to the patient/therapist interface that this chapter has been developed specifically with them in mind, with the presumption that they provide the nursing standing orders, local protocols, and institutional guidelines. The core goal is to provide continuity in prolonged and sequential care, gradually reducing services as recovery proceeds.

The pain-relief techniques that best meet the bulk of requirements within the paradigms of activities of an acute pain service and its duties of care, are those deliverable by catheter. In this setting, the thoracic anesthesiologist becomes special, not only by virtue of expertise in placement but also in dictating the agents and regimens to be deployed. These agents and regimens need to be open for scrutiny by patients, pain services, and anesthesiologists in terms of efficacy, safety, patient tolerance, robustness, and cost.

Many ancillary issues, such as the use of moderate and mild analgesics as coanalgesia, enteral and rectal access, the deployment of antiemetics, and so forth, are not specific to thoracic practice and so will not be discussed at length in this chapter.

Frameworks for Thoracic Nociception and Treatment

Ethical Framework

In an era when a patient's experience of surgery was largely unmodified by analgesia considerations, the thoracotomy was recognizably a severe ordeal. It has since been forgotten that there was evidence of a curious paradox: after major surgery (including thoracotomy), 25% of patients did not appear to

---

TABLE 20-1

Recent Trends in Perioperative Mortality After Lung Cancer Surgery

Authors	Year	Patients	Mortality (%)	Analgesic Technique
Nakahara[3]	1988	All risks	6.4	IV/IM
Licker[5]	1993	All risks	4.8	IV/IM/LEA
Cerfolio[4]	1996	High-risk	2.4	LEA/TEA
Licker[5]	1997	All risks	2.1	TEA

IV, Intravenous; *IM*, intramuscular; *LEA*, lumbar epidural analgesia; *TEA*, thoracic epidural analgesia

require or demand analgesia.[14] The reasons for this phenomenon included sex, national, cultural, psychologic, and genetic factors. It would be unethical to base any study on a presumption that analgesia is unnecessary, but this 25% factor should be borne in mind when making assessments about evidence of analgesic efficacy. The current ethical framework, which leads to the moral impetus to treat, presumes that posterolateral thoracotomy is a highly painful condition, superceded in the magnitude of painfulness only by the thoracoabdominal incisions used for the surgical approach to, for instance, the lower third of the esophagus.[15]

Surgery via sternotomy, lateral thoracotomy, and thoracoscopic ports is regarded as less traumatic, and therefore less painful, than posterolateral thoracotomy. In those clinical situations in which obtaining good-quality analgesia is the critical determinant of survival, it makes sense ethically to advocate the least painful route of access commensurate with ease of surgery. For example, open lung volume reduction surgery, if bilateral, is best conducted via a sternotomy. Those patients having an ASA status of 3 or more, who are likely to be further downgraded by surgery to critical levels of pulmonary function, are safer undergoing minimal thoracoscopic access than open procedures.

Use of small incisions, with their consequent reduction in trauma to soft tissue and muscle, less intercostal space retraction, and less use of rib resection, has led to a perception that there must be a quantitative reduction in generated chest wall nociception. Modern patient expectations of being free of any pain might have masked this perception so that it is not quantifiable. Equally, the shift toward videoscopically assisted minimal-access techniques appears not to have genuinely lessened the amount of nociception perceived in adults, though it might have done so in children.[13,16]

Theoretically, with less nociception arising from chest wall and segmental trauma (e.g., incisional pain), outcome measures such as pain analog scores should be registering less pain overall. In practice, this assumption is not borne out. It is a moot point whether this outcome is due to patients' cultural concepts of painfulness, poor-quality analgesia, or the prominence and dominance of other algesics from pleural irritation (visceral or inflammatory nociception, i.e., nonincisional pain), recently referred to as the phenomenon of *disaggregation*.[13]

Anatomic Framework

Chest wall nociception, whether generated by surgery or trauma, is conducted via the intercostal nerves. Incision starts the process; traumatized tissue, such as skin, soft tissue, and muscle, releases a host of algesic substances that includes hydrogen ions, potassium, acetylcholine, serotonin, bradykinin, and prostaglandins.[17] Rib and intercostal space retraction increases the nocigenic output by damaging costotransverse and costovertebral ligaments. The final anatomic area of significance to intercostal nerve hegemony is the parietal pleura.

Intercostal nerves can be targeted individually or in multiples in the paravertebral or epidural spaces. The advantage of the multiple and central analgesic techniques is that the posterior ramus of the intercostal nerve is also blocked. As this is the route taken by nociception from the posterior intercostal space and

ligaments, it is important that it is blocked in thoracotomy incisions, and it is less of a necessity at sites from thoracoscopy.

The mediastinal pleura and diaphragmatic pleura are other recognized sources of nociogenic factors. The conduits are the vagus nerve and the phrenic nerve, respectively. The usual picture of nociception from these areas—that of nonincisional pain—is of deep-seated, ill-defined, nonlocalizable discomfort, with the addition of the classic pain referred to the shoulder because of diaphragmatic irritation. Chest or pleural drains produce both incisional and nonincisional pain profiles.

A slightly different pain profile, which is reported after operations such as thoracoscopic sympathectomy, suggests that another of the "hard-wired" routes for nociceptive traffic might be the autonomic nervous system (ANS), or that somehow the ANS modulates the transmission of nociceptive traffic. This thinking is in keeping with modern pain theory.[18-20] An understanding of the multiple afferent pathways involved in the etiology of postthoracotomy pain (Table 20-2) leads to an appreciation of why no single analgesic technique can be completely satisfactory and why postthoracotomy analgesia needs to be multimodal (Table 20-3).

Therapeutic Framework

Broadly, two strategies of pain management have evolved, and a mixture of both is often used. The first strategy—the calculated targeting and decreasing afferent transmission by the "hard-wired" routes with local anesthetics—has a long tradition. The second strategy is a multimodal, triple component, balanced strategy of local anesthetics to deal with hard wiring, opioids for nonincisional pain, and nonsteroidal antiinflammatory drugs (NSAIDs) to deal with a "noxious soup" of algesics.

TABLE 20-2
Postthoracotomy Pain Pathways

Pain Source	Afferent Conduction
Incision	Intercostal nerves (4-6)
Chest drains	Intercostal nerves (5-8)
Mediastinal pleura	Vagus nerve
Central diaphragmatic pleura	Phrenic nerve
Ipsilateral shoulder	Phrenic nerve +/− brachial plexus

TABLE 20-3
Multimodal Postthoracotomy Analgesia

Anesthesia Type	Method of Administration
Regional anesthesia	Infiltration, intercostal, intrapleural, extrapleural, paravertebral, epidural
Opioids	Oral, transdermal, subcutaneous, intramuscular, intravenous, epidural, spinal
Nonsteroidal antiinflammatory drugs (NSAIDs)	Oral, rectal, intravenous
Other drugs/modalities	Ketamine, α_2-agonists, GABA-agonists, Transcutaneous electrical nerve stimulation (TENS), cryoanalgesia

Execution of this strategy builds up an analgesic "firewall" in which the gaps can be plugged with simple analgesics. Largely based on an unsophisticated philosophy of interfering as much as possible with the normal biophysiologic responses to pain, it has much appeal for its indiscriminate, "catch-all" approach.

The indiscriminate effects of local anesthetics on nerves that have important efferent and motor functions have comprised the principal disadvantage of the first strategy.[21,22] In the case of the second strategy, adverse effects of pharmacology eclipse technical and technique-related complications.

With a patient population at risk for having adverse effects because of age, comorbidity, and vulnerability to complications, a combination or mixture of the best of both strategies is usually sought. The use of low-dose local anesthetics is sufficient in many cases to prevent motor blocks and sympatholytic effects. The addition of neuraxial opioids prevents many of the nondiscriminatory effects of systemic opioids and tachyphylaxis to the local anesthetics.[23] Synergistic combinations are often more than enough to negate a requirement for complementary analgesic drugs (such as NSAIDs) that have the potential to cause gastrointestinal irritation, bleeding, and renal dysfunction.[24]

Framework for Analgesia Administration

The connection between the patient and the therapy in the early phases after thoracic trauma and surgery is a parenteral catheter. Catheters facilitate bolusing, continuous infusion, and interfacing with automatic and patient-controlled devices. Prolonged efficacy can be achieved with short-acting, pharmacologically specific agents that are rapid in effect, easily adjusted, customized, and inherently safer than long-acting agents.

Intravenous cannulae attached to a delivery system that the patient can access are the simplest and most universal devices for pain management. Although much of any discussion of intravenous routes and patient-controlled analgesia (PCA) systems is common to all trauma and surgical disciplines, it is important for the specialist to have a working knowledge of these because an intravenous regimen potentially will be deployed by default, as a result of informed patient choice, or after any failure of the more complex or specific techniques.[25,26]

Catheter techniques require either direct placement or percutaneous insertion, in which case a variant or adaptation of the catheter-through-the-needle techniques, which commonly are used to secure access to the epidural space, is practiced. The epidural catheter is regarded as the gold standard of pain management. But, in context and for the more minor intrathoracic procedures, there are cogent arguments for considering catheters in the thoracic paravertebral space, in the subarachnoid space, or between the layers of the pleura (including attachment to the diaphragm).

For the "low-tech," low-maintenance, and low-cost schools of thought and practice, there is a limited place for single injections of long-acting analgesics. These have had a significant but limited history within the field.[27,28] The potential of new, long-acting local anesthetics being developed—and possibly biologically packaged—is appealing. Intrathecal morphine, one of the hydrophilic opioids, is first-line therapy for many units and reportedly can be effective for more than 24 hours.

However, these analgesics must be viewed with circumspection. Placement must be close to the neuraxis in the case of local anesthetics, or within the neuraxis in the case of opioids. Total spinal anesthesia of very prolonged duration, or late-onset respiratory depression, are potentially life-threatening consequences.[29]

Pathophysiologic Consequences of Thoracic Pain

The normal pattern of respiration is active inspiration followed by passive expiration. This can be geared up—increasing inspiratory action and force and activating expiration—to generate force for coughing that clears the airway of sputum and the post-traumatic detritus of blood and secretions.

A negative process begins with anesthesia. Various loads are imposed in succession. Supranormal ventilator pressures to protect functional residual capacity, high inspired oxygen concentrations, alternate collapse and reinflation of lungs, and consequences to pulmonary vasculature and right ventricular function, are all enough in their own rights to activate inflammatory cascades.[30] These, added to the effects of surgery (including lung handling and resection), summate to produce lungs stiffened with retained water (usually interstitial but also intraalveolar). To this mix are added the pain and trauma of incision and muscle disruption. In consequence, reflex muscle spasm of the upper abdominal muscles (supplied by intercostal nerves) splints the diaphragm.

The physiologic end result is a restrictive ventilation pattern with dysfunctional and discordant respiratory activity.[31] The ability to cough is seriously diminished, both by a lack of power to generate the necessary muscle force and by poor coordination, which is locally (and sometimes centrally) exacerbated by analgesic therapy.

As the functional residual capacity (FRC) falls, ventilation-perfusion mismatch—due to collapsed alveoli, atelectasis, and interstitial and alveolar lung water—leads to hypoxemia and predisposes the patient to infective complications and pneumonic collapse. Ultimately, carbon dioxide retention occurs, a process hastened by overzealous administration of analgesics, particularly opioids.

The modern archetype is the thoracotomy. A recent meta-analysis of the effects of analgesia on thoracotomy pain confirms that, in general, forced spirometric measures are reduced to a third of preoperative values. The respiratory restorative effect of analgesia is variable, but at best, with optimal analgesia, it can approach only 75% of preoperative values.[11]

With the current demand to operate on patients with overt evidence of respiratory failure—patients who in the past would have been refused surgery—the simplistic concept that there is an obligatory loss of respiratory reserves of 25% that is a function of trauma and the presence of chest drains, and which is only reversible with time and healing, is useful.[32] It provides a measure of how much improvement has to be predicted and of the effort required to ensure optimum analgesia. Again, lung volume reduction surgery is illustrative. For patients with normal pulmonary function, typical management planning allows for a reduction of function of an order of at least a third immediately after the surgical procedure. In the cases of those already verging on respiratory failure, any result less than an equivalent gain in respiratory function as an immediate consequence of surgery, or any shortfall in pain relief, will probably result in morbidity.

Looking for Quality

The current method of gauging systems is to consider the various issues and dynamics from a consumer's perspective. Specifically, this means that the patient is seen as the consumer. A pain service, as the provider, must have goals and targets, set standards to which others can aspire, and help gain the patients' acceptance. Techniques integral to activities of pain services are best examined as though being road tested. Through this process, it is possible to formulate some markers of quality of service.

Finding an evidence base for thoracic analgesia to gauge the quality of the product is a complex exercise. The database has assumed uncontrolled and chaotic proportions, not helped by the human factors that bedevil any studies of pain. Other hindrances include the empiricism and lack of uniform and internationally agreed-upon criteria that facilitate objective analysis of the science. It would be a great help if standard methodologies and standard batteries of tests were used, and it is to be hoped that the thoracic anesthesia world eventually will recognize this.

At one time, upper abdominal surgery was the model for assessing the quality of pain management; with the advent of minimal access techniques, this no longer provides realistic index populations. In comparison, thoracic surgery now has the major populations of worst-case, most-painful scenarios, which are rendered critical by failures in analgesic techniques. Thoracotomy, esophagectomy, and lung volume reduction surgery are typical of situations in which poor analgesia for painful surgery translates as morbidity threatening recovery and life; these types of surgeries could be the basis of index population cohorts of quality. There are also significant populations of patients with moderate discomfort who require immediate postoperative mobility—notably, patients undergoing endoscopic transthoracic sympathectomy.[12,33]

The most direct morbidity of consequence, second only to interference with pulmonary function, is related to failure to cough and its consequences. Protecting and facilitating the ability to cough are the fundamental functions of proactive analgesia regimens, and therefore the prime measure of quality—the discriminatory one that must be impressed on the patient.

Increasingly, it is being suggested that the preservation of gastrointestinal function is also a significant quality issue. Gastrointestinal dysfunction can have consequences for the treatment of coexisting disease, which might be exacerbated and lead to comorbidity in those already weakened by trauma, surgery, or (sometimes) analgesia itself.

Quality, in pain management, requires breadth as well as depth. That is, there must be a range of pain-relieving techniques available, both to accommodate choice and to provide backup in the event of failure. This range of techniques must be available to complement and facilitate all systems designed to deal both with the straightforward case progressing toward rapid recovery and with those patients with little physiologic

reserve who battle from crisis to crisis, even if the surgical intervention has been minimal.

To reiterate, the highest priority after thoracic injury is for patients to be able to cough to clear secretions and recruit and retain alveolar volume. Clearly, many will not be able to achieve this unaided. These patients might require additional help with coughing from physiotherapists; alternatively, they might require active measures, such as mini-tracheostomy to remove retained secretions or noninvasive positive pressure ventilation systems to recruit lung volume.

Patients' Requirements

For patients to make informed and contributory decisions, it is necessary that they be given sufficient information about the balance of risks. Specifically, they must be informed about the risk of morbidity from inadequately treated posttraumatic pain vs. that due to the risks inherent in establishing analgesic regimens. Once again, the single most important issue—and one with which the patient must be fully conversant—is the ability to cough. It is the fulcrum for complications—complications from the failure of analgesia to prevent morbidity and from morbidity brought about by the analgesia itself.

The natural desire for patients to be totally free of pain (as though trauma had never occurred) has to be qualified, as does the desire of therapists to deliver this level of care. Both groups tend to recognize that there will be some discomfort, but the message must be clear that this discomfort is a trade-off for safety and avoiding adverse effects. In particular, patients desire that normal activities—essentially those that make any obligatory bedridden state bearable—at least be maintained. Therefore any pain management system requires sufficient attention to detail to ensure that moving, urinating, and defecation are not unbearable ordeals.[34]

Issues of informed consent and the amount of information to give to patients are a matter of debate, both judicially and internationally.[35,36] For the purposes of definition, however, an adverse effect that occurs in 5% of patients is deemed noteworthy, as is any risk in which a complication of the analgesic technique causes or contributes to major neurologic deficits or fatalities.

The "awake vs. asleep" debate surrounding the insertion of catheters is also an issue of informed consent: patients should be given the freedom to choose and information about the timing of insertion.[37,38] There is evidence that 8% of patients will decline an offer of epidural analgesia after informed discussion.[39] There is no international consensus on whether it is optimal practice to place a thoracic epidural catheter before or after induction of general anesthesia. Points in favor of postinduction placement include better patient comfort, lack of necessity for active patient cooperation, and convenience. A survey of anesthetic practice in the United Kingdom published in 1998 reported that 60% of practitioners " most often" place a thoracic epidural after induction of anesthesia.[40]

In contrast, a North American review of this question in the April 2001 American Society of Anethesiologists (ASA) Newsletter concluded that ". . . the safety of regional anesthesia performed on anesthetized pediatric patients is not readily applicable to adults. Needle and catheter placement at the lumbar level only, appears to be safe. However, techniques performed above the termination of the cord or injection of local anesthetics that have the potential for neurotoxicity, should be avoided."[41]

The practice at the institution with which one of the authors (PS) is affiliated is routinely to place epidural catheter before induction of general anesthesia. Only in very exceptional circumstances (e.g., in the case of a mentally handicapped adult, with a guardian's consent) and with full discussion of the risks is an epidural placed in an anesthetized patient. In those cases, local anesthetics are not administered until the patient regains consciousness. This choice of awake placement is due in part to medico legal concerns but also to a preference for being able to test the catheter and ensure a working thoracic epidural block prior to induction.

Assessing Analgesic Techniques

It is the nature of the case-mix that assessment has to be conducted on patients who are bedridden and at their worst moments—mentally obtunded, physiologically weakened, and feeling uncooperative. These considerations limit testing to the use of bedside interviews and devices, so reproducibility of results may be uncertain (Table 20-4).

Only "broad-brush" discriminators can be obtained from patients acutely injured by surgery or trauma. One suggestion (Conacher and Piper, unpublished, 1998) has been to devote nursing effort to the humanitarian and functional improvement

aspects of analgesia for the first 24 hours, and to conduct population studies, audit, and research later on during recovery (albeit when the acute pain situation is lessening naturally). Index and study groups are then more cooperative; more complex tests (e.g., CO_2 response curves, evoked sensory potentials) can be conducted, and variability factors are reduced and reproducibility improved.[42,43]

It is something of a paradox, perhaps reflecting the state of the art, that most contemporary comparison studies in thoracic analgesia demonstrate few significant differences in variables attributable to good analgesia except in the early and acute phases of institution (less than 12 hours).[44] Any margins in benefit are usually absent after a short time because regimens are adjusted successfully to achieve equianalgesia and pain perception falls.

Subjective Assessment

The subjective assessment most commonly in use is the pain score. Visual analogs, based on a mark on a line from 0 to 10 representing the gamut from no pain to the worst pain imaginable, are popular and have stood the test of time.[45-47] In the context of the acute phases of thoracic surgery, the 4- or 5-point verbal rating systems (no pain, mild pain, moderate pain, severe pain) do, in practice, prove easier to obtain and more reproducible in conditioned populations. More recently, a combined observer/patient verbal ranking scale has been tested.[48]

To be relevant, pain scores should be recorded when the patient is stressed. Customary stresses (dynamics) are arm movement ipsilateral to the injury and coughing.[49] Ultimately, the best discriminator or outcome measure of an analgesic technique for a patient with thoracic nociception is the pain score resulting from the attempt to make a purposeful, productive cough that is preceded by deep inspiration and forced expiration.

A better way for comparison of techniques is to titrate to equianalgesia with pain scores. Indeed, it has been stated that this should be an ethical imperative in research.[34] So far, the method has been used only at the rest level, not tested to the dynamics of movement and coughing.[50]

The advocacy of including pain scores among the vital parameters, and of charting those scores along with temperature and pulse rate, is attributable to the work of Keele.[51] One group, using a 10-hour sequence of pain scores, constructed each individual's pain profile reflecting the pain experience at each of the dynamic levels of rest, on movement, and on coughing. The area under the curve of the profile proved to be the useful summary measure for statistical analysis.[49,52] The reason for suggesting this technique of analysis, as with the ideas of standardizing study and test periods mentioned previously, is to obtain a uniform measure or bench mark. For example, a statistic derived from a 10-hour pain profile on the second day after surgery would be valuable for audit and for between-unit and even international comparisons.

Behavioral Assessment

The only realistically applicable test in this category is opioid sparing or consumption as an indicator of efficacy.[53] Because many patient variables dictate the extent of use of opioids to control breakthrough pain (or as rescue analgesia), values are not particularly robust measures of efficacy; they are capable of

---

TABLE 20-4

Analgesia Systems Assessment

Purpose	Test Battery	Examples
Patient safety	Vital signs	
Detecting adverse effects	Vital signs	
	Subject/observer scoring systems	Sedation scales
		Nausea and vomiting scales
Efficacy	Subjective	Pain analog scales
	Objective	Observer ranking scale*
	Behavioral	Opioid requirements
	Physiologic	Sensory loss testing
		Sympatholytic testing
		Pulmonary function tests
Function	Physiologic	Bromage scale
		Pulmonary function tests
		Stress biochemistry
		Pulmonary radiology
		Electromyography
Audit	Subject/observer scoring systems	Pain analog scales
		Critical incident reporting
Research	Drug research	Controlled trials
	New techniques	Volunteer studies
	Experimental	CO_2 response†
		Somatosensory evoked potentials‡

*Mahon SV, Berry PD, Jackson M, et al: *Anaesthesia* 54:641, 1999.
†Doblar DD, Muldoon SM, Abbrecht PH, et al: *Anesthesiology* 55:423, 1981.
‡Richardson J, Jones J, Atkinson R: *Anesth Analg* 87:373, 1998.

discriminating only such disparate techniques as epidural opioids vs. intravenous opioids.[54]

Physiologic Assessment

The concept of restoration of function was an early idea and was tested on index populations of patients who had undergone upper abdominal surgery.[55] The respiratory restoration factor was based on simple forced pulmonary function measurements. The preoperative and postoperative values of forced expiratory volume in one second (FEV_1) and forced vital capacity (FVC) were compared as recovery progressed. This concept has stood the test of time and remains useful even for thoracic operations, in which confounders (e.g., postoperative respiratory muscle dysfunction and lung resection) are present. Small electronic spirometers make regular assessment very easy and even beneficial, if it is combined with incentive spirometry. Similar information can be obtained with peak expiratory flow rates. Such tests can be subject to meta-analysis, having been in common use for such a prolonged period that there are many historical controls.[11]

Pulmonary function testing has outlived its time as the most useful discriminator of analgesic efficacy because it is consistent only in demonstrating the superiority (or lack thereof) of various analgesic techniques.[56,57] It is now increasingly difficult to demonstrate differences. This suggests that a ceiling has been reached, reflecting factors that are not a function of pain. This point is not being made to limit the value of pulmonary function tests, which are now markers of quality. Any technique in which postoperative values fall short of a 70% threshold of preoperative values should be viewed as likely to fail to meet an acceptable standard or norm in improving patient function.

Modifications of the biochemical effects of stress are achievable with neural blockade and regional anesthesia. This effect is evident with lower abdominal surgery but only partially evident after upper abdominal surgery or thoracic surgery, even if patients are pain free.[58-61] It is intuitive to link these and allied phenomena, in which neuroendocrine activity is altered, directly with pain relief. In general, however, these are not quantitative phenomena. Suppression of immune responses, reduction of catecholamine release, and reduction of catabolism are more closely associated with prophylaxis against trauma and acute lung injury than with analgesia.[62] Changes in markers of these processes (e.g., interleukins) could reflect the secondary benefits of epidural regimens on cardiac performance, hemodynamics, and gastrointestinal function. The information is complementary to rather than discriminatory of analgesic technique and is useful as surrogate indication of functional improvement.[63,64]

The most important assessment of any method of analgesia is whether it can affect outcome. The most important cause of morbidity and mortality after thoracic surgery is respiratory complications (atelectasis, pneumonia, etc.). It is very difficult for the individual anesthesiologist assessing a single patient or group of patients over a short postoperative period to extrapolate his or her impressions of pain control to the outcome for these patients. For this reason, the meta-anlaysis of analgesia techniques and respiratory outcomes done by Ballantyne et al is important.[65] This group found that the most useful surrogate marker for respiratory outcome was postoperative analgesia with movement. This simple evaluation was more valid than pulmonary function tests or other clinical markers in predicting outcome. This information is very useful to the anesthesiologist either when considering a single patient or when evaluating research in the literature.

Thoracic Epidural Analgesia

History

Epidural block developed only recently in the field of thoracic surgery, reflecting all the difficulties associated with the introduction of local anesthetic techniques into a climate in which general anesthesia had become the norm and was regarded as best and safest. Crawford et al reported a series from 1945 to 1952, consisting of 2172 operations conducted with "peridural anesthesia."[66] They noted improvements in the early postoperative period. It took until the 1970s, however, before the technique was considered specifically for postoperative analgesia, initially on high-risk patients and then tentatively for routine patients.[67,68] Other studies demonstrated that although there were still problems and significant risks, these were no longer insurmountable.[69]

The advent of neuraxial opioids provided the impetus to add thoracic epidural analgesia (TEA) to the armamentarium of thoracic anesthesiology and establish it as the gold standard. Bromage et al, in a classic study, demonstrated the remarkable effect of epidural opioids in comparison with local anesthetics in thoracotomy and upper abdominal operations.[70] With increased experience of continuous techniques and the advent of ambulatory and patient-controlled analgesia systems, TEA became generally accepted.[71,72] By 1997, 80% of units performing more than 100 thoracotomies annually were using midthoracic epidural techniques and opioid/local anesthetic synergistic combinations as standard practice.[73]

Anatomy

It is the obliquity of the vertebral spinous processes that directs the percutaneous approaches to the epidural space. The interspinous space is most vertical in the midthoracic (T_4 to T_7) region, with the result that the palpable tip of a spinous process is a landmark indicating the intervertebral space of the next vertebral body (Figure 20-1). Midline approaches to the epidural space aim at an oblique cephalad direction to the needle point, "walking" it off the superior surface of the spinous process of the vertebra below in a cephalad direction.

Paramedian approaches to the epidural space are popular—in part for reasons already stated, and also because of the ease with which catheters can be threaded into the thoracic epidural space. The landmark for needle puncture is approximately 1.0 cm lateral to the spinous process, which leads directly to the lamina of the vertebra below. On bony contact, the needle is directed medially and cephalad to locate the epidural space (Figures 20-2 and 20-3). The use of the higher spaces (T_2 to T_4) are advocated for postthoracotomy pain because patients tend to be nursed sitting up, but it is more common for T_4 to T_6 to be used if TEA is part of the intraoperative anesthesia. Spread in the epidural space is aided by gravity, ensuring that segmental analgesia covers the area from T_2 to T_8 or T_{10}, which includes all the dermatomes likely

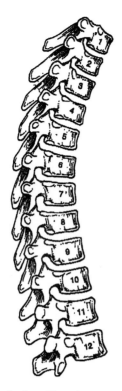

FIGURE 20-1 The inclination of the spinous processes from T_1 to T_{12}. The steepest caudal angulation of the spinous processes is in the midthoracic (T_3 to T_7) region, which is the optimal site for thoracic epidural placement for postthoracotomy analgesia. (From Ramamurthy S: Thoracic epidural nerve block. In Waldman SD, Winnie AP [eds]: *Interventional pain management,* Philadelphia, 1996, WB Saunders.)

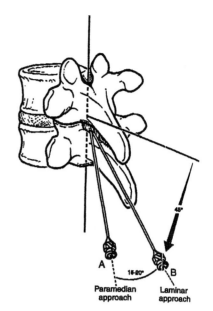

FIGURE 20-2 A, The paramedian approach to the epidural space is favored by most anesthesiologists at the midthoracic levels. The needle is inserted 1 cm lateral to the superior tip of the spinous process and then advanced perpendicular to all planes to contact the lamina of the vertebral body immediately below. The needle is then "walked" up the lamina at an angle rostrally (45 degrees) and medially (20 degrees) until the rostral edge of the lamina is felt. The needle is next advanced over the edge of the lamina seeking for a loss of resistance on entering the epidural space after transversing the ligamentum flavum. **B,** The laminar approach is favored by some practitioners. The needle is inserted right next to the rostral edge of the spinous process and advanced straight, without any angle from the midline. (From Ramamurthy S: Thoracic epidural nerve block. In Waldman SD, Winnie AP [eds]: *Interventional pain management,* Philadelphia, 1996, WB Saunders.)

to crossed by the incision.[74] The spread of local anesthetics in the thoracic epidural space tends to be more caudal than rostral, but this spread depends on the level at which the injection is made (Figure 20-4). At high levels of thoracic epidural injection (above T_3), there is very limited rostral spread, whereas at lower levels, the rostral spread is approximately the same as the caudal spread.[75] The optimal level of placement of an epidural catheter depends on the dermatome levels at which the majority of the pain will be perceived. For most conventional posterolateral thoracotomies (occurring in the fifth or sixth intercostal space), the thoracic epidural can be placed anywhere between T_3 and T_6.

If the patient adopts a hunched sitting position, the intervertebral space is widened, the spinous processes are more horizontal, and the standing operator can work from a more comfortable position. In the midthoracic region, where the ligamentum flavum (Figures 20-5 and 20-6) is thicker than in the cervical region, the epidural space is 1 to 5 mm in depth. In the spontaneously breathing patient, the space is at a negative pressure. Despite this fact, most reports are of the space being sought by loss-of-resistance techniques; only rarely are "hanging drops" used, although many often observe the movement of a bubble in the epidural catheter as confirmation of the correct location.

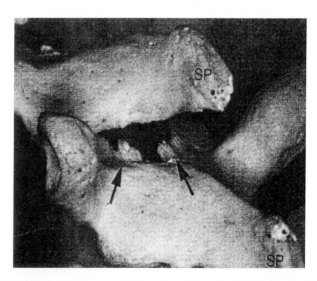

FIGURE 20-3 In some patients, aging and/or osteoarthritis leads to calcified deposits in the ligamantum flavum and osteophytes from the lamina *(dark arrows),* which can be particularly problematic for the paramedian approach to the epidural space. *SP,* Spinous process. (From Ramamurthy S: Thoracic epidural nerve block. In Waldman SD, Winnie AP [eds]: *Interventional pain management,* Philadelphia, 1996, WB Saunders.)

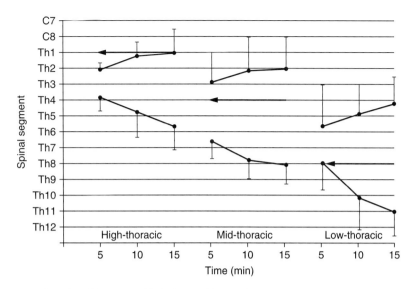

FIGURE 20-4 Extension of the sensory blockade tested by pinprick vs. time after administration of 6 mL of lidocaine 1% in the high (C_8 to T_1), midthoracic (T_2 to T_4), or low thoracic (T_7 to T_9) epidural space. Data represent the mean +/− standard deviation bars. Arrows indicate the level of the epidural puncture. Note that for midthoracic or high thoracic injections, the spread of the block is more caudal than cephalad. (From Visser WA, Liem TH, van Egmond J, et al: *Anesth Analg* 86:332, 1998.)

Adverse Effects

TECHNIQUE-RELATED ADVERSE EFFECTS

The overall incidence of complications because of the technique is 3%. Within this group are included dural perforation, postoperative radicular pain, and transient peripheral nerve lesions (which are possibly unrelated). The incidence of dura perforation increases when the lower thoracic and the lumbar spaces are used.[39] Damage to the spinal cord as a result of needle trauma, or as a sequela of hematoma development, gives cause for concern. The current working figure of permanent neurologic damage, based on about a quarter of a million patients, is 0.07%. Trauma occurs in 3% to 12% of cases, if epidural vein perforation is accepted as a surrogate marker of trauma. This is significant in light of the current debates about low-molecular-weight heparin.[76] Common sense should apply.

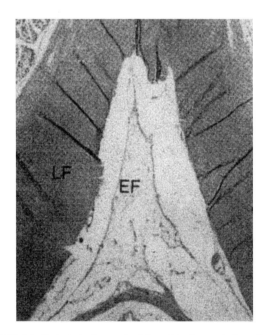

FIGURE 20-5 A photomicrograph of the epidural space in the midthoracic region; posterior is at the top of the photo, and anterior is at the bottom. Note the inverted V-shape of the ligamentum flavum (LF). Note also how minor variations in the needle angulation during paramedian approach to the epidural space can lead to differences in the perceived width of the epidural space. *EF,* Fat in the epidural space. (From Ramamurthy S: Thoracic epidural nerve block. In Waldman SD, Winnie AP [eds]: *Interventional pain management,* Philadelphia, 1996, WB Saunders.)

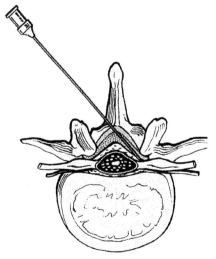

FIGURE 20-6 Diagram of an attempted paramedian approach to the epidural space (in this case at a lumbar level). In this illustration, the epidural needle is angled too medially, leading to a prolonged trajectory through the ligamentum flavum and the potential to injure a nerve root. The epidural space is normally found within the first 1 cm after advancing the needle beyond the lamina. (From Cousins MJ, Veering BT: Epidural neural blockade. In Cousins MJ, Bridenbaugh PO [eds]: *Neural blockade in anesthesia and pain management,* ed 3, Philadelphia, 1998, Lippincott-Raven.)

Irrespective of indications, when the surgery is known to have a potential for resulting in neurologic damage (e.g., coarctation of the aorta, thoracic aneurysms), then TEA should be used with extreme caution.[76,77] The risk of the anesthesiologist being blamed for neurologic damage is significant.

NEURAXIAL BLOCKS AND ANTICOAGULATION

The risk of neurologic dysfunction as a result of hemorrhagic complications of a neuraxial block are estimated to be 1/150,000 for epidural anesthetics and 1/220,000 for spinal anesthetics.[78] Factors associated with increased risk include impaired hemostasis (Table 20-5), difficult needle placement, and multiple punctures. Patients with impaired hemostasis are also at risk during catheter removal. There is a consensus among thoracic surgeons that the incidence of postoperative pulmonary emboli has been decreased by perioperative antithrombus prophylactic programs, which in most institutions include low-dose anticoagulants. Thus placement and removal of epidural catheters in the face of some degree of coagulation impairment is a daily consideration in thoracic anesthesia practice. The American Society of Regional Anesthesia (ASRA) developed a consensus position on neuraxial blockade and anticoagulation in 1998.[79] Some of their recommendations regarding heparin, however, are open to interpretation: "During subcutaneous (mini-dose) prophylaxis there is no contraindication to the use of neuraxial techniques. The risk of neuraxial bleeding may be decreased by delay of the heparin injection until after the block, and may be increased in debilitated patients or after prolonged therapy." Because of this uncertainty, each anesthesiologist and institution need to develop their own protocol that takes into account not only the published guidelines but also local factors relating to timing of patient admission. At the hospital with which one of the authors

is affiliated (PS), the current protocol for a patient with no other risk factors for bleeding is to administer the initial preoperative dose of subcutaneous heparin, 5000 U, 2 hours before epidural placement. Postoperatively, catheters are removed more than 2 hours after the preceding heparin dose. This practice has evolved partially for administrative reasons (to avoid missed heparin doses) and also because it has been shown that no significant serum heparin anti-IIa or anti-Xa levels are detectable more than 2 hours after subcutaneous heparin, 5000 U.[80] For low-molecular-weight heparins (LMWHs), the ASRA guidelines are to delay epidural placement for more than 12 hours for standard doses and more than 24 hours for higher doses (e.g., enoxaparin, 1 mg/kg, twice daily).

REDUCING THE TECHNICAL FAILURE RATE

A review of epidural analgesia has suggested a failure rate ranging from 30% to 50% under clinical conditions.[76] Research studies conducted after learning curves have been overcome, however, have published figures well below 10%. Experience, the use of fluoroscopy and radiocontrast for catheter siting, waiting for the effects of test doses of local anesthetics, and preventing catheter dislocation all help to keep the failure rate to less than 5%—a more respectable figure in keeping with the best of regional techniques.[39,48,81]

AGENT-ADVERSE EFFECTS

The shift in types of adverse effects is illustrated in Table 20-6, as the favored agents evolved from local anesthetics to epidural opioids alone to combinations and ultimately to synergistic combinations.[69,82-84]

Local anesthetics. The adverse effects of local anesthetics are related either to motor blockade (manifesting as muscle weakness) or sympathetic blockade (manifesting as hypotension due to peripheral vasodilatation). Bradycardia can

---

TABLE 20-5

Pharmacologic Activities of Anticoagulants, Antiplatelet Agents, and Thrombolytics

Agent	Effect on Coagulation Variables		Peak Effect	Time to Normal Hemostasis after Discontinuation	Comments
	PT	aPTT			
Intravenous heparin	↑	↑↑↑	Minutes	4-6 hours	Monitor ACT, aPTT, delay heparinization for 1 hour after needle placement
Subcutaneous heparin	–	↑	40-50 minutes	4-6 hours	aPTT could remain normal, anti-Xa activity reflects degree of anticoagulation
Low-molecular-weight heparin	–	–	3-5 hours	12-24 hours	Anti-Xa activity not monitored. Use with caution in patients receiving epidural analgesia
Warfarin	↑↑↑	↑	4-6 days (Less with loading dose)	4-6 days	Monitor PT daily, remove indwelling neuraxial catheter when INR < 1.5
Antiplatelet agents					Bleeding time not reliable
Aspirin	–	–	Hours	5-8 days	Predictor of platelet function
Other NSAIDs				1-3 days	No increased risk with NSAIDs; risk
Glycoprotein IIb/IIIa receptor inhibitors				1-2 weeks	associated with ticlopidine, clopidogrel, and other IIb/IIIa inhibitors unknown
Fibrinolytics	↑	↑↑	Minutes	24-36 hours	Fibrinogen level decreased for 1-2 days Heparin administered in combination Neuraxial block not recommended

From Horlocker TT: Regional anesthesia and anticoagulation: are the risks worth the benefits? In Chaney MA (ed): *Regional anesthesia for cardiothoracic surgery SCA mongraph*, Baltimore, 2002, Lippincott Williams and Wilkins.

PT, Prothrombin time; *aPTT,* activated partial thromboplastin time; *ACT,* activated coagulation time; ↑, clinically insignificant increase; ↑↑, possibly clinically significant increase; ↑↑↑, clinically significant increase; *NSAIDs,* nonsteroidal anti-inflammatory drugs.

TABLE 20-6

The Changing Pattern of Adverse Effects of Thoracic Epidural Analgesia

Adverse Effect	Opioid*	LA†	Mixed	LA/Opioid§	Syngergistic (LA/opioid)‖
	(All) n=1200 (1982) (%)	(TEA) n=54 (1983) (%)	LA/Opioid/ Combinations‡ n=1324 (1987-1993) (%)	(TEA+lumbar) n=42 (1993) (%)	(TEA, Different Subsets) n=106 (1999) (%) (%)
Nausea and vomiting	17	NR	11.2	7	30
Hemodynamic instability	24	70	4.3	19	7.5
Sedation	NR	5	3.3	19	
Unpleasant sensations (numbness or pruritus)	15¶	10	14	14	40
Inadequate analgesia	NR	40	3.8	12	0.1
Urinary retention	15	30		45	All patients catheterized
Respiratory depression	0.1	0	1 case	0	4

*Reiz S, Westberg M: *Lancet* 203, 1980.
†Conacher ID, Paes ML, Jacobson L, et al: *Anaesthesia* 38:546, 1983.
‡Lubenow TR, Faber LP, McCarthy, et al: *Ann Thorac Surg* 58:924, 1995.
§Hurford WE, Dutton RP, Alfille PH, et al: *J Cardiothorac Vasc Anesth* 7:521, 1993.
‖Mahon SV, Berry PD, Jackson M, et al: *Anaesthesia* 54:641, 1999.
¶Pruritus incidence reduced to 1% by use of preservative-free morphine.

follow, because of a vagal preponderance of cardiac control.[85] Hemodynamic changes are limited by careful attention to fluid resuscitation and are reduced with continuous infusions in comparison with intermittent bolusing techniques.

The motor effects of full concentrations of local anesthetics in normal volunteers are documented.[86] Blockade results in an increased functional residual capacity because of a caudad movement of the diaphragm and a decrease in intrathoracic fluid volume. Inspiratory effort, however, is weakened. In the traumatized patient, increased functional residual capacity is of benefit, but weakened inspiratory effort is a disadvantage. It is likely that low-dose local anesthetics come close to achieving an ideal situation: abolishing reflex spasm to allow caudal movement of the diaphragm and recruitment of lung volume, without reducing the power of the intercostal muscles that are necessary for coughing. In practice, motor block is reduced, almost to clinical insignificance, by the use of dilute solutions, without loss of sensory block.

Opioids. All clinically available opioids have been used for TEA.[13,39,73] Comparable epidural doses of several opioids are

shown in Table 20-7. There is a division between adverse effects that are manifestations of systemic absorption and those that are exaggerated or more prominent as result of neuraxial placement: the latter are a function of lipophilicity or hydrophilicity. The systemic side effects of significance are sedation, nausea and vomiting, and changes in gastrointestinal motility. Pruritus, in its facial form, is a systemic effect; the segmental form has a local pathway. Respiratory depression is the most feared consequence of opioid use. It has usually been reported after the use of morphine, a hydrophilic molecule that lingers in the cerebrospinal fluid (CSF) and slowly migrates centrally over a 12- to 24-hour period with normal CSF circulation. Despite the pressures to reduce the surveillance of those treated with neuraxial opioids, a particularly cautious regimen must remain in place if the hydrophilic opioids (meperidine, morphine) are being used.

Advantages of Thoracic Eqidural Analgesia

An optimally functioning epidural is a near-ideal solution, meeting all the clinical and patient expectations, and having an excellent safety record.[39] It is second to none in terms of

TABLE 20-7

Dosage Comparisons for Epidural PCA

Opioid	Concentration	Loading Dose*	Epidural PCA Dose	Lockout (min)	Continuous Rate	4-Hour Limit
Morphine	50 μg/mL	2-4 mg	2-4 mL	10-15	6-12 mL/h	40-70 mL
Hydromorphone	10 μg/mL	0.5-1.5 mg	2-4 mL	6-10	6-12 mL/h	40-70 mL
Fentanyl	5 μg/mL	75-100 μg	2-4 mL	6	6-15 mL/h	40-70 mL
Sufentanil	2 μg/mL	0.5 μg/kg	2-4 mL	6	0.1 μg/kg/h	40-70 mL

From Sinatra RS: Acute pain management and acute pain services. In Cousins MJ, Bridenbaugh PO (eds): *Neural blockade in clinical anesthesia and management of pain*, ed 3, Philadelphia, 1998, Lippincott-Raven.
*Dependent on site of epidural catheter, extent of surgery, and patient physical status.

accrued ancillary benefit over and above analgesia. There is experiential evidence of TEA's demonstrable superiority over other analgesic techniques in terms of effects on pulmonary function, stress reduction, myocardial function, oxygen delivery, and reduction of myocardial irritability, particularly when epidural techniques are used intraoperatively and are extended to cover the postoperative period.[87-90] As with colonic surgery, gastrointestinal function is much less disturbed when TEA is used, and after esophagectomy, patients are more easily mobilized.[91]

The Optimal Combination of Agents

There is little indication for a single agent. Combinations of local anesthetic and opioid are now standard. With these, the advantages of TEA as opposed to lumbar epidural become manifest, particularly in the early postoperative period and in terms of the patient's ability to cough. Many institutions have protocols that are designed to be applicable to all types of surgery. Most, as a result of the debate over volume vs. concentration, have settled for a vehicle of 0.1% bupivacaine for postoperative analgesia in upper abdominal and thoracic procedures.

As of the time of writing, there are new local anesthetics entering the field: Levobupivacaine and ropivacaine at higher doses are less toxic than their predecessors, and the latter causes less motor blockade. At the dilute doses found optimal for postoperative analgesia, however, the advantages of the new agents are likely to be marginal and difficult to prove.

Various opioids, including meperidine, sufentanil, and hydromorphone, have been advocated. These are often dictated by protocol, based on pragmatism, and designed for local circumstance.[73,76] There is no single "best opioid" for epidural analgesia. Each opioid has a different set of pharmacologic properties that determine its effectiveness in a given clinical situation. One of the major properties of the opioids that affects their application for neuraxial analgesia is their lipid solubility (Figure 20-7 and Table 20-7). The more hydrophilic opioids (such as morphine) produce a wider dermatomal band of analgesia but are associated with more minor side effects, such as nausea and vomiting. The more lipophilic opioids (e.g., sufentanil) are faster in onset but might cause central nervous system side effects (e.g., drowsiness from cumulative systemic absorption) when used for prolonged periods. A major proviso is that the catheter be placed to match the area of nociception: The further away, the bigger the failure rate; the bigger the volumes, the greater the hemodynamic instability, and the more significant are the stumbling blocks to achieving equianalgesia.[50,92-95] A sample postthoracotomy analgesic regimen from the hospital with which one of the authors (PS) is affiliated is shown in Table 20-8.

Two recent studies have come to identical conclusions regarding the local anesthetic/opioid ratio. One was a randomized control trial conducted on thoracotomy patients, and the other was a complex statistical method that sorted out twenty combinations for optimization.[48,81] Both found that the addition of fentanyl at 10.0 µg/mL to a base of 0.1% bupivacaine proved most suitable for thoracotomy and upper abdominal surgery and was least disruptive of gastrointestinal function. The optimal ratio for sufentanil is 1.0 µg/mL in bupivacaine 0.1% (Table 20-9).[50,96,97]

The primary reason to favor thoracic vs. lumbar epidurals for postthoracotomy analgesia is that thoracic epidurals permit the use of combinations of local anesthetics and opioids, and these

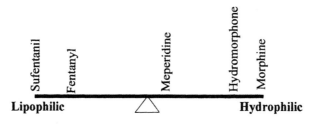

FIGURE 20-7 The neuraxial opioid "teeter-totter." When choosing an opioid to use for epidural analgesia, the anesthesiologist needs to balance the pros and cons of each agent in the clinical context. A major pharmacokinetic factor that determines the effects and side effects of the neuraxial opioids is their lipid solubility. Low-lipid solubility agents (e.g., hydrophilic agents such as morphine) tend to produce a wider band of analgesia with slower onset and offset and more minor side effects. Highly lipid-soluble agents can cause central nervous system effects from systemic absorption when they are used for prolonged periods, and tachyphylaxis can develop. Meperidine has a lipid solubility toward the middle of the range, but the accumulation of active metabolites is a concern. Patient factors to be weighed in choosing a neuraxial opioid include the rostral-caudal width of the analgesia band required (thoracotomy vs. sternotomy vs. thoracoabdominal incision) and the anticipated duration of the epidural infusion.

TABLE 20-8

Sample Analgesic Protocol (Potential Dose Ranges or Alternative Drug Choices in Brackets)

Patient	60 years old, 70 kg, thoracotomy incision fifth intercostal space, normal renal function
Preoperatively	Heparin 5000 U, subcutaneously 2 hours before (1 hour after) epidural placement
Intraoperatively	1) Thoracic epidural catheter placed before induction at T_4-T_5 (range T_3-T_7)
	2) Test dose lidocaine, 2%, 3 mL (2-4 mL), test sensory level at 5 minutes
	3) Following induction of anesthesia, during the period of chest incision, boluses of fentanyl 10 μg/mL plus bupivacaine 0.2% in 2 mL increments as tolerated to a maximum total dose of 10 mL (4-10 mL) guided by blood pressure
	4) Minimal systemic opioids after induction and intubation
	5) Ketorolac 30 mg IV (15-30 mg) before chest closure
	6) Begin postoperative analgesic epidural infusion (see below) intraoperatively 1–2 hours after induction plus p.r.n. boluses of epidural solution (2-3mL) during chest closure guided by blood pressure
Postoperatively	1) Patient-controlled epidural analgesia (PCEA) with fixed infusion rate and p.r.n. boluses TEA infusion: bupivacaine 0.1% (0.1%-0.05%) plus hydromorphone 15 μg/mL*(or morphine 50 μg/mL, or fentanyl 4 μg/mL) at 6 mL/hr (3-8 mL/hr) with boluses 3 mL.(2-4 mL) every 20 minutes p.r.n., 4 hours maximum dose limit 40 mL.
	2) Ketorolac 15-30 mg IV every 12 hours (rectal indomethacin 50-100 mg for 12 hours) × 48 hours
	3) Famotidine 10 mg IV every 12 hours × 48 hours
Monitoring on ward	(Recovery room 0-2 hours, "step-down" monitored ward bed 2-24 hours, then regular ward bed >24 hours)
	1) Activity: check postural blood pressure, pulse and sensory/motor block before getting up
	2) Respiratory rate and sedation scale every hour for 24 hours, then every 2 hours if infusion rate not increased
	3) Pulse, blood pressure every hour
	4) Sensory/motor block every 4 hours for 24 hours, then every 8 hours if infusion rate not increased
	5) Notify acute pain service for
	i) Inadequate pain control
	ii) BP systolic <90, pulse <50, respiratory rate <10
	iii) Sedation score of 3 (somnolent, difficult to arouse)
	iv) Increasing sensory or motor block
Discontinue epidural	Stop infusion at 72 hours (unless chest drains still in place) and observe pain control with oral opioid/antiinflammatory; remove catheter after satisfactory mobilization with oral analgesics

*Opioid is discontinued in epidural solution for refractory pruritis, sedation, or other opioid side effects, and the infusion is changed to ropivacaine 0.2% with similar PCEA infusion/bolus dosing.

TABLE 20-9

Quick Reference, Best Evidence: Analgesic Technique and Agents

Technique	Local anesthetic base	Opioid	Loading/ Bolus Dose	Infusion Rate	Instruction	Adverse Effect	Ref. No.
Thoracic epidural[†]	Bupivacaine 0.1%	Fentanyl 10 μg/mL	5 mL	0.05-0.10 mL/kg/hr	Max. rate 10 mL/hr		
Paravertebral block[‡]	Bupivacaine 0.5%			0.1 mL/kg/hr	Change to 0.25% bupivacaine after 48 hr	Local anesthetic toxicity	
Adult	0.25%						
Infant	See ref #4						
Intrathecal							
Opioid 1[§]	Fentanyl						
Opioid 2[‖]	1.0 μg/kg				Preservative free	Late onset	
	Morphine 15–20 μg/kg				*>70 yr age reduce to 10 μg/kg Inject calculated dose at 1 mL/10 kg or in 10 mL N/Saline	respiratory depression	

*Courtesy of Birmingham Heartlands NHS Hospital Trust UK.
[†]Mahon SV, Berry PD, Jackson M, et al: *Anaesthesia* 54:641, 1999. and Curatolo M, Schnider TW, Petersen-Felix S, et al: *Anesthesiology* 92:325, 2000.
[‡]Richardson J, Lönnqvist PA: *Br J Anaesth* 81:230, 1998 and Cheung SLW, Booker PD, Franks R, et al: *Br J Anaesth* 79:9, 1997.
[§]Sudarshan G, Browne BL, Matthews JNS, et al: *Br J Anaesth* 75:19, 1995.
[‖]Alhashemi JA, Sharpe MD, Harris CL, et al: *J Cardiothorac Vasc Anesth* 14:639, 2000.

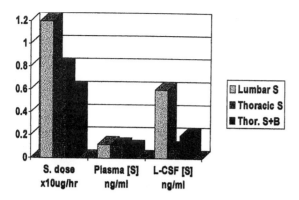

FIGURE 20-8 Differences in the pharmacology of postthoracotomy epidural infusions of lumbar sufentanil (lumbar S), thoracic sufentanil (thoracic S), and thoracic sufentanil plus bupivacaine (thor S + B). Thoracic S + B produced significantly superior analgesia with movement with lower total sufentanil dosage (S dose) and lower plasma levels (Plasma [S]) than the other two techniques. Note that in spite of lower dosage, thoracic S + B patients had higher mean lumbar cerebrospinal fluid (CSF) sufentanil levels than the thoracic sufentanil group, as measured by separate lumbar punctures at 24 and 48 hours postoperatively. This suggests a pharmacokinetic mechanism with local anesthetics that facilitates transfer of epidural opioid into the CSF. (From Slinger PD: *J Cardiothorac Vasc Anesth* 13:350, 1999.)

combinations seem to be synergistic in producing pain relief. The synergy manifest by these combinations is thought to be due in part to facilitation of the transfer of the opioid into the cerebrospinal fluid by the local anesthetic, and this phenomenon is independent of the dosage of the local anesthetic (Figure 20-8).[50] Also, there is evidence that this synergy is due partly to an increase in the affinity of the opioid receptor for the opioid, an increase caused by the local anesthetic (Figure 20-9).[98] This synergism seems to be operational at low doses of local anesthetics and is not increased by higher doses. Thus, it could be

possible to use very low doses of local anesthetics in combination with opioids to avoid the sympathetic-block side effects that are a major drawback of thoracic epidural analgesia.

Respiratory Effects of Thoracic Epidural Analgesia

Initially, it was theorized that TEA could diminish the diaphragmatic inhibition that is known to occur after thoracotomy.[99] Such disinhibition was shown for TEA after upper abdominal surgery.[100] Indeed, a postthoracotomy animal model demonstrated similar disinhibition.[101] A postthoracotomy human study of patients with moderate COPD, however, failed to show any improvement in diaphragmatic contractility by TEA, even though respiratory function (tidal volume) was improved.[102] How TEA can improve respiratory mechanics without improving diaphragm contractility is not easy to explain, but the process might be similar to the known concept of increasing cardiac output without increasing myocardial contractility by changing loading conditions for the ventricle. The diaphragm inserts on the chest wall, and by decreasing chest splinting, the diaphragm can be returned to a mechanically more efficient position on its force-length (Starling) contraction curve without affecting its actual contractility.

It has been shown in volunteers that a thoracic level of epidural blockade increases FRC.[86] This increase is due largely to an increase in thoracic gas volume caused by a fall in the resting level of the diaphragm without a fall in tidal volume. This finding contradicts earlier studies, which found no change in FRC with TEA.[103] The different results are probably related to the more advanced method of the recent work. FRC is considered the most important determinant of oxygenation in the postoperative period.[104]

There has been concern that the nerve block produced by thoracic epidural local anesthetic might have a deleterious effect on respiratory function in patients with severe COPD.

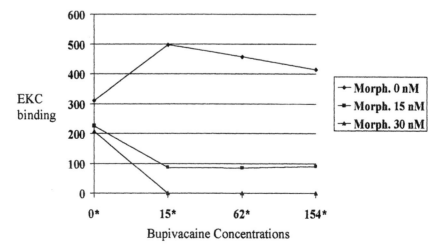

FIGURE 20-9 The effects of spinal morphine and bupivacaine on the binding of EKC (a K-ligand) to opioid receptors in the spinal cords of rats. Bupivacaine produced a tenfold increase in morphine-induced antinociception. This correlated with increased displacement of EKC from spinal K-receptors in the presence of both morphine and bupivacaine (i.e., increased affinity of morphine for the opioid receptors). This synergy occurred at the lowest concentration of bupivacaine studied and was not augmented by increasing the bupivacaine dosage. (From Slinger PD: *J Cardiothorac Vasc Anesth* 13:350, 1999.)

Although the possibility still exists that a thoracic motor block could impair respiratory function, there are clearly no negative effects from the sensory block associated with typical analgesic doses of local anesthetic. Gruber et al studied a group of patients with severe COPD (mean FEV_1 = 27% of predicted values) and found that the sensory block from 10 to 12 mL of 0.25% bupivacaine (mean number of blocked dermatome segments = 8) produced a slight but significant increase in tidal volume and a decrease in lung resistance without any significant effect on other measures of pulmonary mechanics.[105]

Although it is possible to deliver an opioid to the spinal cord receptors via a lumbar catheter in amounts that are adequate for analgesia at rest, the beneficial synergistic effects of local anesthetics on respiratory mechanics require a thoracic catheter. Improvement in respiratory function with combined local anesthetic and opioid TEA has been confirmed in postthoracotomy clinical studies.

Cardiovascular Effects of Thoracic Epidural Analgesia

The leading cardiovascular cause of morbidity and mortality after thoracic surgery is arrhythmias—particularly atrial fibrillation, which occurs in approximately 15% of patients after lung resection surgery.[106] In-hospital mortality increases from 2% to 17% in those postthoracotomy patients who develop arrhythmias. Arrhythmias also correlate with poor long-term outcome. Mean survival in patients 18 months after lung resection for cancer was decreased to 10% in patients who had early postoperative arrhythmias, compared with 57% in those without arrhythmias.[107]

The cause of postthoracotomy arrhythmias is due to the interaction of two factors: strain to the right side of the heart and increased stimulation of the sympathetic nervous system.[108] In theory, TEA can decrease both of these causes of arrhythmia. In animal models of ischemia, TEA has been shown to decrease arrhythmias by decreasing sympathetic tone. In a recent study of prophylactic oxygen administration to decrease postthoracotomy arrhythmias, Backlund et al found no clinically significant episodes of postoperative atrial fibrillation in their control group (those patients who received supplemental oxygen for only the first 24 hours).[109] This compares with an incidence of 30% in a similar control group from a previous study by the same research group.[110] The major difference between the two control groups was that the recent group received TEA and the previous group did not. No statistical conclusions can be reached comparing the two groups from different studies, but the data suggest that the TEA group had lower pressures in the right side of the heart.

Perioperative myocardial ischemia occurs in approximately 5% of postthoracotomy patients—an incidence that would be expected for any type of major surgery in a patient population of this age with a high incidence of smoking. The benefits of TEA as a treatment for myocardial ischemia are well known.[111] The sympathetic blockade from TEA in patients with coronary artery disease decreases both the supply and demand of myocardial oxygen but has no net effect on echocardiographic segmental wall motion, which is the most sensitive indicator of ischemia.[112] This finding is in contrast to the effects of lumbar epidural analgesia (LEA), which can induce segmental wall motion abnormalities in patients with known coronary artery disease because myocardial oxygen supply is decreased but demand is not affected.[113]

There has been a concern that thoracic sympathetic blockade from local anesthetics can cause problematic hypotension in postoperative patients. With the use of synergistic combinations of local anesthetics and opioids—and if the total dose of local anesthetics is limited—this problem can be avoided. Moniche et al, in a study of upper abdominal surgery, found that TEA infusions of bupivacaine 0.25% and morphine, 0.05 mg/mL, at a mean rate of 4 mL/hr, produced superior analgesia to intravenous/intramuscular morphine; there were no differences between groups in blood pressures at rest, whether the patients were standing or walking. The only significant hemodynamic difference between groups was a slightly lower heart rate in the TEA group.[114]

In patients with advanced pulmonary disease, the effects of thoracic sympathetic blockade are a concern because of potential changes in the balance between the pulmonary and systemic vascular resistances. In one case report of a patient with primary pulmonary hypertension, TEA produced a favorable effect on this balance, reducing the pulmonary artery pressure and pulmonary vascular resistance more than the systemic pressure and vascular resistance.[115]

Adjuvants

Several adjuvants for epidural analgesia have been described. Epinephrine, 2 µg/mL, showed clear additive effects on the analgesia produced by a fentanyl/bupivacaine infusion in a group of patients who had either thoracic or abdominal surgery.[116] It is not yet certain whether there is any synergistic effect from the inclusion of epinephrine or whether fewer side effects will result. Other adjuvants include N-methyl-D-aspartate (NMDA) antagonists (ketamine), gamma-aminobutyric acid (GABA) agonists (midazolam), and clonidine, an α_2-agonist, to prolong activity.[81,117-118] Some of these have been the subjects of randomized trials, but there is concern that the improved quality of analgesia might not justify the risk. Neurotoxicity and increased hemodynamic instability are the most prominent of current concerns.[76,81] There is some evidence that clonidine may improve the quality of analgesia in pediatric practice, as children tend to be resistant to the hemodynamic effects.[119] The most exciting possibility on the horizon is the potential combination of ultra–low-dose opioid antagonists with opioids.[120] This research is still in preliminary stages at present.

Somatic Paravertebral Nerve Block

The only serious contenders challenging epidural techniques are those in which analgesic agents are deposited in the thoracic paravertebral space (TPVS). Fundamentally, these are multiple-level intercostal nerve blocks, which have replaced the direct and multiple applications of local anesthetics to intercostal nerves, cryotherapy, and interpleural local anesthetics.[121] It is possible with paravertebral nerve block (PNB) to approach the levels of analgesia and restoration of respiration that are seen with TEA, but only when PVB is used as part of a multimodal package with intravenous opioids and NSAIDs. In addition, much attention and effort are required to ensure effective spread of effect of local anesthetic.[122] Whether PVB can have the same beneficial effects on outcome that have been seen with TEA (Table 20-1) remains to be determined. The common clinical impression is that multimodal analgesia that includes PVB is a very good alternative to TEA.

A percutaneous approach is useful for patients who are not undergoing thoracotomy, and several institutions use this approach routinely for thoracoscopic procedures. Much of the advantage of the technique, however, lies in being able to position catheters at the termination of open thoracic surgery before closure of the chest wall.

The addition of adjuvants to make an analgesic cocktail has been tried but to date is of no advantage. It would seem that the TPVS is little more than an exotic site for a parenteral injection.[123] Adjuvants (apart from epinephrine) are best administered by more traditional routes, either intravenously or epidurally.

History of Paravertebral Nerve Block

The concept of PVB was probably formulated by Sellheim in 1906. Kappis (1912) is regarded as the initiator of the technique, and Laewen gave it the name "paravertebral conduction" anesthesia.[124] It gradually gained in popularity throughout the early twentieth century for the treatment of a variety of conditions ranging from angina pectoris to surgery of the abdomen.[125] After World War II, PVB briefly gained the attention of authorities on regional anesthesia, who considered each paravertebral space as a separate entity, sealed off from above and below, and who until then held the belief that the anesthetic action took place via the epidural space—a concept that later led to the term "partial epidural."[126] PVB continued to be practiced widely in veterinary medicine, but in human medicine it almost disappeared. A paper by Eason and Wyatt suggested that with a different approach to percutaneous access, the technique lent itself both to detection by loss of resistance and easier catheter insertion, and that it was suitable for treating acute postthoracotomy pain.[127] This and other studies clarified the relationships and dynamics of injectates within the paravertebral space.[128-131] Direct communication between ipsilateral paravertebral spaces is the norm, and rarely is action through the epidural space. Sabanathan et al promulgated a direct, open technique. In patients with intact parietal pleura, the catheter is placed by the surgeon before closing the chest.[132]

Anatomy

The exact borders of the thoracic paravertebral space (TPVS) remain somewhat unclear. At a thoracic segmental level, it is wedge-shaped, with the base formed by the lateral surface of a vertebral body and, significantly, by the intervertebral foramen (Figure 20-10). The fascial planes on the vertebral body cross the midline, but it is generally believed that the prevertebral fascia and the anterior longitudinal ligament usually form an impermeable barrier to communication to the contralateral paravertebral space, a barrier breached only by lymphatic channels crossing from left to right.[133] Occasional breaches have been reported.[134] The posterior wall of the TPVS is less rigid, being formed by the inner surface of the vertebral transverse process, the neck of the rib, and attached superior costotransverse ligament. Laterally, the rib and internal intercostal muscle meld with the intercostal space. The anterior wall is the parietal

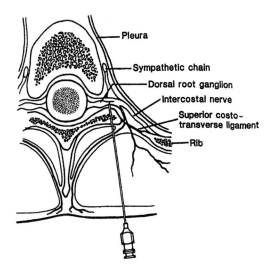

FIGURE 20-10 The percutaneous approach to paravertebral blockade. As it exits the intervertebral foramen, the thoracic somatic nerve enters a small triangular space formed by the vertebral body, the plane of the transverse process, and the pleura. Slight medial angulation of the needle reduces the chance of a pneumothorax. (From Mulroy MF: Peripheral nerve blockade. In Barash PG, Cullen BF, Stoelting RK [eds]: *Clinical anesthesia,* ed 3, Philadelphia, 1997, Lippincott-Raven.)

pleura, and, being malleable (because of the lung it covers), it "enables" the space. Studies on children provide evidence that there is a caudad limit to the paravertebral gutter, possibly created by the psoas muscle.[135] There might also be a cephalad limit; this premise is based on the clinical observations that blockade is rarely detected above the T2 dermatome and on the rarity of markers of cervical sympathectomy, such as Horner's syndrome.[136] The superior costotransverse ligament is the landmark for percutaneous approaches and is important for loss-of-resistance detection, similar to the role that the ligamentum flavum plays as a landmark for the boundaries of the epidural space.

Like the intercostal space, the TPVS is known to contain a rich mesh of blood vessels but not plexuses. The main trunk of the intercostal nerve exits the intervertebral foramen and traverses the space from side to side, linked by rami communicantes to the sympathetic chain that runs caudad-cephalad. Importantly, the posterior ramus of the intercostal nerve lies within the space and usually exits past the medial border of the superior costotransverse ligament.

The complex issues of anatomy and the dynamics of the spread of injectate into the TPVS have been summarized by Richardson and Lönnqvist.[137] Injectate takes the route of least resistance, which will vary in each patient. The usual paths are the following:

1. Cephalad and caudad within the space, for a variable number of adjacent spaces
2. Contiguous to the intercostal space
3. Lateral border of the vertebral body
4. Adjacent to the intervertebral foramen

There is also evidence that the route of least resistance depends on the presence of local factors such as pathologic condition, pleural effusions, rib trauma, epidural venous dynamics, and intrathoracic pressure. The proximity of the neuraxis remains the single most important factor regarding the use of the TPVS as a repository for local anesthetics.

Adverse Effects of Paravertebral Nerve Block
TECHNIQUE-RELATED
Vascular puncture, skin hematoma, and pain at the site of injection all occur on occasion (3.8%). Major vessel damage is unusual, but in circumstances in which intercostal vessels might be enlarged (e.g., coarctation of the aorta or thoracic aneurysms), percutaneous injection is not advised. Pleural puncture with pneumothorax or lung penetration have an incidence of 1.1% and 0.5%, respectively, but there is an eightfold increase in risk when a bilateral block is attempted.[138,139] In the context of thoracic surgery, it is usually a risk of little concern, as chest drainage is routine.

The failure rate is significant. This is due not only to the difficulty of accurate location with percutaneous approaches and uncertain end-points but also to the variety of routes by which injectate can be dispersed from the intercostal nerves.

REDUCING THE FAILURE RATE
Technique failure—defined as a high pain score with no evidence of sensory blockade—reaches 6% to 10% even in the most experienced of hands.[140] The failure rate can be reduced by more accurately locating the space through measuring tissue pressure changes as the needle is advanced; through sonography; by using a nerve stimulator; and by direct catheter insertion.[139-140,142] Skin temperature changes, unilateral platythelia, and somatosensory evoked potentials are indicative of early sympathetic block.[43,143] Methylene blue added to the injectate gives some idea of spread, when viewed at thoracotomy or thoracoscopy. Two injection techniques that bracket the intercostal space being used for surgical access have been advocated: by percutaneous injection preoperatively and when catheters are surgically sited postoperatively.

AGENT-RELATED
Hypotension, due to sympathetic blockade, has an incidence of 4%.[144] Of greater concern is the potential for prolonged continuous infusions to cause local anesthetic toxicity, in part due to the vascularity of the TPVS (and particularly in children). The proximity of the neuraxis means that there is always the risk of total spinal paralysis from perforation of a dural cuff or from catheter trauma.[29]

Advantages of Paravertebral Nerve Block
Once the technique has been learned, PVB can be implemented rapidly before surgery, as soon as the patient is in a thoracotomy position. A block can be instituted quickly that preempts surgical pressor response to skin incision, rib retraction, and intercostal space distraction, and that will leave some remnant of antiincisional nociception for several hours. Similarly, in those undergoing a closed procedure such as videoscopic pleurectomy, an effective PVB suppresses the tachycardia caused by, for instance, pleural stripping. Ideal as a regional analgesia adjuvant to a general anesthetic, it is equally as applicable to those undergoing major thoracic surgery via thoracotomy as it is to someone undergoing a thorascopic procedure such as lung biopsy, pleurectomy, or transthoracic sympathectomy. It is a useful technique for chest trauma, particularly unilateral, and when rib fractures are present. A percutaneous approach can be done in patients for whom surgical access to the paravertebral gutter is difficult or prevented by pathology such as mesothelioma. In pediatric practice, PVB has many devotees because it is technically easier to perform than epidural techniques. It is also convenient for the surgeon, who can site a catheter strategically before wound closure. It is a technique with a few (mostly minor) adverse effects that are easily corrected, and, reportedly, there are no major adverse events.

Percutaneous Approach
Early techniques, in keeping with the concept that the TPVS was a sealed compartment, directed the needle tip in a lateral approach, with emphasis on the target being the intervertebral foramen, and assuming that overshoot would be signaled by contact with the vertebral body (Table 20-10).

The midline bony landmark is the upper border of the spinous process: 2 to 3 cm lateral places the needle over the transverse process or neck of rib that forms the posterior border of the TPVS space some 2 to 3 cm away (Figure 20-10).[127]

Allowance needs to be made for both large and small patients, and the rule-of-thumb distances should be adjusted accordingly. The needle is advanced at right angles to the skin in all planes until contact with bone is made. Close approximation to the intercostal nerve of the rib above as it traverses the paravertebral space is made by angling the needle cephalad and "walking" it over the top of the bony contact. These directions are accurate for the upper part of the thorax, but from T_6 and caudad some hunting for bone contact may be necessary. The end point is loss of resistance—usually the same sensation that is transmitted by entrance into the epidural space through the ligamentum flavum, and a few millemeters beyond the bony contact (Figure 20-11). Any more medial approach increases the risk of entering the epidural space; any more lateral approach, and the TPVS space will be missed and the pleura and lung entered.

Open Technique
An epidural catheter is first passed into the open hemithorax by means of a Tuohy needle through an intercostal space in the lateral chest wall. In order to site the catheter, the surgeon then makes a small incision in the parietal pleura covering the paravertebral gutter and, with blunt dissection, threads the tip of the catheter close to the neurovascular bundle of the next cephalad space (Figures 20-12 and 20-13).[145] An absorbable suture is often used to reseal the wound and limit the leakage of local anesthetic. An alternative technique for open placement of a paravertebral catheter is shown in Figure 20-14.[146] Placement of an open catheter by this alternative technique is also called "extrapleural" or "intercostal" by some authors, and local anesthetic might or might not reach the paravertebral space; there is some confusion and overlap in the literature about these techniques. A thoracoscopic technique of siting the catheter has been described in which passage is made by blunt dissection, with saline injected down the catheter as it is advanced.[147]

Agents for Paravertebral Nerve Block
Only local anesthetics are suitable, and of these, only bupivacaine (either 0.25% or 0.5%) is favored. The epinephrine-containing solutions are advocated because the TPVS space is

---

TABLE 20-10

Quick Guide for Paravertebral Block

TECHNIQUE FOR PERCUTANEOUS APPROACH, APPLICABLE WHEN PATIENT IS IN LATERAL THORACOTOMY POSITION

Preparation	Hand washing, gloves, skin prep, no needle touching
Skin access point	Palpate two fingers breadth (2 cm) lateral to top of spinous process
Needle	Standard epidural type
Procedure	1. With needle axis at right angles to the skin, advance on to bone (1-6 cm depending on body habitus)
	2. Fan out in a sagittal plane if bony contact is not found (more likely a requirement with lower thoracic segments)
	3. Walk over the top of the bony landmark looking for loss of resistance (a.k.a. epidural)
	4. Inject 10-20 mL 0.5% l-bupivacaine with epinephrine
For thoracotomy to improve nociceptive yield	Use two injection (catheter) technique bracketing space for thoracotomy and dividing the calculated dose of local anesthetic; separate injections at $T_{3/4}$ and $T_{7/8}$ ensure a maximum concentration of local anesthetic at $T_{5/6}$ (the space used for surgical access), and a 6-7dermatome spread to block the skin and muscle incisional nociception of a typical posterolateral thoracotomy

CATHETERS FOR INFUSIONS

Best inserted directly at surgery. Can use two-catheter technique.
Use epidural catheters.
Protect with filters as per epidural protocols.
Reinforce information that catheters are not in the epidural space, and use separately identifiable pumps (local practice is to use syringe drivers).

COMPLICATIONS

	Presents with
Toxicity of local anesthetic	Tingling of fingers
	Convulsions
	Hypotension
Epidural infusion	Bilateral numbness and lack of sensation
	Heavy legs, muscle weakness
	Problems with getting a breath
	Hypotension
Pneumothorax	Dyspnea
	Circulatory collapse

INSTRUCTION: IN THE EVENT OF ANY OF THE ABOVE OCCURRING

Stop the paravertebral infusion
Treat the emergency
Inform on-duty anesthesiologist

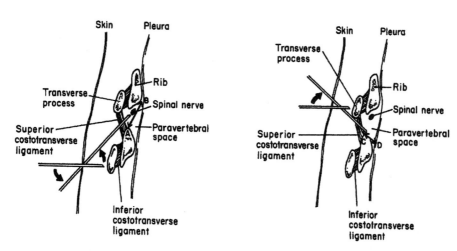

FIGURE 20-11 Paravertebral blockade: variations of technique. The conventional percutaneous approach to the paravertebral space is seen on the left, walking the needle off the superior border of the transverse process, through the costotransverse ligament, then seeking for a loss of resistance. Some authors advocate the technique on the right, walking the needle off the inferior border of the transverse process. The margin of safety to avoid puncturing the pleura, however, is larger when the technique on the left (the distance A to B) is used than with the technique on the right (the distance C to D). (From Chan VWS, Ferrante FM: Continuous thoracic paravertebral block. In Ferrante FM, VadeBoncouer TR [eds]: *Postoperative pain management,* New York, 1993, Churchill Livingstone.)

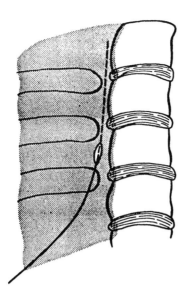

FIGURE 20-12 One method of open placement of a paravertebral catheter intraoperatively. The parietal pleura (stippled) is raised from the posterior chest wall. The epidural catheter is passed into the paravertebral space through a small defect created in the extrapleural (endothoracic) fascia. The proximal end of the catheter is then brought out of the chest through a separate needle puncture in an intercostal space near the chest drains. (From Berrisford RG, Sabanathan SS: *Ann Thorac Surg* 49:854, 1990.)

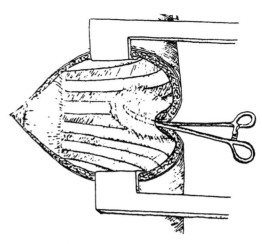

FIGURE 20-14 An alternative method of placing a paravertebral catheter is to create an extrapleural pocket at the posterior end of the surgical incision. The catheter is introduced percutaneously into this pocket under direct vision by a needle placed through an intercostal space directly into the pocket. This "extrapleural" block could function more as a multilevel intercostal block if the pocket is not developed medially to the paravertebral space. (From Watson DS, Panian S, Kendall V, et al: *Ann Thorac Surg* 67:825, 1999.)

regarded as vessel-rich (similar to the intercostal space) and because blood levels in toxic dosages are easily achievable. For catheter techniques, an infusion of 0.25% at the hourly rate of 0.5 to 1.0 mL per segment to be blocked or 0.1 mL/kg/hr, serves well in average adult practice. This amount should be reduced, however, in the smaller, the elderly, and the more frail.[137] In children, a loading dose of 2 to 2.5 mg/kg and a continuous infusion of 0.4 to 0.5mg/kg for 24 hours are regarded as appropriate. The dose and concentration should be halved in the neonate.[148-150]

Subarachnoid (Intrathecal) Injection

A single injection of opioid in the subarachnoid space is a longstanding but infrequently used analgesic technique in thoracic surgery that has recently experienced an increase in interest for cardiac surgery. The advent of microspinal catheter technology was the original impetus to extend continuous techniques to the cardiovascular and thoracic fields. These techniques make possible the use of opioids with short-lived activity profiles due to high octanol-water partition coefficients and lipophilicity, such as fentanyl and sufentanil.[49,151] Inherently, these are safer, more quick to bind to plasma, and more quickly deactivated. They also feature fewer troublesome adverse effects (e.g., pruritus, nausea, and vomiting), less sedation, and a greatly diminished risk of causing late-onset respiratory depression.[151]

Catheters are sited in the lumbar subarachnoid space. Spinal needles are 22-gauge and are sheathed by a larger bore introducer to enable negotiation of the skin and intraspinal ligaments. Once cerebrospinal fluid is seen or aspirated, a fine-bore catheter is placed through the needle. The catheters are very small and require considerable care in placement to avoid kinks that render them unusable.

Adverse Effects

With subarachnoid injection, there is some risk of spinal headache. Generally regarded as small, it is nevertheless quantifiable (less than 10%). In context, the problem is that it might occur at a time when a patient is not progressing as hoped, so it becomes difficult to determine whether the headache is a complication of subarachnoid puncture or masking a systemic complication, particularly if there is concomitant fever.[49] The 28- or 32-gauge catheters proved awkward to use for prolonged infusion with high pressures being generated, and they did

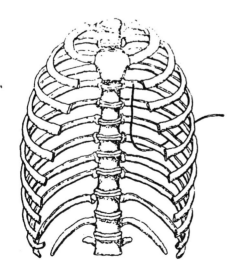

FIGURE 20-13 The optimal final position of a paravertebral catheter. (From Watson DS, Panian S, Kendall V, et al: *Ann Thorac Surg* 67:825, 1999.)

not prove robust, as they ran the risk of fracturing within the patient.[152]

The reputation of the subarachnoid technique, however, has not recovered from reports of permanent neurologic deficit. These catastrophes were related to neurotoxic dextrose–loaded local anesthetics applied continuously to one small part of the neuraxis. Reservations continue even when agents not known to be neurotoxic (such as opioids) are advocated.[153,154]

Caution is required in bolus techniques. Users of morphine need supplies of preservative-free preparations.[155] Hydrophilic agents continue to "move" rostrally for a considerable amount of time: cisternal morphine has been detected up to 12 hours after lumbar injection. Therefore pain relief could be delayed in onset, and there is an ever-present risk of late-onset respiratory depression, particularly if other opioids are added systemically.

Advantages

The ease with which the lumbar subarachnoid space can be found is important. This has advantages in patients with thoracic skeletal deformities or in those situations in which a rapid effect is required—for instance, in the slightly obtunded patient or the disinhibited and distressed patient who requires rescue analgesia, or as a second option before reverting to intravenous opioids. A 1-mL bolus (50 µg) of fentanyl has been used to regain control under just such testing conditions. A single-bolus injection of preservative-free morphine (10 µg/kg) in a 10-mL volume can result in up to 48 hours of analgesia but has a slower onset than fentanyl. Also, lumbar spinal injections or catheter placements can be done quickly and safely in the anesthetized patient in the lateral decubitus position immediately before the surgical incision. Based on the best available evidence at present in the literature, the three favored blocks for postthoracotomy analgesia would be either thoracic epidural, paravertebral, or spinal (Table 20-9). At least one of these blocks should be appropriate in the vast majority of thoracic surgical patients.

Intercostal Blocks

Blocks of the intercostal nerves that supply the dermatomes of the surgical incision(s) are an effective adjunct to methods of postthoracotomy analgesia. These can be done percutaneously or under direct vision when the chest is open. The duration of analgesia is transient (up to 6 to 8 hours with bupivacaine), and the blocks will need to be repeated to have any useful effect on postoperative lung function.[128] Indwelling intercostal catheters are an option and can be used for boluses or infusions, but they can be difficult to position reliably percutaneously, and they are difficult to secure in place.[156]

The intercostal nerves lie consistently between the same anatomical planes, deep to the internal intercostal muscle and superficial to the endothoracic fascia, which in turn are superficial to the parietal pleura. Local anesthetic deposited in the correct plane will block the nerve reliably, even though the course of the nerve often lies in the middle or lower part of the intercostal space and might not be confined to the subcostal groove as classically described.[157] Small boluses (less than 5 mL) tend to remain at the site of injection. Larger boluses can produce a multiple-level intercostal blockade by extension

medially to the paravertebral space or by direct extrapleural superior and inferior spread to adjacent intercostal spaces.[158,159] Systemic uptake of local anesthetic is rapid from the intercostal space compared with other sites of regional anesthesia, and doses must be adjusted with the possibility of systemic toxicity in mind.

It is important to understand fully the anatomy of the intercostal nerve to appreciate the potential usefulness and limitations of intercostal nerve blockade. Note in Figure 20-15 that there are three main sensory divisions—the posterior, lateral, and anterior cutaneous nerves. It is not possible to anesthetize the posterior nerve with an intercostal block. Thus, intercostal blocks are less useful for the traditional posterolateral thoracotomy incision than they are for the lateral or anterolateral incisions now favored by some surgeons. Also, intercostal blocks are useful for chest-drain incision pain and can be used for awake thoracoscopy. It is important that the intercostal nerve be blocked at or posterior to the posterior axillary line so that the lateral cutaneous branch can be anesthetized reliably. This task usually requires turning a supine patient to a lateral or prone position to place the block (Figure 20-16).

Cryoanalgesia and Transcutaneous Electrical Nerve Stimulation

Application of a –60° C probe to the exposed intercostal nerves in the open thorax intraoperatively produces an intercostal block that can persist for up to 6 months. This technique can be moderately efficient for decreasing postoperative pain but is

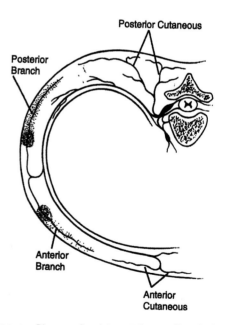

FIGURE 20-15 Diagram of an intercostal nerve. Note the location of the three cutaneous nerves (anterior, lateral, posterior), which is derived from the dorsal nerve ramus. An intercostal block must be placed at or posterior to the posterior axillary line to be certain to block the posterior branch of the lateral nerve. The posterior cutaneous nerve, which supplies the innervation for the posterior end of a traditional posterolateral thoracotomy incision, cannot be blocked with an intercostal block. (From Thompson GE: Intercostal nerve block. In Waldman SD, Winnie AP [eds]: *Interventional pain management*, Philadelphia, 1996, WB Saunders.)

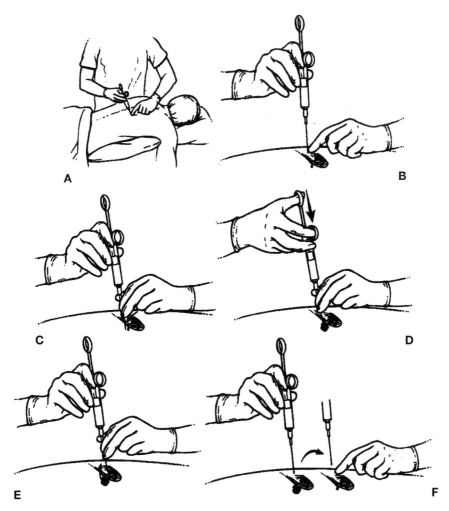

FIGURE 20-16 Performance of intercostal nerve blocks. The needle is introduced perpendicularly to contact the rib **(A, B)**. The shaft of the needle is then grasped with the fingers of the nondominant hand and walked inferiorly off the rib, and then advanced 2–4 mm into the intercostal groove. After aspiration, local anesthetic is injected **(C, D)**. The procedure is then repeated at other levels **(E, F)**. Total bupivacaine dose for a single session of blocks should not exceed 1 mg/kg (e.g., for a 75 kg patient, 3 mL bupivacaine 0.5% with epinephrine 1:200,000 at each of 5 levels). (From Thompson GE: Intercostal nerve block. In Waldman SD, Winnie AP [eds]: *Interventional pain management,* Philadelphia, 1996, WB Saunders.)

associated with an incidence of chronic neuralgia that has led many centers to abandon the procedure.[159,160] It is not certain that the incidence of long-term neuralgia exceeds that seen from the thoracotomy incision itself. One study of long-term postoperative pain in patients who had not received cryoanalgesia found that more than 50% of patients reported pain at the incision for longer than one year following thoracotomy.[161] A randomized study found the pain relief from cryoanalgesia inferior to relief from thoracic epidural fentanyl.[162] Neurolytic agents have been applied directly for postthoracotomy pain, but like cryotherapy, the consequences can be devastating, converting neuralgia into a life-long neuritis. Such practices are not to be commended for postthoracotomy pain.[163]

Transcutaneous electrical nerve stimulation (TENS) can be useful when pain is mild to moderate but is ineffective when pain is severe.[164] At best, it might decrease opioid requirements and limit the side effects of nausea and vomiting.[165,166]

Interpleural Catheters

Originally suggested by Reiestad and Strømskag in 1986, the potential for thoracic analgesia was quickly seen and reported in studies on chest trauma and thoracotomy. Interpleural injections were regarded as an alternative to multiple intercostal nerve injections.[167-169] There are consistent observations, however, that the technique compares unfavorably with other catheter techniques, in terms of both pain relief and improvement in pulmonary function.[11,170] Reasons cited for poor performance include a wide dispersal of local anesthetic throughout the hemithorax and sequestration and loss of agent through chest drains.[169,171] In addition, the semiupright position, assumed as optimum for patients postoperatively, results in pooling in the costophrenic angle.

Although interpleural catheters cannot be recommended, there might be a limited use for interpleural local anesthetics.

Catheters sited on the diaphragm and infused with local anesthetic might be one technique for dealing with phrenic nerve-conducted nociception. A similar technique has been recommended for patients undergoing thoracoscopic sympathectomy.[19]

Systemic Opioids

Systemic opioids alone are effective in controlling background pain, but the acute pain component associated with coughing or movement requires plasma levels that are associated with sedation and hypoventilation in most patients.[54] Even when administered by patient-controlled devices, pain control is generally poor after thoracotomy, and patients report interrupted sleep patterns when serum opioid levels fall below the therapeutic range.[172]

Nonsteroidal Antiinflammatory Drugs

Nonsteroidal antiinflammatory drugs (NSAIDs) are an essential component of multimodal analgesia treatment and have been shown to reduce opioid requirements after the first postoperative day.[24] The perceived problem in the thoracic field is related to the propensity for adverse effects in patients primed by age, comorbidity, or surgery.[173] Gastrointestinal hemorrhage and disturbance, even when NSAIDs are administered rectally or intravenously, is a concern, particularly for esophageal surgery.

The association with renal failure, however, causes a particular concern for some clinicians. Fluid restriction to the point of dehydration is regarded as necessary for pneumonectomy and lung transplantation to prevent the development of postpneumonectomy pulmonary edema. A constant theme in the pathogenesis of this complex condition is disruption of the pulmonary lymphatics so that the capacity to rid the body of excess pulmonary interstitial and intraalveolar fluid is diminished. A state of lymphatic inefficiency and depletion occurs in patients with obstructive airways disease, emphysema, and chronic bronchitis. An acute state can follow deliberate lung collapse, particularly after surgery requiring prolonged one-lung ventilation.[174,175] Provided that situations in which lymphatic dysfunction is present (or likely to occur) are regarded as contraindications, NSAIDs have a role.

Indomethacin, diclofenac, ketorolac, and ketoprofen are the most popular agents.[176,177] These can be deployed for many procedures in thoracic surgery: notably, for many relatively minor procedures (e.g., thoracoscopic sympathectomy, lung biopsy, and pleurodesis) in which there is little incisional nociception, and in children, to whom some of these analgesics can be rectally administered. NSAIDs are rarely effective enough to serve as stand-alone analgesics for major surgery; they are most useful as supplements to other agents for plugging gaps, such as the ill-defined pain of diaphragmatic and pleural irritation (Table 20-11).

Infants and Children

Custom and practice for infants and children has been to use intravenous opioids and to avoid local anesthetic techniques as technically too difficult. In the case of epidural techniques, thoracic approaches are not recommended due to the potential for spinal cord damage; a caudal approach, however, is practicable if the clinician has considerable expertise.[178-180] Both interpleural and paravertebral catheters can be sited easily at surgery and are increasingly popular for continuous analgesia after thoracotomy.[150,181-184] Children appear to be resistant to (or compensate well for) hemodynamic complications but are vulnerable to the toxic effects of prolonged infusion of local anesthetics.[117,119,144] Particular caution is required if bilateral catheters are used.[185]

Acute Postthoracomy Neuralgia

Occasionally, patients are seen after thoracotomy or thoracoscopy with a particularly distressing and intractable pain experience within hours of surgery; a 5% incidence has been reported.[186] Characterized by vague localization, allodynia, and dysesthesia, it has many of the hallmarks of neuritic pain and is peculiarly resistant to the usual regimens of local anesthetics, NSAIDs, and opioids. Intercostal nerve block and PVB with local anesthetics are part of the treatment for these intractable

---

TABLE 20-11

Nonsteroidal Antiinflammatory Drugs

Potential Contraindications to the Use of NSAIDs

Pneumonectomy
Lung transplantation
Lung volume reduction surgery
Any situation in which fluid policy restriction is imposed

Drug	Dose (mg) (In Addition to Opioids, Normal Adults)	Prescription	24-hour Maximum Dose
Ibuprofen	200-400	1× daily oral	1.6-2.4 g
Diclofenac	50	3× daily oral	150 mg
Ketorolac	10-30	3× daily IV	90 mg
Ketoprofen	50	4× daily oral	200 mg
*Rofecoxib	12.5	1× daily oral	25 mg
*Celecoxib	100	2× daily oral	200 mg

*No detailed experience in thoracic practice

situations, as is the early introduction of some of the armamentarium of chronic pain (e.g., diazepam, amitryptyline, and the anticonvulsants carbemazepine and gabapentin).[187] There is no real evidence as yet for the treatment of this rare and distressing scenario, which almost certainly heralds the development of a chronic postthoracotomy neuralgia or neuritis.[188]

Shoulder Pain and Diaphragmatic Irritation

It is has been a consistent observation that the targeting of intercostal nerve-mediated nociception results in other pain being revealed.[8] Some 80% of patients with a functioning and effective epidural complain of ipsilateral shoulder pain. Usually, this is thought to be referred pain from diaphragmatic irritation.[189,190] Other factors, including position during operation and major bronchus transection, have been implicated, although the mechanisms are not clear. Typically, these pains are dealt with by using NSAIDs or by increasing the dose of opioid. As most TEA are sited in the T_4 to T_6 area, there is some room for maneuver in increasing the height of the block to counter nociception from cut major bronchi. Placement of an interpleural catheter on the diaphragm is part of the tradition of the specialty but has not been the subject of serious investigation. There are several reports of the use of nerve blocks.[191] Phrenic nerve infiltration and interscalene brachial plexus block have had a variable success rate but carry a risk of causing significant diaphragm dysfunction.[192] Suprascapular nerve block has been shown to be of no real benefit.[193]

Pain Disaggregation

Observations that nonincisional nociception dominates when incisional pain is treated have become worthy of study, particularly in situations of diaphragmatic irritation, where 80% of a clinical case-mix might be involved. The term *disaggregation* has been applied to the effect of a therapeutic modality that alters the character and the observed and perceived routes of nociception.[13] Other examples include the effects of different types of surgery, with a different balance of nociception depending on whether the dominant source is incisional (as in thoracotomy) or visceral (e.g., after thoracoscopy). Pain is not normally viewed as a quantitative phenomenon, but the observations stemming from a theory of disaggregation suggest that a quantitative-physiologic model and methodology could clarify, for example, preemptive analgesia, the balance of multimodal techniques, and the site of action of interpleurally placed local anesthetics (i.e., intercostal nerve or pleural receptors).

Transition to Chronicity

One of the more attractive notions of so-called preemptive pain theory is that the transition of acute pain syndromes associated with thoracic surgery, to chronic ones such as postthoracotomy neuralgia, are preventable with analgesic regimens that prophylactically block nerves and desensitize peripheral nerve endings and dorsal horn cells of nerves that are then damaged by surgery.[24,194] So far, there is no good evidence to support this theory as a clinical phenomenon.[195] Although it is unrealistic and counterintuitive to believe that such a prophylactic mecha-

nism is to be found, anything that highlights the problem of finding a cure to neural trauma is an advance.

The actual incidence of postthoracotomy pain syndromes is as high as 50% (but generally above 30%) and includes some cases in whom symptomatology could be due to tumor recurrence or invasion.[161,186,188,196] The incidence of those who present with deafferentation discomfort diagnosed as postthoracotomy neuralgia (PTN) as a primary complaint, and who require treatment, has been thought to be in the region of 5% to 10%.[197] Even this figure (and it is probably higher in some institutions) represents a significant morbidity at an international level and has clear implications for resources.

There is epidemiologic evidence that treatment of the acute pain of operation influences the incidence of chronic neuralgia.[198] Although this could be a function of the method of analgesia, those with significant pain on the second postoperative day frequently end up with chronic discomfort irrespective of the type of analgesia, an observation suggesting that a pain profile resistant to treatment could be a marker of nerve damage.

There is some evidence that the incidence of PTN has fallen. This might reflect the abandonment of surgical techniques, such as rib resection, to gain better access at thoracotomy. It might also reflect the abandonment of suturing techniques that cause direct neural trauma or intercostal nerve entrapment, which in turn lead to the putative neuroma that causes the problem. Unfortunately, the shift toward minimal access and thoracoscopic techniques has not translated to any real evidence of a cause for this fall in PTN.[199] The ports forced between ribs to spread the intercostal space exert a radial force on the neurovascular bundle of the upper rib that is sufficient to cause pressure damage to its contents.

Management of Opioid-Tolerant Patients

The opioid-tolerant patient who requires thoracic surgery presents a significant challenge. Postoperative analgesia requires careful planning and frequent reassessment. Patients might be using physician-prescribed opioids for pain related to their thoracic disease or to other chronic pain syndromes. Active abusers of narcotic, or those in a rehabilitation program receiving daily methadone, also are included in this group. Whenever possible, patients should take their regular analgesia or methadone preoperatively; otherwise, substitute opioids must be provided.

Opioid tolerance occurs as a result of loss of active receptor sites from chronic exposure to agonist. Both a decreased number of receptors and desensitization to agonist binding are implicated. Clinically, the opioid doses required to produce adequate postoperative analgesia are increased. A multimodal analgesic regimen that includes the use of NSAIDs and regional analgesia is optimal. A choice must be made regarding the distribution of increased opioid delivery either systemically or through an epidural catheter. Increased narcotic can be provided in the epidural solution, or standard narcotic concentrations can be used in the epidural with additional systemic narcotic. DeLeon-Casasola reports that higher epidural doses of opioid are able to curtail the appearance of narcotic withdrawal in most patients.[200] More frequently, the patient receives a standard or slightly increased concentration of opioid in the epidural infusion and additional systemic opioids to minimize the occurrence of withdrawal. A convenient way to provide drug delivery in patients not immediately able to take oral medication is in the form of a transdermal fentanyl patch. Systemic opioids can be provided alternatively, either as a continuous intravenous infusion or in oral format.

Patient-controlled analgesic techniques are often difficult to manage in these patients, and they can best be managed with fixed dosage regimens that are modified as needed. Ultimately, after dose titration, the patient might be receiving both increased epidural opioid and doses of systemic opioid greater than those given preoperatively, all without significant side effects. DeLeon-Casasola has documented a number of patients in whom epidural bupivacaine-morphine analgesia was inadequate, who then responded to a switch to bupivacaine-sufentanil.[201] Patients in drug rehabilitation programs with methadone might be highly reluctant to modify their methadone doses perioperatively, having struggled to establish a stable dose in the past. They frequently can take their full methadone dose throughout the perioperative period. In addition, continuous peripheral nerve blockade with a paravertebral or intercostal catheter can provide adjunctive analgesia, but these are not routes for opioid delivery, so increased doses of systemic opioids must be delivered.

Supplemental therapies to be considered for these patients include the addition of epinephrine, 5 µg/mL, to the epidural infusion solution, and the addition of low-dose continuous intravenous ketamine infusions.[202] All opioid-tolerant patients require frequent adjustment of analgesic doses. Despite such adjustment, pain scores of 2 to 4 (on a scale of 10) with movement are often the lowest achievable. Opioid-tolerant patients' increased analgesic requirements are for a longer duration postoperatively than is the case for opioid-naïve patients.

Conclusion

There have been immense changes in pain management over the past 20 years. When viewed from a modern (essentially consumerist) perspective of a product (the ability to cough), pain relief is better packaged and delivered than in the past. A far greater percentage of the surgical population gains access to quality service. Such is the scale of change in functional improvements brought about by attention to analgesia that simple pulmonary function testing is now a marker of quality rather than a discriminator. It is also a marker that the improvements in function might have reached a finite point, limited by a tradeoff between pain relief and surgical outcome that no longer can be regarded as simple or straightforward.[64,65,203,204]

The outcomes of thoracic surgery, which have been considered to be a function of pain, are postoperative mobility; duration of hospital stay; the respiratory factors of atelectasis, pneumonia, and respiratory failure; and the development of chronic pain syndromes. Realistically, the first two are not directly connected with the analgesic regimen and are subject to a multiple of extraneous factors. The respiratory factors are regarded as the most critical ones, reflecting morbidity and the potential for fatalities.[204]

Only the use of postoperative epidural analgesia has reached what is defined as a Level 1 evidence base for reducing

pathologic pulmonary consequences of surgical chest trauma. With the same criteria, epidural local anesthetic/opioid synergistic mixtures are superior to either type of agent alone and reduce the adverse effects of each. Only as ingredients of multimodal analgesic stratagems can NSAIDs reduce severe pain.[205,206] Regardless, the days of insulating and compartmentalizing postoperative pain from the whole perioperative process are over.

There is not robust evidence to support the idea that a seamless continuum of analgesia, starting preemptively before the surgical stress and continued postoperatively is an advantage.[206] Intuitively, TEA techniques have the potential to protect against the development of chronic pain syndromes, but whether this is a psychologic prophylaxis or a physical influence representing antinociception is not, as yet, elucidated.

At an operational level, the superiority of a regimen lies, not in the pain relief attained, but in the peripheral and parallel benefits and in the effort required to achieve these.[207] Effective pain relief, as judged by pain scores at rest, is just as achievable with intravenous opioids and paravertebral blocks plus NSAIDs as with TEA. But, given the same major operation (e.g., esophagectomy), those patients who receive TEA have an advantage that makes recovery less likely to be complicated.[206,208] Given a lesser operation, such as a pulmonary resection, the advantages of TEA over other techniques are less obvious. The issue of which technique is best is one of debate and circumstance, usually settled on pragmatic rather than on scientific grounds.[13,73,209]

REFERENCES

1. National Emphysema Treatment Trial Research Group: Patients at high risk of death after lung volume reduction surgery, *New Eng J Med* 345:1075, 2001.
2. Nakahara K, Monden Y, Ohno K, et al: A method for predicting postoperative lung function and its relation to postoperative complications in patients with lung cancer, *Ann Thorac Surg* 39:260, 1985.
3. Nakahara K, Ohno K, Hashimoto J, et al: Prediction of postoperative respiratory failure in patients undergoing lung resection for cancer, *Ann Thorac Surg* 46:549, 1988.
4. Cerfolio RJ, Allen MS, Trastek VF, et al: Lung resection in patients with compromised pulmonary function, *Ann Thorac Surg* 62:348, 1996.
5. Licker M, de Perrot M, Hohn L, et al: Perioperative mortality and major cardio-pulmonary complications after lung surgery for non-small cell carcinoma, *Eur J Cardiothorac Surg* 15:314, 1999.
6. Edge WG, Cooper GM, Morgan M: Analgesic effects of sublingual buprenorphine, *Anaesthesia* 34:463, 1979.
7. Coleman DL: Control of postoperative pain. Non-narcotic and narcotic alternatives and their effect on pulmonary function, *Chest* 92:520, 1987.
8. Conacher ID: Pain relief following thoracic surgery. In Gothard JWW (ed): *Thoracic anaesthesia. Bailliere's Clinical Anaesth* 1:233, 1987.
9. Miguel R, Hubbell D: Pain management and spirometry following thoracotomy: a prospective randomized study of four techniques, *J Cardiothorac Vasc Anesth* 7:529, 1993.
10. Brichon PY, Pison C, Chaffanjon P, et al: Comparison of epidural analgesia and cryoanalgesia in thoracic surgery, *Eur J Cardiothorac Surg* 8:482, 1994.
11. Richardson J, Sabanathan S, Shah R: Post-thoracotomy spirometric lung function: the effect of analgesia, *J Cardiovasc Surg* 40:445, 1999.
12. Kruger M, Sandler AN: Post-thoracotomy pain control, *Curr Opin Anaesth* 112:55, 1999.
13. Conacher ID: Post-thoracotomy analgesia. In Slinger PD (ed): *Thoracic Anesthesia. Anesthes Clin NA* 19/3:611, 2001.
14. Loan WB, Morrison JD: The incidence and severity of postoperative pain, *Br J Anaesth* 39:695, 1967.

15. Black J, Kalloor GJ, Collis JL: The effect of surgical approach on respiratory function after oesophageal resection, *Br J Surg* 64:624, 1977.
16. Furrer M, Rechsteiner R, Eigenmann V, et al: Thoracotomy and thoracoscopy: postoperative pulmonary function, pain and chest wall complaints, *Eur J Thor Cardiovasc Surg* 12:82, 1997.
17. Kidd BL, Urban LA: Mechanisms of inflammatory pain, *Br J Anaesth* 87:3, 2001.
18. Jedeikin R, Olsfanger D, Shachor D, et al: Anaesthesia for transthoracic endoscopic sympathectomy in treatment of upper limb hyperhidrosis, *Br J Anaesth* 69:349, 1992.
19. Gilligan S, Smith MB, Allen PR: Transthoracic endoscopic sympathectomy, *Br J Anaesth* 70:491, 1992.
20. Woolf CJ: Recent advances in pathophysiology of acute pain, *Br J Anaesth* 63:139, 1989.
21. Macintosh RR, Mushin WW: Anaesthetic research in wartime, *Medical Times* 253, 1945.
22. Guz A, Noble MIM, Widdicombe JG, et al: The role of the vagal and glossopharyngeal afferent nerves in respiratory sensation, control of breathing and arterial pressure regulation in conscious man, *Clin Sci* 30:161, 1966.
23. Etches RC, Gammer Tl, Cornish R: Patient-controlled epidural analgesia after thoracotomy: a comparison of meperidine with and without bupivacaine, *Anesth Analg* 83:81, 1996.
24. Murphy DF: NSAIDs and postoperative pain, *Br Med J* 306:1493, 1993.
25. Rowbotham DJ: Advances in pain, *Br J Anaesth* 87:1, 2001 (Editorial).
26. Macintyre PE: Safety and efficacy of patient-controlled analgesia, *Br J Anaesth* 87:36, 2001.
27. Simpson BR, Parkhouse J, Marshall R, et al: Extradural analgesia and the prevention of postoperative respiratory complications, *Br J Anaesth* 33:628, 1961.
28. Kaplan JA, Miller ED, Gallagher EG: Postoperative analgesia for thoracotomy patients, *Anesth Analg* 54:773, 1975.
29. Lekhak B, Bartley C, Conacher ID, et al: Total spinal anaesthesia in association with insertion of a paravertebral catheter, *Br J Anaesth* 86:280, 2001.
30. Jordan S, Mitchell JA, Quinlan GJ, et al: The pathogenesis of lung injury following pulmonary resection, *Eur Resp J* 15:790, 2000.
31. Sabanathan S, Eng J, Mearns AJ: Alterations in respiratory mechanics following thoracotomy, *J Roy Coll Surg Engl* 35:144, 1990.
32. Hagl C, Harringer W, Gohrbrandt B, et al: Site of pleural drain insertion and early postoperative pulmonary function following coronary artery bypass grafting with internal mammary artery, *Chest* 115:757, 1999.
33. Olsfanger D, Jedeikin R, Fredman B, et al: Tracheal anaesthesia for transthoracic endoscopic sympathectomy: an alternative to endobronchial anaesthesia, *Br J Anaesth* 74:141, 1995.
34. Conacher ID: The ethics of acute pain studies in the 21st century, *Pain* 86:321, 2000.
35. Oxman AD, Chalmers I, Sackett DL: A practical guide to informed consent to treatment, *Br Med J* 323:1464, 2001.
36. Skene L, Smallwood R: Informed consent: lessons from Australia, *Br Med J* 324:39, 2002.
37. Wildsmith JAW, Fischer HBI, Grüning T: Regional anaesthesia—before or after general anaesthesia, *Anaesthesia* 54:86, 1999.
38. Reynolds F: Logic in the safe practice of spinal anaesthesia, *Anaesthesia* 55:1045, 2000.
39. Giebler RM, Scherer RU, Peters J: Incidence of neurologic complications related to thoracic epidural catheterization, *Anesthesiology* 86:55, 1997.
40. Romer HC, Russell GN: A survey of the practice of thoracic epidural analgesia in the United Kingdom, *Anaesthesia* 53:1016, 1998.
41. Horlocker TT, Caplan RA: Should regional blockade be performed on anesthetized patients? *ASA Newslett* 65:5, 2001.
42. Doblar DD, Muldoon SM, Abbrecht PH, et al: Epidural morphine following epidural local anesthesia: effect on ventilatory and airway occlusion pressure responses to CO₂, *Anesthesiology* 55:423, 1981.
43. Richardson J, Jones J, Atkinson R: The effect of thoracic paravertebral blockade on intercostal somatosensory evoked potentials, *Anesth Analg* 87:373, 1998.
44. Snijdelaar DG, Hasenbos MA, van Egmond J, et al: High thoracic epidural sufentanil with bupivacaine: continuous infusion of high volume versus low volume, *Anesth Analg* 78:490, 1994.
45. Bond MR, Pilowsky I: Subjective assessment of pain and its relationship to the administration of analgesics in patients with advanced cancer, *J Psychosom Res* 10:203, 1966.
46. Scott J, Huskisson EC: Graphic representation of pain, *Pain* 2:175, 1976.
47. Revill SI, Robinson JL, Rosen M, et al: The reliability of a linear analogue for evaluating pain, *Anaesthesia* 31:1191, 1976.
48. Mahon SV, Berry PD, Jackson M, et al: Thoracic epidural infusions for post-thoracotomy pain: a comparison of fentanyl-bupivacaine mixtures v fentanyl alone, *Anaesthesia* 54:641, 1999.
49. Sudarshan G, Browne BL, Matthews JNS, et al: Intrathecal fentanyl for post-thoracotomy pain, *Br J Anaesth* 75:19, 1995.
50. Hansdottir V, Woestenborghs R, Nordberg G: The pharmacokinetics of continuous epidural sufentanil and bupivacaine infusion after thoracotomy, *Anesth Analg* 83:401, 1996.
51. Keele KD: The pain chart, *Lancet* 255:6, 1948.
52. Matthews JNS, Altman DG, Campbell MJ, et al: Analysis of serial mesurements in medical research, *Br Med J* 300:230, 1990.
53. Nayman J: Measurement and control of postoperative pain, *Ann Roy Col Surg Eng* 61:419, 1979.
54. Shulman M, Sandler AN, Bradley JW, et al: Postthoracotomy pain and pulmonary function following epidural and systemic morphine, *Anesthesiology* 61:569, 1984.
55. Bromage PR: Spirometry in assessment of analgesia after upper abdominal surgery: a method of comparing analgesic drugs, *Br Med J* ii:589, 1955.
56. Hasenbos M, van Egmond J, Gielen M, et al: Postoperative analgesia by epidural versus intramuscular nicomorphine after thoracotomy (PartII), *Acta Anaesthesiol Scand* 29:577, 1985.
57. Slinger P, Shennib H, Wilson S: Postthoracotomy pulmonary function: a comparison of epidural versus intravenous meperidine infusions, *J Cardiothorac Vasc Anesth* 9:128, 1995.
58. Child CS, Kaufman L: The effect of intrathecal diamorphine on the adrenocortical, hyperglycaemic and cardiovascular response to major colonic surgery, *Br J Anaesth* 57:389, 1985.
59. Schulze S, Roikjaer O, Hasselstrøm L, et al: Epidural bupivacaine and morphine plus systemic indomethacin eliminates pain but not systemic response and convalescence after cholecystectomy, *Surgery* 103:321, 1987.
60. Scott NB, Mogensen T, Bigler D, et al: Continuous thoracic extradural 0.5% bupivacaine with or without morphine: effect on quality of blockade, lung function and surgical stress response, *Br J Anaesth* 62:253, 1989.
61. Salomaki TE, Leppaluoto J, Laitinen JO, et al: Epidural versus intravenous fentanyl for reducing hormonal, metabolic and physiologic responses after thoracotomy, *Anesthesiol* 79:672, 1993.
62. Moon MR, Luchette FA, Gibson SW, et al: Prospective, randomised comparison of epidural versus parenteral opioid analgesia in thoracic trauma, *Ann Surg* 229:684, 1999.
63. Kehlet H, Holte K: Effect of postoperative analgesia on surgical outcome, *Br J Anaesth* 87:62, 2001.
64. Lawrence V: Predicting postoperative pulmonary complications: the sleeping giant stirs, *Ann Int Med* 135:919, 2001.
65. Ballantyne JC, Carr JB, deFerranti S, et al: The comparative effects of postoperative analgesic therapies on pulmonary outcome: cumulative meta-analysis of randomised, controlled trials, *Anesth Analg* 86:598, 1998.
66. Crawford OB, Brasher C, Buckingham WW: Peridural anesthesia for thoracic surgery, *Anesthesiology* 27:241, 1957.
67. Shuman RL, Peters RM: Epidural anesthesia following thoracotomy in patients with chronic obstructive airway disease, *J Thorac Cardiovasc Surg* 71:82, 1976.
68. Griffiths DPG, Diamond AW, Cameron JD: Postoperative extradural analgesia following thoracic surgery: a feasibility study, *Br J Anaesth* 47:48, 1975.
69. Conacher ID, Paes ML, Jacobson L, et al: Epidural analgesia after thoracic surgery, *Anaesthesia* 38:546, 1983.
70. Bromage PR, Camporesi E, Chestnut D: Epidural narcotics for postoperative analgesia, *Anesth Analg* 59:473, 1980.
71. Welchew EA: The optimum concentration of epidural fentanyl: a randomised, double-blind comparison with and without 1:200,000 adrenaline, *Anaesthesia* 38:1037, 1983.
72. Logas WG, El-Baz N, El-Ganzouri A, et al: Continuous thoracic epidural analgesia for postoperative pain relief following thoracotomy, *Anesthesiology* 67:787, 1987.
73. Cook TM, Riley RH: Analgesia following thoracotomy: a survey of Australian practice, *Anaesth Int Care* 25:520, 1997.
74. Hasenbos M, van Egmond J, Gielen M, et al: Postoperative analgesia by epidural versus intramuscular nicomorphine after thoracotomy(Part 1), *Acta Anaesthesiol Scand* 29:572, 1985.

75. Visser WA, Liem TH, van Egmond J, et al: Extension of sensory blockade after thoracic epidural administration of a test dose of lidocaine at three different levels, *Anesth Analg* 86:332, 1998.

76. Wheatley RG, Schug SA, Watson D: Safety and efficacy of postoperative epidural analgesia, *Br J Anaesth* 87:47, 2001.

77. Horlocker TT, Wedel DJ: Neuraxial block and low-molecular-weight heparin: balancing perioperative analgesia and thromboprophylaxis, *Reg Anesth Pain Med* 23:164, 1998.

78. Vandermeulen E, Van Aken H, Vermylen J: Anticoagulants and spinal-epidural anesthesia, *Anesth Analg* 79:1165, 1994.

79. Liu SS: ASRA neuraxial anesthesia and anticoagulation consensus statements, *Regional Anesth* 23 (Suppl 2):157-63, 1998.

80. Kassis J, Fugere F, Dube S: The safe use of epidural anesthesia after subcutaneous injection of low-dose heparin in general abdominal surgery, *Can J Surg* 43:289, 2000.

81. Curatolo M, Schnider TW, Petersen-Felix S, et al: A direct search procedure to optimise combinations of epidural bupivacaine, fentanyl, and clonidine for postoperative analgesia, *Anesthesiology* 92:325, 2000.

82. Reiz S, Westberg M: Side effects of epidural morphine, *Lancet* xx:203, 1980.

83. Hurford WE, Dutton RP, Alfille PH, et al: Comparison of thoracic and lumbar epidural infusions of bupivacaine and fentanyl for postthoracotomy analgesia, *J Cardiothorac Vasc Anesth* 7:521, 1993.

84. Lubenow TR, Faber LP, McCarthy, et al: Postthoracotomy pain management using continuous epidural analgesia in 1324 patients, *Ann Thorac Surg* 58:924, 1995.

85. Stanton-Hicks M, Hock A, Stuhmeier KD, et al: Venoconstrictor agents mobilize blood from different sources and increase intrathoracic filling during epidural anesthesia in supine humans, *Anesthesiology* 66:317, 1987.

86. Warner DO, Warner MA, Ritman EL: Human chest wall function during epidural anesthesia, *Anesthesiology* 85:761, 1996.

87. Meisner A, Rolf N, Van Aken H: Thoracic epidural anesthesia and the patient with heart disease: benefits, risks, and controversies, *Anesth Analg* 85:517, 1997.

88. Gramling-Babb PM, Zile MR, Reeves ST: Preliminary report on high thoracic epidural analgesia: relationship between its therapeutic effects and myocardial blood flow as assessed by stress thallium distribution, *J Cardiothorac Vasc Anesth* 14:657, 2000.

89. Von Dossow V, Welte M, Zaune U, et al: Thoracic epidural anesthesia: the preferred anesthetic technique for thoracic surgery, *Anesth Analg* 92:848, 2001.

90. Groban L, Dolinksi S, Zvara DA, et al: Thoracic epidural analgesia: its role in postthoracotomy atrial arrhythmias, *J Cardiothor Vasc Anesth* 14:662, 2000.

91. Flisberg P, Törnebrandt L, Walther B, et al: Pain relief after esophagectomy: thoracic epidural analgesia is better than parenteral opioids, *J Cardiothorac Vasc Anesth* 15:279, 2001.

92. Grant GJ, Zakowski M, Ramanathan S, et al: Thoracic versus lumbar administration of epidural morphine for postoperative analgesia after thoracotomy, *Reg Anesth* 18:351, 1993.

93. Benzon HT: Post-thoracotomy epidural analgesia: lumbar or thoracic placement, *J Cardiothorac Vasc Anesth* 7:515, 1993.

94. Chisakuta AM, George KA, Hawthorne CT: Postoperative epidural infusion of a mixture of bupivacaine 0.2% with fentanyl for upper abdominal surgery. A comparison of thoracic and lumbar routes, *Anaesthesia* 50:72, 1995.

95. Mourisse J, Hasenbos MA, Gielen MJ, et al: Epidural bupivacaine, sufentanil or combination for post-thoracotomy pain, *Acta Anaesthesiolog Scand* 36:70, 1992.

96. Hansdottir V, Bake B, Nordberg G: The analgesic efficacy and adverse effects of continuous epidural sufentanil and bupivacaine infusion after thoracotomy, *Anesth Analg* 83:394, 1996.

97. Wiebalck A, Brodner G, Van Aken H: The effects of adding sufentanil to bupivacaine for post-operative patient-controlled epidural analgesia, *Anesth Analg* 85:124, 1997.

98. Tejwani GA, Rattan AK, McDonald JS: Role of spinal opioid receptors in the antinociceptive interactions between intrathecal morphine and bupivacaine, *Anesth Analg* 84:726, 1992.

99. Dales RE, Dionne G, Leech JA: Preoperative prediction of pulmonary complications following thoracic surgery, *Chest* 104:155, 1993.

100. Pansard JL, Mankikian B, Bertrand M, et al: Effects of thoracic extradural block on diaphragmatic electrical activity and contractility after upper abdominal surgery, *Anesthesiology* 78:63, 1993.

101. Polaner DM, Kimball WR, Fratacci MD: Improvement of diaphragmatic function by a thoracic epidural block after upper abdominal surgery, *Anesthesiology* 79:808, 1993.

102. Fratacci MD, Kimball WR, Wain JC: Diaphragmatic shortening after thoracic surgery in humans, *Anesthesiology* 79:654, 1993.

103. Wahba WM, Craig DB, Don HF, et al: The cardiorespiratory effects of thoracic epidural analgesia, *Can Anaesth Soc J* 19:8, 1972.

104. Craig DB: Postoperative recovery of pulmonary function, *Anesth Analg* 60:46, 1981.

105. Gruber EM, Tschernko EM, Kritzinger M, et al: The effects of thoracic epidural analgesia with bupivacaine 0.25% on ventilatory mechanics in patients with severe chronic obstructive pulmonary disease, *Anesth Analg* 92:1015, 2001.

106. Von Knorring J, Lepantalo J, Lindgren L, et al: Cardiac arrhythmias and myocardial ischemia after thoracotomy for lung cancer, *Ann Thorac Surg* 53:642, 1992.

107. Amar D, Burt M, Reinsel RA, et al: Relationship of early postoperative dysrhythmias and long-term outcome after rescection of non-small cell lung cancer, *Chest* 110:437, 1996.

108. Staats PS, Panchal SJ: Thoracic epidural analgesia for treatment of angina, *J Cardiothorac Vasc Anesth* 11:105, 1997.

109. Backlund M, Laasonen L, Leptantalo: Effect of oxygen on pulmonary hemodynamics and incidence of atrial fibrillation after noncardiac thoracic surgery, *J Cardiothorac Vasc Anesth* 12:422, 1998.

110. Lindgren L, Lepantalo M, Von Knorring J: Effect of verapamil on right ventricular pressure and atrial tachyarrhythmias after thoracotomy, *Brit J Anaesth* 66:205, 1991.

111. Meissner A, Rolf N, Van Aken H: Thoracic epidural anesthesia and patients with heart disease: benefits, risks and controversies, *Anesth Analg* 85:517, 1997.

112. Saada M, Catoire P, Bonnet F: Effect of thoracic epidural anesthesia combined with general anesthesia on segmental wall motion assessed by transesophageal echocardiography, *Anesth Analg* 75:329, 1991.

113. Saada M, Duval AM, Bonnet F: Abnormalities in myocardial wall motion during lumbar epidural anesthesia, *Anesth Analg* 71:26, 1989.

114. Moniche S, Hjortso NC, Blemmer T: Blood pressure and heart rate during orthostatic stress and walking with continuous postoperative epidural bupivacaine/morphine, *Acta Anaesthesiol Scand* 37:65, 1993.

115. Armstrong P: Thoracic epidural anaesthesia and primary pulmonary hypertension, *Anaesthesia* 47:496, 1992.

116. Niemi G, Brevik H: Adrenalin markedly improves thoracic epidural analgesia produced by a low-dose infusion of bupivacaine, fentanyl and adrenalin after major surgery, *Acta Anaesthesiol Scand* 42:897, 1998.

117. Murat I, Delleur MM, Esteve C, et al: Continuous extradural anaesthesia in children, *Br J Anaesth* 69:1441, 1987.

118. Ivani G, Bergendahl HTG, Lampugnani E, et al: Plasma levels of clonidine following epidural bolus injection in children, *Acta Anesthesiol Scand* 42:306, 1998.

119. De Negri P, Ivani G, Visconti C, et al: The dose-response relationship for clonidine added to a postoperative continuous epidural infusion of ropivacaine in children, *Anesth Analg* 93:71, 2001.

120. Crain SM, Shen KF: Antagonists of excitatory opioid receptor functions enhance morphine's analgesic potency and attenuate opioid tolerance/dependence liability, *Pain* 84:121, 2000.

121. Keenan DJM, Cave K, Langdon L, et al: Comparative trial of rectal indomethacin and cryoanalgesia for control of early postthoracotomy pain, *Br Med J* 287:1335, 1983.

122. Richardson J, Sabanathan S, Jones J, et al: Prospective randomised comparison of preoperative and continuous balanced epidural or paravertebral bupivacaine on post-thoracotomy pain, pulmonary function and stress responses, *Br J Anaesth* 83:387, 1999.

123. Jacobson L, Phillips PD, Hull CJ, et al: Extradural versus intramuscular diamorphine, *Anaesthesia* 38:10, 1983.

124. Braun H: Operations on the spinal column and thorax. In Klimpton H (ed): *Local anesthesia*, London, 1924, Henry Klimpton.

125. Mandl F: *Paravertebral block: in diagnosis, prognosis, surgery*, London, 1947, William Henemann.

126. Macintosh RR, Bryce-Smith R: The paravertebral space etc. In *Local analgesia: abdominal surgery*, p34, Edinburgh, 1953, E & S Livingstone.

127. Eason MJ, Wyatt R: Paravertebral thoracic block; a reappraisal, *Anaesthesia* 34:638, 1979.

128. Moore DC, Bush WH, Scurlock HE: Intercostal nerve block: a roentgenographic anatomic study of technique and absorption in humans, *Anesth Analg* 59:815, 1980.

129. Conacher ID, Kokri M: Postoperative paravertebral blocks for thoracic surgery: a radiological appraisal, *Br J Anaesth* 59:155, 1987.
130. Conacher ID: Resin injection of thoracic paravertebral spaces, *Br J Anaesth* 61:657, 1988.
131. Purcell-Jones G, Pither CE, Justins DM, et al: Paravertebral somatic nerve block: a clinical, radiographic and computed tomographic study in chronic pain patients, *Anesth Analg* 68:32, 1989.
132. Sabanathan S, Bickford Smith PJ, et al: Continuous intercostal nerve block for pain relief after thoracotomy, *Ann Thorac Surg* 46:425, 1988.
133. Nel L, Conacher ID, Shanahan D: Lymphatic drainage of the thoracic paravertebral space, *Br J Anaesth* 86:453, 2001.
134. Karmakar MK, Kwok WH, Kew J: Thoracic paravertebral block: radiological evidence of contralateral spread anterior to the vertebral bodies, *Br J Anaesth* 84:263, 2000.
135. Lönnqvist PA, Hildingsson U: The caudal boundary of the thoracic paravertebral space: a study in human cadavers, *Anaesthesia* 47:1051, 1992.
136. Richardson J, Sabanathan S: Thoracic paravertebral analgesia, *Acta Anaesthesiol Scand* 39:1005, 1995.
137. Richardson J, Lönnqvist PA: Thoracic paravertebral block, *Br J Anaesth* 81:230, 1998.
138. Lönnqvist PA, MacKenzie J, Soni AK, et al: Paravertebral blockade: failure rate and complications, *Anaesthesia* 50:813, 1995.
139. Naja Z, Lönnqvist PA: Somatic paravertebral nerve blockade, *Anaesthesia* 56:1181, 2001.
140. Richardson J, Cheema SPS, Hawkins J, et al: Thoracic paravertebral space location: a new method using pressure measurement, *Anaesthesia* 51:137, 1996.
141. Sabanathan S, Smith PJ, Pradhan GN, et al: 1996: Continuous intercostal nerve block for pain relief after thoracotomy, *Ann Thorac Surg* 46:425, 1988.
142. Pusch F, Wilding E, Klimsha W, et al: Sonographic measurement of needle insertion depth in paravertebral blocks in women, *Br J Anaesth* 85:841, 2000.
143. Saito T, Den S, Cheema SPS, et al: A single-injection, multi-segmental paravertebral block—extension of somatosensory and sympathetic block in volunteers, *Acta Anesthiol Scand* 45:30, 2001.
144. Lönnqvist PA, MacKenzie J, Soni AK, et al: Paravertebral blockade: failure rate and complications, *Anaesthesia* 50:813, 1995.
145. Berrisford RG, Sabanathan SS: Direct access to the paravertebral space at thoracotomy, *Ann Thorac Surg* 49:854, 1990.
146. Watson DS, Panian S, Kendall V, et al: Pain control after thoracotomy: bupivacaine versus lidocaine in continuous extrapleural intercostal nerve blockade, *Ann Thorac Surg* 67:825, 1999.
147. Soni AK, Conacher ID, Waller DA, et al: Video-assisted thoracoscopic placement of paravertebral catheters: a technique for postoperative analgesia for bilateral thoracoscopic surgery, *Br J Anaesth* 72:462, 1994.
148. Berde CB: Toxicity of local anesthetics in infants and children, *J. Ped* 122:S14, 1993.
149. Larsson BA, Lönnqvist PA, Olsson GL: Plasma concentrations of bupivacaine in neonates after continuous epidural infusion, *Anesth Analg* 84:501, 1997.
150. Cheung SLW, Booker PD, Franks R, et al: Serum concentrations of bupivacaine during prolonged continuous epidural infusion in young infants, *Br J Anaesth* 79:9, 1997.
151. Hansdottir V, Hedner T, Woestenborghs CE, et al: The CSF and plasma pharmacokinetics of sufentanil after intrathecal administration, *Anesthesiology* 74:264, 1991.
152. Guinard JP, Chiolero R, Mavrocordatos P, et al: Prolonged intrathecal fentanyl analgesia via 32-gauge catheters after thoracotomy, *Anesth Analg* 77:936, 1993.
153. Rigler ML, Drasner K, Krejcie TC, et al: Cauda equina syndrome after continuous spinal anesthesia, *Anesth Analg* 72:275, 1991.
154. Lambert DH, Hurley RJ: Cauda equina syndrome and continuous spinal anesthesia, *Anesth Analg* 72:817, 1991.
155. Alhashemi JA, Sharpe MD, Harris CL, et al: Effect of subarachnoid morphine administration on extubation time after coronary artery bypass graft surgery, *J Cardiothorac Vasc Anesth* 14:639, 2000.
156. Dryden CM, McMenemin I, Duthie DJ: Efficacy of continuous intercostal bupivacaine for pain relief after thoracotomy, *Brit J Anaesth* 70:508, 1993.
157. Hardy PAJ: Anatomical variation in the position of the proximal intercostal nerve, *Br J Anaesth* 61:338, 1988.
158. Crossley AWA, Hosie HE: Radiographic study of intercostal nerve blockade in healthy volunteers, *Br J Anaesth* 59:149, 1987.
159. Fagiano G, Borasio P, Salamino A, et al: Risultat immediati e a distanza del crio-bloco dei nervi intercostali, *Minerva Anestesiol* 51:39, 1985.
160. Mueller LC, Salzer G, Ransmayer G: Intraoperative cryoanalgesia for post-thoracotomy pain relief, *Ann Thorac Surg* 18:15, 1989.
161. Dajczman E, Gordon A, Kreisman H, Wolkove N: Long-term postthoracotomy pain, *Chest* 99:270, 1991.
162. Gough JD, Williams AB, Vaughn RS: The control of post-thoracotomy pain. A comparative evaluation of thoracic epidural fentanyl infusions and cryoanalgesia, *Anaesthesia* 43:780, 1988.
163. Roviaro GC, Varoli F, Fascianella A, et al: Intrathoracic intercostal nerve block with phenol in open chest surgery, *Chest* 90:64, 1986.
164. Benedetti F, Amazanio M, CasadioC: Control of postoperative pain by transcutaneous electrical nerve stimulation after thoracic operations, *Ann Thorac Surg* 63:773, 1997.
165. Stubbing JF, Jellicoe JA: Transcutaneuous electrical nerve stimulation after thoracotomy, *Anaesthesia* 43:296, 1998.
166. Warfield CA, Stein JM, Frank HA: The effect of transcutaneous electrical nerve stimulation on pain after thoracotomy, *Ann Thorac Surg* 39:462, 1985.
167. Rocco A, Reiestad F, GudmanJ, et al: Intrapleural administration of local anesthetics for pain relief in patients with multiple rib fractures, *Reg Anesth* 12:10, 1987.
168. Rosenberg PH, Scheinin BMA, Lepäntalo MJA, et al: Continuous intrapleural infusion of bupivacaine for analgesia after thoracotomy, *Anesthesiology* 67:811, 1987.
169. Ferrante M, Chan WS, Arthur R, et al: Interpleural analgesia after thoracotomy, *Anesth Analg* 72:105, 1991.
170. Bachmann-Mennenga, Biscoping J, Kuhn DFM, et al: Intercostal nerve block, interpleural analgesia, thoracic epidural block or systemic opioid for pain relief after thoracotomy, *Eur J Cardiothorac Surg* 7:12, 1993.
171. Richardson J, Sabanathan S, Shah RD, et al: Pleural bupivacaine placement for optimal postthoracotomy pulmonary function: a prospective, randomised study, *J Cardiothorac Vasc Anesth* 12:166, 1998.
172. Kavanagh BP, Katz J, Sandler AN: Pain control after thoracic surgery. A review of current techniques, *Anesthesiology* 81:737, 1994.
173. Gøtzsche PC: Non-steroidal anti-inflammatory drugs, *Br Med J* 320:1058, 2000.
174. Slinger PD: Perioperative fluid management for thoracic surgery: the puzzle of postpnemonectomy pulmonary oedema, *J Cardiothorac Vasc Anesth* 9:442, 1995.
175. Mehran RJ, Deslauriers J: Late complications: postpneumonectomy syndrome, *Chest Surg Clin North Am* 9:655, 1999.
176. Singh H, Bossard RF, White PF, et al Effects of ketorolac versus bupivacaine coadmistration during patient-controlled hydromorphone epidural analgesia after thoracotomy procedures, *Anesth Analg* 84:564, 1997.
177. Forrest JB, Camu F, Greer IA, et al: Ketorolac, diclofenac, and ketoprofen are equally safe for pain relief after major surgery, *Br J Anaesth* 88:227, 2001.
178. Bosenburg AT, Bland BAR, Schulte-Steinberg O, et al: Thoracic epidural anesthesia via caudal route in infants, *Anesthiol* 69:265, 1988.
179. Gunter JB, Eng C: Thoracic epidural via the caudal approach in children, *Anesthiol* 76:935, 1992.
180. Lejus C, Roussiere G, Testa S, et al: Postoperative extradural analgesia in children: comparison of morphine with fentanyl, *Br J Anaesth* 72:156, 1994.
181. Blanco D, Llamazares J, Rincon R, et al: Thoracic epidural anesthesia via the lumbar approach in children, *Anesthesiology* 84:1312, 1996.
182. Lönnqvist PA: Continuous paravertebral block in children: initial experience, *Anaesthesia* 47:607, 1992.
183. Karmakar MK, Booker PD, Franks R, et al: Continuous extrapleural paravertebral infusion of bupivacaine for post-thoracotomy analgesia in young infants, *Br J Anaesth* 76:811, 1996.
184. Semsroth M, Plattner O, Horcher E: Effective pain relief with continuous intrapleural bupivacaine after thoracotomy in infants and children, *Paed Anaesth* 6:303, 1996.
185. Karmakar MK, Booker PD, Franks R: Bilateral continuous paravertebral block used for postoperative analgesia in an infant having bilateral thoracotomy, *Paed Anaesth* 7:469, 1997.
186. Kalso E, Pertunnen K, Kaasinen S: Pain after thoracic surgery, *Acta Anaesthiol Scand* 36:96, 1992.
187. Harden RN: Complex regional pain syndrome, *Br J Anaesth* 87:99, 2001.
188. Katz J, Jackson M, Kavanagh BP, et al: Acute pain after thoracic surgery predicts long-term post-thoracotomy pain, *Clin J Pain* 12:50, 1996.

189. Burgess FW, Anderson DM, Colonna D, et al: Ipsilateral shoulder pain following surgery, *Anesthesiology* 78:365, 1993.

190. Scawn N, Pennefather SH, Soorae A, et al: Ipsilateral pain after thoracotomy with epidural analgesia: the influence of phrenic nerve infiltration with lidocaine, *Anesth Analg* 93:260, 2001.

191. Ng KP, Chow YF: Brachial plexus block for ipsilateral shoulder pain after thoracotomy, *Anaesth Intens Care* 25:74, 1997.

192. Urmey WF, McDonald M: Hemidiaphragmatic paresis during interscalene brachial plexus block: effects on pulmonary function and chest wall mechanics, *Anesth Analg* 74:352, 1992.

193. Tan N, Agnew NM, Scawn ND, et al: Suprascapular nerve block for ipsilateral shoulder pain after thoracotomy with thoracic epidural analgesia, *Anesth Analg* 94:199, 2002.

194. Woolf CJ, Chong MS: Pre-emptive analgesia—treating postoperative pain by preventing the establishment of central sensitisation, *Anesth Analg* 77:362, 1993.

195. Doyle E, Bowler GM: Pre-emptive effect of multimodal analgesia in thoracic surgery, *Br J Anaesth* 80:147, 1998.

196. Macrae WA: Chronic pain after surgery, *Br J Anaesth* 87:88, 2001.

197. Conacher ID: Therapists and therapies for post-thoracotomy neuralgia, *Pain* 48:409, 1992.

198. Senturk M, Ozcan PE, Tabe GK, et al: The effects of three different analgesia techniques on long-term postthoracotomy pain, *Anesth Analg* 94:11, 1992.

199. Hutter J, Miller K, Moritz E: Chronic sequels after thoracoscopic procedures for benign diseases, *Eur J Cardiothorac Surg* 17:687, 2000.

200. de Leon-Casasola OA, Yarussi A: Physiopathology of opioid tolerance and clinical approach to the opioid-tolerant patient, *Curr Rev Pain* 4:203, 2000.

201. de Leon-Casasola OA, Lema MJ: Epidural bupivacaine/sufentanil therapy for postoperative pain control in patients tolerant to opioid and unresponsive to epidural bupivacaine/morphine, *Anesthesiology* 80:303, 1994.

202. Schmid R, Sandler AN, Katz J: Use and efficacy of low-dose ketamine in the management of acute postoperative pain, *Pain* 82:111, 1999.

203. Boisseau N, Rabary O, Padovani B, et al: Improvement of 'dynamic analgesia' does not decrease atelectasis after thoracotomy, *Br J Anaesth* 87:564, 2001.

204. Warner DO: Preventing postoperative pulmonary complications: the role of the anesthesiologist, *Anesthesiology* 92:1467, 2000.

205. Smith G, Power I, Cousins MJ: Acute pain—is there evidence on which to base treatment, *Br J Anaesth* 82:817, 1999.

206. Riedal BJCJ: Regional anesthesia for major cardiac and noncardiac surgery: more than a strategy for effective analgesia, *J Cardiothorac Vasc Anesth* 15:279, 2001.

207. Buggy DJ, Smith G: Epidural anaesthesia and analgesia; better outcome after major surgery, *Br Med J* 319:530, 1999.

208. Slinger PD: Pro: Every postthoracotomy patient deserves thoracic epidural analgesia, *J Cardiothorac Vasc Anesth* 13:350, 1999.

209. Grant RP. Con: Every postthoracotomy patient deserves thoracic epidural analgesia, *J Cardiothorac Vasc Anesth* 13:355, 1999.

Index

Page numbers followed by f indicate figures; t, tables; b, boxes.

463